2014

中国中医药年鉴

学术卷

周谷城题

主办　国家中医药管理局

承办　上海中医药大学

编审　《中国中医药年鉴（学术卷）》编辑委员会

上海辞书出版社

图书在版编目(CIP)数据

中国中医药年鉴.学术卷.2014卷. /《中国中医药年鉴(学术卷)》编辑委员会编.—上海:上海辞书出版社,2015.3
ISBN 978-7-5326-4355-4

Ⅰ.①中… Ⅱ.①中… Ⅲ.①中国医药学—2014—年鉴 Ⅳ.①R2-54

中国版本图书馆CIP数据核字(2015)第052391号

中国中医药年鉴(学术卷)2014
《中国中医药年鉴(学术卷)》编辑委员会　编
责任编辑/朱荣所　装帧设计/汪　溪

上海世纪出版股份有限公司
辞书出版社出版
200040　上海市陕西北路457号　www.cishu.com.cn
上海世纪出版股份有限公司发行中心发行
200001　上海市福建中路193号　www.ewen.co
苏州越洋印刷有限公司印刷

开本889毫米×1194毫米　1/16　印张33　字数976 000
2015年3月第1版　2015年3月第1次印刷

ISBN 978-7-5326-4355-4/R·62
定价:280.00元

Traditional Chinese Medicine Yearbook of China (Academic Volume) 2014

Responsible Institution

State Administration of Traditional Chinese Medicine

Sponsor

Shanghai University of Traditional Chinese Medicine

Edited by

Editorial Office of Traditional Chinese Medicine Yearbook of China (Academic Volume)

Shanghai Lexicographical Publishing House

学 科 编 辑 （以姓氏笔画为序）

孙晓燕（中药药剂、中药炮制、中药药理）

肖梅华（针灸、推拿、医史文献）

邸若虹（校院长论坛、中医基础理论、名医经验、台港澳中医药、教学与科技研究等）

宋　卫（学术交流、中外交流、动态消息）

张应文（传染科、五官科、新订中医药规范原则等）

袁久林（儿科、外科、骨伤科）

徐丽莉（中药资源、中药质量评价、中药化学）

黄　燕（特载、专论、中药理论、方剂研究等）

鲍健欣（肿瘤、内科、国外中医药）

熊　俊（妇科、气功、护理、养生与保健、民族医药）

薛建维（获奖项目、出版新书目、期刊论文分类目录等）

前　言

由国家中医药管理局主办、上海中医药大学承办的《中国中医药年鉴》是反映我国中医药事业和学术进展的资料工具书。1983年，《中国中医药年鉴》创刊(原名《中医年鉴》)，至今已连续编撰出版了31卷。根据国家中医药管理局的决定，自2003年卷起，《中国中医药年鉴》分行政和学术两卷出版。本书作为学术卷，源于《中国中医药年鉴》中的“学术进展”部分，经栏目调整后单独成书，定名为《中国中医药年鉴(学术卷)》，由国家中医药管理局主办、上海中医药大学承办、上海中医药大学出版社出版，2012年卷起改由上海辞书出版社出版。

2014年《中国中医药年鉴(学术卷)》以上一年度全国公开发行的中医药学术期刊和全国性学术会议中发表的优秀论文为依据，由全国各特约专栏(科)撰稿人进行初选，拟定选目后提交《中国中医药年鉴(学术卷)》编辑部的相关学科编辑筛选论证，列出入选条目，由相关专业的专家撰写。全书经学科编辑初审，副主编、主编复审，《中国中医药年鉴(学术卷)》编辑委员会最终审定。

本书由文字版(纸质)和光盘版两个部分组成。

文字版设有特载、专论、校院长论坛、学术进展、记事、索引等栏目。其中对学术进展的选条，密切追踪各学科重大项目的连续性报道。如基础性研究条目突出反映在中医药理论指导下开展的各项实验研究，侧重理论与实践相结合；临床各科栏目，重点反映中医药对常见病、多发病、疑难疾病的治疗特色和用药经验。理论研究、中药及临床传染科、内科、外科、妇科等栏目引用国家“973”计划、“863”计划、国家自然科学基金、国家科技部、国家中医药管理局等资助项目的论文约850余篇。2014卷《中国中医药年鉴(学术卷)》的目录采用中英文对照。

光盘版设有2013年中医药学术期刊论文目录索引、获奖科研项目、出版(重印)新书目以及中医药期刊杂志一览表等栏目。其中中医药学术期刊论文目录索引约200余万字，具有多途径的检索功能，为读者查询上一年度的中医文献信息提供便利。

诚如王国强副主任所说：“《年鉴》是中医药事业的历史记录，是当代整个行业的一面镜子，是今后各项工作的起点。我们必须要站在这样的高度来认识《年鉴》编纂的重要性。”本着“一切有利于中医事业发展”和“一切便利读者”的宗旨，我们会尽力将反映中医药事业前进足迹的《中国中医药年鉴(学术卷)》编纂和出版工作做得更好，以期成为中医药工作者的挚友。

编　者

2014年9月

Preface

Traditional Chinese Medicine Yearbook of China, sponsored by the State Administration of Traditional Chinese Medicine (SATCM), and compiled by the Shanghai University of Traditional Chinese Medicine (SUTCM), is the reference reflecting the academic advance of Traditional Chinese Medicine. Thirty-one volumes have been consecutively published since its first publication in 1983. It has been published in two volumes annually since 2003, the administration volume and the academic volume. The content of the academic volume is adapted from the academic progress part in the former yearbook with adjusting some columns. Traditional Chinese Medicine Yearbook of China (academic volume), is sponsored by SATCM, compiled by SUTCM, and published by Shanghai University of Traditional Chinese Medicine Press. The Traditional Chinese Medicine Yearbook of China (2013) was published by Shanghai Lexicographical Publishing House.

The Traditional Chinese Medicine Yearbook of China of 2014 (academic volume) includes articles published in TCM journals and presented in TCM congresses in 2013. Editors select and refine items from the list initially recommended by special writers for each column. Professional authors detail each items. The Yearbook is finally published after proofreading by editors, the editor-in-chief, and the editing committee.

Traditional Chinese Medicine Yearbook of China 2013 (academic volume) consists of paper version and CD - ROM.

The paper version includes special reprint, special papers, university president forum, academic progress, news and events, and index. The academic progress focuses on and follows up key projects. The contents of theoretical researches largely reflect the experimental studies and their application in clinic practice in accordance with the TCM theories. The contents of clinic specialties emphasize the specific therapies and prescription experience in commonly-encountered and difficult diseases. There are about 850 articles from the projects sponsored by "National 973 Plan", "National 863 Plan", National Natural Science Foundation of China, Ministry of Science and Technology and SATCM being cited in the categories of Basic Theories of TCM, Chinese Materia Medica, Infectious Diseases, Internal Medicine, External Medicine, and Gynecology. The contents of the Yearbook (academic volume) are written in both Chinese and English.

The CD - ROM includes content indexes of articles of TCM journals 2013, awarded research projects, newly published or reprinted books, and list of TCM journals etc. The content indexes of TCM articles contain 2,000,000 characters with multi-way retrieval function, providing easy access for readers to find the useful TCM literature of 2013.

Wang Guoqiang, the Vice-Minister of Health China, says, "Traditional Chinese Medicine Yearbook of China is the historical recording of TCM career, is the mirror reflecting the status quo of TCM development, and is the starting point of work in future. We need to understand the importance of compiling Traditional Chinese Medicine Yearbook of China on such a high plane." For the benefit of the progress of TCM career and the readers, we will try our best in compiling and publishing Traditional Chinese Medicine Yearbook of China (academic volume) in order to reflect the progress of TCM. We hope that the Yearbook would be the friends of the readers.

Editor

September 2014

目　录

特　载

始终把中西医放在同等位置…………………… 3

专　论

将中医药发展纳入国家战略…………………… 7
大数据绘制当代中医航海图…………………… 9

校院长论坛

研究生课程教学改革的思考与探索 ………… 17

学术进展

一、理论研究 ………………………………… 23
(一) 中医基础理论 ………………………… 23
概述 ………………………………………… 23
阴阳五行学说研究 ………………………… 25
运气学说研究 ……………………………… 26
肺与大肠相表里研究 ……………………… 27
体质学说研究 ……………………………… 28
证候试验研究 ……………………………… 29
证候动物模型研究 ………………………… 31
[附] 参考文献 …………………………… 34
(二) 中药理论 ……………………………… 38
概述 ………………………………………… 38
中药的配伍禁忌应用与机制研究 ………… 40
中药内在属性的关联研究 ………………… 42
[附] 参考文献 …………………………… 43
二、临床各科 ………………………………… 46
(一) 名医经验 ……………………………… 46
李玉奇 ……………………………………… 46
班秀文 ……………………………………… 48
颜德馨 ……………………………………… 50
[附] 参考文献 …………………………… 52
(二) 传染病 ………………………………… 54
概述 ………………………………………… 54
艾滋病的治疗及实验研究 ………………… 56
慢性重型肝炎的治疗及实验研究 ………… 57
慢性乙型肝炎病毒携带者的治疗与研究 ………………………………………… 57
慢性乙型肝炎证型及其相关实验室指标的研究 ………………………………… 58
慢性丙型肝炎的治疗与研究 ……………… 59
肺结核的治疗与研究 ……………………… 60
手足口病的治疗与研究 …………………… 61
[附] 参考文献 …………………………… 62
(三) 肿瘤 …………………………………… 65
概述 ………………………………………… 65
肺癌的治疗及实验研究 …………………… 65
肝癌的治疗与研究 ………………………… 67
癌性贫血的治疗及实验研究 ……………… 68
恶性肿瘤并发抑郁的治疗 ………………… 69
肿瘤多药耐药性的研究 …………………… 69
中医药与微创技术联合治疗恶性肿瘤 …………………………………………… 71
[附] 参考文献 …………………………… 72
(四) 内科 …………………………………… 75
概述 ………………………………………… 75
支气管哮喘的研究 ………………………… 78
慢性支气管炎的治疗 ……………………… 78
慢性阻塞性肺疾病的治疗及实验研究 ………………………………………… 78
肺源性心脏病的中西医结合治疗及实验研究 ………………………………… 79
心肌缺血再灌注的实验研究 ……………… 80
心肌梗死的实验研究 ……………………… 80
动脉粥样硬化的实验研究 ………………… 81
病毒性心肌炎的治疗 ……………………… 82
慢性萎缩性胃炎的治疗及实验研究 ………………………………………… 82
胃癌前病变的治疗及实验研究 …………… 82
腹泻型肠易激综合征的研究 ……………… 83
溃疡性结肠炎的治疗及实验研究 ………… 83
非酒精性脂肪肝的治疗及实验研究 ………………………………………… 84

抗肝纤维化的实验研究 …………………… 85
肝硬化腹水的治疗 …………………… 86
慢性肾脏病的治疗与研究 …………………… 87
抗肾纤维化的实验研究 …………………… 87
慢性再生障碍性贫血的治疗与研究 …………………… 88
免疫性血小板减少症的治疗与研究 …………………… 89
过敏性紫癜的治疗 …………………… 89
2 型糖尿病的治疗及实验研究 …………………… 90
糖尿病肾病的临床与实验研究 …………………… 91
糖尿病周围神经病变的中西医结合治疗及实验研究 …………………… 92
代谢综合征的实验研究 …………………… 93
高尿酸血症的实验研究 …………………… 94
帕金森病的临床与实验研究 …………………… 94
急性脑梗死的治疗 …………………… 95
脑卒中后抑郁的治疗及实验研究 …………………… 95
强直性脊柱炎的治疗与研究 …………………… 96
血管性痴呆的治疗及实验研究 …………………… 96
焦虑症的中西医结合治疗与研究 …………………… 97
[附] 参考文献 …………………… 98
(五) 妇科 …………………… 105
概述 …………………… 105
月经过少的治疗 …………………… 105
阴道假丝酵母菌病的治疗与研究 …………………… 106
子宫颈人乳头瘤病毒感染的治疗 …………………… 106
盆腔炎性疾病、慢性盆腔疼痛的治疗与研究 …………………… 107
先兆流产与复发性流产的治疗及实验研究 …………………… 108
产后缺乳的治疗及实验研究 …………………… 109
多囊卵巢综合征的治疗及实验研究 …………………… 109
卵巢储备功能低下与卵巢早衰的治疗与研究 …………………… 110
绝经前后诸证的治疗与研究 …………………… 111
中医药在辅助生育中的应用 …………………… 112
[附] 参考文献 …………………… 113
(六) 儿科 …………………… 117
概述 …………………… 117
小儿慢性咳嗽的治疗 …………………… 119
小儿支气管肺炎的治疗 …………………… 119
小儿支原体肺炎的治疗 …………………… 120
小儿病毒性心肌炎的治疗 …………………… 121
小儿慢性胃炎的治疗 …………………… 122
小儿功能性便秘的治疗 …………………… 122
小儿特发性血小板减少性紫癜的治疗 …………………… 123
小儿癫痫的治疗 …………………… 123
小儿注意缺陷多动障碍的治疗 …………………… 123
[附] 参考文献 …………………… 124
(七) 外科 …………………… 127
概述 …………………… 127
慢性皮肤溃疡的治疗及实验研究 …………………… 130
带状疱疹的治疗与研究 …………………… 131
湿疹的治疗及实验研究 …………………… 132
荨麻疹的治疗与研究 …………………… 133
黄褐斑的治疗及实验研究 …………………… 134
银屑病的治疗及实验研究 …………………… 135
痤疮的治疗及实验研究 …………………… 136
浆细胞性乳腺炎的治疗与研究 …………………… 137
乳腺增生病的治疗及实验研究 …………………… 138
混合痔的治疗 …………………… 139
深静脉血栓的治疗及实验研究 …………………… 140
糖尿病足的治疗及实验研究 …………………… 141
烧伤的治疗及实验研究 …………………… 142
重症胰腺炎的治疗及实验研究 …………………… 143
男性不育症的治疗及实验研究 …………………… 144
[附] 参考文献 …………………… 145
(八) 骨伤科 …………………… 151
概述 …………………… 151
桡骨远端骨折的治疗与研究 …………………… 152
股骨粗隆间骨折的治疗与研究 …………………… 153
胸腰椎骨折的治疗 …………………… 154
腰肌劳损的治疗与研究 …………………… 155
肩关节周围炎的治疗 …………………… 155
骨质疏松的治疗及实验研究 …………………… 156
骨性关节炎的治疗及实验研究 …………………… 157
颈椎病的治疗与研究 …………………… 158
腰椎间盘突出症的治疗与研究 …………………… 159
[附] 参考文献 …………………… 160
(九) 五官科 …………………… 164
概述 …………………… 164
视网膜静脉阻塞的治疗及实验研究 …………………… 166
糖尿病性视网膜病变的治疗及实验研究 …………………… 167
年龄相关性黄斑变性的治疗及实验研究 …………………… 168

视神经萎缩的治疗 …… 168
干眼症的治疗及实验研究 …… 169
突发性耳聋的治疗及实验研究 …… 169
变应性鼻炎的临床与实验研究 …… 170
慢性鼻窦炎的治疗与研究 …… 171
慢性咽炎的治疗及实验研究 …… 171
口腔扁平苔藓的治疗与研究 …… 172
[附]　参考文献 …… 173
(十) 针灸 …… 177
概述 …… 177
针刺手法及进针量化研究 …… 180
支气管哮喘的针灸治疗及实验研究 …… 181
针灸治疗慢性阻塞性肺疾病的研究 …… 182
糖尿病及其并发症的针灸治疗与实验研究 …… 183
针灸治疗胃病的实验研究 …… 184
肠易激综合征的针灸治疗及实验研究 …… 185
针灸治疗肥胖的临床及实验研究 …… 186
慢性疲劳综合征的治疗 …… 187
中风后肩手综合征的针灸治疗 …… 187
针刺治疗 Bell's 面瘫 …… 188
针刺治疗失眠 …… 189
针刺治疗女性压力性尿失禁 …… 191
针灸治疗类风湿关节炎的实验研究 …… 191
针灸治疗带状疱疹 …… 192
灸法文献研究 …… 193
澄江学派研究 …… 194
[附]　参考文献 …… 195
(十一) 推拿 …… 201
概述 …… 201
推拿手法及其机理的实验研究 …… 202
肩周炎的治疗 …… 204
推拿治疗小儿便秘 …… 204
推拿治疗小儿厌食 …… 205
[附]　参考文献 …… 205
(十二) 气功 …… 207
概述 …… 207
气功机理研究 …… 207
八段锦的临床研究 …… 208
太极拳对人体生理功能影响及机制研究 …… 209
[附]　参考文献 …… 210
(十三) 护理 …… 211
概述 …… 211
中风的护理 …… 212
骨折的护理 …… 213
消化性溃疡的护理 …… 213
[附]　参考文献 …… 214
三、中药 …… 216
(一) 中药资源 …… 216
概述 …… 216
药用植物的遗传多样性研究 …… 218
道地药材形成及其产区变迁的影响 …… 220
采收期对中药材含量的影响 …… 221
硫黄熏蒸对中药材有效成分的影响 …… 222
产地加工对中药材有效成分的影响 …… 223
秦艽的生药学研究 …… 225
[附]　参考文献 …… 226
(二) 中药质量评价 …… 231
概述 …… 231
分子鉴定技术在药用植物研究中的应用 …… 233
电子鼻在中药材品质评价中的应用 …… 234
[附]　参考文献 …… 235
(三) 中药化学 …… 238
概述 …… 238
344 种中草药中的新成分研究 …… 239
62 种中草药中挥发油成分的研究 …… 283
[附]　参考文献 …… 289
(四) 中药药剂 …… 306
概述 …… 306
中药闪式提取的研究 …… 313
中药的酶提取工艺研究 …… 313
中药片剂制备的研究 …… 314
中药脂质体制备的研究 …… 316
[附]　参考文献 …… 317
(五) 中药炮制 …… 323
概述 …… 323
基于多指标评价中药炮制工艺的研究 …… 326
中药炮制品质量控制的研究 …… 326

13种中药炮制前后化学成分的比较 …… 327
11种中药炮制前后药理作用的比较 …… 329
[附] 参考文献 …… 331
(六) 中药药理 …… 335
概述 …… 335
中药干预血管性痴呆的实验研究 …… 339
中药改善神经细胞凋亡的机制研究 …… 340
中药抑制血管生成作用的研究 …… 341
中药调节内质网应激作用的研究 …… 342
中药调控小胶质细胞活化的研究 …… 343
中药调节PI3K/Akt信号通路的研究 …… 344
[附] 参考文献 …… 345
(七) 方剂研究 …… 355
概述 …… 355
小柴胡汤的临床应用与药理作用 …… 356
茵陈蒿汤的药理研究与临床应用 …… 357
金匮肾气丸的药理作用与临床应用 …… 358
四君子汤的药理作用 …… 359
中药复方防治肺癌作用机制的研究 …… 361
中药复方改善缺血性脑损伤的作用机制研究 …… 362
中药复方抗流感作用机理的研究 …… 363
中药复方及其有效成分改善胰岛素抵抗机制的研究 …… 364
[附] 参考文献 …… 365
四、养生保健 …… 371
概述 …… 371
古代医家养生思想研究 …… 372
亚健康状态的基础研究 …… 373
延缓衰老方药的实验研究 …… 374
[附] 参考文献 …… 375
五、医史文献 …… 377
(一) 古籍文献 …… 377
概述 …… 377
《黄帝内经》训诂学研究 …… 378
中医文献研究方法研究 …… 379
[附] 参考文献 …… 380
(二) 医家学派 …… 382
概述 …… 382
近现代伤寒名家学术思想研究 …… 383
温病治法研究 …… 383
盱江医学研究 …… 384
新安医学研究 …… 385
孟河医派学术思想研究 …… 386
朱丹溪治疗脾胃病学术思想研究 …… 387
[附] 参考文献 …… 387
(三) 医史文化 …… 390
概述 …… 390
中医药文化的内涵与核心价值研究 …… 391
中医学身体观研究 …… 392
中医教育史研究 …… 392
卫生用品与医药文化 …… 393
宋代文化名人与医学研究 …… 394
近代西医东渐之研究 …… 394
医事制度研究 …… 395
[附] 参考文献 …… 395
六、民族医药 …… 398
概述 …… 398
藏族医药研究 …… 399
蒙族医药研究 …… 400
蒙药德都红花-7味散治疗肝损伤的实验研究 …… 401
壮族医药研究 …… 401
回医香药研究 …… 402
土家族医药研究 …… 403
民族医药治疗关节炎的临床及实验研究 …… 403
[附] 参考文献 …… 404
七、港澳台中医药 …… 408
香港中医药 …… 408
台湾中医药 …… 410
[附] 参考文献 …… 415
八、国外中医药 …… 420
国外针灸治疗乳腺癌伴随症状的研究 …… 420
国外对气功的研究 …… 420
[附] 参考文献 …… 421
九、教学与科技研究 …… 422
(一) 教学研究 …… 422
中医经典课程教学方法研究 …… 422
临床教学方法研究 …… 424
中医药人才培养模式研究 …… 424
[附] 参考文献 …… 426

(二) 科技研究 …… 428
中西医结合研究的理论与方法学思考 …… 428
中医临床研究方法探讨 …… 429
交叉学科知识在中医药研究中的应用 …… 430
[附]　参考文献 …… 431

记　事

一、学术会议 …… 435
全国中医妇科流派学术研讨会在广州举行 …… 435
骨伤流派传承工作研讨会在北京举行 …… 435
第十一次全国老年医学学术会议在武汉召开 …… 435
中国男科医学大会在北京召开 …… 435
2013 年卷《中国中医药年鉴(学术卷)》编委会暨审稿会议在上海召开 …… 435
关幼波诞辰 100 周年纪念大会暨中医肝病学术研讨会在北京召开 …… 435
海峡两岸中医药研讨会在厦门召开 …… 435
中医男科新进展暨陈文伯学术研讨班在北京举行 …… 435
第八次全国中西医结合男科学术会议在开封举行 …… 435
第九次中医急诊学术研讨会暨急诊分会换届改选会议在连云港举行 …… 435
世界中医药学会联合会神志病专委会成立暨第一届学术年会在哈尔滨举行 …… 436
第十七次全国儿科中西医结合学术会议在杭州萧山举行 …… 436
中国骨科医学大会暨国际骨科专家高峰论坛在北京召开 …… 436
第十二届国际针灸学术研讨会在天津召开 …… 436
首届回医药学术交流会在北京召开 …… 436
2013 中华中医药学会编辑出版年会暨慢病防控优秀论文交流会在张家港举行 …… 436
2013 全国中西医创面修复高层论坛在天津举办 …… 436
首届全国骨科微创外固定关键技术推广应用学习研讨会在北京举行 …… 436
国际气功科学研讨会在上海举行 …… 436
第五届心身医学国际论坛在北京广安门医院召开 …… 436
首届世界脊诊整脊医学联盟大会暨全国脊诊整脊技术学术委员会换届大会在天津召开 …… 437
高健生和庄曾渊从医五十年研讨会在北京中国中医科学院眼科医院举办 …… 437
第 30 次全国中医儿科学术大会在济南举行 …… 437
第十七届全国药史本草学术研讨会在蕲春召开 …… 437
王焘学术思想研讨会在陕西眉县召开 …… 437
国际健康论坛暨《中华医学百科全书》2013 主编年会在北京召开 …… 437
世界中医药学会联合会中药专业委员会换届会议暨保健食品国际学术会议在北京召开 …… 437
世界中医药学会联合会护理专业委员会成立大会暨首届中医护理学术国际研讨会在南京召开 …… 437
泰山学术论坛在济南山东中医药大学举行 …… 437
国医大师陆广莘学术思想研讨会在北京举行 …… 437
全国第十六次中医药文化学术研讨会与中华中医药学会中医药文化分会换届在北京召开 …… 437
二、中外交流 …… 438
ISO 秘书长考察中医药标准化工作 …… 438
韩国正统针灸学会学员到甘肃学习针灸 …… 438
李大宁率团访问美国、巴哈马 …… 438
2013 国际中医药学术交流大会在旧金山市举办 …… 438
第 16 届日中友好针灸研修之旅研讨会在京举办 …… 438
中法中医药合作委员会第五次会议在法国巴黎召开 …… 438

中新签署中医药合作计划书 …………… 438
甘肃与乌克兰基辅州合作培养中医药人才 …………… 438
北京中医药大学与慕尼黑工大续签合作协议 …………… 438
王国强会见吉尔吉斯斯坦代表团 …………… 438
富布赖特项目访问团到陕西中医学院附属医院参观交流 …………… 438
上合组织官员赴陕西中医学院附属医院访问交流 …………… 439
中澳合建国际中医药研究中心 …………… 439
中瑞签署中医药合作计划书 …………… 439
第十三次中韩传统医学协调委员会会议在北京召开 …………… 439
中美开展JCI中医院质量标准研究 …………… 439
王国强会见世卫组织总干事陈冯富珍 …………… 439
中医系列讲座走进墨西哥 …………… 439
第四期亚洲区域中医药教育高级师资研修班在天津中医药大学开班 …………… 439
中吉两国签署中医药领域合作谅解备忘录 …………… 439
王国强率中医药代表团访问俄罗斯 …………… 439
第十届世界中医药大会暨世界中医药学会联合会成立十周年庆典在旧金山举行 …………… 440
马建中会见波兰代表团 …………… 440
以岭医药研究院与英国卡迪夫大学联姻 …………… 440
王国强会见马其顿卫生部代表团 …………… 440
马其顿总统伊万诺夫到成都中医药大学附属医院参观访问 …………… 440
岐黄中医学院在乌克兰医科大学挂牌 …………… 440
马建中率团访问澳大利亚和斐济 …………… 440
世界针联第八届针灸学术大会在悉尼会展中心开幕 …………… 440
中国中医科学院望京医院与墨西哥东南针灸医学协会签署合作协议 …………… 440
2013新加坡国际中医药高层论坛在新加坡大巴窑中医学院举行 …………… 440
黑龙江中医药大学与俄医学院签署合作协议 …………… 441
中国中医科学院与俄罗斯莫斯科州政府开展中医医疗合作 …………… 441

三、动态消息 …………… 442

《东医宝鉴》英译本正式发行 …………… 442
夏桂成荣获“白求恩奖章” …………… 442
2013年全国中医药工作会议在北京召开 …………… 442
首届中国中医药非遗保护发展论坛在太原举办 …………… 442
第七届全国名中医临床经验传承论坛暨中国民间中医医药研究开发协会名中医学术研究专业委员会换届大会在北京举行 …………… 442
果德安荣获美国植物药委员会最高荣誉奖 …………… 442
2012年中医药十大新闻揭晓 …………… 442
82家医院被命名为“全国综合医院中医药工作示范单位” …………… 442
全国标准化工作会议在北京召开 …………… 443
国家食品药品监管局药品审评中心发布《2012年度中国药品审评报告》 …………… 443
王李名珍王定一中西医药研讨会在香港举行 …………… 443
国家卫生和计划生育委员会正式组建 …………… 443
广东率先成立中医药标准化专委会 …………… 443
安徽中医学院更名为安徽中医药大学 …………… 443
国家食品药品监督管理总局正式挂牌 …………… 443
北京中医药大学校友会上海分会成立 …………… 443
针灸名家胡荫培百年纪念会在北京举行 …………… 443
“三棱针”技术规范获中国标准创新贡献奖 …………… 444
2013中国—东盟传统医药高峰论坛和第五届中国(玉林)中医药博览会在玉林市国际会展中心开幕 …………… 444
国家明确中药二氧化硫残留标准 …………… 444
王国强等被任命为国家卫生和计生委副主任 …………… 444
第二届中药质量鉴定技术研修班在澳门举办 …………… 444
针灸国际标准新闻发布会在北京召开 …………… 444
北京中医药大学举行中医内科学

临床学系成立大会 …………………… 444
首家肿瘤专家远程会诊中心在北京安定门中医医院成立 …………………… 444
新疆维吾尔药材及特有植物数据库建成 …………………… 444
首届国际中西医结合慢病管理论坛在香港召开 …………………… 444
世界中医药网络联盟成立大会在北京召开 …………………… 444
第三届 973 中医理论专题专家组在北京成立 …………………… 444
第五届中医药国际贡献奖在北京揭晓 …………………… 444
第一期中医医院职业化管理高级研修班在北京开班 …………………… 444
中美中医药合作战略座谈会在北京召开 …………………… 445
中国药品监督管理研究会在北京成立 …………………… 445
中医学术流派传承工作室启动建设项目会在广州召开 …………………… 445
第五次中医膏方大会在上海举行 ……… 445
中医药文化与产业博览会及"第二届中国道地药材论坛"在北京展览馆举办 …………………… 445
香港食物及卫生局局长访问国家中医药管理局 …………………… 445
全国卫生援外工作暨援外医疗队派遣 50 周年会议在北京召开 ……… 445
第十二届国际现代化中医药及健康产品展览会在香港举行 …………………… 445
中国卫生信息学会中医药信息化专业委员会成立大会暨中医药信息化工作座谈会在石家庄召开 …………………… 445
海峡两岸医卫媒体交流座谈会在北京举行 …………………… 445
全国中医药养生产业发展论坛在北京举办 …………………… 445
教育部高等学校中医学类专业教学指导委员会工作会议在兰州举办…… 445
"弘扬大医精神 抵制不正之风"高峰论坛在北京举行 …………………… 446
2013 年山清世界传统医药博览会暨山清世界药膳烹饪大赛在韩国山清郡东医宝鉴村举行 …………………… 446
全国回医药学术论坛暨中国民族医药学会回医药分会筹备成立大会在吴忠举行 …………………… 446
第四届中医药现代化科技大会在成都召开 …………………… 446
北京中医药大学校友会内蒙古分会在包头成立 …………………… 446
中国针刀医学技术创新联盟在北京成立 …………………… 446
2013 年中医急诊高峰论坛在北京开幕 …………………… 446
国家中医药管理局确定全国名老中医药专家传承工作室建设项目专家名单 …………………… 446
2013 中药上市后再评价国际大会在北京召开 …………………… 447
首届中医佛典高级研修班在北京开班 …………………… 447
王琦获 2013 年何梁何利奖 ……… 447
世界中医药学会联合会成立 10 周年座谈会在北京召开 …………………… 447
全国"中医药科技查新"暨"方剂数据汇交"培训会议在长沙召开 ……… 447
第四届藏医药研修班在北京藏医院结业 …………………… 447
北京中医药大学校友会宁夏分会在银川成立 …………………… 447
首届"世界针灸周"在北京举行 ……… 448
中澳中医药国际联合研究中心获国家级认定 …………………… 448
第六届南方医药论坛在广州举行 ……… 448
北京中医药大学校友会福建分会在厦门成立 …………………… 448
于文明会见香港慈善机构联合代表团 …… 448
《中华大典·医药卫生典·药学分典》出版 …………………… 448
于文明会见香港大学中医药学院院长劳力行 …………………… 448

索　引

主题词索引 …………………… 451

附:《中国中医药年鉴(学术卷)2014》光盘目录

一、2013 年新订中医药规范、原则、标准
1.《国家基本药物目录》(2012 年版)
2.《人感染 H7N9 禽流感诊疗方案(2013 年第 2 版)》
3.《按照传统既是食品又是中药材的物质目录(2013 版)》(征求意见稿)
4.《国家临床重点专科建设项目管理暂行办法》
二、2013 年中医药科研获奖项目
1. 2013 年度·国家科学技术奖励
2. 2013 年中华医学会科技奖获奖项目
3. 2013 年度中华中医药学会科学技术奖获奖项目
4. 2013 年度李时珍医药创新奖
5. 2013 年度中国中西医结合学会科学技术奖获奖项目
三、2013 年中医药出版新书目
四、2013 年中医药期刊杂志一览表
五、2013 年中医药学术期刊论文分类目录

Contents

Special Reprint

Continuous Development of Traditional Chinese Medicine and Conventional Medicine on an equal status ··· 3

Special Papers

Inclusion of Traditional Chinese Medicine Development in National Strategy ··· 7

Charting Course of Traditional Chinese Medicine Development by Big Data in Contemporary Age ··· 9

University President Forum

Reflection and Exploration of Curriculum Reform for Graduates by Using Case from Fujian University of Traditional Chinese Medicine as an Example ··· 17

Academic Progress

1. Theoretical Research ··· 23

1) Basic Theories of TCM ··· 23

Overview ··· 23

Research on Theories of Ying-Yan and Five Phases ··· 25

Research on Theories of Five Periods and Six Qi ··· 26

Research on Theory of Exterior-Interior Relationship between Lund and Large Intestine ··· 27

Research on Theories of Body Constitution ··· 28

Experimental Study of Patterns ··· 29

Research on Animal Models for Patterns ··· 31

Appendix: References ··· 34

2) Theories of Chinese Materia Medica ··· 38

Overview ··· 38

Research on Application and Mechanism of Combinative Contraindications of Herbs ··· 40

Research on Relations of Intrinsic Nature of Herbs ··· 42

Appendix: References ··· 43

2. Clinical Specialties ··· 46

1) Experience of Famous Physicians ··· 46

LI Yuqi ··· 46

BAN Xiuwen ··· 48

YAN Dexin ··· 50

Appendix: References ··· 52

2) Infectious Diseases ··· 54

Overview ··· 54

Treatment and Experimental Study of AIDs ··· 56

Treatment and Experimental Study of Chronic Severe Hepatitis ··· 57

Treatment and Research on HBV Carriers ··· 57

Research on Patterns and Relevant Laboratory Indexes of Hepatitis B ··· 58

Treatment and Research on Hepatitis C ··· 59

Treatment and Research on Pulmonary Tuberculosis ··· 60

Treatment and Research on Hand, Foot and Mouth Disease

(HFMD) ······ 61
Appendix: References ······ 62
3) Oncology ······ 65
Overview ······ 65
Treatment and Experimental Study of Lung Cancer ······ 65
Treatment and Research on Liver Cancer ······ 67
Treatment and Experimental Study of Anemia due to Cancers ······ 68
Treatment of Depression Complicated by Malignant Tumors ······ 69
Research on Multidrug Resistance of Cancers ······ 69
Treatment of Malignant Tumors by Herbs and Minimally Invasive Skill ······ 71
Appendix: References ······ 72
4) Internal Medicine ······ 75
Overview ······ 75
Research on Bronchial Asthma ······ 78
Treatment of Chronic Bronchitis ······ 78
Treatment and Experimental Study of Chronic Obstructive Pulmonary Diseases ······ 78
Treatment and Experimental Study of Cor Pulmonale by Integrative Medicine ······ 79
Experimental Study of Myocardial Ischemia Reperfusion ······ 80
Experimental Study of Myocardial Infarction ······ 80
Experimental Study of Atherosclerosis ······ 81
Treatment of Viral Myocarditis ······ 82
Treatment and Experimental Study of Chronic Atrophic Gastritis ······ 82
Treatment and Experimental Study of Pre-cancerous Lesions of Gastric Cancer ······ 82
Research on Irritated Bowel Syndrome with Diarrhea ······ 83
Treatment and Experimental Study of Ulcerative Colitis ······ 83
Treatment and Experimental Study of Non-Alcoholic Fatty Liver ······ 84
Treatment and Experimental Study of Anti-Hepatic Fibrosis ······ 85
Treatment of Ascites due to Cirrhosis ······ 86
Treatment and Research on Chronic Nephropathy ······ 87
Experimental Study of Anti-Renal Fibrosis ······ 87
Treatment and Research on Aplastic Anemia ······ 88
Treatment and Research on Immune Thrombocytopenia (ITP) ······ 89
Treatment of Allergic Purpura ······ 89
Treatment and Experimental Study of Type-II Diabetes Mellitus ······ 90
Clinical and Experimental Study of Diabetic Nephropathy ······ 91
Treatment and Experimental Study of Diabetic Peripheral Neuropathy by Integrative Medicine ······ 92
Experimental Study of Metabolic Syndrome ······ 93
Experimental Study of Hyperuricemia ······ 94
Clinical and Experimental Study of Parkinson's Disease ······ 94
Treatment of Acute Cerebral Infarction ······ 95
Treatment and Experimental Study of Depression after Apoplexy ······ 95
Treatment and Research on Ankylosing Spondylosis ······ 96
Treatment and Experimental Study of Vascular Dementia ······ 96
Treatment and Research on Anxiety by Integrative Medicine ······ 97
Reference ······ 98
5) Gynecology ······ 105

Overview ·· 105
Treatment of Scant Menstruation ······ 105
Treatment and Research on
Vulvovaginal Candidiasis ············ 106
Treatment of Cervical HPV
Infection ································ 106
Treatment and Research on Pelvic
Inflammation and Chronic
Pelvic Pain ····························· 107
Treatment and Experimental Study of
Threatened and Recurrent
Abortions ······························· 108
Treatment and Experimental Study of
Postpartum Hypogalactia ············ 109
Treatment and Experimental Study of
Polycystic Ovary Syndrome ········ 110
Treatment and Research on Poor Ovary
Reserve Function and Premature
Ovary Failure ·························· 110
Treatment and Research on Symptoms
Before and After Menopause ········ 111
Application of Herbs in Assisted
Reproductive Technologies
(ARTs) ·································· 112
Appendix: References ···················· 113
6) Pediatrics ······························ 117
Overview ································· 117
Treatment of Chronic Coughing in
Children ································ 119
Treatment of Mycoplasmal Pneumonia
in Children ···························· 119
Treatment of Bronchial Pneumonia in
Children ································ 120
Treatment of Viral Myocarditis in
Children ································ 121
Treatment of Chronic Gastritis in
Children ································ 122
Treatment of Functional Constipation
in Children ···························· 122
Treatment of Idiopathic Thrombocytopenic
Purpura (ITP) in Children ········ 123
Treatment of Epilepsy in Children ······ 123
Treatment of Attention Deficit
Hyperactivity Disorder in
Children ································ 123
Appendix: References ···················· 124
7) External Medicine ······················ 127
Overview ································· 127
Treatment and Experimental Study of
Chronic Skin Ulceration ·············· 130
Treatment and Research on Herpes
Zoster ··································· 131
Treatment and Experimental Study of
Eczema ································· 132
Treatment and Research on
Urticaria ································ 133
Treatment and Experimental Study of
Chloasma ······························· 134
Treatment and Experimental Study of
Psoriasis ································ 135
Treatment and Experimental Study of
Acne ···································· 136
Treatment and Research on Plasma
Cell Mastitis ··························· 137
Treatment and Experimental Study of
Cyclomastopathy ······················ 138
Treatment of Combined Hemorrhoids
··· 139
Treatment and Experimental Study of
Deep Venous Thrombosis ··········· 140
Treatment and Experimental Study of
Diabetic Foot ·························· 141
Treatment and Experimental Study of
Burn ···································· 142
Treatment and Experimental Study of
Severe Acute Pancreatitis ··········· 143
Treatment and Experimental Study of
Male Sterility ························· 144
Appendix: References ···················· 145
8) Orthopedics and Traumatology ······ 151
Overview ································· 151
Treatment of Distal Radius Fracture ······ 152
Treatment and Research on
Intertrochanteric Fracture

of Femur ······ 153
Treatment of Fracture of Thoracic and Lumber Vertebrae ······ 154
Treatment and Research on Strain of Lumber Muscles ······ 155
Treatment of Scapulohumeral Periarthritis ······ 156
Treatment and Experimental Study of Osteoporosis ······ 156
Treatment and Experimental Study of Osteoritis ······ 157
Treatment and Research on Cervical Spondylosis ······ 158
Treatment and Research of Prolapse of Lumbar Intervertebral Disc ······ 159
Appendix: References ······ 160
9) Ophthalmology and Otorhinolaryngology ······ 164
Overview ······ 164
Treatment and Experimental Study of Retinal Vein Obstruction ······ 166
Treatment and Experimental Study of Diabetic Retinopathy ······ 167
Treatment and Experimental Study of Age-related Macular Degeneration ······ 168
Treatment of Optic Atrophy ······ 168
Treatment and Experimental Study of Dry Eye Syndrome ······ 169
Treatment and Study of Sudden Deafness ······ 169
Clinical and Experimental Study of Allergic Rhinitis ······ 170
Treatment and Research on Chronic Nasosinusitis ······ 171
Treatment and Experimental Study of Chronic Pharyngitis ······ 171
Treatment and Research on Lichen Planus of Mouth ······ 172
Appendix: References ······ 173
10) Acupuncture and Moxibustion ······ 177
Overview ······ 177
Research on Needling Techniques and Quantitative Measurement of Insertion Methods ······ 180
Treatment and Experimental Study of Asthma by Acupuncture ······ 181
Research on Treatment of Chronic Obstructive Pneumonia by Acupuncture ······ 182
Treatment and Experimental Study of Diabetes and its Complications by Acupuncture ······ 183
Experimental Study of Treatment of Gastric Diseases by Acupuncture ······ 184
Treatment and Experimental Study of Irritated Bowel Syndrome ······ 185
Clinical and Experimental Study of Treatment of Obesity by Acupuncture ······ 186
Treatment of Chronic Fatigue Syndrome ······ 187
Treatment of Hand-Shoulder Syndrome after Stroke by Acupuncture ······ 187
Treatment of Bell's Palsy ······ 188
Treatment of Insomnia ······ 189
Treatment of Female Stress Incontinence by Acupuncture ······ 191
Experimental Study of Treatment of Rheumatoid Arthritis by Acupuncture ······ 191
Treatment of Herpes Zoster by Acupuncture ······ 192
Study of Acupuncture Literature ······ 193
Study of Chengjiang School ······ 194
Appendix: References ······ 195
11) Tuina (Chinese Medical Massage) ······ 201
Overview ······ 201
Experimental Study of Tuina Methods and their Mechanism ······ 202
Treatment of Scapulohumeral Periarthritis ······ 204

Treatment of Constipation in Children by Tuina Therapy ······ 204
Treatment of Infantile Anorexia by Tuina Therapy ······ 205
Appendix: References ······ 205
12) Qigong ······ 207
Overview ······ 207
Study of Mechanism of Qigong ······ 207
Clinical Study of *Ba Duan Jin* Exercise ······ 208
Study of Influence of *Taiji* Exercise on Human Physiological Function ······ 209
Appendix: References ······ 210
13) Nursing ······ 211
Overview ······ 211
Nursing for Stroke ······ 212
Nursing for Facture ······ 213
Nursing for Peptic Ulcer ······ 213
Appendix: References ······ 214
3. Chinese Materia Medica ······ 216
1) Resources of Chinese Materia Medica ······ 216
Overview ······ 216
Research on Genetic Diversity of Medicinal Plants ······ 218
Origins of Authentic Herbs (Dao Di Yao Cai) and Influence of Changes of Production Area ······ 220
Influence of Harvest Time on Quantity of Components of Herbs ······ 221
Influence of Sulfur Fumigation on Effective Components of Herbs ······ 222
Influence of Processing at Place of Production on Effective Components of Herbs ······ 223
Pharmacognostic Study of Radix Gentianae Macrophyllae ······ 225
Appendix: References ······ 226
2) Quality Control of Chinese Materia Medica ······ 231
Overview ······ 231
Application of Molecular Identification Techniques in Studies of Medicinal Plants ······ 233
Application of Electronic Nose in Evaluating Quality of Raw Herbal Materials ······ 234
Appendix: References ······ 235
3) Chemistry of Chinese Materia Medica ······ 238
Overview ······ 238
Research on New Components of 344 Herbs ······ 239
Research on Volatile Oils of 62 Herbs ······ 283
Appendix: References ······ 289
4) Preparation of Chinese Materia Medica ······ 306
Overview ······ 306
Research on Flash Extraction of Herbs ······ 313
Research on Procedures and Techniques of Enzyme Extraction of Herbs ······ 313
Research on Preparation of Herbal Tablet ······ 314
Research on Preparation of Herbal Liposome ······ 316
Appendix: References ······ 317
5) Procession of Chinese Materia Medica ······ 323
Overview ······ 323
Study of Processing Procedures based on Multi-Index Assessment ······ 326
Study of Quality Control of Processed Herbal Products ······ 326
Comparison of Chemical Components of 13 Herbs before and after Procession ······ 327
Comparison of Pharmacological Function of 11 Herbs before and after Procession ······ 329
Appendix: References ······ 331

6) Pharmacology of Chinese Materia Medica ······ 335
Overview ······ 335
Experimental Study of Herbs in Intervening Vascular Dementia ······ 339
Research on Mechanism of Herbs in Alleviating Apoptosis of Neurocytes ······ 340
Research on Herbs in Inhibiting Angiogenesis ······ 341
Research on Herbs in Regulating Stress of Endoplasmic Reticulum ······ 342
Research on Herbs in Regulating and Controlling Activation of Microglia ······ 343
Research on Herbs in Regulating Signal Channel of PI3K/Akt ······ 344
Appendix: References ······ 345
7) Researches on Herbal Formulas ······ 355
Overview ······ 355
Clinical Application and Pharmacological Function of Xiaochaihu Decoction ······ 356
Pharmacological Study and Clinical Application of Yinchenhao Decoction ······ 357
Pharmacological Study and Clinical Application of Jinkuishenqi Pill ······ 358
Pharmacological Function of Sijunzi Decoction ······ 359
Study of Herbal Formulae in Prevention and Treatment of Lung Cancer ······ 361
Study of Mechanism of Herbal Formulae in Alleviating Ischemic Brain Injury ······ 362
Study of Herbal Formulae in Prevention and Treatment of Influenza ······ 363
Study of Herbal Formulae and Effective Components in Diminishing Insulin Resistance ······ 364
Appendix: References ······ 365

4. Healthcare ······ 371
Overview ······ 371
Study of Healthcare Philosophies of Ancient Doctors ······ 372
Fundamental Research on Sub-health Condition ······ 373
Experimental Study of Herbs and Herbal Formulae in Slowing Down Aging Process ······ 374
Appendix: References ······ 375

5. Literature and Medical History ······ 377
1) Ancient Medical Literature ······ 377
Overview ······ 377
Study of Exegetics of *Yellow Emperor's Inner Canon* (Huang Di Nei Jing) ······ 378
Study of Research Methodology of Ancient Chinese Medical Literature ······ 379
Appendix: References ······ 380
2) Schools of Traditional Chinese Medicine ······ 382
Overview ······ 382
Study of Academic Thoughts of Doctors in Cold Damage (Shang Han) School in Modern Times and Contemporary Times ······ 383
Research on Treatment of Warmth Diseases (Wen Bing) ······ 383
Study of Traditional Chinese Medicine in Xujiang Region ······ 384
Study of Traditional Chinese Medicine in Xin'an Region ······ 385
Study of Academic Thoughts of Menghe School for Traditional Chinese Medicine ······ 386
Study of Academic Thoughts of Dr. ZHU Danxi in Treatment of Spleen and Stomach Diseases ······ 387
Appendix: References ······ 387
3) Medical History and Culture ······ 390
Overview ······ 390

Study of Connotation and Core Value of TCM Culture ······ 391
Study of Body Concept in Traditional Chinese Medicine ······ 392
Study of TCM Education History ······ 392
Sanitary Articles and Medical Culture ······ 393
Study of Relations between Culture Celebrities and Traditional Chinese Medicine in Song Dynasty ······ 394
Study of Eastward Spread of Conventional Medicine in Modern Times ······ 394
Study of Medical Systems ······ 395
Appendix: References ······ 395

6. Traditional Medicines of National Minorities ······ 398
Overview ······ 398
Study of Traditional Tibetan Medicine ······ 399
Study of Traditional Mongolian Medicine ······ 400
Experimental Study of Dedu Honghua Qiwei Powder from Traditional Mongolian Medicine in Treatment of Liver Injury ······ 401
Study of Traditional Medicine of Zhuang Nationality ······ 401
Study of Fragrant Herbs in Traditional Medicine of Hui Nationality ······ 402
Study of Traditional Medicine of Tujia Nationality ······ 403
Clinical and Experimental Studies of Treatment of Arthritis by Traditional Medicines of National Minorities ······ 403
Appendix: References ······ 404

7. Traditional Chinese Medicine in Hong Kong SAR, Macao SAR, and Chinese Taiwan ······ 408
Traditional Chinese Medicine in Hong Kong SAR ······ 408
Traditional Chinese Medicine in Chinese Taiwan ······ 410
Appendix: References ······ 415

8. Traditional Chinese Medicine in Foreign Countries ······ 420
Research on Acupuncture Treatment of Accompanying Symptoms of Mammary Cancers in Foreign Countries ······ 420
Study of Qigong in Foreign Countries ······ 420
Appendix: References ······ 421

9. Education and Scientific Researches ······ 422
1) Educational Researches ······ 422
Research on Teaching Methodology of TCM Classical Books ······ 422
Study of Clinical Training Methods ······ 424
Study of Modes of Training TCM Talents ······ 424
Appendix: References ······ 426
2) Scientific and Technological Researches ······ 428
Thoughts on Theories and Methodology of Study of Integrative Medicine ······ 428
Discussion on Clinical Study Methodology of Traditional Chinese Medicine ······ 429
Application of Interdisciplinary Knowledge in Research of Traditional Chinese Medicine ······ 430
Appendix: References ······ 431

Events

1. Academic Conferences ······ 435
National Symposium on TCM Gynecology Schools was Held in Guangzhou ······ 435
Workshop on Inheritance of TCM Traumatology and Orthopedics

Schools was Held in Beijing ········· 435
Eleventh National Congress on Geriatrics was Held in Wuhan ················· 435
China Congress on TCM Andrology was Held in Beijing ······················ 435
Congress Celebrating Century of Master GUAN Youbo's Birth and Symposium on TCM Hepatopathy was Held in Beijing ················· 435
Symposium on Traditional Chinese Medicine between Two Sides of Taiwan Straits was Held in Xiamen ································ 435
Workshop on Progress of TCM Adrology and Symposium on Dr. CHEN Bowen's Academic Thought was Held in Beijing ······················ 435
Editorial Meeting and Manuscript Proofreading Meeting for 2013 Traditional Chinese Medicine Yearbook of China (Academic Volume) was Held in Shanghai ····························· 435
Eighth National Congress on Adrology by Integrative Medicine was Held in Kaifeng ······················ 435
Ninth Symposium on Emergency Medicine of TCM and Electing Meeting of Emergency Medicine of TCM Branch Association was Held in Lianyungang ················· 435
Inauguration Conference of Mental Disease Branch Association, World Federation of Chinese Medicine Societies and First Annual Academic Symposium was Held in Harbin ················· 436
Seventeenth National Congress on Pediatrics by Integrative Medicine was Held in Xiaoshan County, Hangzhou ······ 436
China Congress on Orthopedics and International Summit of Expert Orthopedists was Held in Beijing ································ 436
Twelfth International Symposium on Acupuncture was Held in Tianjin ································ 436
Fist Academic Exchange Seminar on Traditional Medicine of Hui Nationality was Held in Beijing ································ 436
2013 Annual Meeting on Editing and Publishing, China Society of Chinese Medicine, and Seminar for Presenting Excellent Papers on Prevention of Chronic Diseases was Held in Zhangjiagang ··········· 436
2013 National Summit on Wound Repairing by Integrative Medicine was Held in Tianjin ················· 436
First Workshop on Promoting Critical Techniques for External Fixation in Minimally Invasive Skill in Orthopedic Operation was Held in Beijing ······························ 436
International Symposium on Qigong was Held in Shanghai ···················· 436
Fifth International Forum on Psychosomatic Medicine was Held in Guang'anmen Hospital in Beijing ···················· 436
First International Conference of Chiropractic Alliance and Electing Meeting of National Chiropractic Technique and Academic Committee was Held in Tianjin ······························ 437
Symposium in Honor of their 50 - year Profession of Dr. GAO Jiansheng and Dr. ZHUANG Cengyuan was Held in Ophthalmology Hospital, China Academy of Chinese Medical Science ································ 437

Thirtieth National Congress on TCM Pediatrics was Held in Jinan ········ 437
Seventeenth National Symposium on Herbal Medicine History was Held Jichun City ···························· 437
Seminar on Academic Thought of Dr. WANG Tao was Held in Mei County, Shanxi Province ··········· 437
International Forum on Health and 2013 Annual Meeting for Editors-in-chief of Encyclopedia of Traditional Chinese Medicine was Held in Beijing ································ 437
Electing Meeting of Chinese Materia Medica Branch Association, World Federation of Chinese Medicine Societies, and International Congress on Health Foods was Held in Beijing ······················ 437
Inauguration Conference of Branch Association of Nursing and First International Symposium on Nursing of Traditional Chinese Medicine was Held in Nanjing ······ 437
Taishan Academic Forum was Held in Shandong University of Traditional Chinese Medicine in Jinan ································· 437
Seminar on Academic Thought of National TCM Master LU Guangxin was Held in Beijing ················· 437
Sixteenth National Symposium on TCM Culture and Electing Meeting of TCM Culture Branch Association, China Society of Chinese Medicine was Held in Beijing ················· 437

2. International Exchange ····················· 438

Secretary General of International Standard Organization (ISO) Investigated Standardization Work of Traditional Chinese Medicine ······························ 438
Members from Authentic Korean Acupuncture and Moxibustion Academy Studied Acupuncture in Gansu Province ···················· 438
LI Daning, Vice-Commissioner of State Administration of Traditional Chinese Medicine Led Group to Visit USA and Cuba ················ 438
2013 International Conference on Traditional Chinese Medicine was Held in San Francisco, USA ···································· 438
Sixteenth Seminar on Acupuncture Study for Sino-Japanese Friendship was Held in Beijing ······················ 438
Fifth Meeting for Sino-French Committee for Cooperation of Traditional Chinese Medicine was Held in Paris, France ······················ 438
China and Singapore Signed Cooperation Plan for Traditional Chinese Medicine ······························ 438
Cooperation on Training TCM Talents was Developed by Gansu Province of China and Kiev of Ukraine ······ 438
Beijing University of Traditional Chinese Medicine Renewed Agreement with Technical University Munich ································· 438
WANG Guoqiang, Vice-Minister of Health China, Met with Delegation from Kirgizia ································· 438
Delegation Sponsored by Fulbright Programs Visited Affiliated Hospital of Shanxi College of Traditional Chinese Medicine ······ 438
Officers of Shanghai Cooperation Organization Visited Affiliated Hospital of Shanxi College of Traditional Chinese Medicine ······ 439
China and Australia Jointly Established Research Center for Traditional

Chinese Medicine ······················ 439
China and Switzerland Signed Cooperation Plan on Traditional Chinese Medicine ································· 439
Thirteenth Meeting of Sino-Korean Coordination Committee of Traditional Medicine was Held in Beijing ································· 439
China and USA Started Research on Quality Standard for TCM Hospitals for JCI ······················ 439
WANG Guoqiang, Vice-Minister of Health China, Met with Dr. Margaret Chan, Director-General of World Health Organization ······ 439
A Series of Lectures on Traditional Chinese Medicine was Delivered in Mexico ···································· 439
Fourth Training Course for Senior Teachers of Traditional Chinese Medicine in Asia was Held in Tianjin ··································· 439
China and Kirgizia Signed Memorandum of Understanding in Cooperation of Traditional Chinese Medicine ································ 439
WANG Guoqiang, Vice-Minister of Health China, Led Delegation of Traditional Chinese Medicine to Visit Russia ························ 439
Tenth International Congress on Traditional Chinese Medicine and Conference Celebrating 10 Anniversary of World Federation of Chinese Medicine Societies was Held in San Francisco ········ 440
MA Jianzhong, Vice-Commissioner of State Administration of Traditional Chinese Medicine, Met with Delegation from Poland ··············· 440
Research Institute of Shijiazhuang Yiling Pharmaceutical Company Limited Cooperated with Cardiff University, UK ························ 440
WANG Guoqiang, Vice-Minister of Health China, Met with Delegation from Macedonia ······················ 440
Gjorge Ivanov, President of Republic of Macedonia Visited Affiliated Hospital of Chengdu University of Traditional Chinese Medicine ································ 440
Qihuang College of Traditional Chinese Medicine was Opened in Ukraine Medical University ···················· 440
MA Jianzhong, Vice-Commissioner of State Administration of Traditional Chinese Medicine, Led Delegation to Visit Australia and Fiji ··········· 440
Eighth Acupuncture Congress of World Federation of Acupuncture and Moxibustion Societies was Held in Convention Center in Sydney, Australia ································ 440
Wangjing Hospital, China Academy of Chinese Medical Science, Signed Cooperation Agreement with Mexico Eastsouth Medical Association of Acupuncture and Moxibustion ····························· 440
2013 Singapore High-Level Forum on Traditional Chinese Medicine was Held in Singapore College of Traditional Chinese Medicine in Toa Payoh, Singapore ·············· 440
Heilongjiang University of Traditional Chinese Medicine Signed Cooperation Agreement with School of Medicine in Russia ······ 441
China Academy of Chinese Medical Science Developed Cooperation on Clinic of Traditional Chinese Medicine with Government of Moscow Region, Russia ··········· 441

3. News and Events ······························ 442
Donguibogam in English Edition was Officially Published ·················· 442
XIA Guicheng was Awarded Bethune Prize ······································ 442
2013 National Work Conference on Traditional Chinese Medicine was Held in Beijing ························ 442
First Forum on Protection and Development of Intangible Heritage of Traditional Chinese Medicine was Held in Taiyuan ································· 442
Seventh Forum on Inheriting National TCM Masters' Experience and Electing Meeting of Committee of Inheritance of Distinguished TCM Master's Experience, China Folklore TCM Development Association was Held in Beijing ··································· 442
GUO De'an was Awarded Norman Farnsworth Prize by American Botanical Council ····················· 442
Top Ten News of Traditional Chinese Medicine in 2012 was Announced ····························· 442
Eighty Two Hospitals were Awarded Role Model of National General Hospital of Traditional Chinese Medicine ································ 442
National Standardization Workshop was Held in Beijing ······················· 443
Accreditation Center of State Food and Drug Administration Published Report on Evaluation of Drugs in China 2012 ····························· 443
TWGHs Sophia Wang Eddie Wang Integrated Chinese Medicine with Western Medicine Symposium was Held in Hong Kong SAR ··········· 443
National Health and Family Planning Commission of People's Republic of China was Officially Formed ······ 443
Professional Committee for Standardization of Traditional Chinese Medicine was First Established in Guangdong Province ································ 443
Anhui College of Traditional Chinese Medicine was Renamed as Anhui University of Traditional Chinese Medicine ································ 443
China Food and Drug Administration was Officially Launched ·············· 443
Shanghai Branch of Alumni Association of Beijing University of Traditional Chinese Medicine was Established ····························· 443
Conference in Honor of Acupuncture Master HU Yinpei's 100 Birth was Held in Beijing ·················· 443
Standard Protocol for Three-edged Needle was Awarded China Standardization Innovation Prize ························ 444
2013 Sino-ASEAN Summit on Traditional Chinese Medicine and Fifth China (Yulin) Exposition of Traditional Chinese Medicine was Held in International Conference Center in Yulin City ····························· 444
China Defined Standard of Residue of Sulfur Dioxide in Herbs ··············· 444
WANG Guoqiang was Appointed as Deputy General Director of National Health and Family Planning Commission of People's Republic of China ····················· 444
2nd Workshop on Quality Identification Techniques for Herbs was Held in Macau SAR ····························· 444
Press Conference for Launching First International Standard for Acupuncture Needle was Held in Beijing ································ 444
Beijing University of Traditional Chinese

Medicine Celebrated Establishing TCM Internal Medicine Department ··· 444
First Distant Diagnosis Center for Cancer Experts was Launched in Andingmen TCM Hospital in Beijing ··· 444
Database for Unique Plants Used in Traditional Uygur Medicine in Xinjiang Uygur Autonomous Region ··· 444
First International Forum on Chronic Diseases Management by Integrative Medicine was Held in Hong Kong SAR ··· 444
Inauguration Conference of International Network Alliance for Traditional Chinese Medicine was Held in Beijing ··· 444
Third Expert Committee for 973 Project of Theories of Traditional Chinese Medicine was Set up in Beijing ··· 444
Fifth International Contribution Award for Traditional Chinese Medicine was Announced in Beijing ··· 444
First Advanced Workshop for Professional Management of Traditional Chinese Medical Hospital was Launched in Beijing ··· 444
Sino-American Workshop on Strategic Cooperation on Traditional Chinese Medicine was Held in Beijing ··· 445
Seminar on Drug Monitoring Management in China was Formed in Beijing ··· 445
Meeting for Initiating Workshops for Inheriting TCM Academic Schools was Held in Guangzhou ··· 445
Fifth Symposium on Herbal Paste (Gao Fang) was Held in Shanghai ··· 445
TCM Culture and Industry Exposition and Second Forum on Authentic Herbal Material in China was Held in Beijing ··· 445
Director of Food and Health Bureau Hong Kong SAR Visited State Administration of Traditional Chinese Medicine ··· 445
National Meeting for Health Aiding for Foreign Countries and in Honor of 50th Anniversary of Assigning Medical Teams to Foreign Countries was Held in Beijing ··· 445
Twelfth International TCM Modernization and Healthcare Product Exhibition was Held in Hong Kong SAR ··· 445
Inauguration Meeting for Traditional Chinese Medicine Information Branch Association, Chinese Health Information Association and Workshop for Traditional Chinese Medicine Information was Held in Shijizhuang ··· 445
Seminar for Health Media between Two Sides of Taiwan Straits was Held in Beijing ··· 445
National Forum on Development of TCM Healthcare Industry was Held in Beijing ··· 445
Meeting of Committee of TCM Education in Higher Institution, Ministry of Education, was Held in Lanzhou ··· 445
Summit for Advocating Moral as a Master Doctor and Resisting Unhealthy Practice was Held in Beijing ··· 446
2013 World Traditional Medicine Exhibition and Festival and World Competition of Herbal Diet was Held in Donguibogam Village, Sancheong, Korea ··· 446

National Forum on Traditional Medicine of Hui Nationality and Inauguration Conference for Traditional Medicine of Hui Nationality Branch Association, China Society of Traditional Medicine of Minor Races was Held in Wuzhong ········ 446
Fourth International Conference on Modernization of Traditional Chinese Medicine was Held in Chengdu ································ 446
Inner Mongolian Branch of Alumni Association of Beijing University of Traditional Chinese Medicine was Established ······················ 446
China Needle-Knife Technique Innovation Alliance was Formed in Beijing ································· 446
2013 Summit on Emergency Medicine of Traditional Chinese Medicine was Held in Beijing ······················ 446
State Administration of Traditional Chinese Medicine Finalized List of Inheritance Workshops for National TCM Masters ·············· 446
2013 International Congress on Re-evaluation of Marketed Herbal Products was Held in Beijing ······ 447
First Advanced Training Workshop on Buddhist Scriptures for Traditional Chinese Medicine was Held in Beijing ································· 447
WANG Qi was Awarded Ho Leung Ho Lee Prize in 2013 ···················· 447
Workshop for 10th Anniversary of World Federation of Chinese Medicine Societies was Held in Beijing ······ 447
Training Workshop for Innovative Technique of Traditional Chinese Medicine and Cross Reference of Herbal Formula Database was Held in Changsha ···················· 447
Fourth Training Course for Traditional Tibetan Medicine was Held in Beijing Hospital of Traditional Tibetan Medicine ··················· 447
Ningxia Branch of Alumni Association of Beijing University of Traditional Chinese Medicine was Established in Yinchuan ···························· 447
First World Acupuncture Week was Held in Beijing ······················ 448
Sino-Austral International Research Center for Traditional Chinese Medicine was Officially Recognized as a National Level Center ·············· 448
Sixth South China Forum on Traditional Chinese Medicine was Held in Guangzhou ···························· 448
Fujian Branch of Alumni Association of Beijing University of Traditional Chinese Medicine was Established in Xiamen ······························ 448
YU Wenming, Vice-Commissioner of State Administration of Traditional Chinese Medicine, Met with Delegation of Charity Organizations from Hong Kong SAR ·············· 448
Sub-Volume of Chinese Materia Medica, Volume of Chinese Medicine, Chinese Classical Encyclopedia was Published ······························ 448
YU Wenming, Vice-Commissioner of State Administration of Traditional Chinese Medicine, Met with Prof. LAO Lixing, Dean of College of Traditional Chinese Medicine, University of Hong Kong ·········· 448

Index

Subject Index of Traditional Chinese Medicine Yearbook of China (Academic Volume) (2014) ·········· 451

Appendix: CD Contents of The Yearbook f Traditional Chinese Medicine of China (Academic Volume, 2014)

New Formulated Regulations, Principles, and Standards on Chinese Medicine in 2013
National Essential Drug List (2012)
Diagnostic and Treatment Protocol for Human Infected by H7N9 Avian Influenza (2nd edition, 2013)
List of Herbal Materials Traditionally being Used also as Food (draft 2013)
Interim Regulation on Management of National Key Clinical Specialties Project
Research Awards for Traditional Chinese Medicine in 2013
List of 2013 National Science and Technology Prize
List of 2013 China Medical Association Science and Technology Prize
List of 2013 Science and Technology Prize, China Society of Chinese Medicine
List of 2013 LI Shizhen Medical Innovation Prize
List of 2013 Science and Technolgy Prize, Chinese Integrative Medicine Association
List of Newly Published Books of Traditional Chinese Medicine in 2013
List of Journals of Traditional Chinese Medicine in 2013
Classified Contents of Papers of Academic Journals on Chinese Medicine in 2013

特　　载

始终把中西医放在同等位置

陈　竺　全国人大常委会副委员长

众所周知，中医药是中华民族的瑰宝。几千年来，中医药不仅为中华民族的繁衍昌盛作出了巨大贡献，也对世界文明进步产生了积极影响，时至今日仍在为维护人民健康发挥着重要作用。中医药不仅是国家重要的卫生资源，也是优秀的文化资源、有潜力的经济资源和具有原创优势的科技资源。大力发展中医药事业，有利于深化医改、维护人民健康、改善民生，有利于加快转变经济发展方式、推动经济发展，有利于弘扬中华文化、增强国家软实力。

近年来，在中央高度重视下，中医药事业得到了长足发展，初步形成了中医药医疗、保健、教育、科研、产业、文化、对外交流与合作全面发展的新格局，为深化医改、提高人民健康水平和服务经济社会发展作出了贡献。面对经济全球化、文化多元化的当今世界，以及我国经济社会的快速发展，如何加快推进中医药继承与创新，充分发挥中医药特色与优势，使之更顺应医学发展的新趋势、人民群众对健康的新期待、经济社会进步的新要求，值得我们深思。

必须坚持中西医并重方针

中西医并重是我国基本卫生工作方针，也是我国医药卫生事业的显著特征和优势。坚持中西医并重方针，就是要始终把中医药与西医药摆在同等重要的位置，使中医与西医发挥各自优势，相互取长补短，共同为维护和增进人民健康发挥积极作用。虽然近些年来国家扶持中医药发展的力度不断加大，但中医、西医发展依然不平衡，中医药发展相对于卫生事业发展依然比较滞后，一条腿长、一条腿短的局面继续存在。必须毫不动摇、不折不扣地坚持中西医在思想认识上、法律地位上、学术发展上和实践应用上的平等地位，不断创新体制机制，完善政策措施，增加资金投入，增强发展能力，促进中西医协调发展。

发挥中医药在深化医改中的作用

中医药具有临床疗效确切、预防保健作用独特、治疗方式灵活、费用比较低廉的特色和优势。实践已经充分证明，将中医药纳于深化医改全局，发挥中医药简便验廉的优势，不仅有效减轻了群众看病就医的负担，放大了医改的惠民效果，而且丰富和完善了中国特色基本医疗卫生制度，有利于实现深化改革的总体目标。当前，医改已进入攻坚时期，必须按照中央统一部署，抓住关键问题，充分利用好中医药这一独具特色的卫生资源，不断提高中医药的服务能力与水平，切实提高改革成效。与此同时，千百年来，中医药在养生保健、妇幼保健、妇科儿科疾病治疗等方面形成了特色，可以为提高出生人口素质作出更大的贡献。

加快传承创新促中医药学术进步

随着经济社会的深刻变化、科学技术的日新月异、现代医学的快速发展，中医药学术的传承创新发展面临新的机遇和挑战。加快推进学术进步、提高疗效，如何保持特色、突出优势，是当前乃至未来中医药发展的重中之重。只有好的疗效，才能有条件和能力与西医药并重；只有凸显特色优势，才能与西医药优势互补，共同担负起提高人民健康水平的历史重任。必须始终坚持以临床实践为核心，紧紧围绕中医药学术发展的瓶颈性问题，正确认识和处理好继承与创新的关系；在始终遵循中医药原创思维的前提下，充分运用现代科学的新理论、新技术和多学科交叉渗透的思路和方法，特别是注重多中心随机对照研究方法的应用，建立一批中西医学汇聚的转化医学中心，通过协同创新的体制机制，发挥中央和地方的两个积极性，加快中医药学理论与技术的创新；充分利用医改强基层、保基本的优势，和卫生计生部门机构改革的机遇，以省为单位甚至以大区为单位进行前瞻性的大规模队列研究，从而积累必要的科学数据;充分发挥中医药在生命观、健康观、医学模式等方面的特色优势,不断拓展在常见病、多发病、慢性病和疑难病以及预防保健等方面的优势领域,提高中医药的防病治病与养生保健能力。

加快中医药立法使中医药发展有法可依

目前,越来越多的国家对传统医药实行了立法管理,制定颁布了有关传统医药方面的法律法规。我国作为传统医药大国,作为中医药的发源地,中医药还缺乏国家层面的法律保障。令人欣喜的是,中医药法草案已于2011年底报送国务院法制办,并列入了2013年全国人大常委会立法计划一档。我们要共同努力,加快推进中医药立法进程,争取中医药法早日出台,促进中医药依法持续健康发展。

中医药正面临前所未有的发展机遇,衷心希望广大中医药工作者以党的十八大精神为指引,坚定信心,凝心聚力,把中医药这一国之瑰宝传承好、创新好、发展好,让中医药在全面建成小康社会和实现中华民族伟大复兴的征程中作出新的更大贡献!

原载《中国中医药报》2013年7月1日第1版

专　　论

将中医药发展纳入国家战略

任　壮

建议编制实施国家中医药中长期发展规划。明确中医药在国家战略中的地位，提出国家发展中医药的战略方针、战略目标、战略任务、战略步骤以及战略措施。

建议将中医药产业纳入新的战略性新兴产业。

建议加强对中医药工作的领导。成立高规格的国家中医药工作领导小组，加强统筹协调。建立健全地方各级中医药管理机构，强化管理职能。

纳入必要性

中医药在改善民生、转变经济发展方式、弘扬中华文化、建设生态文明等国家大局中作用日益凸显。

记者：国家战略是最高层面的战略，一项事业要纳入其中，首在其"重"。而中医药在一些人的心目中，似乎不太重要。您认为将中医药纳入国家战略必要吗？

王国强：尽管近代以来中医药历经坎坷，甚至屡受质疑或否定，但新中国成立后，党中央、国务院重视中医药事业发展。尤其近年来，国务院发布实施《关于扶持和促进中医药事业发展的若干意见》，中医药迅猛发展，不仅在参与深化医改中发挥着越来越重要的作用，而且在经济、文化、社会、科技、生态、国际交流等方面，日益显示出重要价值。

一是中医药可为深化医改、维护人民健康、改善民生发挥更大作用。中医药临床疗效确切、预防保健作用独特、治疗方式灵活、费用比较低廉，深受群众欢迎，有助于建立政府承受得了、群众负担得起、财政可持续保障、中西医并重的中国特色医疗保障制度和医疗卫生发展模式，实现人人享有基本医疗卫生服务。

二是中医药可为加快转变经济发展方式、推动经济发展发挥更大作用。中医药是我国最具原始创新潜力的科技资源，有助于实施创新驱动发展战略，形成新的经济增长点；中医药相关健康产业，贯穿整个产业链，是潜力巨大的战略性新兴产业。随着中医药走向世界，国际需求日益增长，有助于提高开放型经济和服务贸易水平。

三是中医药可为弘扬中华文化、推进文化强国建设发挥更大作用。中医药是中华民族优秀传统文化，正如习近平总书记所指出的，中医药学凝聚着深邃的哲学智慧和中华民族几千年的健康养生理念及其实践经验，是中国古代科学的瑰宝，也是打开中华文明宝库的钥匙。中医药以人为本，崇尚和谐，体现了中华民族的认知方式和价值取向，是我国文化软实力的重要体现。繁荣发展中医药文化，有助于建设优秀文化传承体系，增强中华文化国际影响力。

四是中医药可为推进生态文明建设发挥更大作用。中医药产业具有环境友好型、资源节约型特征，是典型的绿色产业、生态产业、节约型产业。加强中药资源保护和合理利用，有助于保护生物多样性、生物遗传资源，保护自然生态环境；推动中药材规范化、规模化种植，有助于生态修复；发展中药产业，有助于推进绿色发展、低碳发展。

所以，在当前国内外形势下，将中医药发展纳入国家战略有重要意义，是必要的。

纳入可行性

中医药具备战略意义和新兴产业特征，科技创新体系日趋完善，产业基础良好，服务贸易渐兴。

记者：一项事业要纳入国家战略，不仅因其重要，还须在国家总体战略中能够发挥重要作用，具备可行性。您认为，当前中医药的发展做好这方面准备了吗？

王国强：是的。特别是近年来，在党中央、国务院的高度重视和支持下，中医药工作取得显著成就，形成了中医药"六位一体"科学发展的新格局，为中医药在国家总体战略中发挥作用奠定了基础，蓄积了势能。

一是中医药发展具备战略意义和新兴产业特征。中医药已成为维护人民健康、改善民生的重要战略资源。医改的实践表明,中医药服务在缓解看病就医问题、减轻患者和医保负担、提高人民健康水平等方面发挥了很好的作用,放大了医改的惠民效果。

中医药可提升我国在全球经济竞争中的比较优势。医药产业在国家经济发展中的独特作用已成共识,中医药相关产业则是我国医药产业中独有的特色和优势领域,具有自主知识产权,是典型的民族工业之一,在全球化经济竞争中具有明显的比较优势。

中医药具有新兴产业的基本特征。中医药具有新兴产业的“服务+制造型”的模式,可以集中各种创新要素,推动高技术产品的推出和更新换代。中医药产业发展,可以改变“资源—产品—废品”的简单线性生产方式,变为“资源—产品—再生资源”的循环经济模式,实现资源利用循环化。

中医药已成为许多地方经济社会发展的战略选择。近年来,许多地方将发展中医药作为转变经济发展方式的重要选择,成效显著。西部各省市普遍依托中药材的资源优势,繁荣了中药产业经济,带动地区经济跨越发展,已成为我国西部大开发的重要支撑点。广东省早在 2006 年就提出了中医药强省战略,陕西铜川将发展中医药作为城市转型的方向,安徽亳州、河北安国等地都将中医药产业作为支柱性产业。

二是中医药科技创新体系日趋完善。中医药科技创新平台基本形成。目前,我国已建成 16 家国家中医临床研究基地、8 个“国家工程技术研究中心”、3 个“国家中药工程研究中心”,一大批国家重点研究室,基本形成了中医药科技创新体系。

中医药自主创新能力显著增强。“十一五”期间,有 52 项中医药成果获国家科技奖励,发明专利授权 2.3 万件。中药研发取得重大突破。我国学者因发现用于治疗疟疾的药物青蒿素,获 2011 年美国拉斯克临床医学奖;复方丹参滴丸通过美国 FDA 二期认证,成为我国首个进入美国 FDA 三期临床试验的中成药,展示了中医药巨大开发潜力和前景。

三是中医药产业已具备良好发展基础。国家统计局数据显示,2011 年我国中药工业产值4 178 亿元,同比增长 37%,占医药工业总产值的 27%,中药产业已成为我国快速增长的产业之一。中药产品出口快速增长,2012 年中药出口已达 24 亿多美元。

四是中医药已成为我国服务贸易的重要组成部分和文化传播的重要载体。中医药已传播到 160 多个国家和地区,世界各地从事中医针灸服务的针灸师约 20 万人,每年针灸服务总产值超过 100 亿美元。中医针灸被列入人类非物质文化遗产代表作名录,在一些国家成立了中医孔子学院,成为国际社会了解中国优秀传统文化重要窗。

因此,将中医药发展纳入国家战略有可行性。

怎样纳入

编制实施国家中医药中长期发展规划,纳入新战略性新兴产业,成立高规格国家中医药工作领导小组。

记者:您既是卫生部副部长、国家中医药管理局局长,又是全国政协委员,对将中医药发展纳入国家战略有何具体建议?

王国强:事实上,自 2007 年国务院建立中医药工作部际协调机制以来,中医药得到各方支持,在国家经济社会发展大局中日益发挥作用,形成了良好局面,也为将中医药纳入国家战略奠定了较好基础。

一是建议将中医药发展纳入国家战略,并编制实施国家中医药中长期发展规划。明确中医药在国家战略中的重要地位,提出国家发展中医药的战略方针、战略目标、战略任务、战略步骤以及战略措施,推动中医药为全面建成小康社会作出更大贡献。

二是建议将中医药产业纳入新的战略性新兴产业。中医药产业不仅具备战略性新兴产业的基本特征,也具有了作为战略性新兴产业发展的基本条件,建议将中医药作为战略性新兴产业培育发展。

三是建议进一步加强对中医药工作的领导。成立高规格的国家中医药工作领导小组,加强统筹协调,研究解决中医药发展中的问题,推动各地落实扶持促进中医药发展的政策措施。逐步理顺中医药管理职能,建立健全地方各级中医药管理机构,强化管理职能。

原载《中国中医药报》2013 年 3 月 8 日第 2 版

大数据绘制当代中医航海图

刘保延　中国中医科学院常务副院长，首席研究员

● 利用大数据的继承创新过程，不同于靠抽取小样本产生的精确数据，通过因果关系的分析来回答“为什么”，但可以靠多源混杂全样本，通过相关关系来较好地回答“是什么”，通过数据发声，来帮助人们做出更加准确的决策和对未来的预测。在大数据背景下的继承创新之路，将会使人们从因果思维的束缚中得以解放，通过相关思维，把更多的精力放在提高服务质量和能力上，放在解决发展中的具体问题上。

● 如果能够抢抓机遇，绘制出当代全新概念的中医航海图，将会使蕴含了数千年丰富实践经验的继承创新成果得以激活，使辨证论治个体化诊疗能力、对人体健康状态的预测能力以及防病治病、促进人体健康的服务能力大大提升。大数据支撑下的中医药也必将在当代航海图的指引下，从传统的经验医学转化为循证医学，产生一场脱胎换骨性的变革。

● 中医学理论体系是一种“关系本体”，强调了主客体的一致、互动和相互影响。她尽管还不能很好地从生物学的角度解释“为什么”，但却可以很好地告诉你“是什么”，而正是这些“是什么”已经给人类健康保障做出了巨大贡献，同时也使其流传数千年而不衰。而大数据时代关注相关关系的强劲东风，无疑可以吹散当代科学长期以来追求“因果关系”而笼罩在中医头上的阴影，使中医可以理直气壮地沿着自身规律发展，更加道路自信、理论自信、方法自信。

大数据时代已经到来

2008 年 9 月，*Nature* 出版了一个专刊，讨论大数据存储、管理和分析等问题，昭示着大数据时代的到来。之后麦肯锡公司、*Science* 先后出版大数据报告和专刊。大数据的讨论在中国也风起云涌，中国计算机学会于 2012 年 10 月在大连成立了以中国工程院院士李国杰为首的大数据专家委员会，国家自然科学基金委于 2013 年 3 月在上海举办了第 89 期双清论坛“大数据技术与应用中的挑战性科学问题”。

2009 年，在甲型 H1N1 流感爆发的几周前，互联网巨头谷歌公司的工程师在 *Nature* 杂志发表一篇令人震惊的论文，该文根据互联网上 5 000 万条美国人最频繁检索的词条如“哪些是治疗咳嗽和发热的药物”等，与美国疾控中心在 2003 年至 2008 年间季节性流感传播时期的数据进行比较，发现了 45 条检索词条的组合，再将它们用于一个特定的数学模型所预测的流感发病趋势与 CDC 曾经预测的相关性高达 97%。该论文不仅预测了流感在美国全境的发生，还预测了在不同州或地方的传播趋势，而这样的预测不像疾控中心只能在流感爆发一两周之后才可以做到。大量类似的例子告诉人们，大数据已经在你身边。大数据的运用已经悄然启动了一次重大的时代转型！

什么是大数据，其概念定义至今莫衷一是。2012 年 8 月份国际数据挖掘会议 SIG KDD 的大数据论坛，从数据存储角度认为大数据应该是 10 台服务器也无法存储的数据，这样的数据必须进行在线分析，否则计算机存储无法支持；有专家从数据分析角度认为，数据结构很复杂，现有方法无法处理，必须采用类似谷歌的 Hadoop 平台进行处理的就是大数据。而在 2013 年维克托·迈尔·舍恩伯格和肯尼斯·库克耶出版的《大数据时代》，则从数据利用价值的角度认为“大数据是人们在大规模数据的基础上可以做到的事情，而这些事情在小规模数据的基础上是无法完成的。大数据是人们获得新的认知，创造新价值的源泉，还是改变市场、组织机构以及政府与公民关系的方法”。

总之，笔者体会“大数据”不仅是数据量大，数据结构复杂，而且应该是动态变化、蕴含着丰富使用价值的数据。如今在我们身边具有大数据潜质的信息资源随处可见，目前大多以纸张或模拟信

息媒介的形式存放,但随着数字信息技术、网络技术以及物联网技术的出现和应用,他们大都可以被数据化后而激活,成为拥有巨大创新价值的宝库。而中医药领域浩瀚的古代医籍、大量病历资料与现代科学研究文献,以及随着物联网的广泛应用,人们衣食住行过程以及健康信息监测所产生的数字信息,也都将成为可以有力促进中医药和人类健康事业发展的大数据。

大数据是继承创新的源泉和利器

远在 1855 年,时任美国海军的马修·方丹·莫里利用前人遗留的具有大数据潜质的航海日志,绘制出给航海业带来巨大变化的航海图。航海日志是船长个人的航海经历的记录,但这些经验信息并没有得到应用。而莫里在发现库房中存留的大量航海日志后,他与 20 位从事数据处理的人一起,把破损的航海日志记录的有用信息,通过数据提取,制成表格,整合数据之后,把整个大西洋按经纬度划分成了 5 块,并按月份标出了温度、风速和风向等。于是,这些来自破旧脏乱航海日志的信息,变成了有效的航海路线图。为了不断地提高航海线路的精度,莫里要求航海图的使用者都要将航行经历、使用事先特定的表格继续记录成航海日志,他们再根据航海日志产生的数据不断地修订和完善航海图。航海图使用后使原航行路程缩短了三分之一,并大大减少了航行的危险,此后不仅得到美国海军的使用,而且也被商船大量使用。

尽管谷歌公司预测流感发病趋势与莫里绘制航海图相差了 100 多年,如今存储、管理和利用数据的方式与速度已经发生了革命性的变化,但二者都是在"继承"已经存在的"检索词条"或"航海日志"的基础上,将这些信息数据化,而后利用这些数据创造出了那些记录"航海日志"或在互联网检索的人们不可想象的创新成果。

所以我们可以看到,大数据是继承创新的源泉,也是继承创新的有力工具。利用大数据的继承创新过程,不同于靠抽取小样本产生的精确数据,通过因果关系的分析来回答"为什么",但可以靠多源混杂全样本,通过相关关系来较好地回答"是什么",通过数据发声,来帮助人们做出更加准确的决策和对未来的预测。大数据背景下的继承创新之路,将会使人们从因果思维的束缚中得以解放,通过相关思维,把更多的精力放在提高服务质量和能力上,放在解决发展中的具体问题上,他必将大大推进社会发展的进程和速度。

用大数据绘制中医药的航海图

作为持续发展了数千年的中医药学,以人为中心,以显著的临床效果为基础,将人体状态变化与干预方法相关联,构建了其系统的理论体系,形成了其自身发展道路。继承创新是其发展的主要模式,从临床中来、到临床中去是其发展的主要途径;"名医"是其发展的重要载体和代表,而浩瀚的医籍著作则是中医丰富经验和体悟的真实记载,是中医药理论与新方法、新技术的重要源泉,也是真实记载中医发展历程的"航海日志"。

历代不断有人对这些"航海日志"进行着整理总结和提炼,并已经绘制出了不同层次的"航海图",指引着中医航行的方向。如目前可见的最早系统阐述中医理论的《黄帝内经》、辨证论治鼻祖《伤寒杂病论》都是先贤们在"勤求古训、博采众方",结合临床经验对大量已有中医"航海日志"的梳理中,所绘制的中医"航海图"。这些"航海图",在数千年发展历程中,指引着中医药的发展方向,指导广大中医药"航海者",拯救了无数人的生命,为人类健康做出了巨大贡献。

"航海图"的绘制,关键是靠有效的数据,而从浩瀚医籍提取出特征数据并将其整合升华,变成新的知识,则靠创新思维以及相应的方法和技术。以往中医航海图的绘制,是将大量医籍或临证记录通过摘抄等方法提取特征数据,而后主要是靠"悟性"与渊博的知识来提炼升华而成。但受到古医籍存在方式和个人占有量、阅读量的限制,以及有效数据提取和融合加工能力的制约,绝大多数中医的航海日志的有效信息并没有得到系统提取利用,而对于隐藏在大量混杂数据中的知识,也没能被很好的挖掘出来,中医宝库中大多数的精华并未得到激活和利用。

当代,中医药的数据资源已经有了极大的丰富,除了浩瀚的古代医籍外,现代大量的研究文献(包括现代医学与生物学研究文献)以及动态更新的、多媒体的临床病历资料等,已经形成了真正意义上的"大数据"。而已经被广泛使用的数字信息技术、网络通讯技术、物联网、数据挖掘利用与数据存储与传输技术等,则为绘制当代中医药航海图提供了有力的技术支撑。如果能够抢抓机遇,通过多学科人员的密切合作，组织起中医药大数据产生、管理与利用的专业化队伍，搭建起相应的技术平台，以丰富的文献和临床资源为基础，整合现代医学和生物学等研究的成果，以临床问题为驱动，以数据为导向，借助数据模型，绘制出当代全新概念的中医航海图，将会使蕴含了数千年丰富实践经验的继承创新成果得以激活，使辨证论治个体化诊疗能力、对人体健康状态的预测能力以及防病治病、促进人体健康的服务能力大大提升。大数据支撑下的中医药也必将在当代航海图的指引下，从传统的经验医学转化为循证医学，产生一场脱胎换骨性的变革。

当代中医航海图的绘制已起步

近些年，随着信息技术的不断发展和应用，作为国家队的中国中医科学院，已经从古代医籍、现代文献与临床病历数据化入手，为绘制当代中医的航海图奠定了丰厚基础。

中医古代医籍数字化、数据化与知识库建设工程已经初具规模。

由柳长华研究员牵头的中国中医科学院中医古籍数字化研究团队，整合全国百余位专家，组成专业化古籍整理、校勘、数字化、数据化的研究队伍，形成了“国家中医古籍整理与数字化研究中心”。截至目前，在国家中医药管理局、国家科技部基础条件平台建设等项目支持下，累计完成1 690种中医古籍的图像扫描，约139万余页。完成了其中613种古籍（约6 957万字）的文本识别工作，部分古籍资源实现了图文对照和全文检索功能。建设了800种中医古籍的影像数据库和全文数据库。完成了350种中医古籍（约4 500万字）的深度加工标引工作。此项工作从2000年开始首先形成了“基于知识元的中医古籍计算机知识表示方法”，解决中医古籍数据化的问题，在此基础上研究团队又制定了《中医古籍数字化文本校勘整理规范》《中医古籍疑难字处理规范》《中医古籍图像采集管理规范》《中医古籍图像处理技术标准》《中医古籍元数据规范》《中医古籍知识元标引流程规范》等一系列指导古籍数字化建设的技术标准及系列古籍知识标引手册等，研发了“中医古籍知识加工平台”、“中医古籍叙词表加工系统”、“中医古籍知识库”、“中医古籍阅览系统”等，为中医古籍大规模数字化、数据化建设以及面向临床的知识服务提供了技术保障。解决了中医古籍数字化以及数据化的技术难题。目前，利用古籍数据资源进行数据挖掘的方法正在研究之中。中医古籍数字化、数据化工作以及中医古籍知识库的构建，已经为利用古代医籍绘制当代中医航海图，提供了有力的工具，奠定了雄厚的基础。

中医现代科技数据共享平台，已经成为国家人口健康科学数据共享平台的重要组成部分。

由崔蒙研究员牵头的中国中医科学院中医药信息研究所的研究团队，自1984年开始进行中医药学大型数据库的建设，制定了中医药元数据标准、中医药一体化语言系统等，基于WEB技术等建立以中国中医科学院为中心的中医科技文献共建平台，形成了全国35家单位300多位研究人员组成的中医科技文献数据化建设队伍，创建了中医、中药、针灸、古籍文献类数据库100余个，包括1984年以来的中医药期刊文献数据库、疾病诊疗数据库、各类中药数据库、方剂数据库、民族医药数据库、药品企业数据库、各类国家标准数据库（中医证候、治则、疾病、药物、方剂）等相关数据库。所有的数据库都可以通过中医药数据库检索系统提供中文（简体、繁体）版联网使用；部分数据提供英文版；所有数据库还可以获取光盘版。中医药数据库检索系统可以实现单库与多库选择查询。单表数据库检索可选择最专指的一个数据库进行相应字段的检索。多库可以进行跨库、多类检索。为了充分利用这些科学数据资源，研究团队还建立了数据挖掘方法的整合平台与高性能运算的技术平台。目前，作为国家人口与健康科学数据共享平台的重要组成部分，为全社会国内外用户提供着科学数据的服务。成为利用现代科技文献绘制当代中医航海图的有力工具。

中医临床科研信息共享系统已经初具规模，临床数据采集与海量数据分析利用的技术平台已经在20多家医院搭建。

中国中医科学院临床评价方法的研究团队，从2001年开始在北京市科委重大项目的支持下，就着手建立中医临床科研信息共享的技术体系，解决将临床实际诊疗信息实时数据化以及对复杂海量临床数据的分析利用的问题。到目前为止，“共享系统”已经建立了“数字化中医临床术语应用体系”、“结构化的临床科研一体化数据采集系统”、“临床数据前处理系统”、“中医临床数据仓库系统”、“中医临床数据多维检索查询与展示系统”

与“中医临床数据挖掘系统”。“共享系统”已经在国家临床研究基地等20余家医院进行了搭建并投入使用。中医临床数据仓库已经有了10余万数据化的病历资源,并以此为基础开展各种研究超百项。以“中医临床科研信息共享系统”为技术支撑,以“真实世界临床研究范式”为指引,将临床实际诊疗信息数据化并开展研究的工作已经开始起步。符合中医自身发展规律的中医临床研究方法与技术体系已经初步形成。利用古代文献、现代科技文献以及临床实际诊疗信息等中医数据资源,绘制当代中医航海图的时代工程已经有了坚实基础。时不我待,拥抱大数据,实现中医腾飞的中医梦,必将成为现实。

绘制当代中医航海图的当务之急

要转变观念,尽快从因果关系的渴求中解脱出来,高度关注相关关系,找到不断提高中医疗效、提升服务质量和能力的根本途径。

观念的转变是根本的转变。“大数据时代对我们的生活,以及与世界交流的方式都提出了挑战。最惊人的是,社会需要放弃它对因果关系的渴求,而仅需关注相关关系……这就推翻了自古以来的惯例,而我们做决定和理解现实的最基本方式也将受到挑战。”

中医学理论体系是一种“关系本体”,强调了主客体的一致、互动和相互影响。它以“效”—“阴平阳秘”为尺度,建立了医者主体以及干预措施与患者客体功能状态间直接的、复杂的相关关系,成为一个独特的、系统的、可以有效指导临床实践的理论体系。这一理论体系是一个复杂的巨系统,她尽管还不能很好地从生物学的角度解释“为什么”,但却可以很好地告诉你“是什么”,而正是这些“是什么”已经给人类健康保障做出了巨大贡献,同时也使其流传数千年而不衰。而大数据时代关注相关关系的强劲东风,无疑可以吹散当代科学长期以来追求“因果关系”而笼罩在中医头上的阴影,使中医可以理直气壮地沿着自身规律发展,更加道路自信、理论自信、方法自信。大张旗鼓地全力以赴通过相关关系,去寻找更加有效的方法、方药,提高解决临床难题的能力和水平,而不急于投入巨大的精力和资源,利用精确的“小数据”去回答“为什么”。当然如果中医学既能告诉“是什么”,同时又能很好的回答“为什么”,中医药学将会成为人们渴望的新医学!

搭建平台,激活周围潜在的大数据,加大中医数据资源的建设,使蕴藏在临床实践中的创新能量最大限度的释放出来

如果要将具有继承创新特点的古今“航海日志”,转变成能够有效服务于中医临床实践的“当代中医航海图”,除了要改变观念以外,还要通过数字信息技术,激活我们周围具有潜在价值的信息,快速扩充中医药数据资源,并在人工智能、数据挖掘等方法的支持下,人机结合,借助“悟性”使中医药大数据变成预测健康状态发展趋势、辅助诊疗决策的有力工具,提升中医服务能力和水平。加快建设国家中医药数据中心,建立数据共享机制,围绕重大疾病采集大数据,尝试整合临床诊疗与医学研究数据。

丰富的中医、中西医结合临床资源是我国独有的宝库,也是许多人梦寐以求的资源。如果能发挥“举国体制”的优势,将有一定实力的中医医院的临床信息数据化并汇集起来,形成可以共享的临床数据资源,将会大大加快中医利用大数据发展的速度。可以借鉴国家临床研究基地临床科研信息共享系统建设的经验,按照临床科研一体化研究范式,围绕重大疾病建立数据分中心与国家临床数据中心。可以组织通过国家临床研究基地、重点专科等带动相应的科室或医院,在统一的标准规范下,进行数据的采集、汇聚与共享、分析等。国家数据中心不只是数据的汇聚地,也是数据化技术、数据分析利用技术的提供地,大数据项目的研究中心与多学科人才的培训基地。不久前,李嘉诚基金会与政府共同支持的英国首个综合运用大数据技术的医药卫生科研中心在牛津大学成立。英国首相卡梅伦在揭牌仪式上说,这一中心的成立有望给英国医学研究和医疗服务带来革命性变化,它将促进医疗数据分析方面的新进展,帮助科学家更好地理解人类疾病及其治疗方法。这是一个很值得关注的案例。

在目前的中医临床研究中,临床诊疗数据只是其中重要的一部分。为了更全面地从基础医学、临床医学和预防医学角度进行研究,要整合临床病历和相关医学研究数据,为中医辨证论治个体化诊疗体系提供基础原理支持和更深入的科学认识。要建立医学健康信息数据库,整合并融合古代文献数据、现代科技文献数据以及HIS、RIS、PACS、病理、用药等临床理化检测数据和基因表达、SNP、蛋白质组学、代谢组学以及新药临床试验等医学生物学研究数据，这样利用大数据所开展的研究，不但能回答“是什么”，同时也可以回答“为什么”了。

大力发展物联网技术，提高中医大数据采集的便捷性和准确性

大力发展物联网技术，提高数据采集、存储、传输的规范性、正确性和广泛性。随着物联网技术的广泛应用，可以实时自动采集人们衣食住行过程的各种信息，同时可以通过穿戴式采集系统实时收集大量的人体健康状态的变化信息，提高信息采集的完整性、便利性、正确性，同时降低成本。物联网技术不仅在信息采集，而且在临床干预方面也很重要，比如可以提醒病人按个性化时间进行用药，提高药物疗效等。

充分利用数字信息技术，大力发展中医诊疗仪器设备，使其成为中医临床信息的重要组成部分，如果这些信息能够与临床诊疗信息融合，必将为提升中医诊疗水平提供有力的支撑。目前在模拟航天训练项目中中医四诊仪的应用，通过远程采集症状、脉诊、舌诊等信息的综合分析，为航天员远程健康状态的自动检测与干预提供了新的经验和数据。

深入推进研究大数据分析处理技术，建立适合中医数据复杂特点的挖掘框架。

抽提中医数据分析中的需求，发展智能信息处理技术，有针对性地提高中医信息处理的效果。从数据分析角度看，中医数据存在多维、非线性、动态等特点，针对中医特点研究开发智能信息处理技术，如数据预处理、数据挖掘、模式分析、分类、聚类等技术，从大量临床数据中发掘隐藏在现象背后的知识，可以发掘以往靠人无法找出的规律。而且专家经验也在与时俱进，通过计算机可以自动、实时跟踪医生的思路变化，总结最新的辨证思路和用药经验，提高青年名中医的培养效率。利用智能信息处理技术，才能挖掘出中医辨证论治个体化诊疗规律，才能结合互联网技术，实时采集人和外界环境的信息，实现个体化医学。

创建体制和机制，为数据化和海量数据资源管理利用的系统工程保驾护航，才可能源源不断地从那些最不可能的地方提取出有价值的数据并形成大数据

要形成中医药大数据，要使浩瀚的中医药古籍数据化、使数十万现代研究报告数据化、使每天就诊患者病历数据化，变成用之不竭的数据资源，有以下 4 个方面的问题需要解决：第一，需要投入资金、投入大量的人力、物力；第二，只有将大家的数据资源汇集起来，建立国家、地区层次的中医药数据中心、分中心，中医药的大数据才可能很快地产生，而且可以有序地管理和高效合理地利用；第三，既然数据变成为有巨大价值的资源，资源利用的权限、使用的方法、资源相关的伦理问题、隐私保护、知识产权保护问题等均会很快成为发展的拦路虎；第四，数据资源的建设和利用，是一个在高技术支撑下的系统工程，如何建立工程实施的流程、保障工程顺畅运行、保质保量完成工程目标等等，这些均需要相应的法律、法规或管理的办法与运行的机制。其中，专业化的机构是一个核心，而产、学、研紧密结合的运行机制也是成功与否的关键。

在中医药领域开展大数据研究，要特别重视多学科人才的培养，要构建中医药大数据研究人员的知识体系，要能清晰认识中医药创新发展面临的关键问题，要有临床经验，还要了解甚至掌握计算机、数据结构、数据分析挖掘模型等知识和技术。要勇于吸纳跨学科人才，促进企业和研究机构的结合，为中医数据分析、挖掘提供充足的技术工具。具体来说可以考虑尽快设立大数据研究生班，吸收中医和数据科学领域的专业研究人员，培养既懂中医，熟悉临床，也擅长数据采集、分析的复合型人才。

原载《中国中医药报》2013 年 6 月 5 日第 3 版

校院长论坛

研究生课程教学改革的思考与探索

——以福建中医药大学为例

福建中医药大学校长　陈立典

一、研究生课程教学改革的背景及动因

研究生教育在高等教育中占有重要地位。在招生规模持续扩大的背景下，研究生教育质量越来越成为全社会关注的焦点。课程是教学的基本单元，课程教学是实现研究生培养目标的重要手段，也是研究生培养质量高低的重要标志。中医药研究生教育起步较晚，其课程设置和教学模式多参照西医院校。随着国家对高层次人才综合素质要求的提高，原有的研究生教育教学理念、专业课程设置、课程内容及教学方法已难以适应新形势的要求。总体而言，目前的中医药研究生培养存在医学基础知识不扎实、临床适应能力差、人文素质弱、学生学习动力不足等问题，其根源在于研究生课程教学仍以被动灌输为主，严重影响了教与学的积极性，制约和阻碍着中医药研究生教育质量的提高。

福建中医药大学是一所具有50多年办学历史的省属重点建设高校。现有2个博士学位授权一级学科，2个博士后科研流动站，14个博士点、41个硕士点，有研究生1 349人。随着学校研究生规模的扩大，走以质量提升为核心的内涵式发展道路，全面提高研究生培养质量成为学校当前的首要任务，被列为学校“十二五”发展规划的一项重要任务。基于此，在学校党委的正确领导和校领导的直接参与下，2010年5月，学校开始启动了以“提高研究生培养质量，建设高水平有特色的教学研究型大学”为最终目的，以“完善专业课程体系、更新教育教学模式、提高学生自主拓展学习能力”为主要目标的研究生课程教学改革。

二、研究生课程教学改革的探索与实践

学校研究生课程教学改革的探索与实践经历了5个主要阶段。

第一阶段：寻找共识、确定方案

在学校党政的直接指导下，通过赴兄弟院校调研，召开研究生导师、任课教师及学生代表座谈会及对近几年来学校研究生课程教学评教结果进行综合分析等活动，探寻影响学校研究生课程教学质量的制约因素，在此基础上制定了课程教学改革的初步方案。

随后，学校召开多场研究生课程教学改革专题会议，宣讲研究生课程教学改革的理念、目标、内容及实施办法。同时，深入各培养单位开展了30多场座谈会，向研究生导师、相关专家传达改革精神，介绍具体做法，并征询意见和建议。通过一系列有效举措，使各研究生培养单位从“要不要改革”的迷茫和彷徨中统一到“改革势在必行”的认识上，达成了齐心协力推进改革的共识，并在反复论证的基础上制定了研究生课程教学改革方案。

第二阶段：外延切入，推进公共课改革

1. *转变公共必修课教学方式*　大力推进思想政治、哲学等公共必修课程的改革，在遵守教育部相关政策的前提下，与时俱进地对教学内容和教学方式进行合理调整。采取教师讲解、学生讨论及外聘专家讲座等灵活多样的方式进行教学，在一定程度上解决了相关课程内容枯燥乏味、教学形式单一的问题，提高了学生学习的积极性和主动性。

2. *试行分班式的英语教学*　按照学生入学时是否通过大学生英语六级考试进行分班教学，做到因材施教，并在课程中设置以提高研究生英语综合素养为目的的“通识英语”教育课程(含英语口语、英语听说及读写能力等内容)。同时，聘请外校著名专家到校讲学，开设高水平英语讲座，以促进我校研究生英语教师教学水平的提升，也扩大学生视野。

3. *增设《医学信息检索》选修课*　以增强学

生自我学习能力为目标，增加实践操作部分，全部课程在图书馆电子阅览室中完成。

4. 加强研究生科研实践能力的培养　博士研究生在福建中西医结合研究院细胞生物学、蛋白组学、分子生化学、基因组学等 4 个实验平台轮转，并要求通过严格的出站式考核，以确保每位博士研究生都能掌握先进的科研实验技术。整合全校科研实验资源，为硕士研究生开放基因组实验技术、形态学等 13 个平台。每位研究生可根据自己的研究方向和兴趣爱好选择到相关平台轮转学习，为自己的课题设计及科研打基础。

第三阶段：结合实际，推动专业核心课程改革

为帮助学生夯实专业基础知识，提高创新能力和综合素质，并充分发挥研究生个人的才能和特长。经充分讨论、反复凝练，学校按照导师的研究方向设置课程，并依托导师或研究团队讲授、辅导和研究生自学相结合的方式，引导每个专业打造一门让学生终身受益的核心课程。核心课程的考核采用试卷、文献阅读记录(心得)和专业小论文等灵活多样的形式。通过专业核心课程的建设，我校研究生培养既融入专业特色，体现学校的特色和优势，又彰显了学生的个性化特点。

第四阶段：内涵提升，打造研究生课程库

学校通过召开教师、博士生、硕士生座谈会，发放调查问卷，进行研究生随机抽样调研等形式，充分征求师生对研究生课程库建设的意见和建议。同时，建立健全了研究生课程申报、遴选和审批流程，由各学院任课教师申报课程，并及时召开系列课程遴选会议。各课程主任通过遴选报告会汇报课程设置理念、课程内容及教学方法等，评审专家进行现场点评，并就如何开设好研究生系列课程提出建设性意见及建议。

在此基础上，学校对全校研究生专业课程进行梳理，明确了硕士研究生阶段课程内容的特点和层次，淘汰内容陈旧的课程，新增必要的课程 25 门，使研究生课程库的课程总数达 128 门，形成基础、人文等系列课程模块，打通了各专业的必修课程与选修课程，从而构建了开放、互通的研究生课程库。

第五阶段：及时总结，巩固改革成果

为及时总结经验，巩固研究生课程教学改革成果，学校开展了以下工作：一是于课程教学改革开展 6 周后，做了初步总结，并及时发出通知要求各学院、任课教师将课程教学改革结合到具体教研室活动中，要求他们在教研过程中解决存在的问题。二是召开研究生教学改革阶段性经验交流会，安排中医诊断学、针灸推拿学(康复方向)等 2 个专业举行研究生课程教学改革交流报告会，为各研究生培养单位开展课程教学改革工作进行示范。三是以 2011 级、2012 级研究生为对象，开展改革效果和存在问题的问卷调查，并召开教师和研究生代表座谈会，了解改革后的研究生课程教学效果。四是启动学校研究生教育改革科研项目立项征集工作，共立项 33 个项目，加强了课程教学改革理论研究，为深化改革提供了进一步的理论支撑。

三、研究生课程教学改革的成效

1. 确立了新的研究生教育理念

在改革过程中，逐步树立了以学生发展为中心的教学思路，构建了以学生素质为核心的知识结构，实现了教学过程师生的良好互动。同时，实现了教师角色的 3 大转变，即由书本知识的传授者转变为学生学习和成长的促进者、合作者、参与者；由教学秩序的管理者转变为学生自我管理和自主发展的引导者；由教学大纲的具体实施者转变为学生发展和教学实践的研究者。

2. 建构了新的课程教学模式

通过改革，学校研究生课程教学已普遍实行"教师讲授、学生分组讨论、重点答疑与问题引导下的学生自主解答"的教学模式。新的课程教学模式压缩了课堂教学的学时，将学位课程的教师讲授控制在 36 学时以内，选修课控制在 18 学时以内。这使博士研究生 1 个学期的课程学习平均周学时由原来的 24 学时减少到 18 学时以内，硕士研究生平均周学时由 28 学时减少到 20 学时以内，真正把研究生从课堂中解放出来，给了学生更大的自我拓展、自主学习的时间与空间。

3. 优化了研究生教育课程体系

学校 2 个博士点、18 个硕士点均对原有课程设置作了较大调整，优化了各专业的课程体系，初步形成了具有学校特色的基础、人文等系列课程模块，打造了专业核心课程，增强了课程设置的科学性。

4. 调动了师生教与学的积极性

随着课程体系的不断优化，面授学时数的减少，研究生不仅自由支配时间增多，获得了更大的自我发展空间，而且直接参与评教、参与申报国家自然科学基金项目等活动，进一步调动了学生积极性，学习氛围更加浓厚。

5. 提高了研究生外语、科研实力

研究生英语教学在精简课时的基础上对内容作较大调整，增加了博士口语、硕士医学英语等课程，提高了学生外语应用的能力。允许研究生根据自己的研究方向和兴趣爱好，选择相关平台轮转学习，以更好地掌握科学实验研究的基本方法和技能。同时，指导和帮助在校博士生申报国家自然科学基金项目，通过课题申报实践来有效提升学生的科研能力。

6. 提高了研究生人文素养

学校开展了一系列人文素质和专业知识讲座，组织研究生参加院士、知名专家的专题报告。通过《我们为何读经典》、《阴阳五行学说与中医学思维模式》、《音乐欣赏》、《京剧欣赏》、《创意摄影》等讲座丰富学生的人文素养，提高学生的综合素质。

7. 提升了研究生教育管理水平

各专业已制定了围绕专业培养目标的知识基准，建立了研究生专业知识基准考核制度，并改革了课程考核方式，修订了《福建中医药大学研究生课程考试管理办法》，规范了研究生各类别课程考试的管理。在学生评教上，优化了教学评教指标体系，实现评教的网络化和信息化。

四、研究生课程教学改革的体会

1. 改革需要教育理念更新

理念是行动的先导。在改革过程中我们发现：相当部分的教职员工对此次改革理念、目标、意义的理解未完全到位，没能在专业培养方案、培养目标、课程设置、课程教学目的与教学模式、专业知识基准等方面形成系统的科学认识，使改革浮于表面，难以进一步深入。各学位点及教学单位尚未完全投入到改革实际行动中，存在走过场的心理，尚未能将改革的具体工作融入到学位点建设及教研室活动中。因此，要切实推进研究生课程教学改革，还须思想再解放一点，胆子再大一点，步子再快一点，精力再投入一点。

2. 改革需要管理制度创新

现有的研究生课程教学评教机制和绩效考核制度还不能真正对课程教学改革起到实质性推动作用，研究生科研平台轮转学习尚未建立起完善的管理规章制度等问题，急需制度创新予以指导和保障。

3. 改革需要投入足够的人力

目前能适应研究生课程教学改革要求，承担改革任务的教师还较少，尚不能很好地满足教学改革的需要。甚至，部分课程负责人都没能尽到课程负责人应尽的责任，未按要求认真组织对课程目标、课程内容、教学方法、教师队伍及课程组织实施等进行集体讨论，使得所负责的课程改革流于形式。

4. 改革需要专业指导

中医药研究生课程教学改革尚处摸索和总结阶段，中医药研究生课程教学改革工作没有现成的、成熟的经验可供借鉴，缺乏坚实的理论指导。如各专业制定的专业基准尚需有关专家充分论证，考核还未形成更成熟科学的方法等，还须更多更专业的指导。

学术进展

一、理 论 研 究

（一）中医基础理论

【概述】

2013年，中医基础理论研究的活跃领域是病因病机和证候动物模型，在疾病病因、病机、证候、治疗等方面的研究成果给人留下深刻印象，尤其是“973”中医基础理论专项的实施对证候动物模型研究起了促进作用。在诊断学研究领域，除了脉象仪的应用研究有切实的成果表达之外，如何将现代仪器运用于中医诊断，也有新的探索。汉族与少数民族的中医临床病、证、治疗特点的比较研究值得鼓励。邢玉瑞对10余年来中医理论发生学研究作了总结。其他在运气学说研究、经络学说研究、肺与大肠相表里研究、治则治法研究、辨证论治理论研究、证候实质研究等领域也均有所成就。

运气学说的研究仍在论证规律和探索概念之中。自上世纪60年代，五运六气理论开始运用气象医学模式进行研究，融入统计学、流行病学等多学科知识。王利锋等从近50年文献资料整理中发现，五运六气理论与医学气象模式研究尚未形成统一的量化标准，60年周期的研究成为一种趋势，以气象学为主多学科研究五运六气理论已成为主要途径。宾炜等探讨了运气学说中岁气客气关系的矛盾，认为司天、在泉应是协同主司全年气候变化的岁气，作用时间是全年，而不是客气之一。时间医学方面，陈玉萍、徐颖等均采用动物实验方法，探索了褪黑素合成限速酶（芳香烷基胺-N-乙酰基转移酶、羟基吲哚-氧-甲基转移酶）mRNA表达与季节、中医时间医学理论的关系。徐颖等还研制了四季模拟系统，用人工方式模拟季节，为本领域研究提供了重要的技术手段。

经络学说研究方面，为了解释大肠经红外辐射轨迹的形成机制，吴祖星等观察电针前后及电针合谷穴时，大肠经深部组织氧分压、微循环血流灌注量、温度的反应，发现电针可使大肠经的氧利用率提高。

肺与大肠相表里理论的研究，主要仍是以动物实验方法寻找肺病理和肠道病理的因果关系和相关性。唐洪屈所在课题组相继建立了肺病（过敏性哮喘）、肺肠合病（过敏性哮喘合便秘）模型，发现肺病可能影响到肠。2013年该课题组建立了肺系疾病慢性支气管炎模型，观察肺部疾病是否可传变至大肠及传变的时间节点。惠毅等观察肺病（慢性支气管炎）大鼠在胃肠动力方面的变化，探寻肺病及肠病理传变机制。郑秀丽等观察肺病、肠病、肺肠合病3种不同病理状态下大鼠肺部和肠道的菌群情况，探讨肺肠菌群变化的相关性。应该指出，肺病理和肠道病理关系的特异性，仍属“肺与大肠相表里”理论研究中的薄弱环节。

病因病机研究一直是较活跃的领域。对疾病的病因病机不断有新的发现，其中不少有较坚实的实践和理论基础，值得重视。程园园、汪四海、张继烈等分别论述了骨关节炎（骨痹）、强直性脊柱炎合并骨代谢失衡、高血压这3种以往更注重肝肾疾病从脾论治的观点。程园园等认为骨关节炎最根本的病机是本虚标实，又以本虚为主，本虚则以脾虚为先，标实则以痰湿为主，故在治疗上应重视从脾论治。汪四海等提出脾虚贯穿于强直性脊柱炎骨代谢异常的始终，前期以脾虚为基础，后期则出现脾肾两虚，从而提出了采用益气健脾法治疗的观点。张继烈等指出，高血压的病机一般认为与肝肾两脏有关，不建议使用补气温阳药。但张氏在40多年的临床实践中发现：早期高血压多为脾气虚，慢慢发展为肝肾阴虚、肝阳上亢。因此许多高血压患者都可以使用补脾益气药，这既能减少并发症的发生率、减轻并发症的症状，又可减少西药降压药的用量与副作用。韩艳武、陈瑛等强调了内伤与本虚在甲型H1N1流感或肺部感染中的重要性。韩艳武等采用回顾性病例研究的方法,比较分析了770例甲型H1N1流感确诊病例中无内伤基础病组和5类不同内伤组的临床资料,归纳各自的证候特点及病因病机。结果发现不同内伤基础病对于本病临床特征及预后具有一定影响。陈瑛等发现肺部感染的发病根源在于本气先虚,与肺、脾、肾密切相关,老、弱、幼儿因其特点,更易于感邪致病,从本气先虚着手论治肺部感染有重要临床意义。杨朝阳等应用气血津液状态辨识系统测试版开展毒瘾的中医病理因素研究。分别对公安组(较轻,192例)和司法组(较重,167例)进行观察,发现痰是毒品成瘾的主要病理因素,虚实夹杂是毒品成瘾的证候学特点。两组在阴虚、血虚、阳虚、痰、湿等病理因素方面有显著差异,且司法组的程度大于公安组。刘正华分析了现代生存方式下青壮年妇女下寒上热(下真寒、上假热)证的病因病机,有其简单而重要的生物学原理。于琦等研究了古今对温病病因病机认识的差异,发现古代病因病机主要集中在湿邪、湿热、暑邪、风热、外感、饥饿、治疗失误,现代病因病机主要集中在血瘀、疫毒、六淫、邪气、寒邪、肝风内动、热入心营等。

诊断学研究方面,近年脉象仪的应用研究取得了切实成果。2013年,闪增郁等采用高精度智能机械手中医脉诊信息采集分析系统,对平人大暑、处暑和秋分的脉图模型及其参数变化规律进行比较研究,发现夏、秋季脉图参数有明显变化,秋季的处暑和秋分比较脉图参数变化较小,认为脉位和频域参数在分类中的作用明显大于时域参数。吴宏进等采用DDMX－100型单道脉象仪采集了677例健康人群寸口关部脉象信息,探讨了健康人群体表面积、身体质量指数对采脉压力及脉图参数的影响。结果发现体表面积较大及超重人群的左心室射血功能和动脉血管壁顺应性不及体表面积相对较小、非肥胖人群。认为临床诊脉时要考虑性别、体表面积、体质指数等因素对脉象的影响。朱丽萍等用DDMX－100型单道脉象仪采集健康大学生(男性28例,女性26例)两手关部脉象信息,发现男性以平脉、滑脉为多见,女性以平脉或平弦脉为多见。男女右手动脉血管壁的紧张性与外周阻力均低于左手。男性左心室的射血功能及动脉管壁顺应性均优于女性。林雪娟等选择青年学生表证患者114例和健康青年学生255名,运用基于薄膜型气体传感器阵列技术的医用电子鼻采集口腔呼气的气味图谱,以响应曲线的振幅和上升斜率作为曲线特征,分析表证患者及其寒热病性的图谱特征。结果发现表证患者口腔呼气的气味较健康人浓烈,且表热证患者气味变化较表寒证患者更明显。认为电子鼻技术的发展可为中医嗅诊客观化研究提供手段和方法。近年来出现许多监测微循环的新技术,高伟等采用旁流暗视野技术观察97例不同舌色的严重脓毒症患者舌下微循环差异,认为舌下微循环与内脏微循环变化基本一致。

治则治法研究方面,陈小野曾提出了“气虚证的非定位性”、“肾虚证的非定位性”等观点,2013年则进一步指出,如果肠化、特别是大肠型肠化成为胃黏膜主要而稳定的生物学特征,则需要补肾。其原理是:① 虚证的病理以逆向重演生物个体发育和生物进化过程为主要特点。② 胚胎乃生命之原始,虚证病理逆向重演至胚胎阶段正是“虚极及肾”。③ 整体“虚极”是对整体而言的肾虚证。局部“虚极”是对局部而言的肾虚证。④ 胃黏膜肠化的实质是胚胎化。与小肠型肠化比较,大肠型肠化的胚胎化更为彻底。所以,胃黏膜的肠化、特别是大肠型肠化占主导地位而稳定,即是“胃的肾虚证”。王付针对“为医皆知附子温壮阳气,少有问津附子亡损阳气”,指出“附子何以亡阳,因其味辛性热也。味辛太过多耗散,性热太过多伤气,即辛热合体太过则亡损阳气。”这会对一些滥用附子现象有纠偏作用,也促使学者深化思考阳气的本质。

辨证论治理论研究方面,中医以往运用于运动医学有可圈点的成绩。陈清光等研究高强度训练对女运动员临床表型的影响,并对中医四诊客观化评价方法进行了探讨。认为高强度训练女运动员处于运动疲劳状态,以肝郁、气虚证为主,而采用临床表型和中医四诊客观化评价是可行的。近年新疆地区汉族与维吾尔族临床病、证、治疗特点的比较研究有良好的开端。以往研究表明,新疆不同民族代谢性疾病的患病率表现出民族差异,哈萨克族高血压患病率高于全国水平,维吾尔族糖尿病高发,而汉族高尿酸血症高发。王燕等报道,课题组在乌鲁木齐、喀什地区共收集397例汉族与维吾尔族高尿酸血症患者,运用因子分析方法提取支配高脂血症诊断信息的公因子,以确定高尿酸血症中医分型。结果发现,397例高尿酸血症患者中医证型可分为痰浊阻滞、气虚、脾虚、湿热、肾虚、水湿停留、血瘀7类。高尿酸血症患者以虚证居多,尤以肾虚(41.81%)突出。汉族与维吾尔族比较,气虚、湿热、水湿停留、血瘀罹患率均较高,而脾虚、肾虚罹患率则较低。课题组前期对高尿酸血症的研究发现,新疆汉族尿酸水平和高尿酸血症的检出率高于维吾尔族,维吾尔族又高于哈萨克族,各民族男性均大于女性。根据国家卫生与计划生育委员会制定的《人感染H7N9禽流感诊疗方案(2013年第1版、第2版)》,中医药辨证论治在禽流感防治中的作用受到肯定并得到推荐。陈晓蓉等研究了18例新型H7N9禽流感的中医证候特点。发现新型人感染H7N9发病直接入气分、营分多见,或为卫气同病,卫分证不明显。

证候实质研究是中西医结合科研的一类标志性工作,上世纪七八十年代形成高潮,嗣后的研究呈零散态势,近年来结合新的实验指标,为此项工作注入了新的活力。张颖等探讨了105例吸毒人群获得性免疫缺陷综合征(AIDS)患者中医证型与CD_4^+ T淋巴细胞的关系。发现吸毒人群AIDS患者的中医证型分布与CD_4^+ T淋巴细胞计数分段密切相关。初起实证为主,随着疾病进程继发痰饮、瘀血等病理产物,虚实交错,变证丛生。后期人体正气损伤严重,累及津、血、精,气血阴阳俱虚,故虚证较多见。王春芳等探讨了276例HIV/AIDS患者证型与T淋巴细胞亚群的关系。发现HIV/AIDS中医证型与T细胞亚群有一定的关系,初步表现出由虚证—虚实夹杂证—实证之间免疫损害逐渐加深的趋势。金贺等探讨了缺血性中风急性期甲状腺激素表达异常患者证候规律及血管病变特点。结果发现甲状腺激素水平异常组风证、火证、阴虚阳亢证发生频率较高,甲状腺激素水平正常组与异常组的TCD(经颅多普勒)和颈动脉B超结果无明显统计学差异。徐万忠等探讨了80例慢性肾衰竭维持性血液透析患者血瘀证积分与内皮素(ET)、NO的相关性。发现血液透析患者血瘀证积分与ET呈正相关关系,认为可以根据血瘀证积分判断患者内皮损伤和凝血功能的情况。

证候动物模型研究比较活跃,近年"973"中医基础理论专项的实施对这一工作起了促进作用。徐晶晶等在前期研究中发现,经过一段时间的D-半乳糖(D-Gal)皮下注射,大鼠会出现明显的多尿症状,包括总尿量增多和排尿次数增加两方面。从而建立了D-Gal致肾虚多尿动物模型,并进一步考察了不同剂量D-Gal对该动物模型尿量的影响,测定了与膀胱储尿和排尿功能密切相关的尿动力学参数。肖凌等研究D-Gal诱导衰老阳虚大鼠的生化指标改变和应激蛋白HSP70表达,发现D-Gal诱导的衰老大鼠应激蛋白HSP70表达降低,导致超氧化物歧化酶(SOD)活性降低,进一步导致高脂血症及行为认知水平降低,且与阳虚证动物模型表征相符。维吾尔医学的异常黑胆质证动物模型研究已有长足进展,特别是哈木拉提·吾甫尔课题组的工作。阿衣古丽·玉努斯等在建立异常黑胆质证大鼠模型的基础上,对异常黑胆质证及正常大鼠血清进行代谢组学研究,分析两组大鼠血清差异代谢组分。结果发现异常黑胆质证大鼠存在糖、脂肪、蛋白质及磷酸肌酸代谢紊乱。景兴文等观察了气虚血瘀证大鼠子二代大脑中动脉栓塞(MCAO)脑缺血耐受性及细胞外信号调节激酶(ERK)信号转导通路改变,研究其是否存在缺血性脑卒中遗传易感性。结果发现MCAO气虚血瘀证大鼠子二代与正常同龄SD大鼠相比,对脑缺血的耐受性及修复能力降低,其机制可能与其ERK信号转导通路异常有关。

中医方法学研究方面,中医理论发生学研究10余年来较为集中。乔文虎等介绍了发生学方法的由来、界定及引入中医学研究中的过程,全面、系统地总结了中医理论的发生学研究现状,包括藏象学说、精气血神理论、经络学说、病因病机理论、中医相关哲学理论、中医理论发生与先秦诸子的比较、诊法与方药理论的发生学研究七个方面。认为中医理论发生学研究中存在的问题主要有缺乏总体规划,研究很不均衡;研究水平不高,创新急需加强;逻辑思维混乱,推理过程错误;理论诠释错误,文献引证不准等四个方面。同时指出,中医理论的发生学研究不能替代中医理论的创新研究,而应该与之紧密结合,以促进中医理论的现代发展。

(陈小野)

【阴阳五行学说研究】

李维娜等认为《黄帝内经》中阴阳学说主要运用了形象思维模式、逻辑思维模式、数学思维模式等方法,具有整体可分性、唯物辩证性及发展进步的性质,是认识自然、认识人体、诊断疾病、治疗疾病的指导思想,具有广泛科学性,既是古代哲学的思辩方法,更是现代针对复杂的人体和疾病以及其他事物巨系统的复合思维模式。既注意事物的宏观整体性,又注意其微观可分性,强调各部分之间的相互关联。李秀美等讨论了太极图里的"无极、太极、阴阳"三大哲学元素,认为中国古典哲学潜在着精确的思维模型和数学模型及数学模型公式,揭示了宇宙万物以统一的思维模型和数学模型及数学模型公式而演化的宇宙全息论本质。人体任何相对独立的全息元均符合这一统一理论的解释。阴阳是任何哲学元素潜在或显在的哲学思维模型,反映了同源演化的物质系两个构成相对待意义上的演化趋势与分类。阴阳成立的条件是"中时空位"的唯一存在,并且阴阳演化的潜在属类相等。阴阳比较的前提是纳于到统一的比较范畴中。阴阳分类有同属阴阳、异属阴阳两种。

孙振等运用发生学的方法,从"五"、"行"、"五行起源"、"五行演化"以及五行在中医理论的形成过程等方面,从根源上探讨中医学五行学说的发生和发展过程。指出"五"源于对数字"五"的崇拜。"行"字的来源,有"运动"、"运作"、"行施"等意义,表示大自然中气的运行和运动方式。"五行"的应用源于"万物有灵"、"图腾观念"和"祖先崇拜"。五行学说应用于中医学源自《黄帝内经》,对中医理论起到了很大的指导作用,依据五行的物质特性描述出了五脏的生理功能、五脏之间的相互关系、五脏病变的相互影响等,与人体的生理、病理以及诊断和治疗方面的应用。陈润东指出五行学说的局限性体现在把系统的要素规定为五个,以原则来裁剪事实,而不是让原则来反映事实。事实上系统不同,其内在的要素数量也有异,不可能千篇一律为五。"五"的死框限制了人们对系统内在要素的搜索与考察,也不利于认识系统的本质。此外,把系统内在要素之间的相互作用看作是定向的生克、乘侮关系,固然有一定的合理性,但仍不足以全面地反映复杂多变的实际情况。五行系统的反馈回路非螺旋式运动,具有循环论的倾向。陈氏以《神农本草经》的药物分类为依据,提出了"六行学说"的分类方法,就是在五行这五气当中加入"石"这一行。并认为《伤寒论》就是尊神农氏药分六类而形成六经辨证理论体系。

刘润兰等应用控制论原理和方法探讨五行生克制化的科学内涵及其所反映的生命规律。认为五行的相生相克,可视为信息的输入或输出,是控制系统和受控对象之间"促静"和"促动"两种相互矛盾信息的相互作用;五行生克是信息的多路多级控制,任何子系统都可对其他四个子系统发生或接受生克两方面影响;用状态空间方法分析五行生克的周期性可知,五行系统在不同的时间内,其状态是不同的,具有时间概念上的不可逆性;五行系统五个子系统之间的联系"如环无端",构成了闭合回路,各行之间作用有生有克,是一种内稳定器模型。五行学说实际上描述的是一个人与自然、社会相通的开放巨系统,人体五行结构不是"实物中心论模型"而是"功能中心论模型",它表征和模拟了生命复杂系统的功能过程和调控机制。

(邱若虹)

【运气学说研究】

郭梅珍等探讨了"七篇大论"与《素问》之间的关系,认为"七篇大论"所涉及的内容自成体系,独创五运六气历法,采取干支甲子演绎法,对 60 年为 1 周期的气象变化规律进行预测,并且阐述不同时段气候变化对生物界带来的影响,特别是对人类生命活动的影响,对疾病发生、发展产生的影响,进一步对临床诊断及用药进行指导。陈蓓等认为《黄帝内经》以天人合一、阴阳五行理论为指导,强调人体生命运动、病理状态具有时间周期性及节律性,疾病的诊断和治疗应顺应天时,形成了关于时间生理学、时间病理学、时间诊断学、时间治疗学、时间养生学在内的诸多理论,构建了中医时间医学的理论框架,是中医时间生物医学的起源之书。吴凡伟等认为在临床实践中,审查病机时不仅要看患者的症状表现,还要综合考虑天时、地理环境以及人文、社会等因素。自然界的气候变化有盛衰、太过或不及之分,其变化会引起人体气血、阴阳、脏腑的虚实、盛衰变化。同时要正确看待运气学说,不可拘泥。

李俊龙等根据《素问·六元正纪大论》相关记载,指出 2012(壬辰)年为太阳寒水司天年,通过观察与记录 2012 年的天气变化与临床就诊疾病分析,来考证五运六气对疾病的影响。发现 2012 年就诊最多的疾病分别为感冒、心悸、眩晕、鼽窒、抑郁等,均与寒冷气候有密切关系。彭薇淇等认为中医时间医学是中医学不可分割的一部分,从宏观角度上反映着人体生理活动和脏腑活动的节律。现代胃肠动力学发现胃肠道的消化、运动能力也有相对固定的时间节律性。其中，移行性复合运动与卫气的运行相一致，均有夜伏昼出的特点，而结肠的集团运动节律与阴阳变动的昼夜节律亦有很大的相似性，胃肠的节律运动与十二经脉气血流注的昼夜节律在某种程度上是相符合的。

刘文波认为中医学是一门时相医学，构建时相医学的理论核心体系是五运六气学说。运气学说是在天人合一思想的指导下，将人置于天地时空大环境下，从宇宙宏观背景中加以观察和思考，从天地人三才一体的角度，衡量宇宙某一时空形成的特定环境对人类健康的影响。在三才一体观思想的指导下，运气学说把病候、气候、物候放在同一坐标水平上研究，对于寻找病因病机提供了一个可靠的时空模型。刘氏指出《黄帝内经》中时间和空间的概念是用三阴三阳来表示的，即太阳、阳明、少阳、太阴、少阴、厥阴，并且三阴三阳是对立统一的，一阳对一阴，二阳对二阴，三阳对三阴。三阴三阳形成了一个开放的、动态的宇宙运行规律模型。临床中根据患者症状表现，利用时相医学理论，可以推导出患者所处的“时空”，指导治疗用药。郭春风等认为六气之一的燥，并非导致干燥综合征的非自然界的燥邪，认为干燥综合征的燥邪多由外邪引发或内伤导致人体五行相生相克规律紊乱。病机表现在燥、虚、疲三个方面。运用五运六气理论分析其病因病机，以中土不运为其本，木火金水失调为其标。土载四行，为万物之母，土居中而运四方，中土不运则中土不安。郭氏基于五运六气学说，通过对病因病机的分析，总结出补土运中法、敛金润燥法、疏木通瘀法、引火归原法等五种治法。各法以补土运中法为必用之法，如出现其他症状，再考虑结合其他治法。土为中轴，木火金水四维为轮。治轴以运轮，治轮以运轴，相互为用，方可效如桴鼓。同时，也应根据四季变化选择适当的治法。如秋季燥气主令，患者干燥症状剧烈，可加用敛金润燥法。“时辰药理学”，是研究根据机体自身的节律变化，选择合适的用药时机，以达到最小剂量、最佳疗效、最小毒性，来改善病人的生存质量。李江等从生物节律与时辰药理学、时辰疗法与时辰药理学两方面来说明人体的身体变化、生理周期与时间有着重要的关系。指出依从性是时辰用药治疗的关键。

（于　峥）

【肺与大肠相表里研究】

张敏等从相合的含义、肺与大肠相合的内在机制、作用体现3个方面，对肺与大肠相合理论进行初步探讨，认为肺与大肠相合的内在机制是相同而合与相异而合，这两方面相互促进，互为基础，同中有异，异中有同，因而具有内在相互吸引的力量，内聚而相合。肺与大肠在来源上，均同源于元气；在形态上，具有相类似的色白、中空结构；在时间上同应秋，同属阳明燥气，同气相求，相互感应，通过经脉络属行气，二者具有同源、同构、同气的生理基础，相同而合。同时，肺与大肠之间上下部位相对，阴阳相异，具有内在相互吸引的力量，相异而合。肺与大肠之间相同与相异的部分相互促进，同中有异，异中有同，相合而为用，协同发挥主排浊、主出入、司开合的功能。陈丽斌等从同气相求的概念、肺与大肠同气相求的深层内涵及表里构建3个方面，对肺与大肠相表里理论的构建进行探讨，总结出肺与大肠相表里的内在机制在于二者的同气相求，同气与相求两方面互为基础，相互作用。肺与大肠异位同源、异属同性，在气机升降、营卫生成与敷布、津液代谢及时空相应、经脉络属等方面相互感应、联系是其同气相求的重要内容。马师雷等探讨了在泄泻的病理过程中肺脏对于大肠腑的影响，阐述从肺论治泄泻的辨证思路，分析了清源洁流治湿泄、逆流挽舟治风泄、宣肺化痰治痰泄、清肺润燥治热泄、温肺补气治虚泄等治疗方法。孟庆岩等指出肺通调水道功能与大肠主津功能在生理上相辅相成，病理上相互影响。一方面，肺宣发肃降、布散津液、濡润肠道；另一方面，肺通调水道，使体内津液平衡，保证大肠燥化有度，大肠传导糟粕的功能才能正常发挥。大肠主津功能正常，一方面将重吸收的水液上输心肺，促进肺的宣发肃降；另一方面，保证肠道润滑，大便成形，使腑气通畅，保证肺气运行正常。病理上，外邪侵袭或者肺气虚耗，导致肺失通调水道，邪气下移，进而影响大肠传导功能，引起便秘或腹泻。大肠主津的功能异常，水液代谢失衡，腑气不通，也会影响肺气功能，出现咳嗽喘闷等症。认为津液代谢在“肺与大肠相表里”理论中发挥着重要作用。

郑秀丽等建立了肺病（过敏性哮喘）、肠病（便秘）、肺肠合病（过敏性哮喘合便秘）3种大鼠模型，分别进行肺部和肠道菌群的菌落计数与种类鉴定。实验发现在病理状态下，肺、肠菌群的变化具有一定的相关性和同步性，即肺病可引起肠道菌群的同步变化，肠病亦可引起肺部菌群的同步变化,且肺病对肠道菌群的影响较大,而肠病对肺部菌群的影响较小。肺肠合病对肺部和肠道菌群均有显著影响,其菌群变化比单纯肺病组和单纯肠病组显著。郑氏还通过实验发现大鼠肠病(便秘)模型肺和结肠组织病理形态同步改变,而其他四脏无明显变化。模型大鼠结肠组织和肺组织中八肽胆囊收缩素、降钙素基因相关肽、P物质、血管活性肠肽均出现显著变化($P<0.05$,$P<0.01$),而在心、肝、脾、肾却无显著差异。认为肠病对肺的影响具有一定程度的特异性。

于宁等从肺的功能探讨了从肺论治肠易激综合征的理论基础。指出肺的生理功能失调是导致肠易激综合征的重要原因。肺的气机逆乱可以导致腹胀、腹痛、腹泻、大便性状及习惯改变等。增强肺通调水道的功能,可以改善肠易激综合征腹泻、便秘的症状。肺主治节的功能与大肠变化、传导的功能密切相关,肺失治节会引起排便习惯改变等症状。朱立等采用家兔结肠黏膜组织致敏与三硝基苯磺酸-乙醇模型相结合的免疫复合法复制溃疡性结肠炎(UC)大鼠模型,并与正常大鼠对照。结果模型组大鼠急、慢性期均表现为体重下降,黏液便、稀便,部分大鼠出现呼吸困难,气促、喘鸣等症状。与正常组比较,模型组大鼠急性期最大通气量、用力肺活量、0.2秒率和平均用力呼气流速以及慢性期吸气阻力、呼气阻力、最大通气量、用力肺活量和平均用力呼气流速均显著降低($P<0.05$,$P<0.01$),0.2秒率显著升高($P<0.05$),且病理显示有间质性肺炎及肺间质纤维化改变。两组肝肾功能均在正常范围,肝肾组织病理观察未见明显病变。认为溃疡性结肠炎可以特异性引起肺支气管病损,肺损伤是本病的肠外表现之一。盛益华等通过实验研究发现肺组织中Bcl-2和Bax蛋白表达异常并诱导肺组织细胞凋亡可能是UC肺损伤的分子机制之一。认为以干预细胞凋亡信号转导途径为中心,对明确UC肺损伤细胞凋亡的发生机制和"肠病及肺"的现代生物学机制将有较好的启示作用。刘恩顺等观察肺肠相关在急性肺损伤/急性呼吸窘迫综合征证候表现中的具体形式及其演变规律。采用临床流行病学调查的方法,收集患者127例,于第1、3、7 d 3个访视点观察记录临床症状并判断肺与大肠证候类型,采用spearman相关方法,分析证候学资料。结果发现,在第一访视点,痰热壅盛与肠热腑实正相关。在第二访视点,痰热壅盛与肠热腑实正相关;肺气虚与肠燥津亏、肠道气滞正相关、与肠热腑实负相关;肺热炽盛与肠道气滞正相关。在第三访视点,痰热壅盛与肠热腑实正相关;肺气虚与肠热腑实负相关;肺阴虚与肠燥津亏正相关。认为肺肠相关急性肺损伤/急性呼吸窘迫综合征在临床证候中具有特定的表现形式,并随病情发展呈现一定的演变规律。

(邸若虹)

【体质学说研究】

李海峰等把《内经》体质相关诸多要素分为外围要素与核心要素。外围要素包括社会地位、生活的地域环境、年龄、肥瘦、肤色、脏腑位置、勇怯、耐痛度等,是导致体质差别的主要影响因子和区别不同体质的外部指标。核心要素为气血、阴阳、脏腑等,是判别不同体质的主要核心指标。认为《内经》在论述不同体质时,应用多层次多维度的众多指标,在整体观的指导下,形成了一整套综合性全方位的体质辨别系统。王昊等认为中医人格体质论立足对人格、体质内涵的深入认识,基于先秦时期唯物的"形神观",提出了对人类特征的整体认识。充分体现了"形神合一"的整体观思想,同时按照阴阳五行来划分人格、体质,也是一种"辨证论治"、"因人制宜"的医学原则,形成了独具特色的身心医学及中医的健康观。从生理机制上去阐述人格心理现象,不仅符合唯物论原则,而且利于将人格、体质与中医的"病"、"证"结合,从而从健康及疾病发生的个体内在因素更深刻地认识疾病的发生、发展及转归。

吴小秋等运用流行病学的调研方法,对147例2型糖尿病患者进行问卷调查,分析其体质分布特点。发现主要体质类型为阴虚质(24.5%),其他依次为血瘀质(14.3%)、气虚质(13.0%)、痰湿质(12.2%)、平和质(8.8%)、阳虚质(6.8%)、湿热质(10.2%)、气郁质(6.1%)、特禀质(4.1%)。阴虚质与其他体质类型比较,均$P<0.01$。胰岛素抵抗指数痰湿质水平最高,胰岛素敏感指数痰湿质水平最低,与其他各体质类型比较,均$P<0.01$;胰岛β细胞功能阴虚质水平最低,与其他各体质类型比较,均$P<0.05$或$P<0.01$。同时,各体质类型患者的糖尿病危险因素如吸烟、饮酒、体质量指数、腰臀比及空腹血糖、空腹C肽、空腹胰岛素、糖化血红蛋白、血脂、炎症因子等均有统计学差异($P<0.05$或$P<0.01$)。认为2型糖尿病患者的体质类型与胰岛素抵抗指

数、胰岛素敏感指数等均具有一定的关系。高泓等观察了不同体质人群在糖调节受损中的比例及1年后糖尿病的转化率，探讨糖调节受损患者的体质特点。收集134例糖调节受损病例，根据《中医体质分类与判定》标准将患者进行中医体质分类。1年后，随访受试者，并进行相关临床实验室检查，统计不同体质受试者的糖尿病年转化率。结果134例糖调节受损患者中，痰湿质患者所占比例最大，随后依次为：阴虚质、湿热质、气虚质、血瘀质、气郁质；在1年之后的复查中，糖尿病年转化率由高到低依次为：湿热质、痰湿质、气郁质、阴虚质、气虚质。认为在罹患糖调节受损的患者中，痰湿体质、阴虚体质、气虚体质、湿热体质占多数；其中，痰湿体质和湿热体质的糖调节受损患者更倾向于转化为糖尿病，可能与肥胖引起胰岛素抵抗，使糖代谢异常加速，最终导致糖尿病的发病有关。

辛海等研究了社区慢性病人群体型与中医体质的分布特点。按照体质量指数(BMI)将人的体型分为正常、超重、肥胖和消瘦4种体型，通过应用中医9种体质量表，调查北京市东城区8个社区慢性病人群的体型和中医体质分布特点，了解9种体质在4种体型的分布特征。结果，平和质在超重和肥胖体型中分布较多，在消瘦体型中分布较少；气虚质在消瘦体型和正常体型中分布较多，在超重和肥胖体型中分布较少；阳虚质在消瘦体型中分布最少，在超重体型中分布较多。阴虚质在消瘦体型分布最多，在超重和肥胖体型中分布较少($P<0.05$)；相关分析结果提示，BMI数值与平和质呈正相关，与气虚质、阳虚质呈负相关($P<0.01$)。认为慢性病患者中消瘦体型多为阳虚质、阴虚质和气虚质，超重体型多见平和质和阳虚质，肥胖体型中平和质较多。杨惠民等研究了北京地区汉族中老年人原发性血脂异常患者的体质分布状况及中老年人原发性血脂异常与中医体质的相关性。收集了226例亚临床组病例和216例并发症组病例的临床及体质信息，并分别分析两组人群的体质分布特点，并作中老年人原发性血脂异常与患者中医体质的相关性多元Logistic回归分析。结果：① 中老年人原发性血脂异常亚临床组与并发症组在体质的构成上差异显著($P<0.0001$)，各偏颇体质都是以兼夹体质为主。② 以体质类型因素对中老年人原发性血脂异常并发症发病进行二值多元Logistic回归分析，在$P<0.05$水平，最终进入回归方程的中医体质类型是：气虚质(X2)与血瘀质(X7)。认为气虚质与血瘀质为中老年原发性血脂异常患者出现冠状动脉粥样硬化性心脏病、动脉粥样硬化性血栓性脑梗死的危险因素。余敏英等研究了原发性血脂异常平和质和湿热质者在ApoE基因型和等位基因分布上有差异。发现ApoE基因型ε4/ε4和等位基因ε4具有更明显的湿热体质倾向，可能更易于形成湿热体质血脂异常或其与湿热体质血脂异常关联的可能性大。ApoE基因型ε3/ε3和等位基因ε3具有更明显的平和质倾向，可能更易于形成平和质血脂异常或其与平和质血脂异常关联的可能性大。

（邱若虹）

【证候试验研究】

廖凌虹运用证素辨证法得出1134名体检者各证素积分，将228例“痰”证素积分≥70分者归为痰证组，286名所有证素积分均<70分者归为健康对照组。痰证组中，体质量、体质指数、丙氨酸氨基转移酶和谷酰转肽酶高于对照组($P<0.05$)，载脂蛋白A_1和高密度脂蛋白水平均低于对照组($P<0.05$)。提示代谢异常是“痰”主要病理基础之一，载脂蛋白A_1等差异指标可作为“痰”证病理的潜在共性指标。刘燕鸿以103例慢性阻塞性肺疾病稳定期患者为观察对象，根据痰证素积分，按照痰的严重度分为3级。各级间痰证素积分、诱导痰中性粒细胞百分比及巨噬细胞百分比均有统计学意义($P<0.01$)，且痰证素积分与诱导痰中性粒细胞百分比呈高度正相关($P<0.01$)，与巨噬细胞百分比呈高度负相关($P<0.01$)；诱导痰嗜酸性粒细胞百分比1、2级显著高于3级($P<0.05$)，且痰证素积分与嗜酸性粒细胞百分比呈负相关($r=-0.309, P<0.01$)。王彩娟观察了153例脑卒中痉挛性瘫痪患者，发现痰瘀证组血小板、凝血酶、血脂水平、颈动脉内中膜增厚程度均明显高于非痰瘀证组。

徐万忠选取80例维持性血液透析血瘀证患者，观察该病血瘀证患者内皮素(ET)、NO情况。发现血瘀证组ET、ET/NO值高于非血瘀证组($P<0.05$)，NO值显著低于非血瘀证($P<0.01$)；血瘀证积分与ET、NO有相关性($P<0.05$)；与ET值呈正相关($P<0.01$)。段俊国将89例2型糖尿病视网膜病变(DR)分为无阳虚证

组和有阳虚证组,应用气相色谱-飞行时间质谱技术进行血浆代谢组学检测。发现DR有阳虚证组和无阳虚证组在临床前期和非增殖期基本重叠,而增殖期和非增殖期基本分离,重叠较少。认为阳虚可能影响机体能量代谢,诱导引起DR增殖性改变的新生血管因子相关基因表达,使DR从非增殖期转化为增殖期。

殷婷婷采用超高效液相色谱/飞行时间质谱联用技术,对61例强直性脊柱炎(AS)患者、29例痛风性关节炎(GA)患者及44名健康志愿者的血清样本进行脂质组学研究。发现AS湿热证组与AS非湿热证组血清脂质指纹图谱存在明显差异,其中甘油磷脂酰胆碱类(GPC)和甘油三酯(TG)差异较明显。与健康对照组相比,GA湿热证组和AS湿热证组共同表现的溶血甘油磷脂酰胆碱类(Lyso-GPC)明显下降。提示Lyso-GPC(18∶2)、Lyso-GPC(16∶0)和Lyso-GPC(18∶1)可能为风湿性疾病湿热证脂质代谢的共性指标。孙萌发现脾气虚证HIV/AIDS淋巴细胞线粒体膜电位偏低,特别是在热应激条件下(40℃孵育1 h)明显下降,认为本病脾气虚证患者在发热情况下能量代谢功能下降。马振将60例非糖尿病性维持性血液透析患者平分为脾肾阳虚型与非脾肾阳虚型。发现脾肾阳虚组肾小球滤过率(eGFR)值明显低于非脾肾阳虚组($P<0.05$),而氨基末端B型脑钠肽前体(NT-proBNP)水平显著高于非脾肾阳虚组($P<0.01$);经直线相关性分析,eGFR与NT-proBNP之间存在负相关。张颖探讨了105例吸毒人群AIDS患者中医证型与CD_4^+ T淋巴细胞的关系。发现CD_4^+ T淋巴细胞计数在50～200 μL之间时,以气阴两虚、肺肾不足型多见;计数在201～350 μL之间时,以气阴两虚、肺肾不足型和肝肾阴虚、湿毒蕴结型多见;计数在351～500 μL之间时,以脾肾亏虚、湿邪阻滞型多见;计数在501～650 μL之间时,以肝郁气滞火旺型多见。

王春芳分析了276例HIV/AIDS患者T淋巴细胞亚群与中医证型之间的关系。结果,痰湿内蕴证与其他证型在$CD_4/CD_{45}RO$、CD_4/CD_{28}、CD_8/CD_{38}、CD_8/CD_{95}方面差异显著($P<0.05$),阴虚火旺证在$CD_4/CD_{45}RO$、CD_8/CD_{25}方面与气血亏虚证、脾肾两虚证差异明显($P<0.05$),而气血亏虚证、气血亏虚兼血瘀证、脾肾两虚证间各免疫指标差异较小,无统计学意义。刘怀珍对300例2型糖尿病血脂异常患者进行观察,发现痰湿阻遏证最多(105例),其次是气阴两虚证(84例);血瘀脉络证型患者TG升高较其他证型更明显($P<0.01$);痰湿阻遏型患者三酰甘油升高较其他证型明显($P<0.05$)。王宏献探讨了同型半胱氨酸(HCY)及C反应蛋白(CRP)与糖尿病肾病(DN)中医证候的关系。发现单纯糖尿病组、早期DN组和临床DN组血清HCY、CRP水平逐渐升高($P<0.01$)。糖尿病肾病阴虚燥热证、气阴两虚证、脾肾气虚证、阴阳两虚证血清HCY水平逐渐升高,而血清CRP水平则表现为脾肾气虚、阴阳两虚、气阴两虚、阴虚燥热依次升高。寒湿证、湿热证、痰瘀证、瘀证各组间血清HCY水平逐渐升高,血清CRP水平则表现为瘀证、痰瘀证、寒湿证、湿热证依次升高($P<0.01$)。认为血清HCY和CRP水平与2型糖尿病及DN相关,且在不同证型间有显著区别。陈素华以245例DN患者作为研究对象,探讨了DN彩色多普勒超声诊断与辨证分型的关系。发现随着DN患者病情的加重,肾动脉收缩期峰值流速、舒张末血流速度及平均血流速度逐渐下降,搏动指数及阻力指数逐渐增加,而辨证分型按照气阴两虚、阴阳两虚、阳衰瘀阻的规律发展。可见以上指标与证型分布关系密切。

何淑寅探讨了原发性高血压患者中医证型与B型脑钠肽及未来10年脑卒中风险的相关性。发现血清BNP水平与未来10年脑卒中风险显著相关,EH患者BNP水平上升1 pg/ml,脑卒中发生率升高0.5%;血清BNP水平:痰湿壅盛组>阴阳两虚组>阴虚阳亢组>肝火亢盛组;10年脑卒中发生率:痰湿壅盛组>阴阳两虚组>肝火亢盛组>阴虚阳亢组(9.90%±10.35%)。吴炜景发现广东地区胃溃疡患者以脾胃湿热证多见,其幽门螺杆菌感染率、细胞毒素相关抗原(CagA)基因阳性率明显高于肝脾不和证组、脾胃虚寒证组、瘀毒内阻证组($P<0.05$)。谢春娥以192例胃痛患者为对象,发现不同证型幽门螺杆菌(Hp)的检出率不同,脾胃湿热型及肝气犯胃型胃痛患者的Hp检出率最高,分别为28.3%、25.4%;Hp阳性的胃痛患者黄腻苔及红舌的检出率最高,明显高于Hp阴性的患者。刘南发现急性冠脉综合征常见证候为痰浊闭塞证、气滞血瘀证、阴血虚证、阳气虚证。痰浊闭塞证及气滞血瘀证的超敏C反应蛋白、白细胞介素-6、单核细胞趋化蛋白-1、基

质金属蛋白酶-9、内脂素、丝裂原活化蛋白激酶浓度均显著高于阴血虚证及阳气虚证($P<0.05$)。痰浊闭塞证与气滞血瘀证间、阴血虚证与阳气虚证间均无显著差别($P>0.05$)。

刘文兰分析了180例慢性乙型肝炎患者血清可溶性细胞间黏附分子-1(sICAM-1)与舌色、证候和年龄之间的关系。发现本病患者以暗、紫舌多见,随年龄增高、病程延长,暗、紫舌明显增多,50岁以上患者以紫舌为主,提示舌色与患者病程密切相关。紫舌患者较淡白舌、淡红舌、暗舌患者血清sICAM-1显著增高($P<0.05$),提示紫舌的形成机制与血清sICAM-1增高相关。血清sICAM-1与肝郁脾虚证候积分显著相关($P<0.05$),提示肝郁脾虚是形成肝脏微循环障碍的重要证候因素。

杨聘探讨了96例轻度认知功能障碍(MCI)中医证型与HCY水平的相关性。发现MCI组HCY水平较健康对照组明显升高($P<0.05$);脾肾两虚型、痰湿阻络型HCY水平均高于湿热壅滞型、气阴两虚型、肝肾阴虚型($P<0.05$),但两型HCY水平无明显差异($P>0.05$)。提示HCY的异常增高是MCI的一个危险因素,可以考虑将其作为脾肾两虚、痰湿阻络证型的客观辨证指标之一。娄彦梅通过对366例原发性血脂异常患者的研究,发现本病患者心血管危险以低中危为多见,气滞血瘀证所占比例最大,典型相关分析显示痰浊瘀阻证与冠心病风险评估呈正相关,患者的年龄与心气虚证呈正相关。

张静观察了61例肝豆状核变性(HLD)患者,发现HLD患者脾静脉内径均增宽,湿热内蕴型与痰湿阻络型间差异显著($P<0.05$)。HLD患者门静脉最大血流速度、脾静脉最大血流速度均减慢($P<0.05$),不同证型间无显著性差异($P>0.05$)。HLD患者门静脉血流量、脾静脉血流量与对照组差异显著($P<0.05$),湿热内蕴型与痰湿阻络型间差异显著($P<0.05$)。

陈镇秋分析了74例股骨头坏死患者,发现肾虚血瘀型血清200/S、30/S、3/S、Arbe、EPT5项指标计数值均高于痰瘀蕴结型与气滞血瘀型($P<0.05$);痰瘀蕴结型血清胆固醇(CHOL)、载脂蛋白B(ApoB)、载脂蛋白A(ApoA)、HLD与气滞血瘀型和肾虚血瘀型比较差异显著($P<0.05$,$P<0.01$)。潘碧琦通过分析160例发性痛风患者,发现湿阻型、热毒型的血尿酸显著高于阴虚型($P<0.05$,$P<0.01$);湿阻型、痰浊型及气虚型TG显著高于血瘀型($P<0.01$);热毒型CRP显著高于阴虚型($P<0.05$);各证型患者CHOL、高密度脂蛋白、低密度脂蛋白等均无显著性差别($P>0.05$)。

(柏　冬)

【证候动物模型研究】

魏盛等探讨了异病同证动物模型的造模方法。分别使用两种动物,建立了抑郁症、经前期综合征(PMS)、肠易激综合征(IBS)、原发性高血压(EH)4种疾病肝气郁证动物模型。抑郁症肝气郁证大鼠模型:参照孤养加慢性不可预测性温和刺激法、社会挫败应激法造模。抑郁症肝气郁证猕猴模型:参照母子分离饲养加社会压力应激方法造模。PMS肝气郁证大鼠模型:应用孕激素撤退法及埋藏行为应激法制备PMS大鼠模型,经动物行为学测试鉴别分化出肝气逆、肝气郁证型。PMS肝气郁证猕猴模型:挑选同笼打斗低地位猕猴配合择时挤压造模法制备。IBS肝气郁证大鼠模型:按照铁桶限制运动加冷水刺激法复制。EH肝气郁证大鼠模型:选用自发性高血压大鼠应用孤养加慢性束缚应激法、慢性社会挫败应激法造模。EH肝气郁证猕猴模型:筛选中老年自发性高血压猕猴以社会压力应激建立高血压肝气郁证猕猴模型。模型动物证候表征采集:大鼠证候表征采集应用图像模式识别技术对舌象、唇象、爪象、耳轮、尾尖、眼球、皮毛图片进行特征提取并定量分析(如颜色和纹理比较)配合动物行为学检测(如旷场实验、糖水偏好、强迫游泳、社会逃避、埋藏行为等)。猕猴证候表征采集则应用视频跟踪系统及远程遥测技术监控猕猴表情行为并结合量表评定猕猴情绪得分,运用猕猴多导生理监测芯片采集猕猴呼吸、心跳、皮肤电等与情绪改变密切相关生理指标,配合运用猕猴面部表情与肢体形态识别计算机原型系统定性评判。上述表征信息是证候模型较直接、关键的指标,以期锁定模型证候归属。模型动物生物指标采集:① 微透析取样技术采集脑组织液或其他部位体液,采集血液、尿液,HPLCMS测定代谢指纹,以正常动物为对照,比较模型动物与正常动物代谢指纹差异,寻找特异性生物标记物,辅助完成模型评价。② 采集动物血液、尿液标本HPTLC、放射免疫方法检测与疾病相关关键生物学指标波动变化,比较正常对照组、造模组及造模给药组间差异。

③ 取病变组织标本,固定,染色,显微镜下观察其病理组织学改变。④ 其他特异性检测:如 IBS 大鼠模型的腹壁撤退反射评分、腹壁肌电活动,抑郁症肝气郁证动物模型的皮质醇抑制实验等。上述生物指标采集检测工作主要锁定模型动物的疾病归属。应用逍遥散作为上述同病异证动物模型的统一干预药物,考察药物干预前后模型动物指标波动变化,反证模型可靠性及稳定性。拟定的异病同证动物模型造模方法中较多采用了目前国际医学界常用的社会挫败(针对大鼠)及社会压力(针对猕猴)应激,基本上排除了躯体应激对实验动物的伤害及对实验结果的干扰,符合动物伦理学及动物实验的一般要求。

李长禄等建立了肾虚型老年痴呆大鼠模型,采用灌胃给予氢化可的松(15 mg/kg)复合侧脑室注射β-淀粉样蛋白(25～35) 10 μg 的方法,复制肾虚型老年痴呆动物模型,每 5 d 记录 1 次大鼠的体质量,通过体质量变化、自主活动、免疫学指标以及血浆中睾酮和皮质酮含量的变化,评价该模型肾虚的形成情况;通过奖励性操作式条件反射任务和水迷宫实验结合脑组织病理学的变化,评价该模型学习记忆的变化。结果与对照组比较,肾虚组和肾虚型老年痴呆组大鼠体质量增长缓慢,自主活动度显著降低,胸腺和脾指数显著降低,血清中睾酮和皮质酮含量显著降低。在水迷宫实验和奖励性操作式条件反射任务中,与对照组比较,肾虚型老年痴呆大鼠的学习记忆能力显著受损。从而证实灌胃给予氢化可的松(15 mg/kg)复合侧脑室注射β-淀粉样蛋白(25～35) 10 μg可以用于复制肾虚型老年痴呆模型,既可以使大鼠产生一系列肾虚表现,又可以造成其学习记忆功能障碍。孙瑜嫣等观察了肾虚质大鼠白细胞介素-2(IL-2)水平变化对 CD_4^+ T 细胞和 CD_8^+ T 细胞的影响。采用"猫吓鼠"的方法造成肾虚质孕鼠,将肾虚质孕鼠所产雄性子鼠 16 只随机平分为模型组及药物组,随机选取正常组孕鼠所产雄性子鼠 8 只作为空白组,模型组和药物组的 16 只子代鼠于每日定时进行恐吓,空白组不予恐吓,持续 1 个月;同时药物组给予桂附地黄丸混悬液,空白组和模型组给予等量生理盐水。采用 ELISA 法检测大鼠血清 IL-2 含量的变化,运用流式细胞仪检测脾脏 T 淋巴细胞亚群 CD_4^+、CD_8^+ 百分率的变化。结果,与空白组相比,模型组 IL-2 的含量降低,CD_4^+ 百分率下降,CD_8^+ 百分率升高;与模型组比,药物组 IL-2 的含量、CD_4^+ 百分率升高,CD_8^+ 百分率降低,差异均无统计学意义。所以提出肾虚质大鼠 IL-2 的水平与 T 细胞免疫功能具有相关性。徐晶晶等摸索了 D-半乳糖(D-Gal)致肾虚多尿动物模型的合适剂量。方法:将筛选后的 SD 大鼠随机分为 4 组,分别为正常对照组,D-Gal 125、150、175 mg/kg · d 剂量组;采用 D-半乳糖连续注射 8 周,停止注射后继续观察 1 周,以 24 h 总尿量及水负荷 5 h 后尿量为直接观测指标,同时采用尿动力仪检测膀胱储尿及排尿功能以探索 D-Gal 致肾虚多尿动物模型的合适剂量。结果,从各组大鼠 24 h 总尿量及水负荷 5 h 后尿量观察,D-Gal 150 mg/kg · d 剂量组增加尿量作用更显著。从尿动力参数观察,D-Gal 150 mg/kg · d 剂量组对大鼠膀胱漏尿点压、腹压漏尿点压、顺应性、最大膀胱排尿压、残余尿量、排尿效率的影响更显著,且其改变趋势与衰老动物尿动力学的变化相符。认为 D-Gal 150 mg/kg · d 剂量组在对尿液的生成、膀胱储存及排泄功能的影响方面更符合衰老所致肾虚多尿动物模型的制备。樊新荣等通过实验建立了前列腺增生症肾虚血瘀证大鼠动物模型。方法:采用去势手术、激素注射加冰浴方法制作良性前列腺增生(BPH)肾虚血瘀证大鼠模型,观察前列腺湿重、前列腺指数和血清前列腺特异性酸性磷酸酶含量,观察模型大鼠病理组织形态学。结果,模型组大鼠全血黏度、血浆黏度、红细胞聚集指数和卡松黏度均明显高于空白组和假手术组;模型组血清前列腺酸性磷酸酶(PAP)的含量升高,并且模型组大鼠前列腺组织病理组织学观察可见小血管扩张、充血,符合瘀血的病理表现。付小卫等分析中医防治骨质疏松症(OP)研究中动物模型的选用。指出啮齿目动物是运用最广泛且最实用经济的一类模型,但因其体型较小,不易多次取血、活检等,所以不太合适作为骨质疏松症模型。其次为兔形目,越来越多的为临床重视,运用也越来越广泛。食肉目动物比格犬虽然骨骼重建与人类相似,但是对骨组织生长代谢对雌激素的依赖性相对较小,特别是其卵巢和子宫切除并不足以引起明显的骨丢失,所以不适合做此实验。偶蹄目动物主要为小型猪和绵羊、山羊等,可多次取血、活检。山羊与绵羊有许多相似的之处,已被证明是合适的 OP 模型动物。但应注意的是,羊是反刍类动物,胃肠道系统与人不同,不适合口服给药,需要时可采取建立胃瘘管进行给药。施旭光等建立了脾气虚证4种造模方法并进行比较，筛取最接近脾气虚证的造模方法。选用SD大鼠分别采用酒醋硝黄饲料法、酒硝黄灌胃法、大黄灌胃法和利血平法复制脾气虚证模型，造模成功后，比较各模型组与正常对照组大鼠体质量、脾指数、胸腺指数以及血清肌酸激酶(CK)与淀粉酶(AMS)活性之间的差异。结果，与正常对照组比较，喂饲酒醋硝黄饲料组大鼠的体质量、脾指数、胸腺指数、CK与AMS活性均显著降低($P<0.05$)，其他3组各项指标均有不同程度降低。认为酒醋硝黄饲料法为4种造模方法中最理想、有效、接近中医脾气虚证候的大鼠模型的造模方法。杨宇峰等探讨了脾气虚证代谢综合征大鼠模型的复制方法。运用健康雄性SD大鼠40只，体质量180±20 g，随机分为空白对照组(n＝10)和模型组(n＝30)。模型组单日喂食甘蓝15～20 g/只，游泳至耐力极限；双日高糖高脂膳食持续喂养，共计12周。结果，造模结束后模型组出现高胰岛素血症、胰岛素抵抗，符合脾气虚证代谢综合征的评估标准。刘建鸿等对肝郁脾虚证模型大鼠免疫细胞分化和增殖变化规律进行研究。采用夹尾激怒、束缚应激、过度疲劳与饮食失节的复合方法复制肝郁脾虚证动物模型。检测空白对照组和模型2、6、9周组雄性大鼠外周血象、骨髓象和骨髓细胞增殖周期。结果，外周血象显示：与空白对照组比较，模型大鼠2周组白细胞和中性粒细胞数量升高($P<0.05$，$P<0.01$)，9周组淋巴细胞数量降低($P<0.05$)。骨髓象显示：与空白对照组比较，模型大鼠2周组成熟中性粒细胞升高、淋巴细胞比例降低($P<0.05$)，9周组淋巴细胞比例升高($P<0.05$)。骨髓细胞周期显示：与空白对照组比较，模型大鼠2周组S期和G_2/M期升高($P<0.05$)，2周、6周组增殖指数升高($P<0.05$，$P<0.01$)。李聪等通过建立肝郁-脾虚-肝郁脾虚证模型，用来观察大鼠胰腺内、外分泌变化。方法分别采用慢性束缚应激法、过度疲劳＋饮食失节法、慢性束缚＋过度疲劳＋饮食失节法复制肝郁、脾虚和肝郁脾虚证大鼠模型，测定各模型大鼠十二指肠中的胰蛋白酶、胰脂肪酶、胰淀粉酶和血中胰岛素、胰高血糖素、生长抑素及血糖水平。结果，与正常组比较，肝郁模型组大鼠小肠液中胰脂肪酶和胰淀粉酶均显著升高，脾虚模型组和肝郁脾虚模型组胰脂肪酶和胰淀粉酶均显著降低，3个模型组的胰蛋白酶均显著降低；肝郁模型组大鼠血糖显著升高，胰高血糖素和生长抑素呈降低趋势，脾虚模型组和肝郁脾虚模型组大鼠的血糖和胰高血糖素均显著降低，生长抑素显著升高，3个模型组的胰岛素均显著增高。认为肝郁、脾虚、肝郁脾虚三证模型大鼠均存在胰脏功能的异常，但同中有异。肝郁脾虚证大鼠胰腺内、外分泌功能状态与脾虚证模型基本相同。

谢波等探讨了不同冷冻时间对寒凝血瘀证动物模型建立的影响。方法：将雌性大鼠随机分为空白组、5 d组、10 d组、15 d组、20 d组。除空白组外，其余大鼠置于0℃冰水中15 min，1次/d，各组分别冷冻相应天数，造成寒凝血瘀模型。观察血常规、卵巢和子宫指数和血液流变指标。结果，与空白组比较，造模5 d和10 d组大鼠红细胞显著降低，活化部分凝血酶时间显著延长；造模5 d组还可见血浆黏度、低转速全血黏度和红细胞聚集指数的显著降低，红细胞变形能力的显著增加，血红蛋白显著降低，子宫指数可见显著减少。造模10 d组还可见中性粒细胞百分比的显著增加，凝血酶时间的显著缩短。造模10 d和15 d虽然均可见红细胞压积的显著减少，但是造模10 d组可见红细胞变形指数的降低，而造模15 d却见其变形指数的显著增加，凝血酶时间的显著缩短，血浆黏度的显著增加，另外活化部分凝血酶时间也有缩短的趋势。而当造模时间延长到20 d，反而可见凝血酶原时间和活化部分凝血酶时间的显著延长。造模10 d和15 d可见大鼠出现凝血功能增强，并且15 d组血液流变学异常最明显。该造模方法为中医寒凝血瘀证的研究提供新的思路。袁颖等建立气虚血瘀证大鼠模型，并观察气虚血瘀证大鼠模型血液流变学及Th_1/Th_2平衡的变化，用于探讨气虚血瘀证的病理机制。方法：采用限食＋强迫游泳＋皮下注射肾上腺素方法制备气虚血瘀证大鼠模型，观察模型大鼠体重、胸腺指数、脾指数、血液流变学变化，应用ELISA方法测定血清中干扰素-γ(IFN-γ)、白细胞介素-4(IL-4)含量。结果，与空白对照组相比，模型组体重下降，血液流变学指标升高，胸腺、脾指数降低，血清IFN-γ含量降低，IL-4含量升高。认为气虚血瘀证大鼠存在一定免疫功能缺陷，Th_1/Th_2细胞平衡向Th_2细胞偏移，可能是本证的病理机制之一。

(于　峥)

[附] 参 考 文 献

A

阿衣古丽·玉努斯,哈木拉提·吾甫尔,帕丽旦·麦麦提,等.基于异常黑胆质证载体大鼠模型血清代谢组学研究[J].中华中医药杂志,2013,28(8):2251

B

宾炜,黎敬波,林嬿钊,等.议析运气学说中岁气客气关系的矛盾[J].长春中医药大学学报,2013,29(1):1

C

陈蓓,李艳.《黄帝内经》时间医学理论研究[J].辽宁中医药大学学报,2013,15(2):126

陈丽斌,纪立金,高思华.基于"同气相求"理论探索肺与大肠的表里构建[J].中华中医药杂志,2013,28(12):3483

陈清光,陆灏,许家佗,等,高强度训练女运动员的临床表型及评价方法研究[J].中华中医药杂志,2013,28(5):1500

陈润东.从《神农本草经》谈谈"六行学说"分类法[J].新中医,2013,45(3):191

陈素华.糖尿病肾病彩色多普勒超声诊断及中医辨证分型[J].贵阳中医学院学报,2013,35(3):54

陈小野.胃黏膜肠化当补肾[J].中国中医基础医学杂志,2013,19(1):92

陈晓蓉,陆云飞,杨宗国,等.新型H7N9禽流感中医证候特点分析[J].中华中医药杂志,2013,28(7):1929

陈瑛,阮永队,马春玲.从本气先虚论肺部感染[J].河南中医,2013,33(7):1018

陈玉萍,马淑然,王乐鹏,等,中医"肝应春"调控机制与下丘脑褪黑素合成限速酶芳香烷基胺-N-乙酰基转移酶mRNA表达相关性的研究[J].中华中医药杂志,2013,28(5):1556

陈镇秋,何伟,魏秋实.股骨头坏死中医证型与血液学指标的相关性研究[J].中华中医药杂志,2013,28(7):2205

程园园,刘健,万磊,等.骨关节炎发病与脾气亏虚的关系探讨[J].中国中医基础医学杂志,2013,19(7):742

D

段俊国,罗向霞,许国旺,等.DR病情进展与阳虚病机关系的研究[J].西部中医药,2013,26(8):1

F

樊新荣,颜苗,何清湖.前列腺增生症肾虚血瘀证大鼠动物模型的建立与评价[J].中国中医基础医学杂志,2013,19(3):257

付小卫,宋长恒,王如然,等.关于中医防治骨质疏松症研究中动物模型的选用[J].中国中医基础医学杂志,2013,19(3):266

G

高泓,何宝明,高黝,等.134例糖调节受损人群的中医体质临床观察研究[J].成都中医药大学学报,2013,36(2):42

高伟,张蓓蓓,张家留,等.不同舌色严重脓毒症患者舌下微循环差异的临床研究[J].江苏中医药,2013,45(9):31

郭春风,尚国旗,宫妍,等.从五运六气论治干燥综合征[J].新中医,2013,45(6):184

郭梅珍,张留超.论述运气"七篇大论"与《素问》的关系[J].中国中医基础医学杂志,2013,19(2):122

H

韩艳武,张伟,王融冰,等,不同内伤基础甲型H1N1流感的中医病因病机初探[J].中华中医药杂志,2013,28(5):1418

何淑寅,符德玉,祖亮华.高血压病中医证型与B型脑钠肽及脑卒中风险的相关性初探[J].中华中医药杂志,2013,28(1):281

惠毅,杨宇,唐洪屈,等.从肺病模型大鼠胃肠动力学角度探讨"肺病及肠"病理传变机制[J].中国中医基础医学杂志,2013,19(1):50

J

金贺,王佳艳,李宗衡,等.缺血性中风急性期甲状腺激素表达异常患者证候规律及血管病变特点的初步研究[J].中国中医基础医学杂志,2013,19(2):160

景兴文,刘福友,陈维.气虚血瘀证大鼠子二代大脑中动脉栓塞脑缺血耐受性及ERK信号转导通路的实验研究[J].新中医,2013,45(1):132

L

李聪,谢鸣,赵荣华.肝郁-脾虚-肝郁脾虚证模型大鼠胰腺内、外分泌变化的比较观察[J].广州中医药大学学报,2013,30(5):729

李海峰,陈正,赵心华.《内经》多层次的体质辨别系统[J].中国中医基础医学杂志,2013,19(7):722

李江,刘治中,王建升,等.运用时辰药理学规范住院患者临床用药[J].中国中医基础医学杂志,2013,

19(7)：758

李俊龙，李燕. 2012(壬辰)年太阳寒水司天[J]. 中国中医基础医学杂志，2013，19(4)：455

李维娜，李炳茂.《黄帝内经》阴阳学说的科学性[J]. 河北中医，2013，35(8)：1236

李秀美，王全年. 模型中医学的阴阳观[J]. 时珍国医国药，2013，24(6)：1437

李长禄，王红梅，王立为. 肾虚型老年痴呆大鼠模型的复制[J]. 安徽中医学院学报，2013，32(3)：62

廖凌虹，李灿东，汪欣，等. 514 例体检者生化指标与中医痰证的相关性分析[J]. 中华中医药杂志，2013，28(7)：2078

林雪娟，李灿东，吴青海，等. 基于电子鼻技术的表证患者气味图谱研究[J]. 中华中医药杂志，2013，28(1)：52

刘恩顺，孙增涛，苏景深，等. 基于肺与大肠相表里的 ALI/ARDS 证候特征的临床研究[J]. 天津中医药，2013，30(1)：14

刘怀珍，吴守锋，谈佳佳. 2 型糖尿病血脂异常患者的中医证候学特点探究[J]. 中国中医药现代远程教育，2013，11(5)：1

刘建鸿，岳嘉，段永强，等. 肝郁脾虚证模型大鼠免疫细胞分化和增殖变化规律研究[J]. 中国中医药信息杂志，2013，20(1)：43

刘南，曹伟锋，余锋. 急性冠脉综合征中医辨证分型与丝裂原活化蛋白激酶、内脂素等炎症因子的相关性[J]. 广州中医药大学学报，2013，30(5)：615

刘润兰，陶功定. 从控制论看《内经》五行生克制化与反馈调节[J]. 世界中西医结合杂志，2013，8(5)：433

刘文波. 运气学说的临床指导意义探讨[J]. 中医药临床杂志，2013，25(6)：552

刘文兰，刘汶，车念聪，等. 慢性乙型肝炎患者血清 sICAM - 1 与舌色和证候关系的研究[J]. 中华中医药杂志，2013，28(8)：2444

刘燕鸿，洪敏俐，黄小华，等. 慢性阻塞性肺疾病中医痰证素与气道炎症的相关性研究[J]. 中华中医药杂志，2013，28(2)：507

刘正华. 浅析青壮年妇女下寒上热证的病因病机和治疗[J]. 四川中医，2013，31(4)：36

娄彦梅，李峰，韩萍，等. 原发性血脂异常心血管危险分级及血脂指标与中医证候相关性[J]. 中华中医药杂志，2013，28(6)：1893

M

马师雷，田甜，李鸿涛，等. 从"肺与大肠相表里"探讨调肺在泄泻治疗中的作用[J]. 中医杂志，2013，54(8)：653

马振，朱云利. 脾肾阳虚型非糖尿病性维持性血液透析患者与残余肾功能和氨基末端 B 型脑钠肽前体的相关性研究[J]. 中医研究，2013，26(6)：16

孟庆岩，张庆祥，高思华. 从"津液相关"探讨肺与大肠相表里[J]. 北京中医药大学学报，2013，36(11)：729

P

潘碧琦，潘建科，刘军，等. 痛风辨证分型与痛风危险因素的相关性研究[J]. 新中医，2013，45(7)：33

彭薇淇，尚文皤，李泽鹏. 试探中医时间医学与胃肠动力学的内在联系[J]. 世界中医药，2013，8(4)：460

Q

乔文彪，邢玉瑞，李翠娟. 中医理论发生学研究述评(二)[J]. 陕西中医学院学报，2013，36(1)：1

S

闪增郁，陈燕萍，黄大威，等. 平人大暑、处暑、秋分脉图参数的比较研究[J]. 中医杂志，2013，54(8)：684

盛益华，王新月，闫昕，等. 从溃疡性结肠炎大鼠肺损伤细胞凋亡机制探讨"肺与大肠相表里"[J]. 世界华人消化杂志，2013，21(13)：1171

施旭光，王闽予，吴美音，等. 脾气虚证 4 种造模方法的比较研究[J]. 广州中医药大学学报，2013，30(2)：196

孙萌，刘颖，王克林，等. 脾气虚型 HIV/AIDS 患者淋巴细胞线粒体功能状态在常温和热应激条件下的改变情况[J]. 中国中医基础医学杂志，2013，19(7)：777

孙瑜嫣，孙理军，党照丽，等. 肾虚质大鼠 IL - 2 水平变化对 CD_4^+ T 细胞和 CD_8^+ T 细胞的影响[J]. 中医药导报，2013，19(8)：9

孙振，丁小龙，王全年. 从发生学角度探讨中医五行学说理论的形成[J]. 山东中医杂志，2013，32(3)：147

T

唐洪屈，王宝家，郑秀丽，等. 肺病及肠大鼠动物模型的建立及评价[J]. 四川中医，2013，31(3)：46

W

汪四海，刘健，张金山. 从脾论治强直性脊柱炎骨代谢失衡理论探讨[J]. 中华中医药杂志，2013，28(8)：2233

王彩娟，陆红研，焦久存，等. 脑卒中痉挛性瘫痪患者痰瘀证与颈动脉彩超及部分血液指标关系的临床观察[J]. 四川中医，2013，31(2)：57

王春芳，徐立然，符林春，等. HIV/AIDS 中医证型与 T 淋巴细胞亚群关系的研究[J]. 中华中医药杂志，2013，28(9)：2560

王付. 附子亡阳论[J]. 中医药通报，2013，12(1)：18

王昊，王克勤，薛崇成，等. 中医人格体质论的内涵探析[J]. 中医杂志，2013，54(7)：551

王宏献，柴可夫. 同型半胱氨酸及 C 反应蛋白与糖尿

病肾病中医证候关系研究[J]. 中华中医药杂志,2013,28(3):778

王利锋,苏颖. 近 50 年五运六气理论与相关气象资料研究概述[J]. 长春中医药大学学报,2013,29(3):542

王燕,赵长海,王先敏,等. 新疆地区汉族与维吾尔族高尿酸血症证候类型特点因子分析[J]. 中国中医基础医学杂志,2013,19(3):320

魏盛,乔明琦. 从肝论治异病同证动物模型造模与评价的理论思考[J]. 山东中医药大学学报,2013,37(2):94

吴凡伟,杜震生. 五运六气学说临床运用举隅[J]. 中医药信息,2013,30(3):8

吴宏进,张志枫,许家佗,等. 677 例健康人群体表面积、体质指数与采脉压力及脉图参数的关系探讨[J]. 中华中医药杂志,2013,28(5):1361

吴炜景,李立平,林延超,等. 广东地区胃窦溃疡患者幽门螺杆菌 CagA 基因型与中医证型相关性分析[J]. 中华中医药杂志,2013,28(6):1803

吴小秋,罗玉韵,徐进华,等. 2 型糖尿病中医体质特点及与胰岛素抵抗、分泌的关系[J]. 广州中医药大学学报,2013,30(3):312

吴祖星,陈铭,杨广印,等. 大肠经的能量代谢特征[J]. 福建中医药大学学报,2013,23(3):4

X

肖凌,王静芝,翁鑫宇,等. 衰老阳虚大鼠生化指标及 HSP70 表达的研究[J]. 中华中医药学刊,2013,31(1):101

谢波,邓海山,喻斌,等. 寒凝血瘀证大鼠模型的优化筛选研究[J]. 南京中医药大学学报,2013,29(3):262

谢春娥,薛晓轩,刘晶,等. 胃痛辨证分型及舌象与幽门螺杆菌感染的关系分析[J]. 中华中医药杂志,2013,28(8):2287

辛海,吴剑坤,金玫,等. 1 350 例社区慢性病人群的体型与中医体质分布特点[J]. 中华中医药杂志,2013,28(6):1719

邢玉瑞,田丙坤. 中医理论发生学研究述评(一)[J]. 陕西中医学院学报,2012,35(5):1

邢玉瑞. 中医理论发生学研究述评(三)[J]. 陕西中医学院学报,2013,36(2):1

邢玉瑞. 中医理论发生学研究述评(四)[J]. 陕西中医学院学报,2013,36(3):1

邢玉瑞. 中医理论发生学研究述评(五)[J]. 陕西中医学院学报,2013,36(4):6

邢玉瑞. 中医理论发生学研究述评(六)[J]. 陕西中医学院学报,2013,36(5):1

邢玉瑞. 中医理论发生学研究述评(七)[J]. 陕西中医学院学报,2013,36(6):6

徐晶晶,邱琼华,赖焕玲,等. D-半乳糖致肾虚多尿动物模型研究[J]. 广州中医药大学学报,2013,30(3):386

徐万忠,李思,张昱. 维持性血液透析患者血瘀证积分与 ET、NO 的相关性研究[J]. 中医临床研究,2013,5(3):1

徐颖,许筱颖,郭霞珍. 季节变化对仓鼠褪黑素合成限速酶羟基吲哚-氧-甲基转移酶 mRNA 表达的影响[J]. 中华中医药杂志,2013,28(5):1306

Y

杨朝阳,苏志扬,蔡美美,等. 基于中医健康状态气血津液辨识法的毒瘾中医病理因素研究[J]. 世界中医药,2013,8(1):15

杨惠民,赵宇捷. 北京地区汉族中老年人原发性血脂异常与中医体质相关性研究[J]. 中华中医药杂志,2013,28(1):96

杨聘. 轻度认知功能障碍中医证型与同型半胱氨酸的相关性研究[J]. 新中医,2013,45(4):22

杨宇峰,滕飞,石岩. 脾气虚证代谢综合征大鼠模型的复制[J]. 中国中医基础医学杂志,2013,19(4):392

殷婷婷,赵春杰,张英泽,等. 风湿性疾病湿热证实质的脂质组学研究[J]. 中华中医药杂志,2013,28(1):210

于宁,翟双庆. 从肺论治肠易激综合征的理论探析[J]. 中华中医药杂志,2013,28(12):3494

于琦,崔蒙,李园白,等,基于文献研究的中医温病病因病机认识的时代变迁[J]. 中华中医药杂志,2013,28(8):2245

余敏英,黄李平,凌江红,等. 湿热体质与平和体质原发性血脂异常者 ApoE 基因多态性研究[J]. 辽宁中医药大学学报,2013,15(1):84

袁颖,郭忻,金素安,等. 气虚血瘀证大鼠模型血液流变学及 Th1/Th2 平衡研究[J]. 辽宁中医杂志,2013,40(6):1244

Z

张继烈,鞠鲤亦. 从数字看高血压与脾气虚[J]. 中国中医药现代远程教育,2013,11(16):126

张静,蔡永亮,陈怀珍,等. 不同证型肝豆状核变性患者门静脉血流动力学改变研究[J]. 新中医,2013,45(1):84

张敏,纪立金,高思华. 肺与大肠"相合"的理论探讨[J]. 中华中医药杂志,2013,28(10):2840

张颖,马建萍,马秀兰,等. 105 例吸毒人群 AIDS 患者中医证型与 $CD4^+$ T 淋巴细胞关系的探讨[J]. 中华中医药杂志,2013,28(4):1115

郑秀丽,杨宇,唐洪屈,等. 从肺与大肠的特异相关性探讨"肺与大肠相表里"[J]. 中华中医药杂志,2013,

28(5)：1492

郑秀丽，杨宇，郑旭锐，等.从肺肠菌群变化的相关性探讨“肺与大肠相表里”[J].中华中医药杂志，2013，28(8)：2294

朱立，王新月，杨雪，等.从溃疡性结肠炎大鼠肺损伤看“肺与大肠相表里”的特异性[J].中国中西医结合杂志，2013，33(3)：346

朱丽萍，吴宏进，张志枫，等.54例不同性别健康大学生“寸口”脉象及脉图参数分析[J].上海中医药大学学报，2013，27(2)：28

(二)中药理论

【概述】

中药理论研究涉及药性(气味、归经、毒性、升降沉浮)、配伍、禁忌、炮制、效用等方面。2013年,有关中药理论研究的报道,既有传统的文献整理和理论探讨,也有利用现代方法的分析归纳,内容丰富。

1. 药性理论的研究

(1) 气味的研究　谢素萍等报道,中药性状气味与功效气味既有相似之处,又有显著差异。前者是中药嗅之可闻、尝之可得的客观属性,是闻与尝的感觉。后者是根据药物作用于人体后发生的不同反应和治疗效果而作出的概括性归纳,是前者的发展,同时又具有药物临床疗效的实际功能。余坚报道,酸味中药的功效主要为敛肺止咳、回阳固脱、敛津止汗、涩肠止泻、敛涩固肛、涩精止遗、固冲止血、开胃生津、清利咽喉。邓家刚等报道,平性药性理论研究分成四个阶段:春秋战国至东汉时期是理论萌芽阶段,晋隋唐时期是理论形成阶段,宋金元时期是理论发展阶段,明清时期是理论丰富与完善阶段。崔利锐等报道,中药四性理论研究需要进一步深入,一要确立科学的研究思路;二要提出理论假说,并对理论假说进行证实与证伪;三要搭建高水平的多学科融合平台;四要宏观研究与微观研究相结合;五要文献研究、实验研究、临床研究相结合。

(2) 归经的研究　邓凯文等报道,特定的中药成分群对特定的经络脏腑有选择性的作用,体现"物"性;经络脏腑的功能状态以一定的证候表现出来,体现"象"性;一定功能的经络脏腑对特征中药成分群有反作用,可用于探知和表征经络脏腑,体现"候"性,三者实为"物-象-候"印迹关系。杨雪梅等整理了《中华本草》所载8 980味中药的五脏归经分类关联规则32条,并总结了5种不同类别中药功效的五脏归经趋向。张靖等以《中国药典》(2010年版)收录、中医临床常用方药及上市中成药中有毒中药为研究对象,系统总结其性味归经、化学成分、药理作用,并从抗癌研究与应用角度探讨其与归经的关系。李芳等以药物归经学说为理论依据,结合方剂的组方配伍规律,应用层次分析法(AHP)及向量理论,构建方剂"归经强度"数学模型。

(3) 毒性的研究　关卿报道,中医药古籍早有毒性记载,中药有毒、无毒以及毒性强弱都是相对的,受到品种因素、炮制因素、配伍因素、剂量因素以及剂型、煎服方法等因素的影响。朱梦莺报道,中药导致肾功能损伤,包括误治引起肾脏损害和药物性肾损害,前者属于辨证不明而采用了错误的治法,后者是没有注意用药方法。徐义高报道,毒性中药有独特疗效,但由于配伍不当、炮制欠佳或剂量过大等原因,则毒副反应随之增多,影响中药的信誉和临床应用。

(4) 升降浮沉的研究　韩翠翠等报道,升降浮沉理论经历萌芽和实践、金元时期创立和发展、明清时期丰富和普及、近现代研究和认识等4个发展阶段,并提出药物的气味厚薄、质地等因素决定药物的升降浮沉,而药物的用药部位、炮制、配伍等因素影响药物的升降浮沉,临床应用主要依据病因病机,还需考虑病位、病势、四时等因素。黄建忠报道,升降浮沉理论是反映药物在人体内发挥作用的趋向,以脏腑气机升降出入的生理特点为指导,以能顺应脏腑气机发生障碍时出现的疾病指导选方用药。

仲宗亮等报道,生大黄能明显促进小鼠小肠排空,对血液循环系统有促进作用,对中枢神经有一定兴奋作用,表现出向上向外趋势,为升浮药。清半夏对消化系统影响不明显,对血液循环系统有促进作用,对中枢神经具有明显抑制作用;常山对消化系统活动有明显抑制作用,对血液循环系统有促进作用,对中枢神经系统效果不明显,清半夏和常山两者表现出向下向内趋势,为沉降药。赵春梅报道,具有升散之性的常用中药如柴胡、升麻、羌活、荆芥穗、防风等,在升阳益气和升散除湿方面的作用明显。俞仲毅等报道,中药升降浮沉理论研究现状并不乐观,主要表现为:明确升降浮沉归属的药物数量有限,大多混乱不统一;理论研究无突破;实验研究严重缺乏等,导致中药升降浮沉缺少合理的研究假说。

（5）药性的综合研究　王哲等采用数据挖掘技术研究药性与功能、主治之间的相关性，建立了中药药性-药味-归经、药性-药味-归经-功能以及药性-药味-归经-功能-主治间较密切的频繁项目集，并计算出相关支持度及支持率。杨雪梅等以《中华本草》收载药物为例，分析了四气、五味、归经、毒性之间的关联性。王兰等报道，通过基于藏象思维模型建立药性组合与脏腑精、神、元气、气、血、阴、阳关系的复杂系统模型，揭示了药性组合的作用特征，有助于中药药性理论与藏象学说整体关联的研究，并提供了药性理论发展应用的新思路。王晓燕报道，数学建模策略在中药药性物质基础的研究中得到了应用，如从 64 种建模策略中选出 17 种判别良好的模型，选出 4 种适宜模型，统计模拟选出 PLS 作为目前最适宜的中药药性特征标记识别模型。

2. 配伍理论的研究

位亚丽等报道，中药配伍理论体系应当包括七情和合、配伍宜忌、君臣佐使以及中药配伍的现代药理学、药效学、毒理学等研究。邓家刚等报道了平性药的配伍规律，认为平性药在组方配伍方面有两大特点，一是少为君臣，重在和合；二是多为佐使，调和辅助。从 1 307 首古今方剂中所筛选出的君臣佐使常用平性药和主干平性药，为临床组方用药及研究提供了有益的参考。闫军堂等报道，经方中“角药”的配伍有同类相须、异类相使、阴阳配伍、气血配伍、寒热并用、升降相因、开阖并施、散敛兼顾、润燥相随、攻补同施、动静结合、刚柔相济、表里兼顾、气味配伍 14 个方面。赵正奇等报道，茯苓配伍用药时应注意在中气下陷、虚寒精滑、阴虚而无湿热者及孕妇(对气血虚弱所致的堕胎、滑胎而言)等情况下慎用或忌用。临床运用茯苓不能单独局限于其健脾利湿、宁心安神的功效，还需考虑其淡渗下泄有碍脾阳之升发，不能因其可食用而大量应用。盛华刚报道，目前方剂组分配伍研究仅局限于少数组分，组分配伍多采用单个药效指标评价法来确定最佳配伍比例，研究组分的层次不一致等问题急需解决，并认为对组分配伍的研究已逐步扩大到单味药中的组分配伍和标准物质的组分配伍。秦丹等报道，应用数据挖掘软件 Enterprise Miner 关联规则法，分析七情配伍中相使药对的药性组合规律。结果表明，相使药对的常见药性组合模式包括：温辛脾-温辛肝、温辛脾-温辛脾、温辛胃-温辛脾、寒苦肝-寒苦肺、温辛脾胃-温辛肝脾等。

在药对配伍研究方面，张明德报道了白芍药因配伍的不同而分别具有养血敛阴、柔肝止痛、平抑肝阳、化阴和营等多种功效。英洪友等报道，麻黄常用药对的配伍与相关的证治规律，认为麻黄的常用配伍中药为甘草、防风、川芎、当归、杏仁等，常见的相关主治病症为咳嗽、中风、伤寒等。王付研究了经方中柴胡药对的配伍关系、用量调配、临床运用，认为柴胡药对因配伍不同则治疗作用不同，配伍用药是柴胡治病的最佳选择。罗年翠研究表明，当归-黄芪、当归-白芍药药对偏于补血，当归-赤芍药、当归-川芎和当归-桃仁药对偏于活血，当归-熟地黄药对补血、活血作用均较强。何瑶等综述了近年来附子甘草配伍药对减毒增效作用机制研究进展，提出了一些新的研究思路。陈金锋等报道，酸枣仁-五味子药对醇水双提物具有一定镇静催眠作用，其机制可能与调节单胺类神经递质有关。杨艳等对大剂量使用芍药与甘草配伍的解痉作用进行了研究。结果表明，改变白芍药与炙甘草配伍比例，增大白芍药配伍用量，可以直接影响回肠平滑肌收缩频率及张力变化率，使肠蠕动变慢，解痉作用加强，进而增强缓急止痛效果。杨慧波等对生川乌与不同比例生半夏配伍镇痛作用进行了研究。结果表明，随着生半夏比例的增加，生川乌的镇痛作用减弱，且有一定的剂量依赖关系。张荣等研究不同比例甘草诃子配伍制草乌对其次乌头碱含量的影响。结果表明，草乌-甘草、草乌-诃子合煎后，次乌头碱含量均低于草乌单煎，且在相同配伍比例下，草乌-诃子合煎液中的次乌头碱含量低于草乌-甘草合煎液。认为甘草、诃子与草乌共煎均有减轻草乌毒性的作用。谢炜等研究了柴胡-白芍药不同比例配伍应用的抗惊厥作用。结果表明，柴胡-白芍药配伍应用具有良好的抗惊厥的作用，其抗惊厥作用优于单用柴胡或白芍药，其中以柴胡-白芍药 2∶1 配伍比例的抗惊厥作用最好。

3. 禁忌理论的研究

李晓鹤等报道，反药同方中存在归经相同、性味相反的药性组合，常根据辨证取其中 1 味药的非相反药性组合为主，而相反药性组合相互制约，具有一定的保护作用。杨环等报道，治疗中风病的方剂中有许多含“十八反”的药物同用，其中以半夏-附子使用最多。田文全报道,附子、半夏配伍应用确实客观存在,但附子、半夏配伍能增强毒性,因此不应废弃"相反"之说而随便应用。衡晴晴等报道,中药"十八反"中"藻戟遂芫俱战草"的研究目前主要集中在急性毒性、长期毒性,而很少对特定部位的实验研究,且存在药物基原、给药方式、配伍比例等实验条件不统一现象,应该加以改善。程显怡等报道,近年来十八反中"半蒌贝蔹及攻乌"尚未对所属的全部药对逐对进行系统研究,毒理学研究采用正常动物的较多,而用病理模型的较少;化学研究用液相测定毒性成分含量变化的较多,而对机制的研究较少;对反药药对单独配伍研究较多,而对其在中药复方中的配伍效应研究较少。并提出"十八反"中"半蒌贝蔹及攻乌"不是绝对配伍禁忌。李世哲报道,乌头汤与生半夏、川贝母配伍均会对抗氧化活性有一定的抑制作用,其中与川贝母的配伍降低作用最为明显。

4. 炮制理论的研究

杨明等从文化理念、哲学思想的角度,探讨了传统中药炮制的文化起源、思维模式、道法术,追溯了中药炮制的形成与演绎、凝练与提升及其核心价值等文化历史,总结了中药炮制以整体、客观、动态、平衡、适度等哲学思想为指导的基本原则。李广峰等报道,中药炮制可以改变药性、增加疗效、降低毒性、提高患者顺应性以及引药归经等,并认为中药炮制是依据辨证施治用药的需要和药物自身性质以及调剂、制剂的不同要求所采取的一项制药技术,中药必须经过炮制之后才能入药,保证药物的稳定性,更好发挥药物的疗效。查小芹等报道半夏经炮制后,能降低毒性,缓和药性,消除副作用;正品半夏及其炮制品的药理作用有显著的不同,生半夏具有催呕作用、清半夏以燥湿化痰为主、姜半夏以温中化痰和降逆止呕为主、法半夏偏以祛寒痰及调脾和胃。杨洁报道,姜制法对中药作用的影响以及生姜药对配伍中生姜的作用,揭示了方剂中药物配伍与炮制的关系,为临床合理调配方剂、制备更多姜制中药提供借鉴。

5. 效用理论的研究

李具宝等报道,近10年来虫类药临床应用已涉及呼吸、消化、泌尿、神经、风湿免疫、妇科、男科、皮肤科等多种疾病,其同病机为经脉痹阻。但因虫类药具毒性或峻烈之性,且剂量难以掌握,容易引起药疹瘙痒等过敏反应,在临床的应用也受到了限制。虫类药多辛温燥烈、易伤津液,对于阴虚阳亢、血虚发痉、生风者应慎用,或与养阴药配伍使用。李卫祥报道,丹参在治疗冠心病、小儿肺炎、糖尿病并发末梢神经炎、慢性肾炎、高血压、血管性头痛、消化性溃疡、细菌性阴道病、改善肝硬化患者肝功能等方面的作用明显。辛淑杰等分析了80例应用和未应用何首乌的同种疾病患者临床资料。结果表明,何首乌在保肝、增强免疫力、抗衰老、抗炎、抗肿瘤、抗诱变、镇痛及在心血管系统等方面均具有显著疗效。徐义高研究了黄芩与滑石、白蔻仁、通草、桑白皮、知母、麦冬、金银花、连翘、牛蒡子、板蓝根、生地黄、白茅根、白术、当归、青蒿等配伍的临床应用,表明黄芩用量为3～10 g,清热多生用,安胎多炒用,止血多炒炭用,清上焦热多酒炒用;枯芩(即生长年久的宿根)善清肺火,条芩(生长年少的子根)善清大肠之火、泻下焦湿热。王晓红报道,大黄在临床应用中的新用途,主要表现为治疗蛔虫性肠梗阻、肠胀气、清洁肠道、急性胆囊炎、胆道出血等。

此外,还有一些中药中毒反应及量效关系的报道。如张红燕等综述1994～2012年间山豆根引起中毒反应,主要表现为用于治疗急慢性咽炎、扁桃体炎及慢性肝炎后,个别用于肿瘤术后、脱发等。常见的毒副反应主要为消化系统、神经系统及呼吸系统症状,其部分症状经停药或及时治疗可完全缓解,预后良好,一旦出现全身肌张力障碍,临床药物治疗效果不佳,预后不良。张仕玉等报道采用均数、百分位数和极差等统计方法处理,结果半夏的剂量80%分布在6～15 g之间,与《中国药典》(2010版)法定剂量的完全符合率为54.7%,高于法定剂量为45.3%,故认为半夏在汤剂中的剂量以6～15 g为宜。陆华通过比较12种苗药和中药的药名、药性、功能、主治以及用法等,认为苗药与中药在药名上有很大的区别,苗药的药用部位比中药广泛,苗药的主治比中药更丰富。苗药与中药在药性、功能以及主治上,既有诸多相似之处,也有许多不同点。

(陈仁寿　程　旺)

【中药的配伍禁忌应用与机制研究】

"十八反、十九畏"是中医临床用药配伍禁忌的重要组成部分,然而历代医家对此问题争议颇多,临床报道也屡见不鲜。但在古今文献中,不乏此类配伍的应用,现代实验研究也对其配伍进行了相关研究。

1. 古今临床应用文献研究

李怡文等对 2009 年版《医保目录》中成药部分含"十八反"、"十九畏"药对的成方制剂进行整理，分别从这些含反药药对成方制剂的收载情况、反药药对出现频率、处方药味数、剂型用法以及现代临床的应用方面进行了归纳分析。结果，《医保目录》中成药部分共收录成方制剂 987 个品种，其中含反药配伍的成方制剂 9 个，包括含"十八反"药对的品种 5 个，含"十九畏"药对的品种 4 个。其用药特点为探讨反药配伍的临床使用规律，指导临床合理安全使用"十八反"、"十九畏"提供了思路。杨环等运用关联规则等方法分析古代及近现代含"十八反"药物治疗中风病方剂的配伍和治疗特点，得到古今中风病"十八反"反药同方方剂共 173 首(古方 111 首，近现代方 62 首)，相反药对以半夏-附子使用最多，共 76 首。古今含"十八反"药物治疗中风方剂高频药物存在显著差异($P<0.05$)。古今治疗中风均重视治痰，但古方用药偏于熄风通络化痰，近现代方用药偏于益气健脾化痰。刘佳等整理了甘草与海藻组合的临床研究文献共计 149 篇，发现该药对主要治疗中医外科疾病，乳癖为最多，其次是内科瘿病，再次是妇科子宫肌瘤，其它各科记载较少。两者临床组合同用多以未经炮制加工的生品以 1∶2 的比例配伍使用，多加工制成汤剂，口服使用，但因文献之间异质性太高无法进行疗效的定量综合分析，安全性尚不能确定。刘氏等还分析了甘草与甘遂反药组合的临床研究文献共计 119 篇，主要治疗中医内科疾病，有 62 篇，其他各科依次为外科 5 篇、骨伤科 3 篇、皮肤科 2 篇，两药同用多以生甘草、醋甘遂的炮制形式，以 1∶1 的比例，汤剂或口服使用，但其安全性尚不能确定。

2. 实验研究

(1) 药效研究　① 半蒌贝蔹及攻乌：刘春芳等研究了制川乌与生半夏不同配比和剂量变化对小鼠镇痛、抗炎、祛痰、镇咳作用的影响。结果表明，制川乌与生半夏配伍能降低制川乌的镇痛和抗炎作用，增强生半夏的祛痰作用，其作用强度随配比和剂量的不同而改变。谭淑芳等研究了制川乌分别与川贝母、浙贝母配伍对小鼠镇痛、祛痰、镇咳的作用。结果表明，制川乌与川贝母配伍能增强制川乌的镇痛作用并降低川贝母的祛痰镇咳作用，其作用强度随配比和剂量的不同而改变，制川乌与浙贝母配伍对浙贝母的镇咳作用无影响。杨慧波等研究不同比例生半夏与生川乌配伍对镇痛作用的影响。结果表明，随着生半夏比例的增加，生川乌的镇痛作用减弱，且有一定的剂量依赖关系。李世哲等研究了乌头汤中加入半夏、贝母对抗氧化活性的影响，结果乌头汤与生半夏、川贝母配伍均对抗氧化活性有一定的抑制作用，能降低其抗氧化活性，其中与川贝母的配伍降低作用最为明显。王楚盈等研究了制川乌与瓜蒌配伍对大鼠慢性心衰模型的影响，发现适当剂量两药共煎液，高、中、低剂量组均可改善慢性心衰大鼠血流动力学指标，高剂量组上调 Bcl-2 抑制凋亡基因的表达，提高 Bcl-2/Bax 比值，表明其对慢性心力衰竭大鼠心肌具有保护作用。② 藻戟遂芫俱战草：李怡文等研究了大鼠甲状腺肿大模型肝脏系统，对不同配伍比例海藻与甘草配伍的海藻玉壶汤的反应，与模型组相比，多组均可显著降低 ALT 水平和 AST 水平，认为该相反药对在肝脏系统未发现明显的毒副作用，需进行不同剂量、不同炮制品种的进一步研究。王茜等研究了甘遂半夏汤中醋甘遂、炙甘草不同配伍比例对腹水模型大鼠的生物效应影响。结果表明，在增加腹水大鼠的尿量，降低腹水干扰素-α(TNF-α)，血管内皮生长因子(VEGF)水平等方面均有显著意义，并用中药组方优化软件得出当醋甘遂与炙甘草以 1∶15 配伍时，可能有较好的利水及抗细胞因子作用。

(2) 药物代谢研究　诸参辛芍反藜芦：朱冠秀等采用 Cocktail 底物探针法结合 HPTLC 测定北沙参与藜芦对代谢酶 P_{450} 同工酶活性的影响。结果表明，与空白组相比，藜芦组、北沙参组对大鼠 CYP_2C_9 酶具有诱导作用，合用组对大鼠 CYP_1A_2、CYP_2C_9 酶具有显著诱导作用；与藜芦组相比，合用组对大鼠 CYP_3A_4 酶具有抑制作用，对 CYP_1A_2、CYP_2C_9 酶具有诱导作用；与北沙参组相比，合用组对大鼠 CYP_3A_4 酶具有抑制作用，对 CYP_1A_2 酶具有诱导作用，对 CYP_2C_9、CYP_2C_{19} 无明显影响。所以，北沙参与藜芦配伍前后对部分 CYP 亚型的酶活性影响具有差异，可能会使藜芦中的毒性成分在体内的代谢特征发生改变，使配伍前后毒性具有差异，产生中药间相互作用，但需进一步通过代谢研究并综合分析，以进一步阐明作用机制。

(3) 毒性研究　柳海艳等用昆明小鼠的急性毒性实验观察甘遂半夏汤中一对反药组合甘遂与甘草，以累计半数致死量的方法评价毒性大小。结果，该方去甘遂与甘草反药组合中的一味或两味未显示出蓄积毒性，两味反药组合在复方中应用其 LD_{50}(n)值有增加趋势，说明复方中的其他药物可能在一定程度上可升高甘遂与甘草反药组合的 LD_{50}(n)值。

对相反药对的文献挖掘、临床用药分析，以及实验机制的研究，是从另一层面开展配伍的研究，对完善中药配伍理论、探寻实质、指导临床应用均具有重要意义，故应当结合药理、毒理以及循证医学领域系统的研究结果，更加全面的阐述中药配伍禁忌理论。

(朱靓贤　陈德兴)

【中药内在属性的关联研究】

近年来，利用数据挖掘技术对中药内在性效、成分、药理、基原、药材特性间的关联研究已成了新的研究热点。

1. 中药药性与功效关联研究

杨雪梅等对《中华本草》中 8 356 味具有四气属性、8 366 味具有五味属性的中药，在等级编码基础上，采用 spearman 等级相关法，对四气与五味之间的相关性进行分析。结果，四气与辛、甘或苦、淡，与脾、胃、肾三经或大肠、心、膀胱、胆、小肠、肺六经，与毒性之间存在正负不同的相关性；在 PG0.01 显著水平，酸味与肝、大肠、胃三经，苦味与寒性及肝、大肠、胆三经、毒性，甘味与热性及肾、肺、脾等经，辛味与热性和脾、胃、肝、肺四经及毒性，咸味与肾、肝、心、肺四经，淡味与寒性及膀胱、小肠经，涩味与大肠经均存在正相关。杨氏等还对《中华本草》所载 8 980 味中药，采用 IBM SPSS Clementine 14.1 数据挖掘平台，选择 Apriori 模型挖掘分类关联规则进行分析。结果，具有发散风寒、温中、止痛等功能的中药多属温性，具有补肺功能的中药多属平性，具有清热燥湿、清热泻火、除烦功能的中药多属寒性。此外，挖掘出涉及五脏归经的分类关联规则 32 条，涉及甘、辛、苦 3 种药味的分类关联规则 21 条，总结出 5 种不同类别中药功效的五味趋向。

2. 中药性效与成分药理关联研究

张靖等以《中国药典》(2010 年版)收录、临床常用方药以及上市中成药中有毒中药为研究对象，系统总结其性味归经、化学成分、药理作用，着重从抗癌角度探讨其与归经的关系，为有毒中药治疗癌症研究提供了参考。于红艳等以《中国药典》(2010 年版)，《中药学》等为信息来源，利用改进的 Apriori 计算法，建立了药性-药理作用、药性-主治、药性-西医病名、药性-功能、药性-药味、药性-归经、药性-化学成分等频繁项目集，统计出中药药性与其他属性间的支持度和支持率，如药性“温”与药味“辛”支持度为 117，支持率为 10.57%。杨萍等通过对《中国药典》(2010 年版)所载归肺经中药从四气、五味、归经、功效、化学成分和药理作用等方面进行统计分析，得出 250 味归肺经中药中寒凉性药物占 50.4%，温热性占 28.4%；五味中以苦味居多，其次是甘味和辛味；功效以清热、祛湿、化痰为主；化学成分以苷类最多，其次是黄酮类、糖类、挥发油类；药理作用主要是抗菌、抗病毒、祛痰、镇咳、平喘。认为归肺经中药多苦寒、多含苷类成分，具有清热、化痰止咳平喘、抗菌、抗病毒作用。冯帅等通过建立基于 18 种氨基酸含量的寒热药性数学 Fisher 判别函数分析，60 种中药的寒热药性判别正确率达到 82%。以 SVM 为最佳模型得出氨基酸 HPTLC 分析的寒性标记为：Glu、Gly、Arg、Thr、Ala、Tyr、Val、Ile 和 lys，热性标记为：Asp、Ser、His、Pro、Met、Cys、Leu、Phe 和 Trp。表明 18 种氨基酸含量与中药寒热药性具有一定的相关性。

3. 中药性效与基原药材关联研究

曹佳等报道来源于同一科亲缘植物药网络结构呈聚集状态，同类药性在网络中普遍相连，同时存在“药性空洞”现象。并以毛茛科和伞形科植物的药性特征与化学成分物质基础的关系为例，证明了聚集程度紧密的同科亲缘药物的药性相似，而不同亲缘科的植物药只要其化学成分相近且其重叠的化学成分特异性强，其药性也非常有可能相近。田方等报道用四格表卡方检验法和相关分析法来探讨药用植物地理成分及海拔与中药功效的相关性，结果发现清热药在青藏高原成分中比例较高、行气药在华中成分中比例较高、解表药在蒙新荒漠成分中比例较高，具有显著性差异。且清热药等与海拔呈正相关、温里药等与海拔呈负相关。史雪等通过分析《中华本草》收载的 40 味禾本科利水药物，发现以谷类为主，性味属甘寒者最多、甘平者其次，且禾本科利水药大多是治疗水液代谢病症的食药两宜品种。翟华强等以118味寒凉药、114味温热药作为研究对象，应用SPSS 18.0统计软件分析药材的“形、色、嗅、味”等形态学特征，结果表明，两者的形态学特征均有一定规律，寒凉药以圆柱形、黄色、气微、微苦、质脆者为多，温热药以圆柱形、红色、气香、味辛、质地坚硬者为多。

4. 中药内在属性关联规则方法学研究

王哲等以《中国药典》(2010版)和《中药学》《中华本草·精选本》《中药药理学》《新编中药志》等书为数据来源，结合临床用药经验及相关规范用语，创建了中药药性理论及其功能主治等相关数据模型，建立了中药药性-药味-归经、药性-药味-归经-功能以及药性-药味-归经-功能-主治间较密切的频繁项目集，并计算出相关支持度及支持率。王晓燕等研究了数学建模策略在中药药性物质基础研究中的应用，并尝试建立一套客观且可重复的建模思路与方法。从64种建模策略中选出17种判别良好的模型，继而考察其可视化表达能力，选出4种适宜模型，最后经统计模拟，选出PLS作为目前最适宜模型。认为中药药性与其发挥作用的物质基础之间难以找到现成的公式或规律来表达二者关联，可用穷举策略，经数据库建立、数据预处理、建模策略选择和评价4步筛选适宜的中药药性特征标记识别模型。王氏等又研究了中药物质成分与寒热药性的相关性，寻找适合解释此相关性的统计模式识别方法，发现采用统计模式识别方法可以从HPTLC图谱信息中筛选出识别中药药性的物质基础，即中药药性特征标记。肖小河等报道以系统观为指导，以物质基础、生物效应和作用靶标为寒热药性的三大要素，融合多学科交叉的方法构建基于传统功效的中药寒热药性表征方法，基本能揭示寒热药性的科学内涵。

(陈仁寿　程　旺)

[附] 参考文献

C

曹佳，王耘. 基于化学成分关系药物网的亲缘植物药药性研究[J]. 中国中药杂志，2013，38(3)：453

陈金锋，高家荣，季文博，等. 酸枣仁-五味子药对镇静催眠作用及机制研究[J]. 中药药理与临床，2013，29(4)：128

程显怡，张志明，马骏. 十八反中“半蒌贝蔹及攻乌”反与不反的研究[J]. 西部中医药，2013，26(4)：117

崔利锐，王鹏，欧阳兵. 试论中药四性理论现代研究发展趋势[J]. 山东中医药大学学报，2013，37(4)：275

D

邓家刚，郭宏伟，郝二伟. 平性药理论渊源探析[J]. 中华中医药学刊，2013，31(5)：967

邓家刚，孙冰，郝二伟，等. 基于数据库的平性药组方配伍规律研究[J]. 中国实验方剂学杂志，2013，19(8)：347

邓凯文，贺福元. 中药归经研究的现状及“穴药”法的提出[J]. 中国中药杂志，2013，38(10)：1643

F

冯帅，刘杨，李峰. 氨基酸含量与寒热药性的多元统计分析[J]. 世界科学技术(中医药现代化)，2013，15(4)：672

G

关卿. 中药毒性及其影响因素[J]. 内蒙古中医药，2013，32(13)：86

H

韩翠翠，俞仲毅. 中药升降浮沉理论沿革及应用纂要[J]. 上海中医药大学学报，2013，27(2)：16

何瑶，章津铭，高飞，等. 附子甘草配伍减毒增效作用机制研究进展及展望[J]. 中药与临床，2013，4(3)：62

衡晴晴，徐立. 中药十八反“藻戟遂芫俱战草”的毒理学研究进展[J]. 中国实验方剂学杂志，2013，19(11)：348

黄建忠. 试析中药的升降浮沉理论[J]. 中国民族民间医药，2013，22(9)：50

L

李芳，顾作林，袁同山，等. 方剂归经量化研究方法初探[J]. 北京中医药大学学报，2013，36(6)：370

李广峰. 探讨中药炮制的目的及作用[J]. 中国民族民间医药，2013，22(9)：22

李具宝，刘文琴，汤小虎，等. 虫类药的临床应用现状分析[J]. 上海中医药杂志，2013，47(3)：66

李世哲，陈瑞战，齐瑶，等. 配伍禁忌半夏、贝母对乌

头汤抗氧化活性的影响[J]. 中国实验方剂学杂志，2013，19(8)：198

李卫祥. 丹参的药理作用与临床应用[J]. 北方药学，2013，10(3)：34

李晓鹤，王耘，乔延江. 基于药性组合的"反药"同方应用特征研究[J]. 世界科学技术(中医药现代化)，2013，15(3)：613

李怡文，钟赣生，柳海艳，等.《国家基本医疗保险、工伤保险和生育保险药品目录》含十八反十九畏药对的成方制剂及临床应用分析[J]. 中国实验方剂学杂志，2013，19(9)：353

李怡文，钟赣生，柳海艳，等. 基于均匀设计的海藻玉壶汤中海藻与甘草不同比例配伍对甲状腺肿大大鼠模型肝脏功能及病理形态的影响[J]. 中华中医药杂志，2013，28(5)：1295

刘春芳，谭淑芳，王丹华，等. 基于均匀设计法的制川乌与生半夏配伍药效研究[J]. 中国中药杂志，2013，38(13)：2169

刘佳，费宇彤，钟赣生，等. 十八反中甘草甘遂临床同用的文献特征分析[J]. 中医杂志，2013，54(21)：1863

刘佳，费宇彤，钟赣生，等. 十八反中甘草海藻反药组合临床同用文献的文献特征分析[J]. 中华中医药杂志，2013，28(5)：1449

柳海艳，王茜，钟赣生，等. 甘遂半夏汤中甘遂甘草反药组合加减应用的急性毒性研究[J]. 科技导报，2013，31(25)：48

陆华. 苗药与中药药性理论分析[J]. 光明中医，2013，28(6)：1264

罗年翠，丁雯，钱大玮，等. 当归补血—活血药对功效取向研究[J]. 中国实验方剂学杂志，2013，19(4)：240

Q

秦丹，吴嘉瑞，杨瑞，等. 基于关联规则的相使药对"药性组合规律"数据的挖掘研究[J]. 国际中医中药杂志，2013，35(6)：526

S

盛华刚. 中药组分配伍模式的研究进展[J]. 中国实验方剂学杂志，2013，19(16)：349

史雪，郭瑞华.《中华本草》收载具有利水功效的禾本科药物的药性规律研究[J]. 江西中医药，2013，44(4)：57

T

谭淑芳，刘春芳，王春生，等. 基于均匀设计法评价制川乌与川贝、浙贝反药配伍组合的镇痛和祛痰镇咳作用[J]. 中国中药杂志，2013，38(16)：2706

田方，焦多礼，陈学林，等. 药用植物地理成分及海拔与中药功效的相关性研究[J]. 时珍国医国药，2013，24(7)：1746

田文全. 附子半夏配伍应慎用[J]. 辽宁中医药大学学报，2013，15(4)：147

W

王楚盈，张超，张琦，等. 制川乌与瓜蒌相反配伍对慢性心衰大鼠血流动力学及其机制研究[J]. 中药新药与临床药理，2013，24(1)：59

王付. 经方柴胡药对探索与实践[J]. 中医药通报，2013，12(2)：17

王兰，王耘，乔延江. 药性组合与脏腑关系的复杂系统模型研究[J]. 世界科学技术(中医药现代化)，2013，15(3)：531

王茜，钟赣生，王宏蕾，等. 甘遂半夏汤中甘遂与甘草不同比例配伍对癌性腹水模型大鼠生物效应影响的研究[J]. 中国实验方剂学杂志，2013，19(4)：177

王晓红. 中药大黄在临床应用中的新功效[J]. 亚太传统医药，2013，9(7)：159

王晓燕，李峰. 中药药性特征标记模式识别建模研究[J]. 辽宁中医杂志，2013，40(8)：1665

王晓燕. 中药药性物质基础研究中数学建模思路探讨[J]. 中国实验方剂学杂志，2013，19(15)：337

王哲，张佩江. 中药药性间的相关性研究[J]. 中国现代应用药学，2013，30(8)：859

位亚丽，王志国. 中药配伍理论研究[J]. 世界中医药，2013，8(5)：509

X

肖小河，郭玉明，王伽伯，等. 基于传统功效的中药寒热药性研究策论[J]. 世界科学技术(中医药现代化)，2013，15(1)：9

谢素萍，闫晓宏，徐桔叶. 浅谈中药性状气味与功效气味[J]. 内蒙古中医药，2013，32(11)：52

谢炜，郑跃辉，陈伟军，等. 柴胡-白芍不同比例配伍应用的抗惊厥作用[J]. 中国实验方剂学杂志，2013，19(18)：184

辛淑杰. 何首乌的药理作用、临床应用及不良反应[J]. 北方药学，2013，10(7)：36

徐义高. 对毒性中药的正确认识与合理应用[J]. 北方药学，2013，10(8)：105

徐义高. 黄芩的配伍与临床应用[J]. 内蒙古中医药，2013，32(26)：35

Y

闫军堂，刘晓倩，马小娜，等. 经方中"角药"的配伍应用特点[J]. 中华中医药学刊，2013，31(2)：364

杨环，范欣生，卞雅莉，等. 古今治疗中风病"十八反"反药同方配伍研究[J]. 世界科学技术(中医药现代化)，

2013,15(1):105

杨慧波,许柳,张树峰,等.生川乌与不同比例生半夏配伍镇痛作用研究[J].时珍国医国药,2013,24(3):637

杨洁.浅谈姜制法与姜的药对配伍[J].西部中医药,2013,26(4):12

杨明,张定堃,钟凌云,等.对传统中药炮制文化与哲学的思考[J].中国中药杂志,2013,38(13):2223

杨萍,车立娟,金素安,等.归肺经中药的药性、化学成分及药理作用分析[J].上海中医药大学学报,2013,27(4):80

杨雪梅,赖新梅,陈梅妹,等.《中华本草》药性数据中的五味规律[J].中国中医药信息杂志,2013,20(3):26

杨雪梅,赖新梅,陈梅妹,等.基于分类关联规则的中药功效与药味关联关系研究[J].中国中医药信息杂志,2013,20(1):31

杨雪梅,赖新梅,陈梅妹,等.挖掘中药功能组合判定五脏归经的规律[J].福建中医药大学学报,2013,23(2):49

杨雪梅,林端宜,赖新梅,等.《中华本草》药性数据中的四气规律[J].中国中药杂志,2013,38(9):1438

杨雪梅,林端宜,赖新梅,等.挖掘中药功能组合判定四气药性的规律[J].中国中药杂志,2013,38(10):1624

杨艳,李东华,王洋,等.大剂量使用芍药与甘草配伍解痉作用的研究[J].时珍国医国药,2013,24(2):347

英洪友,张凌凌,朱邦贤,等.数据挖掘法探究麻黄药对配伍与证治规律[J].上海中医药杂志,2013,47(7):15

于红艳,许成刚.关联挖掘技术在中药药性及其他属性间关系的应用研究[J].中国实验方剂学杂志,2013,19(14):343

余坚.酸味中药临床效用分析[J].上海中医药杂志,2013,47(1):59

俞仲毅,韩翠翠.中药升降浮沉研究相关问题探讨[J].上海中医药大学学报,2013,27(3):7

Z

查小芹,高存亮.浅析半夏的炮制与临床应用[J].内蒙古中医药,2013,32(12):77

翟华强,王燕平,黄璐琦,等.寒凉类中药材"形、色、嗅、味"特征初步分析[J].中国中药杂志,2013,38(7):1091

翟华强,王燕平,黄璐琦,等.温热类中药材"形、色、嗅、味"特征初步分析[J].中国中药杂志,2013,38(8):1255

张红燕,丁天红,李军.山豆根临床应用及毒性反应概述[J].西部中医药,2013,26(3):121

张靖,张瑶,王彦丽,等.有毒中药抗癌作用及其与归经的相关性研究进展[J].中草药,2013,44(13):1852

张明德.白芍之药对效用探析[J].湖南中医杂志,2013,29(8):105

张荣,李晓波,段美美.不同比例甘草诃子配伍制草乌对其次乌头碱含量的影响[J].时珍国医国药,2013,24(8):2025

张仕玉,陶春晖,周祯祥,等.基于现代中医名家临床用药的半夏剂量研究[J].中华中医药学刊,2013,31(5):1007

赵春梅.对升散之性中药的妙用浅识[J].内蒙古中医药,2013,32(11):141

赵正奇,翁靖,叶新苗.论茯苓配伍之不宜[J].内蒙古中医药,2013,32(14):52

仲宗亮,张盼盼,金国泰,等.实验探讨生大黄、清半夏、常山的升降浮沉药性[J].湖南中医杂志,2013,29(7):128

朱冠秀,王宇光,马增春,等.北沙参与藜芦配伍对大鼠体内细胞色素 P450 酶活性的影响[J].中药药理与临床,2013,29(3):107

朱梦莺.肾毒性中药浅析[J].北方药学,2013,10(5):108

二、临 床 各 科

(一) 名 医 经 验

【李玉奇】

李玉奇，辽宁中医药大学教授，博士生导师。国家人事部、卫生部遴选全国首批500名老中医之一，国医大师。享受首批国务院政府特殊津贴，中华中医药学会终身理事。曾任辽宁省卫生厅中医处处长、辽宁中医药大学副校长兼附属医院院长、辽宁省肿瘤医院常务副院长、辽宁省中医学会会长、辽宁省药品评审委员会副主任委员、辽宁省老年科技工作者联合会副会长、沈阳药科大学中药系兼职教授。从医60余年，擅长内、妇、儿三科，尤精于脾胃病的治疗。

1. 脾胃病

王晓戎等探讨了李氏治疗脾胃病用药经验。① 善用黄芪。凡脾胃气虚证者皆重用之，并针对不同胃病，予以巧妙配伍。如浅表性胃炎配柴胡、升麻、枳壳、苦参、黄连以益胃升阳，升清降浊；浅表-萎缩性胃炎则伍石斛、知母、桃仁、鳖甲以益气养阴，活血化瘀；萎缩性胃炎合天冬、莪术、桃仁、白花蛇舌草以益气养阴，祛腐生新；消化性溃疡则佐炮姜、小茴香、白及、乌贼骨、煅瓦楞以温胃弥疡，逐腐祛瘀。② 重视升降。如浅表性胃炎，以黄芪、升麻、柴胡等升发脾阳，又配以苦参、黄连、枳壳等苦降胃气，使清升浊降。胆汁返流性胃炎为气虚不能约束幽门引起幽门失控，仍以黄芪、山药、升麻、柴胡健脾升阳，配以枳壳、黄连苦降胃气。③ 用药平和。提倡用药平和，切勿辛热或苦寒太过，不利于保护胃气阴津。反对用附子理中丸、八宝瑞生丹等治浅表性胃炎。如补气常用党参、黄芪、白术、茯苓、薏苡仁等，而慎用红参、野山参等温热峻补；补阴取石斛、知母、枸杞子、山萸肉等，而恐熟地黄、龟板、沙参、麦冬等过于滋腻。即使寒甚，也慎用附子、干姜，虑其"壮火食气"，而多用小茴香、炮姜等温而不燥之味，以图"少火生气"。脾胃郁热或湿热，喜用连翘、焦栀子、滑石、蒲公英、豆豉、百合等甘苦微寒之品，而弃大黄、芒硝、黄芩、龙胆草等防峻下或苦寒太过，化燥伤阴。便秘也喜用桃仁、杏仁、郁李仁、皂角子、黑芝麻之类润下药。

2. 便秘

汤立东等论述了李氏治疗便秘的经验。分为脾约与大肠郁滞2个证型。脾约证为燥结伤阴，泻药耗气，久则造成气阴两伤，善以补中益气之法升提中焦脾胃之气，上补肺以通调水道，中补脾以运化升清，下补肾以滋阴养液，益津亏之本，润肠之艰涩，升清降浊，通腑利肠。药用黑芝麻、炒杏仁、火麻仁、桃仁等，意在润燥而不伤气，尤适于体弱而不胜攻伐之人。对湿热蕴结，肠道传导失常之黏滞型便秘，治以清热燥湿，行气健脾之法。以苦参燥湿清热，茯苓、苍术健脾化湿，厚朴、槟榔、沉香行气通腑，利水消肿。

3. 消渴病

张会永总结了李氏治疗消渴病的经验。治疗重点于"润燥生津"。泻心火阳热之势，滋肾中真水之亏；除胃肠燥热之邪，济少阴津液之涸。津生而后阴救，使"道路散而不结，津液生而不枯，气血利而不涩"。具体归纳为：清燥救肺、润燥救脾胃、除燥生肾水，按不同主症辨治，分而论之。① 口渴多溲。为肾水不能上涵君火，而君火刑于肺金，燥伤肺津所致。治以清燥救肺生津。药用苦参、槐花、胡黄连、葛根、冬瓜仁、藕节、泽兰、枇杷叶等。② 饥饿无度。为大肠龙雷火热，移热于胃，脾阴无力救胃，胃气衰微，欲得食而自救。治当润燥生津以救脾胃。药用苦参、黄连、槐花、当归、桑白皮、五灵脂、浮萍、鹿角霜等。除消渴外，很多疾患常伴饥饿无度症，多因胃中伏火，肾水亏乏引发，其擅用黄连泻肠胃燥热除其所因，山药滋脾肾之阴补其不足。③ 身形消瘦。多因脾阴为燥火所伤，脾气大衰，胃不得助，无力化谷，筋脉失养而致骨削肉脱；肺金受刑，饮一溲一，甚则饮一溲二，精微遗失殆尽，精血内竭见形如枯槁。燥火亢盛，水火不济，肾水干涸，燥伤肾阴出现小便如膏、如脂等。治宜救肾水将涸之急。药用山药、鸡内金、石莲子(捣)、菟丝子、五味子、茯苓、泽泻、黄连等。李氏提出消渴病的治疗禁忌，其本为燥伤阴竭，而不宜大下通利，徒伤津液，反助燥邪；不宜过于活血，损伤气血加重内燥；不宜妄投辛温，伤津耗液；不宜过用苦寒，助邪败胃。对变症的辨治：① 男子遗精阳痿，女子绝经、月经不调等症，为肾水渐涸、肾精匮乏之象。治当固精补肾、填精益髓。药用山药、桑螵蛸、蚕砂、牡蛎、芡实、桑椹子、黑芝麻、当归等。② 心悸怔忡，多因燥伤阴津，肾水不能上济心火，阴火独亢，暗耗心血，心阴不足。治宜补心阴，宁心神。药用苦参、远志、五味子、西洋参、川芎、炒枣仁、柏子仁、竹茹等。③ 青盲内障，消渴病后期肾阴不足，必累及于肝木，致肝阴血不足，加之虚火上扰清窍所致。治宜养肝柔肝、滋阴降火。药用密蒙花、菊花、枸杞子、蒺藜、珍珠母、山药、生地黄、牡丹皮等。

4. 肝硬化腹水

高尚社总结了李氏治疗肝硬化腹水的经验。认为其病机为肝郁脾虚，耗气损津，阴液干涸，恶血内留，水湿内聚。核心为阴亏、血瘀、湿聚三者俱存。其治贵在顺其"肝体阴而用阳"之性，补肝体助肝用，当以滋养肝阴，活血化瘀，利水渗湿为法，切不可再行攻伐。强调标本兼治，补中有攻，攻中寓补，利湿之中有养阴之义，止血之中寓化瘀之功。虚火去则血热清，血热宁则血溢止；瘀血去则络脉通，水湿除则腹水消。组方特点：① 滋补肝体，养血育阴。多选用阿胶、文蛤、当归相伍。② 凉血止血，化瘀通络。常配伍生槐花、生侧柏、生蒲黄。③ 开门逐邪，化湿利水。善用浮萍、白茅根、泽泻，使利中有清，清中有养，湿去热清，真阴得保。

5. 水气病

刘林等总结了李氏治疗水气病的经验。治以祛邪为先，不宜过度峻猛，也不宜过分柔和，应有适当法度。泄浊解毒为核心疗法，并列举了 8 种疗法。① 泄浊解毒、益气养血。治营血亏虚，症见面色苍白或晦暗无华，口唇爪甲苍白，身疲乏力，气短心悸、嗜卧懒言、食少纳呆，舌淡脉细无力。药用大黄、苦参、败酱草、藿香、佩兰、砂仁、郁李仁、人参等。② 泄浊解毒、清营凉血。治复感外邪，症见发热、口干口渴、咳嗽、咳痰色黄。药用大黄、郁李仁、生地黄、败酱草、鱼腥草、玄参、胡黄连、栀子等。③ 泄浊解毒、凉血止血。治湿浊化热，扰动营血，血热妄行，症见尿血、出血。药用大黄、蒲公英、败酱草、郁李仁、牡丹皮、生地黄、黄连、栀子等。④ 泄浊解毒、补脾和胃。治湿浊内阻中焦，脾不升清，胃失降浊，浊气上逆，症见恶心呕吐，食少纳呆，大便稀溏。药用大黄、郁李仁、败酱草、藿香、佩兰、砂仁、白蔻仁、半夏等。⑤ 泄浊解毒、化气行水。治脾肾气衰、肾阳不足、湿浊毒邪内盛，三焦气化不行水，症见全身水肿、小便量少，畏寒肢冷。药用大黄、郁李仁、败酱草、佩兰、葶苈子、王不留行、防己、淫羊藿等。⑥ 泄浊解毒、开窍醒神。治湿浊毒邪内蕴日久，充斥表里，上蒙清窍、内闭心神，症见神昏或嗜眠、呼吸深大，谵语摸床，搓空理线。药用大黄、郁李仁、元明粉、败酱草、佩兰、藿香、白蔻仁、石菖蒲等，并灌服苏合香丸。⑦ 泄浊解毒、养阴柔肝。治湿浊化热动风，症见四肢抽搐，筋惕肉瞤。药用大黄、郁李仁、佩兰、栀子、败酱草、天竺黄、胆南星、白芍药等。⑧ 泄浊解毒、通关利尿。治湿浊内阻，三焦闭塞，肾关不开，水道不通，症见小便不通，尿量极少，全身水肿，恶心呕吐。药用大黄、郁李仁、佩兰、苦参、王不留行、葶苈子、商陆、杏仁等。

6. 热入血室

刘林等总结了李氏治疗热入血室的经验。其为原因不明之发热，每以日晡发热为多，为感邪后邪热传经入里，邪伏阴分所致。常用青蒿鳖甲汤化裁治疗。鳖甲入阴分，滋阴退热，入络搜邪；青蒿芳香，清热透络，引邪外出，有先入后出之妙；柴胡和解少阳，为少阳之引经药；胡黄连、地骨皮、生地黄清热凉血，上清肺中浮火，下去肝肾虚热；牡蛎入肝肾经，敛阴止汗；桃仁散结化瘀，润肠通便。全方以养阴凉血透热为法，意在清热又不伤阴。

7. 再生障碍性贫血

张会永介绍了李氏治疗再生障碍性贫血经验。分为 3 个阶段，疗程数年，或长达数十年，甚则终身。① 清利骨髓湿热。药用青蒿、银柴胡、牡丹皮、葛根、仙鹤草、槐花、藕节、茜草、水牛角、胡黄连、石斛、知母、羊骨髓少许。重用青蒿为君，清骨蒸，能引诸药入里，透邪外出；银柴胡走络脉，与青蒿相须，直达血分；仙鹤草、槐花清血分热邪；藕节、茜草、水牛角、牡丹皮凉血止血；黄连走气分，胡黄连入血分，加胡黄连加强清营凉血之功；石斛、知母清热养阴；尤以羊骨髓为药引，以髓走髓，直达病所。② 祛腐化燥。药用大黄、桃仁、当归、䗪虫、生地黄、海藻、败酱草、牡丹皮、山药适量。大黄祛腐生新，桃仁、䗪虫入络搜剔，海藻散结，亦能化瘀，败酱草、牡丹皮祛腐除败，清除余热，生地黄清热润燥，再以山药顾护胃气，防大黄下利太过。③ 救阴复脉。药用龟甲、鳖甲、石斛、鱼鳔胶、秦艽、地骨皮、乌梅、知母、麦冬、牡蛎。其借用吴鞠通三甲复脉汤，重用龟甲、鳖甲、牡蛎，生津复脉，以石斛、知母、麦冬润燥生津，乌梅酸甘化阴，秦艽、地骨皮清骨中余热，唯以鱼鳔胶补髓生血，为其独到经验。

（李永健）

【班秀文】

班秀文，壮族，广西中医学院主任医师、教授。1990 年，被国家人事部、卫生部及国家中医药管理局确认为全国名老中医，全国老中医药专家学术经验继承工作指导老师，国医大师。享受国务院政府特殊津贴，中华中医药学会终身理事。曾任全国中医妇科专业委员会委员、中华医史学会理事、广西科协常委、广西中医药学会副会长、广西中医药学会妇科委员会主任委员、《广西中医药》主编、澳大利亚自然疗法学院客座教授、广西壮族自治区政协委员、第六届全国人大代表，及广西中医学院各家学说教研室、壮医研究室主任。1989 年被授予广西壮族自治区和全国优秀教师的光荣称号。

1. 肝脾肾为本，五脏并重

李永亮总结了班氏"肝脾肾为本，五脏并重"的学术思想。五脏之中，尤重肾、肝、脾三脏对妇科疾病的影响，并注重心、肺病变与妇科疾病的关系。治疗上主张辨证应审慎，用药要专精，崇尚肝肾之说，擅用花类药物。对月经病变，主张治病求本，疏肝、健脾和胃、滋肾并用，重点治肾，兼顾肝脾，注重活血通络与调节肾藏泻功能的结合。对崩漏的治疗，注重三因制宜，根据时间、地域、气候及患者体质特点的不同来辨证施治，急则治其标，即塞流；缓则治其本，即澄源、复旧。多选用止血不留瘀的药物，如田七、三七、苏木、茜草、大蓟、小蓟、益母草、泽兰等，认为炭类止血药应少用或慎用。另外，班氏主张要做好预防工作，体现了"大医治未病"的思想。在药物的选择上，喜用合欢花、素馨花、佛手花等花类药物。

班氏重视调补肝肾在妇科病的应用，谢佳伶对其从经、带、胎、产四个方面进行了总结。月经病，以疏肝调气为主，兼以养肾扶脾。带下病，以温肾健脾为主，兼以疏肝清热，分脾虚、肝郁化火、阳虚、阴虚带下 4 个证型施治。妊娠病，以补肾安胎为主，兼以健脾益气，柔肝养血。产后病，既补养气血扶正以固本，又活血通络化瘀以去其标，而补虚化瘀、调补肝肾仍是其重要法则。

林寒梅等介绍了班氏治疗胎漏、胎动不安经验。肾虚血瘀为其基本病因病机，采取补肾益气、活血通脉法。以安胎防漏汤（菟丝子、覆盆子、杜仲、白芍药、熟地黄、党参、白术、棉花根、炙甘草）为主方，加活血通脉、化瘀止血之壮药三七、扶芳藤等，取得良好疗效。

2. 提出"经带并病"

刘玉筠等总结了班氏"经带并病"的学术思想。月经病可诱发带下病，带下病亦可诱发月经病，或两者同时发病，称之为经带并病。其病因多为六淫、七情、外伤、劳倦、房事不洁、术后创伤、感染等，导致脏腑、奇经、胞宫功能失常。此外，痰湿、瘀血等病理产物的相互影响也是致病的重要因素。治疗时强调分清经病、带病的先发继发，孰轻孰重，注意两者的相互影响，灵活采用治经及带、治带及经或经带并治。湿浊带下严重时，则需治带调经；经病致带下异常者，治经为主，兼顾治带。从病性而言，虚证以治经为主，从经治带，实证以治带为主，从带治经，且重视湿瘀并治。瘀血常与湿邪相互影响，气机愈滞，经脉愈瘀，劳累、生冷或感受外湿秽毒之邪易致复发，较为难治，须徐图论治。当用燥湿化瘀法，常用鸡血藤、忍冬藤、夜交藤等藤类药。并根据病性的寒热虚实和湿瘀的轻重主次，灵活运用。临床上大致分为 4 个证型施治。① 脾虚证。强调补脾除湿并行，治以益气摄血、健脾除湿，选用补气升阳之举元煎加土茯苓合《内经》乌鲗骨丸。湿聚成痰，则补气行气并行，用苍附导痰丸健脾燥湿，化痰调经；湿聚化热，酌加黄柏、连翘、苦参、薏苡仁；痰湿闭阻经络，经闭不行者，则气血并治，酌加活血引经的当归、川芎、牛膝、枳实。② 肾虚证。强调肾阴肾阳分治，治拟温肾健脾，固摄温化，用附子汤合缩泉丸。若肝肾阴虚，湿流下注，则清补兼施，予滋补肝肾之阴、清热利湿的基础上选用止血止带之品，常用知柏地黄丸或二至丸加减。③ 肝郁脾虚证。强调健脾疏肝各侧重，或健脾化湿为主，兼以疏肝清热；或养血柔肝，兼健脾利水。常用方有异功散、完带汤、当归芍药汤、逍遥散等。④ 湿热血瘀证。强调利湿化瘀解虫毒，治拟清热利湿，活血化瘀，用当归芍药散合四妙散酌加马鞭草、鱼腥草、连翘、救必应等苦寒燥湿、化瘀解毒之品。此外，对实证的带下过多、阴痒之症，其注重与外治法配合，采用肝经清热祛湿解毒之品进行外洗或熏洗。

3. 重视情志与妇科病的关系

刘玉筠等总结了班氏擅长从情志论治妇科病的经验。① 重视情志致病，提倡防治结合。本着“是以善医者，先医其心而后医其身”之宗旨，重视情志对疾病作用，更强调预防。② 调气和血，兼顾心肝脾三脏。认为气郁最为常见，临证多用柴胡、香附、郁金、川芎、白芍药、乌药、素馨花、玫瑰花等，常选逍遥散、柴胡疏肝散以疏肝解郁、调畅气机。兼以补心养血、安神定志，如归脾汤、四物汤之类。如阴不制火，虚热上扰神明之心肾不交，当滋阴养血，加入养阴清热药以标本同治，用归芍地黄丸加减。如兼脾胃受损，脾气虚衰，化源不足，予白术、黄芪、茯苓、莲肉、山药健脾益气；气化不行，水湿内生，则用党参、茯苓、苍术、白术、陈皮、薏苡仁，方如参苓白术散、完带汤。③ 和其阴阳，以平为期。女子体质柔弱，情绪易于波动，选方用药以平和为佳。清热不可过用苦寒，疏肝解郁勿过耗散，温燥不可伤阴，补虚不腻不滞邪，化瘀不伤血本。④ 情志久郁，勿忘痰瘀。妇女情志久郁，易使气机紊乱，血停为瘀，津凝为痰，必致络脉瘀阻或湿聚痰生。治疗上活血通络、祛湿化痰贯穿始终。根据不同的病因灵活采用或温化、或凉散、或益气、或燥湿、或滋补等，以祛有形之实邪，又时时不忘顾护正气。⑤ 身心并治，综合调理。临证诊疗不惟重药疗，尤重疗人之心。了解患者之所思所虑，与其交流要耐心倾听，观察其内心感受及心理反应，分析原因予积极疏导，树立尽早治愈的信心，而达到药力所不及之效。并采用以情胜情、劝说开导、移情易性、静养等法，消除患者的消极情绪。

4. 针药并用治疗妇科病

张璐砾等总结了班氏针药并用治疗妇科病的经验。首先，针灸常选用任脉、五脏之俞穴，如任脉常用中极、关元、气海等穴。其次，先后天并重，兼以疏肝，如治疗经行吐衄，证属元气虚损，脾虚不能统血之变，宜健脾益气以摄血，以归脾汤加减治之，并加用温和灸肝俞、脾俞、肾俞、关元、足三里、三阴交等穴位。再次，疏通气血，分型选穴。① 寒证型：有外邪袭表，宜解肌发汗，调和营卫，以桂枝汤为主，酌加小茴香、乌药、吴茱萸等；若冲任损伤、小腹冷痛证型较重者，宜温经散寒，以吴茱萸汤去牡丹皮、麦冬，加乌药、小茴香治之。针灸取关元、归来、上髎等穴，用较粗毫针强刺激，留针 15～30 min，加灸 5～10 min，同时直接灸三阴交 3～5 壮。② 热证型：以芩连四物汤加香附、延胡索、桃仁、红花治之，有颧赤潮热、心烦不寐实热者，以养阴清热为主，酌加活血行气类，用保阴煎去续断，加牡丹皮、延胡索、香附、桃仁治之。针灸取中极、水道、中髎、三阴交、大椎等穴，单针不灸，行针强而久刺激，留针 30 min；实热宜以任脉穴与五脏俞穴为主，如气海、归来、心俞、肝俞等穴，仍单针不灸，惟行针宜轻得气而止，留针 10～20 min。③ 虚证型：以补血益气为主，用八珍汤加炙黄芪等，若四肢冷感，虚而更虚者，以十全大补汤加补骨脂、龙眼肉；若腰腿酸痛、疲乏无力、脉弦、脉细，致肾阴亏损不能涵木，又宜肝肾并治，用清肝汤加川楝子、桑寄生。针灸取中极、气海、归来、水道、足三里、肾俞、肝俞、脾俞、下髎、三阴交等穴，每天轮换选用 3～5 穴，单灸不针，隔蒜灸 5～10 壮为宜，痛止后，隔天灸 3～5 穴，并加隔蒜灸神阙 10～20 壮，以达元气。④ 实证型：有气滞、血瘀之分。前者以顺气行滞，宜加味乌鸡汤加川楝子、郁金治之。若心烦易怒、神志不安者，宜逍遥散加川楝子、紫苏叶治之；如月经超前，脉弦数者，宜丹栀逍遥散加香附、白薇治之。后者以活血行瘀，新瘀未久者，宜桃红四物汤加乌药、延胡索、穿破石、泽兰治之；久瘀正虚者，宜攻补并施以抵当丸加党参、当归、鸡血藤、龟甲、阿胶、牡丹皮等治之。针灸取中极、归来、气海、气海俞、下髎、地机、三阴交等穴，单针不灸，气滞者加针膻中、肝俞；血瘀者加针膈俞、心俞、阳陵泉；行针宜强刺激,留针 30～50 min,若瘀久正虚者,行针宜轻,针后加隔蒜灸足三里、大椎各 5～10 壮。班氏认为,针药并用不但能标本兼治,还能寒热虚实同调,疏通经络、宣导气血。

(邸若虹)

【颜德馨】

颜德馨,主任医师,教授,国医大师。曾任中国中医药学会理事,国家中医药管理局科技进步奖评审委员会委员,铁道部专家委员会委员、中医专业组组长,上海铁道中心医院主任医师,上海市中医药工作咨询委员会顾问,上海市医学领先专业专家委员会委员,上海中医药大学、上海市中医药研究院专家委员会委员,上海中医药大学客座教授,成都中医药大学名誉教授,上海师范大学客座教授,长春中医学院客座教授,美国中国医学研究院学术顾问,台湾中医针灸学会、中国医药研究会学术顾问等职。

任壮概况了颜氏的学术思想。首倡中医治病“八法”之外的“衡法”,提出“气为百病之长,血为百病之胎”、“久病必有瘀,怪病必有瘀”的学术观点及调气活血为主的“衡法”治则。“八纲辨证”虽无气血二字,但气血内容贯穿于其中,认为气血是临床辨证的基础,也是疑难病证的辨证基础。衡法具有平衡和权衡之意,其以活血化瘀药为主,配以行气、益气药组合而成,能调畅气血,平衡阴阳,发挥扶正祛邪、固本清源的作用,适用于阴阳表里寒热虚实等多种疾病。衡法分为升降气机、降气平逆、补气升阳、清热活血等 10 余种治则与方法,对冠心病、白血病、肝硬化等都有较好疗效。颜氏还将气血学说和“衡法”治则应用于抗衰老领域。指出人体衰老的主要机制为气血失调,内环境失衡,而内环境失衡则是由于瘀血的存在。调整气血以延缓衰老,与过去补肾、健脾等抗衰老的理论截然不同。

曹田梅等阐述了颜氏对活血化瘀理论的发展和贡献。其从症状、体征、实验室检查、病史、适应证等方面对血瘀证的诊断进行了补充,下列症状与体征均可归于瘀血证范畴。① 发热。不超过 38℃,低热绵绵,不定期发热,无规律发热;自感心胸发热;局部发热;局部皮肤发热,但非潮热。② 疼痛。痛有定处。③ 出血。不论颜色是否发黑,出血必有瘀血。④ 胀满。如《金匮》所言“腹不满,其人言我满,为有瘀血”。⑤ 但欲漱口不欲咽。⑥ 抓痒。皮肤瘙痒,抓出血方止,为有瘀血,血出风泄而痒止。⑦ 多梦、健忘。⑧ 毛发干燥、干枯。突然发生的的毛发干枯,发为血之余,和瘀血有关。⑨ 面色发暗。尿毒症、大出血的病人面部可见红色或褐色斑,以及脸色青紫暗红、眼球色暗、两颧潮红或暗红、红丝赤缕、酒渣鼻、鼻红起疱等均为瘀血面部体征。⑩ 皮肤板滞、肌肤甲错,是典型的瘀血症状,或突然起鸡皮疙瘩,及老年人的皮肤粗糙也属有瘀血。其他体征,如伸舌青紫、颈部淋巴结痰核肿块、胸部皮肤的变化、腹部膨隆(肝硬化腹水)、爪甲青紫等均为瘀血之征;病史和实验室检查方面,如存在手术、外伤、久病等病史,不必具备典型瘀血症候,皆有内在瘀血,而部分患者病史、症状、体征无瘀血表现,但实验室检查结果如血液流变异常、甲皱微循环改变、肾盂积水、脑血流图异常、高血脂,抗“O”高等亦可认为有瘀血。其善用活血化瘀法治疗各类疑难病证,擅长活用王清任《医林改错》诸方。尤其是血府逐瘀汤的应用,如治慢性咽炎,用此方桔梗加倍;治妇女不育,原方加紫石英(治宫寒)、韭子、蛇床子;原方生地黄改为熟地黄,加紫石英、蛇床子、韭子治男科一切难治病;加桑叶、桑白皮治面部色素沉着及鼻部疾病;加磁珠丸、生铁落治疗长期失眠、神经衰弱、神经官能症、精神分裂症;加生半夏治癫痫;加升麻治疗失音,声带闭合不全。

1. 慢性胆囊炎

高尚社报道了颜氏治疗慢性胆囊炎的经验。认为本病的病机关键是肝胆湿热,治宗六腑以通为用,宜疏肝利胆、调畅气机,以应肝喜条达之性,顺胆腑贵在通降之机。用药首选柴胡、枳壳、陈皮 3 味药,诸药相伍,升降相宜、行散并举、胆胃同调。肝气舒、胆腑利、胃气和,诸症自愈。

2. 糖尿病

韩天雄等介绍了颜氏治疗糖尿病的经验。认为本病初、中期多在太阳、阳明,后期常在厥阴、少阴,肝肾阴亏是其本,肺胃燥热乃其标。中焦脾胃是津液输布的枢纽,亦是消渴起病的关键。瘀血贯穿于糖尿病的始末,是糖尿病的病理产物。治疗上打破视糖尿病为“虚症”,以补肾为主的治则,而强调“脾统四脏”之说,抓住健脾和活血化瘀来解决“胰岛素依赖”和并发症问题。① 运脾行津,治脾治胰。提出“脾胰同源”之说,以运脾法治疗胰的病变,善用苍术健中运脾,使脾气健运,不治渴而渴自止。② 活血化瘀，调畅气血。常用益气健脾，活血化瘀之补阳还五汤加减。对糖尿病并发症治疗亦重视活血化瘀，如糖尿病酮症以燥热、血瘀、浊邪互结为病机，方用温清饮合四妙丸；糖尿病肾病以气阴两虚夹瘀证为多，方用防己黄芪汤、六味地黄丸、四物汤化裁；周围神经障碍病机多为气虚血瘀，方用黄芪桂枝五物汤；视网膜病变多属肝肾阴虚挟瘀证，方用杞菊地黄丸合芍药甘草汤，眼底出血不止加止血药；脉管炎、疮疽证为燥热挟瘀，方用五味消毒饮加丹皮、赤芍药，久不收口加黄芪。其自拟“消渴清”治疗本病，方中苍术健脾运脾，激发胰岛功能，以之为君；知母养阴清热，生津润燥，以之为臣，并可缓解苍术之燥性，刚柔相济，促使药性平和，汇固本清源为一体，解决糖尿病阴虚内热常见症状；蒲黄专入血分，以清香之气，兼行气分，故能导瘀结，降血脂，有效预防糖尿病合并症；地锦草清热凉血，化瘀通络，有降糖的作用，二药合用为佐；黄连清热燥湿，泻火解毒，用其为使。诸药合用，苦甘化阴，共奏养阴生津、健脾活血之功。对胃热炽盛，瘀热内结之消渴尤为有效。

3. 肝硬化腹水

高氏报道了颜氏治疗肝硬化腹水的经验。其病机多为肝肾阴虚，血瘀水停。根据虚中夹实的病机特点，从滋养肝肾、化瘀利水、健脾育阴、利水调气论治。组方用药兼顾5个方面。① 滋养肝肾，补体助阳。善用《柳洲医话》一贯煎(北沙参、麦冬、当归、生地黄、枸杞子、川楝子)以养肝体助肝用。② 软坚散结，化瘀利水。多配伍生鳖甲、丹参、猪苓、茯苓、泽泻等。③ 调畅气机，降气利水。选用小茴香、葶苈子为佐药，辛温与辛凉相辅相成，降气行水之中寓温和之妙义。④ 导邪外出。选用十枣丸、制大黄为佐药，从二便分消利水。⑤ 培土制水。健脾益气，养阴利水，并辅以食疗，以图缓效。

4. 脑梗死

高氏报道了颜氏治疗脑梗死的经验。认为本病为肝肾不足，气阴本亏，肝阳夹痰浊上扰，清窍受蒙，脉络受阻所致。治宜平肝化瘀、清化湿热、疏通经脉。用药组方重在疏通脉道，推陈出新，自拟脑梗灵，药用水蛭、通天草、石菖蒲、蒲黄、海藻、葛根等。若痰热炽盛，用大黄通腑泄热，尝谓“撤热有釜底抽薪之功，降火有导龙入海之力，入血分能凉血止血，散瘀醒脑，与芳香开窍有异曲同工之妙”。若肝阳亢盛，则投以滋阴潜阳之剂，如羚羊角粉、山羊角、生石决明、天麻等，以平上冲之逆气，潜其阳，降其气。

5. 冠心病心绞痛

胡晓贞等阐述了颜氏治疗胸痹的用药特点。指出本病基本病机是本虚邪实。本虚指气血阴阳不足，尤以阳虚为多，心脉失于充养，是本病发生的基础。邪实指瘀血、痰浊、气滞、阴寒等邪气痹阻心脉，是胸痹发生的直接诱因。其治一是从阳气不振，瘀血内凝论治。善用附子温阳解凝、化瘀泄浊，配合桃仁、红花、蒲黄诸药，标本兼顾。二是从脾运不健，升降失司论治。常以李东垣清暑益气汤合二陈汤为主，根据病情或配入枳壳、桔梗，一降一升，调畅气机；或配入川芎、牛膝一升一降，流行血脉，上下输布；或配入葛根升胸中清气、降香降上焦之浊气。三是从痰浊阻滞，饮凝胸中论治。以瓜蒌薤白通阳为主，选加半夏、茯苓、陈皮、枳壳、桔梗。常用药物配伍：① 附子配生脉散。附子振阳，生脉饮养阴，共成复脉之功。② 三七粉配血竭粉。均具化瘀生新之长，相须同用，其功倍增。治疗心痛如针刺，痛处固定不移，舌质紫黯、有瘀点或瘀斑，脉沉弦或沉涩以瘀阻心脉为主要表现者多有捷效。③ 桔梗配枳壳。辛开苦泄，一升一降，降已而还升，具开滞消痹，宣展气机之功。胸痹因痰湿内因，或因肝郁不舒，阻滞气机者，均可用以调畅气机。

高氏总结了颜氏治疗冠心病心绞痛的临床经验。认为本病病机多为心气不足，营血亏损，心脉不通。治以益气固本、活血逐瘀为大法，常用补阳还五汤。并强调以下几方面：① 补益元气，温通心阳。常选黄芪、党参相伍，补益元气，振奋心阳，使气以推血，温以煦脉，气血和畅，诸症自解。② 活血化瘀，益心通脉。用丹参、川芎、赤芍药相伍，活血与行气同用，逐瘀与养血并举。活中有补，散中有养，气顺血活，脉通络畅。③ 和营通脉，化瘀止痛。用参三七、血竭相伍，和营通脉，化瘀止痛。④ 顺通气机，升达清阳。用葛根、降香，清升浊降，气机顺通，脉和络畅，诸症自降。⑤ 顺通腑气，化瘀行滞。配伍决明子、山楂，顺腑气以畅气机，化瘀血而通脉络，气调血和，络通脉畅。⑥ 芳香开窍，布达清阳。善用石菖蒲，其气薄清芬，芳香通利。一可开心窍，通心神，避秽恶，利清阳；二可辟秽涤痰而卫宫域，宣心思之结而通神明；三可燥脾湿、化湿浊、调壅滞、和中州。

6. 头痛

高氏报道了颜氏治疗头痛的临证经验。认为脉络瘀阻、风潜清窍为本病主要病机。从治风先治血入手，以活血化瘀、通络止痛为大法，以化瘀升清为要。① 活血养血，通络止痛。选用四物汤为基础方，以生地黄易熟地黄，以赤芍药易白芍药，使熟四物汤变生四物，由温养变为清养，从而使其功效更为轻灵通达，通络止痛之功更胜。瘀去络通，脑络得濡，其痛自除。② 活血破瘀，通络止痛。多配伍桃仁、红花，破血逐瘀，通络止痛，瘀祛络通，脑窍清利，其痛自止。③ 搜风祛邪，通络止痛。选用羌活、川芎，为治疗头痛、头风重要药对。④ 虫类逐瘀，通络止痛。用石楠叶、露蜂房、乌梢蛇、全蝎、蜈蚣等，共奏搜风驱邪、通络止痛之功。组方用药邪正兼顾，活中有补，散中有养，抓住"风邪夹瘀，久病入络"这一关键病机，治法以搜风驱邪、活血逐瘀、通络止痛为首务。

7. 抑郁症

高氏总结了颜氏治疗抑郁症的临床经验。本病多因肝郁情志不畅，气血失于调达，血瘀心脉脑络，神明失主而致。治以清脑化瘀，以宁其神，善用血府逐瘀汤加减治疗。用药特点一是活血化瘀，净心醒脑。多选用赤芍药、川芎、桃仁、红花、丹参、川牛膝等，治中有养，攻中宜补，瘀去络通，窍清心净，神明复位，其症自愈。二是升达清阳，调畅气机。配伍柴胡、桔梗、枳壳，清阳升则浊阴降，滞气开而痞满降，升降相宜，腑气通利。三是清心泻火，醒窍安神。多用黄连、石菖蒲、生甘草，可清心泻火，安神定志，又可化痰开窍，醒脑安神。心火得清，痰浊得除，清窍畅利。

（李永健）

［附］ 参 考 文 献

C

曹田梅，张李兴，颜新. 化瘀法探源及国医大师颜德馨对活血化瘀理论的创新贡献[J]. 深圳中西医结合杂志，2013，23(5)：292

G

高尚社. 国医大师颜德馨教授辨治慢性胆囊炎验案赏析[J]. 中国中医药现代远程教育，2012，10(5)：7

高尚社. 国医大师颜德馨教授辨治脑梗死验案赏析[J]. 中国中医药现代远程教育，2012，10(6)：5

高尚社. 国医大师颜德馨教授治疗抑郁症验案赏析[J]. 中国中医药现代远程教育，2012，10(23)：3

高尚社. 国医大师李玉奇教授治疗肝硬化腹水验案赏析[J]. 中国中医药现代远程教育，2013，11(2)：6

高尚社. 国医大师颜德馨教授治疗冠心病心绞痛验案赏析[J]. 中国中医药现代远程教育，2013，11(7)：1

高尚社. 国医大师颜德馨教授治疗头痛验案赏析[J]. 中国中医药现代远程教育，2013，11(16)：3

高尚社. 国医大师颜德馨教授治疗肝硬化腹水验案赏析[J]. 中国中医药现代远程教育，2013，11(22)：6

H

韩天雄，颜琼枝. 国医大师颜德馨教授辨治糖尿病经验[J]. 浙江中医药大学学报，2012，36(10)：1067

胡晓贞，颜乾麟. 颜德馨教授论胸痹证病机与治法[J]. 中国中医急症，2012，21(6)：901

L

李永亮，戴铭，张亚萍. 班秀文教授治疗妇科疾病学术思想探析[J]. 中华中医药杂志，2011，26(4)：730

林寒梅，庞秋华，班胜. 班秀文活血通脉安胎经验[J]. 山东中医杂志，2013，32(3)：199

刘林，王垂杰，郭恩绵. 李玉奇教授治疗水气病经验[J]. 世界中医药，2013，8(6)：644

刘林，王垂杰，王辉. 李玉奇治疗热入血室经验[J]. 中医杂志，2013，54(2)：102

刘玉筠，戴铭，董岚，等. 班秀文教授从情志论治妇科病经验[J]. 中医学报，2013，28(10)：1476

刘玉筠，员晓云，戴铭，等. 班秀文教授论治经带并病学术思想探析[J]. 时珍国医国药，2013，24(11)：2776

R

任壮. 国医大师颜德馨[J]. 中医学报，2011，26(12)：1429

T

汤立东，王学良，王垂杰，等. 李玉奇教授治疗便秘经验[J]. 世界中医药，2013，8(8)：932

W

王晓戎，马继松. 国医大师李玉奇治疗脾胃病临证用药经验探析[J]. 辽宁中医杂志，2011，38(7)：1281

X

谢佳伶. 八桂中医学术流派之班氏妇科[J]. 中医临床研究，2011，3(12)：106

Z

张会永. 国医大师李玉奇先生治疗消渴病临床经验[J]. 中华中医药杂志，2011，26(12)：2882

张会永. 李玉奇治疗再生障碍性贫血经验[J]. 中医杂志，2013，54(12)：998

张璐砾，戴铭，刘玉筠，等. 班秀文针药并用治疗妇科病经验[J]. 中医杂志，2013，54，(17)：1453

(二) 传 染 病

【概述】

2013 年发表的国家法定传染病范畴文献约 1 000篇，其中病毒性肝炎的临床及实验研究约 73%，其余为艾滋病、流行性感冒、手足口病、肺结核、脑炎、细菌性痢疾、腮腺炎等病症的治疗与研究。

1. 艾滋病(AISD)

王阶等对 287 例未接受过任何治疗的人类免疫缺陷病毒(HIV)/AIDS 患者检测外周血CD_4^+ T 细胞计数、免疫异常激活标志物及血浆病毒载量，分析 AIDS 患者的免疫异常激活水平及其与 CD_4^+ T 细胞计数、疾病进展的相关性。发现 CD_4^+ T细胞计数越低的患者，其免疫异常激活水平越高，慢性免疫激活与 CD_4^+ T 细胞计数呈显著的负相关。中药具有多靶点，双向调节的作用特点，优势在于强调调整机体的免疫功能状态，而免疫异常激活则有可能是中医药干预 HIV/AIDS 的重要切入点。(详见专条)

2. 病毒性肝炎

雷陵等将 80 例 HBeAg 阴性慢性乙型病毒性肝炎(CHB)中病毒低水平复制(5.0×10^2 拷贝 / ml≤HBV DNA 水平≤10^4拷贝/ml，ALT≤2×ULN)患者随机平分为两组，均予西医一般常规(护肝、支持及对症)疗法，治疗组加服扶正益肝颗粒(香菇、绞股蓝、黑木耳、柴胡、虎杖等)。经治 52 周，治疗组与对照组综合有效率分别为 70.0%(28/40)、40.0%(16/40)，血清 HBV DNA 阴转率分别为 37.5%(15/40)、15.0%(6/40)，组间比较，$P<0.01$，$P<0.05$。赵庆等研究 CHB 中医证候的蛋白质组学规律，发现 5 个证型患者与正常人比较，存在多个蛋白质表达差异，其中免疫球蛋白 J 链(IG－J)与 CHB 患者肝纤维化改变有较强的相关性。IG－J 表达在 5 个 CHB 证候组中均有规律的上调，且组间比较，$P<0.05$。其中以瘀血阻络证组肝功能损害和免疫紊乱最为严重，其次为肝肾阴虚证、脾肾阳虚证、肝郁脾虚证、湿热中阻证。

对慢性重型肝炎的治疗及实验研究、慢性乙型肝炎病毒携带者的治疗与研究、慢性乙型肝炎证型及其相关性实验室指标的研究以及慢性丙型病毒性肝炎的治疗与研究见专条。

苏立稳等将 80 例失代偿期乙型肝炎肝硬化患者平分为两组，均予综合治疗并服恩替卡韦(ETV)0.5 mg/次，1 次/d，治疗组加服复方肝欣合剂(白术、蚤休、半枝莲、虎杖、黄芪、茯苓等)。经治 6 个月，两组患者肝功能较治疗前明显改善，而治疗组患者的肝功能指标的改善及 Child－Pugh 评分降低、HBV DNA 的转阴率均优于对照组(均 $P<0.05$)。李野平等对 7 例中西医治疗前后行 2 次肝脏大体形态学和组织学检查的乙肝肝硬化患者，采用描述性方法分析中药(扶正化瘀胶囊、丹参注射液及辨证治疗 4 例)、西药(核苷类似物治疗 1 例)及中西药结合(核苷类似物联合扶正化瘀胶囊、丹参注射液及辨证治疗 2 例)对肝脏大体形态学及组织学的变化的影响。与治疗前相比，在肝脏大体形态学改变方面，1 例小结节肝脏表面结节基本消失，6 例结节形态未见明显变化；在组织学改变方面，肝脏纤维化程度的改变，以中西药结合治疗后纤维化程度减轻最明显，其次为中药，西药治疗无变化；在肝脏受损的坏死程度方面，西药治疗后坏死程度减轻最明显，其次为中药、中西药结合治疗。

3. 甲型流感

孙丽梅等将 79 例甲型H1N1流感轻症患者随机分为中药组(61 例)与西药组，分别予服小柴胡汤加味、磷酸奥司他韦胶囊。经治 5 d，中药组患者发热、咳嗽、咯痰等流感样症状消失时间明显短于西药组($P<0.05$)，头痛、咽痛、恶寒等流感样症状消失时间，咽部红肿、扁桃体肿大等体征恢复正常时间以及白细胞恢复正常时间、甲型H1N1流感病毒核酸转阴时间与西药组比较，$P>0.05$。

向燕等研究表明，冰香散(野菊花、茴香、冰片等)滴鼻、雾化均能显著降低小鼠感染甲型H1N1流感病毒后的肺指数，与模型组比较，$P<0.05$；冰香散滴鼻组中 CD_4^+ T 细胞和 CD_4^+/CD_8^+ 比值与

模型组比较显著升高($P<0.05$ 或 $P<0.01$)，当采用雾化方式给药时，其结果与模型组比较无显著性差异。表明冰香散不同给药途径(滴鼻、雾化)的抗病毒免疫机制有所不同。何婷等研究表明，荆芥挥发油、薄荷酮及胡薄荷酮治疗方式给药能显著降低病毒感染小鼠肺组织病毒滴度，显示出体内抗病毒作用，但预防给药效果不明显。体内抗病毒感染机制与提高感染小鼠干扰素(IFN-α、IFN-β)、IL-2 水平，抑制 IL-6、INF-α 分泌有关；细胞模型结果提示药物通过 Toll 样受体 $(TLR)_3$ 和 TLR_7 信号通路影响 IFN-β 的表达。刘蓉等研究表明，桂枝挥发油与桂皮醛能提高流感病毒性肺炎小鼠的死亡保护率，其抗病毒作用机制与激活 TLR_7 信号通路、促进 IFN 的分泌有关。

刘琪等研究表明，疏风宣肺抗流感方(金银花、连翘、牛蒡子、蝉蜕、荆芥等)和解表清里抗流感方(炙麻黄、生石膏、黄芩、杏仁、生甘草等)中、低剂量组能较明显地降低小鼠的肺指数，与模型组比较，$P<0.05$；能减轻小鼠肺组织病变。李荣荣等研究表明，麻黄细辛附子汤干预肾阳虚外感模型小鼠后能够明显地延长小鼠的平均生存时间，升高小鼠体温，改善体征，对小鼠流感肺炎症状的减轻、机体非特异性免疫功能的增强具有一定的效果。

李湘潋等研究表明，茶黄素衍生物能明显地抑制H5N1假病毒的感染力，其可能通过与血凝素 HA_2 亚基结合而抑制禽流感病毒的感染，同时能够在一定程度上抑制病毒的神经氨酸酶活性，提示茶黄素衍生物是通过多靶点发挥抗H5N1亚型禽流感病毒的作用。

4. 疫病预警

童佳兵等对建国以来 60 年重大传染病防治实践采用多因子综合和动态变化分析的方法，进行回顾性对照和前瞻性预测研究，利用数据库挖掘技术寻找新的关联，归纳出可能导致传染病的“高危”指标，揭示其证候规律，结合“天人相应”“三因制宜”等理论，构建传染病中医药预测预警诊治智能辅助系统，形成中医药防治传染病的应急预案，促进了重大传染病防治能力的提高。

刘忠第等利用北京地区 1970～2004 年之间的 35 年痢疾发病数据和同期气象数据，进行相关和回归的统计学分析，探讨痢疾发病与 3 年前及当年气象因素之间的相关性。研究表明，痢疾发病与 3 年前的气温、风速和相对湿度具有显著相关性($P<0.05$)，“3 年化疫”理论对于痢疾发病的预测具有一定指导意义。

汤巧玲等收集北京地区 1970～2004 年之间的 35 年猩红热发病人数及相对应气象资料(包括日平均气温、降雨量、相对湿度、水汽压、风速)，按六气分段并进行描述性分析和相关分析，筛选相关性高的气象因子，建立多元逐步回归方程，并对方程进行检验后发现，猩红热的发病集中于冬春之季，与气温、相对湿度、风速共 13 个气象因子具有相关性($P<0.05$)。该研究提示猩红热的发病与六气及气象密切相关，利用前一年不同时段的气象变化规律可以预测后一年猩红热的发病情况。

张轩等收集北京地区 1970～2004 年之间的 35 年气象数据和伤寒副伤寒发病数据，采用描述性统计分析 Spearman 相关分析和 BP 人工神经网络分析，研究伤寒、副伤寒发病与当年及 3 年前气象因素的相关性后发现，伤寒、副伤寒发病在各年度呈不均衡分布，在六气时段内集中在三之气、四之气高发。其发病与当年及 3 年前的平均气温、平均风速和平均相对湿度具有显著相关性($P<0.05$)。在气象预测模型中，3 年前的平均风速和平均相对湿度是重要影响因素，当年的平均相对湿度是重要影响因素。

此外，对肺结核、手足口病的治疗与研究已立专条。董梦久等将 75 例流行性乙型脑炎患者随机分为两组，治疗组 30 例患者在对照组的综合治疗及护理基础上加用醒脑静注射液静脉滴注，经治 15 d，治疗组在降温(5.40 ± 1.30)d、平均昏迷时间(5.64 ± 1.03)d、平均缓解抽搐时间(2.20 ± 1.17)d 均短于对照组，且恶化和后遗症较少，其疗效明显优于对照组($P<0.05$)。艾军等应用德尔菲法通过 3 轮专家问卷调查论证，研究制定出《麻疹中医诊疗指南》，将麻疹中医辨证论治方法，分为顺证：邪犯肺卫证，邪入肺胃证，气阴耗伤证；逆证：麻毒闭肺证，麻毒攻喉证，邪陷心肝证等 6 个主要证候。并提出了证候、治法、主方及常用药建议，对促进中医的规范化标准化有着积极意义。熊益居等对 9 例流行性腮腺炎并发前庭神经元炎患者，以普济消毒饮合清眩汤加减(黄芩、黄连、柴胡、升麻、荆芥、防风等)煎服，紫金锭调醋成糊剂分别涂于腮腺、睾丸处以及病毒唑静

脉滴注、苯海拉明深部肌内注射等治疗14 d,9 例患者均治愈出院,随访 2 个月无复发。

(赵　雷　张　玮)

【艾滋病的治疗及实验研究】

徐立然等随机设盲 1 200 例无症状期 HIV 感染者作为受试者,依据诊断标准和纳入标准要求,随机入组 1 199 例。治疗组(入组 796 例、完成 622 例)予相应证型中药制剂(无证可辨或气虚证予服益艾康胶囊、气阴两虚证予服艾宁颗粒、湿热内蕴证予服唐草片、气虚血瘀证予服艾奇康胶囊、痰瘀互结证予服金龙胶囊),对照组(入组 403 例、完成 325 例)予相应证型中药制剂的模拟剂。经治 18 个月,治疗组患者随着整体症状和体征的改善,生存质量得到显著提高;而对照组生存质量显著下降,组间生存质量有极显著差异($P<0.01$)。

吴欣芳等将 228 例 HIV/AIDS 患者,随机平分为两组,均予 HAART 治疗,治疗组加服免疫 1 号方(西洋参、冬虫夏草、紫花地丁等),对照组予免疫 1 号方安慰剂。治疗 6 周,评价两组患者治疗后 CD_4^+ T 细胞计数的变化及其免疫重建有效率。对于 CD_4^+ T 细胞在 200～350 个/μL 的患者,治疗组免疫重建有效率优于对照组($P<0.05$)。刘震等将经 HAART 治疗 1 年以上的免疫重建不全患者随机分为两组,均予 HAART 治疗,治疗组加服免疫 2 号方。经治 6 个月,治疗组与对照组免疫重建有效率分别为 34.5%(40/116)、21.4%(25/117),组间比较,$P<0.05$。两组患者的 CD_4、CD_{45}RA、CD_{45}RO 细胞绝对计数均能显著提高($P<0.05$),治疗组 CD_8、CD_{28} 相对计数较对照组显著提高($P<0.05$)。

岑玉文等对 164 例 AIDS 合并肺部感染患者随机分为两组,均予针对相应病原体的抗肺部感染西医基础治疗,实验组 111 例按辨证分为痰热壅盛、肺肾两亏、痰湿阻肺 3 个证型分别予清金化痰汤、补肺汤合七味都气丸、小青龙汤合二陈汤加减治疗。经治 4 周,实验组证候治愈率和显效率均优于纯西医对照组($P<0.05$),尤其对于缓解发热(但热不寒)和头痛 2 个主要症状上具有明显优势。

王阶等对 287 例未接受过任何治疗的 HIV/AIDS 患者检测外周血 CD_4^+ T 细胞计数、免疫异常激活标志物及血浆病毒载量,分析 AIDS 患者的免疫异常激活水平及其与 CD_4^+ T 细胞计数、疾病进展的相关性。发现 CD_4^+ T 细胞计数越低的患者,其免疫异常激活水平越高,慢性免疫激活与 CD_4^+ T 细胞计数呈显著的负相关。中药具有多靶点、双向调节的作用特点,优势在于强调调整机体的免疫功能状态,而免疫异常激活则有可能是中医药干预 HIV/AIDS 的重要切入点。

王阶等采集 37 例 AIDS 免疫重建不全患者治疗前后的外周血 PBMC,采用人类 TCRVβ 基因 CDR3 多样性定量检测,基因扫描作图并计算 Vβ 家族中每个家族不同大小 CDR3 区片段的分布,同时以 15 例 HIV 抗体阴性健康献血员做对照。经中药免疫 2 号方(西洋参、黄芪、地丁草等)等治疗后各家族单寡克隆情况有不同程度的改善和恢复。其中 9、11、21、22 等 4 个家族的 D 值,两组治疗后均比治疗前下降,治疗组下降幅度较对照组在 21、22 的 2 个家族更为显著($P<0.05$)。治疗组显著降低第 18 家族 D 值,而对照组则显著增加($P<0.05$)。提示中医药可能促进 T 细胞部分受体基因重排,丰富受体库,帮助机体免疫细胞有效识别病毒,减少 T 细胞凋亡。

熊兴江等回顾经典名方在 AIDS 治疗中的运用,国内外关于经典名方的临床与实验研究已显示出一定优势,约 30 余首经典名方在 AIDS 的治疗上显示出一定疗效,如理中汤、四君子汤、四物汤、复脉汤、八珍汤、人参养荣汤等。还对 AIDS 典型症状、机会性感染及各系统并发症的方证特征及其经典名方证治规律进行了探索,如 AIDS 发热以柴胡证和桂枝证出现的频率较高,AIDS 抑郁症以柴胡加龙骨牡蛎汤、逍遥散等柴胡类方为其常见方证,AIDS 腹泻以半夏泻心汤方证出现的频率极高等,其高频出现的现象可能与疾病的自然转归有关,可能也是辨证论治在相对固定化阶段而具有“专病专方”特征有关。刘巍等临床研究认为,AIDS 发热的治疗唯尽早将邪气透达于体外,才可减轻对正气的损害。

王健等从理论层面和文献 2 个方面分析、比较中西药治疗 AIDS 的疗效作用点之异同,探讨免疫功能病毒载量与症状等的相关性。临床结果表明,中医治疗 AIDS 更多的实际情况是免疫功能改善,症状减轻,生活质量提高,但病毒载量不会很快降低。长期而持续的免疫功能稳定或改善能否使病毒载量不上升或逐步下降,有待于今后大样本、长时间临床观察进行证实。

高国建等对近 20 年来中药复方在促进艾滋

病免疫重建方面的相关研究进行梳理后发现，中药复方在AIDS免疫重建方面有独特的作用，具有安全性和可控性较高，长期使用毒副作用小，产生耐药性的几率小。存在的问题是国内的中医药治疗艾滋病试点项目少、规模小，不能满足AIDS患者的治疗需要；对AIDS的治疗尚未形成系统统一规范的辨证论治认识和评价标准；缺少中医药疗法进行随机对照盲法重复均衡大样本的临床试验研究；中药剂型的规范化和药物的质量问题；中医药人员队伍中的医师水平参差不齐等。

陈静等采用SIVmac239病毒株静脉接种健康中国恒河猴复制中国恒河猴AIDS动物模型，观察猴HIV感染后动物模型亚急性期内T淋巴细胞亚群变化、病毒载量变化情况，结果表明中国恒河猴艾滋病动物模型与国外印度恒河猴艾滋病动物模型亚急性期相似，此为中国恒河猴应用于AIDS模型研究的标准化建立补充了更详尽的亚急性期变化内容。

（赵　雷　张　玮）

【慢性重型肝炎的治疗及实验研究】

马文峰等将60例慢性乙型病毒性肝炎（CHB）肝衰竭患者随机分为单纯西药常规治疗的对照组（23例）和配合辨证论治及大黄乌梅汤灌肠治疗的实验组。结果实验组的整体疗效明显优于对照组，两组治疗8周后，患者血清内毒素水平及血清总胆红素（TBiL）、直接胆红素（DBiL）、凝血酶原时间（PT）、凝血酶原活动度（PTA）水平比较，$P<0.05$。浦忠平等将96例重度CHB患者随机平分为两组，均予常规护肝疗法，治疗组加服肝炎一号方（茵陈蒿、平地木、垂盆草、泽泻、茯苓、生山楂等）。经治1个月后，两组患者证候、肝功能指标均有改善，治疗组与对照组总有效率分别为91.7%（44/48）、66.7%（32/48），组间比较，$P<0.05$。

樊冬梅等将58例慢性重型肝炎患者随机分为两组，均予西医内科基础用药，观察组加服凉血解毒方（水牛角、茵陈、叶下珠、茜草、白背叶根、田基黄等），经治4周后，观察组与对照组总有效率分别为78.6%（22/28）、66.7%（20/30）。两组患者治疗前血浆内毒素、sCD_{14}、TLR4 mRNA水平比较无显著性差异，有可比性，治疗后观察组血浆内毒素、sCD_{14}、TLR4 mRNA水平较治疗前降低，与对照组比较，$P<0.05$。提示凉血解毒方作用机制可能与干预慢性重型肝炎患者内毒素受体通路有关。石清兰等及龙富立等将110例慢性重型肝炎患者随机平分为两组，均予对症支持和常规基础西药，治疗组加服解毒化瘀颗粒（茵陈、白花蛇舌草、赤芍药、大黄、石菖蒲、郁金）。治疗前两组患者外周血单个核细胞（PBMC）TLR4均呈高表达状态，经治4周后，治疗组患者外周血PBMCTLR4表达明显低于对照组（$P<0.05$）。治疗组患者在治疗后第2、4、8周血清中TNF-α、IL-6、IL-12水平较对照组明显下降，而IL-10在治疗后第4、8周与对照组比较有显著增高（均$P<0.05$）。提示解毒化瘀颗粒对LPS（脂多糖，为细胞内毒素化学成分）/TLR4信号传导通路有调控作用，能降低慢性重型肝炎患者血清促炎因子水平，提高抗炎因子水平，对LPS介导的机体炎症反应具有一定防治作用。

胡建华等通过检索1911～2012年中国期刊全文数据库（CNKI）关于中医药、中西医结合诊治慢性重型肝炎文献，总结慢性重型肝炎病因病机、辨证分型及治疗研究进展，提出慢性重型肝炎病因病机中“毒、瘀、虚”是关键；辨证分型较多，但实质均以“毒、瘀、虚”为核心，毒常见热毒、湿毒、湿热之毒、痰浊之毒等证，虚常见阴虚、气虚、阳虚等；治疗重点也是针对“毒、瘀、虚”，常用清热解毒、活血化瘀、益气养阴温阳之法，同时强调针对阴阳病性论治。

王轩等研究表明，以温阳解毒化瘀颗粒（茵陈、白术、丹参、薏苡仁、附片、赤芍药等）干预肝衰竭肠源性内毒血症（ITEM）模型大鼠24小时，与模型组比较，能明显降低大鼠门静脉内毒素水平（$P<0.05$），明显增加肠道sIgA分泌（$P<0.05$），减轻肝组织病变。提示增加肠道sIgA分泌是该制剂改善ITEM机制之一。

（周希禛　张　玮）

【慢性乙型肝炎病毒携带者的治疗与研究】

林巧等报道46例慢性乙肝病毒（HBV）携带者，其中27例予服用益肾固本方（山茱萸、熟地黄、旱莲草、女贞子、泽泻、黑芝麻），19例未予任何药物治疗作对照。动态随访24周后，检测$CD4^+$ T细胞中干扰素调节因子（IRF）-4^+细胞比例，益肾固本方组IRF-4^+细胞群峰值偏移程度小于对照组，IRF-4mRNA表达量显著低于对照组（$P<0.05$）。表明益肾固本方可以抑制HBV携带者IRF-4基因转录和蛋白表达水平，对于纠正Th_1/Th_2细胞失衡、打破免疫耐受具有

重要意义。

陈英杰等将400例HBeAg阳性HBV携带者平分为两组,分别予服补肾健脾方(淫羊藿、怀牛膝、杜仲、菟丝子、白术、黄芪等)与安慰剂。经治52周后,补肾健脾方组患者的血清细胞因子IL-2和IFN-γ显著上升,TNF-α、IL-4和IL-10则明显下降($P<0.01$),治疗前后的各细胞因子差值比较以及血清HBV-DNA载量较基线下降的比例均优于安慰剂组($P<0.01$)。陈氏等将300例e-抗原阳性HBV携带者随机分为两组,分别予服补肾清透方(印度叶下珠、菟丝子、淫羊藿、女贞子、旱莲草、柴胡等)与安慰剂。经治52周后,补肾清透方组(200例)患者血清HBV-DNA水平、HBeAg均值下降显著优于安慰剂组($P<0.01$),且作用呈时间依赖趋势。

吴银亚等收集200例慢性HBV携带者分为HBeAg阳性与HBeAg阴性两组各100例,辨证分析"湿、热、瘀、虚"证候的分布特点。结果两组均以气虚证为主,湿证、血虚证和阳虚证均较少,而HBeAg阳性组热证多于HBeAg阴性组($P<0.05$),HBeAg阴性组瘀证和阴虚证多于HBeAg阳性组($P<0.05$)。提示慢性HBV携带者在慢性病程中以气虚证为主,HBeAg阳性与HBeAg阴性兼夹有湿热瘀证的不同,阳性者热证居多,而阴性者瘀证居多。

郭新新等对125例慢性HBV携带者采用中医体质量表探讨其体质类型分布及其特点,发现慢性HBV携带者体质类型按照平和质、阳虚质、气郁质、湿热质、气虚质、痰湿质、血瘀质、阴虚质和特禀质从高到低分布;有60%人出现复合体质,出现的频率从高到低依次为湿热质、气虚质、气郁质、阳虚质、痰湿质、血瘀质、阴虚质、平和质和特禀质。黄少妮等探讨HBV携带者中医体质类型分布规律及特点研究,发现乙肝"大三阳"型(HBsAg、HBeAg、HBcAb 3项均阳性)的中医体质分布特点为:气郁质>阳虚质>气虚质>湿热质>平和质=痰湿质=阴虚质>血瘀质>特禀质;其中气郁质居首位,占23.3%(10/23),气郁质、阳虚质、气虚质和湿热质占74.4%(32/43)。在"小三阳"型(HBsAg、HBeAb、HBcAb 3项均阳性)的中医体质分布为:气虚质=阳虚质>血瘀质>气郁质>平和质=痰湿质=湿热质>阴虚质>特禀质;其中气虚质、阳虚质、瘀血质和气郁质占69.64%(39/56)。王志强等对43例慢性HBV携带者体质类型与T淋巴细胞亚群的相关性进行研究后发现,CD_4^+、CD_8^+ T细胞及CD_4^+/CD_8^+比值的差异可以在一定程度上反映不同中医体质慢性HBV携带者免疫状态,并指导慢性HBV携带者的临床防治。

姜桂宁等对236例慢性HBV携带者的中医证候及证候要素分布规律研究后发现,慢性HBV携带者病位的证候要素主要为肝、脾、肾,病例的证候要素主要为气滞、阴虚、湿热、湿阻、血瘀、阳虚,主要证型有肝肾阴虚型、脾虚湿阻型、肝胆湿热型、肝郁气滞型、无症可辨型、血瘀型和脾肾阳虚型。

聂凡等总结了近10年来国内外学者对导致HBV携带者肝脏病理学改变的相关因素如患者年龄、血清ALT水平、血清PCⅢ、血清HBV-DNA载量、血清HBeAg表达、基因型,以及肝内HBsAg、HBcAg表达与分布等研究进展,尽管某些因素与肝脏病理学上的改变还存在分歧和争论,但并不影响人们继续深入探讨它们之间的关系,对临床诊断及其防治有一定的指导意义。

(周希祯　张　玮)

【慢性乙型肝炎证型及其相关实验室指标的研究】

陈潇雨等将555例肝胆湿热证与肝郁脾虚证慢性乙型病毒性肝炎(CHB)患者的证候学调查信息和理化指标作为研究对象,采用特征属性筛选与C5.0决策树算法等数据挖掘技术,构建CHB肝胆湿热证与肝郁脾虚证的信息分类模型,筛选出与肝胆湿热和肝郁脾虚分类相关的(苔白、舌红、舌胖、膝软、苔厚、脉细、HBeAb等)7项重要属性及8条分类规则,并达到了96.9%的分类准确率,对中医诊断学的客观化研究具有重要意义。

刘一博等收集31例CHB肝气郁结证患者及对照组肝血瘀证患者16例与健康人组30例,通过GC/MS(气相色谱/质谱)技术检测各组人员生物学标志物及内源性代谢谱,找到了肝气郁结证与健康者之间的差异性代谢物质(包括丙酸、丙二酸、嘧啶、吲哚胺、5-恶唑胺、萘啶等),提示中医证候是有其生物学物质基础的,而代谢组学是对其研究的工具之一。

杨华升等收集74例慢性乙型重型肝炎(CSHB)住院患者的辨证分型、相关实验室指标与并发症情况,对CSHB患者的脉象、舌象及常见症状的频次进行分析研究。结果显示,CSHB

的证型以气虚瘀黄证(25.7%)阳虚瘀黄证(16.2%)湿热发黄证(27.0%)瘀热发黄证(21.6%)较为常见,阴虚瘀黄证(9.5%)发生率较低。按照5个证型辨证,TBiL、PT、中性粒细胞比例(NAUT%)、Hb等实验室指标及腹水、肝性脑病、细菌性腹膜炎等并发症的发生率在各型间均无显著性差异($P>0.05$),5个证型合并为虚、实两型统计分析,则虚证组NAUT%及腹水发生率高于实证组($P<0.05$)。提示CSHB的证型与实验室指标及并发症之间有一定的相关性,临床应该首重虚实辨证。

冯建英等对虚实不同证型的90例CHB患者检测体内HBV特异性的细胞毒性T淋巴细胞(CTL)、T淋巴细胞亚群及病毒复制水平,探讨其与机体特异性细胞免疫及病毒复制的关系。结果表明,实证组患者特异性CTL细胞的阳性率高于虚证组($P<0.05$);两组CD_4^+ T细胞水平均较正常组下降,虚证组下降更明显($P<0.05$),CD_4^+/CD_8^+值由高到低依次为正常组、实证组、虚证组,虚证组CD_8^+ T细胞水平较正常组、实证组均有所升高($P<0.05$);两组患者病毒复制程度不同,实证组高病毒载量患者约为62.2%,虚证组仅为40%,较前者明显减少($P<0.05$)。

李红山等选择初次治疗的CHB肝胆湿热证和肝郁脾虚证患者各30例,探讨各证型与临床免疫指标的关联性。结果表明,肝胆湿热型患者CD_3^+ T细胞水平在初次、随访8周和16周时均明显升高,与肝郁脾虚型相应数值相比,$P<0.05$;两组患者初次、随访8周和16周时CD_4^+ T细胞水平相比,肝胆湿热组高于肝郁脾虚组(P均<0.05);初次IgM含量相比,肝胆湿热组低于肝郁脾虚组($P<0.05$),随访8周和16周时相比无差异性。两组患者CD_8^+ T细胞、IgA、IgG水平比较均无差异性。

杨丽莎等对慢性HBV感染免疫耐受、免疫清除和免疫不全状态患者各200例,采用免疫学分类、辨证分型及临床流行病学调查等方法研究其证型分布的特点。结果表明,3种不同免疫状态间的证型分布具有差异性,免疫耐受状态组以肝郁脾虚为主,免疫清除状态组以湿热内蕴为主,免疫不全状态组以肝肾阴虚为主。为中西医结合防治慢性HBV感染的临床诊断及疗效评价提供了理论依据。

艾香英等对80例CHB患者辨证分型并行肝组织病理活检,探讨证型与肝组织病理改变的关系。结果表明,患者的肝组织病理改变程度为肝郁脾虚证<肝胆湿热证<肝肾阴虚证,各证型肝组织的炎症分级和纤维化分期比较有显著性差异($P<0.01$)。从肝郁脾虚证到肝胆湿热证再到肝肾阴虚证,肝组织病理损害呈逐渐加重的趋势。

胡大庆等对90例$1\times ULN\leqslant ALT\leqslant 2\times ULN$、血清HBV-DNA均为阳性的轻症CHB患者辨证分型(肝郁脾虚证50例、湿热中阻证18例、肝肾阴虚证13例、瘀血阻络证9例)并行肝脏活组织穿刺病理检查,研究其与肝病理相关性。结果,轻症CHB患者肝组织病理检查炎症坏死≥G2者占80.0%(72/90),纤维化≥S2者占45.6%(41/90),满足正规的抗病毒治疗条件;可将肝组织病理作为判断是否抗病毒治疗的主要依据。轻症CHB患者的证型与肝组织病理活动度有一定的关系,而瘀血阻络型病理程度比其余证型可能更为严重。

高月求对CHB中医证候规律研究思路进行探讨,认为中医证候规律研究只有以提高临床疗效为目标,以证—方—效这一中医临床诊治思维方式为纲,才更具指导意义。而将CHB作为研究对象,建立中医四诊信息结构化数据采集平台、规范信息采集和统计分析,开展中医证型诊断标准的临床再验证等基础性研究,可为中医证候规律研究提供良好的思路。

邓华亮等梳理近年来CHB证候分型及相关研究文献,分析证候规范化研究中存在的问题,并在此基础上提出以证候要素理论为指导,基于病证结合建立中医证候量化诊断标准的思路,以期建立CHB中医辨证新的诊断模式。

(刘一博　张　玮)

【慢性丙型肝炎的治疗与研究】

怀平艾等将50例慢性丙型肝炎(CHC)患者随机分成两组,均予皮下注射聚乙二醇干扰素α-2a及口服利巴韦林,治疗组26例加服小柴胡汤(柴胡、黄芩、党参、半夏、炙甘草)。治疗48周,两组在显效率和总有效率比较,$P>0.05$;停药后6个月,两组持续有效完全应答分别为46.2%(12/26)、16.7%(4/24),组间比较,$P<0.01$。赵瑞敏等将100例CHC患者随机平分为两组,均予皮下注射聚乙二醇干扰素α-2a及口服利巴韦林,治疗组加服苦参素胶囊。经治180 d,治疗组与对照组总有效率分别为86.0%(43/50)、

72.0%(36/50),组间比较,$P<0.05$。田凌云等将62例CHC患者随机分为两组,均予聚乙二醇干扰素α-2a皮下注射及利巴韦林口服,治疗组32例加服(太子参、茯苓、佛手、炒白术、五味子、黄芪等)。经治48周,两组完全应答(ALT复常及HCV RNA转阴)分别为24例、15例,总应答率分别为93.8%(30/32)、80.0(24/30),组间比较,$P<0.05$。

沈健等将60例难治性CHC患者随机、双盲平分为两组,治疗组予服丙肝冲剂(黄芪、白术、虎杖、苦参、栀子、胡黄连),对照组予服丙肝冲剂原方药量的1/10。治疗48周,治疗组与安慰剂组HCV RNA下降率分别为33.3%(10/30)和10.0%(3/30),组间比较,$P<0.05$。

许文君等对28例CHC患者予聚乙二醇干扰素联合利巴韦林治疗后的中医证候资料进行分析,发现患者治疗前后中医症状积分变化有明显差异($P<0.01$);治疗前的证型分布为正虚邪恋证>肝郁脾虚证＝肝肾阴虚证>湿热中阻证＝脾肾阳虚证>瘀血阻络证,治疗后为肝郁脾虚证>正虚邪恋证>脾肾阳虚证>湿热中阻证＝肝肾阴虚证。肝郁脾虚证患者明显比治疗前增多($P<0.01$)。

董慧琳等总结了陈建杰治疗CHC经验,提出伏邪致病的病因学理论和邪恋正虚的病机特点。应用"伏邪理论"指导其治疗,根据病情,针对干扰素使用前后患者的不同特点辨证施治,强化中医辨证与西药治疗的结合,在治疗过程中,紧扣"正虚邪恋"的特点,以祛邪为主,兼顾扶正,疗效独特。李燚光等总结薛博瑜诊疗CHC经验,认为热毒瘀结、肝脾损伤为病机重点,以凉血解毒、调养肝脾为治疗基本大法,方选犀角地黄汤合四逆散之类,取得较好临床疗效。

刘旭等认为目前关于CHC病因病机的探讨主要有湿热疫毒、阴邪湿毒、邪气伏藏3种学说,但这3种学说不能对其进行完整的阐述,为完善病因病机理论,其通过探寻古代典籍,纳入"主客交"学说,CHC的辨证分型以正虚邪恋型为多见,这是CHC区别于CHB的重要特征,比其他类病毒性肝炎更适于用"主客交"学说来阐明。

张富永等认为CHC与CHB有各自独立系统的发病机制、病理学诊断、临床表现和治疗方法,二者在中医证治上是不同的,有必要对其进行区别比较,使临床诊治不致混淆。并从病因病机、证型、治疗3个方面对二者进行了区别比较。

于晓雯等认为现阶段中医药治疗CHC对提高免疫应答,抗病毒药物不良反应及改善代谢紊乱等方面有一定优势。对有标准化治疗禁忌、不能耐受标准化治疗不良反应或无经济条件者,中药治疗可起支柱作用。

(张　玮　王晶晶)

【肺结核的治疗与研究】

刘峋松等选择全国14家医院共1 404例符合西医初治继发性肺结核和中医肺痨(肺阴亏虚、气阴两虚、阴虚火旺证候)诊断标准的患者随机平分为两组,均予常规化疗(异烟肼、利福平、吡嗪酰胺、乙胺丁醇),试验组加服中药(根据证候分别予滋阴润肺免煎颗粒、肺泰胶囊、双百口服液)。经治6个月,试验组在减少治疗中因药物引起的肝损伤及其他不良反应的发生率明显低于对照组($P<0.01$)。且在症状总积分、中医证候疗效及安全性评价分层分析等与对照组比较,均$P<0.01$。刘忠达等将400例患者随机平分为两组,均予常规抗痨化疗,治疗组予辨证(分为肺阴虚、阴虚火旺、气阴两虚3个证型分别)施治。经治2个月后,治疗组与对照组的痰菌阴转率分别为100%(75/75)、96.8%(61/63),$P>0.05$;两组病灶吸收率分别为66.5%(133/200)、55.5%(111/200),空洞闭合有效率分别为69.8%(44/63)、49.1%(28/57),白细胞降低发生率分别为29.0%(58/200)、42.0%(84/200),肝功能损害发生率分别为23.0%(46/200)、38.5%(75/200)。组间比较,均$P<0.01$。杨晓云将60例气阴两虚夹瘀证患者随机平分为两组,均予常规化疗,治疗组予加服参苓白术散加减(党参、黄精、北沙参、茯苓、白术、陈皮等)。治疗2个月后,治疗组和对照组的证候改善率分别为73.3%(22/30)、40.0%(12/30);痰结核分枝杆菌涂阳阴转率分别为57.9%(11/19)、37.5%(6/16);X线胸片病灶改善率分别为56.6%(17/30),50.0%(15/30)。组间比较,均$P<0.05$。任郭侠等将80例空洞型患者随机平分为两组,均予标准化疗,治疗组加丹参注射液静脉滴注。治疗30 d,治疗组与对照组总有效率分别为87.5%(35/40)、62.5%(25/40),两组空洞愈合率比较,$P<0.01$。唐晓琦等将100例复治菌阳性患者随机平分为两组,均予常规化疗,治疗组加服加减保真汤(黄芪、党参、白术、茯苓、天门冬、麦门冬等),经治2个月,治疗组痰菌

转阴情况、X线病灶吸收情况均明显优于对照组（$P<0.01$）。周杰等将324例气阴两虚型初治继发性患者随机分为两组，均予常规化疗，治疗组172例予服双百口服液（百合、百部、南沙参、麦冬、地黄、人参等）。治疗1～6个月期间，两组痰菌转阴率及空洞闭合率比较，$P>0.05$；愈显率及有效率、肺部阴影吸收率和毒副反应情况等治疗组与对照组相比，$P<0.01$或$P<0.05$。

邓俊等将640例初治、涂阳患者随机分为两组，均予常规短程化疗，治疗组323例加服补中益气丸。经治6个月，两组痰菌阴转率分别为98.1%(317/323)、90.2%(286/317)，组间比较，$P<0.01$；结核菌素试验阳性率分别为83.59%(270/323)，44.48%(141/317)，组间比较，$P<0.01$。两组治疗后CD_3^+、CD_4^+及CD_4^+/CD_8^+值均升高，而治疗组显著优于对照组（$P<0.01$）。王园等报道1 205例继发性患者，其中591例单纯采用化疗方案作为对照，治疗组加服虫草抗痨胶囊。初治患者治疗6个月，复治患者治疗9个月，总有效率分别为78.8%(466/591)、94.5%(580/614)，组间比较，$P<0.05$。治疗组CD_3^+、CD_4^+及CD_4^+/CD_8^+值均显著升高，CD_8^+值显著降低（$P<0.05$或$P<0.01$）。黄春合等将68例患者随机平分为两组，均予常规化疗，治疗组加服滋阴利肺汤（沙参、黄芪、怀山药、桑白皮、桔梗、百部等）。经治6个月，两组患者血清IL-6、IL-10和TNF-α水平均有明显下降（$P<0.01$或$P<0.05$），而治疗组明显优于对照组（$P<0.01$或$P<0.05$）。周玲霞等将116例耐多药患者随机平分为两组，均予常规抗痨，治疗组加服养阴润肺益气健脾汤（黄芪、生晒参、百合、白及、百部、黄精等），经治6个月，治疗组与对照组总有效率分别为91.4%(53/58)，75.9%(44/58)，$P<0.05$；两组患者血T淋巴细胞亚群CD_3^+、CD_4^+、CD_4^+/CD_8^+及血IL-12、干扰素水平较治疗前均有不同程度上升、CD_8^+水平较治疗前均有不同程度下降（$P<0.05$），且治疗组上升、下降幅度明显优于对照组（$P<0.05$）。

朱江春等对110例继发性患者按中医体质类型分类、量化，计算频率，结合临床表现探讨其证候规律。其发病节气以春季始逐渐上升，清明、谷雨季节达到高峰，夏、秋、冬季发病低。辨证为肺阴虚45例，阴虚火旺34例，气阴两虚25例，其他证型6例。阴虚型出现空洞、合并胸膜病变发生率低、病变单纯（$P<0.05$）。

（刘一博　张　玮）

【手足口病的治疗与研究】

钟雪梅等以口服清热散瘟口服液（金银花、连翘、大青叶、大黄、牛蒡子、射干等）治疗手足口病(HFMD)47例，并以口服利巴韦林颗粒治疗的44例作对照。经治3 d，两组的显效率分别为63.8%(30/47)、56.8%(25/44)，总有效率分别为93.6%(44/47)、86.4%(38/44)。姚光将80例重症HFMD患儿随机平分为两组，分别予静脉滴注利巴韦林、服用黄栀花口服液（黄芩、金银花、大黄、栀子）。经治5 d，中药组与西药组的总有效率分别为90.0%(36/40)、80.0%(32/40)，组间比较，$P<0.05$。中药组在热退、皮疹消退及易惊消退时间方面均短于西药组（$P<0.05$或$P<0.01$）。赵健雄等将90例重症HFMD患儿随机平分为两组，均予西医常规对症、支持治疗，观察组予静脉滴注热毒宁注射液、中药（水牛角、金银花、石菖蒲、川贝母、连翘、生地黄等）煎服和（生大黄、生栀子、黄连、板蓝根、藿香）保留灌肠。经治7 d，观察组在患者体温恢复正常、皮疹疱疹消退、口腔溃疡愈合及住院时间等均明显缩短于对照组（均$P<0.05$）。

姜燕等将200例HFMD口腔溃疡患儿随机平分为两组，均予静脉滴注喜炎平，治疗组予儿童型开喉剑喷剂匀喷口腔，对照组予锡类散喷涂患处。经治3～5 d，治疗组与对照组总有效率分别为95.0%(95/100)、70.0%(70/100)，组间比较，$P<0.05$。口腔溃疡愈合时间治疗组(4.0±1.5 d)显著短于对照组(6.2±2.3 d)。

王晶等从中国生物医学文献、中国期刊全文、中文科技期刊全文、万方等数据库检索2012年5月以来喜炎平注射液配合西药常规治疗HFMD的随机对照试验(RCT)进行了系统评价。有24篇RCT满足纳入标准，共2 974例患者。Meta分析结果显示，喜炎平注射液加用常规治疗组治疗HFMD总有效率优于单用常规治疗组；退热时间和皮疹消退时间均短于常规治疗组；其不良反应表现轻微，使用安全。喜炎平联合西药常规治疗可以提高HFMD的疗效，但由于该系统评价纳入研究均为中文文献且质量较差，研究间的异质性很大，上述结论尚需更多高质量的临床试验加以证实，从而为喜炎平注射液循证临床决策奠定基础。梁锦枝等从中国生物医学文献、中国期刊全文、中文科技期刊全文、万方等数据库检索从建库至 2013 年 2 月痰热清注射液治疗 HFMD 的疗效进行评价。有 39 篇满足纳入标准,其中痰热清与利巴韦林组纳入研究 12 篇,痰热清联合利巴韦林与利巴韦林组纳入研究 27 篇,共 3 289 例患者。Meta 分析结果显示,痰热清与利巴韦林相比,痰热清治疗 HFMD 的有效率更高,患者的退热时间、疱疹消退时间以及治愈时间比利巴韦林治疗更短。痰热清联合利巴韦林与利巴韦林相比,联合用药在总有效率、退热时间、疱疹消退时间以及治愈时间上更有优势。痰热清联合利巴韦林与单用痰热清治疗 HFMD 临床疗效均优于单用利巴韦林。

(王俐琼　张　玮)

[附] 参考文献

A

艾军,汪受传,戴铭,等. 麻疹中医辨证论治方法专家调查研究报告[J]. 辽宁中医杂志,2013,40(4):622

艾香英,符林春,谭行华,等. 慢性乙型肝炎患者中医证型与肝组织病理改变的相关性研究[J]. 中医学报,2013,28(4):577

C

岑玉文,谭行华,张坚生,等. 中西医结合疗法改善艾滋病合并肺部感染患者中医症候的随机对照研究[J]. 中国中药杂志,2013,38(15):2448

陈静,李茂清,符林春,等. 中国恒河猴 SIVmac239 艾滋病模型亚急性期的实验观察[J]. 中国中药杂志,2013,38(15):2463

陈潇雨,马利庄,胡义扬. 基于决策树方法的慢性乙型肝炎中医证候分类[J]. 上海中医药大学学报,2013,27(1):40

陈英杰,李慧贞,童光东,等. 补肾清透方对 e-抗原阳性乙肝病毒携带者的抗病毒疗效[J]. 中国实验方剂学杂志,2013,19(7):283

陈英杰,周大桥,童光东,等. 补肾健脾方对 HBeAg 阳性乙肝病毒携带者的免疫调节作用[J]. 中医临床研究,2013,5(12):1

D

邓华亮,王玉娟,张少军. 慢性乙型肝炎中医证候规范化研究的思考[J]. 山东中医药大学学报,2013,37(3):182

邓俊,武学华,薛玉琴,等. 补中益气丸治疗肺结核 323 例临床观察[J]. 新中医,2013,45(8):31

董慧琳,聂红明,陈逸云,等. 陈建杰教授应用"伏邪理论"诊治慢性丙型肝炎的经验[J]. 中西医结合肝病杂志,2013,23(1):54

董梦久,李耘,刘志勇,等. 醒脑静注射液治疗重型流行性乙型脑炎临床观察[J]. 光明中医,2013,28(4):682

F

樊冬梅,陶双友,陈斌. 凉血解毒方干预慢性重型肝炎疗效及内毒素受体通路研究[J]. 中国实验方剂学杂志,2013,19(2):295

冯建英,邵建国,陈琳,等. 慢性乙型肝炎中医虚实辨证与机体特异性细胞免疫及病毒复制的关系探讨[J]. 辽宁中医药大学学报,2013,15(8):136

G

高国建,邹雯,刘颖,等. 中药复方促进艾滋病免疫重建研究综述[J]. 中国中药杂志,2013,38(15):2523

高月求. 慢性乙型肝炎中医证候规律研究思路探讨[J]. 上海中医药大学学报,2013,27(2):5

郭新新,车念聪,王志强,等. 125 例慢性乙肝病毒携带者中医体质类型分布特征研究[J]. 中西医结合肝病杂志,2013,23(1):47

H

何婷,汤奇,曾南,等. 荆芥挥发油及其主要成分抗流感病毒作用与机制研究[J]. 中国中药杂志,2013,38(11):1772

胡大庆,施卫兵,王金萍,等. 轻症慢性乙型肝炎的中医证型与病理相关性研究[J]. 山西中医,2013,29(4):51

胡建华,李晓东,姚乃礼,等. 中医药诊治慢性重型肝炎研究进展述评[J]. 中西医结合肝病杂志,2013,23(2):125

怀平艾,郝芳. 小柴胡汤联合聚乙二醇干扰素 α-2a 治疗慢性丙型肝炎的临床研究[J]. 世界中西医结合杂志,2013,8(8):801

黄春合,梁烨,李天资,等. 滋阴利肺汤治疗肺结核患者炎症因子变化及其临床意义[J]. 贵阳中医学院学报,2013,35(2):16

黄少妮,贺松其. 乙型肝炎病毒携带者中医体质类型分布规律及特点研究[J]. 新中医,2013,45(10):38

J

姜桂宁,孙建光,孙程程.236例慢性HBV携带者中医证候及证候要素分布规律研究[J].山东中医杂志,2013,32(7):455

姜燕,李晓菊.开喉剑喷剂佐治手足口病口腔溃疡疗效观察[J].中国中医药信息杂志,2013,20(6):67

L

雷陵,刘志勇,夏启芝.扶正益肝颗粒对HBeAg阴性慢性乙型肝炎病毒低水平复制的影响[J].中西医结合肝病杂志,2013,23(4):199

李红山,朱德东,傅琪琳,等.慢性乙型肝炎不同中医证候机体免疫功能的动态变化[J].中华中医药学刊,2013,31(11):2391

李荣荣,杨勇,容蓉,等.麻黄细辛附子汤对肾阳虚外感模型小鼠的干预作用[J].中国实验方剂学杂志,2013,19(3):226

李湘溦,刘叔文,杨洁.茶黄素衍生物抗甲型流感病毒的作用研究[J].中草药,2013,44(17):2437

李野平,王岭,张均倡,等.以肝脏大体形态学联合组织学变化探讨中西医治疗乙肝肝硬化的效果[J].时珍国医国药,2013,24(7):1738

李燚光,华忠,薛博瑜.薛博瑜教授运用犀角地黄汤合四逆散治疗慢性丙型肝炎经验[J].辽宁中医药大学学报,2013,15(2):192

梁锦枝,罗钦宏,方乙生,等.痰热清注射液治疗手足口病疗效评价的Meta分析[J].中国循证医学杂志,2013,13(12):1446

林巧,刘腊香,张国良,等.益肾固本法对慢性HBV携带者外周血干扰素调节因子-4表达的影响[J].中西医结合肝病杂志,2013,23(3):136

刘嵋松,孙良梅,王胜圣,等.中西医结合疗法治疗初治继发性肺结核病的临床疗效及安全性评价[J].中国中医药信息杂志,2013,20(9):6

刘琪,顾立刚,周旭澎,等.疏风宣肺及解表清里方药对流感病毒感染小鼠肺损伤的保护研究[J].中华中医药杂志,2013,28(7):2132

刘蓉,苟玲,于柳,等.桂枝挥发油与桂皮醛对病毒性肺炎小鼠死亡保护作用及TLR/IFN信号机制研究[J].中药药理与临床,2013,29(4):33

刘巍,王阶.透邪在艾滋病发热中的运用[J].中国中药杂志,2013,38(15):2513

刘旭,张富永,王立娟,等.从"主客交"学说浅谈慢性丙型肝炎的中医证治[J].黑龙江中医药,2013,42(1):6

刘一博,张玮,张永煜,等.慢性乙型肝炎肝气郁结证患者血液代谢指纹图谱研究初探[J].中西医结合肝病杂志,2013,23(1):7

刘震,王阶,林洪生,等.中药免疫2号方对艾滋病患者免疫重建的研究[J].中国中药杂志,2013,38(15):2458

刘忠达,张尊敬,李权,等.中西医结合治疗肺结核临床研究[J].中华中医药学刊,2013,31(4):758

刘忠第,张轩,贺娟.基于"3年化疫"理论探讨气象因素与北京地区痢疾发病的关系[J].北京中医药大学学报,2013,36(4):258

龙富立,毛德文,盛庆寿,等.解毒化瘀颗粒对慢性重型肝炎患者血清细胞因子的影响[J].中西医结合肝病杂志,2013,23(1):11

M

马文峰,周小舟,孙新锋,等.中药治疗肝衰竭患者内毒素血症及其检测方法[J].中西医结合肝病杂志,2013,23(2):107

N

聂凡,童光东,周大桥.导致慢性HBV携带者肝脏病理学改变的相关因素[J].中西医结合肝病杂志,2013,23(1):61

P

浦忠平,花海兵.肝炎一号方治疗重度慢性乙型肝炎48例[J].实用中西医结合临床,2013,13(3):19

R

任郭侠,董琪,张熙祎.丹参滴注液辅助治疗空洞型肺结核40例[J].陕西中医,2013,34(1):35

S

沈健,陈建杰,商斌仪,等.丙肝冲剂治疗难治性丙型肝炎研究[J].现代中西医结合杂志,2013,22(18):1947

石清兰,袁果,毛德文,等.解毒化瘀颗粒对慢性重型肝炎患者外周血单个核细胞Toll样受体4表达调控的研究[J].中西医结合肝病杂志,2013,23(2):76

苏立稳,赵凯丰,王国华.恩替卡韦联合复方肝欣合剂治疗失代偿期乙型肝炎肝硬化临床研究[J].中西医结合肝病杂志,2013,23(2):86

孙丽梅,王军,苏海涛,等.小柴胡汤加减治疗甲型H1N1流感61例[J].山东中医杂志,2013,32(6):399

T

汤巧玲,马师雷,刘宏伟,等.北京地区1970～2004年猩红热发病与六气及气象因子的相关性研究[J].北京中医药大学学报,2013,36(5):333

唐晓琦,徐文琦,成小娇.加减保真汤配合抗痨强化期治疗复治菌阳肺结核的疗效[J].中医临床研究,2013,5(8):88

田凌云,吴哲,邓桂元,等.中药联合派罗欣及利巴韦林治疗慢性丙型肝炎32例[J].中西医结合肝病杂志,2013,23(4):247

童佳兵,李泽庚,刘健,等.基于建国以来中医疫病预测预警的研究方法与思路探讨[J].中医药临床杂志,2013,25(1):6

W

王健,邹雯,刘颖.中西药治疗艾滋病疗效作用点比较分析[J].中国中药杂志,2013,38(15):2504

王阶,汤艳莉,李勇,等.中医干预对艾滋病免疫重建不全患者TCRVβ基因CDR3区克隆片断的影响[J].中国中药杂志,2013,38(15):2424

王阶,吴欣芳,李勇,等.HIV/AIDS免疫异常激活及其与疾病进展的相关性研究[J].中国中药杂志,2013,38(15):2429

王晶,任吉祥,谢雁鸣,等.喜炎平注射液治疗手足口病的系统评价[J].中国中药杂志,2013,38(18):3215

王轩,陈斌,彭杰,等.温阳解毒化瘀颗粒对肝衰竭内毒素血症大鼠肠道sIgA的影响[J].中西医结合肝病杂志,2013,23(3):157

王园,戴恩来,贾忠.虫草抗痨胶囊配合化疗治疗继发性肺结核614例回顾性分析[J].中医杂志,2013,54(15):1304

王志强,车念聪,郭新新,等.慢性乙肝病毒携带者中医体质类型与T淋巴细胞亚群相关性研究[J].中西医结合肝病杂志,2013,23(2):79

文晓涛,毛德文,张荣臻.慢性乙型肝炎重症化倾向期证候规律及治疗方案研究[J].长春中医药大学学报,2013,29(1):39

吴欣芳,王阶,李勇.免疫1号方联合HAART对HIV/AIDS患者免疫功能重建的干预研究[J].中国中药杂志,2013,38(15):2453

吴银亚,谭善忠,沈建军,等.慢性乙型肝炎病毒携带者中医证候分布特点[J].中医药信息,2013,30(5):20

X

向燕,徐培平,符林春,等.冰香散挥发油对流感病毒感染鼠的预防作用及T淋巴细胞亚群的影响[J].广州中医药大学学报,2013,30(2):214

熊兴江,杨晓忱,刘巍,等.经典名方与艾滋病治疗[J].中国中药杂志,2013,38(15):2510

熊益居,杨建平.中西医结合治疗流行性腮腺炎并发前庭神经元炎9例[J].福建中医药,2013,44(4):28

徐立然,杨小平,郭会军,等.中医药辨证施治对HIV感染者生存质量影响的初步探讨[J].中国中药杂志,2013,38(15):2480

许文君,李秀惠,李红艳,等.聚乙二醇干扰素联合利巴韦林对慢性丙型肝炎患者中医辨证分型的影响[J].北京中医药,2013,32(4):269

Y

杨华升,勾春燕,李晶滢,等.慢性乙型重型肝炎中医辨证分型与实验室指标及并发症相关性分析[J].中西医结合肝病杂志,2013,23(2):70

杨丽莎,梁志清,范剑薇,等.慢性HBV感染不同免疫状态中医证型特点的研究[J].南京中医药大学学报,2013,29(4):324

杨晓云.参苓白术散加减治疗老年性肺结核气阴两虚夹瘀证30例总结[J].湖南中医杂志,2013,29(5):45

姚光.黄栀花口服液治疗重症手足口病40例疗效观察[J].中医儿科杂志,2013,9(1):46

于晓雯,薛博瑜.难治性丙型肝炎中西医治疗研究[J].长春中医药大学学报,2013,29(1):97

Z

张富永,陈逸云,刘旭,等.慢性丙型肝炎与慢性乙型肝炎中医证治比较研究[J].湖南中医杂志,2013,29(5):5

张轩,祖丽胡玛尔·艾尼瓦尔,刘忠第,等.基于运气理论探讨伤寒副伤寒与气象因素的相关性并建立预测模型[J].北京中医药大学学报,2013,36(5):797

赵健雄,何玉明,马孝涛,等.清热解毒开窍醒神法治疗重症手足口病90例[J].中国实验方剂学杂志,2013,19(17):316

赵庆,魏嵋,刘友平,等.免疫球蛋白J链与慢性乙肝中医证候肝纤维化相关性研究初探[J].辽宁中医药大学学报,2013,15(5):115

赵瑞敏,张志强.苦参素联合聚乙二醇化干扰素α-2a和利巴韦林治疗慢性丙型肝炎50例[J].中医研究,2013,26(7):37

钟雪梅,张艳玲,郑崇光,等.清热散瘟口服液治疗小儿手足口病[J].中国实验方剂学杂志,2013,19(7):345

周杰,王胜圣,于春江,等.双百口服液治疗初治继发性肺结核172例临床观察[J].世界中西医结合杂志,2013,8(8):784

周玲霞,黄金鹏,楼敏.中西医联合治疗耐多药肺结核病的临床疗效观察[J].中华中医药学刊,2013,31(4):942

朱江春,许兰竹.继发性肺结核发病季节、中医体质与证候及合并空洞、胸膜病变系统综述[J].实用中医内科杂志,2013,27(12上):1

（三）肿　瘤

【概述】

2013 年公开发表的中医药防治恶性肿瘤的相关文献近 1 700 篇。其中，实体瘤研究论文约占 77.5%，血液系统恶性肿瘤约占 22.5%。本年度有关支气管肺癌、肝癌、癌性贫血、恶性肿瘤并发抑郁的治疗与研究，以及预防肿瘤多药耐药的研究、中医药与微创技术联合治疗恶性肿瘤等详见专条。

1. 病种研究

在实体瘤研究方面，按照实体瘤病种排名，发表论文篇数依次为肺癌、乳腺癌、胃癌、肝癌、食管癌、结直肠癌、胰腺癌、膀胱癌、甲状腺癌。总体分析可以看出，中医界关注与研究最多的前五位肿瘤（肺癌、乳腺癌、胃癌、肝癌、食管癌）与《2013 年中国肿瘤登记年报》病种基本一致。在血液肿瘤研究方面，改变了既往以增效为主的研究思路，而关注更多的是如何预防骨髓肿瘤性疾病如骨髓增生异常综合征向急性白血病转化速度与转化率，重点对西医尚缺乏疗效的难治与复发白血病及老年性白血病的中医药综合治疗，并把提高老龄人群急性白血病患者生活质量、稳定病情作为重点研究内容之一。在淋巴系统肿瘤如恶性淋巴瘤、多发性骨髓瘤等研究方面，更多地主张扶正为主的治疗，强调通过中医药干预措施来提高患者免疫功能或机体自稳状态，争取免疫系统的功能恢复和增强免疫监视效果。

2. 临床研究

尽管肿瘤发生和死亡率居高不下，但与肿瘤诊断检测技术进展相比，除手术能够治愈性切除早期无转移的肿瘤病灶外，对于中晚期恶性肿瘤的治疗尚没有取得实质性进展。相反，手术切除后与中晚期患者过度放化疗等密集的治疗并没有使患者在群体治疗中受益。同时，肿瘤本身以及密集治疗带来的相关并发症，如癌性相关抑郁状态、癌性疼痛、化疗厌食导致的恶病质、癌性乏力症状、癌性贫血、癌性相关失眠、吗啡控制癌痛导致的便秘、肿瘤高凝状态以及放化疗导致的骨髓抑制、末梢神经病变、皮疹等已经构成癌症患者产生新的“痛苦”状态，这些“痛苦”状态可严重影响患者生存质量，并使生存时间缩短。因此，目前已有趋势重新审视中医药在治疗癌症或控制癌症进展中的优劣势，并基于中医药治疗肿瘤特点和现实，把主要研究方向定位于控制肿瘤及其治疗相关并发症，将稳定中晚期患者肿瘤病灶、提高患者生存质量与延长生存时间作为治疗的终点事件，并组织全国或区域性大协作实践上述研究目标。如北京市科委在京组织由 8 家三级甲等中医医院牵头，并联合在京的三级甲等西医医院与部分区县级医院实施的科技重大科技攻关项目“中医药提升恶性肿瘤疗效系统研究”，明确将“中医药治疗乳腺癌疲乏症临床研究”（首都医科大学北京市中医医院）、“中医药治疗胃癌贫血与高凝状态的临床研究”（北京中医药大学东直门医院）、“中医药治疗胃瘫等恶性肿瘤术后并发症的临床研究”（北京中医药大学东方医院）、“恶性肿瘤疼痛及胸、腹腔积液中医药外治法规范化临床研究”（卫生部中日友好医院）、“放射性皮肤损伤等恶性肿瘤治疗相关不良反应外治法规范化临床研究”（中国中医科学院广安门医院）5 大肿瘤及其治疗相关并发症列为重点研究内容。

3. 基础研究

本年度，中医药防治肿瘤基础研究文献多集中在中医药综合抗肿瘤效应机制研究如诱导肿瘤细胞凋亡、调节免疫机制、针对肿瘤基因的调控研究、中医药的增效与减毒等。但有两个值得关注的热点研究正在悄然崛起，一是选择肿瘤表观遗传学指标，探讨中医药抗肿瘤效位靶点；二是针对肿瘤高甲基化的特点，研究中医药调控肿瘤甲基化过程与去甲基化治疗。由于此类研究刚刚起步，尽管研究尚处于初浅层次，但预测可能形成今后中医药抗肿瘤研究的热点方向之一。

（陈信义）

【肺癌的治疗及实验研究】

乔新梅等将 80 例辨证为瘀阻肺络证的小细胞肺癌患者随机平分为两组，治疗组应用 EP 方案化疗联合血府逐瘀汤治疗,对照组单纯 EP 方案化疗。经治 4 个月,治疗组缓解率及控制率分别为 85.0%(34/40)、57.5%(23/40),对照组分别为 62.5%(25/40)、32.5%(13/40),组间比较,均 $P<0.05$。卢利员等将 92 例晚期非小细胞肺癌(NSCLC)患者分为中药(北沙参、麦冬、百部、鱼腥草、山海螺、太子参等)+化疗(采用含铂方案)组 31 例、单纯化疗组 31 例、单纯中药组 30 例。经治 3 个月,三组缓解率分别为 45.2%(14/31)、41.9%(13/31)、20.0%(6/30),稳定率分别为 80.6%(25/31)、54.8%(17/31)、80.0%(24/30),组间比较,均 $P<0.05$。中药+化疗组出现的Ⅲ度至Ⅳ度骨髓抑制明显低于单纯化疗组($P<0.05$)。束家和等将 70 例 NSCLC 患者随机平分为两组,治疗组以养正消积胶囊(黄芪、莪术、女贞子、人参、灵芝、绞股蓝等)联合 GP 方案化疗,对照组单纯用 GP 方案化疗。经治 42 d,治疗组总有效率为 48.6%(17/35),对照组为 31.4%(11/35),组间比较,$P<0.05$。陈志刚等将 106 例晚期 NSCLC 患者随机分为两组,均予多西紫杉醇+顺铂方案化疗;治疗组 54 例加用艾迪注射液(黄芪、人参、刺五加、斑蝥等)静脉滴注。经治 12 周,总有效率分别为 64.8%(35/54)、48.1%(25/52),组间比较,$P<0.05$。黄新宇将 98 例晚期 NSCLC 患者分为治疗组(GP 方案化疗联合复方苦参注射液静脉滴注+全身热疗)50 例与对照组(GP 方案化疗)48 例。经治 2 个月,有效率分别为 58.0%(29/50)、37.5%(18/48),组间比较,$P<0.05$。刘礼荣等将 74 例不可手术的肺腺癌患者随机平分为对照组(GP 方案化疗)与观察组(GP 方案化疗联合鸦胆子油乳注射液静脉滴注)。经治 42 d,观察组与对照组有效率分别为 56.8%(21/37)、37.8(14/37),组间比较,$P<0.05$。

顾恪波等总结分析孙桂芝治疗肺癌的常用方剂千金苇茎汤、清燥救肺汤、百合固金汤。在千金苇茎汤的基础上伍以金荞麦化痈排脓,助脾胃、除湿气。因肺癌常见气阴两虚之证,病因多源于燥热之邪,加之鳞癌、小细胞癌常用放射疗法,易于损伤津液,故多用清燥救肺汤随证治之。百合固金汤可清热解毒、凉血止血、养阴涵阳,适用于肺鳞癌及小细胞癌的阴虚血热证。李柏颖总结宋康治疗肺癌的经验。正虚邪实是其辨证总纲,热毒是主要致病邪气。根据患者体质的强弱,热毒的轻重,常选用三叶青、山海螺、白花蛇舌草、藤梨根、野荞麦根、虎杖等;顾护脾胃是扶正要诀,常以参苓白术散为基础化裁以达到生化气血、增强抗病能力的目的;同时根据患者的具体情况采用化痰、活血、利水等方法,驱除痰瘀水湿。郑健等介绍庞德湘治疗肺癌擅用药对,常用泽漆配石见穿,桂枝配泽漆,瓜蒌配薤白,浙贝母配牡蛎,白芥子配制天南星,仙鹤草配白及,附子配细辛,青蒿配鳖甲,蜂房配红豆杉,补骨脂配自然铜,全蝎配蜈蚣。

杨小兵等采用回顾性研究方法调查晚期 NSCLC(207 例ⅢB 和Ⅳ期)患者的证型分布规律,结果显示,气虚痰湿证占 76.3%,气阴两虚证占 9.2%,气滞血瘀证、阴虚毒热证及热毒炽盛证分别占 5.8%、5.8%、2.9%。

艾叶盛等以苦寒泻下法建立小鼠脾气虚证 Lewis 肺癌模型,随机分为模型组,黄芪建中汤高(1.32 g/ml)、中(0.66 g/ml)、低(0.33 g/ml)剂量组,环磷酰胺组。灌胃给药 15 d 后,与模型组比较,黄芪建中汤中高剂量组、环磷酰胺组胸腺指数、CD44/β-actin 比值、nm23-mRNA/β-actin 比值均升高($P<0.05$,$P<0.01$)。提示黄芪建中汤对脾气虚证肺癌小鼠肿瘤的转移具有一定的抑制作用,其机制可能与提高胸腺指数、下调 CD44-mRNA 及上调 nm23 的表达有关。张宏方等将大鼠随机分组灌胃给药 5 d,制备调衡方(生黄芪、生山药、白花蛇舌草、西洋参、天花粉、莪术等)大(32 g/kg)、中(18 g/kg)、小(9 g/kg)剂量含药血清,正常血清。又将细胞分为 5 组,即正常血清组(不含药血清组),大、中、小剂量含药血清组,中剂量含药血清+AG490(JAK-STAT 信号通路特异性抑制剂)干预组,分别孵育 Lewis 肺癌细胞株 24 h 后,检测结果显示,与不含药血清组比较,Lewis 肺癌细胞经调衡方大、小剂量含药血清作用后,细胞内 stat3、stat5 蛋白表达均显著下降(均$P<0.01$)。提示调衡方含药血清能显著抑制 Lewis 肺癌细胞增殖,促进其凋亡,其机制可能与下调 stat3、stat5 的基因表达,抑制细胞信号转导通路有关。曹洋等对邓铁涛治疗肺癌验方——金福安汤(生南星、生半夏、太子参、苇茎、生薏仁、桃仁等)进行研究,培养 A549 细胞,随机分为空白对照组,金福安汤高(4.29 g/d)、中(2.145 g/d)、低(0.429 g/d)剂量组,环磷酰胺组,分别予含空白血清和含药血清培养液干预。

结果与空白对照组比较，各给药组A549细胞OD值均显著降低（均$P<0.01$），金福安汤各剂量组OD值且呈剂量相关性。金福安汤中剂量组A549细胞p120ctn磷酸化程度较空白对照组显著降低，中、高剂量组A549细胞的黏附能力较空白对照组增强，各剂量组A549细胞的迁移能力较空白对照组减弱（均$P<0.05$）。提示金福安汤具有较强的抑瘤作用，呈药物剂量相关性，其可抑制p120ctn磷酸化，从而抑制癌细胞的迁移。丁纪元研究古方息贲丸（厚朴、黄连、干姜、桂枝、巴豆霜、白茯苓等）抗肺癌作用。将Lewis肺癌小鼠分为模型组，环磷酰胺组，息贲丸高（0.013 g/g）、中（0.039 g/g）、低（0.026 g/g）剂量组，灌胃给药15 d。结果显示，息贲丸高、中、低剂量组的抑瘤率分别为56.47%、47.84%、44.96%。与模型组比较，息贲丸各剂量组中Caspase-3的表达升高，Caspase-8表达降低（均$P<0.01$）。李秀荣等制备六神丸含药血清，体外分为对照组、六神丸组（5%、10%、15%浓度）、顺铂（DDP）组、联合用药组（10%六神丸药血清+DDP组）干预肺癌A549细胞，与对照组比较，六神丸药血清各浓度组、DDP组、联合用药组的Caspase-3阳性率均明显升高，联合用药组的Caspase-3阳性率明显高于六神丸各浓度组及DDP组（均$P<0.05$）；六神丸含药血清各浓度组、DDP组及联合用药组的Survivin相对灰度值均明显降低，联合用药组的Survivin相对灰度值明显低于六神丸各浓度组及DDP组（均$P<0.05$）。提示六神丸具有诱导肺癌A549细胞凋亡的作用，与顺铂联合应用可产生协同作用，其机理与上调Caspase-3表达和下调Survivin表达有关。李妍等将Lewis肺癌瘤源小鼠随机分为模型组、环磷酰胺组、姜黄素组，灌胃给药13 d，与模型组比较，姜黄素组瘤组织TGF-β_1、Smad3表达均降低（均$P<0.05$），Smad7表达增加（$P<0.01$）。提示姜黄素对于小鼠Lewis肺癌原发瘤的生长具有一定的抑制作用，并能抑制肿瘤组织微血管形成，其作用靶点可能与其上调Smad7和下调Smad3蛋白表达，从而减少TGF-β_1在肺癌血管生长过程中的过度表达有关。易亚乔等以体外培养肺腺癌细胞系A549细胞，MTT法检测桔梗总皂苷对其增殖的影响，并以Giemsa染色法观察细胞形态学变化，流式细胞术检测桔梗总皂苷对A549细胞周期的影响。结果显示，不同浓度（50、40、30、20、10、5、2.5 μg/ml）的桔梗总皂苷能明显抑制人肺腺癌A549细胞的增殖，其抑制作用随药物浓度的增加而增强，呈剂量依赖关系（$P<0.05$）。不同浓度的桔梗总皂苷均能促细胞凋亡，细胞周期被阻滞于G_0/G_1期，其凋亡率随药物浓度增高而增加（$P<0.05$）。

（田劭丹）

【肝癌的治疗与研究】

韩克起等将原发性肝癌患者93例随机分为两组，治疗组47例以扶正解毒方（生黄芪、炒白术、石见穿、石上柏、石打穿、猫人参等）并随症加减联合肝动脉栓塞化疗（TACE）治疗，对照组单纯以TACE治疗。经治4周，两组中位生存期分别为17个月、11个月；1年生存率分别为74.5%（35/47）、69.6%（32/46），组间比较，$P<0.05$；中位疾病进展时间分别为158 d、87 d，组间比较，$P<0.05$。陈强松等将60例晚期原发性肝癌患者平分为两组，均予对症支持疗法（兰索拉唑、苦参素氯化钠、多烯磷脂胆硷、联苯双脂丸、肌苷、维生素K_1、葡醛内酯、盐酸普萘洛尔、人血白蛋白或血浆等），治疗组加用健脾抑瘤汤（黄芪、党参、土炒白术、茯苓、陈皮、白花蛇舌草等）治疗。疗程均为60 d，治疗组与对照组总改善率分别为83.3%（25/30）、60.0%（18/30），组间比较，$P<0.05$。Zhai XF等将小肝癌切除术后患者随机分为以华蟾素注射液静滴联合解毒颗粒（猫人参、石见穿、山慈菇、鸡内金）口服的中药组188例与TACE组191例，经治6个月，除中药组3例、TACE组1例未完成治疗外，中药组复发67例，TACE组87例，组间比较，$P<0.05$；无复发的中位生存期中药组为46.89个月，TACE组为34.49个月；第1、2、3年的中药组复发率分别为17.7%（33/185）、33.0%（61/185）、43.5%（80/185），TACE组分别为28.8%（55/190）、42.5%（81/190）、54.0%（103/190），组间比较，均$P<0.05$。

何立丽等总结孙桂芝治疗肝癌经验，其在肝脏“体阴用阳”理论的指导下，常用三甲汤、化纤通络方、益气柔肝方、辛散止痛方和藤虎汤等进行辨病辨证治疗。夏宁俊总结章永红辨治肝癌经验，其病机特点为本虚标实，本虚主要为脾胃虚弱、肝阴亏虚及肾精不足，标实主要为气滞、血瘀、水湿、癌毒，治疗首当辨清虚实之异，强调健运脾胃、保护胃气贯穿治疗始终。肖跃红认为肝癌病机的本质因素是正气亏虚，关键因素是癌毒内发，促进因素是血瘀、痰湿、热毒、气滞,治疗以扶正祛邪、辨证论治为主。

杨素芳等基于365例肝癌患者的62项中医四诊信息,采用主成分法分析患者围介入治疗前的中医证型,得出5类四诊信息群并对应5种证型,分别为脾虚证、肝郁证、湿热证、血瘀证和阴虚证。杨小兵等对151例原发性肝癌患者进行证候分析,发现其证型出现率由高到低分别为湿瘀互结证、肝郁脾虚证、气滞血瘀证、湿热蕴结证及肝肾阴虚证,结合各证型的生存期分析,发现肝郁脾虚证预后较好,而肝肾阴虚证预后最差。

方肇勤等以MTT法观察肝癌常用代表方(清热解毒方+行气活血方+健脾益气方)及其清热(半枝莲、白花蛇舌草、蒲公英)、活血(柴胡、八月札、丹参、桃仁、赤芍药、茵陈等)、健脾(白术、薏苡仁、黄芪、白芍药、神曲、云苓等)等拆方联合G418对人肝癌细胞株SMMC-7721肝癌细胞及转染MTs iRNA质粒肝癌细胞增殖的抑制作用。并与转染表达绿荧光蛋白质粒进行对照。结果显示,代表方及不同拆方具有不同程度的抑制肝癌细胞增殖作用,且存在量效关系,联合G418用药后作用显著增强($P<0.05$)。G418给药1 d后撤药,2 d后肝癌细胞出现增殖加速;代表方、清热方、活血方、健脾方等联合G418后撤药2 d,细胞增殖仍不活跃(均$P<0.05$)。提示不同治法中药联合G418用药具有显著抑制肝癌细胞恶性增殖,并减缓停药后细胞增殖反跳的作用。陈培丰等建立小鼠H_{22}肝癌模型,随机分为空白对照组,龙葵(龙葵正丁醇萃取物)高(4.550 g/kg)、中(2.275)、低(1.1375 g/kg)剂量组,5-氟尿嘧啶(5-Fu)组,空白对照组及龙葵各剂量组予灌胃给药,5-Fu组予腹腔注射给药。10 d后显示,与空白对照组比较,龙葵中剂量组的胸腺指数、脾脏指数显著增高(均$P<0.05$),5-Fu组显著性降低($P<0.01$)。与空白对照组比较,龙葵中剂量组和5-Fu组血清IFN-γ、TNF-α含量增加($P<0.05$,$P<0.01$)。龙葵高、中、低剂量组的抑瘤率分别为28.96%、44.36%、37.91%,5-Fu组为46.74%。提示龙葵正丁醇萃取物对小鼠H_{22}肝癌移植瘤的生长具有一定的抑制作用,以中剂量效果最佳,其机理可能与改善荷瘤机体细胞因子异常,调节机体免疫功能有关。张斌等将大鼠随机分为正常组、模型组、中药组,后两组以DEN诱导建立肝癌模型,中药组予健脾解毒方剂(生黄芪、白术、猪苓、八月札、石见穿、野葡萄藤等)灌胃12周。结果显示,中药组死亡率为17.5%,16~20周腹水发生率为44.4%;模型组死亡率为42.5%,16~20周腹水发生率为87.5%,组间比较,均$P<0.05$。

(顾　瞻)

【癌性贫血的治疗及实验研究】

张弦以八珍汤随证加减治疗恶性肿瘤放、化疗后骨髓抑制患者30例,设对照组30例予西药对症治疗,经治14 d,治疗组中医症状疗效总有效率为90.0%(27/30),对照组为50.0%(15/30),组间比较,$P<0.05$。治疗组WBC计数下降幅度较对照组小($P<0.05$)。蒋立峰等将66例恶性肿瘤患者随机平分为两组,均予常规化疗方案,治疗组加服当归补血汤。经治4周,治疗组血红蛋白数显著高于对照组,Ⅲ+Ⅳ度白细胞血小板及血红蛋白减少的人次明显低于对照组(均$P<0.05$)。临床症状、生活质量情况的改善均优于对照组(均$P<0.05$)。赵增虎等将72例中、晚期非小细胞肺癌随机分为两组,均予吉西他宾+顺铂化疗方案治疗,治疗组35例加服益气补血片(人参、当归、黄芪、大枣、制何首乌、陈皮等)。经治9周,治疗组红细胞计数、血小板计数高于对照组(均$P<0.05$),两组骨髓抑制率分别为40.0%(14/35)、81.1%(30/37),组间比较,$P<0.05$。林洪生等将118例非小细胞肺癌化疗患者随机分为两组,对照组56例单纯化疗,治疗组加服生血丸(鹿茸、黄柏、炒白术、山药、紫河车等),疗程均为42 d。两组证候疗效总有效率分别为37.5%(21/56)、74.2%(46/62),组间比较,$P<0.01$。化疗期间两组血象均出现不同程度下降,对照组下降幅度较治疗组更为明显(均$P<0.01$)。唐丽雯等选取60例肿瘤患者随机分为两组,治疗组自化疗第1 d起服用健脾补肾膏方(龟板胶、鳖甲、党参、枸杞子、女贞子、旱莲草等)及中药汤剂(按不同病种常规辨证分型论治),对照组单纯予中药汤剂,疗程均为21 d。结果治疗组发生Ⅲ~Ⅳ度骨髓抑制的频次较对照组明显减少($P<0.01$),化疗后2周,治疗组外周血血红蛋白下降幅度比对照组小($P<0.05$)。

黄云胜将72例晚期恶性肿瘤患者随机分为治疗组与对照组,均予常规对症支持治疗,治疗组加用艾迪注射液(黄芪、人参、刺五加、斑蝥等)联合参麦注射液静脉滴注。经治30 d,治疗组血红蛋白、红细胞计数较治疗前有显著提高（$P<0.01$），并优于对照组（$P<0.01$）。郑召鹏等将61例晚期非小细胞肺癌患者随机分为两组，对照组单纯化疗，治疗组同时予黄芪多糖静脉滴注，连续给药10 d。结果治疗组4周期化疗按时、足量完成率为84.4%（27/32），对照组为62.1%（18/29），组间比较，$P<0.05$。治疗组骨髓抑制发生率为31.3%（10/32），对照组为58.6%（17/29），组间比较，$P<0.05$，且治疗组未出现重度（Ⅲ、Ⅳ度）骨髓抑制。李潇等将98例辨证为气血两虚证的中晚期恶性肿瘤伴有贫血患者随机分成两组，均予常规治疗，治疗组50例加服复方阿胶浆（阿胶、红参、熟地黄、党参、山楂等）。经治4周，两组患者红细胞、血红蛋白水平均较治疗前升高；其中在化疗患者中第3、4周此两项指标治疗组优于对照组。非化疗患者中治疗组第3、4周此两项指标较治疗前升高，对照组第4周此两项指标较治疗前升高，治疗组优于对照组（均$P<0.05$）。治疗组在改善临床症状方面优于对照组。

曹娟等建立H_{22}小鼠腹水模型，随机分为模型组、当归补血汤组，灌胃给药10 d，并设正常组对照。结果与正常组相比，模型组红细胞数及血红蛋白含量明显减少（均$P<0.05$），与模型组比较，当归补血汤组红细胞数、血红蛋白均有所上升（$P<0.05$），提示当归补血汤可有效修复骨髓造血干细胞延缓其凋亡速度。

（侯　丽　郭晓青）

【恶性肿瘤并发抑郁的治疗】

陈震宏等将107例乳腺癌术后焦虑抑郁患者随机分为两组，均予常规化疗，治疗组54例加服疏络散结汤（太子参、香附、夏枯草、百合、怀小麦、当归等）。治疗2个月，两组患者抑郁自评量表、焦虑自评量表积分均较治疗前明显降低（均$P<0.05$），以治疗组更为显著（均$P<0.05$）。杨玉兴等将112例消化系统癌症并发抑郁症患者随机分为消痰解郁方（法半夏、制南星、柴胡、陈皮、当归、白术等）治疗组、中药（逍遥丸）对照组及西药（盐酸氟西汀）对照组，经治6周，治疗组、中药对照组、西药对照组总有效率分别为82.5%（47/57）、53.6%（15/28）、70.4%（19/27），治疗组与中药对照组比较有显著性差异（$P<0.05$），与西药对照组比较无显著性差异（$P>0.05$）。各组汉密顿抑郁量表总分均降低，其中治疗组最低（$P<0.01$，$P<0.05$）。贾玫等将肿瘤相关性抑郁患者随机分为艾迪注射液（黄芪、人参、刺五加、斑蝥等）治疗组52例与复方苦参注射液对照组55例。治疗14 d，总有效率分别为40.0%（22/55）、28.8%（15/52），组间比较，$P<0.05$。

吕晓皑等将112例乳腺癌阈下抑郁患者随机平分为两组，均予常规乳腺癌药物治疗，治疗组加用中医团体情志疗法，为期8周，每周1次。结果与对照组比较，治疗组抑郁自评量表分值下降，生命质量测定量表分值升高（$P<0.01$，$P<0.05$）。胡淑贤等将120例首次接受化学治疗的乳腺癌改良根治术后患者均分为莫扎特音乐干预组（莫扎特音乐化疗）、梁祝音乐干预组（梁祝音乐化疗）、对照组（单纯化疗）。音乐干预每日2次，每次60 min，共42 d。结果治疗后莫扎特音乐干预组化疗后抑郁自评量表、焦虑自评量表分值均降低，但无显著性差异（均$P>0.05$），梁祝音乐干预组两自评量表亦降低，且有显著性差异（均$P<0.05$）。

（贾　玫）

【肿瘤多药耐药性的研究】

1. 血液系统肿瘤

刘思等研究解毒化瘀方（青黛、川芎、莪术、山慈姑、丹参、虎杖等）对HL60/VCR白血病细胞耐药株多药耐药的影响。制备含解毒化瘀药的高（9 g/kg）、中（6 g/kg）、低（3 g/kg）剂量兔血清培养HL60/VCR白血病细胞耐药株并进行检测。结果显示，多药耐药基因P-糖蛋白（P-gp）在HL60/VCR细胞中呈高表达，在HL60细胞中呈低表达，经不同剂量的解毒化瘀方含药血清处理后，HL60/VCR细胞P-gp的表达均明显降低（均$P<0.05$）。提示含解毒化瘀药的兔血清逆转HL60/VCR白血病细胞耐药株耐药性与下调P-gp的表达有关。王博等通过四甲基偶氮唑蓝（MTT）法研究白花蛇舌草活性成分之一熊果酸（UAHD）对白血病K562/ADM细胞株的生长抑制作用及诱导凋亡情况。结果显示，不同浓度的UAHD（1.25 mg/ml、2.5 mg/ml、5 mg/ml、10 mg/ml）作用于K562/ADM细胞株24 h抑制率分别为：7.2%、10.6%、16.0%、75.6%，48 h抑制率分别为：33.0%、39.0%、51.1%、61.6%，72 h抑制率分别为：34.1%、52.2%、72.7%、64.9%。作用于K562/ADM细胞株48 h细胞凋亡率分别为：3.2%、8.8%、17.8%、23.5%。不

同浓度的UAHD作用后，K562/ADM细胞株内谷胱甘肽(GSH)含量下降，谷胱甘肽-S转移酶(GST)活性先升高后下降，谷胱甘肽过氧化物酶(GSH-PX)活性先升高后下降，丙二醛(MDA)含量随UAHD浓度及作用时间的增加而增加。以上各组指标均具有较明显的剂量和时间的依赖性(均$P<0.05$)。提示UAHD能够诱导K562/ADM细胞凋亡，凋亡的机制与细胞内氧化应激反应有关。陈英玉等采用MTT法检测急性白血病HL-60/ADR细胞对大黄素以及8种临床常用化疗药物的耐药性，结果显示，大黄素对HL-60/ADR耐药株和相应HL-60细胞敏感株的IC_{50}值接近，对阿霉素(ADR)、柔红霉素(DNR)、依托泊苷(VPl6)、长春新碱(VCR)、阿糖胞苷(Ara-C)、高三尖杉酯碱(HHT)、米托蒽醌(MTZ)和吡柔比星(THP)呈现不同程度耐药。小剂量大黄素对8种药物耐药逆转倍数介于1.58～4.12之间，其中对ADR的耐药细胞逆转效果最好($P<0.05$)。与单药组比较，大黄素与ADR联合用药组MRPl、TOPOⅡB、GSTπ、BCL-2耐药相关基因mRNA和蛋白表达水平下调明显，细胞内ADR和DNR蓄积水平增加，胞浆和胞核DNR分布增加，该作用与大黄素呈浓度依赖性。提示大黄素具有逆转HL-60/ADR细胞多药耐药作用，可能与其下调耐药相关基因表达水平、增加细胞内化疗药物蓄积和促进细胞凋亡作用有关。王相朦等以MTT法检测ADM对耐ADM的急性髓系白血病HL-60细胞株(HL-60/ADM)耐药情况及雷公藤甲素(TPL)对其增殖抑制作用，检测IC_{20}浓度TPL联合不同浓度的ADM对HL-60/ADM的增殖抑制作用和两者之间的相互作用。结果显示，ADM对野生株HL-60细胞和ADM耐药细胞株24 h的IC_{20}值分别为(0.28±0.35)umol/L和(22.03±0.22)umol/L，耐药细胞株的耐药倍数为78.68。TPL作用于HL-60/ADM细胞48 h的IC_{20}值为(43.06±1.06)umol/L。48 h的IC_{20} TPL可使ADM对HL-60/ADM的IC_{20}值下降，逆转耐药倍数为1.82倍($P<0.01$)。在抑制率小于60%的情况下，ADM与TPL有协同作用。两者联合可明显下调缺氧诱导因子-1(HIF-α)HIF-α及CXC趋化因子受体4蛋白的表达。提示IC_{20} TPL可逆转耐药急性髓系白血病细胞的耐药性，其分子机制与下调HIF-α通路有关。

2. 肺癌

史妍婷等研究补中益气汤含药血清对肺腺癌顺铂耐药细胞株(A549/DDP)顺铂耐药的逆转作用及对哺乳动物雷帕霉素靶蛋白(mTOR)表达的影响。制备补中益气汤高(11.34 g/kg·d)、中(5.67 g/kg·d)、低(2.83 g/kg·d)剂量血清，将A549、A549/DDP细胞体外分为顺铂(DDP)组，空白血清＋DDP组，含药血清高剂量＋DDP组，含药血清中剂量＋DDP组，含药血清低剂量＋DDP组，细胞对照组。结果显示，与DDP组比较，补中益气汤不同浓度含药血清作用于A549/DDP后IC_{50}，及耐药倍数均有显著降低($P<0.05$)，以中剂量组最为显著($P<0.01$)，A549/DDP中mTOR的染色吸光度及荧光强度均明显减弱，mTOR蛋白表达水平明显降低(均$P<0.01$)。提示补中益气汤能增强A549/DDP对顺铂的敏感性，并可通过降低细胞生存通路中mTOR的表达而有效逆转肺腺癌细胞的顺铂耐药。

3. 乳腺癌

李海燕等通过MTT等方法检测药物对细胞增殖的影响及P-gp表达的变化，研究苦参碱与粉防己碱合用对人乳腺癌MCF-7细胞多药耐药性的影响。结果显示，苦参碱作用耐药和敏感细胞的IC_{50}相近。苦参碱单独处理MCF-7/DOX耐药细胞，可以微弱地降低其耐药性，并且与粉防己碱有协同作用；苦参碱与多柔比星合用，可以增加多柔比星对MCF-7/DOX耐药细胞的生长抑制作用，且与粉防己碱有协同作用；苦参碱和粉防己碱、多柔比星合用处理细胞，MCF-7/DOX耐药细胞株P-gp表达水平下降。提示苦参碱与粉防己碱合用具有协同作用，能逆转人乳腺癌MCF-7细胞的多药耐药性，降低P-gp的表达。姜真等采用MTT法检测不同浓度(20 mg/L、40 mg/L、80 mg/L)的天花粉蛋白对MCF-7/ADR细胞增殖的影响。结果显示，天花粉蛋白有明显的抑制MCF-7/ADR细胞增殖的作用，存在剂量—效应和时间—效应关系。各浓度天花粉蛋白作用48 h后，MCF-7/ADR细胞凋亡率随药物浓度增加而增加($P<0.05$)。20 mg/L天花粉蛋白作用2 d后，MCF-7/ADR中的ALDH1蛋白表达开始下降，作用5 d后未

检测到 ALDH1 蛋白的表达。提示天花粉蛋白可逆转 MCF－7/ADR 耐药性，与其下调 ALDH1 蛋白表达，抑制乳腺癌干细胞富集，诱导 MCF－7/ADR 细胞凋亡、抑制其增殖相关。

4. 结肠癌

马克龙等研究千金藤碱逆转人结肠癌耐药细胞株 LoVo/5－Fu 对 5－氟尿嘧啶(5－Fu)耐药性的机制，以 MTT 等方法检测千金藤碱和化疗药物对结肠癌细胞的细胞毒性，及 HO－1 和 NQ01 基因的 mRNA 和蛋白表达水平。结果显示，LoVo/5－Fu 细胞对 5－Fu 耐药性最高，千金藤碱对 LoVo 和 LoVo/5－Fu 细胞增殖均有抑制作用，千金藤碱(2.5～10.0 ug/ml)可降低 LoVo/5－Fu 细胞 5－Fu 的 IC_{50} 值($P<0.05$)，且在此浓度范围内，IC_{50} 值降低的程度与剂量成正相关。LoVo/5－Fu 细胞中 HO－1 和 NQ01 的 mRNA 和蛋白表达水平明显高于 LoVo 细胞($P<0.05$)，而经 10.0 ug/ml 千金藤碱与 5－Fu 联合处理后，两者表达水平均明显降低($P<0.05$，0.01)。提示千金藤碱可抑制结肠癌细胞增殖，增加结肠癌耐药细胞株 LoVo/5－Fu 对 5－Fu 的敏感性，与其抑制结肠癌细胞中 HO－1 和 NQ01 的表达水平有关。

5. 肝癌

凌博凡等以流式细胞仪检测肝癌细胞 bel－7402、肝癌耐药细胞 bel－7402/5－Fu 细胞表面 P－gp、MDR 相关蛋白的表达率及细胞内罗丹明 123(Rho123)的蓄积浓度。并以 MTT 法测定不同浓度(0.5 mg/ml、1 mg/ml、2 mg/ml、4 mg/ml)健脾化瘀方(白术、茯苓、茵陈、半枝莲、重楼、丹参等)对 bel－7402/5－Fu 细胞增殖的抑制。结果显示，bel－7402/5－Fu 细胞表面 P－gp 表达率高于 bel－7402 细胞，细胞内 Rho123 蓄积浓度低于 bel－7402 细胞。提示健脾化瘀方可显著抑制细胞生长，并呈量效关系。可能通过降低 P－gp 的表达来实现逆转肝癌耐药细胞的多药耐药。陈旭征等研究解毒消癥饮(白花蛇舌草、夏枯草、山慈菇、苦参)乙酸乙酯提取物(EE－JXY)减低肝癌细胞株 Huh7 对小剂量 5－Fu 化疗耐药的机制。以 EE－JXY 联合小剂量 5－Fu 体外干预人肝癌细胞株 Huh7，并进行相关检测。结果显示，小剂量 5－Fu 对 Huh7 细胞的增殖有抑制作用，但同时 Huh7 肝癌细胞株中侧群(SP)细胞的比例也有所升高，且 ATP 结合盒转运蛋白 G2(ABCG2)、八聚体结合转录因子 4(Oct4) mRNA 的表达亦上调。EE－JXY 可增强小剂量 5－Fu 对 Huh7 细胞增殖的抑制能力，同时 SP 含量下降，ABCG2、Oct4 mRNA 的表达下调。提示 EE－JXY 可通过降低肝癌干细胞相关基因 ABCG2 mRNA 和 Oct4 mRNA 水平及 SP 的比例，增强 Huh7 细胞对小剂量 5－Fu 的化疗敏感性。

(许亚梅)

【中医药与微创技术联合治疗恶性肿瘤】

1. 与经动脉化疗栓塞联合

曾普华等将 65 例中晚期原发性肝癌患者随机分为两组，试验组 35 例予益气化瘀解毒方(黄芪、人参、白术、女贞子、八月札、莪术等)加减联合鸦胆子油乳经血管介入治疗，对照组单纯行化疗栓塞治疗。均 8 周内行 2 次化疗栓塞治疗。结果与对照组比较，试验组肝区疼痛、乏力、食欲不振、腹胀等主要症状评分均下降($P<0.01$)，生活质量及免疫功能均有所改善($P<0.05$，$P<0.01$)。试验组 VEGF、bFGF 表达均低于对照组(均 $P<0.05$)。董明娥以六君子汤合三子养亲汤随症加减联合 EP 改良方案(根据肿瘤部位的不同，选择性的将导管留置于肿瘤相关的供血动脉，灌注化疗药物)治疗中晚期非小细胞肺癌 60 例，对照组单纯行 EP 改良方案。治疗 12 周，治疗组与对照组总有效率分别为 85.0%(51/60)、76.7%(46/60)，组间比较，$P<0.05$。毒副反应方面，治疗组恶心呕吐的发生率为 46.7%，骨髓抑制发生率为 20.0%，肝肾功能损伤(轻度)发生率 6.7%，便秘发生率 11.7%，脱发发生率 10.0%。对照组分别为 60.0%、30.0%、11.7%、21.7%、16.7%。两组外周周围毒性发生率均为 0。曲金荣等将 160 例原发性中晚期肝癌患者予肝动脉化疗栓塞术治疗，随机分为单纯介入治疗组(对照组)、康艾注射液(人参、黄芪、苦参素)联合介入治疗组(康艾组)、参芪扶正注射液(黄芪、党参)联合介入治疗组(参芪组)、蟾酥注射液联合介入治疗组(蟾酥组)，均 60 d 内行 2 次肝动脉化疗栓塞术治疗。结果显示，与对照组比较，各联合治疗组 AFP 均显著下降(均 $P<0.01$)，以参芪组最低($P<0.01$)。生活质量改善率分别为 37.5%(15/40)、70.0%(28/40)、67.5%(27/40)、60.0%(24/40)，

组间比较,$P<0.01$。

2. 与氩氦刀联合

刘建刚等将76例病理诊断为Ⅲ期和Ⅳ期的晚期恶性肿瘤患者随机平分为氩氦冷冻治疗组与氩氦冷冻联合中药(党参、黄芪、茯苓、白术、柴胡、郁金等)治疗组。治疗4周后,与氩氦冷冻治疗组比较,氩氦冷冻联合中药治疗组的CD_3^+、CD_4^+、NK细胞水平及CD_4^+/CD_8^+略有升高($P>0.05$),8周后上述指标则显著升高(均$P<0.05$)。

3. 与射频消融联合

刘华等将40例晚期肝癌患者随机平分为两组,均行伽玛刀及对症支持、护肝治疗,1次/d,共12～18次;治疗组加服扶正口服液(西洋参、黄芪、何首乌、熟地黄、枸杞子、白术等)。结果治疗组出现Ⅰ度骨髓抑制8例,Ⅱ度骨髓抑制2例,对照组出现Ⅰ度骨髓抑制13例,Ⅱ度骨髓抑制4例,Ⅲ骨髓抑制2例。组间比较,$P<0.05$。

(左明焕)

[附] 参考文献

A

艾叶盛,包素珍.黄芪建中汤抑制脾气虚证肺癌小鼠肿瘤转移的实验研究[J].山西中医学院学报,2013,14(2):16

C

曹娟,黄宇枚.当归补血汤治疗癌性贫血的实验研究[J].江西中医学院学报,2013,25(6):69

曹洋,陈文华,周京旭,等.金福安汤对人肺腺癌A549细胞生物学行为的影响[J].中医杂志,2013,54(3):241

陈培丰,潘磊,高聚伟,等.龙葵正丁醇萃取物对肝癌H22荷瘤小鼠的抑瘤作用及其免疫功能的影响[J].中国中医药科技,2013,20(2):141

陈强松,陈奕,裴润琼,等.健脾抑瘤汤治疗晚期原发性肝癌30例临床观察[J].世界中西医结合杂志,2013,8(4):368

陈旭征,黎金浓,胡丹,等.解毒消癥饮逆转氟尿嘧啶诱导的肝癌干细胞耐药的机制研究[J].中华细胞与干细胞杂志,2013,3(4):191

陈英玉,李静,胡建达,等.大黄素对HL·60/ADR耐药细胞多药耐药逆转作用的研究[J].中国实验血液学杂志,2013,21(6):1413

陈震宏,许盈,舒敬德,等.疏络散结汤治疗乳腺癌术后焦虑抑郁疗效观察[J].上海中医药杂志,2013,47(7):55

陈志刚,卢宏达.中西医结合治疗非小细胞肺癌[J].中国实验方剂学杂志,2013,19(11):322

D

丁纪元.息贲丸对Lewis肺癌小鼠Caspase 3/8基因表达的影响[J].中华中医药学刊,2013,31(3):646

董明娥.六君子汤三子养亲汤联合介入治疗中晚期肺癌60例[J].陕西中医,2013,34(6):705

F

方肇勤,梁超,任红艳.肝癌常用治法复方抑制肝癌细胞恶性增殖的机制研究[J].中国中医基础医学杂志,2013,19(1):34

G

顾恪波,王逊,何立丽,等.孙桂芝教授治疗肺癌常用方剂浅析[J].世界中西医结合杂志,2013,8(2):187

H

韩克起,谢国群,陈洁,等.中药联合肝动脉栓塞化疗术治疗中晚期肝癌临床疗效观察[J].中国中西医结合消化杂志,2013,21(2):57

何立丽,顾恪波,王逊,等.孙桂芝运用"体阴用阳"理论论治肝癌经验[J].辽宁中医杂志,2013,40(11):2216

胡淑贤,石搏黄,可欣,等.不同类型音乐对缓解乳腺癌患者化疗焦虑、抑郁的效果研究[J].中国妇幼保健,2013,28(2):359

黄新宇.复方苦参注射液联合全身热疗治疗晚期非小细胞肺癌50例观察[J].浙江中医杂志,2013,48(9):697

黄云胜.艾迪联合参麦注射液治疗晚期癌症患者肿瘤相关性贫血的临床研究[J].江西中医药,2013,44(1):35

J

贾玫,田杰,李潇,等.艾迪注射液改善肿瘤相关性抑郁临床观察[J].北京中医药大学学报(中医临床版),2013,20(15):310

姜真,孙长岗,庄静,等.天花粉蛋白对人乳腺癌耐药细胞株 MCF-7/ADR 及干细胞标志物 ALDH1 蛋白表达的实验研究[J]. 潍坊医学院学报,2013,35(3):185

蒋立峰,刘怀民. 当归补血汤防治肿瘤化疗后骨髓抑制临床观察[J]. 中医学报,2013,28(4):475

L

李柏颖. 宋康教授治疗肺癌经验介绍[J]. 浙江中西医结合杂志,2013,23(2):82

李海燕,陈阳,何琪杨. 苦参碱与粉防己碱逆转人 MCF-7 细胞耐药性的作用与机制[J]. 中国实验方剂学杂志,2013,19(18):275

李潇,陈信义,侯丽,等. 复方阿胶浆治疗癌性贫血的临床研究[J]. 北京中医药大学学报(中医临床版),2013,20(6):27

李秀荣,李慧杰,王秀娟. 六神丸对肺癌 A549 细胞 Caspase-3 及 Survivin 表达的影响[J]. 中医学报,2013,28(4):469

李妍,杨维泓,徐玉芬,等. 姜黄素对 Lewis 肺癌小鼠 TGF-β1 信号转导通路的影响[J]. 中华中医药学刊,2013,31(1):138

林洪生,杨宗艳,张培彤,等. 生血丸治疗非小细胞肺癌脾肾阳虚证化疗所致血象下降的临床疗效观察[J]. 中华中医药杂志,2013,28(8):2491

凌博凡,王瑞平,邹玺,等. 健脾化瘀方对肝癌 bel-7402/5-Fu 细胞表面耐药蛋白影响的研究[J]. 世界中西医结合杂志,2013,8(2):120

刘华,李杳瑶,王理槐. 扶正口服液防治伽玛刀治疗原发性肝癌毒副反应临床观察[J]. 中国中医药信息杂志,2013,20(10):65

刘建刚,韦巍,张积仁. 氩氦冷冻联合中药治疗肿瘤对机体细胞免疫功能的影响[J]. 现代中西医结合杂志,2013,22(22):2411

刘礼荣,吴海弟. 鸦胆子油乳联合 GP 方案治疗肺腺癌的临床研究[J]. 中医学报,2013,28(7):927

刘思,姚宇红. 解毒化瘀方逆转 HL60/VCR 白血病细胞耐药株多药耐药机制研究[J]. 实用中医药杂志,2013,29(4):241

卢利员,黄斌,李永浩,等. 益气养阴消积饮结合化疗治疗晚期非小细胞肺癌的临床疗效观察[J]. 北京中医药大学学报,2013,36(3):192

吕晓皑,高秀飞,王蓓,等. 应用中医团体情志疗法"治未病"调治乳腺癌术后阈下抑郁[J]. 中华中医药学刊,2013,31(4):819

M

马克龙,汪远金,汪天明,等. 千金藤碱对结肠癌细胞 5-氟尿嘧啶耐药性的逆转作用和对 HO-1 和 NQ01 表达的影响[J]. 江西中医学院学报,2013,25(2):59

Q

乔新梅,赵金岭. 血府逐瘀汤联合化疗治疗瘀阻肺络证小细胞肺癌 40 例疗效观察[J]. 新中医,2013,45(2):55

曲金荣,王青山,张敏,等. 康艾、参芪扶正、蟾酥注射液与介入联合治疗原发性中晚期肝癌的近期疗效观察[J]. 河北医药,2013,35(11):1728

S

史妍婷,井欢,王莹,等. 补中益气汤含药血清逆转 A549/DDP 的顺铂耐药及对 mTOR 表达的影响[J]. 中国实验方剂学杂志,2013,19(9):215

束家和,周荣耀,吴丽英,等. 养正消积胶囊联合化疗治疗中晚期非小细胞肺癌 35 例临床观察[J]. 世界中医药,2013,8(4):465

T

唐丽雯,林丽珠. 健脾补肾膏方治疗化疗后骨髓抑制的临床疗效观察[J]. 广州中医药大学学报,2013,30(5):628

W

王博,武利强,叶宝东,等. 白花蛇舌草熊果酸诱导白血病耐药 K562/ADM 细胞凋亡及其作用机理的研究[J]. 中华中医药学刊,2013,31(4):921

王相朦,陈菲莉,柳约,等. 雷公藤甲素体外逆转急性髓系白血病耐药性[J]. 白血病(淋巴瘤),2013,22(9):542

X

夏宁俊,章永红. 原发性肝癌中医辨治心得[J]. 中医杂志,2013,54(14):1237

肖跃红. 原发性肝癌的中医病机及防治探讨[J]. 中国中医基础医学杂志,2013,19(6):617

Y

杨素芳,林永廉. 基于主成分法分析原发性肝癌围介入治疗前的中医证型辨证要点[J]. 时珍国医国药,2013,24(1):190

杨小兵,龙顺钦,吴万垠,等. 原发性肝癌中医证型分布及生存期差异研究[J]. 中国中西医结合杂志,2013,33(7):911

杨玉兴,魏品康,修丽娟,等. 消痰解郁方治疗消化系统癌症并发抑郁症随机对照临床研究[J]. 中国中医药信息杂志,2013,20(2):12

易亚乔,伍参荣,葛金文,等. 桔梗总皂苷对人肺腺癌 A549 细胞抑制作用研究[J]. 中华中医药杂志,2013,28(7):2135

Z

Zhai XF, Chen Z, Li B, et al. Traditional herbal medicine in preventing recurrence after resection of small hepatocellular carcinoma: a multicenter randomized controlled trial [J]. Journal of Integrative Medicine, 2013, 11(2): 90

曾普华,郜文辉,潘敏求,等. 益气化瘀解毒方加减联合鸦胆子油乳经血管介入治疗中晚期原发性肝癌的临床研究[J]. 辽宁中医杂志,2013,40(1): 18

张斌,李琦,殷佩浩,等. 中药健脾解毒方剂对二乙基亚硝胺诱导大鼠肝癌的预防作用[J]. 华南国防医学杂志,2013,27(5): 305

张宏方,吴芳,环诚,等. 调衡方对 Lewis 肺癌细胞增殖及 JAK-STAT 信号通路的影响[J]. 辽宁中医药大学学报,2013,15(3): 16

张弦. 八珍汤治疗恶性肿瘤放、化疗后骨髓抑制 30 例临床观察[J]. 湖南中医杂志,2013,29(4): 51

赵增虎,王超搏,任成波,等. 益气补血片防治非小细胞肺癌 GP 方案化疗引起骨髓抑制的临床研究[J]. 河北中医,2013,35(8): 1214

郑健,周少玲,庞德湘. 庞德湘运用药对治疗肺癌经验[J]. 中医杂志,2013,54(5): 435

郑召鹏,杨卫兵,李宁,等. 注射用黄芪多糖预防非小细胞肺癌化疗后骨髓抑制的疗效观察[J]. 中草药,2013,44(2): 208

(四)内 科

【概述】

2013年公开发表的中医药治疗内科疾病的期刊论文约10 000余篇。其中消化系统约占21.7%,循环系统约占18.6%,新陈代谢系统约占14.6%,神经系统约占11.7%,呼吸系统约占11.7%。其余依次为精神系统、泌尿系统、结缔组织免疫系统、血液系统、内分泌系统、中医急症等。内容涵盖了中医临床研究、中西医结合治疗与研究、实验研究及专家经验总结等。

2013年国家自然科学基金项目的立项课题中,内科项目有176项,以实验研究为主,依次为消化系统、新陈代谢系统、循环系统、呼吸系统、神经系统、精神系统、结缔组织免疫系统、泌尿系统、内分泌系统、血液系统等。

1. 中医急症

文献近80篇,主要集中在脓毒症的研究,约占28.8%,其余依次为急性呼吸窘迫综合征、休克、呼吸衰竭等。

高戎等以盲肠结扎穿孔法(CLP)建立脓毒症大鼠模型,随机分为阴性对照组、CLP组、CLP+人参皂苷Rg5组。检测结果显示,与CLP组比较,CLP+人参皂苷Rg5组的血浆及肺组织高迁移率族蛋白1、TNF-α水平明显降低(均$P<0.05$),且肺组织W/D、MPO活性、NF-κB活性及肺组织损伤评分均明显低于CLP组(均$P<0.05$)。提示人参皂苷Rg5可下调炎性介质,减少肺水肿,减轻肺损伤程度,对脓毒血症引起的急性肺损伤具有一定保护作用。

2. 呼吸系统

文献约1 100余篇,其中支气管哮喘约占10%,急慢性支气管炎、支气管扩张各约占7.1%,肺炎约占6.0%。其余依次为感冒、肺间质纤维化、咳嗽变异性哮喘、慢性阻塞性肺疾病、慢性咳嗽、急性肺损伤、胸膜炎、外感发热等疾病。有21项课题获2013年国家自然科学基金资助。

周宝银等将咳嗽变异性哮喘患者随机分为两组,均予沙美特罗替卡松粉吸入剂治疗,治疗组40例加用桃红止嗽散(桃仁、红花、蜜炙紫菀、百部、白前、陈皮等)随证加减。经治8周,显效率分别为82.5%(33/40)、67.7%(23/34),组间比较,$P<0.05$。

李风雷等运用计算机、人工检索方法,从万方医学文献数据库、维普医学文献数据库、中国学术期刊全文数据库、中国生物医学文献数据库,对近15年文献进行收集整理,运用频数描述方法进行分析,结果显示,咳嗽变异性哮喘的病性证素以风出现频次最高,其次为气虚、热、火、寒。病位均在肺,偶可累及肝和肾;两病性证素组合时,风+寒、风+热的组合频次较高,其病位主要在肺;其余病性证素组合出现频次较低。陈丽等收集、筛选1989年以来国内公开发表的《中国药典》(2010版)所载抗肺纤维化单味中药文献进行统计分析,结果显示,在46味具有抗肺纤维化的中药中,活血化瘀药有8味,归胆经的有6味,与其在药典中所占比例比较,均有统计学差异($P<0.05$)。提示归胆经、膀胱经以及补虚药、活血化瘀药、收涩药均是抗肺纤维化效应的重要影响因素。

有关支气管哮喘、慢性支气管炎、慢性阻塞性肺疾病等的治疗与实验研究详见专条。

3. 循环系统

文献约1 750余篇,其中高血压病约占21.6%,冠心病约占20.7%,心绞痛约占15.1%,心力衰竭约占13.9%。其余依次为心律失常、动脉粥样硬化、心肌病、心肌缺血、肺源性心脏病、病毒性心肌炎、心肌梗死、心脏神经官能症等。除临床治疗与研究外,另有对中药作用机理的实验研究、中医证候研究等。有25项课题获2013年国家自然科学基金资助。

夏文进等将200例高血压病患者按中医辨证分为肝火亢盛证、痰湿壅盛证、阴虚阳亢证、阴阳两虚证,用循环酶法检测高血压病患者与健康对照组血浆同型半胱氨酸(Hcy)水平。结果显示,与健康对照组比较,高血压病患者各个中医证型血浆Hcy水平均显著升高(均$P<0.01$)。肝火亢盛证、痰湿壅盛证血浆Hcy水平显著高于阴虚阳

亢证、气虚痰浊证(均$P<0.01$)。

有关肺源性心脏病、心肌缺血、心肌梗死、动脉粥样硬化、病毒性心肌炎的实验研究等详见专条。

4. 消化系统

文献约2 050余篇,其中胃炎约占18.2%,结肠炎约占11.2%,便秘约占7.7%,脂肪肝占5.6%,肠易激综合征约占5.0%。其余依次为功能性消化不良、肝纤维化、消化性溃疡、肝硬化腹水、胆汁返流性胃炎等。有38项相关课题获2013年国家自然科学基金资助。

冯雯等将大鼠分为正常组,模型组,枳术通便汤(生白术、枳壳、生地黄、黄芪、当归、厚朴等)高(26 g/kg)、低(13 g/kg)剂量组,除正常组外,其余各组以大黄建立慢传输型便秘(STC)大鼠模型,灌胃给药14 d。结果显示,与正常组比较,模型组的墨汁推进长度缩短,黑染肠管长度/总长度下降(均$P<0.01$),与模型组比较,枳术通便汤高、低剂量组的墨汁推进长度有所增加,黑染肠管长度/总长度上升(均$P<0.01$)。光镜下STC大鼠结肠黏膜慢性炎症改变,有少量中性粒细胞浸润,肌层排列紊乱,肌间神经丛神经细胞空泡变性,与模型组比较,枳术通便汤高、低剂量组的结肠结构有所改善,以高剂量组改善更为明显。电镜下STC大鼠结肠神经元胞体肿胀变形,细胞器结构破坏,与模型组比较,枳术通便汤高、低剂量组的结肠肌间神经丛有不同程度的改善。

有关慢性萎缩性胃炎、胃癌前病变、腹泻型肠易激综合征、溃疡性结肠炎、非酒精性脂肪肝、抗肝纤维化、肝硬化腹水的治疗与研究等详见专条。

5. 泌尿系统

文献约630余篇,其中肾炎约占20.5%,肾衰约占12.9%,结石约占9.5%,肾病综合征约占9.2%。其余依次为血尿、IgA肾病、尿路感染、高尿酸血症肾病等。有8项相关课题获2013年国家自然科学基金资助。

李玉卿等采用5/6肾切除造模,随机分为模型组与溺毒清合剂(黄芪、制大黄、淫羊藿、丹参、附片、牡蛎)高(1.5 g/ml)、低(0.75 g/ml)剂量组,灌胃给药8周。结果显示,与模型组比较,各给药组TGF-β总光密度值均下降以厄贝沙坦组最为显著(均$P<0.05$);血肌酐水平均下降,以溺毒清高剂量组最为显著(均$P<0.05$)。提示溺毒清合剂可通过降解Ⅳ型胶原等细胞外基质而抑制残肾组织肾小球硬化,从而延缓慢性肾衰进展,与厄贝沙坦有相近的肾脏保护作用。傅晓骏通过5/6肾切除法制造慢性肾功能衰竭模型大鼠,并随机分为病理组、沉香(沉香粉水煎剂)组。灌胃给药8周后,与病理组相比,沉香组血白细胞降低,血红蛋白和红细胞升高(均$P<0.05$),血管紧张素Ⅰ、Ⅱ水平均降低($P<0.05$,$P<0.01$)。提示沉香粉可在一定程度上降低血管紧张素Ⅰ、Ⅱ,改善肾脏的血液动力学变化,进而延缓慢性肾衰竭的进展。

有关慢性肾脏病、抗肾纤维化的研究详见专条。

6. 血液系统

文献约120余篇,其中贫血约占43.3%,紫癜约占30.8%。其余依次为白细胞减少症、骨髓增生异常综合征等。有8项相关课题获2013年国家自然科学基金资助。

赵琳等将30例骨髓增生异常综合征(MDS)患者随机平分为复方参鹿颗粒(山红参须、鹿角片、炙龟板、菟丝子)治疗组与安特尔胶丸对照组,疗程均为3个月,观察治疗前后骨髓细胞免疫表型变化。另取骨科骨折手术患者(排除影响造血系统疾病与用药史)10例为正常对照组。结果显示,与正常对照组比较,骨髓增生异常综合征患者骨髓造血干/祖细胞存在CD_{13}、CD_{33}、CD_{34}、CD_{117}、HLA-DR高表达,而CD_{15}表达减少(均$P<0.05$)。与对照组比较,治疗组CD_{13}、CD_{33}、CD_{34}、CD_{117}的表达均降低(均$P<0.05$)。两组治疗后CD_{15}的表达均有所增高($P<0.05$)。提示复方参鹿颗粒可能具有促进骨髓造血干/祖细胞的正常增值分化,改善MDS病态造血的作用。

马俊丽等将70例MDS患者均予补肾健脾中药。治疗组40例加服青黄散(含雄黄0.16 g/d),对照组30例则未服用青黄散或其他砷制剂,并设10例正常组进行对照。经治6个月,治疗组总有效率为75.0%(30/40),伴随正常克隆与+8异常克隆患者的疗效明显好于其他异常克隆类型($P<0.05$)。治疗组全血及血浆砷浓度均明显高于对照组及正常组;治疗组全血砷浓度明显高于血浆砷浓度,有效患者的全血砷浓度亦明显高于

治疗失败者(均$P<0.05$)。治疗组疗效好的正常核型和+8异常克隆患者与疗效较差的其他异常核型患者的血砷浓度比较无显著性差异($P>0.05$),治疗组线粒体电位与对照组比较,亦无显著性差异(均$P>0.05$)。提示MDS患者口服青黄散后,砷被人体少量吸收,并进入细胞内发挥作用。MDS患者对青黄散的治疗反应与全血砷浓度具有相关性,青黄散治疗MDS的克隆选择性与全血砷浓度以及线粒体$\Delta\psi m$变化没有相关性。

关于慢性再生障碍性贫血、免疫性血小板减少症、过敏性紫癜的治疗与研究详见专条。

7. 内分泌系统

文献约115余篇,其中甲状腺炎约占32.2%,特发性水肿约占20.0%,肥胖约占19.1%。其余依次为甲状腺功能亢进、甲状腺功能减退等。有4项相关课题获2013年国家自然科学基金资助。

吕秀群等将63例亚急性甲状腺炎患者随机分为两组,观察组32例用放血疗法联合银翘散加减治疗,对照组用消炎痛、强的松等治疗。疗程均为2周,总有效率分别为90.6%(29/32)、67.7%(21/31),组间比较,$P<0.05$。不良反应发生率分别为9.4%(3/32)、35.5%(11/31),组间比较,$P<0.05$。

8. 新陈代谢系统

文献约1 380余篇,其中糖尿病约占70.4%,糖尿病肾病约占20.0%,糖尿病周围神经病变约占9.9%。其余依次为痛风性关节炎、高尿酸血症、代谢综合征、糖尿病胃轻瘫、高血脂症等。有29项相关课题获2013年国家自然科学基金资助。

罗迪检索中国知网、维普数据库,收集中医药有效治疗糖尿病胃轻瘫文献,建立中医用药文献研究数据库,采用Excel 2003软件进行统计描述。检索得到有关文献178篇,其中中药为102味,使用频次1 851次;根据药物使用频率,其种类依次为补气药、理气药、消食药、化痰药、补阴药;其归经以脾、胃、肝、肾为主。本病病机为本虚标实,脾虚为本,痰湿和瘀血为标。

王志宏等以高糖高脂高盐饲料长期喂饲建立代谢综合征(MS)大鼠模型,随机分为模型组、洛伐他汀组、苍白二陈汤(苍术、白术、陈皮、茯苓、半夏、甘草)组。灌胃给药4周后,与模型组比较,苍白二陈汤组血清TG、TC、LDLc和ox-LDL水平均降低,动脉粥样硬化指数及主动脉ICAM1表达量亦降低(均$P<0.05$)。

有关2型糖尿病、糖尿病肾病、糖尿病周围神经病变、代谢综合征、高尿酸血症的治疗与研究详见专条。

9. 神经系统

文献约1 100余篇,其中中风约占32.4%,头痛约占12.5%。其余依次为眩晕、帕金森病、癫痫、脑卒中后抑郁、面神经麻痹、慢性疲劳综合征、面神经炎等。有20项相关课题获2013年国家自然科学基金资助。

朱孔利等将大鼠随机分为空白对照组、癫痫模型组(戊四氮腹腔注射+0.9%NaCl溶液)、灵芝孢子粉组(戊四氮腹腔注射+灵芝孢子粉),灌胃给药28 d。结果显示,癫痫模型组与灵芝孢子粉组均达到癫痫模型"点燃"标准。与空白对照组比较,癫痫模型组大脑皮质及海马生长抑素免疫反应阳性细胞数明显增多,大脑皮质及海马ATP酶含量均降低,海马5-羟色胺(5-HT)含量明显降低(均$P<0.05$)。与癫痫模型组比较近,灵芝孢子粉组大脑皮质及海马SS免疫反应阳性细胞数减少,大脑皮质及海马ATP酶活性升高,海马5-HT含量增多(均$P<0.05$)。提示灵芝孢子粉可能通过调节神经递质水平、影响能量代谢等途径改善各脑区的神经电生理功能,抑制神经元异常放电,保护神经元,减轻对神经细胞的损伤。

有关帕金森病、急性脑梗死、脑卒中后抑郁的治疗与研究详见专条。

10. 结缔组织免疫系统

文献约300余篇,其中类风湿关节炎约占32.0%,风湿性关节炎约占19.7%、强直性脊柱炎约占15.7%。其余依次为重症肌无力、系统性红斑狼疮等。有11项相关课题获2013年国家自然科学基金资助。

邹君等采用弗氏完全佐剂制备类风湿关节炎模型,将大鼠随机分为模型对照组,赤霓根总皂苷(TSTR)高(160 mg/kg·d)、中(80 mg/kg·d)、低(40 mg/kg·d)剂量组,雷公藤多苷阳性对照组。灌胃给药 21 d 后,与模型组比较,TSTR 各剂量组大鼠血清 RANKL 水平均显著降低($P<0.05$ 或$P<0.01$)。血清 OPG 水平均显著升高($P<0.05$ 或$P<0.01$);OPG/RANKL 比值显著升高($P<0.05$ 或$P<0.01$)。提示赤雹根可能有阻止骨破坏的作用。

有关强直性脊柱炎的治疗与研究详见专条。

11. 精神系统

文献约 800 余篇,其中失眠约占 22.3%,抑郁症约占 17.4%,痴呆约占 12.6%。其余依次为焦虑症、痴呆、精神分裂症等。有 18 项课题获 2013 年国家自然科学基金资助。

尹冬青等从 CNKI 数据库中检索并研究近 20 年来抑郁症的相关文献后发现,其常见证候有肝郁脾虚、心脾两虚、气滞血瘀、肝郁气滞、肝郁痰阻、心肾不交等 6 个;证候要素 17 个,其中病性类证素 11 个,病位类证素 6 个。证素的组合形式主要有 4 种,其中二证、三证组合最常见。

有关血管性痴呆的研究、焦虑症的治疗与研究详见专条。

(余小萍 吴 欢)

【支气管哮喘的研究】

赵四林等将 80 例支气管哮喘临床缓解期肾虚证患者随机均分为两组,治疗组予加味二仙丸(淫羊藿、仙茅、巴戟天、蛤蚧粉、五味子等),对照组予固肾定喘丸。疗程均为 6 个月,并随访 1 年。结果两组患者血清白介素-2(IL-2)、干扰素-γ(IFN-γ)水平均升高,血清白介素-4(IL-4)水平及外周血嗜酸性粒细胞阳离子蛋白水平均下降,治疗组更著(均$P<0.05$),两组血清 IL-13 水平比较,$P>0.05$。治疗组在治疗结束后 3、6、12 个月随访期间的发作次数少于对照组($P<0.05$)。

窦迎婷等用卵清蛋白致敏复制支气管哮喘大鼠模型,随机分为模型组,地塞米松组,氯化二联苯碘组,疏风通络方(蝉蜕、荆芥、僵蚕、地龙、丹参、黄芩等)高(40 g/kg)、中(20 g/kg)、低(10 g/kg)剂量组。灌胃给药 10 d 后,与模型组比较,各给药组血清及支气管肺泡灌洗液的 ICAM-1 及 VCAM-1 水平均下降,疏风通络方高剂量组优于中、低剂量组及氯化二联苯碘组(均$P<0.01$)。提示疏风通络方能显著抑制哮喘大鼠黏附分子 ICAM-1 和 VCAM-1 的表达,阻抑嗜酸性粒细胞跨膜迁移,抑制气道嗜酸性粒细胞(EOS)的浸润,减轻气道炎症反应。张慧琪等以相同方法造模并随机分组,观测肺组织 EOS 浸润情况。与模型组比较,给药组肺组织 EOS 浸润程度均有所减轻,以地塞米松组更著。疏风通络方各剂量组中以高剂量组为著。提示疏风通络方可减少肺组织 EOS 浸润,可能是其平喘作用机制之一。杨珺超等建立支气管哮喘小鼠模型,随机分为模型组、醋酸泼尼松组、温补肾阳汤(生地黄、熟地黄、菟丝子、补骨脂、淫羊藿、巴戟天)组、温补肾阳汤+醋酸泼尼松(剂量减半)组。灌胃给药 14 d 后,与模型组比较,各给药组骨髓悬液 EOS 计数明显减少,外周血 IL-5 及肺组织干细胞因子(SCF)表达明显降低(均$P<0.01$);与温补肾阳汤组比较,温补肾阳汤+醋酸泼尼松组及醋酸泼尼松组小鼠的骨髓悬液 EOS 计数、外周血 IL-5 及肺组织 SCF 表达下降更低($P<0.05$)。提示温补肾阳汤与醋酸泼尼松有一定的协同作用,联合使用可减少激素的用量。

(屈 岚)

【慢性支气管炎的治疗】

吴小娜等将 60 例慢性支气管炎迁延期患者随机均分为两组,观察组予服芪冬益肺汤(生黄芪、麦冬、太子参、白术、防风、桑白皮等),对照组予复方地茯口服液。经治 1 个月,观察组与对照组证候疗效总有效率分别为 90.0%(27/30)、63.3%(19/30),组间比较,$P<0.05$;咳嗽、咳痰、喘息、胸闷憋气等主要症状的改善以治疗组为优($P<0.05$)。沈芝琴将 60 例慢性支气管炎稳定期患者随机均分为两组,均予氨茶碱缓释片,治疗组加服养阴润肺汤(南沙参、北沙参、麦冬、法半夏、金荞麦)。经治 4 周,治疗组与对照组总有效率分别为 73.3%(22/30)、60.0%(18/30),组间比较,$P<0.05$;肺功能疗效总有效率分别为 76.7%(23/30)、66.6%(20/30),组间比较,$P<0.05$。舒金堂等将 304 例患者随机分为两组,治疗组 160 例口服截咳糖浆(紫菀、百部、桔梗、白前、荆芥、陈皮等),待咳嗽、咳痰诸症稍退后加服复方松及片(松香、白及、党参、焦白术、百部、桔梗等),对照组口服阿莫西林胶囊,咳甚痰多者加服咳必清、必嗽平。经治 1 个月,总有效率分别为 92.5%(148/160)、63.9%(92/144),组间比较,$P<0.05$。

(刘 芳)

【慢性阻塞性肺疾病的治疗及实验研究】

罗春凤等将 93 例肺肾气虚型慢性阻塞性肺

疾病(COPD)稳定期患者随机分为两组,均予西药常规治疗,对照组48例加服中药安慰剂,治疗组加服纳气通络方(黄芪、山茱萸、补骨脂、沉香、干姜、细辛等)。疗程均为3个月,有86例(治疗组44例、对照组42例)完成临床观察。两组第1秒用力呼吸容积(FEV1)、FEV1与用力肺活量(FVC)比值(FEV1/FVC)及FEV1占预计值百分比(FEV1%)升高(均$P<0.05$),治疗组改善程度优于对照组(均$P<0.05$)。圣乔治呼吸量表(SGRQ)各项评分均降低(均$P<0.05$),且治疗组较对照组明显($P<0.05$)。随访9个月内感冒次数与COPD急性发作的次数,治疗组明显少于对照组($P<0.05$)。张文江等将瘀毒阻络型稳定期COPD患者随机分为两组,均采用西医常规治疗,治疗组加服祛瘀解毒方(川芎、赤芍药、当归、苏子、金银花、丝瓜络)。疗程均为4周,治疗组与对照组总有效率分别为87.1%(27/31)、60.0%(18/30),组间比较,$P<0.05$。在咳嗽、咯痰、胸闷痛、呼吸困难、皮肤晦暗等证候积分降低幅度优于对照组($P<0.05$或$P<0.01$)。韩健等将COPD急性加重期患者随机分为两组。治疗组进入PP(符合方案数据分析)360例,对照组300例。均予西医常规治疗,治疗组加服肺舒颗粒(西洋参、蛤蚧、黄芪、金银花、蒲公英、炙枇杷叶等)。经治28 d后,治疗组西医疗效及中医证候比较均优于对照组(均$P<0.05$);两组IL-8、TNF-α均较治疗前下降,而治疗组更著(均$P<0.05$)。

王成阳等以烟熏加脂多糖气管滴入法建COPD肺气虚证大鼠模型随机分为模型组,六味补气胶囊(人参、黄芪、益智仁、陈皮、肉桂)高(0.16 g/kg)、低(0.04 g/kg)剂量组,金水宝胶囊组,脾氨肽组,并设正常组对照。灌胃给药14 d,与正常组比较,模型组大鼠肺组织树突状细胞(DC)表达的阳性面积增加、平均光密度增强($P<0.01$);与模型组比较,各给药组DC阳性面积减小($P<0.05$,$P<0.01$)、平均光密度不同程度降低,各给药组间比较,$P>0.05$。王英等以香烟暴露联合细菌感染法建COPD大鼠模型随机分为模型组、补肺健脾(党参、黄芪、白术、茯苓、浙贝母等)组、补肺益肾(人参、黄芪、枸杞子、山萸肉等)组、益气滋肾(人参、黄精、熟地黄、枸杞子、五味子)组与氨茶碱组,并设健康对照组。于第9~20周给药,与健康对照组比较,模型组右心室肥大指数(RVHI)升高。第20、32周时,与模型组比较,各给药组RVHI均降低(均$P<0.01$);补肺健脾组、补肺益肾组、益气滋肾组大鼠RVHI较氨茶碱组显著降低($P<0.05$,$P<0.01$);模型组大鼠肌节长度较对照组缩短($P<0.05$),补肺健脾组较模型组增长($P<0.01$);模型组大鼠心脏组织细胞因子表达高于其余各组($P<0.01$);补肺健脾组、补肺益肾组、益气滋肾组大鼠内皮素-1(ET-1)表达较氨茶碱组明显降低($P<0.01$)。刘治坤等以香烟烟雾暴露及气道内滴入脂多糖联合造模随机分为模型组、中药(芪蛭益肺颗粒:黄芪、半夏、水蛭等)治疗组,并设正常组对照。结果模型组第30 d基质金属蛋白水解酶-9(MMP-9)表达低于正常组,第60 d高于正常组(均$P<0.05$);与模型组比较,中药组在第30 d基质金属蛋白水解酶抑制剂-1(TIMP-1)表达下调($P<0.05$);MMP-9/TIMP-1比值第30、40 d中药组均较模型组提高(均$P<0.05$)。

(刘 芳)

【肺源性心脏病的中西医结合治疗及实验研究】

张绍芬将慢性肺源性心脏病急性期患者72例随机分为两组,均予西医基础治疗,治疗组予加服加味桂枝茯苓丸(桂枝、茯苓、赤芍药、桃仁、牡丹皮、麻黄等)。经治14 d,治疗组与对照组总有效率分别为97.2%(35/36)、83.3%(30/36),组间比较,$P<0.05$。刘婷等将慢性肺源性心脏病急性期痰瘀证患者随机平分为两组,均予抗感染、止咳、平喘、祛痰、利尿、抗心衰等对症治疗。观察组加服泻肺宁心汤(葶苈子、海浮石、瓜蒌仁、苦杏仁、桃仁、地龙等)。经治14 d,观察组与对照组总有效率分别为93.8%(45/48)、77.1%(37/48),组间比较,$P<0.05$。观察组的氧分压、血氧饱和度、NO均升高,二氧化碳分压、平均肺动脉压(mPAP)、ET-1及主要症状体征评分下降均优于对照组(均$P<0.01$)。王建忠等将80例患者随机平分为两组,均予西医基础治疗,治疗组加服沉蛤定喘合剂(蛤蚧粉、沉香、红参、茯苓、知母、川贝母等)。经治60 d,两组的临床症状体征总积分均有改善($P<0.01$),治疗组咳痰、胸闷、气短的改善尤为明显,改善程度优于对照组($P<0.05$);两组6 min步行试验距离、肺动脉平均压均改善,治疗组优于对照组(均$P<0.05$)。

韩冰等以野百合碱腹腔注射建立大鼠肺心病模型随机分为模型组,艾叶油高(1.8 g/kg)、低(0.2 g/kg)剂量组,并设正常对照组。灌胃给药

21 d，与正常组比较，模型组平均右心室压(mRVP)、mPAP、最大肺动脉压力(Max mPAP)均显著升高($P<0.05$ 或 $P<0.01$)；肺湿重(wW)、右心室游离壁(RV)、左心室加心室间隔(LV＋S)质量、肺指数(LI)、RVHI 均增加(均 $P<0.01$)。与模型组比较，艾叶油高、低剂量组的 mRVP、mPAP、Max mPAP 均显著降低($P<0.05$ 或 $P<0.01$)；艾叶油高剂量组的 wW、RVHI 显著降低($P<0.05$)。提示艾叶油可在一定程度上抑制肺心病模型大鼠的右心衰竭，且呈现剂量依赖性。

(屈　岚)

【心肌缺血再灌注的实验研究】

欧喜燕等以腹腔异丙肾上腺素注射造模，随机分为模型组、三苦滴丸(三七∶苦碟子)2∶8 高剂量组、3∶7 高剂量组、4∶6 高剂量组，2∶8 中剂量组、3∶7 中剂量组、4∶6 中剂量组，2∶8 组低剂量、3∶7 组低剂量、4∶6 低剂量组给药组。灌胃给药 7 d，与模型组比较，三苦滴丸各比例组心电图 ST 段变化、血清乳酸脱氢酶(LDH)、肌酸激酶(CK)、MDA 含量均降低($P<0.05$，$P<0.01$，$P<0.001$)，心肌组织中超氧化物歧化酶(SOD)活性提高($P<0.05$，$P<0.01$)，其中三苦滴丸 2∶8 组各剂量的作用效果及发挥时效最佳。王永刚等建立大鼠心肌缺血再灌注模型随机分为模型组，人参与丹参 2∶1 配伍组、2∶0 配伍组、0∶1 配伍组，设假手术组对照。灌胃给药 28 d，与假手术组比较，模型组总抗氧化能力(T－AOC)、还原性谷胱甘肽(GSH)、SOD、血管内皮生长因子(VEGF)及碱性成纤维细胞生长因子(bFGF)含量均降低($P<0.05$)。与模型组比较，2∶1 组、2∶0 组、0∶1 组总抗氧化能力(T－AOC)、GSH、SOD、VEGF 及 bFGF 含量均升高(均 $P<0.05$)，以 2∶1 组的变化最著($P<0.05$)。方瑜等研究九龙藤总黄酮(BCF)对急性心肌缺血的作用，将大鼠随机分为生理盐水组，模型组，维拉帕米组，BCF 高(240 mg/kg)、中(120 mg/kg)、低(60 mg/kg)剂量组。灌胃给药 7 d 显示，BCF 能剂量依赖性地抑制心肌缺血 15 s、1 min 心电图 ST 段抬高，减小 HR、降低左心室内压最大上升速率、左心室内压最大下降速率及 LVEDP 升高的幅度，增加血清 T－AOC，改善 Na^+、K^+－ATP、Ca_2^+、Mg_2^+－ATP 酶活性，减少心肌损伤标志物 CK－MB、cTnI、MyoG 的漏出($P<0.05$ 或 $P<0.01$)。提示 BCF 对急性心肌缺血具有明显的保护作用，其机制可能与抗氧化、抑制钙超载、减轻心肌损伤有关。郭齐等以结扎大鼠心脏冠状动脉前降支法建大鼠心肌缺血损伤模型，随机分为模型组，复方丹参片对照组，丹芍配伍高(丹皮酚 100 mg/kg＋ 芍药苷 25 mg/kg)、中(丹皮酚 50 mg/kg＋芍药苷 12.5 mg/kg)、低(25 mg/kg＋芍药苷6.25 mg/kg)剂量组。灌胃给药 5 d，与模型组比较，丹芍配伍各剂量组心电图(ST 段抬高及 T 波高耸)的变化程度显著减轻(均 $P<0.05$)，梗死占全心面积的百分比降低，血清中 AST、CK、LDH、MDA 的含量均降低，血清 SOD 活性、GSH－Px 的含量升高。提示丹芍配伍可通过保护心肌细胞膜、清除氧自由基，提高抗氧化酶活性以及抗脂质过氧化来改善心肌缺血的损伤状况。李雪丽等研究双参宁心方(人参总皂苷、丹参总酚酸、延胡索总生物碱)对大鼠心肌缺血/再灌注损伤能量代谢的影响，建模型后随机分为模型组，曲美他嗪组，双参宁心方高(90 mg/kg)、中(45 mg/kg)、低(22.5 mg/kg)剂量组。灌胃给药 5 d，与模型组比较，双参宁心方各剂量组血清 CK－MB 活性降低，心肌 ATP 含量及能荷水平升高($P<0.05$ 或$P<0.01$)。

(刘　霖)

【心肌梗死的实验研究】

孙涛等研究钙调神经磷酸酶(CaN)、T 细胞活化因子 3($NFAT_3$)蛋白表达对心肌梗死(MI)后大鼠心室重构的影响及益心泰(黄芪、红花、泽泻、猪苓等)对其的干预作用。造模后随机分为模型组、益心泰组、开博组、复方丹参滴丸组，并设假手术组。灌胃给药 8 周后，与假手术组比较，模型组左、右心室质量指数均增加，CaN、$NFAT_3$蛋白表达明显升高($P<0.01$)；与模型组比较，各给药组左、右心室质量指数均降低，CaN、$NFAT_3$蛋白表达均降低，($P<0.01$)。提示益心泰可能通过抑制 CaN、$NFAT_3$蛋白表达干预心肌梗死后心室重构。刘玥等研究芪参益气方(黄芪、丹参、三七、降香)对 MI 大鼠心肌细胞凋亡、梗死面积和心肌组织胶原容积分数的影响。建大鼠模型后随机分为单纯 MI 组、MI 后芪参益气组方干预治疗组，并设假手术对照组。灌胃给药 4 周，与假手术组相比，MI 各组 Bcl－2 蛋白表达水平均明显降低($P<0.05$)，Bax 蛋白表达水平、心肌组织胶原容积分数(CVF)增高($P<0.01$)，与单纯 MI 组相

比，芪参益气组方干预组 Bcl 2 蛋白表达水平升高（$P<0.05$），梗死面积、心肌细胞凋亡指数、Bax 蛋白表达水平、CVF 降低（均 $P<0.05$）。提示芪参益气组方可能通过抑制凋亡、抗心肌纤维化等来减轻心肌梗死后的心室重构。黄绍湘等研究安心颗粒（人参、桂枝、瓜蒌、水蛭、茯苓等）对实验性 MI 大鼠心脏的促血管新生作用。以冠状动脉左前降支结扎法造模并随机分为模型组（B 组）、麝香保心丸组（C 组）、安心颗粒高（1.6 g/kg/d）、中（0.8 g/kg·d）、低（0.4 g/kg·d）剂量组（D1、D2、D3 组），并设假手术组（A 组）。灌胃 4 周后，A 组未见明显的心肌梗死区域。与 B 组比较，D1、D2、D3 组的梗死面积比较均显著减少，与 C 组作用相似；D1、D2、D3 组心肌梗死边缘区的平均血管面密度均明显增多（$P<0.05$ 或 $P<0.01$）。郜俊清等研究补气化痰方（黄芪、瓜蒌、薤白、半夏）对大鼠 MI 模型心功能及血管新生作用的影响。以结扎冠状动脉前降支近端造模随机分为治疗组（黄芪瓜蒌薤白半夏汤组）、中药对照组（瓜蒌薤白半夏汤组）、西药对照组（科素亚组）、模型组。灌胃给药 30 d，与模型组及其他给药组比较，治疗组大鼠心脏超声心脏超声射血分数（EF）下降缓慢（均 $P<0.05$），CD_{31} 染色数目增加。提示补气化痰方可能促进梗死后血管新生从而改善心脏功能。王永刚等研究双参通冠方（丹参、人参、红景天、降香以 5∶2∶3∶1 比例组成）对实验性大鼠 MI 模型冠状动脉血流量的影响。以结扎左冠状动脉主干支造模随机分为模型组，双参通冠方 SSTG 高（0.5 g/ml）、低（0.25 g/ml）剂量组，硝酸异山梨酯组，并设假手术对照组。灌胃给药 2 周，与假手术组比较，模型组 HR、左室收缩压（LVSP）均升高，左室舒张末压（LVEDP）、左室内压最大下降速率（LV Dp/dt mix）降低（均 $P<0.05$）。与模型组比较，各给药组 HR、平均动脉压（MAP）、LVSP 均降低，LVEDP、LV Dp/dt mix（均 $P<0.05$）。与双参通冠方低剂量组比较，双参通冠方高剂量组及硝酸异山梨酯组 HR、MAP、LVSP 均降低，LVEDP、LV Dp/dt mix 升高（均 $P<0.05$）。提示双参通冠方具有一定的降压作用，可以增加冠脉血流量，改善心肌缺血状态。陈铁龙等观察不同剂量冠心合剂（黄芪、蒲黄、五灵脂）对大鼠急性 MI 边缘区细胞凋亡的作用途径。结扎冠状动脉左前降支造模随机分为模型组，冠心合剂高（28 g/kg·d）、中（14 g/kg·d）、低（7 g/kg·d）剂量组，并设正常组对照。灌胃 7 d，与模型组比较，冠心合剂组心肌细胞凋亡明显减少，Fas、FasL、Caspase－8、Caspase－3 的蛋白表达量减少（$P<0.05$ 或 $P<0.01$），以冠心合剂高剂量组最为明显。贾云芳等探讨心肝胃同治法对心梗大鼠 MI 面积及食量的影响。以结扎冠状动脉左前降支造模随机分为模型组，消心痛组，心肝胃同治方（丹参、檀香、延胡索、乳香、没药、龙眼肉等）高（13.5 g/kg·d）、低（6.75 g/kg·d）剂量组。灌胃 2 周后，与模型组比较，各给药组梗死范围均明显缩小（均 $P<0.05$），心肝胃同治高、低剂量组均优于消心痛组（均 $P<0.05$），与消心痛组比较，心肝胃同治高剂量组食量明显增大（$P<0.05$）。

（夏一春　何立人）

【动脉粥样硬化的实验研究】

徐冰等观察四妙勇安汤活性部位配伍方（N8、N16、N18）对载脂蛋白 E 基因缺陷（ApoE－/－）小鼠动脉粥样硬化（AS）斑块形成的影响。将 ApoE－/－小鼠随机分为模型组，四妙勇安汤活性部位配伍方 N8、N16、N18 组，辛伐他汀组、罗格列酮组。给药 16 周，与模型组比较，N8 组、N16 组的斑块面积与管腔面积比值（PA/LA）明显减少（$P<0.01$），N8、N16、N18 各组的血清 TC、TG、LDL 水平均降低（$P<0.01$ 或 $P<0.05$）。章怡祎等研究冠心康（生黄芪、全瓜蒌、薤白、制半夏、益母草、丹参）对 ApoE－/－基因敲除 AS 小鼠血管壁保护及斑块的稳定作用及心脏时钟基因的调节。在 12 h 光照/黑暗条件下，将 ApoE－/－小鼠随机分为模型组、冠心康组、辛伐他汀组，并设正常组对照。灌胃 19 周，与正常组比较，模型组心脏时钟基因昼夜表达节律显著改变，提示 Bmal1、Per2 存在昼夜表达异常。与模型组相比，冠心康组的心脏 Per2 基因在下午 16 点表达显著升高，在上午 8 点及午夜 0 点表达显著降低；冠心康组的心脏 Bmal1 基因在早上 8 点及午夜 0 点表达含量均显著升高，其基因表达水平与正常组较为相似。提示冠心康对 ApoE－/－基因敲除 AS 小鼠心脏时钟基因 Bmal1、Per2 基因表达节律存在干预作用。杨清峰等研究疏肝活血法对老龄 AS 模型大鼠血管内皮功能保护及改善 AS 作用。将高脂饲料喂养的大鼠随机分为模型组，疏肝活血方（郁金、川芎、白芍药、人参、甘松等）高（1.5 g/kg）、低（0.75 g/kg）剂量组。灌胃给药 14 周，与模型组

比较,疏肝活血方高、低剂量组的 PGI_2、NO、TC、TG、LDL－C 水平均升高,TXB_2 水平均降低($P<0.05$ 或 $P<0.01$);高剂量组的 HDL－C 水平明显升高($P<0.05$),主动脉血管中膜钙盐沉积及泡沫细胞、平滑肌细胞增生均减少。提示疏肝活血方能改善模型大鼠的内皮功能,改善脂质代谢紊乱,减轻大鼠 AS 斑块病变程度,并存在量效关系。

(夏一春　何立人)

【病毒性心肌炎的治疗】

任晓晨等认为,病毒性心肌炎的证候特点,邪气停留的层次,及其发展变化趋势都与伤寒六经辨证中少阳证十分相似,其发病过程基本符合六经传变规律。从六经辨证入手,以和解少阳,调畅少阳为主要治法,以小柴胡汤为基本方随症加减取得一定疗效。

陈少禹将 82 例患者随机平分为两组,均予能量合剂、辅酶 A、三磷酸腺苷及维生素 C。治疗组加用补气运脾汤(茯苓、白芍药、板蓝根、当归、白术、炙甘草等)。28 d 为 1 个疗程。经治 3 个疗程,治疗组与对照组总有效率分别为 92.7%(38/41)、68.3%(28/41),组间比较,$P<0.05$。陈玉琴将 86 例患者随机分为两组,均予常规西药治疗,治疗组 48 例加服五味消毒饮合生脉饮汤剂(金银花、野菊花、忍冬藤、紫花地丁、当归、蒲公英等)。经治 1 个月,总有效率分别为 92.3%(48/52)、82.4%(28/34),组间比较,$P<0.05$。田满荣等将 76 例患者随机平分为两组,治疗组予服透邪清心汤(金银花、连翘、薄荷、荆芥、牛蒡子、桔梗等),对照组予能量合剂、维生素 C 及 1,6－二磷酸果糖。经治 14 d,治疗组与对照组总有效率分别为 89.5%(34/38)、65.8%(25/38),组间比较,$P<0.05$。何晓茵将 60 例患者随机平分为两组,均予西医常规治疗,治疗组加用心达康胶囊(主要成份为沙棘果实中提取的醋柳黄酮)。经治 4 周,治疗组与对照组总有效率分别为 93.3%(28/30)、63.3%(19/30),组间比较,$P<0.05$。两组心肌酶水平均明显降低,治疗组更显著(均 $P<0.05$)。

(夏一春　何立人)

【慢性萎缩性胃炎的治疗及实验研究】

林平等选择慢性萎缩性胃炎(CAG)中医诊断为"胃痛""胃痞"患者各 60 例,以证素辨证方法对其证候表现统计分析后显示,胃痛和胃痞主要病位证素(胃、脾、肝)、病性证素(气滞、阳虚、气虚、湿)相同,证素组合频率较高的有肝、脾、胃气滞加气虚,胃气虚,脾胃湿,脾胃阳虚,肝、脾、胃气滞。提示胃痛、胃痞的证素特点和发病规律基本相同,病变实质为虚实夹杂,虚证以脾气虚弱加脾阳不足为主,实证以胃气不降、气机郁滞、湿邪阻滞为主。

吕建兴将 68 例患者随机平分为两组,治疗组予丹红注射液静脉滴注和半夏泻心汤随证加减口服,对照组予胶体果胶及阿莫西林胶囊口服。经治 60 d,治疗组与对照组总有效率分别为 91.2%(31/34)、70.6%(24/34),组间比较,$P<0.05$。HP 清除总有效率分别为 94.1%(32/34)、70.6%(24/34),组间比较,$P<0.05$。邓耀松将 180 例患者随机分为治疗组与对照组,分别予养阴活胃合剂(鸡内金、枳实、丹参、莪术、炒白术、白茅根等)与西药常规治疗。经治 2 个月,治疗组与对照组总有效率分别为 94.4%(84/89)、87.9%(80/91),组间比较,$P<0.05$。

张会存等以幽门弹簧配合高盐热淀粉糊灌胃法制备大鼠模型随机分为模型组、替普瑞酮组、黄芪水煎剂组、三七粉冲剂组、黄芪＋三七组。灌胃 1 个月后,与模型组相比,各给药组大鼠的胃黏膜热休克蛋白 70(HSP70)及 HSP70 转录因子 GAF 的表达均显著升高(均 $P<0.05$)。黄芪组 HSP70 表达高于三七组($P<0.05$),但组间 HSP70 转录因子 GAF 的表达无统计学差异。提示黄芪、三七及其配伍可明显改善萎缩性胃炎大鼠胃黏膜状态;通过诱导并增加转录因子 GAF 的表达,促进 HSP70 的表达,可能是黄芪、三七治疗萎缩性胃炎的作用途径之一。

(张正利)

【胃癌前病变的治疗及实验研究】

韩慧等将 82 例慢性萎缩性胃炎(CAG)伴胃黏膜异型增生属血瘀热毒证患者随机分成治疗组与对照组,分别予服善胃Ⅰ号方(丹参、三棱、莪术、姜黄、地鳖虫、半枝莲等)与猴头菌片。经治 6 个月,治疗组与对照组总有效率分别为 85.3%(29/34)、29.2%(14/48),组间比较,$P<0.05$。治疗组增殖细胞核抗原(PCNA)的表达水平较对照组明显降低($P<0.05$)。

王志坤等探讨小归芍化浊解毒方(冬凌草、藤梨根、紫豆蔻、黄连、半夏、瓜蒌等)对胃癌前病变(PLGC)的作用和机制。以 N－甲基－N－硝基N－亚硝基胍配合饥饱失常造模随机分为 B(模型)

组、C(小归芍化浊解毒方15 g/ml剂量)组、D(小归芍化浊解毒方10 g/ml剂量)组、E(胃复春对照)组,并设A(空白)组对照。灌胃给药24周,与E组比较,C组胃黏膜肠化和异型增生改善明显,胃黏膜组织再生基因表达水平降低($P<0.05$)。C、D组胃组织增殖细胞核抗原的表达明显降低,血清胃蛋白酶原含量升高(均$P<0.05$)。提示该方能够逆转胃癌前病变并对胃癌的形成有抑制作用。其机制可能与抑制致癌基因,升高保护因子有关。

高绍芳等以幽门弹簧插入复合法造模随机分为模型组,维甲酸治疗组,化浊解毒和胃方(茵陈、藿香、佩兰、茯苓、黄连、半枝莲等)高(20 g/kg)、中(10 g/kg)、低(5 g/kg)剂量组,并设空白组对照。灌胃给药16周后,与空白组比较,模型组胃黏膜组织缺氧诱导因子-1α(HIF-1α)、血管内皮生长因子(VEGF)的表达增高(均$P<0.05$)。与模型组比较,各给药组HIF-1α、VEGF表达均降低(均$P<0.05$);与维甲酸组比较,化浊解毒和胃方高、中剂量组两者的表达降低更为显著(均$P<0.05$)。谢晶日等研究欣胃颗粒(黄芪、焦白术、沙参、石斛、白花蛇舌草、三棱等)对PLGC大鼠信号传导及转录活化因子(STAT3)、酪氨酸磷酸化STAT3(p-STAT3)信号通路ST的影响。以N-甲基-N-硝基N-亚硝基胍造模随机分为模型组、欣胃颗粒高(5.016 g/kg)、中(2.508 g/kg)、低(1.254 g/kg)剂量组,维酶素对照(维酶素)组。灌胃12周后,欣胃颗粒各剂量组大鼠活动度、进食水量、体重等一般状态好转,与模型组比较,STAT3、p-STAT3表达水平增高,欣胃颗粒高、低剂量组的STAT3、p-STAT3表达均水平降低(均$P<0.05$)。提示欣胃颗粒可干预PLGC进一步发展,并且改善胃黏膜病理状态,可能通过下调STAT3、p-STAT3的表达以达到对抗PLGC的作用。

(刘　霖)

【腹泻型肠易激综合征的研究】

沈淑华等探讨腹泻型肠易激综合征(IBS-D)的证型及证候要素的分布规律。检索1989年1月至2012年6月IBS-D的相关文献,得40篇合格文献,建立数据库,统计分析显示,IBS-D累积频率达90%的证型依次是肝郁脾虚证、脾气虚证、肝旺脾虚证、肝郁气滞证、脾肾阳虚证、脾虚湿盛证、大肠湿热证和肾阳虚证;病位证素依次是脾、肝和肾;病性证候要素依次是气虚、气郁、阳虚和湿阻。吴皓萌等对237例IBS患者从性别、年龄、病程及检测睾酮(T)和雌二醇(E_2)等对其证型分布的影响。结果显示,病程≤1年和1～3年中多见肝郁脾虚证、肝郁气滞证,3年和5～10年中多见脾胃虚弱证、脾肾阳虚证,病程对肠燥津伤证的分布则无明显影响。年龄≤44岁组多见肝郁脾虚证、肝郁气滞证、脾肾阳虚证。男性以肝郁脾虚证、脾胃虚弱证比例最大,女性以肝郁脾虚证、肝郁气滞证比例最大(均$P<0.05$)。与正常组比较,各证型女性患者E_2均值均降低,脾肾阳虚证最低(均$P<0.05$)。

黄适等通过番泻叶加束缚应激刺激法制备IBS-D大鼠模型随机分为模型组,安肠汤(柴胡、白芍药、木香、牡丹皮、法半夏、白术等)高(26 g/kg)、中(13 g/kg)、低(6.5 g/kg)剂量组,得舒特组,正常组对照。灌胃给药2周,与正常组比较,模型组大鼠结肠及下丘脑辣椒素受体1(TPRV1)的表达面积和光密度均明显增强($P<0.01$)。与模型组比较,安肠汤各剂量组、得舒特组的结肠及下丘脑TPRV1表达面积明显降低(均$P<0.01$)。张洁等基于脑-肠互动理论,观察健脾安神方(白术、白芍药、广木香、陈皮、防风、夜交藤等)对IBS-D模型大鼠的影响。以母子分离情志干预法协同直肠刺激法造模并随机分组。灌胃2周,与模型组比较,健脾安神方组大鼠粪便含水量、小肠推进率降低,腹部回缩反射的阈值升高(均$P<0.05$)。提示健脾安神中可降低内脏高敏感性,改善腹泻症状。丛军等以束缚应激加大黄泻下及结直肠扩张法造模随机分为模型组,肠吉泰(陈皮、炒防风、炒白术、炒白芍药、炙乌梅等)高(2.0 g/ml)、中(1.0 g/ml)、低(0.5 g/ml)剂量组,匹维溴铵组。灌胃2周后,与模型组比较,除肠吉泰低剂量组外,各给药组大鼠的下丘脑促肾上腺皮质激素释放激素(CRH)、P物质(SP) mRNA表达均降低($P<0.05$,$P<0.01$),与匹维溴铵组比较,肠吉泰高、中剂量组大鼠结肠SP mRNA降低($P<0.05$,$P<0.01$),与模型组比较,各给药组大鼠的大便频次显著降低、大便性状明显改善(均$P<0.05$)。提示肠吉泰可通过调节大鼠下丘脑CRH、SP mRNA表达及结肠SP mRNA表达,改善肠动力紊乱及内脏痛觉敏感状态。

(张正利)

【溃疡性结肠炎的治疗及实验研究】

田志刚等将98例溃疡性结肠炎(UC)患者随

机分为两组,治疗组予中药(附子、干姜、补骨脂、鹿角霜、五倍子、肉豆蔻等)内服及(白及、苦参、黄芩、黄连、连翘、红藤等)灌肠,对照组予吡哌酸加黄连素口服。经治 14 d,治疗组与对照组总有效率分别为 98.0%(48/49)、77.6%(38/49),组间比较,$P<0.05$。许风莲将 100 例患者随机平分为治疗组与对照组,分别予失笑散加味(五灵脂、蒲黄、三七、白及、乳香、没药)保留灌肠与柳氮磺胺吡啶片口服。经治 3 周,治疗组与对照组总有效率分别为 92.0%(46/50)、68.0%(34/50),组间比较,$P<0.05$。张伦等将 60 例患者随机平分为治疗组与对照组,分别予健脾清热活血类方药(救必应、三七、白芍药、马齿苋、黄芪、党参等)与美沙拉嗪。经治 9 个月,治疗组与对照组总有效率分别为 76.7%(23/30)、53.3%(16/30),组间比较,$P<0.05$。

许代福等对 150 例 UC 患者的证型与内镜检查结肠黏膜溃疡面积、色泽、水肿、覆苔等变化关系进行分析。结果显示,脾胃虚弱组溃疡白色阳性率显著高于脾胃湿热组、阴血亏虚组($P<0.05$),气滞血瘀组溃疡白色阳性率与脾胃虚弱组比较无显著性差异($P>0.05$)。溃疡面积各组比较无显著性差异($P>0.05$)。表面覆苔气滞血瘀组以黄苔、白苔为主,脾胃湿热组以黄苔为主,脾胃虚弱组、阴血亏虚组以白苔为主。脾胃虚弱组水肿阳性率出现最高,阴血亏虚组水肿阳性率出现最低。水肿阳性率阴血亏虚组与脾胃湿热组、气滞血瘀组、脾胃虚弱组比较有显著性差异($P<0.05$)。提示 UC 脾胃湿热证、脾胃虚弱证结肠镜下的表现存在一定的特异性。

范恒等以 2,4,6-三硝基苯磺酸(TNBS)灌肠建模型大鼠随机分为模型组,美沙拉嗪组,复方苦参汤(苦参、地榆、青黛、白及、甘草等)大(0.67 g/L)、中(0.34 g/L)、小(0.17 g/L)剂量组,并设空白对照组。灌胃给药 15 d,与空白对照组比较,模型组的大鼠结肠黏膜组织 Bc l-2、β-arrestin1 和 δ 阿片受体(DOR)表达明显升高($P<0.05$)。与模型组比较,美沙拉嗪组和复方苦参汤各剂量组的大鼠结肠黏膜组 Bcl-2-arrestin1、DOR 表达均显著下降(均$P<0.05$),但美沙拉嗪组和复方苦参汤各剂量组之间比较,$P>0.05$。提示复方苦参汤可改善 UC 大鼠的结肠组织病理学改变,可能通过对 DOR-β-arrestin1-Bcl-2 信号通路活化环节的干预,促进肠黏膜中 T 细胞凋亡,减轻溃疡性结肠炎的症状。李艳香等以 TNBS/乙醇溶液灌肠法建大鼠模型随机分为正常对照组、模型组、抗风湿中药复方组(白头翁、穿山龙、败酱草、徐长卿、仙鹤草、地榆等)、柳氮磺胺吡啶组。灌肠给药 15 d,与正常对照组比较,模型组血清 TNF-α 含量显著升高($P<0.05$),与模型组比较,柳氮磺胺吡啶组、抗风湿中药复方组血清 TNF-α 含量均下降(均$P<0.05$),组间比较,$P>0.05$。提示抗风湿中药复方能改善溃疡性结肠炎大鼠的营养状况,增加体重,降低 TNF-α 的含量,从而调节免疫反应,抑制炎性细胞,修复受损肠黏膜,减轻炎症,促进溃疡愈合。刘杰民等以同样方法造模随机分为健脾益肠散(黄芪、太子参、焦白术、茯苓、芡实、败酱草等)高(204 g/kg)、中(136 g/kg)、低(68 g/kg)剂量组,柳氮磺吡啶组,模型组,正常组对照。灌胃 21 d,与正常组比较,模型组疾病活动指数(DAI)评分、结肠组织损伤程度评分(CMDI)显著升高(均$P<0.01$)。与模型组比较,健脾益肠散高剂量组 DAI 评分及 CMDI 降低,中剂量组 DAI 评分明显降低($P<0.05$,$P<0.01$);健脾益肠散高剂量组与柳氮磺吡啶组上述指标比较无显著性差异($P>0.05$)。提示健脾益肠散能有效缓解 UC 大鼠症状,改善结肠组织学损伤,且以高剂量效果为佳。张纨等以上述方法造模随机分为模型组,兰茵风扬化浊解毒方(藿香、佩兰、茵陈、泽泻、厚朴、苍术)高(20.0 g/kg)、低(5.0 g/kg)剂量组,柳氮磺胺吡啶组。治疗 14 d 后,与模型组比较,兰茵风扬化浊解毒方高、低剂量组、柳氮磺胺吡啶组 DAI 评分均减低,CD_4^+/CD_{29}^+ T 细胞亚群数量、IL-8 含量均降低,IL-10 含量均升高(均$P<0.05$)。其中与柳氮磺胺吡啶组比较,兰茵风扬化浊解毒方高剂量组 CD_4^+/CD_{29}^+ T 细胞亚群数量降低明显($P<0.05$)。提示兰茵风扬化浊解毒方,可能通过下调促炎症因子,上调抑炎症因子,抑制 CD_4^+/CD_{29}^+ T 细胞亚群的表达起到抗炎和调节免疫的作用。

(鲍健欣)

【非酒精性脂肪肝的治疗及实验研究】

贺建国将 117 例非酒精性脂肪肝(NAFLD)患者随机分为治疗组 60 例与对照组 57 例,分别予调脂复肝汤(陈皮、半夏、白术、姜黄、泽泻、茯苓等)与水飞蓟宾胶囊治疗。经治 3 个月,总有效率分别为 83.3%(50/60)、43.9%(25/57),组间比较，$P<0.01$。宋清武等把 90 例辨证属痰饮病之中阳不足的 NAFLD 患者随机分为两组。在强调合理膳食谱和每日 30 min 有氧运动的基础上，治疗组 48 例予加味苓桂术甘汤（茯苓、白术、桂枝、荷梗、泽泻等），对照组予服多烯磷脂酰胆碱胶囊。经治 3 个月，总有效率分别为 91.7%（44/48）、69.0%（29/42），组间比较，$P<0.01$。

刘旭东等用祛湿活血方（柴胡、丹参、大黄、荷叶、茵陈、虎杖等）干预高脂高糖饲料诱导的 NAFLD 大鼠 8 周，设模型组、维生素 E 组、牛磺熊去氧胆酸组、吡格列酮组对照。与模型组比较，各给药组血清 TNF-α 水平均不同程度降低，但无显著性差异（$P>0.05$）。与维生素 E 组、牛磺熊去氧胆酸组、吡格列酮组比较，祛湿活血方组脂联素（APN）水平明显升高（$P<0.01$）。提示祛湿活血方对 NAFLD 的防治作用可能不是通过对 TNF-α 的调节而是通过对 APN 表达的调节而实现。张玲燕等对高脂饲料诱导的 NAFLD 大鼠予清脂护肝方（党参、淫羊藿、红花、川芎、赤芍药、生黄芪等）灌胃 6 周后，与模型组比较，清脂护肝方高（20.70 g/kg·d）、中（10.35 g/kg·d）、低（5.18 g/kg·d）剂量组的肝纤维化标志物肝组织匀浆Ⅳ型胶原及血清层黏连蛋白均明显降低（均 $P<0.05$，$P<0.01$），肝细胞脂肪变性程度也明显减轻（$P<0.01$）。与优缓平片组比较，清脂护肝方中、高剂量组肝细胞脂肪变性积分明显降低（$P<0.05$，$P<0.01$）。提示清脂护肝方具有良好的抗纤维化及减轻肝细胞脂肪变性作用。郝志民等对高脂饮食饲料诱导的 NAFLD 大鼠予新加越鞠丸（川芎、香附、神曲、白术、莪术、虎杖等）灌胃 4 周后，与模型组比较，新加越鞠丸组较模型对照组血清 APN 含量明显升高，瘦素含量明显下降（$P<0.05$）。何道同等以高脂高糖饲料喂饲造模随机分为模型组（M 组）、罗格列酮组（R 组）、柴胡—人参药对组（Y 组）。给药 4 周后，与 M 组比较，Y 组大鼠肝细胞脂肪病变明显减轻，R 组脂肪变性改善程度不明显；Y 组血清 TC、TG、LDL-C、FBG、FINS、IRI 水平显著降低（$P<0.05$ 或 $P<0.01$），HDL-C 水平未见明显变化。提示柴胡—人参药对能够改善 NAFLD 大鼠肝细胞脂肪变性和炎症程度，降低其血清 TC、TG、LDL-C 和肝脏 TG 水平，降低胰岛素和瘦素抵抗。陈剑明等对高脂饲料诱导的 NAFLD 大鼠随机分为模型组，芍药苷高（200 mg/kg·d）、中（100 mg/kg·d）、低（50 mg/kg·d）剂量组，双环醇组，正常组对照。灌胃给药 14 周，与正常组相比，模型组大鼠表现出内脏型肥胖，胰岛素敏感性及血清 APN、肝组织内 AMPK 磷酸化水平均显著下降（$P<0.05$，$P<0.01$）；同时脂质合成基因 SREBP-1c 和 FAS 的 mRNA 表达量显著增多；与模型组比较，芍药苷各剂量组、双环醇组的胰岛素抵抗得到改善（$P<0.05$，$P<0.01$），血清 APN 水平上调（$P<0.05$，$P<0.01$），各给药组大鼠内脏型肥胖减轻，肝组织内 AMPK 磷酸化水平提高（$P<0.05$，$P<0.01$），以芍药苷高剂量组为著（$P<0.05$）；芍药苷各剂量组 SREBP-1c 基因表达水平显著下降（$P<0.05$，$P<0.01$），FAS 基因表达水平下降，以高、中剂量组为著（均 $P<0.01$）。提示芍药苷的作用机制可能与激活 AMPK 和抑制肝细胞脂质合成途径有关。

（田华捷　徐列明）

【抗肝纤维化的实验研究】

Bai T 等研究百里香醌的抗肝纤维化作用及潜在的作用机制。体内实验采用硫代乙酰胺腹腔注射建小鼠肝纤维化模型，以百里香醌（20、40 mg/kg）干预后发现，其能够有效对抗肝纤维化和减少炎性细胞的浸润；明显地降低小鼠肝组织Ⅰ型胶原、α-平滑肌肌动蛋白（α-SMA）以及金属蛋白酶组织抑制物-1（TIMP-1）的水平。体外实验以不同浓度的百里香醌预处理培养肝星状细胞（HSC）1 h 后，加入脂多糖（LPS）24 h 后显示，百里香醌能够有效减少 T-HSC/Cl-6 的细胞活性，明显降低由 LPS 刺激后Ⅰ型胶原以及α-SMA 的表达，抑制 TLR4/MyD88 信号通路的激活以及 NF-κB 的核转导活性。董妙先等以 40% CCl_4 橄榄油混悬液皮下注射建模型大鼠随机分为 CCl_4 组、大黄素+CCl_4 组，并设空白对照组。灌胃给药 12 周，与空白对照组比较，CCl_4 组大鼠肝脏组织胶原面积显著性增加（$P<0.05$）；与 CCl_4 组比较，大黄素+CCl_4 组肝脏组织胶原面积显著减少（$P<0.05$）。与空白对照组比较，CCl_4 组大鼠肝脏组织 Smad3 mRNA 和蛋白表达显著性增加（均 $P<0.05$）；大黄素+CCl_4 组肝组织 Smad3 mRNA 和蛋白表达则显著性减少（均 $P<0.05$）。提示大黄素可能通过调控 Smad3 的表达来逆转肝纤维化。边艳琴等以腹腔注射二甲基亚硝胺（DMN）造模随机分组给药 4 周后显示，

与正常组比较，模型组的肝体比值显著降低($P<0.01$)。与模型组比较，茵陈蒿汤组、甘露消毒丹组的肝体比值明显升高($P<0.01$，$P<0.05$)；可显著改善肝组织病理，降低肝组织羟脯氨酸(Hyp)含量($P<0.01$)；茵陈蒿汤可显著改善肝功能($P<0.05$，$P<0.01$)；甘露消毒丹显著降低血清总胆红素含量($P<0.01$)，但对血清ACT、AST等作用不明显。提示茵陈蒿汤的疗效果优于甘露消毒丹。傅向阳等以DMN腹腔注射造模随机分为模型组、水飞蓟宾(SIL)组、荔枝核总黄酮(SLTF)高(400 ml/kg·d)、中(200 ml/kg·d)、低(100 ml/kg·d)剂量组。灌胃6周后，与模型组比较，SIL组、SLTF各剂量组的肝功能与肝纤3项指标(LN、HA、PCⅢ)均有改善(均$P<0.05$)，SLTF高剂量组疗效优于SIL组和SLTF中、低剂量组。以模型组比较，SIL组和SLTF高、中剂量组的血小板衍生生长因子(PDGF)、TNF-α mRNA表达均显著降低，以SLTF高剂量组最著(均$P<0.05$)。陈少丽等以腹腔注射猪血清造模随机分为模型组、下瘀血汤(大黄、桃仁、䗪虫)组、组分处方(大黄素、苦杏仁苷与䗪虫提取物)组，设正常组对照。口服给药4周，与正常组相比，模型组大鼠肝组织α-SMA、转化生长因子-β1(TGF-β1)、PDGF受体(PDGF-βR)mRNA的表达均显著升高(均$P<0.05$)；与模型组比较，下瘀血汤组、组分处方组大鼠肝组织α-SMA、TGF-β1、PDGF-βR mRNA的表达显著下调(均$P<0.05$)；与组分处方组相比，下瘀血汤组下调α-SMA、TGF-β1、PDGF-βR mRNA的表达更加明显(均$P<0.05$)。提示下瘀血汤与组分处方通过抑制α-SMA、TGF-β1、PDGF-βR mRNA的表达而发挥抗肝纤维化作用，且下瘀血汤优于组分处方。张俊杰等以腹腔注射1% DMN造模随机分为模型组、桃核参术汤(桃仁、桂枝、大黄、甘草、莪术、白术等)组。灌胃6周后，与模型组比较，桃核参术汤组血浆肾素活性水平、血管紧张素Ⅱ水平显著下降(均$P<0.01$)。Yang T等用HPTLC-ESI/MSn方法检测大鼠含扶正化瘀方血清中吸收和代谢的丹参成分。发现了丹参11个入血成分和2个代谢产物。其中丹参酚酸B、咖啡酸和迷迭香酸能明显抑制培养的人肝星状细胞株的增殖，下调α-SMA的表达。表明其是扶正化瘀方抗肝纤维化的有效成分。

(姜　娜　徐列明)

【肝硬化腹水的治疗】

范杰将60例肝硬化腹水患者随机分为两组，均予护肝、利尿、补充白蛋白及对症治疗，观察组38例加附子楮实汤(制附子、楮实子、干姜、桂枝、吴茱萸、黄芪等)随证加减煎服。治疗6周后，有效率分别为88.9%(32/36)、50.0%(12/24)。陈广梅将56例阴虚型肝硬化腹水患者随机分为两组，均予西医内科综合治疗，治疗组34例加服养阴活血利水方(北沙参、太子参、楮实子、山药、薏苡仁、白术等)。经治8周后，总有效率分别为91.2%(31/34)、68.2%(15/22)。治疗组在改善肝功能、降低胆红素、提高血浆白蛋白、减少腹水时间及中医证候积分减少等方面均优于对照组。张佩江将112例肝硬化腹水患者随机分为两组。在一般治疗(如低盐、高热量、高蛋白、易消化饮食、卧床休息等)的基础上均予西医保肝、利尿、补充白蛋白及新鲜血浆的治疗，治疗组加用腹水1号颗粒(柴胡、桂枝、茯苓、泽泻、丹皮、山茱萸等)随证加减煎服，对照组则予腹水1号颗粒模拟剂(由蔗糖和淀粉组成)。治疗28 d，并随访12个月。结果治疗组与对照组总有效率分别为91.1%(51/56)、73.2%(41/56)，组间比较，$P<0.05$。6个月后随访期治疗组患者复发率和死亡率明显低于对照组($P<0.05$)。许文君将肝硬化腹水湿热蕴结证患者随机分为治疗组40例与对照组38例，分别予清肝利肠方(生大黄、生地黄、厚朴、赤芍药、蒲公英、茵陈)灌肠联合西药基础治疗与单纯西药治疗。经治3周，总有效率分别为87.5%(35/40)、63.2%(24/38)，组间比较，$P<0.05$。齐盛将100例肝硬化腹水患者随机分为两组，治疗组60例用疏肝运脾汤(柴胡、茯苓、黄芪、薏苡仁、桂枝、丹参等)随症加减，对照组用常规西药。经治60 d，总有效率分别为91.7%(55/60)、65.0%(26/40)，组间比较，$P<0.05$。何义华将120例肝硬化腹水患者随机平分为两组，均予基础治疗，治疗组加用黄芪五苓散(黄芪、茯苓、猪苓、白术、泽泻、桂枝)随证加减煎服。经治12周，治疗组与对照组总有效率分别为91.7%(55/60)、76.7%(46/60)，组间比较，$P<0.05$。吴永斌将128例难治性肝硬化腹水患者随机平分为两组，均予保肝、利尿、限制水钠摄入、输注血浆及白蛋白等常规治疗，并予奥曲肽降低门脉压力，治疗组中药(大黄、三棱、芒硝、冰片，研末醋制成糊状)贴脐，每2 d1帖，7帖为1个疗程。经治2周后，

治疗组与对照组总有效率分别为 84.4%(54/64)、45.3%(29/64),组间比较,$P<0.01$。两组腹围均减少,24 h 尿量及尿钠含量均增多,以治疗组更著($P<0.05$)。

(蒋式骊　徐列明)

【慢性肾脏病的治疗与研究】

尹雪皎总结孙伟运用络病理论治疗慢性肾脏病(CKD)经验,认为慢性肾脏病属本虚标实之证,以肾虚为本,外感、湿热、瘀血为标。病因病机为"肾络失和",治当益肾清利、和络泄浊,"和络"为关键,虚则扶正理虚、养脏和络,实则祛邪通络。

丁世永等将 70 例慢性肾小球肾炎少阳病患者随机平分为小柴胡汤治疗组和肾炎康复片对照组,疗程均为 4 周。治疗组的中医证候、主要症状改善程度明显优于对照组($P<0.05$,$P<0.01$)。与对照组比较,24 h 尿蛋白定量明显减少($P<0.05$),辅助性 T 细胞 1 型/2 型、IL－17 及细胞因子 RANTES 均有不同程度降低($P<0.05$,$P<0.01$),IL－4 明显升高($P<0.05$),提示小柴胡汤可通过调节患者机体免疫紊乱而改善炎症,起到减轻蛋白尿的作用。丁怀顺等将 60 例慢性肾脏病 2～4 期并属湿热内蕴证患者随机平分为两组,治疗组予服解毒降浊汤(蒲公英、黄柏、土茯苓、生大黄、姜竹茹、白豆蔻等),对照组予服肾衰宁。经治 8 周,治疗组与对照组总有效率分别为 83.3%(25/30)、60.0%(18/30),组间比较,$P<0.05$。且治疗组中医证候积分较对照组明显下降($P<0.01$)。王永钧等将 315 例患者随机分为两组,均予基础治疗,中药辨证组 158 例予苯那普利模拟剂并辨证为肾气阴两虚、肾络瘀痹、风湿扰肾、湿热内蕴 4 个证型,分别予补益气阴(血)方(生黄芪、太子参、当归、女贞子)、肾络瘀痹方(积雪草、丹参、桃仁、制大黄)、祛除风湿方(雷公藤、汉防己、鬼箭羽)、清化湿热方(虎杖、川连、土茯苓、六月雪);西药组 157 例予苯那普利及中药组方模拟剂。经治 24 周,与西药组比较,中药辨证组的肾小球滤过率估算值(eGFR)升高明显($P<0.01$),Scr 下降($P<0.01$)。中药辨证组 29 例由 3 期减轻至 2 期,12 例由 3 期进展至 4 期,西药组 27 例由 3 期进展至 4 期。不良反应中药辨证组 16 例,西药组 32 例。王东等将 81 例患者随机分为两组,中药组 60 例辨证为脾肾气阴两虚、脾肾气阳两虚证,分别予服气阴两虚方(太子参、女贞子、山萸肉、生黄芪)、脾肾气阳两虚方(淫羊霍、党参、生黄芪、覆盆子);西药组予服氯沙坦。经治 24 周,总有效率分别为 93.3%(56/60)、76.2%(16/21),两组的中医证候积分值均明显改善($P<0.01$ 或$P<0.05$),中药组较西药组下降更为明显($P<0.05$)。张长明等将 215 例患者随机分为抗纤灵方(丹参、熟大黄、桃仁、当归、川牛膝)组 110 例与氯沙坦对照组 105 例,均予基础治疗。经治 16 周,总有效率分别为 77.3%(105/110)、51.4%(92/105),组间比较,$P<0.05$。治疗组腰酸、乏力、纳呆、肌肤甲错评分及总积分下降均明显优于对照组(均$P<0.05$)。曹蓓等将 67 例慢性肾小球肾炎血尿患者随机分为两组,均予西医常规治疗,治疗组 34 例加服血尿宁(太子参、炙黄芪、白茅根、山茱萸、白及、炒蒲黄等),对照组加服肾炎康复片。经治 6 个月,总有效率分别为 91.2%(31/34)、45.5%(15/33),组间比较,$P<0.05$。与对照组比较,治疗组尿沉渣红细胞计数明显减少,纤维蛋白原含量降低(均$P<0.05$)。李庆珍等将 78 例 CKD2～3 期患者在常规治疗(包括优质低蛋白饮食、控制血压、纠正贫血等)基础上随机分为两组,治疗组加用益肾化湿颗粒(人参、黄芪、白术、茯苓、泽泻、半夏等)。经治 8 周,与对照组比较,治疗组 24 h 尿蛋白定量、血 Scr 水平、hs－CRP、IL－6 水平明显下降($P<0.05$)。提示益肾化湿颗粒可减轻 CKD2～3 期患者的微炎症状态,有利于延缓 CKD 进展。

(何立群)

【抗肾纤维化的实验研究】

邹赟等以 5/6 肾切除(Plat 法)建慢性肾衰竭大鼠模型随机分为模型组、健脾清化方组(党参、生黄芪、草果仁、苍术、黄连、制大黄)和氯沙坦组,并设假手术组对照。灌胃给药 60 d,与假手术组比较,模型组大鼠血清肌酐和尿素氮均有明显上升,肾组织匀浆中 SOD 活性降低,MDA 含量升高,肾组织中 AT1 蛋白表达显著上调,p47phox mRNA 表达显著增加(均$P<0.05$)。与模型组比较,健脾清化方组、氯沙坦组的血清肌酐、尿素氮含量降低,肾组织匀浆中 SOD 活性上升,MDA 含量下降,肾组织中 AT1 蛋白表达显著下调,p47phox mRNA 表达显著降低(均$P<0.05$)。与氯沙坦组比较,健脾清化方组肾组织 SOD 活性明显升高,($P<0.05$),肾组织中 AT1 蛋白及 p47phox mRNA 表达下降趋势明显,但无显著性

差异($P>0.05$)。提示健脾清化方可通过降低ATⅡ及NADPH氧化酶的表达,从而改善慢性肾衰竭大鼠的氧化应激反应,延缓肾纤维化进程。邹氏以同样方法研究健脾清化方对慢性肾衰肾纤维化大鼠磷酸化p38丝裂原活化蛋白激酶(p38MAPK)介导的炎症因子的调控作用。结果与模型组比较,健脾清化方组、科素亚组肾组织TNF-α、IL-10及p38MAPK蛋白表达均明显下降($P<0.05$)。提示健脾清化方可通过阻止p38MAPK信号通路的活化,继而动态调控致炎因子TNF-α与抑炎因子IL-10的表达,改善慢性肾衰炎症状态。王东等将大鼠随机分组给药灌胃3 d,并体外培养大鼠肾组织骨髓来源的成纤维细胞(FBS)。结果显示,与正常血清组比较,TGF-β_1组α-SMA、CollagenⅠ及α-SMAmRNA、CollagenⅠmRNA表达水平明显增强($P<0.05$或$P<0.01$),与TGF-β_1组比较,TGF-β_1+福辛普利组、TGF-β_1+抗纤灵(丹参、酒大黄、牛膝、桃仁、当归)组的α-SMA、CollagenⅠ及α-SMAmRNA、CollagenⅠmRNA表达水平均降低($P<0.05$或$P<0.01$)。提示抗纤灵方药物血清可从基因及蛋白两个水平有效降低骨髓来源的成纤维细胞α-SMA的表达,抑制其表型转化,从而抑制肾间质纤维化。王氏进一步研究抗纤灵方中的有效单体,采用体外培养肾成纤维细胞株与系膜细胞株并随机分组,以MTT法观察24 h中药单体对两种细胞株的作用以及ELISA法对TGF-β_1的分泌情况。结果与空白对照组相比,加入TGF-β_1刺激因子可以促进两种细胞株的活化($P<0.05$),以及TGF-β_1的分泌($P<0.01$),丹参素、丹酚酸、齐墩果酸、苦杏仁苷、大黄素、大黄酚等抗纤灵中药有效单体可以抑制活化的细胞株增殖和TGF-β_1的分泌($P<0.05$或$P<0.01$)。说明抗纤灵中药单体可以抑制活化的肾成纤维细胞株和系膜细胞株的增殖,有效防治肾纤维化,其作用机制可能与抑制TGF-β_1的分泌有关。周萍等以单侧输尿管梗阻建立肾间质纤维化模型随机分为模型组,黄芪丹参高(25.00 g/kg)、中(12.50 g/kg)、低(6.25 g/kg)剂量组。灌胃给药2周,与模型组比较,黄芪丹参中剂量组血清Cr水平下降($P<0.05$),各给药组血清尿素氮(BUN)水平、尿α1-微球蛋白含量明显降低(均$P<0.05$)。黄芪丹参各剂量组的肾纤维化抑制因子par-3蛋白增高,并随剂量的增大而增高($P<0.01$)。提示黄芪丹参"药对"可通过促进par-3的表达,从而保护肾小管功能,减轻肾间质纤维化的进展,并呈一定的量效关系。梁敏等以单侧输尿管结扎造模随机分为单侧输尿管结扎(UUO)组、单侧输尿管结扎合槲皮素组,并设假手术组对照。灌胃给药14 d后显示,假手术组肾脏结构正常,肾小管排列紧密整齐,小管基底膜光滑。UUO组和UUO合用槲皮素组可见部分肾小管不同程度扩张萎缩及坏死,大量单核细胞与淋巴细胞浸润,小管间质区面积扩大,小管基底膜不同程度断裂增厚。与UUO组比较,UUO合用槲皮素组的肾皮质相对间质容积、胶原含量均有下降($P<0.05$)。UUO组、UUO合用槲皮素组的肾脏HSP47值分别为21.89±1.31、17.55±0.39,E-钙粘素值分别为2.12±0.25、2.77±0.19,组间比较均有显著性差异(均$P<0.05$)。提示槲皮素对大鼠肾皮质相对间质容积、胶原含量及肾脏HSP47、E-钙粘素的影响可能是其抗肾纤维化的机制之一。

(何立群)

【慢性再生障碍性贫血的治疗与研究】

陈海琳等将91例慢性再生障碍性贫血(CAA)患者随机分为两组,治疗组分别辨证为脾肾阳虚证组31例服用生血Ⅰ号合剂(黄芪、党参、当归、淫羊藿、巴戟天、丹参等),脾肾阴虚证组30例服用生血Ⅱ号合剂(黄芪、党参、当归、女贞子、何首乌、丹参等);对照组服用复方皂矾丸。经治6个月,治疗组中医证候改善明显优于对照组($P<0.05$),依赖红细胞悬液输注者比率较对照组明显减少($P<0.05$),依赖血小板悬液输注者减少率大于对照组($P<0.05$),感染发生率较对照组明显下降($P<0.05$)。曾英坚将33例CAA患者随机分成两组,均予环孢素、十一酸睾酮胶囊、细胞刺激因子为主治疗,治疗组18例加用愈障生血汤(淫羊藿、补骨脂、鹿角胶、龟板胶、黄精、黄芪等)。经治6个月,治疗组总有效率为88.9%(16/18),对照组为60.0%(9/15)。治疗组WBC、Hb、BPC均较治疗前明显改善,且优于对照组,血小板输注总量明显少于对照组(均$P<0.05$),两组转化生长因子β_1(TGF-β_1)均较治疗前明显降低(均$P<0.05$),治疗组更为明显($P<0.05$)。

胡令彦等将70例CAA患者随机分为两组,均予安雄或康力龙治疗,治疗组(辨证为脾肾阴虚证与脾肾阳虚证)45 例加用健脾补肾方(黄芪、女贞子、太子参、白术、白芍药、炒丹皮等)并随证加减(脾肾阴虚证加生地黄、黄柏、鳖甲等,脾肾阳虚证加补骨脂、淫羊藿等)。经治 2 个月,与治疗前比较,脾肾阳虚组 Th17 及 IL－17、IL－6 水平均有下降($P<0.05$),脾肾阴虚组仅 IL－16 水平明显下降($P<0.05$),对照组仅 Th17 水平明显下降($P<0.05$)。提示健脾补肾方对 CAA 患者 Th17 失衡的改善作用可能存在于细胞因子层面。通过调整相关细胞因子水平主要是 IL－6,减少 Th17 升高产生的对造血祖细胞或干细胞的破坏而导致的骨髓衰竭变化。王海霞等将 79 例非重型再生障碍性贫血(NSAA)患者随机分为两组,并设正常组 20 例,治疗组 40 例予愈障颗粒(生地黄、熟地黄、菟丝子、枸杞子、鸡血藤、女贞子等),对照组 39 例用西药常规治疗,疗程均为 6 个月。结果与正常组比较,两组患者的骨髓小粒中血管内皮生长因子(VEGF)的表达均明显降低(均$P<0.05$),与对照组比较,治疗组 VEGF 表达明显增高($P<0.05$)。提示愈障颗粒治疗 NSAA 的作用机制可能是通过影响骨髓细胞间通信来实现恢复骨髓的造血功能。

王琰等采用实时荧光定量聚合酶链反应检测 52 例不同证型(肾阳虚、肾阴虚、肾阴阳两虚)获得性再生障碍性贫血患者外周血单个核细胞中端粒保护蛋白 1(POT1)mRNA 表达,设正常对照组 20 例。结果与正常对照组比较,获得性再障患者的 POT1 mRNA 表达明显减低($P<0.05$),肾阴虚型 POT1 mRNA 表达水平低于肾阳虚型,肾阴阳两虚型最低,并与年龄有明显相关性($P<0.05$),提示 POT1 参与了获得性再障的发病过程,其在外周血单个核细胞的表达水平与获得性再障的中医证型有一定相关性。

(胡明辉　周永明)

【免疫性血小板减少症的治疗与研究】

曾英坚将 50 例免疫性血小板减少症(ITP)患者随机分为中药组 20 例、联合组 15 例和西药组 15 例。中药组以疏风凉血补肾方(防风、蝉蜕、苍耳子、水牛角、生地黄、赤芍药等)随症加减治疗,联合组以疏风凉血补肾方加强的松治疗,西药组以强的松为主治疗。经治 12 周,中药组患者血小板计数明显上升($P<0.01$),且优于西药组($P<0.05$),与联合组相似;中药组骨髓巨核细胞总数降低、产板巨核细胞比例上升($P<0.01$),与联合组相似,而西药组治疗前后无明显差异。与西药组比较,中药组、联合组治疗后 TGF－β_1 值降低(均$P<0.05$)。任娟等将 64 例激素依赖性 ITP 患者随机平分为两组,均予服强的松片,治疗组加用仙连颗粒(仙鹤草、连翘、生地黄、黄芪、茜草、淫羊藿等)。经治 4 个月,治疗组与对照组总有效率分别为 87.5%(28/32)、62.5%(20/32),组间比较,$P<0.01$。

刘清池等选取 ITP 患者 64 例随机平分为两组,治疗组予地黄止血胶囊(生地黄、茜草、牡丹皮、水牛角、太子参、三七等)合升板汤(紫珠、炒栀子、鹿茸草、紫草、地锦草、连翘等)治疗,对照组予服醋酸泼尼松片,设正常组 30 例。经治 8 周后,与正常组比较,ITP 患者外周血 T 淋巴细胞亚群 CD_4^+、$CD_4^+CD_{25}^+$ 及 CD_4^+/CD_8^+ 均降低,CD_8^+ 升高(均$P<0.05$),CD_3^+ T 淋巴细胞及 NK 细胞比例的变化无显著性差异($P>0.05$)。中药治疗组治疗后 CD_4^+、$CD_4^+CD_{25}^+$ 及 CD_4^+/CD_8^+ 明显升高,CD_8^+ 明显降低,与治疗前比较差异均有统计学意义($P<0.05$),NK 细胞比例与治疗前比较无明显差异($P>0.05$);西药对照组仅 $CD3^+$、CD_8^+ 与治疗前比较,$P<0.05$,CD_4^+、$CD_4^+CD_{25}^+$、CD_4^+/CD_8^+ 及 NK 细胞比例与治疗前比较,均$P>0.05$。提示 ITP 发病机制与免疫功能失调有关,凉血解毒中药治疗 ITP 的作用机制可能与其对 CD_3^+ T 淋巴细胞亚群的调节作用有关。郭锦荣等采用双向电泳、质谱分析等蛋白质组学技术建立 ITP 患者、激素敏感型及激素抵抗型 ITP 患者血清全蛋白双向凝胶电泳图谱,分析各组之间差异的蛋白质位点,并观察生血灵冲剂(黄芪、党参、当归、生地黄、熟地黄、牡丹皮等)对激素抵抗型 ITP 患者蛋白质表达的调节作用。结果与激素敏感型患者比较,ITP 激素抵抗型患者存在蛋白质纤维二糖水解酶高表达、外切纤维二糖水解酶低表达($P<0.05$)。经生血灵治疗后,ITP 激素抵抗型患者蛋白质表达水平有所改善($P<0.01$)。提示纤维二糖水解酶相对高表达、外切纤维二糖水解酶相对低表达,可能是 ITP 患者产生激素抵抗的重要机制,也可能是激素治疗无效的重要原因;生血灵可通过调节蛋白质表达水平而逆转激素抵抗。

(鲍计章　周永明)

【过敏性紫癜的治疗】

周密将 78 例过敏性紫癜(HSP)患者随机分

为两组，均用西医常规治疗，治疗组40例加用脱敏煎(防风、银柴胡、乌梅、五味子)。结果总有效率分别为95.0%(38/40)、76.3%(29/38)，组间比较，$P<0.05$。吴文英将208例患者随机平分为两组，均予消除致病因素、抗组胺药、改善血管通透性药物、糖皮质激素及对症治疗，治疗组加用加味桃红四物汤(桃仁、红花、生地黄、当归、赤芍药、丹参等)随症加减治疗。经治20 d，治疗组与对照组总有效率分别为86.5%(90/104)、64.4%(67/104)，组间比较，$P<0.05$。贾先红将60例辨证为风热伤络证HSP患者随机分成两组，治疗组31例予清火消斑汤(黄连、紫草、连翘、竹叶、玄参、丹参等)随症加减，对照组29例予常规治疗。经治4周，总有效率分别为80.7%(25/31)、58.6%(17/29)，组间比较，$P<0.05$。杜锐玲将80例辨证为湿浊内蕴型HSP患者随机平分为两组，对照组采用西医常规治疗，治疗组予三仁汤并随症加减煎服。经治4周后，治疗组与对照组总有效率分别为95.0%(38/40)、77.5%(31/40)，组间比较，$P<0.05$。宁亚军等将60例患者随机平分为两组，对照组予西医常规治疗，治疗组从脾胃辨证分脾胃虚、脾胃实热、不典型虚实寒热及脾胃阴虚4个证型，分别予服方1(人参、白术、茯苓、炙甘草、桂枝、白芍药等)、方2(生石膏、知母、黄芩、黄连、黄柏、栀子等)、方3(党参、白术、茯苓、炙甘草、桂枝、白芍药等)、方4(北沙参、麦门冬、玄参、生地黄、白薇、地骨皮等)治疗。经治4周，治疗组与对照组总有效率分别为86.7%(26/30)、63.3%(19/30)，组间比较，$P<0.05$。

(孙伟玲　周永明)

【2型糖尿病的治疗及实验研究】

李惠林等将60例2型糖尿病湿热蕴脾证患者平分为两组，均服二甲双胍片，治疗组加用三仁汤(苦杏仁、厚朴、法半夏、白豆蔻、薏苡仁、滑石等)随症加减煎服。经治3个月，治疗组与对照组总有效率分别为93.3%(28/30)、73.3%(22/30)，组间比较，$P<0.05$。与对照组比较，治疗组湿热蕴脾证候积分明显下降($P<0.05$)，FPG、餐后2 hPG、HbA1c、TG、TC、BMI均明显下降($P<0.01$或$P<0.05$)。黄婷等将60例脾虚湿困证肥胖糖尿病患者平分为两组，均予服二甲双胍片或格列齐特Ⅱ基础治疗，治疗组加用藿朴夏苓汤(藿香、厚朴、苍术、茯苓、猪苓、党参等)随证加减煎服，经治8周，治疗组与对照组总有效率分别为86.7%(26/30)、63.3%(19/30)，组间比较，$P<0.05$。唐奇志等将120例2型糖尿病患者随机分为治疗组与对照组。分别用姚氏芪薏四君子汤(黄芪、薏苡仁、党参、白术、茯苓、炙甘草)与二甲双胍治疗。经治1年，与对照组比较，治疗组BMI、HbA1c、LDL-C、TC、TG、纤维蛋白原(Fib)、HOMA-IR、Leptin、FINS均下降，HDL-C、凝血酶原时间(PT)、活化部分凝血酶时间(APTT)、APN水平均上升(均$P<0.05$)。朱蕴华等将具备中医“热”证素特点的60例患者随机分为两组，均予西药原降糖方案，治疗组加服清化颗粒(黄芩、黄连、葛根等)，对照组加服安慰剂。经治12周，与对照组比较，治疗组HbA1c、MDA明显下降，稳态模式评估指数HOMA2%B、SOD明显上升(均$P<0.05$)。王永刚等将123例气阴两虚证患者随机分为两组，均予常规降糖西药配合安慰剂，治疗组62例加服四黄降糖颗粒(黄芪、生地黄、大黄、黄连、鬼箭羽)。经治6个月，与对照组比较，治疗组FPG、餐后1 hPG、餐后2 hPG、HbA1c均下降($P<0.01$或$P<0.05$)。且在改善中医证候方面优于对照组($P<0.05$)。周潮等将420例初发2型糖尿病患者随机分为两组，治疗组279例寅时服用调气降糖丸(麦冬、黄芪、黄芩、郁金、僵蚕、女贞子等)，巳时服用益脾降糖丸(黄芪、山药、茯苓、白术、泽泻、砂仁等)，酉时服用糖肾康(生地黄、山茱萸、木瓜、巴戟天、附子、西洋参等)，对照组予服二甲双胍。经治3个月，与对照组比较，治疗组FPG、餐后2 hPG、胰高血糖素明显下降(均$P<0.01$)，空腹、餐后1h胰岛素水平均降低(均$P<0.05$)。

杨海燕等将255例患者根据HbA1c水平分为血糖控制良好(HbA1c≤6.5%)、血糖控制一般(6.5%<HbA1c<7.5)、血糖控制差(HbA1c≥7.5%)三组。比较三组患者生存质量，并分别比较脾胃气虚、气阴两虚、肺胃燥热、肝肾阴虚、湿热中阻5个证的HbA1c水平。结果糖尿病不同HbA1c水平生存质量各个维度得分，除躯体角色功能外，差异无统计学意义($P>0.05$)。气阴两虚证HbA1c水平高于脾胃气虚证，偏阴虚组HbA1c水平高于偏阳虚组($P<0.05$，$P<0.01$)。戴立恒等将100例患者分为阴虚热盛证组、气阴两虚证组、阴阳两虚证组，设30例正常对照组。结果和正常对照组相比，阴虚热盛证、气阴两虚证、阴阳两虚证患者的C-肽分泌均延迟，分泌数

值减低，呈依次下降趋势；空腹血糖呈依次上升趋势（均$P<0.05$）；3个证型之间比较，空腹胰岛素、HOMA－IR依次降低（均$P<0.05$）。

常柏等将大鼠120只随机分为正常对照组，模型组，抵挡汤（桃仁、水蛭、虻虫、大黄）早、中、晚期干预组，辛伐他汀组与罗格列酮组，除正常对照组外其余各组以高脂饲料喂养及尾静脉注射链脲佐茵素（STZ）造模，灌胃给药均24周。结果与模型对照组比较，抵挡汤早期干预组、辛伐他汀组大鼠血清IL－4水平升高；抵挡汤早期干预组、抵挡汤中期干预组、罗格列酮组大鼠血清IL－13水平升高（均$P<0.05$）；抵挡汤早期干预组、抵挡汤中期干预组、罗格列酮组大鼠主动脉TNF－αmRNA表达均降低（均$P<0.05$）。提示抵挡汤早期干预可通过调节炎性介质的释放而抑制糖尿病大血管炎症反应，改善糖尿病大血管炎症病变。付丽媛等以腹腔注射小剂量STZ加高糖高脂饲料建立模型，随机分为模型组、二甲双胍组、健脾增液汤组（黄芪、山药、苍术、茯苓、生地黄、玄参等）、健脾化湿汤组（黄芪、山药、苍术、茯苓）、增液汤组（生地黄、玄参、麦冬）。灌胃给药8周，与模型组比较，二甲双胍组、健脾增液汤组、健脾化湿汤组TC、TG、血游离脂肪酸（FFA）均下降（均$P<0.01$），以健脾增液汤组尤为显著，增液汤组各项指标无显著性差异。田春雨等以高脂加注射STZ造模，随机分为模型组、罗格列酮阳性对照组、双益降糖方（黄芪、山茱萸、桑白皮、黄连、葛根、佩兰）高（4.0 g/kg·d）、低（1.0 g/kg·d）剂量组，设正常对照组。治疗4周，与模型组比较，双益降糖方高、低剂量组，罗格列酮组餐后0.5、2 h血糖明显降低（均$P<0.05$）；双益降糖方低剂量组、罗格列酮组空腹血糖明显降低（均$P<0.05$）。各治疗组糖耐量、糖化血红蛋白、血脂明显降低（均$P<0.05$），血清胰岛素升高（均$P<0.05$）。双益降糖方低剂量组、罗格列酮阳性对照组之间比较未见显著性差异。张先慧等以高能量饲料建立模型小鼠，随机分为模型组、辛开（柴胡、清半夏、生姜）组、苦降（黄连、黄芩、枳实、熟大黄）组、辛开苦降（柴胡、黄芩、黄连、清半夏、枳实、熟大黄等）组、马来酸罗格列酮组。灌胃给药4周，与模型组比较，苦降组、马来酸罗格列酮组血糖明显降低（均$P<0.05$），各给药组小鼠胰岛素浓度均降低，胰岛素敏感指数均升高（均$P<0.05$），但组间比较，$P>0.05$。马来酸罗格列酮组CHO、TG、LDL值均降低，苦降组、辛开苦降组TG值降低（均$P<0.05$）。提示辛开苦降方及其拆方可以降低血清胰岛素浓度，增强胰岛素的敏感性，辛开苦降方还可降低小鼠TG含量，改善脂代谢紊乱状态。江明金等以链脲佐菌素加高糖、高脂饲料造模随机分为模型组，罗格列酮组，胡芦巴碱低（5 mg/kg）、中（15 mg/kg）、高（45 mg/kg）剂量组，另设正常对照组。灌胃给药8周，与模型组相比，胡芦巴碱中、高剂量组，罗格列酮组FBG、HbA1c、FINS水平均下降，ISI、肝糖原和肌糖原水平、海马neuritin mRNA及蛋白表达水平均上升（均$P<0.01$）；胡芦巴碱中、高剂量组TC、TG明显下降（均$P<0.01$），罗格列酮组无显著变化。任岩海等以高脂高糖饲料加小剂量STZ造模随机分为模型组，桑叶多糖高（1.0 g/kg·d）、中（0.5 g/kg·d）、低（0.25 g/kg·d）剂量组。灌胃给药12周，与模型组相比，桑叶多糖各剂量组血糖均显著降低（均$P<0.01$），以高剂量组最为著；TG、CH、LDL均显著降低（$P<0.01$），HDL均升高（均$P<0.05$）。王春梅等以高脂联合STZ造模随机分为模型组，松针提取物高（800 mg/kg）、中（400 mg/kg）、低（200 mg/kg）剂量组。灌胃4周后，与模型组比较，松针提取物各剂量组空腹血糖、血清总胆固醇、甘油三酯、血清NO、MDA水平均降低，SOD活性均增高（$P<0.05$或$P<0.01$）。以高剂量组最显著。提示松针提取物可通过减轻脂质过氧化、提高抗氧化酶活性而改善2型糖尿病大鼠的抗氧化能力。

（张　丹）

【糖尿病肾病的临床与实验研究】

樊威伟等将糖尿病肾病（DN）患者100例随机平分为两组，均予基础治疗，治疗组加用糖肾康胶囊（黄芪、女贞子、旱莲草、赤芍药、丹参、冬虫夏草），对照组加用贝那普利。经治2个月，与对照组比较，治疗组24 h尿蛋白定量下降（$P<0.01$），血栓调节蛋白含量降低（$P<0.05$）。提示糖肾康胶囊具有血管内皮保护作用，其机制可能与减轻高凝、防止尿蛋白外漏、延缓肾小球硬化及改善微循环有关。王洪武等选取气阴两虚兼夹血瘀证的早期糖尿病肾病（EDN）患者65例，以糖微康胶囊（黄芪、枸杞子、大黄、水蛭等）治疗3个月，运用聚合酶链反应—限制性内切酶片段长度多态性法检测相关指标。结果显示，患者血清血浆同型半胱氨酸（Hcy）明显升高，阳性率达到83.1%；中药

干预后血清 Hcy 水平明显下降,阳性率为 44.6%($P<0.01$)。MTHFR C677T 基因突变 44 例,突变率达到 67.7%。基因多态性则无变化。提示糖微康胶囊对 MTHFR 并无逆转基因型突变的作用,但可能通过改善 MTHFR 基因 C677T 突变造成的 MTHFR 活力下降,而使血清 Hcy 的含量降低。方朝晖等将 EDN 患者随机平分为两组,均予缬沙坦为基础的西医综合治疗,治疗组加用丹蛭降糖胶囊(太子参、生地黄、菟丝子、牡丹皮、水蛭、泽泻)。经治 8 周,两组 MCP-1,NF-κB,TGF-$β_1$及尿微量白蛋白排泄率(UAER)均明显下降(均$P<0.05$),与对照组比较,治疗组治疗后 MCP-1,NF-κB,TGF-$β_1$及 UAER 均明显降低($P<0.05$ 或$P<0.01$)。提示丹蛭降糖胶囊可降低尿白蛋白排泄率,延缓肾脏损伤,从而下调患者血 MCP-1,NF-κB 及 TGF-$β_1$的水平,阻断炎症介质的表达,抑制炎症反应,改善 EDN 微炎症状态。

奚悦等以高脂高糖饲料加链脲佐菌素造模随机分为模型对照组(B 组)、益气活络方(黄芪、生地黄、茺蔚子等)治疗组(C 组),并设空白对照组(A 组)。灌胃给药 6 周,与 A 组比较,B 组的24 h 尿蛋白量明显升高,肾小球中 nephrin 阳性表达的细胞数降低($P<0.01$,$P<0.05$)。与 B 组比较,C 组 24 h 尿蛋白量降低($P<0.05$),肾小球中 nephrin 阳性细胞显著增多,肾皮质中 nephrin mRNA 表达水平显著上调(均$P<0.05$)。提示上调 nephrin 基因及蛋白的表达水平可能是益气活络方减少尿蛋白的机制之一。王天文等以注射链脲佐菌素造模随机分为模型对照组,糖肾芪(黄芪、生地黄、水蛭、土鳖虫、匙羹藤叶、青风藤等)高(28.0 g/kg)、中(14.0 g/kg)、低(7.0 g/kg)剂量组,糖脉康颗粒组,糖适平+卡托普利组。灌胃给药 12 周,与模型组比较,糖肾芪高剂量组尿糖在(+++)以上的发生率下降($P<0.05$),其余各给药组变化不显著。糖肾芪高、中剂量组,及两个阳性药组空腹血糖 4、8、12 周均显著降低($P<0.05$ 或$P<0.01$)。各给药组糖化血红蛋白含量、血清肌酐含量均显著降低(均$P<0.05$)。糖肾芪高、中剂量及两个阳性药组大鼠 PAS 阳性区域占肾小球面积百分比均降低($P<0.05$ 或 $P<0.01$),其中糖肾芪高剂量组较为明显。提示糖肾芪可控制血糖、降低 24 h 尿蛋白量及尿蛋白排泄率、降低血清肌酐;可抑制及降低肾小球系膜增宽增厚,延缓 DN 的进展。潘永梅等以注射链脲佐菌素造模随机分为对照组、活血化瘀通络(丹参、川芎、地龙、水蛭、全蝎)组、正常组。灌胃给药 16 周,与正常组比较,对照组大鼠 BMP-7 及其 mRNA 表达明显减少,肾脏指数、FBG、HbAlc、尿微量白蛋(U-Alb)水平明显升高,肾小球基底膜(GBM)明显增厚(均$P<0.05$)。与对照组比较,活血化瘀通络组大鼠 BMP-7 及其 mRNA 表达明显增加,KI、U-Alb 以及 GBM 厚度明显降低(均$P<0.05$)。李敏州等采用高脂饲料喂养制备 DN 模型小鼠随机分为模型组、芪卫颗粒(黄芪、生地黄、鬼箭羽、大黄等)组、缬沙坦胶囊组,设正常组。灌胃给药 12 周。进行检测。结果显示,与正常组比较,模型组肾组织 TGF-$β_1$、TIMP-1 表达、磷酸化 Smad2(P-Smad2)、磷酸化 Smad3(P-Smad3)、整合素连接激酶(ILK)及 ILK mRNA 表达均明显增加,MMP-9、Smad7 表达明显下降(均$P<0.01$)。与模型组比较,芪卫颗粒组及缬沙坦胶囊组 TGF-$β_1$、P-Smad2、P-Smad3、ILK 及 IL KmRNA 表达显著减少($P<0.05$ 或 $P<0.01$),Smad7 表达明显增加($P<0.01$),与缬沙坦胶囊组比较,芪卫颗粒组 P-Smad3 表达增加($P<0.05$)。提示芪卫颗粒可能通过下调 TGF-$β_1$、P-Smad2、P-Smad3、ILK 的表达,上调 Smad7 的表达,影响 TGF-$β_1$/Smads 信号通路,从而延缓 DN 肾脏纤维化。王辉等将链脲佐菌素诱导的模型大鼠随机分为模型组、开博通组、虎杖—益母草配伍组、虎杖—黄芪配伍组。灌胃给药 8 周,与模型组比较,虎杖—黄芪组、虎杖—益母草组在用药第 4~8 周血糖、TG 水平均明显降低(均$P<0.05$),两组全血黏度、血浆黏度明显减轻,其中虎杖—益母草组的血浆黏度减轻程度更为明显($P<0.01$)。

(刘　霖)

【糖尿病周围神经病变的中西医结合治疗及实验研究】

高友安将 210 例糖尿病周围神经病变(DPN)患者随机分为两组,均予甲钴胺静脉滴注和胰岛素强化疗法,治疗组加服当归四逆汤(当归、桂枝、白芍药、通草、丹参、细辛等)。经治 1 个月,治疗组与对照组总有效率分别为 87.6%(92/105)、69.5%(73/105),组间比较,$P<0.05$。李增祥等将 70 例 DPN 患者随机分为两组,均予西医常规治疗,治疗组加服身痛逐瘀汤(桃仁、红花、

秦艽、川芎、羌活、当归)。经治60 d,治疗组与对照组总有效率分别为91.4%(32/35)、77.1%(27/35),组间比较,$P<0.05$。治疗组在正中神经及腓总神经功能改善方面优于对照组(均$P<0.05$)。王坤玲等将65例患者随机分为两组,均予降糖处理和甲钴胺片剂口服,治疗组予加服疏肝清热通络方(柴胡、郁金、大黄、黄芩、黄连、芍药等)。经治8周,治疗组与对照组总有效率分别为97.1%(34/35)、90.0%(27/30),组间比较,$P<0.05$。治疗组NTSS-6评分、神经传导速度均优于对照组($P<0.05$)。季海锋等将60例患者随机平分为两组,均予常规治疗,观察组加服通痹活血汤(薏苡仁、生黄芪、怀山药、葛根、鸡血藤、当归等)治疗。经治8周后,观察组与对照组总有效率分别为70%(21/30)、53.3%(16/30),组间比较,$P<0.05$。杨德良将患者随机分为两组,均予常规治疗,治疗组37例加服滋水荣木通络汤(熟地黄、山茱萸、山药、白芍药、木瓜、乌梅等)。经治2个月,总有效率分别为91.9%(34/37)、75.0%(27/36),组间比较,$P<0.05$。

沈祥峰等以链尿佐菌素加柠檬酸钠缓冲液腹腔注射大鼠造模随机分为模型组,运脾和络颗粒(黄芪、苍术、赤芍药、金银花、汉防己、当归等)高(12 g/kg)、中(6 g/kg)、低(3 g/kg)剂量组,甲钴胺组,糖脉康组。灌胃给药24周,与模型组比较,运脾和络颗粒高、中剂量组,糖脉康组的坐骨神经组织脑源性神经营养因子(BDNF)的蛋白与基因表达明显上调($P<0.05$),以运脾和络颗粒组高剂量组最为明显。张会欣等将小鼠造模并随机分为模型组,周络通胶囊(黄芪、桂枝、当归、生地黄、细辛等)高(6.85 g/kg)、中(4.43 g/kg)、低(1.71 g/kg)剂量组,设正常对照组。灌胃给药12周后,与正常对照组比较,模型组运动神经传导速度明显下降,TGF-β_1、TGF-βRI、TGF-βRII及Smad3表达明显上升(均$P<0.01$)。与模型组比较,周络通各剂量组运动神经传导速度均提高($P<0.05$,$P<0.01$),TGF-β_1、TGF-βRI、TGF-βRII及Smad3 mRNA表达均降低($P<0.05$,$P<0.01$)。提示周络通可通过抑制TGF-β_1/Smad3信号通路,减少细胞外基质积聚,降低神经髓鞘增厚,来改善糖尿病周围神经病变。

(张 丹)

【代谢综合征的实验研究】

田金英、李娟等对红景天、蛹虫草、大黄配伍组成的中药复方(FF16)治疗代谢综合征(MS)的作用机理进行系列实验,分别对其治疗肥胖症、控制血糖、改善肝脏脂质堆积、调节糖代谢紊乱、对糖尿病大鼠肾脏保护作用进行研究后发现,FF16可显著控制以高脂饮食造模的IRF肥胖小鼠和2型糖尿病KKAy肥胖小鼠的体重增长;降低KKAy小鼠血清TC水平、增加血清HDL-C含量、减小脂肪指数;可显著控制KKAy小鼠的餐后血糖和空腹血糖水平;使其葡萄糖负荷后的血糖峰值和AUC明显降低。使IRF小鼠葡萄糖耐量试验AUCIPGTT较IRF组降低22.3%;能显著增加IRF小鼠的胰岛素敏感性,使胰岛素耐量试验AUCITT降低22.1%,HOMA-IR指数降低49.5%。使IRF小鼠肝脏Akt磷酸化水平升高116.4%,GSK3β磷酸化水平升高24.9%。可显著降低IRF小鼠的肝脏指数,改善肝细胞脂肪变性。其能够改善IRF小鼠肝脏微循环障碍,使红细胞流速和红细胞切变速率分别增加了62.5%、49.7%,肝窦开放数增加70.0%,白细胞滚动数目显著减少。其还可显著改善IRF小鼠肝脏中胰岛素信号通路相关蛋白IRS-2、脂代谢相关蛋白HSL的异常表达。体外酶学实验显示,FF16可明显抑制分子靶点α-葡萄糖苷酶的活性。另外,FF16能够明显降低1型糖尿病大鼠血糖、血脂水平;降低肾脏指数和血尿素氮水平,增加尿肌酐排出,降低尿酶活性和尿蛋白水平;使血清和肾脏中SOD活性升高、MDA含量降低。

郭妍等研究中药新药LW-AFC(由六味地黄汤活性成分群配伍组成)对MS的作用。以高热量饲料造模小鼠随机分为模型组,二甲双胍组,LW-AFC高(3.2 g/kg)、中(0.8 g/kg)、低(0.2 g/kg)剂量组,并设正常对照组。灌胃给药6周,与正常对照组比较,模型组腹型肥胖相关指标内脏脂肪质量(VFM)及内脏脂肪系数(VFC)、空腹血清TC、LDL-C、FBG增高($P<0.01$),肝细胞呈弥漫性小泡性脂变,日均摄食量增高($P<0.01$),促食欲肽下丘脑神经肽Y(NPY)、抑食欲激素瘦素及抵抗素增高($P<0.05$)。与模型组比较,LW-AFC各剂量组TC、LDL-C、FBG,HOMA-IR、C肽均降低、HDL-C均升高($P<0.05$,$P<0.01$)。二甲双胍组与LW-AFC低剂量组肝细胞小泡性脂变减轻,LW-AFC中、高剂量组小泡性脂变改善明显,肝细胞恢复放射状排

列。提示LW-AFC对模型小鼠糖脂代谢紊乱及肝脏病理损伤具有改善作用。并且LW-AFC高、低剂量与二甲双胍可降低小鼠的日均摄食量和促食欲肽NPY水平($P<0.05$),LW-AFC高剂量显著增高抑食欲激素瘦素的水平($P<0.01$)。不同剂量的LW-AFC还可降低血清脂肪因子抵抗素和TNF-α、IL-6的水平($P<0.05$,$P<0.01$)。

姜楠等用以方测证法探讨糖代谢异常的MS大鼠可能出现的中医证型。将大鼠随机分为模型组及A、B、C、D组,分别用大柴胡汤(A组,9.4 g/kg)、黄连温胆汤(B组,10.4 g/kg)、知柏地黄丸(C组,15.1 g/kg)、血府逐瘀汤(D组,7.8 g/kg)干预。灌胃给药3周,与模型组比较,A~D组体重、血压、FBG均无显著差异,A、B、D组TG水平显著降低($P<0.05$或$P<0.01$),B组HDL-C显著升高($P<0.05$),A~D组FINS和HOMA-IR显著降低(均$P<0.01$)。提示糖代谢异常的MS大鼠可能同时存在肝胃郁热证、痰热互结证、阴虚热盛证、血瘀脉络证4种证型。各证型并不单独存在,而是病理因素相互夹杂,混合在一起组成复合证型,出现于糖代谢异常的MS大鼠中。

(刘　霖)

【高尿酸血症的实验研究】

吴生元等以酵母饲料加腺嘌呤造大鼠模型随机分为模型对照组、苯溴马隆组、健脾渗湿方(党参、茯苓、白术、三七、白芥子、金钱草等)组,并设正常对照组。灌胃给药14 d,与正常对照组比较,模型对照组肾脏中OAT3蛋白表达水平有所降低;与模型对照组比较,苯溴马隆组、健脾渗方组OAT3蛋白表达水平显著上调。提示上调尿酸盐转运蛋白OAT3,可能是健脾渗湿法治疗高尿酸血症的作用机制之一。李欣等以腺嘌呤与乙胺丁醇联合造模随机分为模型组,别嘌呤醇组,上中下通用痛风汤(苍术、黄柏、制南星、木防己、威灵仙、羌活等)高(20 g/kg)、中(10 g/kg)、低(5 g/kg)剂量组。灌胃给药21 d,与模型组比较,上中下通用痛风汤各剂量组的血尿酸水平显著降低(均$P<0.05$),且低于别嘌呤醇组($P<0.05$)。上中下通用痛风汤中剂量组黄嘌呤氧化酶(XOD)明显降低;高、中剂量组腺苷脱氨酶(ADA)明显降低;各剂量组血清BUN及Cre水平均显著降低,且低于别嘌呤醇组(均$P<0.05$)。提示上中下通用痛风汤可能通过降低XOD、ADA酶活性来降低血尿酸水平,并对肾脏有保护作用。周琦等以尿酸酶抑制剂奥替拉西钾诱导高尿酸血症小鼠模型随机分为模型组,别嘌呤醇组,穿山龙总皂苷高(600 mg/kg)、中(300 mg/kg)、低(60 mg/kg)剂量组。灌胃给药7 d后,与模型组比较,穿山龙总皂苷各剂量组的血清尿酸值(SUA)水平均显著降低,血清黄嘌呤氧化酶(XOD)、腺苷脱氨酶(ADA)活性降低,肾组织阴离子转运体1(OAT1) mRNA的表达量上调(均$P<0.05$)。体外实验结果显示,穿山龙总皂苷各剂量均可显著抑制与微晶型尿酸钠(MSU)进行孵育的多形核白细胞(PMNL)中β-GD和LDH的释放率(均$P<0.05$)。提示穿山龙总皂苷可能通过抑制XOD和ADA降低尿酸的生成,提高OAT1的表达从而促进尿酸的排泄。具有降高尿酸血症血尿酸及抗炎作用。

(徐光耀)

【帕金森病的临床与实验研究】

顾超等收集1998~2011年“万方数据库知识服务平台”帕金森病中医证型和方药研究的相关文献,归纳统计主要证型和常用药物。结果证型以肝肾亏虚(18.1%)、气血不足(15.4%)、气血瘀滞(14.3%)、肾精不足(13.5%)、阴虚动风(11.6%)等5种最为常见,占总频次的72.9%。实证以痰、瘀、风为主,虚证以肾虚及气血两虚为主。处方39首,常用方剂有大定风珠、导痰汤、天麻钩藤饮、大补阴丸、人参养荣汤等。用药110种,按功能归为15类,补益药列首位,活血药、安神药次之,3类药使用频次占60.5%,再次为开窍药、化痰药等。提示帕金森病以心、肝、脾、肾四脏虚为本,以风、火、痰、瘀为标,临证可从肝、肾、风、痰、瘀论治。

董其谦等以6-羟基多巴(6-OHDA)单侧内侧前脑束注射法造模随机分为模型组、养脾阴组(白芍药、甘草、肉苁蓉等),另设假手术对照组。灌胃给药8周,与模型组比较,第4、第8周养脾阴组向健侧旋转的圈数明显减少($P<0.01$)。与假手术组比较,模型组纹状体多巴胺(DA)、二羟苯乙酸(DOPAC)、高香草酸(HVA)含量显著降低(均$P<0.05$);与模型组比较,养脾阴组纹状体DA、DOPAC、HVA含量明显升高($P<0.05$或$P<0.01$)。提示养脾阴法可能对多巴胺能神经元具有神经保护作用。吴娜等通过6-OHDA立体定向至大鼠前脑内侧束建立帕金森病模型随机

分为模型组、西药(左旋多巴甲酯/苄丝肼)组、西药+天芪平颤颗粒(天麻、黄芪、熟地黄、白芍药、当归等)、大剂量组(中剂量组每味药剂量增加20%)、西药+天芪平颤颗粒中剂量组、西药+天芪平颤颗粒小剂量组(中剂量组每味药剂量减少20%)。灌胃给药4周,与模型组及西药组比较,西药+天芪平颤颗粒各剂量组的峰旋转次数均减少,以西药+天芪平颤颗粒大剂量组最为显著(均$P<0.05$)。与西药组比较,西药+天芪平颤颗粒大、中剂量组的磷酸化DARPP-32表达水平均未出现明显降低,磷酸化ERK1/2表达量均未出现明显上升(均$P<0.05$)。提示天芪平颤颗粒可能通过上调磷酸化DARPP-32的表达,抑制ERK通路的异常激活以达到减少PD大鼠剂峰异动行为。金泽等以脑立体定位注射6-OHDA建立大鼠PD模型随机分为模型组、洋金花高(0.036 g/kg)、中(0.018 g/kg)、低(0.009 g/kg)剂量组、美多芭组,同时设假手术组。灌胃给药3周,与模型组比较,各给药组纹状体内MDA含量均有明显降低(均$P<0.01$),其中美多芭组、洋金花高、中剂量组降低显著,组间比较,$P>0.05$;各给药组纹状体内SOD活性均明显增加(均$P<0.05$),其中美多芭组、洋金花高剂量组增加显著,组间比较,$P>0.05$。各给药组纹状体内GSH、GSH-Px均明显增加(均$P<0.05$),其中洋金花中剂量组增加最为明显。提示洋金花可能是通过减轻脂质过氧化反应,增强抗氧化防御机制,减少氧化应激,进而保护神经元,起到治疗PD的作用。

(张　洁)

【急性脑梗死的治疗】

黄月芳等将160例急性脑梗死风痰瘀血痹阻证且属于高同型半胱氨酸血症患者随机平分为两组,均予常规西医治疗,治疗组加服化痰通络汤合牵正散(半夏、化橘红、红花、丹参、川芎、党参等)。经治3周,治疗组与对照组总有效率分别为85.0%(68/80)、75.0%(60/80),组间比较,$P<0.01$。且在证候的改善、同型半胱氨酸的下降方面均优于对照组(均$P<0.05$)。张社峰等将239例急性脑梗死患者进行辨证并随机分为两组,均给予基础治疗;治疗组152例辨证属风火上扰、风痰火亢、痰热腑实、气虚血瘀、阴虚风动5个证型者均予中风防治灵Ⅰ号(太子参、制首乌、大黄、决明子、胆南星、水蛭等),属风痰瘀阻、痰湿蒙神2个证型者均予中风防治灵Ⅱ号口服(法半夏、陈皮、茯苓、炒白术、泽兰、泽泻等);对照组根据证型分别给予灯盏生脉胶囊及脑安胶囊口服。经治90 d,总有效率分别为90.1%(137/152)、79.3%(69/87),组间比较,$P<0.05$。治疗组的神经功能缺损评分下降较对照组更明显($P<0.01$)。麻志恒等将86例急性脑梗死风痰瘀阻证患者随机分为两组,均予西医常规治疗,观察组44例加服桃红三虫汤(桃仁、红花、水蛭、全蝎、僵蚕、川芎),对照组加服血滞通胶囊。经治8周,总有效率分别为90.9%(40/44)、83.3%(35/42),组间比较,$P<0.05$。且观察组TG、TC、全血黏度、血球压积、纤维蛋白原均较对照组明显降低($P<0.05$或$P<0.01$)。亓慧敏等将121例急性脑梗死伴有高同型半胱氨酸患者随机分为两组,治疗组予胆蒲通脉胶囊(石菖蒲、胆南星、三七、全蝎、红花、土元等),对照组予同等量的淀粉胶囊口服。经治4周,总有效率分别为93.5%(58/62)、88.1%(52/59),组间比较,$P<0.05$。且治疗组血浆同型半胱氨酸水平较对照组明显降低($P<0.05$)。张瑞等将76例患者随机平分为两组,均予常规治疗,治疗组加服通络醒脑颗粒(天麻、郁金、生大黄、地龙、浙贝母、水蛭等)。经治14 d,治疗组、对照组总有效率分别为86.8%(33/38)、71.1%(27/38)。组间比较,$P<0.05$。

(张　洁)

【脑卒中后抑郁的治疗及实验研究】

史先芬等将105例脑卒中后抑郁患者随机分为两组,均予服黛力新,治疗组55例加服加味奔豚汤(李根白皮、半夏、川芎、当归、白芍药、葛根等)。经治2个月,总有效率分别为95.4%(52/55)、76.0%(38/50),组间比较,$P<0.05$。林卿等认为肝郁痰结是脑卒中后抑郁的主要病机,将64例患者随机分为两组,均予脑血管病常规治疗和基本康复训练。治疗组加服柴桂温胆汤(北柴胡、黄芩、姜半夏、桂枝、赤芍药、白芍药等),对照组加服盐酸氟西汀。经治6周,治疗组与对照组总有效率分别为87.5%(28/32)、68.8%(22/32),组间比较,$P<0.05$。治疗组汉密尔顿抑郁量表评分、神经功能缺损程度评分均优于对照组(均$P<0.05$)。李钢以精乌胶囊(何首乌、黄精、女贞子、墨旱莲)治疗40例,设对照组30例予以谷维素。经治56 d,总有效率分别为92.5%(37/40)、43.3%(13/30),组间比较,$P<0.05$。两组

患者治疗后抑郁症状均有明显改善,HAMD评分均降低,治疗组更为明显(均$P<0.01$)。

张伟骏等以双侧颈总动脉永久性结扎造模随机分为模型组、涤痰开窍组(半夏、胆南星、石菖蒲、远志)、补肾益气组(人参、黄芪、何首乌、枸杞子、熟地黄)、活血祛瘀组(丹参、川芎、赤芍药、郁金)、氟西汀组、假手术组。灌胃给药28 d,与模型组比较,涤痰开窍组、补肾益气组,活血祛瘀组、氟西汀组的海马CA3区神经元锥体细胞数目均有上调($P<0.05$),与阳性药氟西汀组比较,涤痰开窍组CA3区神经元锥体细胞数目上调($P<0.05$)。提示中医不同治法对脑卒中后抑郁症大鼠海马神经元均有保护作用,以涤痰开窍法为优。王娣等将脑缺血后抑郁状态大鼠模型随机分为模型组、中药组、西药组。中药组、西药组分别予颐脑解郁方(刺五加、郁金等)、盐酸氟西汀灌胃共6周,另设正常组、假手术组对照。结果与正常组比较,模型组大鼠皮层及海马发光值降低,三磷酸肌醇(IP_3)含量明显升高($P<0.01$)。中药组、西药组大鼠的皮层及海马发光值升高,而IP_3含量均较模型组明显下降(均$P<0.01$)。与西药组相比,中药组皮层IP_3含量无显著差异($P>0.05$),中药组海马IP_3含量升高(均$P<0.05$)。与正常组比较,模型组、假手术组大鼠的海马及皮层子蛋白激酶C(PKC)含量明显升高($P<0.05$,$P<0.01$);与模型组比较,中药组、西药组大鼠的海马及皮层PKCα含量均明显下降(均$P<0.01$)。提示脑缺血后抑郁症的发病可能与磷脂酰肌醇(PI)通路有关;颐脑解郁方对PI通路有干预作用,可能是其治疗脑缺血后抑郁症的作用靶点。

(奚 骏)

【强直性脊柱炎的治疗与研究】

张俊莉等将110例强直性脊柱炎(AS)患者随机平分为两组,均予柳氮磺吡啶片加尼美舒利分散片,治疗组予加服盘龙七片(当归、丹参、重楼、盘龙七、竹根七、羊角七等)。经治12周后,两组腰背晨僵时间缩短,关节疼痛度评分、关节功能评分、ESR、CRP均下降(均$P<0.01$),其中治疗组在改善腰背晨僵时间、关节疼痛度方面优于对照组(均$P<0.05$),在治疗第4、第12周时,治疗组非甾体类消炎药减量人数多于对照组。范利锋等将100例湿热毒痹型活动期AS患者随机平分为两组,均予口服美洛昔康分散片及柳氮磺吡啶片,连续治疗12周。治疗组加用清热凉血膏(玄参、金银花、黄柏、苍术、薏苡仁、白芍药等)塌渍疗法,同时予红外线照射,治疗30 d。结果治疗组总有效率为96.0%(48/50),对照组为70.0%(35/50),组间比较,$P<0.01$。两组临床症状均明显改善,外周关节疼痛度评分、腰背痛评分均下降,晨僵时间缩短,以治疗组为优(均$P<0.05$)。韩福祥等以祛痛散(青风藤、海风藤、防风、土茯苓、川牛膝、金狗脊等)外敷治疗早中期AS寒湿痹证患者35例,设伤湿止痛膏外敷对照组。经治6个月,两组总有效率分别为97.1%(34/35)、86.7%(26/30),组间比较,$P<0.05$。

汪四海等认为AS病机为脾气亏虚,肝失濡养,肾失所藏,则筋骨失养,痹证乃生。脾虚证贯穿于AS骨代谢异常的始终,肝脾肾亏虚与AS发病密切相关,脾虚为其根本,认为采用益气健脾法治疗AS及干预AS骨代谢失衡具有实际意义。李仲贤等基于文本挖掘技术研究AS"理法方药"的相应规律,结果显示,AS证候以肾阴虚、肝肾阴虚为主,其次为肝肾亏虚、血瘀证;治以活血化瘀、温补肾阳、祛风通络为多,方药多选补肝肾、益气血、活血通络、温经散寒之品。

(黄陈招)

【血管性痴呆的治疗及实验研究】

程善廷等以归芎疗痴汤(当归、赤芍药、川芎、白术、茯苓、熟地黄等)治疗血管性痴呆(VD)患者40例,设对照组予服奥拉西坦胶囊。经治12周,以简易精神状态检查量表(MMSE)评价,治疗组与对照组总有效率分别为75.0%(30/40)、45.0%(18/40);以简易痴呆筛查量表评价,总有效率分别为82.5%(33/40)、50.0%(20/40),组间比较,均$P<0.05$。王东梅等将60例VD肾精亏虚证患者随机平分为两组,治疗组予服地黄益脑胶囊(熟地黄、生地黄、淮山药、川芎、当归、何首乌藤等),对照组予服脑复康片。经治8周,治疗组与对照组总有效率分别为80.0%(24/30)、53.3%(16/30),组间比较,$P<0.05$。孟凡莲等将92例VD肾虚血瘀证患者平分为两组,治疗组予服通络益脑丸(黄芪、何首乌、石菖蒲、肉苁蓉、红花、川芎等),对照组予服尼莫地平片及银杏叶片。经治3个月,治疗组与对照组总有效率分别为82.6%(38/46)、60.9%(28/46),组间比较,$P<0.05$。舒宏等将70例患者随机平分为圣济二精颗粒(黄精、枸杞子)治疗组和脑复康胶囊对照组。经治60 d,中医证候积分疗效总有效率分

别为94.3%(33/35)、82.9%(29/35)，组间比较，$P<0.05$。付毅敏等以醒智颗粒(人参、葛根、丹参、石菖蒲、天竺黄、茯苓等)治疗轻中度VD肝肾阴虚、痰浊瘀阻型的患者38例，设尼莫同组对照，疗程均为12周。治疗组与对照组总有效率分别为84.2%(32/38)、60.5%(23/38)，组间比较，$P<0.05$；且治疗组MMSE、ADL评分改善较对照组更明显(均$P<0.05$)。

张海燕等用喂食高脂饲料继以采用双侧颈总动脉夹闭再灌注方法复制动脉粥样硬化VD大鼠模型随机分为模型组，五脏温阳化瘀汤(附子、干姜、巴戟天、桂枝、半夏、石菖蒲等)高(5.0 g/kg)、中(2.5 g/kg)、低(1.25 g/kg)剂量组，脑复康阳性对照组。灌胃给药4周，与模型组比较，五脏温阳化瘀汤高、中剂量组从第3 d开始Morris水迷宫的逃避潜伏期明显缩短($P<0.01$)。五脏温阳化瘀汤各剂量组大鼠Nrf2在脑细胞核内表达显著增强，在细胞质中含量降低，HO-1蛋白表达显著增强($P<0.01$或$P<0.05$)。提示五脏温阳化瘀汤可能通过激活Nrf2蛋白通路来改善动脉粥样硬化VD大鼠学习记忆能力。刘春丽等以永久性结扎双侧颈总动脉法建立VD大鼠模型随机分为模型组，松果菊苷(ECH)高(45 mg/kg)、中(30 mg/kg)、低(15 mg/kg)剂量组，阳性药加兰他敏组(GAL)。腹腔注射给药4周，与模型组比较，ECH各剂量组、GAL组3～5 d的逃避潜伏期明显缩短($P<0.05$或$P<0.01$)，且第6 d穿越平台次数亦显著增加($P<0.05$或$P<0.01$)；ECH各剂量组、GAL组皮层、海马中的SOD、胆碱乙酰转移酶(ChAT)、胆碱酯酶(AChE)活性增高($P<0.05$或$P<0.01$)，MDA含量下降($P<0.05$或$P<0.01$)。提示ECH可能通过清除皮层、海马中自由基、减少脂质过氧化反应来改善脑缺血后自由基损伤所致的酶合成障碍，使ChAT、AChE活性增加，从而提高VD大鼠的学习记忆能力。段小花等以永久性双侧颈总动脉结扎法制作VD大鼠模型并随机分组，灌胃给药8周后，与模型组比较，天麻乙酸乙酯提取物高剂量(7.29 g/kg·d)组、尼莫地平组大鼠海马CA1区锥体细胞数目明显增多($P<0.01$)，天麻乙酸乙酯提取物低剂量(0.81 g生药/kg·d)组大鼠海马区CA1区锥体细胞数目则无明显变化。提示天麻乙酸乙酯提取物能明显改善脑缺血模型大鼠脑组织海马CA1区锥体细胞的病理改变。

(黄陈招)

【焦虑症的中西医结合治疗与研究】

赵洪运对64例焦虑症惊恐发作患者随机平分为两组，均予服氟哌噻吨美利曲辛片，治疗组加服安神定惊汤(龙骨、珍珠母、磁石、茯神、合欢皮、远志等)。经治8周，治疗组与对照组总有效率分别为93.8%(30/32)、81.3%(26/32)，组间比较，$P<0.05$。郭宇新将120例汉密顿焦虑量表(HAMA)总分≥21分的广泛性焦虑症未治患者平分为三组，A组予丁螺环酮片，B组予九味镇心颗粒(人参、酸枣仁、五味子、茯苓、远志、延胡索等)，C组予九味镇心颗粒加丁螺环酮片。经治6周后，C组的HAMA评分分值下降幅度均大于A、B两组($P<0.05$)，A、B两组间比较，$P>0.05$。李红琴等将63例焦虑症患者随机分为两组，均予服黛力新，治疗组32例加服中药(党参、茯神、当归、阿胶、麦冬、甘草等)。经治6周，总有效率分别为90.6%(29/32)、71.0%(22/31)，组间比较，$P<0.05$。刘飞将患者随机平分为两组，辨证组分为肝郁气滞证、痰热上扰证、心胆气虚证，分别予柴胡疏肝散加减、黄连温胆汤加减、平补镇心丹加减治疗。西药组单纯予罗拉。经治6周后，辨证组有效率为86.8%(33/38)、西药组为76.3%(29/38)，组间比较，$P<0.05$。

耿东等通过统计59篇文献中证候及证候要素的频数、频率来探讨焦虑症所涉及的中医证候的分布特征。结果频次出现在10次以上的证候有肝气郁结，心胆气虚，阴虚火旺，痰热内扰，心脾两虚，气郁化火。病位类证候要素6个，依次为心、肝、肾、脾、胆、胃；病机、病性类证候要素出现频率在10%以上的有气滞、火热、气虚、阴虚。耿氏以四诊信息采集表对200例广泛性焦虑症患者中医症状及证候要素分布特征进行研究后发现，前十位症状依次为急躁易怒、心情郁闷、胸闷喜太息、乏力疲倦、心慌多梦、短气、头身困重、神疲懒言、口干咽燥、口苦，证候要素依次为气滞、气虚、火热、血虚、阴虚、痰证、血瘀。初步推断广泛性焦虑症的病位为心、肝等脏腑，以气虚、气滞的表现为主，疾病属性以虚实夹杂为主。

(奚　骏)

[附] 参 考 文 献

B

Bai T, Yang Y, Wu YL, et al. Thymoquinone alleviates in fl ammation-associated liver fi brosis via TLR4 signaling pathway [J]. China Journal of Traditional Chinese Medicine and Pharmacy, 2013, 28(5): 1541

边艳琴,曹红燕,董姝,等,与甘露茵陈蒿汤消毒丹对二甲基亚硝胺诱导肝纤维化大鼠模型的方证比较研究[J]. 中华中医药杂志,2013,28(5): 1396

C

曹蓓,王琛,何立群. 血尿宁治疗慢性肾小球肾炎血尿的临床观察[J]. 上海中医药杂志,2013,47(2): 34

常柏,李巧芬,李春深,等. 抵挡汤早期干预对 2 型糖尿病大鼠血清 IL-4、IL-13 水平及主动脉 TNF-αmRNA 表达的影响[J]. 四川中医,2013,31(3): 48

陈广梅,赵红兵,何晶,等. 养阴活血利水方治疗阴虚型肝硬化腹水的临床疗效观察[J]. 四川中医,2013,31(2): 68

陈海琳,孙伟玲,周永明,等. 健脾补肾活血法联合小剂量雄激素治疗慢性再生障碍性贫血的临床观察[J]. 中医药信息,2013,30(4): 113

陈剑明,张声生,郭前坤,等. 芍药苷对非酒精性脂肪肝大鼠模型的疗效与保护机制研究[J]. 中华中医药杂志,2013,28(5): 1376

陈丽,刘永琦,李朝霞,等. 单味中药抗肺纤维化效应的规律分析及其 Logistic 回归模型[J]. 中华中医药杂志,2013,28(1): 247

陈少丽,都广礼,鲁艳平,等,下瘀血汤全药与组分处方对免疫性肝纤维化大鼠肝组织 α-SMA、TGF-β1、PDGF-β RmRNA 表达影响的比较研究[J]. 中华中医药学刊,2013,31(10): 2227

陈少禹. 补气运脾汤联合能量合剂治疗慢性病毒性心肌炎随机平行对照研究[J]. 实用中医内科杂志,2013,27(9): 21

陈铁龙,祝光礼,赫小龙,等. 冠心合剂减少大鼠心肌梗死边缘区凋亡及对 Fas、FasL、Caspase-8、Caspase-3 蛋白表达的影响[J]. 中华中医药学刊,2013,31(11): 2453

陈玉琴. 五味消毒饮合生脉饮治疗病毒性心肌炎的临床疗效观察[J]. 中医临床研究,2013,5(8): 102

程善廷,魏岳斌,王嘉锋. "归芍疗痴汤"改善血管性痴呆患者认知能力 40 例临床观察[J]. 江苏中医药,2013,45(2): 36

丛军,蔡淦,林江,等. 肠吉泰对腹泻型肠易激综合征大鼠 CRH、SPmRNA 表达的影响[J]. 上海中医药杂志,2013,47(5): 81

D

戴立恒,施文甫,梁金荣,等. 初发 2 型糖尿病胰岛功能与中医证型相关性研究[J]. 湖北中医杂志,2013,35(9): 18

邓耀松. 观察养阴活胃合剂对萎缩性胃炎的中医疗效观察[J]. 中医临床研究,2013,5(4): 85

丁怀顺,王家胜,白其昌,等. 解毒降浊汤对 CKD 肾功能减退治疗作用的观察[J]. 中医药临床杂志,2013,25(7): 606

丁世永,郑平东,何立群,等. 小柴胡汤改善慢性肾小球肾炎患者炎症及减轻蛋白尿的作用研究[J]. 中国中西医结合杂志,2013,33(1): 21

董妙先,邹宇,刘玉章,等,大黄素对肝纤维化大鼠肝脏组织 Sm ad3 表达的影响[J]. 中华中医药杂志,2013,28(2): 529

董其谦,王修敏,郑国庆. 养脾阴法对早期帕金森病大鼠模型行为学、纹状体多巴胺及其代谢产物的影响[J]. 中华中医药学刊,2013,31(2): 358

窦迎婷,刘贵颖. 疏风通络方对哮喘大鼠外周血和肺泡灌洗液黏附分子 ICAM-1 和 VCAM-1 的影响[J]. 中国中医急症,2013,22(5): 693

杜锐玲,杜新芬. 三仁汤治疗过敏性紫癜(湿浊内蕴型)临床疗效观察[J]. 四川中医,2013,31(5): 95

段小花,吴霜,王莉莉,等. 天麻乙酸乙酯提取物对血管性痴呆大鼠海马 CA1 区锥体细胞的影响[J]. 中华老年心脑血管病杂志,2013,15(2): 197

F

樊威伟,车树强,徐英,等. 糖肾康胶囊对糖尿病肾病血管内皮保护作用的临床观察[J]. 中国中医基础医学杂志,2013,19(4): 426

范恒,张丽娟,钟敏. 复方苦参汤对溃疡性结肠炎 DOR-β-arrestin1-Bcl-2 信号转导通路的干预作用[J]. 世界华人消化杂志,2013,21(8): 647

范杰,黄静祎,冯幸,等. 附子楮实汤治疗肝硬化腹水的疗效观察[J]. 光明中医,2013,28(5): 936

范利锋,张永红,翁庚民. 清热凉血膏治疗活动期强直性脊柱炎临床研究[J]. 山东中医杂志,2013,32(2): 83

方朝晖,程森华,吴倩,等. 丹蛭降糖胶囊对早期糖尿病肾病患者血 NF-κB 和尿白蛋白排泄率的影响[J]. 世界科学技术(中医药现代化),2013,15(5): 891

方瑜,孙瑶,简洁.九龙藤总黄酮对垂体后叶素致大鼠急性心肌缺血的保护作用[J].中国药理学通报,2013,29(11):1592

冯雯,范一宏,徐国萍,等.枳术通便汤对慢传输型便秘大鼠结肠结构的影响[J].中国中医药科技,2013,20(1):33

付健阳,张晓琳,田金英,等.红景天、蛹虫草、大黄配伍治疗代谢综合征的实验研究Ⅵ——对糖尿病大鼠肾脏保护作用[J].中国中药杂志,2013,38(22):3961

付丽媛,杨进,王灿晖,等.健脾增液汤对肥胖2型糖尿病大鼠脂肪—胰岛素轴的影响[J].中药药理与临床,2013,29(4):141

傅向阳,喻勤,罗伟生,等.荔枝核总黄酮对大鼠肝纤维化血小板衍生生长因子、肿瘤坏死因子的影响[J].广州中医药大学学报,2013,30(5):685

傅晓骏.中药沉香粉对慢性肾衰大鼠血清ATⅠ、ATⅡ的影响[J].浙江中医杂志,2013,48(2):123

付毅敏,顾友谊,王绪云,等.醒智颗粒治疗血管性痴呆38例[J].中国中医药现代远程教育,2013,11(3):20

G

高戎,徐建如,李仁奇,等.人参皂苷Rg5对脓毒血症大鼠急性肺损伤的保护作用[J].现代生物医学进展,2013,13(11):2062

高绍芳,王彦刚,李佃贵,等.化浊解毒和胃方对胃癌前病变大鼠血管生成机制的影响[J].中国中西医结合杂志,2013,33(11):1515

高友安.加味当归四逆汤联合甲钴胺和胰岛素强化疗法治疗糖尿病周围神经病变的临床效果观察[J].中医临床研究,2013,5(2):16

郜俊清,陈弢,于宏梅,等.补气化痰方对大鼠心肌梗死模型心功能及血管新生的研究[J].辽宁中医药大学学报,2013,15(8):89

耿东,郭蓉娟.广泛性焦虑症中医症状及证候要素的临床调研[J].北京中医药大学学报,2013,36(6):421

耿东,郭蓉娟.基于现代文献的焦虑症中医证候研究[J].北京中医药大学学报,2013,36(7):484

顾超,袁灿兴.帕金森病的中医证型分布和用药规律探析[J].上海中医药杂志,2013,47(7):12

郭锦荣,鲍计章,周永明.生血灵对激素抵抗型免疫性血小板减少症蛋白质表达的影响[J].山西中医,2013,29(3):40

郭齐,王志国,杨傲然,等.丹皮酚和芍药苷配伍对急性心肌缺血模型大鼠的保护作用[J].时珍国医国药,2013,24(1):45

郭妍,迟晓丽,马渊,等.六味地黄汤活性成分组方LW-AFC对高热量饲料诱导小鼠代谢综合征的改善作用[J].中国药理学与毒理学杂志,2013,27(3):367

郭宇新.九味镇心颗粒联合丁螺环酮治疗焦虑症临床观察[J].内蒙古中医药,2013,32(22):48

H

韩冰,应茵,丁晓霁,等.艾叶油治疗肺心病模型大鼠肺动脉高压的实验研究[J].浙江中西医结合杂志,2013,23(9):700

韩福祥,秘兴锋,杨维波,等.祛痛散外敷治疗早中期强直性脊柱炎的临床观察[J].中国实用医药,2013,8(25):181

韩慧,袁红霞.善胃Ⅰ号方对血瘀热毒型胃癌前病变PCNA的影响[J].辽宁中医杂志,2013,40(1):87

韩健,张伟.从气道炎症因子研究肺舒颗粒对慢性阻塞性肺疾病急性加重期的疗效机制[J].中华中医药杂志,2013,28(7):2202

郝志民,赵云昇,朱维平,等.新加越鞠丸对非酒精性脂肪肝大鼠脂联素及瘦素影响的实验研究[J].世界中西医结合杂志,2013,8(3):237

何道同,陈珺明,宋海燕,等.柴胡人参药对对非酒精性脂肪性肝病大鼠胰岛素抵抗和瘦素的影响[J].中西医结合肝病杂志,2013,23(2):98

何晓茵.心达康胶囊治疗病毒性心肌炎30例[J].中医杂志,2013,54(7):611

何义华,李力强,宾建平,等.黄芪五苓散治疗肝硬化腹水临床观察[J].新中医,2013,45(3):45

贺建国.调脂复肝汤治疗非酒精性脂肪肝60例疗效观察[J].新中医,2013,45(5):50

胡令彦,周永明,陈英坤,等.健脾补肾方对再生障碍性贫血患者外周血Th17及相关细胞因子水平的影响[J].云南中医学院学报,2013,36(3):4

黄绍湘,李峰,路超,等.安心颗粒对大鼠心肌梗塞模型血管新生作用的影响[J].陕西中医,2013,34(4):493

黄适,张涛,郑东林,等.安肠汤对腹泻型肠易激综合征大鼠结肠及下丘脑中TPRV1的影响[J].广西中医药,2013,36(4):61

黄婷,卢巧英.藿朴夏苓汤加减治疗肥胖2型糖尿病30例[J].浙江中医杂志,2013,48(8):564

黄月芳,楼招欢,陈坚翱.化痰通络汤合牵正散对风痰瘀血痹阻证急性脑梗死患者同型半胱氨酸的影响及临床疗效观察[J].中华中医药杂志,2013,28(6):1907

J

季海锋,孙玉周,李立伟.通痹活血汤治疗糖尿病周围神经病变临床观察[J].中国中医急症,2013,22(4):622

贾先红,任玉乐.清火消斑汤治疗过敏性紫癜31例临床观察[J].新中医,2013,45(2):40

贾云芳,侯仙明,王文智,等.心肝胃同治法对心梗大

鼠心肌梗死面积及食量的影响[J]. 中国中医基础医学杂志,2013,19(6): 642

江明金,莫志贤,周吉银,等. 胡芦巴碱对2型糖尿病大鼠糖脂代谢及海马 neuritin 表达的影响[J]. 中国新药与临床杂志,2013,32(2): 113

姜楠,张冰冰,蒲纪,等. 糖代谢异常代谢综合征大鼠中医证型的以方测证法研究(Ⅰ)[J]. 中国实验方剂学杂志,2013,19(17): 211

金泽,王玉琳,姜珊珊,等. 洋金花对帕金森病大鼠脑纹状体组织 SOD、GSH-Px 影响的研究[J]. 中医药信息,2013,30(2): 87

L

李风雷,李建生,王明航,等. 成人咳嗽变异性哮喘中医证素分布规律文献研究[J]. 中医学报,2013,28(4): 488

李钢. 精乌胶囊治疗脑卒中后抑郁40例[J]. 中国中医药现代远程教育,2013,11(16): 21

李红琴,曹利民,胡志诚,等. 中西医结合治疗广泛性焦虑症临床观察[J]. 浙江中西医结合杂志,2013,23(2): 107

李惠林,刘玲,赵恒侠,等. 三仁汤治疗湿热蕴脾型肥胖2型糖尿病疗效观察[J]. 新中医,2013,45(6): 108

李娟,张晓琳,刘育英,等. 红景天、蛹虫草、大黄配伍治疗代谢综合征的实验研究Ⅳ——改善肝脏脂质堆积作用[J]. 中国中药杂志,2013,38(11): 1789

李敏州,高彦彬,马鸣飞,等. 芪卫颗粒对 KK-Ay 小鼠肾组织 TGF-β1/Smads 信号转导通路的影响[J]. 中医杂志,2013,54(13): 1141

李庆珍,刘佩佩,宋卫国,等. 益肾化湿颗粒对慢性肾脏病2～3期患者微炎症状态的影响[J]. 医学信息,2013,26(7): 225

李欣,邹佳宏,秦昊,等. 上中下通用痛风汤治疗高尿酸血症的实验研究[J]. 中国实验方剂学杂志,2013,19(14): 284

李雪丽,刘建勋,郭宇洁. 双参宁心方对大鼠心肌缺血/再灌注损伤能量代谢的影响[J]. 中国中药杂志,2013,38(17): 2874

李艳香,贾艳秋,朱叶珊. 改良愈疡方对溃疡性结肠炎大鼠 TNF-α 的影响[J]. 四川中医,2013,31(8): 44

李玉卿,张忠贤,费德升,等. 溺毒清合剂对慢性肾衰竭大鼠纤维化指标的影响[J]. 中华中医药学刊,2013,31(2): 350

李增祥,李朝. 身痛逐瘀汤加减治疗糖尿病周围神经病变疗效观察[J]. 四川中医,2013,31(6): 112

李仲贤,郑光,展俊平,等. 基于文本挖掘技术探索强直性脊柱炎"理—法—方—药"相应规律[J]. 兰州工业学院学报,2013,20(2): 23

梁敏,李强盛,湛昌文. 槲皮素对 UUO 模型大鼠肾纤维化的影响[J]. 数理医药学杂志,2013,26(5): 522

林平,黄小燕,施婧瑶,等. 慢性胃炎的证素特点[J]. 福建中医药大学学报,2013,23(9): 7

林卿,李成. 柴桂温胆汤治疗中风后抑郁疗效观察[J]. 辽宁中医药大学学报,2013,15(7): 231

刘春丽,陈虹,姜勇,等. 松果菊苷对血管性痴呆大鼠行为学、氧自由基以及胆碱能神经递质代谢速率的影响[J]. 中国药理学通报,2013,29(7): 1035

刘飞. 中医辨证结合药物疗法治疗焦虑症的临床观察[J]. 贵阳中医学院学报 2013,35(3): 104

刘杰民,蔺晓源,纪云西. 健脾益肠散对溃疡性结肠炎大鼠的作用研究[J]. 中国中医急症,2013,22(3): 348

刘清池,高习华,王淑珍,等. 凉血解毒法对免疫性血小板减少症患者T淋巴细胞亚群的调节作用[J]. 河北中医,2013,35(5): 652

刘婷,王欣,李培培,等. 泻肺宁心汤对肺心病急性期血管内皮功能和炎性因子的影响[J]. 中国实验方剂学杂志,2013,19(22): 279

刘旭东,邓鑫,张红星,等. 祛湿活血方对非酒精性脂肪性肝病大鼠血清肿瘤坏死因子-α 和脂联素的调节[J]. 中西医结合肝病杂志,2013,23(4): 231

刘玥,齐新,刘克强. 芪参益气组方对心肌梗死大鼠心肌细胞凋亡和胶原容积的影响[J]. 天津中医药,2013,30(8): 488

刘治坤,张前,李宝萍,等. 芪蛭益肺颗粒对慢性阻塞性肺疾病模型大鼠小气道上皮 MMP-9、TIMP-1 表达的影响[J]. 北京中医药大学学报,2014,36(5): 322

罗春凤,陈婉,赵丽红,等. 纳气通络方联合西药治疗肺肾气虚型慢性阻塞性肺疾病稳定期临床研究[J]. 上海中医药杂志,2013,47(9): 41

罗迪. 基于文献统计的糖尿病胃轻瘫中医用药规律研究[J]. 辽宁中医药大学学报,2013,15(8): 157

吕建兴. 半夏泻心汤联合丹红注射液治疗萎缩性胃炎随机平行对照研究[J]. 实用中医内科杂志,2013,27(7): 68

吕秀群,刘得华. 放血疗法联合银翘散治疗亚急性甲状腺炎疗效观察[J]. 新中医,2013,45(2): 42

M

麻志恒,施志琴,张汉新,等. 桃红三虫汤治疗急性脑梗死患者疗效分析[J]. 中国实验方剂学杂志,2013,19(3): 286

马俊丽,曲文闻,胡晓梅,等. 含砷中药复方青黄散治疗骨髓增生异常综合征的克隆选择性与砷体内效应的相关性研究[J]. 中国中医药信息杂志,2013,20(6): 8

马鸣飞,高彦彬,王金羊,等. 芪卫颗粒调节 USF2 及其下游信号分子表达对 KK-Ay 小鼠糖尿病肾病的干预

作用[J].中华中医药杂志,2013,28(5):1321
孟凡莲,马忠金,尹广利.通络益脑丸治疗血管性痴呆46例临床观察[J].中医药导报,2013,19(1):60

N

宁亚军,王文禹,蒋中秋.自拟方从脾胃论治过敏性紫癜临床分析[J].河北医学,2013,19(8):1267

O

欧喜燕,张永和,李驰坤,等.三苦滴丸抗急性心肌缺血拆方研究[J].中国实验方剂学杂志,2013,19(12):155

P

潘永梅,陈志强,马赟,等.活血化瘀通络方对糖尿病肾病大鼠肾脏骨形态蛋白7表达的影响[J].中医杂志,2013,54(19):1672

Q

亓慧敏,边俊莉.胆蒲通脉胶囊对急性脑梗死患者高同型半胱氨酸的影响[J].光明中医,2013,28(6):1188
齐盛.疏肝扶阳运脾汤治疗肝硬化腹水60例[J].中国中医药现代远程教育,2013,11(4):33

R

任娟,张滢,王祥麒,等.仙连颗粒治疗激素依赖性特发性血小板减少性紫癜临床研究[J].中医学报,2013,28(4):565
任晓晨,阚香玲.和解少阳法治疗病毒性心肌炎初探[J].四川中医,2013,31(6):37
任岩海,刘洪凤,韩智学,等.桑叶多糖对2型糖尿病大鼠血糖血脂的影响[J].中医药学报,2013,41(1):20

S

沈淑华,黄宣,吕宾,等.腹泻型肠易激综合征证型及证候要素的文献研究[J].中华中医药杂志,2013,28(5):1538
沈祥峰,柴可夫.运脾和络颗粒对糖尿病周围神经病变大鼠坐骨神经脑源性神经营养因子表达的影响[J].中华中医药杂志,2013,28(9):2569
沈芝琴.养阴润肺汤防治慢性支气管炎稳定期患者的临床研究[J].中国医药指南,2013,11(30):179
史先芬,吴自光.加味奔豚汤治疗中风后抑郁55例疗效观察[J].中医临床研究,2013,5(12):29
舒宏,丁春,周毅,等.圣济二精颗粒治疗血管性痴呆临床疗效观察[J].湖北中医杂志,2013,35(2):9
舒金堂,吴君华.截咳糖浆联合复方松苃片治疗老年慢性支气管炎临床观察[J].湖北中医杂志,2013,35(2):46
宋清武,李慧臻.加味苓桂术甘汤治疗非酒精性脂肪性肝病的临床研究[J].四川中医,2013,31(8):60
孙涛,郭志华,毛湘屏,等.益心泰对心肌梗死大鼠心室重构及CaN、$NFAT_3$蛋白表达的影响[J].湖南中医药大学学报,2013,33(7):23

T

唐奇志,张燕华,陈聪,等.姚氏芪薏四君子汤对2型糖尿病胰岛素抵抗的影响[J].新中医,2013,45(9):91
田春雨,刘志霞,王亚,等.双益降糖方对2型糖尿病大鼠糖、脂代谢的影响[J].中国实验方剂学杂志,2013,19(9):177
田金英,陈玲,张晓琳,等.红景天、蛹虫草、大黄配伍治疗代谢综合征的实验研究Ⅱ——治疗肥胖症作用[J].中国中药杂志,2013,38(9):1411
田金英,陈玲,张晓琳,等.红景天、蛹虫草、大黄配伍治疗代谢综合征的实验研究Ⅲ——控制血糖作用[J].中国中药杂志,2013,38(10):1570
田满荣,王响,杨红梅.以"透邪外出"为主治疗急性病毒性心肌炎38例临床观察[J].国医论坛,2013,28(5):35
田志刚,王秀娟.中药内服配合灌肠治疗慢性溃疡性结肠炎49例[J].中国中医药现代远程教育,2013,11(16):29

W

汪四海,刘健,张金山.从脾论治强直性脊柱炎骨代谢失衡理论探讨[J].中华中医药杂志,2013,28(8):2233
王成阳,李泽庚,刘向国,等.六味补气胶囊对COPD肺气虚证模型大鼠树突状细胞的影响[J].北京中医药大学学报,2013,36(11):779
王春梅,杜兴旭.松针提取物对Ⅱ型糖尿病大鼠的抗氧化作用[J].北华大学学报,2013,14(4):426
王娣,唐启盛,赵瑞珍,等.颐脑解郁方对脑缺血后抑郁大鼠PI通路上重要调节因子的干预作用[J].北京中医药大学学报,2013,36(4):242
王东,吴同茹,谢婷婷,等.中医辨证治疗慢性肾脏病蛋白尿的多中心前瞻性临床研究[J].南方医科大学学报,2013,33(4):502
王东,张江,谢婷婷,等.抗纤灵有效单体对活化的肾成纤维细胞株和系膜细胞株的影响[J].中华中医药杂志,2013,28(9):2554
王东,张长明,王云满,等.抗纤灵方药物血清对骨髓来源成纤维细胞表型转化的影响[J].中医杂志,2013,54(5):420
王东梅,王立军.地黄益脑胶囊治疗血管性痴呆30例临床观察[J].中医药学报,2013,41(1):115
王海霞,王安全,田丛丛,等.愈障颗粒对非重型再生

障碍性贫血患者骨髓小粒中 VEGF 表达的影响[J]. 陕西中医学院学报,2013,36(3):92

王洪武,林兰,倪青,等. 益气养阴中药对早期糖尿病肾病同型半胱氨酸、亚甲基四氢叶酸还原酶多态性的干预作用[J]. 中华中医药杂志,2013,28(10):2877

王辉,叶同生,陈素华,等. 虎杖不同配伍对糖尿病肾病大鼠糖、脂代谢及血液流变学指标的影响[J]. 中国实验方剂学杂志,2013,19(12):181

王建忠,王亚宽,王希珏. 沉蛤定喘合剂治疗厦性肺源性心脏病临床研究[J]. 中国中医急症,2013,22(7):1142

王坤玲,侯兵. 疏肝清热通络方治疗 2 型糖尿病周围神经病变 35 例临床观察[J]. 中医药导报,2013,19(7):34

王丽,张晓琳,李莫涵,等. 红景天、蛹虫草、大黄配伍治疗代谢综合征的实验研究Ⅴ——调节糖代谢紊乱作用机制研究[J]. 中国中药杂志,2013,38(12):1972

王天文,钟代华,黄文涛,等. 糖肾芪(齐)对链脲佐菌素致糖尿病肾病模型大鼠的影响[J]. 中国实验方剂学杂志,2013,19(19):295

王琰,徐瑞荣,崔思远,等. 端粒保护蛋白 1 在不同证型获得性再生障碍性贫血患者中的表达及相关性研究[J]. 中国中医药信息杂志,2013,20(8):18

王英,李亚,李建生,等. 调补肺肾三法对慢性阻塞性肺疾病大鼠右心室重构的影响和远后效应[J]. 中医杂志,2013,54(5):415

王永刚,钟伟,于远望,等. 人参与丹参配伍对心肌缺血再灌注模型大鼠抗氧化和血管内皮细胞因子的影响[J]. 世界中西医结合杂志,2013,8(7):669

王永刚,钟伟,于远望,等. 双参通冠方对实验性大鼠心肌梗死模型冠脉血流量的影响[J]. 辽宁中医杂志,2013,40(10):2143

王永刚,周晓俊,尤金枝,等. 四黄降糖颗粒改善 2 型糖尿病患者中医证候临床观察[J]. 陕西中医学院学报,2013,36(2):41

王永钧,何立群,孙伟,等. 中药辨证组方对慢性肾脏病 3 期的肾保护作用——315 例多中心、前瞻性、双盲、随机对照试验[J]. 世界中医药,2013,8(9):1001

王志宏,季旭明,吴智春,等. 苍白二陈汤对代谢综合征大鼠血脂水平和主动脉 ICAM1 表达的影响[J]. 中华中医药学刊,2013,31(6):1243

王志坤,李博林,刘启泉,等. 小归芍化浊解毒方对胃癌前病变大鼠胃蛋白酶原及胃黏膜组织再生基因表达的影响[J]. 中国老年学杂志,2013,33(24):6240

吴皓萌,徐志伟,敖海清. 肠易激综合征中医证候分布与常见指标关系的研究[J]. 中华中医药杂志,2013,28(9):2534

吴娜,宋璐,杨新新,等. 天芪平颤颗粒对帕金森病大鼠异动症行为学及信号转导蛋白表达的影响[J]. 上海中医药大学学报,2013,27(1):55

吴生元,彭江云,万春平,等. 健脾渗湿方对高尿酸血症大鼠模型尿酸盐转运蛋白 OAT3 调控作用的研究[J]. 风湿病与关节炎,2013,2(12):22

吴天敏,陈金水,曾细阳. 软脉灵口服液对 ApoE 基因敲除小鼠动脉粥样硬化斑块内血管新生的影响[J]. 中国中医药信息杂志,2013,20(9):37

吴文英. 桃红四物汤加味治疗过敏性紫癜临床疗效观察[J]. 河北医学,2013,19(8):1269

吴小娜,王燕. 芪冬益肺汤治疗慢性支气管炎迁延期的临床研究[J]. 中国社区医师,2013,15(6):215.

吴永斌,王修锋. 奥曲肽联合中药脐贴治疗难治性腹水 64 例临床观察[J]. 江苏中医药,2013,45(5):60

X

奚悦,马贤德,李敬林. 益气活络方对糖尿病肾病大鼠 nephrin 表达的影响[J]. 安徽医科大学学报,2013,48(4):375

夏文进,吴敏,王洪,等. 高血压病患者不同中医证型与血浆同型半胱氨酸水平相关性研究[J]. 中华中医药学刊,2013,31(1):164

谢晶日,孙芳,梁国英. 欣胃颗粒对胃癌前病变大鼠 STAT3、p-STAT3 信号通路的影响[J]. 中国中西医结合杂志,2013,33(1):65

徐冰,聂波,徐颖,等. 基于 ApoE-/-小鼠动脉粥样硬化模型的四妙勇安汤活性部位配伍规律研究[J]. 辽宁中医杂志,2013,40(6):1250

许代福,郑波,李智红. 溃疡性结肠炎中医证型与结肠镜象相关性研究[J]. 实用中医药杂志,2013,29(1):4

许风莲. 失笑散加味保留灌肠治疗溃疡性结肠炎急性期 50 例[J]. 中国中医急症,2013,22(4):576

许文君,李秀惠,勾春燕,等. 清肝利肠方灌肠治疗肝硬化腹水 40 例临床观察[J]. 北京中医药,2013,32(7):522

Y

Yang T, Shen D, Wang Q, Tao Y, et al. Investigation of the absorbed and metabolized components of Danshen from Fuzheng Huayu recipe and study on the anti-hepatic fibrosis effects of these components[J]. Journal of Ethnopharmacology, 2013, 148(2): 691

杨德良. 中西医结合治疗糖尿病周围神经病变 37 例观察[J]. 实用中医药杂志,2013,29(5):365

杨海燕,金艳蓉,杨红,等. 2 型糖尿病糖化血红蛋白水平与生存质量及中医证型相关性研究[J]. 中国中医药信息杂志,2013,20(6):11

杨珺超,宋康,王媛,等. 温补肾阳汤对哮喘小鼠 EOS

分化的干预作用[J]. 中国中医药科技,2013,20(4):340

杨清峰,刘瑞霞. 疏肝活血法对老龄动脉硬化模型大鼠血管内皮功能的影响[J]. 吉林中医药,2013,33(7):711

尹冬青,田金洲,时晶,等. 15196例抑郁症中医证候及证候要素特点的文献研究[J]. 中华中医药学刊,2013,31(2):279

尹雪皎,孙伟. 孙伟运用络病理论治疗慢性肾脏病经验[J]. 河南中医,2013,33(3):342

Z

曾英坚. 疏风凉血补肾方治疗慢性特发性血小板减少性紫癜临床研究[J]. 中国中医药信息杂志,2013,20(7):15

曾英坚. 愈障生血汤治疗慢性再生障碍性贫血输血依赖临床研究[J]. 新中医,2013,45(3):58

张海燕,唐农,葛金文,等. 五脏温阳化瘀汤对动脉粥样硬化血管性痴呆大鼠海马组织Nrf2蛋白通路的影响[J]. 云南中医学院学报,2013,36(3):8

张会存,史瑞,李健,等. 黄芪、三七对萎缩性胃炎大鼠胃黏膜HSP70及其转录因子GAF表达的影响[J]. 世界华人消化杂志,2013,21(7):559

张会欣,赵韶华,王宏涛,等. 周络通胶囊对糖尿病周围神经病变小鼠坐骨神经TGF-β1/Smad3信号通路的影响[J]. 中成药,2013,35(4):652

张慧琪,刘贵颖,尹新中,等. 疏风通络方对哮喘大鼠肺组织嗜酸细胞浸润影响随机平行对照研究[J]. 实用中医内科杂志,2013,27(3):76

张洁,刘月禅,何小琦,等. 健脾安神法对腹泻型肠易激综合征大鼠胃肠动力的作用[J]. 广东医学,2013,34(15):2299

张俊杰,林庚庭,滕飞,等. 桃核参术汤对肝纤维化过程中肾素-血管紧张素系统的影响[J]. 中华中医药杂志,2013,28(4):930

张俊莉,董军胜. 盘龙七片治疗强直性脊柱炎的临床观察[J]. 中国中医骨伤科杂志,2013,21(5):52

张玲燕,李民,邵建国,等. 清脂护肝方对非酒精性脂肪肝大鼠肝组织病理及纤维化指标的影响[J]. 上海中医药杂志,2013,47(8):78

张伦,黄紫锋,罗露露. 基于NF-κBp65变化及溃疡愈合质量探讨健脾清热活血类方药干预溃疡性结肠炎随机对照研究[J]. 广州中医药大学学报,2013,30(4):463

张佩江,赵文霞. 中西医结合治疗肝硬化腹水112例临床研究[J]. 中国中医基础医学杂志,2013,19(4):476

张瑞,陈小兵,唐宇平. 通络醒脑颗粒治疗急性脑梗死患者临床疗效及对炎性因子的影响[J]. 新中医,2013,45(9):21

张绍芬. 加味桂枝茯苓丸(汤剂)治疗慢性肺源性心脏病急性期36例临床疗效观察[J]. 中医临床研究,2013,5(8):76

张社峰,王松龄,赵彦青,等. 中风防治灵Ⅰ号、Ⅱ号联合治疗急性脑梗死152例[J]. 中医研究,2013,26(4):20

张纨,王志坤,董林林. 兰茵风扬化浊解毒方对溃疡性结肠炎大鼠免疫调控机制的影响[J]. 中国实验方剂学杂志,2013,19(1):236

张伟骏,裘涛. 不同治法对卒中后抑郁症大鼠海马CA3区神经元保护作用研究[J]. 中华中医药学刊,2013,31(6):1356

张文江,姚明江,张旭丽. 祛瘀解毒方治疗慢性阻塞性肺疾病稳定期临床观察[J]. 中国中医急症,2013,22(8):1323

张先慧,张艳红,胡照娟,等. 辛开苦降方对初发2型糖尿病KKay小鼠胰岛素抵抗及脂质代谢的影响[J]. 北京中医药,2013,32(4):243

章怡祎,刘萍,励冬斐,等. 冠心康对ApoE基因敲除动脉粥样硬化小鼠心脏时钟基因昼夜节律的影响[J]. 中华中医药学刊,2013,31(8):1680

张长明,周家俊,何立群,等. 抗纤灵方治疗慢性肾脏病3期患者110例临床研究[J]. 中医杂志,2013,54(3):214

赵洪运. 安神定惊汤治疗焦虑症惊恐发作疗效观察[J]. 中国中医药信息杂志,2013,20(1):74

赵琳,邱仲川,陈珮,等. 复方参鹿颗粒对相对低危骨髓增生异常综合征患者骨髓细胞免疫表型的影响[J]. 新中医,2013,45(4):104

赵四林,王伟. 加味二仙丸对支气管哮喘临床缓解期患者血清白细胞介素及干扰素-γ的影响[J]. 中国中医药信息杂志,2013,20(4):16

周宝银,陈坤,何卉,等. 祛风活血化瘀止咳疗法治疗咳嗽变异性哮喘临床观察[J]. 中国中医急症,2013,22(5):779

周潮,佟杰,杨荣阁,等. 辨证分时论治2型糖尿病及对胰岛功能的影响[J]. 陕西中医,2013,34(4):410

周密. 脱敏煎加减联合西药治疗过敏性紫癜40例[J]. 陕西中医,2013,34(6):722

周萍,李均,阳小敏,等. 黄芪丹参“药对”干预肾纤维化抑制因子par-3的量效关系研究[J]. 上海中医药杂志,2013,47(5):77

周琦,张翀,于栋华,等. 穿山龙总皂苷对高尿酸血症的降尿酸及细胞抗炎作用研究[J]. 中华中医药杂志,2013,28(5):1444

朱孔利,张士岭,王淑秋,等. 灵芝孢子粉对癫痫大鼠脑组织中SS、5-HT和ATP酶的影响[J]. 上海中医药杂志,2013,47(4):75

朱蕴华,陶枫,金昕,等. 清化颗粒对具备“热”证素特征 2 型糖尿病患者糖代谢、胰岛功能和氧化应激水平的疗效观察[J]. 世界科学技术(中医药现代化),2013,15(4):753

邹君,刘永平,顾士栋,等. 赤雹根总皂苷对类风湿性关节炎大鼠血清 OPG/RANKL 水平的影响[J]. 中国实验方剂学杂志,2013,19(8):218

邹赟,朱祎,邵命海,等. 健脾清化方对 5/6 肾切除大鼠 ATⅡ/NADPH 氧化应激通路的干预作用[J]. 中南大学学报(医学版),2013,38(8):779

邹赟,朱祎,王东. 健脾清化方对肾衰大鼠磷酸化 p38 丝裂原活化蛋白激酶介导的炎症因子的调控作用[J]. 上海中医药大学学报,2013,27(3):73

(五)妇　科

【概述】

2013年在国内主要刊物发表的中医、中西医结合妇产科论文近900篇。内容涉及理论研究、临床研究和实验研究。尤以临床研究文献居多，反映了目前中医妇科学界的学术水平。

1. 理论研究

李应存、柳长华阐释了敦煌医学卷子中的妇产科内容，并与《千金方》的相关内容进行比较。谢辉辉等分析了古代对于妊娠禁忌药的划分方法。张建伟对古今文献中有关"天癸"的月节律进行研究。袁霞从古代文献溯源"女子胞"的含义。陈钢等从古今文献探讨"带脉"的功能。赵晓娟、王稳平从理论和临床两方面分析了"热入血室"的沿革与现代含义。

2. 临床研究

在临床研究文献中，有关痛经的报道历年均较多。对于原发性痛经的病机与证候特征，多数文献从气滞血瘀和寒凝血瘀论述，治疗则以中药内服为主，亦有针灸、脐疗、按摩等法，或内治与外敷相配合。对于子宫内膜异位症所致的痛经，相关文献近50篇。临床研究包括中医周期治疗、中药消癥助孕、内治与外治配合、中西医结合、保守性手术后预防复发等。亦有针对子宫内膜异位症患者焦虑抑郁状态进行中药调治的报道。

对异位妊娠的非手术治疗是临床研究的热点之一。中医治疗主要着眼于输卵管妊娠，但异位妊娠非手术治疗的药物杀胚仍是临床难点问题，对杀胚中药的研究尚有待完善。此外，对于少见的子宫疤痕妊娠非手术治疗亦有报道。

对于子宫肌瘤、子宫腺肌病和卵巢囊肿的中医治疗，是历年文献比较多的领域。多数采用经典方药如桂枝茯苓丸、大黄牡丹皮汤等治疗，亦有使用现代中药验方治疗的报道，或中西医结合治疗。

对于输卵管和盆腔因素不孕的中医治疗，也是临床研究的热点。治疗方法包括中药内服、中药外敷、宫腔注药，以及宫腔镜或腹腔镜手术配合中药内外合治。

3. 实验研究

模型是进行中医证候学、中药药理学研究的重要工具。模拟临床病理特征、中医证候特点建立适合的动物模型，包括病理模型、证候模型和病—证结合模型，或采用细胞模型，均可以弥补临床研究之不足，阐明治疗之机理。研究造模方法SOP以及模型系统评价是探讨中医药作用机制的重要环节。李炜等根据妇科疾病的特点，建立大鼠气滞血瘀证的模型评价体系。韩霞建立着床障碍小鼠模型，探讨补肾药对子宫血管内皮生长因子（VEGF）和金属基质蛋白酶9（MMP－9）mRNA表达的影响。对于卵巢功能衰退的造模方法，则有采用免疫抑制剂、化疗药物等药物损伤模型及自身免疫损伤模型等。

（罗颂平）

【月经过少的治疗】

杨鉴冰等认为月经过少有肾虚、血虚、气滞、血瘀、痰郁及手术六类因素，肾虚血瘀是其基本病机。治疗以补益肾精、化瘀调经为主，采用分期调周法，以补肾育宫汤（当归、熟地黄、山萸肉、枸杞子、茯苓、菟丝子等）加减治疗。侯小艳总结孟安琪治疗月经过少的经验。认为肾精虚损，痰湿阻滞冲任，血海满盈不足所致，虚实夹杂。治以补肾化痰，方以补肾化痰调经汤（熟地黄、当归、山药、杜仲、菟丝子、枸杞子等）加减治疗，疗效显著。

于海英等运用苍附导痰汤加减（鸡血藤、苍术、香附、枳壳、当归、桃仁等）治疗34例患者，连服3个月经周期，总有效率为94.1%(32/34)。刘娜等以桃红四物汤（桃仁、红花、当归、白芍药、川芎、熟地黄等）加减治疗33例患者，经治3个月经周期，总有效率为93.9%(31/33)。李顺景采用增量水车汤（熟地黄、白芍药、当归、川芎、桃仁、红花等）内服加外敷治疗宫腔手术后月经过少患者，治疗3个月经周期，有效率为91.8%(45/49)。林楠等将70例人工流产后月经减少患者随机均分为两组，治疗组予坤泰胶囊（熟地黄、黄连、白芍药、黄芩、阿胶、茯苓）联合生物反馈电刺激治疗,对照组予雌激素-孕激素序贯治疗。治疗3个月经周期,两组总有效率分别为82.9%(29/35)、62.9%(22/35),组间比较,$P<0.05$。治疗后子宫内膜厚度比较,治疗组优于对照组($P<0.05$)。李元琪等将绝经过渡期肾虚血瘀证月经过少患者40例随机均分为两组。治疗组予益肾续经汤(肉苁蓉、熟地黄、川牛膝、鸡血藤、何首乌、黄芪等),对照组予戊酸雌二醇合甲羟孕酮序贯周期治疗。3个月经周期后,两组有效率分别为95.0%(19/20)、80.0%(16/20),组间比较无显著差异。但治疗组在改善经色暗红、腰骶酸痛、头晕耳鸣及小腹胀痛方面明显优于对照组($P<0.01$)。李娟等采用补肾化瘀汤(桃仁、当归、丹参、熟地黄、白芍药、川芎等)治疗人流术后月经过少患者60例,经治6个月经周期,总有效率为91.7%(55/60)。

(谢津津　陈静静)

【阴道假丝酵母菌病的治疗与研究】

邓敏端等将80例复发性外阴阴道假丝酵母菌病(RVVC)患者随机均分为两组,进行强化及巩固治疗半年。中西医结合治疗组加用中药周期疗法治疗两个月,共有69例完成远期随访。结果治疗组复发率为36.1%(13/36),平均复发时间为(8.6±2.8)个月,对照组分别为70.0%(23/33)、(2.7±2.3)个月,组间比较,均$P<0.05$。高玉林将280例患者随机均分为两组,均予盐酸特比奈芬阴道泡腾片阴道用药,观察组配合中药(黄柏、苦参、栀子、蛇床子、枯矾、冰片等)水剂灌洗。经治14 d,观察组治愈率为94.3%(132/140),有效率为98.6%(138/140),复发率为3.6%(5/140),对照组分别为73.6%(103/140)、85.0%(119/140)、12.9%(18/140)。组间比较,均$P<0.05$。丁丽仙等将60例患者随机均分为两组,观察组在经前1周及经净2 d各口服萆薢渗湿汤(萆薢、薏苡仁、黄柏、赤茯苓、牡丹皮、泽泻等)1周,连服2个月经周期,对照组不服药。结果,治疗组治疗后平均反复发作率为3.1%,对照组为10.6%,组间比较,$P<0.05$。治疗组平均复发次数和复发天数均少于对照组($P<0.05$)。高学娟等将100例复发性念珠菌性阴道炎患者随机均分为两组,治疗组予青云粉胶囊(煅西月石、冰片、青黛),对照组予制霉菌素栓。7 d为1个疗程,连用3个月经周期,治疗组与对照组总有效率分别为90.0%(45/50)、94.0%(47/50),组间比较,$P>0.05$;复发率分别为26.0%(13/50)、48.0%(24/50),组间比较,$P<0.05$。任桂华等将80例复发性霉菌性阴道炎患者随机均分为两组,治疗组自拟加味桂芍四妙汤(桂枝、白芍药、茯苓、苍术、白术、黄柏等)加减内服配合中药(黄柏、白鲜皮、苦参、百部、蛇床子、甘草)熏蒸外洗,对照组口服酮康唑胶囊,外用制霉菌阴道栓治疗。7～10 d为1个疗程,连续治疗3个疗程。治疗组与对照组总有效率分别为85.0%(34/40)、65.0%(26/40),组间比较,$P<0.05$。治疗组停药3、6、12个月后复发率分别为0、10.3%(3/29)、27.5%(8/29),对照组分别为10.0%(2/20)、35.0%(7/20)、45.0%(9/20),组间比较,均$P<0.05$。牛秀兰自拟参柏外用方(大黄、苦参、蛇床子、地肤子、黄柏、川椒等)治疗77例霉菌性阴道炎,治疗7 d,治愈率为96.1%(74/77),总有效率为97.4%(75/77)。黄梅对50例糖尿病霉菌性阴道炎采用内外合治,辨证选择萆薢渗湿汤(脾虚湿热证)、龙胆泻肝汤(肝胆湿热证)及知柏地黄汤(阴虚内热证),外用以蛇床子、苦参、黄柏、艾叶、川椒、薄荷等熏蒸治疗。7 d为1个疗程,连用3个月经周期,总有效率为90.0%(45/50)。

胡吉升等观察中草药煎剂对念珠菌的抑菌作用。研究表明,黄芩、黄连、黄柏、虎杖对念珠菌体外试验具有较强的抑菌作用,且黄连的MIC值最低,抑菌效果最好。陈妮妮等研究发现,RVVC的主证以湿热下注证为最多,其次为脾虚、肾阳虚型,兼夹证中以兼夹肝郁证者最多,复合证以肝经湿热和脾虚肝郁证为主。在体质分布中,偏颇体质以气郁质、阳虚质、湿热质较多见。

(李亚迪)

【子宫颈人乳头瘤病毒感染的治疗】

袁林等将100例伴有人乳头瘤病毒(HPV)感染的宫颈上皮内瘤变(CIN)患者随机均分为两组,治疗组予二黄散(雄黄、黄连)宫颈用药,对照组不予任何治疗。7 d为1个疗程,均治疗3个疗程。治疗组第3、6、9个月CIN Ⅰ转阴率分别为75.0%(36/48)、81.3%(39/48)、85.4%(39/48),HPV转阴率分别为47.9%(23/48)、52.0%(25/48)、60.4%(29/48);对照组组第3、6、9个月CIN Ⅰ转阴率分别为26.7%(12/45)、36.6%(15/41)、40.0%(16/40),HPV转阴率分别为13.3%(6/45)、17.1%(7/41)、20.0%(8/40),组间比较,均$P<0.05$或$P<0.01$。治疗组患者治疗后白细胞介素(IL)-2水平升高,IL-4及IL-10水平均

无明显变化但干扰素-γ(IFN-γ)水平升高,与治疗前及对照组比较,$P<0.01$。其治疗机制可能通过调节 Th_1/Th_2 的免疫平衡清除 HPV 病毒,且通过调节 Th_1 细胞因子 IFN-γ 在宫颈病变发展过程中的作用可能较 IL-2 更为重要。贾沄等将 42 例患者随机分为两组,治疗组 27 例应用中药(紫草、鱼腥草、金银花、大黄、大青叶、败酱草等)阴道灌洗治疗,对照组 15 例应用爱宝疗栓治疗。7 d 为 1 个疗程,经治 3 个疗程,治疗组 HR-HPV 转阴率为 88.5%(24/26)、总有效率为 100%(26/26),对照组分别为 15.4%(2/13)、46.2%(6/13)。王君将 50 例宫颈糜烂合并 HPV 感染患者随机分为两组,对照组 24 例单纯接受红外线治疗,治疗组 26 例接受红外光治疗、阴道上药(保妇康栓)和口服中药(柴胡、当归、白芍药、白术、茯苓、炙甘草等)治疗。经治 20 d,两组宫颈糜烂面比较,治疗组治愈 20 例,显效 6 例,对照组分别为 19 例、4 例;HPV 荧光定量改变结果比较,治疗组治愈 23 例,显效 3 例,对照组分别为 14 例、8 例。窦保凤等将 86 例患者随机分为两组,治疗组 44 例予加减四妙汤(黄芪、苍术、黄柏、薏苡仁、当归、茯苓等),对照组予保妇康栓阴道上药。经治 4 周,两组总有效率分别为 95.5%(42/44)、83%(35/42),组间比较,$P<0.05$。张天繁等采用保妇康凝胶(莪术油、冰片等)治疗 80 例,对照组不予任何治疗。经治 30 d,治疗组与对照组 HR-HPV 转阴率分别为 75.0%(60/80)、5.0%(1/20),组间比较,$P<0.05$。阙彦臻将 239 例患者随机分为两组,治疗组 157 例予保妇康栓阴道用药 3 个月,对照组不予任何药物。治疗组在第 4、第 8 个月的总有效率分别为 70.7%(111/157)、82.3%(123/157),对照组分别为 39.0%(32/82)、50.0%(41/82),组间比较,均 $P<0.001$。

(李亚迪)

【盆腔炎性疾病、慢性盆腔疼痛的治疗与研究】

朱文涛等介绍了中药治疗盆腔炎性疾病后遗症循证药物经济学评价技术要点,包括研究类型,目标人群选择,中西医诊断标准,干预措施及对照药选择,药物经济学试验样本公式估算,样本量应该达到具有统计学意义的最小样本量,研究时限,成本,健康产出的效果指标、效用指标与效益指标,评价方法之最小成本分析、成本效果分析、成本效用分析等。李莉阐述了桂派中医妇科"湿瘀并重"的理论基础,总结了湿瘀并治法在盆腔疼痛证的临床应用。治疗痛经,以温肾健脾、化瘀利湿、行气止痛法,较单用行气活血法明显。治疗盆腔炎,主张一药多用、顾护中州、相反相成。白杰介绍了金季玲以桂枝茯苓丸加减治疗盆腔炎性疾病后遗症的经验,同时选用清康灌肠液保留灌肠和心理疏导。

蔡蘅等对 100 例患者采用四黄粉(大黄、黄芩、黄连、黄柏)外敷,复方毛冬青灌肠,中成药静滴,以及辨证施治。脾虚湿瘀型以完带汤和盆炎方加减(丹参、赤芍药、当归、茯苓、白术、党参等),肾阳虚型以内补丸加减(附子、补骨脂、淫羊藿、茯苓、菟丝子、黄芪等),湿热瘀阻型以止带方加减,气滞血瘀型以盆炎方加减(当归、牡丹皮、丹参、赤芍药、香附、木香等),寒湿凝滞型以少腹逐瘀汤加减。治疗 2 周,总有效率为 100%。王素改采用补肾清解汤(金银花、连翘、黄连、赤芍药、延胡索、丹皮等)治疗 66 例,10 d 为 1 个疗程;对照组口服康妇炎胶囊,20 d 为 1 个疗程。均治疗 3 个疗程,结果治疗组与对照组总有效率分别为 93.9%(62/66)、84.8%(56/66),组间比较,$P<0.05$。

黄叶芳等将 66 例患者随机分为花红胶囊(一点红、白花蛇舌草、地桃花、白背桐、鸡血藤、桃金娘等)组 24 例、花红颗粒组 18 例和抗生素组 20 例,治疗 14 d。结果,治疗 7 d,花红颗粒组愈显率高于抗生素组($P<0.05$);治疗 14 d,花红胶囊组愈显率高于抗生素组($P<0.05$)。花红胶囊组、花红颗粒组在治疗第 7 d、第 14 d 均优于抗生素组($P<0.05$),在局部体征改善、阴道分泌物检查及盆腔积液和炎性肿块方面与抗生素组具有相似的疗效($P>0.05$)。张雅静等将 300 例患者随机均分为两组,对照组予氧氟沙星合奥硝唑治疗,治疗组予康复消炎栓和金刚藤胶囊。治疗 1 个月后,治疗组与对照组总有效率分别为 94.7%(142/150)、56.0%(84/150),组间比较,$P<0.05$。葛静等采用盆炎净颗粒(忍冬藤、益母草、川芎等)结合康妇消炎栓(苦参、败酱草、紫花地丁等)治疗 74 例,对照组 73 例口服西药。治疗 14 d,治疗组总有效率为 90.5%(67/74),对照组为 78.1%(57/73),组间比较,$P<0.05$。张丽英将 196 例患者随机均分为两组,均予常规西医疗法,治疗组加服中药(红藤、败酱草、香附、延胡索、蒲公英、土茯苓等)和中药(红藤、黄芪、败酱草、蒲公英、鱼腥草、当归等)灌肠。治疗 14 d 后,治疗

组总有效率为 98.0%(96/98),复发率为 2.1%(2/96),对照组分别为 80.6%(79/98)、20.3%(16/79),组间比较,均$P<0.05$。对照组患者腹痛消失、包块消失、白带正常、体温正常和住院时间均明显优于治疗组($P<0.05$)。吴金萍将 180 例患者随机均分为两组,对照组口服西药,治疗组加服中药(生地黄、赤芍药、木香、丹皮、丹参、茯苓等)。经治 4 周,治疗组与对照组有效率分别为 94.4%(85/90)、77.8%(70/90)。

黄远芹等采用中药(赤芍药、三棱、莪术、牛膝、牡丹皮、车前子等)灌肠配合微波治疗,对照组仅采用中药灌肠。治疗 10 d 后,治疗组与总有效率分别为 98.8%(79/80)、88.8%(71/80),组间比较,$P<0.05$。李莉采用中药(金银花、连翘、桃仁、黄柏、益母草、薏苡仁等)灌肠联合理疗治疗 2 周,总有效率为 98.0%(49/50),明显优于中药灌肠组 88.0%(44/50)及理疗组 78.0%(39/50)($P<0.05$)。许亦韬等将 172 例患者随机均分为两组,均予服红藤合剂(红藤、冬瓜子、紫花地丁、蒲公英、忍冬藤、元胡等),15 d 为 1 个疗程。观察组加用红藤汤(红藤、败酱草、蒲公英、紫花地丁、鸭拓草)灌肠,10 d 为 1 个疗程。均治疗 2 个疗程,治疗组总有效率为 84.9%(73/86)、复发率为 32.1%(9/28),对照组分别为 69.8%(60/86)、57.1%(8/14),组间比较,均$P<0.05$。邢风琴等自拟妇春 I 号(金银花、菊花、泽泻、山药、薏苡仁、续断等)联合医经佳热疗袋治疗 338 例,治疗 45 d 后,重度 157 例,总有效率为 98.1%(154/157);中度 112 例,轻度 69 例,总有效率均为 100%。

(郝晓丽)

【先兆流产与复发性流产的治疗及实验研究】

王思慧等调查难免流产患者绒毛染色体核型结果与中医证型分布情况。结果显示,绒毛染色体正常及异常组均以肾虚型、脾肾两虚型为主,绒毛染色体异常与先天禀赋相关,后天因素对绒毛染色体畸变也起着不可忽视的作用。叶平等研究发现自然流产患者最常见的体质为阳虚质,其次为气郁质,为利用中医体质分型干预性防治自然流产提供了有效的临床依据。周群等研究发现,阴虚质、气虚质和阴虚兼肝郁质为反复自然流产的好发体质。

张雪等回顾性分析 2005 年 1 月至 2011 年 1 月期间以中药安胎为主的 401 例先兆流产病例,其中补肾法以寿胎丸加减(川断、桑寄生、菟丝子、杜仲、党参、白术等)安胎的成功率为 68.0%(123/181),活血补肾法以补肾安胎结合活血药(上述补肾药基础上加当归、丹参、赤芍药)安胎的成功率为 85.0%(187/220),组间比较,$P<0.05$。两组方法治疗成功的病例血绒毛膜促性腺激素(β-HCG)浓度上升情况及血孕酮(P)的平均值差异均无统计学意义($P>0.05$)。赵青以寿胎丸加减(菟丝子、桑寄生、续断、阿胶、党参、白术等)治疗胎漏胎动不安患者,有效率为 84.0%(42/50)。刘筱茂将脾肾阳虚型滑胎患者随机均分为两组,对照组予西医常规治疗,治疗组予服胎宝汤(当归、川芎、白芍药、熟地黄、黄芩、黄芪等)。经治 2 周,治疗组与对照组的总有效率分别为 79.3%(46/58)、66.7%(38/57),组间比较,$P<0.05$。两组患者证候积分均较治疗前显著改善($P<0.05$),有效患者的 P 及 β-HCG 均较治疗前显著升高($P<0.05$),且治疗组均优于对照组(均$P<0.05$)。

李静益等总结傅萍治疗封闭抗体低下性复发性自然流产的经验。认为正气不足为发病之先导,肾阳虚为发病之本,兼及心、肝、脾失调,病位在冲任胞宫,变化在气血阴阳。于孕前服益肾毓麟汤(菟丝子、当归、川芎、枸杞子、巴戟天、熟地黄等)3~6 个月后,复查封闭抗体,待各项指标正常后再考虑受孕。徐峻苗等将 111 例封闭抗体低下复发性流产患者随机分为 3 组,中药组(41 例)孕前予益肾毓麟汤(熟地黄、菟丝子、覆盆子、当归、川芎、枸杞子等)加减调治,中药联合免疫组(38 例)同时接受配偶淋巴细胞免疫治疗,空白组(32 例)孕前未采取任何调治措施。结果,中药组和中药联合免疫组治疗后抗 CD_3-BE、抗 CD_4-BE 均有所上升,其中抗 CD_4-BE 较治疗前显著上升($P<0.05$),两组封闭效率上升无明显差异($P>0.05$)。中药组和中药联合免疫组成功妊娠率均高于空白组($P<0.05$)。成功妊娠组抗 CD_4-BE 较治疗前显著上升($P<0.05$),抗 CD_8-BE 较治疗前显著下降($P<0.05$),中药组较中药联合免疫组更为显著($P<0.05$)。李伟莉等采用补肾安胎冲剂(菟丝子、桑寄生、续断、太子参、白术、黄芩等),合黄体酮肌肉注射,治疗 30 例复发性流产患者并与 30 例正常早期妊娠者对照。治疗 2 周,治疗组妊娠成功率为 80.0%(24/30)。与对照组比较,治疗组治疗前血清血管内皮生长因子(VEGF)显著降低($P<0.01$),受体-可溶性 fms

样酪氨酸激酶-1(sFlt-1)显著增高($P<0.01$)。治疗后VEGF显著升高($P<0.01$),sFlt-1显著降低($P<0.01$)。崔火仙将90例复发性流产患者随机分为两组,治疗组采用补肾育胎汤(菟丝子、续断、覆盆子、枸杞子、黄芪、党参等),对照组用叶酸片。孕前均治疗3个月,治疗组妊娠成功率为88.9%(44/50),活产率为83.3%(42/50),对照组分别为55.6%(22/40)、55.6%(22/40),组间比较,均$P<0.05$。

熊程俏等将45只小鼠随机分为模型组、阳性对照药组、中药组,观察小鼠蜕膜VEGF及VEGF受体2($VEGFR_2$)的表达及补肾安胎冲剂(菟丝子、续断、桑寄生、熟地黄、太子参、阿胶等)的干预作用。结果,模型组的流产率高于正常妊娠组及中、西药对照组($P<0.01$)。与模型组比较,中药组蜕膜VEGF、$VEGFR_2$表达升高($P<0.01$),与西药组无显著性差异。雷磊等将50只反复自然流产小鼠随机分为模型组和寿胎丸高、中、低剂量组,观察寿胎丸(菟丝子、续断、桑寄生、阿胶)对子宫蜕膜蛋白表达的影响。结果,与正常组比较,模型组子宫锐膜热休克蛋白27、a-烯醇化酶表达明显升高,转铁蛋白、膜联蛋白A_2表达明显降低($P<0.01$)。与模型组比较,寿胎丸高、中、低剂量组锐膜热休克蛋白27、a-烯醇化酶表达均降低,膜联蛋白A_2表达均升高,寿胎丸高剂量组子宫锐膜转铁蛋白表达升高($P<0.01$);寿胎丸中、低剂量组锐膜转铁蛋白表达差异无统计学意义($P>0.05$)。

(陈静静)

【产后缺乳的治疗及实验研究】

张琼等将160例初产妇随机均分为两组,观察组产后早期(3 d内)进行乳房按摩结合中药(皂角刺、丝瓜络、通草、红花、川芎、赤芍药等)内服,对照组按常规行母乳喂养指导。结果观察组产妇乳房肿胀程度明显轻于对照组,且开始泌乳时间早于对照组,48 h内泌乳量明显多于对照组($P<0.05$)。李春香自拟通乳汤(炒当归、炒党参、生地黄、熟地黄、麦门冬、黄芪等)治疗103例,对照组采用正确指导给新生儿哺乳湿热敷双乳及按摩、拍打乳房等常规治疗。治疗5 d,治疗组治愈率为92.2%(95/103),对照组为70.9%(73/103),组间比较,$P<0.01$。毋妙红等采用催乳汤(黄芪、党参、当归、麦门冬、川芎、柴胡等)并配合辅助疗法如提倡母婴同室、早接触、早吸吮、加强产后营养及指导产妇正确的喂哺姿势和婴儿含接姿势,做好乳房保健等,治疗90例,经治7 d,总有效率为90.0%(81/90)。李香萍自拟通乳汤(蒲公英、全瓜蒌、金银花、连翘、皂角刺、王不留行等)配合蒲公英煎汤热敷及乳房按摩治疗产后乳汁淤积40例,对照组用50%硫酸镁湿热敷,之后排空乳房,及按摩乳房。治疗3 d,两组总有效率分别为97.5%(39/40)、73.3%(22/30),组间比较,$P<0.01$。康红玲将300例产妇随机均分为两组,均食肉汤和鱼汤,治疗组加服生化催乳汤(黄芩、当归、王不留行、漏芦、通草、穿山甲等)。治疗9 d,治疗组和对照组总有效率分别为95.3%(143/150)、82.7%(124/150),组间比较,$P<0.05$。祁慧治疗56例气血虚弱型产后缺乳,采用通乳丹合四物汤加减(党参、炙黄芪、麦冬、当归、通草、穿山甲等),治疗7 d,总有效率为94.6%(53/56)。刘胜春等采用通乳络方(炙黄芪、当归、党参、炒白术、川芎等)治疗45例,并与生乳汁糖浆治疗45例作对照。经治3 d,治疗组与对照组总有效率分别为97.8%(44/45)、77.8%(35/45),组间比较,$P<0.01$。吴金萍将116例患者随机均分为两组,均予维生素E、B_1 5 d,治疗组加服中药(党参、黄芪、当归、熟地黄、麦门冬、白术等)3剂。结果,治疗组与对照组总有效率分别为93.15(54/58)、69.0%(40/58),组间比较,$P<0.05$。张淑英等用醒脾通络散(藿香、佩兰、白芷、王不留行、丝瓜络、漏芦等)加减治疗117例,经治3 d,总有效率为97.4%(114/117)。何文艳等将36例气血不足产后乳汁不行者随机分为两组,均于分娩后30 min内进行乳房按摩,治疗组于分娩后12 h服健脾养胃汤(党参、白术、黄芪、茯苓、半夏、陈皮等),同时进行母乳喂养。经治20 d后,治疗组泌乳量显著多于对照组($P<0.01$)。

陶莉莉等研究发现,广东人产后服用的"姜醋"(猪脚、生姜、甜醋、鸡蛋)可促进乳腺腺泡腔及导管扩大增生,减少乳腺小叶间脂肪结缔组织。且动物实验显示,母鼠的血清催乳素水平、泌乳量显著增加。

(谢津津 陈静静)

【多囊卵巢综合征的治疗及实验研究】

刘新敏等探讨多囊卵巢综合征(PCOS)血清激素异常与中医证候的相关性。结果显示,出现频次最多证候是肝肾阴虚证、肾阴虚火旺证、肝胃郁热证、脾虚胃热证。其中,高睾酮出现频次最多的是肾阴虚火旺证，高促黄体素出现频次最多的是肝肾阴虚证，高胰岛素出现频次最多的是肝胃郁热证。高睾酮与肾阴虚火旺证、高促黄体素与肝肾阴虚证和肾阴虚火旺证、高胰岛素与肝胃郁热证和脾虚胃热证均呈显著正相关($P<0.01$)。张丹英等研究PCOS证型分布及与焦虑抑郁的关系后发现，PCOS患者中肾虚型发病率最高，其次为肝郁型、痰湿型，血瘀型。与正常人比较，焦虑与抑郁的检出率显著增高($P<0.0001$)。肝郁组患者比非肝郁组焦虑、抑郁检出率高($P<0.0001$)，而其他三组之间检出率无显著性差异。徐芳等研究发现补肾化痰方(黄芪、淫羊藿、苍术、茯苓、丹参)中各单味药对PCOS治疗的贡献大小为黄芪>苍术>淫羊藿>茯苓>丹参。徐琬梨研究认为PCOS的主要病理因素以阳虚和痰湿内盛为主，且常相合为病，所涉及五脏病位主要在肾，病性以虚实夹杂为主。肖雯晖等研究发现“怒”是PCOS重要的致病因素，肝郁证是其最基本的病理变化，提出运用“以情胜情”的心理学方法防治。祁冰等总结了中医药防治PCOS的优势及特色，包括中医药调体预防青春期PCOS、生育期治疗PCOS排卵障碍提高妊娠率、孕期预防及控制妊娠糖尿病、妊娠期高血压疾病发生、预防和治疗PCOS远期并发糖尿病及心血管疾病。陶金红等总结了朱南孙以肾为重论治PCOS的经验。治疗原则包括益肾养经、不忘健脾，调经促孕、注重肝肾，补肾活血、化瘀澄源。

管蓬蓬等探讨补肾调周法联合饮食生活方式对PCOS的干预作用。行经期活血调经，重在祛瘀，用五味调经汤加减；经后初期滋阴养血，以阴扶阴，用归芍地黄汤加减；经后中期滋阴养血，佐以助阳，用加减归芍地黄汤，加入助阳之品；经后末期滋阴助阳，阴阳并调，用补天五子种玉汤加减；经间排卵期补肾活血，重在促新，用促排卵汤加减；经前前半期补肾助阳，扶助阳长，方用右归饮加减；经前后半期助阳理气，补理兼施，方用毓麟珠合越鞠丸加减。谢京红等研究发现，PCOS患者母亲异常月经史、家族早秃病史及发病前情绪影响为该病的相关因素。运用多囊饮(菟丝子、白芍药、淫羊藿、柴胡、龙胆草、巴戟天等)治疗30例，治疗6个月，有效率为86.7%(26/30)，妊娠率为62.5%(10/16)，月经改善率为83.3%(25/30)，治疗前后差异均有统计学意义(均$P<0.05$)。梁静等将98例患者随机分为两组，治疗组50例采用复方多囊调经汤(菟丝子、淫羊藿、肉苁蓉、丹皮、泽兰、苍术等)，对照组予服二甲双胍。治疗3个月经周期，总有效率分别为88.0%(44/50)、54.2%(26/48)，组间比较，$P<0.05$。与治疗前比较，两组患者血清胰岛素(INS)、促黄体生成素(LH)、睾酮(T)水平均降低，雌激素(E_2)水平均升高。中药组治疗后双侧卵巢体积缩小，卵泡数减少($P<0.05$)，而对照组双侧卵巢体积、卵泡数均无明显差异($P>0.05$)。王昕等以补肾健脾、祛痰化瘀为治疗原则，运用抑囊助孕汤(紫河车、熟地黄、淫羊藿、山药、白术、姜半夏等)治疗52例患者，经治3个月经周期，总有效率为92.6%(26/27)，明显优于对照组的84.0%(21/25)。

赵莉娜等研究发现，补肾调经汤(紫石英、仙茅、淫羊藿、肉苁蓉、熟地黄、山茱萸等)可通过降低PCOS模型大鼠空腹血糖、胰岛素及雄激素值，纠正低脂联素血症的途径来改善胰岛素抵抗及脂代谢异常。童星丽等研究发现，奠基方(熟地黄、当归、山萸肉、白芍药、菟丝子、紫河车等)可明显增加PCOS大鼠卵巢颗粒细胞E_2的分泌量，降低P的分泌量。

(郝晓丽)

【卵巢储备功能低下与卵巢早衰的治疗与研究】

陈赟等总结夏桂成辨治卵巢功能功能低下性不孕症经验。认为卵巢功能低下的女性，心(脑)-肾-子宫轴失调，其本为肾的阴阳失调，以肾虚偏阴、癸水不足为主，心肝郁火为标。辨证要点在肾阴亏虚、阴虚火旺，但常兼阳虚、气郁等，日久可夹痰夹瘀。治以补肾宁心调周为基础，阴虚火旺证，方选清心滋肾汤(钩藤、莲子心、黄连、青龙齿、合欢皮、茯苓神等)；心火阳虚证，方选清心健脾汤(钩藤、莲子心、青龙齿、茯苓神、党参、炒白术等)；夹痰证，方选清心滋肾汤合越鞠丸(钩藤、莲子心、黄连、青龙齿、茯苓神、怀牛膝等)，夹瘀证，方选清心滋肾汤合血府逐瘀汤(钩藤、莲子心、黄连、青龙齿、川郁金、怀牛膝等)。

胡颖等研究发现，左归丸加减方对月经恢复和血清激素水平的改善与单纯的西药人工周期疗法相似。左归丸加减结合西药人工周期对月经恢复和血清激素水平的改善优于单纯的西药人工周期治疗。刘秀云研究发现，左归丸对化疗导致的卵巢早衰大鼠有一定的治疗作用。崔晓萍等将120例卵巢早衰患者随机均分为中药组、中西药结合组、西药组。中药组经后期予滋阴促卵1号方(熟地黄、山药、山萸肉、黄芪、枸杞子、菟丝子等),经前期予助阳排卵2号方(熟地黄、山药、山萸肉、附子、肉桂、菟丝子等)。均治疗3个月经周期,中药组总有效率为87.5%(36/40),中西医结合组为95.0%(37/40),两组间比较差异无统计学意义,但均明显优于西药组的75.0%(30/40)。中药组及中西医结合组能明显改善患者症状、下调FSH水平,上调抑制素B水平,升高E_2水平,改善卵巢血流再灌注。刘凤兰等将140例卵巢早衰患者随机均分为两组,对照组予安宫黄体酮联合倍美力治疗,治疗组采用补肾健脾调肝活血法(山药、熟地黄、淫羊藿、龟板胶、鹿角胶、山萸肉等)。治疗6个月后,两组总有效率分别为98.6%(69/70)、85.7%(60/70),组间比较,$P<0.05$。治疗组FSH、E_2的水平变化均明显优于对照组($P<0.05$)。杨慧等将80例卵巢早衰患者随机分为两组,治疗组50例予补肾柔肝方(熟地黄、山茱萸、枸杞子、菟丝子、鹿角胶、肉苁蓉等)治疗,对照组30例予常规西药治疗。治疗6个月后,两组FSH水平降低($P<0.05$),E_2水平升高($P<0.05$),但组间比较差异均无统计学意义($P>0.05$)。治疗组治疗后CD_4细胞较本组治疗前及对照组治疗后均增加($P<0.05$),CD_8细胞减少($P<0.05$),CD_4/CD_8比值提高($P<0.05$)。两组治疗后主要症状改善率比较差异无统计学意义($P>0.05$)。杨家林等采用圣愈五子汤(枸杞子、菟丝子、覆盆子、车前子、五味子、黄芪等)加减治疗54例卵巢早衰患者。治疗6~12个月后,总有效率为92.6%(50/54)。治疗后患者血清E_2明显升高,FSH、LH明显降低,潮热汗出、带少、阴道干涩、腰痛、脱发等主要症状明显改善。

张荣等研究发现,卵巢低反应患者临床所出现中医证型按出现频率由高到低为肝郁肾虚、肾气阴两虚、脾肾阳虚、其它证型。肾气阴两虚证患者年龄、周期取消率高于其他证型患者,肾气阴两虚证患者HCG日E_2水平和获卵数低于其他证型患者。其将80例患者随机均分为两组,均采用拮抗剂方案,观察组在促排卵前按中药月经周期疗法治疗3个月经周期,对照组直接进行体外受精-胚胎移植助孕。结果,观察组AFC、HCG日E_2水平、获卵数、MⅡ卵率高于对照组,bFSH水平、周期取消率低于对照组(均$P<0.05$),bAMH水平、妊娠率高于对照组、bFSH/bLH值低于对照组,但差异均无统计学意义(均$P>0.05$)。余丽梅等报道44例卵巢储备功能下降肾阴不足相火旺患者,予服自拟滋阴清热育卵方(龟板、熟地黄、生地黄、知母、黄柏、白芍药等),连续治疗3个月,总有效率为85.3%(38/44)。白云等采用龟鹿调经汤(龟甲、鹿角霜、熟地黄、山茱萸、当归、川芎等)治疗卵巢储备功能低下64例,经治3个月经周期后,总有效率为81.3%(52/64)。杨宏敏等研究认为,逍遥丸可能通过增加卵巢颗粒细胞FSHR蛋白及其mRNA的表达,使FSH更好发挥促进卵泡发育、排卵的作用,并通过调节FSHR、cAMP、P450芳香化酶、E_2水平促进卵巢颗粒细胞的内分泌功能。来玉芹等将80例卵巢储备功能低下患者随机均分为两组,均予服中药(脾肾两虚兼血瘀证用五子衍宗丸四物二仙汤加减,肝肾阴虚证用一贯煎合六味地黄汤加减),治疗组联合穴位埋线(取肝俞、肾俞、卵巢穴、三阴交、关元穴)。经治2个月,治疗组与对照组痊愈率分别为52.2%(21/40)、30.0%(12/40),组间比较,$P<0.05$。两组治疗前后FSH、FSH/LH值、窦卵泡记数、症状体征积分比较有显著性差异($P<0.05$),治疗组症状体征积分及治愈率与对照组比较有显著性差异($P<0.05$)。

(杨利林)

【绝经前后诸证的治疗与研究】

杨敏等研究发现,围绝经期综合征舌象的形成与舌苔脱落细胞具有内在联系,舌苔脱落细胞能够在一定程度上反映肾虚、肝郁病理变化。血脂等指标变化与本病证素的形成有关。而肝郁、肾虚是本病主要中医病理特点,且受年龄、月经情况等因素的影响。邵祺腾等研究发现,更年期妇女以太阳、少阴、太阴人格特征明显,体质以阴寒质、阳虚质、气虚质、偏湿质、血虚质为主,其人格、体质存在一定相关性。张娅等研究发现,围绝经期失眠症的基本证型为肝郁脾虚证、脾肾阳虚证、肾虚肝郁证、肾阴阳两虚证、心胆气虚证和心脾两虚证,各证型在月经和主要失眠症状构成情况上有其自身特点。秦莉花等研究绝经综合征焦虑、抑郁的相关因素后发现,焦虑发生的因素中影响程度由高到低依次为重度病情、大学及大学以上学历、体型偏瘦、中度病情,而体型胖、FSH值对焦虑的的发生没有影响。单纯焦虑症状发病率高于单纯抑郁症状发病率,总焦虑症状的发病率高于总抑郁症状发病率,焦虑、抑郁的发病率以焦虑合并抑郁的发病率最高。肾阴虚、肾阳虚中焦虑、抑郁出现的总频率及单纯焦虑、抑郁出现的频率均比较接近。孟安琪等从肾脑平衡失调理论入手,阐述慢性应激导致海马神经元凋亡,进而影响围绝经期抑郁症的发生发展。严春玲等从肝的生理病理阐述水不涵木、肝旺肾虚的病机立论,并以此为依据,进一步论证泻肝滋肾,"调其阴阳,以平为期"的治法。方晶晶研究发现,围绝经期症状主要有疲倦乏力、腰膝酸软、烘热汗出、焦躁易怒等,异常质中以燥红质为主。刘爱玲等探讨了绝经前后诸症分型论治与主证主方论治模式。要考虑两种模式产生的原因、特征及适宜性疾病,以辨病为前提和基础,先辨病再辨证,辨病与辨证相结合。只有从区域性和趋同性人群的证治案例中筛选和凝炼名家的辨证模式和证治经验,才能对临床有更好的指导价值。

赵嘉勇等将60例患者随机均分为治疗组和对照组,分别予安泰汤(党参、黄芪、当归、山萸肉、酸枣仁、砂仁等)和更年安片治疗。经治8周,两组总有效率分别为86.7%(26/30)、60.0%(18/30),组间比较,$P<0.01$。两组治疗后症状总结分均较治疗前减少($P<0.05$),E_2水平较明显升高,FSH、LH水平降低,且治疗组更为明显($P<0.05$)。刘芳等将76例患者随机均分为两组,试验组口服稳心颗粒(党参、黄精、三七、琥珀、甘松),对照组口服维生素B_1、谷维素。经治4周,试验组与对照组总有效率分别为92.1%(35/38)、73.7%(28/38),组间比较,$P<0.05$。闫凤乐等以青蒿鳖甲汤合四逆散加减治疗48例围绝经期不寐患者,并与32例西药组对照。治疗4周,两组总有效率分别为91.7%(44/48)、90.6%(29/32),无显著差异($P>0.05$)。治疗组在潮热、夜梦频多,长期便秘、悲伤欲哭等症状改善方面明显优于对照组($P<0.05$)。闫燕自拟滋水平肝宁心汤(熟地黄、山萸肉、山药、枸杞子、女贞子、旱莲草等)治疗90例患者,经治8周,总有效率为93.3%(84/90)。许凤全等将164例围绝经期抑郁症患者随机均分为两组,对照组予服盐酸氟西汀,治疗组予服补肾疏肝化瘀汤(仙茅、淫羊藿、女贞子、墨旱莲、柴胡、枳壳等)。经治8周,治疗组总有效率为90.2%(77/82),对照组为58.5%(56/82),组间比较,$P<0.05$。两组治疗后HAMD积分、KMI评分及中医证候积分与治疗前比较均降低($P<0.05$),且治疗组优于对照组($P<0.05$)。

(郝晓丽)

【中医药在辅助生育中的应用】

陈嫣等将60例参加体外受精-胚胎移植(IVF-ET)失败患者随机均分为两组,均予控制性卵巢刺激方案治疗,观察组在此基础上采用中药补肾活血调周法,经期用桃红四物汤加减,经后期用逍遥散架加减,经前期用五子衍宗汤加减。治疗3个月经周期,观察组患者临床症状得到有效改善,与对照组比较有显著差异($P<0.05$)。观察组E_2、血清抑制素B、抗苗勒激素水平、取卵数、优质卵率、受精率、优质胚胎率均明显高于对照组,FSH水平明显低于对照组(均$P<0.05$)。周璐等观察发现,补肾活血调周法能改善子宫内膜厚度,改善子宫内膜血流,提高子宫内膜容受性,从而有助于着床,提高IVF-ET成功率。李楠等将60例促排卵周期宫腔内人工授精(IUI)患者随机分为两组,治疗组在对照组治疗方案的基础上加用中药行周期治疗,月经第5 d开始服用育泡饮(紫河车、菟丝子、熟地黄、枸杞子、当归、黄芪),至IUI日停。IUI术后服用健黄饮(淫羊藿、菟丝子、川断、熟地黄、黄芪、山药)。结果,治疗组治疗后较对照组HCG注射日子宫内膜厚度明显增加($P<0.05$)。治疗组临床妊娠率为34.6%(9/26),周期妊娠率为19.6%(9/46),对照组分别为11.8%(4/34)和6.1%(4/66),组间比较,$P<0.05$。孙云将160例患者随机均分为两组,均接受常规IVF-ET方案促排卵治疗,观察组移植前1个月经周期加服补胞汤(菟丝子、枸杞子、黄精、鸡血藤、何首乌、熟地黄等)至移植周期取卵日。结果,观察组胚胎着床率为42.2%(65/154)、临床妊娠率为60.0%(48/60)、活产率为56.3%(45/80),对照组分别为26.1%(42/161)、38.8%(31/80)、30.0%(24/80),组间比较,$P<0.05$。观察组先兆流产证候积分明显低于对照组($P<0.05$)。周茂溪等将复苏移植周期中子宫内膜发育不良的肾虚血瘀型不孕患者随机均分为两组,观察组在对照组基础上加服血流方(桃仁、当归、赤芍药、白芍药、生地黄、熟地黄等)。经治3个月经周期,观察组临床妊娠率为62.5%(24/40)、生化妊娠率为65.0%(26/40),对照组分别为22.5%(9/40)、25.0%(10/40),组间比较,$P<0.01$。治疗后两组患者内膜厚度及类型、子宫内膜下血流参数比较有显著差异($P<0.05$)。

陈莉等将51例肾阳虚型不孕患者随机分为

两组，对照组27例采用常规宫腔内人工授精方案，观察组根据月经周期加服复方玄驹胶囊（玄驹、淫羊藿、蛇床子、枸杞子等）至授精后14 d。结果总有效率分别为83.3%（20/24）、22.2%（6/27），组间比较，$P<0.01$。授精日成熟卵泡个数、卵泡直径、子宫内膜厚度两组相比无显著差异，但观察组子宫内膜厚度优于对照组。张建伟将66例因输卵管因素行IVF-ET的患者随机均分为中药+控制性超排组和超排组，均予肌注果纳芬及HCG，前者加服二至天癸颗粒（女贞子、旱莲草、枸杞子、菟丝子、当归、白芍药等）。结果中药+控制性超排组HCG注射日E2及E2/卵子水平显著高于超排组（$P<0.05$），两组中重度卵巢过度刺激综合征（OHSS）发生率无显著性差异（$P>0.05$）。提示二至天癸颗粒能明显提高IVF周期卵巢对超促排卵药物的反应性，而未增加OHSS发生的危险性。江媚等总结肖承悰治疗子宫内膜容受性低之经验。认为本病的主要病机是肾虚血瘀，兼心血不足，治疗在补肾的同时注重活血通络，自拟二补助育汤（骨碎补、补骨脂、巴戟天、桑寄生、川断、川牛膝等）在增加子宫内膜容受性低患者的内膜厚度、改善症状以及提高雌激素水平等方面取得满意的效果。

（杨利林）

［附］ 参考文献

B

白杰，金季玲. 金季玲治疗盆腔炎性疾病后遗症经验[J]. 国医论坛，2013，28(3)：32

白云，施晓玲. 龟鹿调经汤治疗卵巢储备功能低下64例分析[J]. 辽宁中医药大学学报，2013，15(3)：14

C

蔡蘅，叶润英. 100例盆腔炎性疾病后遗症慢性盆腔痛中医证型与中医特色治疗[J]. 辽宁中医杂志，2013，40(7)：1366

陈钢，蒋方建，盛昭园，等. 带脉功能探析[J]. 山西中医，2013，29(5)：1

陈莉，孙琴，沈涛，等. 肾阳虚型不孕女性行宫腔内人工授精术中补加复方玄驹胶囊的临床疗效[J]. 医学研究生学报，2013，26(6)：589

陈妮妮，郑燕飞，魏爱平. 复发性外阴阴道假丝酵母菌病的中医证候与体质相关性探讨[J]. 中华中医药杂志，2013，28(3)：829

陈嫣，孙亦婷，徐彩华. 补肾活血调周法对反复体外受精—胚胎移植失败患者卵巢储备功能改善作用的临床研究[J]. 中国中医药科技，2013，20(1)：8

陈赟，钱菁，夏桂成. 夏桂成教授辨治卵巢功能低下性不孕症经验探析[J]. 北京中医药大学学报，2013，36(2)：129

崔火仙. 补肾育胎汤防治复发性流产50例疗效观察[J]. 浙江中医药大学学报，2013，37(6)：709

崔晓萍，李晓莉，武淑慧，等. 抗卵巢早衰序贯方对POF患者卵巢血流再灌注及卵巢储备能力的影响[J]. 陕西中医学院学报，2013，36(4)：98

D

邓敏端，杨秀文，黎庆梅，等. 复发性外阴阴道假丝酵母菌病中药周期治疗与阴道局部Th_{17}细胞免疫功能的关系[J]. 齐齐哈尔医学院学报，2013，34(20)：2977

丁丽仙，孟昱琼. 萆薢渗湿汤干预性治疗外阴阴道假丝酵母菌病30例临床观察[J]. 现代中医药，2013，33(2)：24

窦保凤，张金格，刘彬. 加味四妙汤对宫颈人乳头瘤病毒感染患者疗效研究[J]. 辽宁中医杂志，2013，40(6)：1141

F

方晶晶. 杭州地区110例围绝经期妇女中医体质类型分布研究[J]. 甘肃中医学院学报，2013，30(2)：95

G

高学娟，姚成香，段志芳. 青云粉胶囊治疗复发性念珠菌性阴道炎50例[J]. 浙江中医杂志，2013，48(1)：35

高玉林. 中西医结合治疗外阴阴道假丝酵母菌病临床研究[J]. 中医学报，2013，28(8)：1249

葛静，谢磊，刘晶，等. 盆炎净颗粒结合康妇消炎栓治疗盆腔炎性疾病后遗症[J]. 中国实验方剂学杂志，2013，19(3)：30

管蓬蓬，周惠芳. 补肾调周法联合饮食生活方式干预对多囊卵巢综合征治疗的研究[J]. 辽宁中医药大学学报，2013，15(7)：178

H

韩霞. 补肾安胎中药对着床障碍小鼠子宫VEGF和MMP-9mRNA表达的影响[J]. 陕西中医，2013，34(4)：

497

何文艳,柯贤鹏,张晓峰.健脾养胃汤配合乳房按摩治疗产后乳汁不行疗效观察[J].实用中医药杂志,2013,29(9):717

侯小艳,孟安琪.孟安琪教授治疗肾虚痰湿型月经过少经验总结[J].辽宁中医药大学学报,2013,15(4):200

胡吉升,胡志敏,童中胜,等.17味单味中药煎剂对阴道致病念珠菌的体外抑菌试验研究[J].湖北中医杂志,2013,35(6):23

胡颖,许良智,谭卓林.左归丸加减治疗卵巢早衰的系统评价[J].中华中医药杂志,2013,28(8):2305

黄梅.中药内外合治糖尿病妇女霉菌性阴道炎50例临床观察[J].中国民族民间医药,2013,22(11):77

黄叶芳,袁野,陆华.花红胶囊及花红颗粒治疗慢性盆腔炎(湿热瘀结证)的临床观察[J].西部中医药,2013,26(2):4

黄远芹.清热活血消癥汤灌肠配合微波治疗慢性盆腔炎80例[J].陕西中医,2013,34(6):714

J

贾沄.抗病毒中药阴道灌洗用于宫颈13种高危型人乳头瘤病毒感染的研究[J].国际中医中药杂志,2013,35(5):397

江媚,刘雁峰,吕艳莹.浅谈肖承悰教授中药治疗子宫内膜容受性低之经验[J].环球中医药,2013,6(1):22

K

康红玲.自拟生化催乳汤治疗产后缺乳150例临床观察[J].实用中西医结合临床,2013,13(3):37

L

来玉芹,韦立红,郭钦源,等.中药配合埋线治疗卵巢储备功能低下80例观察[J].实用中医药杂志,2013,29(4):250

雷磊,李慧芳,谭展望,等.寿胎丸对反复自然流产模型小鼠子宫蜕膜蛋白表达的影响[J].中国中医药信息杂志,2013,20(7):42

李春香.自拟通乳汤治疗产后缺乳103例临床观察[J].浙江中医杂志,2013,48(9):681

李静益,傅萍.傅萍治疗封闭抗体低下性复发性自然流产的经验[J].浙江中医杂志,2013,48(6):401

李娟,丁志云."补肾化瘀汤"治疗人流术后月经过少60例[J].江苏中医药,2013,45(7):30

李莉.桂派中医妇科湿瘀并治法在盆腔疼痛证的临床应用[J].湖北中医药大学学报,2013,15(2):46

李莉.中药灌肠联合理疗治疗复发性盆腔炎50例[J].中国实验方剂学杂志,2013,19(7):330

李楠,金哲,刘艳霞.补肾调周法对促排卵周期宫腔内人工授精患者子宫内膜厚度及形态影响的临床研究[J].北京中医药,2013,32(6):431

李顺景.增量水车汤治疗宫腔术后月经过少49例[J].中医研究,2013,26(2):35

李伟莉,胡瑞华.补肾安胎冲剂对复发性流产患者血清血管内皮生长因子及其可溶性受体-1的影响[J].安徽中医学院学报,2013,32(1):20

李炜,段金廒,刘培,等.采用雌性SD大鼠探索建立适宜于气滞血瘀证妇科疾病特点的模型评价体系[J].中国中药杂志,2013,38(8):1211

李香萍.通乳汤治疗乳汁淤积40例[J].浙江中医杂志,2013,48(6):39

李应存,柳长华.敦煌医学卷子中与《千金方》有关的妇产科内容释要[J].西部中医药,2013,26(2):41

李元琪,黎烈荣.益肾续经汤治疗绝经过渡期月经过少临床观察[J].安徽中医学院学报,2013,32(2):42

梁静,孙维峰,周建龙.复方多囊调经汤治疗多囊卵巢综合征的机制研究[J].华南国防医学杂志,2013,27(6):397

林楠,钟菀杞.坤泰胶囊联合生物反馈电刺激治疗人工流产后月经减少临床观察[J].上海中医药杂志,2013,47(7):75

刘爱玲,雷红.中医妇科绝经前后诸症分型论治与主证主方论治模式探讨[J].长春中医药大学学报,2013,29(4):757

刘芳,赵步长,黄俊山,等.稳心颗粒对围绝经期综合征患者神经症状的干预作用[J].世界中医药,2013,8(9):1062

刘凤兰.补肾健脾调肝活血法治疗卵巢功能早衰70例[J].陕西中医,2013,34(7):771

刘娜,刘汉章.补肾疏肝法治疗月经过少33例临床观察[J].中国民族民间医药,2013,22(14):134

刘胜春,赵学刚,祝佩芹,等.通乳络方治疗产后缺乳90例观察[J].中成药,2013,35(3):641

刘筱茂.胎宝汤治疗脾肾阳虚型滑胎疗效观察[J].山东中医杂志,2013,32(5):315

刘新敏,刘睿,艾莉,等.基于血清异常激素的多囊卵巢综合征中医证候研究[J].环球中医药,2013,6(1):12

刘秀云,秦佳佳.左归丸对大鼠化疗导致的卵巢早衰防治作用的研究[J].深圳中西医结合杂志,2013,23(1):5

M

孟安琪,侯小艳,高超,等.围绝经期抑郁症从肾脑而论[J].中国中医基础医学杂志,2013,19(5):503

N

牛秀兰.参柏外用方治疗霉菌性阴道炎77例[J].江西中医药,2013,44(2):26

Q

祁冰,侯丽辉,郝松莉,等.中医药防治多囊卵巢综合征的优势及特色[J].中华中医药学刊,2013,31(2):256

祁慧.自拟通乳丹合四物汤治疗产后缺乳56例临床观察[J].长春中医药大学学报,2013,29(2):306

秦莉花,陈晓阳,李晟,等.基于数据挖掘的绝经综合征焦虑、抑郁的相关因素研究分析[J].时珍国医国药,2013,24(6):1431

秦莉花,王小云,陈晓阳,等.绝经综合征患者情志、中医证候的聚类分析[J].中国老年学杂志,2013,33(5):1996

阙彦臻.保妇康栓治疗宫颈人乳头瘤病毒感染的疗效观察[J].海峡药学,2013,25(4):186

R

任桂华,张静.加味桂芍四妙汤配合中药外洗治疗复发性霉菌性阴道炎临床观察[J].时珍国医国药,2013,24(6):1467

S

邵祺腾,杜渐,李黎,等.更年期妇女中医人格、体质特征分析[J].中医杂志,2013,54(17):1466

孙云.移植前应用补胞汤对体外受精—胚胎移植结局的影响[J].新中医,2013,45(4):61

T

陶金红,康美杰,朱南孙,等.朱氏妇科从肾论治多囊卵巢综合征[J].新中医,2013,45(2):179

陶莉莉,孙冬梅,陈玉兴,等."姜醋"对产后缺乳大鼠的治疗作用[J].江西中医学院学报,2013,25(1):60

童星丽,赵娟,谈勇.奠基方含药血清对类多囊卵巢综合征大鼠卵巢颗粒细胞分泌功能影响的研究[J].山西中医学院学报,2013,14(2):21

W

王芳.丹莪妇康煎膏对子宫内膜异位症患者焦虑抑郁情绪的影响[J].国际中医中药杂志,2013,35(1):49

王君.红外光联合中药治疗宫颈糜烂合并HPV感染疗效观察[J].辽宁中医药大学学报,2013,15(6):164

王思慧,傅萍,姜萍.300例难免流产患者绒毛染色体与中医证型研究[J].中华中医药学刊,2013,31(11):2539

王素改.补肾清解汤治疗湿热瘀滞型慢性盆腔炎66例临床观察[J].实用中西医结合临床,2013,13(2):37

王昕,陈旭."补肾健脾、祛痰化瘀"法辨证论治多囊卵巢综合征[J].辽宁中医药大学学报,2013,15(6):5

毋妙红,范晓惠,南丽娟.催乳汤治疗产后缺乳90例[J].中国民间疗法,2013,21(6):28

吴金萍.中西医结合治疗盆腔炎性疾病90例临床观察[J].中国民族民间医药,2013,22(11):66

吴金萍.中西医药治疗产后乳汁不足或缺乳的临床观察[J].中国民族民间医药,2013,22(10):98

X

肖雯晖,张婷,裘秀月,等.七情因素与多囊卵巢综合征中医证型及性激素水平相关性研究[J].中华中医药学刊,2013,31(8):1714

谢辉辉,徐建亚,汪受传.古人关于妊娠禁忌药划分方法初步总结[J].辽宁中医药大学学报,2013,15(9):153

谢京红,韩冉,张瑶.多囊饮治疗多囊卵巢综合征临床研究[J].中医学报,2013,28(10):1531

邢风琴,刘爱民.妇春Ⅰ号联合医经佳热疗袋治疗盆腔炎性疾病后遗症338例[J].河北中医,2013,35(6):841

熊程俏,李伟莉.反复自然流产小鼠蜕膜VEGF、VEGFR2的表达及中药干预研究[J].中医药临床杂志,2013,25(2):164

徐芳,马明,刘扬,等.补肾化痰方治疗多囊卵巢综合征的药物组成研究[J].辽宁中医杂志,2013,40(9):1758

徐峻苗,傅萍.中医药孕前调治对封闭抗体低下性复发性流产的影响[J].中华中医药学刊,2013,31(6):1311

徐琬梨.多囊卵巢综合征中医证素分布及组合规律的文献研究[J].中华中医药杂志,2013,28(9):2720

许风全,张莹,张琳园.补肾疏肝化瘀汤治疗围绝经期抑郁症82例临床研究[J].河北中医,2013,35(3):333

许亦韬,项迎春.红藤合剂口服联合红藤汤灌肠治疗慢性盆腔炎86例疗效观察[J].海峡药学,2013,25(3):155

Y

闫凤乐,周岳君.滋肾疏肝法治疗围绝经期妇女不寐48例的临床观察[J].浙江中医药大学学报,2013,37(5):546

闫燕.自拟滋水平肝宁心汤治疗围绝经期综合症90例疗效观察[J].国医论坛,2013,28(1):31

严春玲,王辉皪,刘普勇,等.从水不涵木辨治更年期综合征[J].新中医,2013,45(3):7

杨宏敏,宋翠森,周楠,等.逍遥丸含药血清对人卵巢颗粒细胞内分泌功能的影响[J].中医杂志,2013,54(21):1850

杨慧,苏健,靳慧云,等.补肾柔肝方治疗卵巢早衰50例临床观察[J].河北中医,2013,35(3):339

杨家林,刘艺,彭卫东.中药补肾养血治疗卵巢早衰54例[J].辽宁中医杂志,2013,40(1):1

杨鉴冰，王改梅，屈小会. 月经过少的中医诊疗思路[J]. 陕西中医，2013，34(6)：734

杨敏，李灿东，李红，等. 围绝经期综合征中医病理特点的相关研究[J]. 光明中医，2013，28(10)：1993

杨敏，李灿东，李红，等. 围绝经期综合征中医易患因素的临床研究[J]. 光明中医，2013，28(2)：278

杨敏，李灿东，梁文娜，等. 围绝经期综合征中医证素与血脂血糖等的相关研究[J]. 福建中医药大学学报，2013，23(4)：1

杨敏，李灿东，林雪娟，等. 围绝经期综合征证、舌与脱落细胞的相关性研究[J]. 福建中医药大学学报，2013，23(2)：1

叶平，王欢欢，叶骞，等. 465例自然流产患者中医体质类型分布特点的临床研究[J]. 中华中医药学刊，2013，31(10)：2215

于海英，李军. 苍附导痰汤治疗月经过少[J]. 山西中医，2013，29(3)：3

余丽梅，陈爱妮，陈慧依. 自拟滋阴清热育卵方治疗卵巢储备功能下降44例[J]. 广西中医药，2013，36(2)：25

袁林，徐又先，陈静，等. 中药二黄散对伴有HPV感染的CINⅠ患者宫颈局部微环境的影响[J]. 中药药理与临床，2013，29(3)：187

袁霞. 女子胞浅谈[J]. 陕西中医，2013，34(2)：252

Z

张丹英，俞超芹，刘益群，等. 多囊卵巢综合征证型分布及与焦虑抑郁的关系[J]. 山东中医药大学学报，2013，37(4)：300

张建伟，胡文英. 基于文献的天癸月节律研究[J]. 环球中医药，2013，6(1)：42

张建伟. 补肾对控制性超排卵周期HCG日E_2、E_2/卵子水平及OHSS的影响[J]. 辽宁中医药大学学报，2013，15(1)：32

张丽英. 中西医结合治疗急性盆腔炎98例疗效观察[J]. 山东中医杂志，2013，32(3)：188

张琼，陆容辉，金月芳. 产后早期乳房按摩结合中药预防乳房肿胀及促进泌乳的疗效观察[J]. 海峡药学，2013，25(4)：147

张荣，邓伟民. 卵巢低反应患者中医症候分布研究[J]. 辽宁中医药大学学报，2013，15(11)：98

张荣，邓伟民. 中药月经周期疗法治疗卵巢低反应的效果[J]. 广东医学，2013，34(18)：2873

张淑英，李开侠，王爽，等. 醒脾通络散治疗产后缺乳117例临床分析[J]. 河北中医药学报，2013，28(2)：28

张天繁，段丽芹，徐红燕. 保妇康凝胶治疗宫颈HPV感染80例临床分析[J]. 实用中西医结合临床，2013，13(1)：64

张雪，须义贞，王采文. 两种中医治则治疗先兆流产401例回顾分析[J]. 辽宁中医杂志，2013，40(8)：1599

张雅静，段申群. 康妇消炎栓联合金刚藤胶囊治疗盆腔炎性包块150例[J]. 陕西中医，2013，34(3)：264

张娅，黄俊山，吴松鹰，等. 围绝经期失眠症中医证候分布及其特点[J]. 中医杂志，2013，54(18)：1574

赵嘉勇，孟宏，郝晋东，等. 安泰汤治疗心肾不交型围绝经期综合征临床疗效观察[J]. 中国中医基础医学杂志，2013，19(3)：292

赵莉娜，韩亮，胡晓华. 补肾调经汤对多囊卵巢综合征模型大鼠胰岛素及脂联素的影响[J]. 中国民族民间医药，2013，22(12)：53

赵青. 寿胎丸加减治疗胎漏胎动不安50例疗效观察[J]. 中国民族民间医药，2013，22(10)：92

赵晓娟，王稳平. 热入血室之浅析[J]. 陕西中医，2013，34(3)：385

周斌，林雪，马丽，等. 虚燥更平散对更年期高血压病大鼠血管重塑的影响[J]. 中华中医药杂志，2013，28(9)：2733

周璐，徐才华，孙一红. 补肾活血调周法改善反复体外受精—胚胎移植失败患者子宫内膜容受性临床观察[J]. 中华中医药学刊，2013，31(1)：154

周茂溪，冯雪花，李玉，等. 血流方对肾虚血瘀型冻融胚胎移植患者子宫内容受性影响[J]. 辽宁中医药大学学报，2013，15(10)：183

周群，严玮. 反复自然流产与中医体质的相关性研究[J]. 浙江中医杂志，2013，48(7)：488

朱文涛，李磊，张霄潇. 中药治疗盆腔炎性疾病后遗症(慢性盆腔炎)循证药物经济学评价技术要点[J]. 世界科学技术(中医药现代化)，2013，15(3)：461

(六) 儿　科

【概述】

2013年度公开发表的中医儿科学术论文约1 800篇，内容涉及各系统儿科常见病。

1. 新生儿常见疾病

吴肖妮等以茵陈退黄汤(茵陈蒿、矮地茶、虎杖、白茅根、大黄、栀子等)灌肠治疗新生儿高胆红素血症50例，5～7 d为1疗程。对照组用双面蓝光照射，口服巴比妥、维生素 B_2、妈咪爱口服，溶血加入免疫球蛋白静注，用1～2 d。结果总有效率治疗组与对照组分别为100%、94.0%(47/50)；治疗组第1 d胆红素及日均胆红素下降幅度均优于对照组($P<0.05$，$P<0.01$)，治疗后血清胆红素水平、平均住院时间均少于对照组($P<0.01$)。马燕杰等以茵陈大黄汤(茵陈、大黄)治疗母乳性黄疸49例，对照组口服乳酸菌素片、思密达。5 d为1疗程，治疗组胆红素日平均下降值大于对照组($P<0.05$)，血清胆红素下降至正常时间短于对照($P<0.05$)；治愈率治疗组与对照组分别为85.7%(42/49)、53.1%(26/49)，组间比较，$P<0.01$。

2. 呼吸系统疾病

对小儿外感发热、毛细支气管炎、咳嗽变异性哮喘、哮喘等进行了深入研究。小儿慢性咳嗽、小儿支气管肺炎、小儿支原体肺炎的治疗详见专条。

齐晓国等以退热2号方(生麻黄、紫苏叶、柴胡、浮萍、连翘、甘草等)治疗小儿外感发热30例，对照组口服布洛芬混悬液，两组均对症用抗生素(或抗病毒药)。治疗12～48 h，治疗组与对照组总有效率分别为96.7%(29/30)、73.3%(22/30)。徐文平以健脾益肺方(黄芪、太子参、百合、桂枝、白术、制半夏等)治疗小儿反复呼吸道感染非急性感染期40例，对照组口服转移因子液。疗程12周，治疗组与对照组总有效率分别为95.0%(38/40)、77.5%(31/40)，组间比较，$P<0.05$；治疗后发作次数及每次发作天数均少于对照组($P<0.01$)；两组主要症状积分均较治疗前降低($P<0.01$)，但治疗组低于对照($P<0.01$)；治疗后 CD_3^+、CD_4^+、CD_8^+ ＋及 CD_4^+/CD_8^+、IgG、IgA等指标改善均优于对照($P<0.01$ 或 $P<0.05$)。范晖等以舒喘方(黄芪、白术、茯苓、毛冬青、防风、五味子等)治疗小儿哮喘缓解期20例，对照组用沙美特罗替卡松气雾剂。治疗半年，两组显效均为5例，有效分别为11例和8例。陈伟斌等以辛苍汤(辛夷、苍耳子)鼻腔灌洗治疗哮喘缓解期68例，对照组用无菌生理盐水灌洗，隔天1次。经治1～2个月，外周血及灌洗液中的IFN-γ、IL-4水平两组治疗前后自身及同时间点组间比较，$P<0.05$。

3. 消化系统疾病

消化系统疾病的研究有所突破，如厌食、便秘、肠系膜淋巴炎的治疗均有特色。小儿慢性胃炎、功能性便秘的治疗详见专条。

杜晨光等以运脾消食方(焦三仙、炒白术、半夏、陈皮、鸡内金、使君子、三棱、胡黄连、佩兰等)治疗小儿厌食49例，对照组口服小儿健脾化积液。经治8周，总有效率治疗组和对照组分别为95.9%(47/49)、77.5%(31/40)，组间比较，$P<0.01$；摄食量、面色积分、血清Zn含量、体重两组治疗前后均有明显改善，组间比较，$P<0.01$。刘丽平以厌食合剂(苍术、白术、佛手、陈皮、枳实、山楂)治疗小儿厌食30例，对照组用沙棘干乳剂。4周为1疗程，总有效率治疗组与对照组分别为93.3%(28/30)、73.3%(22/30)，组间比较，$P<0.05$。胡长宇以运脾化湿方(炒白术、苍术、茯苓、泽泻、太子参、神曲等)治疗轮状病毒性肠炎60例，对照组用思密达。7 d为1疗程，治疗组治愈率60.0%(36/60)、总有效率96.7%(58/60)，均明显优于对照组的33.3%(20/60)、83.3%(50/60)($P<0.05$)；且在缓解发热、呕吐、腹痛等症状，及大便培养转阴率均优于对照组($P<0.05$)。肖蓉等以健脾开胃饮(太子参、白术、砂仁、陈皮、麦芽、鸡内金等)治疗迁延性泄泻(脾虚型)30例，对照组口服思连康。10 d为1疗程，总有效率治疗组与对照组分别为83.3%(25/30)、76.7%(23/30)。邵征洋等以调中饮治疗功能性消化不

良儿童 40 例,对照组口服吗叮啉。2 周为 1 疗程,两组病例治疗前血清 GAS、SS 水平无显著差异,治疗后 GAS 上升、SS 下降,且中药组较西药组指标变化显著($P<0.05$)。于乐等以疏肝健脾汤(芒果核、薏苡仁、茯苓、麦芽、厚朴、延胡索等)治疗小儿功能性腹痛 69 例,对照组口服四磨汤。总有效率治疗组和对照组分别为 91.3%(63/69)、67.7%(44/65)。张慧等自拟消痰通络汤(制半夏、陈皮、茯苓、枳实、白芍药、党参等)治疗小儿肠系膜淋巴结炎 64 例,对照组口服阿莫西林等。5 d 为 1 疗程,总有效率治疗组与对照组分别为 95.3%(61/64)、78.1%(50/64),组间比较,$P<0.05$。

4. 泌尿系统疾病

肾病综合征、肾小球肾炎、血尿和遗尿等仍是本年度研究的重点。

张霞等以参苓白术散加减(人参、黄芪、白术、山药、莲子、薏苡仁等)治疗肾病综合征肺脾气虚证 20 例,对照组常规西药治疗。30 d 为 1 疗程,总有效率治疗组明显优于对照组。邱继春等以五草五炭汤(马鞭草、仙鹤草、血余炭、棕榈炭、紫草、益母草等)治疗小儿肾小球性血尿 50 例。经治 4～8 周,临床治愈 36 例,总有效率为 88.0%(44/50)。朱俏怡等以疏凿饮子加减(羌活、槟榔、大腹皮、茯苓皮、通草、泽泻等)沐足治疗小儿肾性水肿 30 例。5 d 为 1 疗程,治愈 25 例,总有效率为 93.3%(28/30)。赵晋元以补肾活瘀消白汤(生黄芪、丹参、赤芍药、当归、川芎、红花等治疗小儿慢性肾炎蛋白尿 25 例,对照组常规西药治疗。4 周为 1 疗程,总有效率治疗组和对照组分别为 92.0%(23/25)、56.0%(14/25)。刘佳玲等以补肾止遗配方颗粒(益智仁、山萸肉、乌药、熟地黄、生地黄、山药等)联合敷脐疗法(桂枝、干姜、五倍子,麻黄)治疗小儿遗尿肾气不足证 25 例,对照组用缩泉丸颗粒。治疗 4 周,总有效率治疗组和对照组分别为 96.0%(24/25)、78.3%(18/23);治疗组在睡眠深度疗效方面及尿量清多、精神不振、形寒肢冷、面色淡白及脉沉迟无力等次要症状改善方面均优于对照组。

5. 神经系统疾病

本年度在抽动秽语综合症、小儿面瘫的研究方面取得了较大的进展。儿童癫痫的治疗详见专条。

李伟元等中西医结合阶梯法治疗小儿抽动症 50 例,按照耶鲁综合抽动严重程度量表分级。一级:用逍遥散和归脾丸加减(太子参、白术、茯苓、陈皮、天竺黄、白僵蚕等),眨眼加菊花;鼻部抽动加苍耳子;摇头加天麻;肢体抽动加宽筋藤;多动加牡蛎、珍珠母、龙骨。二级:配合耳穴治疗,肝、脾、交感、内分泌、神门。三级:加捏脊疗法、刺四缝穴。四级:用哌替啶、安坦口服。治疗 12 周,临床痊愈 25 例,总有效率 96.0%(48/50);一、二、三、四级治疗前后抽动积分均明显减轻($P<0.01$);四级治疗后出现食欲减退、乏力、头昏、嗜睡等副作用,降级治疗后减轻至消失。王英华等以清心化痰颗粒(竹黄、钩藤、黄芩、郁金、石菖蒲、竹茹等)治疗抽动秽语综合症风痰上扰证 83 例,对照组口服泰必利。经治 6 个月,总有效率治疗组和对照组分别为 78.3%(65/83)、55.0%(44/80);治疗组抽动、秽语消失时间分别优于对照组。郭飞等以针刺(合谷、攒竹、地仓、颊车、阳白、翳风等)结合自拟方(僵蚕、白附子、全蝎、黄芪、白术、防风等)治疗小儿风寒型周围性面瘫急性期 48 例,对照组用西药常规治疗。15 d 为 1 疗程,总有效率治疗组与对照组分别为 96.0%(46/48)、72.9%(35/48),组间比较,$P<0.05$。

6. 血液系统疾病

儿童特发性血小板减少性紫癜详见专条。

张金举以固表消癜汤(黄芪、防风、槐花、胡麻仁、赤芍药、丹皮等)治疗小儿过敏性紫癜 40 例,对照组用常规西药(强的松、抗过敏、对症)治疗。连服 7～14 d,总有效率治疗组与对照组分别为 95.0%(38/40)、77.5%(31/40),组间比较,$P<0.05$;且皮疹、肾脏损害、腹痛消失时间及大便潜血转阴时间均短于对照组($P<0.05$)。张君等以紫丹颗粒(紫草、牡丹皮、白芍药、牛膝、生地黄、旱墨莲等)治疗过敏性紫癜肾损害 124 例,对照组予服维生素 C、芦丁,有中、重度消化道出血(或血管神经水肿)口服醋酸泼尼松片。治疗 4 周,总有效率治疗组和对照组分别为 100%、98.4%(122/124)。杨红蓉等以健脾化瘀方(苍术、乌梅、花椒、蒲黄、五灵脂、延胡索等)治疗腹型过敏性紫癜 89 例,对照组 87 例加用双嘧达莫片、匹多莫德分散片。经治 6 个月后,治疗组治疗前 D-二聚体升高 85 例,对照组升高 81 例,治疗后两组均恢复正

常。两组患者治疗后同时间比较差异无统计学意义($P>0.05$)。

(高修安　朱锦善)

【小儿慢性咳嗽的治疗】

卢敬东以小青龙汤加减治疗小儿慢性咳嗽外邪里饮证41例,脾胃虚弱兼见神疲乏力、便溏者加苍术、茯苓;表证不明显者,麻黄减量。对照组用止嗽清肺口服液。经治2周,总有效率治疗组和对照组分别为92.6%(38/41)、76.9%(30/39),组间比较,$P<0.01$。杨芝贵以清肺止咳汤(生石膏、生地黄、黄芩、连翘、牛蒡子、前胡等)治疗儿童感染后慢性咳嗽53例,对照组用地氯雷他定分散片、盐酸氨溴索片。经治14 d,总有效率治疗组和对照组分别为81.1%(43/53)、69.8%(37/53),组间比较,$P<0.05$。郭德利等以冬花汤(款冬花、川贝母、麦门冬、甘草、冰糖)治疗顽固性咳嗽98例,久咳肺阴虚者加太子参,去麦冬;伴发热、口干欲饮者,加生石膏;伴喉中痰鸣者,加杏仁;干咳无痰者,加橘红。结果服药5剂痊愈者31例,服药10剂痊愈者56例,10剂以上痊愈者11例。郭文英等以沙参麦门冬汤加减治疗慢性咳嗽300例,喷嚏、流清涕、鼻塞,加辛夷花、苍耳子;恶寒怕冷,加防风、荆芥;头痛、全身酸痛,加羌活、白芷;恶心反胃,加竹茹、生姜。连服7～14剂,其后改服香砂六君子汤善后。结果总有效率为98.0%(294/300)。邓雪自拟沙参芩栀汤(沙参、黄芩、栀子、生大黄、竹叶、薄荷等)治疗小儿顽固性咳嗽33例,痰黏难咳,加瓜蒌皮、葶苈子;发热口渴,加生石膏;咳嗽频剧、胸胁疼痛,加青皮、郁金;夜寐不安,加柏子仁、茯苓。经治10 d,总有效率为93.9%(31/33)。利艳等以玄麦甘桔汤(玄参、麦门冬、生地黄、知母、桔梗、甘草等)治疗小儿阴虚咳嗽42例,结果总有效率为90.5%(38/42),平均治疗时间为6.5 d。

胡宝珍以病证相结合治疗156例慢性咳嗽患儿,主方用瓜蒌、杏仁、款冬花、白前、炙紫苑、炙百部等,咳嗽变异性哮喘证见夜间咳嗽多,或刺激性咳,活动后加剧的加白僵蚕、地龙、川贝母、炙麻黄;上气道综合征证见鼻塞流涕、鼻痒喷嚏或频繁清喉者加白芷、辛夷、蝉衣、三叶青,辨证为风热者加黄芩,风寒者加细辛;胃食道反流见反酸嗳气烧心者加代赭石、莱菔子、制半夏、旋复花;近期有明确的呼吸道感染史,咽痒、喉痒后阵咳,刺激性干咳或伴少量白色黏痰,加用沙参、麦冬、桑叶;痰湿咳嗽痰多,加半夏、橘红、茯苓;喉间痰鸣量多者加苏子、葶苈子、黄芩、桑白皮;阴虚咳嗽,干咳无痰者,加北沙参、制玉竹、石斛;气虚咳嗽,咳嗽无力,痰稀色白,神疲,自汗者,加太子参、黄芪、五味子;痰出不畅,伴胸闷者,加桔梗、枳壳。经治1周,总有效率为96.8%(151/156)。

崔华自拟方(陈皮、桔梗、荆芥、前胡、百部、白果等)治疗小儿肝火犯肺型慢性咳嗽38例,对照组口服愈美颗粒,两组均可根据病情选用抗生素、抗过敏等治疗。经治14 d,总有效率治疗组和对照组分别为84.2%(32/38)、63.3%(19/30),组间比较,$P<0.05$;治疗组起效时间和症状消失时间均短于对照组(均$P<0.05$)。

(刘　瑜　高修安)

【小儿支气管肺炎的治疗】

赵兴宗以清宣合剂(炙麻黄、杏仁、生石膏、黄芩、荆芥穗、板蓝根等)雾化吸入治疗小儿支气管肺炎风热闭肺证患儿80例,对照组用静注或口服头孢呋辛酯或阿奇霉素、对症治疗。经治7 d,治疗组治愈率、显效率分别为66.3%(53/80)、27.5%(22/80),对照组分别为53.8%(43/80)、30.0%(24/80),组间比较,$P<0.05$。张宏玲以滚痰丸合二陈汤治疗小儿肺炎脾虚痰湿证28例,痰甚者加全瓜蒌、胆南星、天竺黄,夹食痰者加莱菔子、枳壳、神曲,纳差、大便稀薄者加炒白术、炒白扁豆、炒山药。经治21 d,总有效率89.3%(25/28)。

肖臻等常规西药治疗的基础上,分期辨证结合外治法(敷贴、微波中医外治法)治疗小儿肺炎100例。急性期:风热闭肺者以清肺汤加减(桑叶、桑白皮、菊花、鱼腥草、前胡、杏仁等)和痰热清静脉滴注,痰热闭肺者以清肺涤痰汤加减(炙麻黄、桃仁、杏仁、生石膏、苏子、葶苈子等)和痰热清静脉滴注;恢复期:痰瘀互阻者以祛瘀化痰汤加减(黄芪、丹参、桃仁、全蝎、矮地茶、浙贝母等)和丹参注射液静脉滴注,脾虚痰蕴者以扶正化痰汤加减(黄芪、茯苓、白术、半夏、陈皮、海浮石等)和黄芪注射液静脉滴注,气阴两虚者以养阴化痰汤加减(沙参、太子参、麦门冬、玉竹、枇杷叶、川贝母等)和参麦注射液静脉滴注。敷贴药(细辛、白芥子、干姜等)亦采用分期取穴,急性期敷于天突、大椎穴,恢复期敷于膻中、神阙穴,1次/d。微波照射肺俞、膏肓穴20 min,1次/d。对照组有单用分期辨证结合西药常规治疗(内治)和单用西药常规治疗两组。结果治疗组总疗效、中医证候急性期和恢复期的愈显率分别为 100%、95.0%(95/100)和 78.0%(78/100),内治对照组分别为 90.0%(90/100)、82.0%(82/100)和 54.0%(54/100),西药对照组分别为 81.0%(81/100)、74.0%(74/100)和 27.0%(27/100);治疗组与内治对照组比较,内治对照组与西药对照组比较,均 $P<0.01$。姚文萍分证论治小儿支气管肺炎 150 例,风热闭肺证予银翘散加减,痰热闭肺证予麻杏石甘汤合葶苈大枣泻肺汤加减,风寒闭肺证予三拗汤合二陈汤加减,痰浊壅肺证予小青龙汤合三子养亲汤加减,对照组用西医常规治疗。经治 7 d,总有效率治疗组和对照组分别为 98.0%(147/150)、88.0%(132/150),组间比较,$P<0.05$;治疗组退热、咳喘缓解及肺部湿啰音消失时间均较对照组明显缩短($P<0.05$ 或 $P<0.01$)。贺辉以桂枝加厚朴杏子汤治疗小儿支气管肺炎患儿 30 例,高热者加石膏、柴胡、黄芩,痰多者加橘红、半夏、茯苓,喘重者加葶苈子、地龙、麻黄,有过敏史者加地龙、乌梅等,同时予病毒唑针、青霉素静脉滴注,庆大霉素、地塞米松、糜蛋白酶粉针、利巴韦林注射液雾化吸入等常规西药,设两对照组分别单用中药和西药治疗。结果,总有效率治疗组 93.3%(28/30),西药对照组分别为 80.0%(24/30)、76.7%(23/30),治疗组疗效明显优于两对照组(均 $P<0.01$)。阴丽霞以参芪十一味颗粒(人参、黄芪、当归、天麻、熟地黄、泽泻等)治疗小儿支气管肺炎 112 例,对照组用青霉素、或红霉素抗感染,氨茶碱解除支气管痉挛、氨溴索化痰治疗。经治 7 d,总有效率分别为 92.9%(104/112)、76.9%(80/104),组间比较,$P<0.05$。马黎以清养肺汤(人参、白术、茯苓、麻黄、杏仁、浙贝母等)治疗小儿支气管肺炎 68 例,对照组用盐酸头孢替安静脉滴注(连用 5 d)。经治 10 d,总有效率治疗组和对照组分别总有效率为 97.1%(66/68)、88.2%(60/68),组间比较,$P<0.05$;治疗组退热、咳嗽消失及住院时间均较对照组明显缩短(均 $P<0.01$)。

王海铭等使用清肺敷脐散(半枝莲、炒谷芽、蛇莓、马鞭草等)治疗小儿肺炎风热犯肺证 30 例,对照组用布地奈德、复方异丙托溴胺高压雾化吸入,痰热清静脉点滴(细菌性肺炎加头孢呋辛钠,支原体肺炎加阿奇霉素)等西医常规疗法治疗。经治 1 周,治疗组咳嗽缓解时间、总病程及总住院时间方面较对照组明显缩短(均 $P<0.05$),两组总有效率无统计学差异($P>0.05$)。高东培以痰热清雾化吸入治疗小儿支气管肺炎 42 例,对照组予氨溴索雾化吸入,均每日 2 次。经治 5 d,总有效率分别为 95.2%(40/42)、80.0%(32/40),组间比较,$P<0.05$;治疗组症状、体征缓解时间均较对照组缩短(均 $P<0.05$)。周卫东以中医经皮给药(金银花、杏仁、生石膏、麻黄、蒲公英、鱼腥草等)治疗小儿肺炎 50 例,对照组根据病原体的种类选择相应的抗病毒类、头孢类以及亲青霉素类抗生素治疗,并予补液。经治 5 d,总有效率分别为 98.0%(49/50)、84.0%(42/40),组间比较,$P<0.05$。

杨琳等运用金荞麦片治疗小儿支气管肺炎肺热证 46 例,对照组采用常规抗感染等治疗。经治 7 d,显效率治疗组和对照组分别为 84.8%(39/46)、65.2%(30/46),组间比较,$P<0.05$;治疗组发热、咳嗽、气促及肺部细湿啰音恢复正常时间明显短于对照组(均 $P<0.05$)。贾春香以痰热清注射液治疗小儿支气管肺炎 36 例,对照组用常规西药治疗。经治 7 d,总有效率治疗组和对照组分别为 94.4%(34/36)、75.0%(27/36),组间比较,$P<0.05$;治疗组发热、咳嗽咳痰症状改善及肺部湿性啰音消失时间均较对照组明显缩短(均 $P<0.01$)。李成德以补肺养阴汤(太子参、麦门冬、五味子、桑白皮、地骨皮、牛蒡子等)治疗小儿支气管肺炎恢复期气阴两虚兼痰浊停滞证 40 例,经治 5 d,治愈 32 例,总有效率为 97.5%(39/40)。顾国祥等以黄芪止嗽饮(黄芪、太子参、法半夏、陈皮、炙百部、炙紫菀等)治疗小儿迁延性肺炎气阴两虚证 84 例。经治 10 d,治愈 59 例,总有效率为 95.2%(80/84)。杜君威等以加味香砂六君子颗粒治疗肺脾气虚证肺炎喘嗽患儿 60 例,对照组口服小儿肺咳颗粒(人参、茯苓、鸡内金、地骨皮、北沙参、麦门冬等)。经治 14 d,治疗组患儿 CD_3、CD_4、CD_8、CD_4/CD_8 较对照组无显著性差异($P>0.05$)。

(高修安　刘　瑜)

【小儿支原体肺炎的治疗】

李丽丽等分证治疗 41 例支原体肺炎急性期患儿,风热闭肺证用银翘散合麻杏石甘汤加减,痰热闭肺型用五虎汤合葶苈大枣泻肺汤加减;对照组用阿奇霉素序贯疗法。结果治疗组住院、退热、咳嗽消失、肺部啰音消失及胸片吸收消散时间均短于对照组(均$P<0.05$);对照组感染后脾虚综合征、迁延性咳嗽、复发例数均明显多于治疗组(均$P<0.05$)。叶志光等分证治疗112例小儿肺炎支原体感染后咳嗽,外感咳嗽证用三拗汤合止嗽散加减,痰热阻肺证用清金化痰汤加减,肺脾两虚证用参苓白术散加减,阴虚邪恋证用沙参麦冬汤加减,对照组用阿奇霉素序贯治疗。连用3周,总有效率分别为95.5%(107/112)、77.8%(70/90),组间比较,$P<0.05$;治疗组在治疗后1、2、3周的咳嗽消失率均优于对照组(均$P<0.05$)。

史竞懿等以清肺通络汤(桑白皮、地骨皮、矮地茶、地龙、桃仁、杏仁等)治疗儿童支原体肺炎20例,与对照组均予乳糖酸阿奇霉素静脉滴注。经治1周,两组全血低切黏度、血浆黏度、聚集指数均有明显下降(均$P<0.001$);且以治疗组为著($P<0.001$,$P<0.05$);两组红细胞压积均明显下降且以治疗组为著($P<0.001$,$P<0.05$)。陈玉琴以双花芩贝煎剂(金银花、栝蒌、沙参、黄芩、桑叶、川贝母等)治疗小儿支原体肺炎80例,对照组用阿奇霉素序贯治疗。服用7 d,总有效率治疗组和对照组分别为92.5%(74/80)、84.2%(64/76),组间比较,$P<0.05$。吴铁峰等用加味麻杏石甘汤(炙麻黄、石膏、杏仁、甘草、瓜蒌皮、芦根等)治疗小儿支原体肺炎63例,肺热偏盛者加黄芩、鱼腥草,对照组用阿奇霉素序贯治疗。经治3周,总有效率分别为93.7%(59/63)、78.3%(47/60),组间比较,$P<0.05$。刘鹏以清肺止咳汤(炙麻黄、炒黄连、僵蚕、炙旋覆花、射干、黄芩等)治疗小儿支原体肺炎42例,与对照组均予阿奇霉素序贯、对症治疗。经治1~2周,总有效率治疗组和对照组分别为95.2%(40/42)、88.1%(37/42),组间比较,$P<0.05$。且治疗组的体温复常、咳嗽消失及肺部啰音消失时间均短于对照组(均$P<0.01$)。王志敏以理肺化痰汤(麻黄、川贝母、杏仁、黄芩、鱼腥草、桑白皮等)治疗小儿支原体肺炎45例,对照组给予常规对症及阿奇霉素序贯治疗。经治14 d,总有效率治疗组和对照组分别为91.1%(41/45)、75.6%(34/45),组间比较,$P<0.05$。且治疗组的退热、咳嗽消失及肺部啰音消失时间均明显短于对照组(均$P<0.05$)。李旺辉等以清肺化痰通络类中药(炙麻黄、川贝母、生石膏、苏子、杏仁、桑白皮等)治疗小儿支原体肺炎42例,对照组用阿奇霉素治疗。经治3周,总有效率治疗组和对照组分别为92.9%(39/42)、75.8%(31/42),组间比较,$P<0.05$;治疗组的肺部体征及咳嗽消失、发热消失、胸部X片恢复正常时间均短于对照组(均$P<0.05$)。任桂华等以久嗽支原康(蜜炙桑白皮、炒杏仁、蜜炙麻黄、橘红、姜半夏、阿胶珠等)治疗支原体感染性久嗽患儿30例,对照组口服阿奇霉素干混悬剂。经治4周,总有效率治疗组和对照组分别为93.3%(28/30)、70.0%(21/30),组间比较,$P<0.05$。朱永琴等以活血化瘀药(丹参、桃仁、川芎、赤芍药,每方使用2味)治疗儿童支原体肺炎痰热闭肺证30例,对照组用阿奇霉素针静脉滴注,同时服用自拟方(麻黄、杏仁、前胡、黄芩、鱼腥草、桑白皮等)。结果显效率治疗组和对照组分别为93.3%(28/30)、83.3%(25/30),组间比较,$P<0.05$;治疗组的热退、肺部罗音消失及住院时间均短于对照组(均$P<0.05$)。张丁录以健脾益气活血汤(黄芪、白术、党参、茯苓、丹参、桃仁等)联合糖皮质激素(强的松或地塞米松口服)治疗小儿支原体肺炎36例,对照组用阿奇霉素序贯治疗。经治10 d,显效率治疗组和对照组分别为91.7%(33/36)、74.9%(21/28),组间比较,$P<0.01$;治疗组住院天数、胃肠道反应、咳嗽消失及X线肺部炎症吸收时间均少于对照(均$P<0.01$)。

来曼丽以宣肺止咳汤(麻黄、杏仁、射干、桔梗、法半夏、百部等)治疗小儿支原体肺炎60例,与对照组均予炎琥宁静脉滴注。结果治疗组患儿咳嗽、咳痰、气喘、肺部罗音缓解时间均明显短于对照组(均$P<0.05$)。陈晓梅等以喜炎平注射液静脉滴注治疗小儿支原体肺炎28例,与对照组均给予常规剂量阿奇霉素序贯治疗(先静脉滴注后口服)。经治5 d,治疗组痊愈17例,总有效率为96.4%(27/28),对照组分别为12例和85.7%(24/28)。张月仙以热毒宁静脉滴注治疗儿童支原体肺炎39例,与对照组均给予阿奇霉素序贯疗法。经治7 d,治疗组总有效率为97.4%(38/39),对照组为79.4%(31/39),组间比较,$P<0.05$;治疗组发热消失、咳嗽消失及肺部干湿罗音消失时间均短于对照组(均$P<0.05$)。

(高修安　刘　瑜)

【小儿病毒性心肌炎的治疗】

李靖等分证治疗小儿病毒性心肌炎54例:犯肺侵心证予银翘散加减,犯脾胃侵心证予葛根黄芩汤加减,犯血脉侵心证予生脉散合炙甘草汤加减,对照组用卧床休息、能量合剂静脉滴注等西医常规治疗。经治2周,治愈率治疗组和对照组分别为88.9%(48/54)、77.8%(42/54),组间比较,$P<0.05$。两组Bardhan指数及肌酸激酶同工酶(CK-MB)、羟基丁酸脱氢酶(HBDH)水平均显著降低(均$P<0.05$),治疗组更为显著($P<0.05$)。王晓岚分证治疗本病30例,热毒侵心证用银翘散加减,气阴两虚证用炙甘草汤加减,对照组用静脉滴注能量合剂,口服维生素C片、肌苷片、辅酶Q_{10}等基础治疗。经治4周,总有效率治疗组和对照组分别为86.7%(26/30)、63.3%(19/30),组间比较,$P<0.05$。治疗组在降低中医证候积分,改善ST-T段异常、过早博动,提高心脏射血分数方面均优于对照组(均$P<0.05$)。

徐忠明等以益心解毒活血通脉方(黄芪、人参、金银花、连翘、虎杖、丹参等)治疗本病35例,对照组用西医常规治疗。经治14 d,总有效率治疗组和对照组分别为91.5%(32/35)、65.7%(23/35),组间比较,$P<0.05$。两组24 h动态心电图及治疗前后心电图比较均有明显改善(均$P<0.05$),且以治疗组更著($P<0.05$);CK-MB检测均显著降低(均$P<0.01$),且以治疗组为著($P<0.05$)。王丛礼等以心肌舒一号颗粒(五味子、党参、黄芪、炒酸枣仁等)治疗本病70例,对照组口服辅酶Q_{10}、维生素B_1、肌苷、维生素C等。结果总有效率分别为94.3%(66/70)、72.7%(48/66),组间比较,$P<0.05$。常玲以自拟方(苦参、丹参、玄参、赤芍药、炙甘草、生地黄等)治疗本病78例,对照组用果糖静脉滴注,具有急性期感染者加穿琥宁,心悸等症状加重时加复方丹参滴丸口服。经治4周,总有效率治疗组和对照组分别为92.3%(36/39)、69.2%(27/39),组间比较,$P<0.05$。

刘保红等在常规西药治疗(绝对休息,予镇静、吸氧、高营养高热量饮食,大剂量维生素C、能量合剂、细胞色素C静脉滴注及辅酶Q_{10}等口服)的基础上加用参芪扶正注射液治疗本病31例,对照组用常规西医治疗。经治2周,总有效率治疗组和对照组分别为90.3%(28/31)、80.0%(24/31)。张耿昌等以生脉注射液、大剂量维生素C、磷酸肌酸钠静脉滴注治疗本病49例,对照组给予卧床休息、清淡饮食、利巴韦林、吸氧、1.6-二磷酸果糖、辅酶A等。经治14 d,总有效率治疗组和对照组分别为91.8%(45/49)、67.3%(33/49),组间比较,$P<0.05$。治疗组组治疗后心肌酶及肌钙蛋白Ⅰ的改善优于对照组(均$P<0.05$),心电图的总有效率95.9%(47/49)明显高于对照组69.4%(34/49)($P<0.05$)。

(刘　瑜　高修安)

【小儿慢性胃炎的治疗】

姜毅等以平幽养胃汤(黄连、半夏、干姜、桂枝、党参、炒白术等)治疗小儿幽门螺旋杆菌性胃炎脾胃湿热证35例,对照组口服克拉霉素、麦滋林。经治4周,除胃脘疼痛以外,治疗组腹胀痞满、食少纳呆、恶心呕吐、大便不调、口黏不渴等症状缓解均优于对照组($P<0.01$);两组胃镜及黏膜病理改变比较结果情况相近($P>0.05$);治疗后治疗组幽门螺旋杆菌清除率高于对照组($P<0.01$)。元国红等以健脾扶正活血散(黄芪、连翘、党参、山药、白术、丹参等)治疗小儿慢性胃炎肺脾两虚证30例,对照组口服复方黄芪健脾口服液(黄芪、炒莱菔子、炒白术、炒山楂、炒山药、桑叶等)。结果总有效率治疗组和对照组分别为93.3%(28/30)、70.0%(21/30),组间比较,$P<0.05$。

肖蓉等以益气养阴法(太子参、黄芪、茯苓、麦门冬、乌梅、山药等)治疗慢性胃炎患儿20例,与对照组均服用口服黏膜保护剂、H_2受体拮抗剂及胃动力药,每周服用3～4 d。经治2个月,总有效率治疗组和对照组分别为90.0%(18/20)、75.0%(15/20)。

刘洁等介绍闫永彬临床经验,以安痛三仁汤(杏仁、滑石、通草、白蔻仁、淡竹叶、薏苡仁等)治疗慢性胃炎脾胃湿热,疗效显著。

(高修安　刘　瑜)

【小儿功能性便秘的治疗】

刘丽等以五行辨证(抑木扶土法:方用柴胡疏肝散、逍遥散加减;金水相生法:方用增液汤加紫菀、桑白皮、杏仁、紫苏子、牛蒡子等;益火补土法:方用理中汤加肉桂、附子、麻子仁等;培土生金法:方用补中益气汤合补肺汤加桔梗、紫菀、太子参、天门冬、黄精等)治疗儿童功能性便秘70例,对照组用双歧杆菌乳杆菌三联活菌片。经治2周,随访1个月,总有效率分别为92.85%(65/70)、66.7%(20/30),组间比较,$P<0.05$。范涛等介绍常克以金润注水合方(桑白皮、地骨皮、知母、天花粉、麦冬、五味子等)治疗本病肺热阴亏证患者,对照组口服乳果糖。经治1个月,总有效率

治疗组和对照组分别为90.0%(27/30)、65.5%(19/29)。组间比较,$P<0.05$。可喜来等以一捻金胶囊(大黄、牵牛子、槟榔、人参等)和乳果糖口服液治疗本病50例,对照组均调节饮食、训练排便、适量活动等。经治12 d,总有效率分别为88.0%(44/50)、50.0%(15/30),组间比较,$P<0.01$。刘小燕等自拟健脾通便方(生白术、白芍药、生地黄、当归、枳实、莱菔子等)治疗本病80例。经治10 d,观察20 d,总有效率为95.0%(76/80)。

王利然用加味增液汤(玄参、生地黄、麦冬、火麻仁、肉苁蓉等)直肠滴注治疗本病42例,对照组口服金双歧。经治14 d,总有效率治疗组和对照组分别为90.5%(38/42)、76.2%(32/42),组间比较,$P<0.05$。田云龙介绍了韩新民以润肠通便汤(木香、槟榔、炒枳实、苦杏仁、决明子、连翘等)配合推拿疗法(先揉双侧天枢穴80～100次,再顺时针摩腹3～5 min)治疗本病的临床经验。

(刘　瑜　高修安)

【小儿特发性血小板减少性紫癜的治疗】

杨云红等以仙鹤草汤(仙鹤草、五味子、枸杞子)治疗小儿原发性血小板减少性紫癜172例,对照组用强的松。经治3个月,总有效率治疗组和对照组分别为95.3%(164/172)、73.1%(98/134),组间比较,$P<0.01$。王文学以自拟方(陈皮、仙鹤草、生地炭、花生衣、当归、阿胶等及云南白药冲服,气虚失血者加白术、党参,加大黄芪用量,兼见外感风热症加银翘散,阴虚火旺者加黄柏、知母,血热妄行者加牡丹皮、紫草,血瘀明显者加三七粉、桃仁、丹参等)配合西药常规治疗本病。经治1个月,总有效率98.2%(55/56)。王红玲等从外感论治(金银花、连翘、荆芥、薄荷、大青叶、侧柏叶等。出血明显者加十灰散,阴虚者加龟板胶、鹿角胶、女贞子,无明显出血者加茜草、牡丹皮,腹泻者加炮姜)儿童特发性血小板减少性紫癜,约50%的患者在6周内血小板可自行恢复正常,病情缓解。而对病情较重、出血明显,血小板计数$<30\times10^9$/L者,加用小剂量丙种球蛋白,疗效满意。

(刘　瑜　高修安)

【小儿癫痫的治疗】

马喜凤等运用平痫汤免煎颗粒(丹参、郁金、石菖蒲、远志、胆南星、地龙等)治疗小儿癫痫35例,对照组24例用鲁米那片。经治1年,治疗组总体疗效总有效率为91.4%(32/35),发作频率疗效总有效率为85.7%(30/35),发作持续时间疗效总有效率为91.4%(32/35);对照组分别为62.5%(15/24)、54.2%(13/24)、87.5%(30/35)。路岩莉等以熄风胶囊(紫河车、石菖蒲、全蝎、天麻、僵蚕、白矾等)治疗具有中央颞区棘波的小儿良性癫痫19例,对照组18例用卡马西平。以6个月为1个观察周期,总有效率分别为84.2%(16/19)、83.3%(15/18)。两组患儿脑电图痫样放电频度在清醒、慢波睡眠和快波睡眠阶段均较治疗前明显减少($P<0.01$),局灶性放电频数均明显减少、局灶性放电部位均有明显改变。孔吉良等以化浊解毒调肝汤(田基黄、红景天、绞股蓝、鳖甲、三棱、虎杖等)治疗小儿癫痫62例,对照组用西医抗癫痫药物常规治疗,观察两组患儿入院前1个月及治疗2个月后每日平均发作频率及临床疗效。结果治疗组治疗前后发作频率分别为(6.49±5.13)和(1.31±1.10)($P<0.05$),对照组分别为(6.75±5.10)和(3.70±3.11)($P>0.05$);总有效率治疗组和对照组分别为95.2%(59/62)和69.4%(43/62),组间比较,$P<0.05$。

(高修安　刘　瑜)

【小儿注意缺陷多动障碍的治疗】

张帆等以静意方(党参、炒白术、远志、石菖蒲、珍珠母、琥珀粉)治疗注意缺陷多动障碍脾虚痰蒙、心肝火旺证患儿99例,对照组有单用利他林及静意方联合利他林。治疗3个月后,静意方组、利他林组、联合组中医证候疗效分别为79.8%(79/99)、51.4%(19/37)、82.5%(33/40),治疗6个月后分别为98.0%(97/99)、83.8%(31/37)、100%(40/40),静意方组和联合组中医证候疗效明显高于同时间利他林组($P<0.05$,$P<0.01$);治疗3、6个月后各组注意力评分和Cornners父母评定量表各因子评分均较治疗前明显降低(均$P<0.01$),而治疗后6个月各组评分低于治疗后3个月(均$P<0.01$);静意方组和联合组治疗后6个月注意力评分和冲动评分明显优于利他林对照组($P<0.05$,$P<0.01$)。丁惠玲等以泻心宁神汤(黄连、黄芩、半夏、白蒺藜、野百合、珍珠母等)治疗儿童多动症心肝火旺证90例,对照用利他林。经治8周,总有效率分别为95.6%(86/90)、90.0%(27/30),组间比较,$P>$

0.05;中医证候疗效有效率分别为 95.6%(86/90)、83.3%(25/30),组间比较,$P<0.05$。

张弛等以健脾平肝颗粒(柴胡、炒白芍药、炒枳壳、炙甘草、浮小麦、石菖蒲等)治疗儿童注意力缺陷多动症脾虚肝亢证 28 例,对照组用多参数生物反馈仪治疗,每次 30 min,每周 5 次。治疗 60 d,总有效率分别为 96.4%(27/28)、81.8%(18/22)。

(刘 瑜 高修安)

[附] 参考文献

C

常玲.中西医结合治疗小儿病毒性心肌炎疗效观察[J].中医临床研究,2013,5(10):91

陈伟斌,黄勋,姚敏.辛苍汤鼻腔灌洗对哮喘儿童缓解期细胞因子的调控作用[J].浙江中医药大学学报,2013,37(3):272

陈晓梅,张燕萍.阿奇霉素联合喜炎平治疗小儿支原体肺炎 28 例临床疗效观察[J].实用中西医结合临床,2013,13(5):5

陈玉琴.双花芩贝煎剂联合阿奇霉素治疗小儿支原体肺炎的疗效与安全性[J].中医临床研究,2013,5(10):83

崔华.中药治疗小儿肝火犯肺型慢性咳嗽 38 例[J].河南中医,2013,33(11):1954

D

邓雪.泻心救肺法治疗小儿顽固性咳嗽 33 例[J].中医儿科杂志,2013,9(3):14

丁惠玲,景晓平,王霞芳.泻心宁神汤治疗儿童多动症(心肝火旺型)临床观察[J].辽宁中医杂志,2013,40(8):2040

杜晨光,丁培杰,曹颖,等.运脾消食方治疗小儿厌食症临床观察[J].辽宁中医药大学学报,2013,15(8):146

杜君威,杨丽珍,侯秀刚.加味香砂六君子颗粒对肺脾气虚型肺炎喘嗽患儿的疗效观察[J].中医药信息,2013,30(2):52

F

范晖,刘建汉.中西医结合治疗缓解期儿童支气管哮喘临床研究[J].中医学报,2013,28(8):1112

范涛,罗芯怡,常克.金润注水合方治疗小儿便秘(肺热阴亏证)30 例临床观察[J].四川中医,2013,31(8):102

G

高东培.痰热清注射液雾化吸入辅助治疗小儿支气管肺炎 42 例疗效观察[J].中国中西医结合儿科学,2013,5(3):231

顾国祥,李志武,杨丽霞,等.黄芪止嗽饮治疗小儿迁延性肺炎气阴两虚证 84 例[J].中医儿科杂志,2013,9(1):41

郭德利,苗爱荣,赵显芳.冬花汤治疗小儿顽固性咳嗽的疗效观察[J].中国民族民间医药,2013,22(12):90

郭飞,卢振产,邱彦昭.针药结合治疗小儿风寒型周围性面瘫急性期 48 例临床观察[J].中医儿科杂志,2013,9(4):40

郭文英,任体祥.沙参麦门冬汤加减治疗儿童慢性咳嗽 300 例临床观察[J].云南中医中药杂志,2013,34(3):36

H

贺辉.桂枝加厚朴杏子汤配合西药治疗小儿支气管肺炎 30 例[J].河南中医,2013,33(7):1029

胡宝珍.小儿慢性咳嗽的辨病和辨证治疗[J].浙江中西医结合杂志,2013,23(7):569

胡长宇.运脾化湿疗法治疗小儿腹泻 60 例[J].中医杂志,2013,54(1):65

J

贾春香.痰热清注射液治疗小儿支气管肺炎疗效观察[J].新中医,2013,45(7):99

姜毅,张伟.平幽养胃汤治疗幽门螺旋杆菌性小儿胃炎(脾胃湿热型)70 例临床研究[J].中医药学报,2013,41(3):122

K

可喜来,燕小伟.一捻金胶囊联合乳果糖口服液治疗婴幼儿功能性便秘的临床研究[J].中医临床研究,2013,5(8):16

孔吉良,商爱江.化浊解毒调肝汤辅助治疗小儿癫痫疗效分析[J].吉林中医药,2013,33(6):595

L

来蔓丽.宣肺止咳汤联合炎琥宁注射液治疗小儿支原体肺炎 60 例[J].中国中医药现代远程教育,2013,11(15):26

李成德.补肺养阴汤治疗气阴两虚兼痰浊停滞型小儿支气管肺炎恢复期 40 例[J].中医研究,2013,

26(5)：49

李靖，史军有. 中西医结合治疗小儿病毒性心肌炎54例疗效观察[J]. 甘肃中医学院学报，2013，30(3)：59

李丽丽，刘薇薇，陈慧，等. 中西医结合治疗小儿肺炎支原体肺炎优势及远期疗效分析[J]. 辽宁中医杂志，2013，40(10)：2082

李旺辉，徐晓娟，宋莉莉. 清肺化痰通络法治疗小儿支原体肺炎42例[J]. 陕西中医，2013，34(7)：787

李伟元，邓丽莎，莫珊，等. 中西医结合阶梯法治疗小儿抽动障碍疗效观察[J]. 广州中医药大学学报，2013，30(2)：157

利艳，李慧梅. 玄麦甘桔汤治疗小儿阴虚咳嗽42例疗效观察[J]. 中国民族民间医药，2013，22(10)：108

刘保红，刘继军，李友梅. 参芪扶正注射液治疗小儿病毒性心肌炎疗效观察[J]. 中国民族民间医药，2013，22(2)：61

刘洁，李艳艳，闫永彬. 安痛三仁汤治疗小儿慢性胃炎浅析[J]. 中医临床研究，2013，5(1)：57

刘丽，邢燕茹，李宗起，等. 运用中医五行理论辨证治疗儿童功能性便秘70例[J]. 浙江中医杂志，2013，48(1)：38

刘丽平. 厌食合剂治疗小儿厌食症30例疗效观察[J]. 中国中西医结合儿科学，2013，5(3)：245

刘玲佳，王俊宏. 补肾止遗配方颗粒联合敷脐疗法治疗小儿遗尿症肾气不足型25例临床观察[J]. 中医杂志，2013，54(23)：2021

刘鹏. 清肺止咳汤联合西药治疗小儿支原体肺炎42例[J]. 中国中医药科技，2013，20(1)：98

刘小燕，刘彩琴. 自拟健脾通便方治疗小儿功能性便秘80例疗效观察[J]. 现代中医药，2013，33(4)：47

卢敬东. 小青龙汤加减治疗小儿外邪里饮证慢性咳嗽41例[J]. 河北中医，2013，35(2)：227

路岩莉，晋黎，孙丹. 熄风胶囊治疗小儿良性癫痫19例临床观察[J]. 中医杂志，2013，54(2)：121

M

马黎. 清养肺汤联合盐酸头孢替安静脉滴注治疗小儿支气管肺炎68例[J]. 中医研究，2013，26(7)：35

马喜凤，张士卿. 平痫汤治疗小儿癫痫35例[J]. 中医杂志，2013，54(4)：336

马燕杰，马耀军，厚晔. 中西医结合治疗母乳性黄疸49例疗效观察[J]. 新中医，2013，45(2)：77

Q

齐晓国，王晓艾，丛丽. 中药退热2号方治疗小儿急性上呼吸道感染发热30例疗效观察[J]. 甘肃中医学院学报，2013，30(2)：60

邱继春，王艳，罗晶晶，等. 五草五炭汤治疗小儿肾小球性血尿50例疗效观察[J]. 中国中西医结合儿科学，2013，5(3)：221

R

任桂华，张静. 久嗽支原康治疗小儿支原体感染性久嗽临床观察[J]. 湖北中医杂志，2013，35(6)：37

S

邵征洋，连俊兰，詹璐，等. 调中饮对功能性消化不良儿童血浆胃肠激素的影响[J]. 中医儿科杂志，2013，9(5)：26

史竞懿，姜之炎，卞菊. 清肺通络汤对儿童肺炎支原体肺炎血液流变学影响的研究[J]. 天津中医药，2013，30(6)：331

T

田云龙，韩新民. 韩新民教授治疗儿童功能性便秘经验[J]. 中医儿科杂志，2013，9(3)：3

W

王丛礼，洪丽君，程春华. 心肌舒一号颗粒治疗病毒性心肌炎70例[J]. 中医儿科杂志，2013，9(1)：50

王海铭，康静. 清肺敷脐散联合西医常规疗法治疗小儿肺炎临床观察[J]. 山西中医，2013，29(4)：22

王红玲，韩倩，王祥麒，等. 从外感论治儿童特发性血小板减少性紫癜[J]. 中医学报，2013，28(9)：1412

王文学. 小儿紫癜56例中西医结合治疗临床分析[J]. 实用中西医结合临床，2013，13(5)：6

王晓岚. 中西医结合治疗小儿急性病毒性心肌炎30例临床观察[J]. 新中医，2013，45(5)：86

王英华，何小仁. 清心化痰颗粒与泰必利治疗儿童抽动—秽语综合症(风痰上扰型)疗效比较[J]. 浙江中医药大学学报，2013，37(4)：398

王志敏. 理肺化痰汤联合西药治疗小儿肺炎支原体肺炎45例疗效观察[J]. 中国中西医结合儿科学，2013，5(1)：41

王利然. 加味增液汤直肠滴入治疗小儿功能性便秘42例疗效观察[J]. 中国中医药科技，2013，20(1)：74

吴铁峰，吴继红，耿喜荣，等. 加味麻杏石甘汤合阿奇霉素治疗小儿支原体肺炎[J]. 浙江中西医结合杂志，2013，23(3)：238

吴肖妮，俞学铭，田真，等. 茵陈退黄汤灌肠治疗新生儿高胆红素血症的临床研究[J]. 浙江中医杂志，2013，48(4)：249

X

肖蓉，范维聪. 益气养阴法治疗儿童慢性胃炎20例临床观察[J]. 中医儿科杂志，2013，9(3)：22

肖蓉，马新蕾. 健脾开胃饮治疗脾虚型泄泻(迁延性

腹泻)30 例疗效观察[J]. 中医儿科杂志,2013,9(4)：25

肖臻,姜之炎,徐彬彬,等. 中医分期辨证联合外治疗法治疗小儿肺炎的多中心临床观察[J]. 浙江中医药大学学报,2013,37(6)：688

徐文平. 健脾益肺方治疗非急性感染期小儿反复呼吸道感染 40 例临床研究[J]. 新中医,2013,45(11)：71

徐忠明,王肖原,李素芳,等. 益心解毒活血通脉方治疗小儿病毒性心肌炎 70 例临床观察[J]. 中国中医药科技,2013,20(2)：179

Y

杨红蓉,郭培京,张娜,等. 健脾化瘀方治疗腹型过敏性紫癜 89 例临床观察[J]. 中医杂志,2013,54(6)：503

杨琳,向希雄. 金荞麦片治疗小儿支气管肺炎(肺热证)46 例[J]. 中国中西医结合儿科学,2013,5(2)：148

杨云红,赵爱珠,赵鹏飞. 仙鹤草汤治疗小儿原发性血小板减少性紫癜 172 例[J]. 陕西中医,2013,34(9)：1164

杨芝贵. 清肺止咳汤治疗儿童感染后慢性咳嗽 53 例临床观察[J]. 河北中医,2013,35(7)：985

姚文萍. 中西医结合治疗小儿支气管肺炎 150 例疗效观察[J]. 中医儿科杂志,2013,9(4)：16

叶志光,曾庆祥,丘文静,等. 中西医结合治疗小儿肺炎支原体感染后咳嗽疗效观察[J]. 现代中西医结合杂志,2013,22(11)：1177

阴丽霞. 参芪十一味颗粒辅治小儿支气管肺炎的临床疗效观察[J]. 中医临床研究,2013,5(17)：6

于乐,李蔷华. 疏肝健脾汤治疗儿童功能性腹痛 69 例临床观察[J]. 新中医,2013,45(11)：70

元国红,周莹. 健脾扶正活血散治疗小儿慢性胃炎 30 例[J]. 陕西中医,2013,34(3)：276

Z

张弛,琚伟,马炳祥,等. 脑电生物反馈联合健脾平肝颗粒治疗脾虚肝亢型儿童注意力缺陷多动症 28 例[J]. 中医研究,2013,26(5)：33

张丁录. 糖皮质激素联合健脾益气活血汤治疗小儿肺炎支原体肺炎 36 例[J]. 光明中医,2013,28(3)：578

张帆,顾明达,朱盛国,等. 静意方治疗注意缺陷多动障碍儿童 99 例临床观察[J]. 中医杂志,2013,54(8)：673

张耿昌,刘建华,江少青. 生脉、大剂量维生素 C 联合磷酸肌酸钠治疗小儿病毒性心肌炎疗效观察[J]. 亚太传统医药,2013,9(7)：160

张宏玲. 滚痰丸合二陈汤治疗小儿肺炎脾虚痰湿型咳嗽 28 例[J]. 中医儿科杂志,2013,9(1)：30

张慧,胥冬梅,厚晔. 中西医结合治疗小儿肠系膜淋巴结炎 64 例疗效观察[J]. 新中医,2013,45(3)：79

张金举. 中西医结合治疗小儿过敏性紫癜 40 例疗效观察[J]. 新中医,2013,45(10)：73

张君,张少卿,王绍洁,等. 紫丹颗粒对过敏性紫癜患儿肾损害的影响[J]. 中医杂志,2013,54(16)：1380

张霞,刘志新,赵文华. 参苓白术散加减治疗小儿肾病综合征(肺脾气虚型)20 例疗效观察[J]. 中国中西医结合儿科学,2013,5(4)：297

张月仙. 阿奇霉素与热毒宁联合治疗儿童支原体肺炎[J]. 中国民族民间医药,2013,22(10)：101

赵晋元. 补肾活瘀消白汤联合西药治疗小儿慢性肾炎蛋白尿对照观察[J]. 中国中西医结合儿科学,2013,5(3)：275

赵兴宗,李秀美. 清宣合剂雾化吸入治疗小儿支气管肺炎 80 例[J]. 中国中医药现代远程教育,2013,11(13)：27

周卫东. 中医经皮给药治疗小儿肺炎 50 例[J]. 中医研究,2013,26(2)：30

朱俏怡,陈熳妮,周春姣. 中药沐足治疗小儿肾性水肿 30 例疗效观察[J]. 新中医,2013,45(6)：91

朱永琴,王艳,邬思远. 活血化瘀药佐治儿童痰热闭肺型支原体肺炎[J]. 中华中医药学刊,2013,31(5)：1200

(七) 外　　科

【概述】

2013年有关外科的文献约2 500篇,以临床报道为主,实验研究主要集中在慢性皮肤溃疡、乳腺增生病、前列腺增生、糖尿病足、急性胰腺炎、烧伤等。除了中药内服、外用和手术疗法,也有部分运用针灸推拿等治疗外科疾病的报道。

1. 疮疡

临床治疗的文献以褥疮及慢性皮肤溃疡居多,其次为皮肤丹毒、化脓性疾病、骨髓炎等,实验研究则集中在慢性皮肤溃疡。

韩炎艳等将116例浅表溃疡期褥疮患者随机均分为两组,给予莫匹罗星配合常规护理疗法,治疗组在此基础上加用如意金黄膏,换药2次/d。结果治疗组有效率91.4%(53/58)、对照组69.0%(40/58),组间比较,$P<0.05$。石世华等将60例下肢丹毒患者随机等分为两组,治疗组用青霉素静脉滴注(连用5~7 d)联合五味消毒饮加减(金银花、蒲公英、紫花地丁、野菊花、紫背天葵、苦参等),6~8层脱脂纱布湿敷患处(2次/d,每次60 min,7~10 d为1个疗程),对照组用青霉素治疗及50%硫酸镁溶液湿敷(方法同中药),症状痊愈后停止治疗。结果治疗组治愈时间为6.17±2.51 d,对照组为9.85±3.67 d,两组比较,$P<0.05$。治疗后两组临床症状积分(治疗组2.18±0.26,对照组5.13±1.37)均明显低于治疗前(治疗组16.46±3.29,对照组15.95±.78),治疗组明显低于对照组($P<0.05$)。

李玉清报道,张灿玾认为痈疽治疗首辨阴阳,阳证宜清热解毒、活血散瘀、消肿止痛,阴证宜温补托毒;临诊常用四妙汤,无论阴证、阳证,已溃、未溃,均可加减使用,且常重用金银花。

慢性皮肤溃疡的治疗及实验研究详见专条。

2. 皮肤病

相关文献仍居外科之首,约占35%。主要是带状疱疹、湿疹、银屑病、痤疮、湿疹、黄褐斑、荨麻疹、手足癣、扁平疣、白癜风等的临床治疗,也有皮肤瘙痒症、尖锐湿疣、特应性皮炎、脱发等报道。

彭勇等将192例特应性皮炎患者随机分为两组,均予尿素乳膏外用,治疗组用健脾祛风方(苍术、白术、薏苡仁、茯苓、山药、白鲜皮等),对照组口服西替利嗪。经治4周,治疗组与对照组总有效率分别为82.1%、(92/95)、61.9%(90/97),组间比较,$P<0.05$。治疗后,两组患者的SCORAD积分(治疗组24.82±6.57,对照组44.65±7.21)较治疗前(治疗组56.74±9.83,对照组57.81±9.69)均降低($P<0.05$),且治疗组的SCORAD积分低于对照组($P<0.05$)。治疗后,两组患者的皮肤角质层含水量均增加($P<0.05$),皮肤pH值降低($P<0.05$);且上述指标治疗组与对照组相比,$P<0.05$。高尚璞等运用活血补肾合剂(黄芪、党参、地黄、玄参、麦冬、丹参等)治疗91例肝肾阴虚型女性脱发患者,设40例健康成人女性作为正常对照组(不用药),疗程3个月。结果治疗组总有效率为93.4%(85/91);腰膝酸软、失眠多梦、头皮出油和头皮痒痛积分降低($P<0.05$);治疗组治疗前血清雌二醇/睾酮比值(E_2/T)(28.52±12.84)低于对照组(53.86±22.98)($P<0.05$),治疗后(40.64±20.17)较治疗前提高($P<0.05$),但仍低于对照组($P<0.05$)。

带状疱疹、湿疹、荨麻疹、银屑病、黄褐斑、痤疮的治疗与研究,详见专条。

3. 乳腺病

以急性乳腺炎、乳腺增生病、浆细胞性乳腺炎、乳腺癌为主,也可见乳房异常发育、乳汁郁积症等临床治疗,实验研究主要集中在乳腺增生病。

罗艳等将64例急性乳腺炎患者随机均分为两组,试验组以阳和汤口服,对照组以青霉素静脉滴注。经治7 d,试验组与对照组总有效率分别为96.9%(31/32)、81.3%(26/32)。试验组治疗后外周血CD_4^+淋巴细胞百分率降低($P<0.05$),CD_8^+淋巴细胞百分率明显升高($P<0.05$),CD_4^+/CD_8^+比例明显降低($P<0.05$);对照组治疗后外

周血 CD_4^+ 百分率降低，CD_8^+ 百分率升高，CD_4^+/CD_8^+ 比例降低($P>0.05$)。凌文津等用揉推排乳手法治疗 120 例郁滞期急性乳腺炎患者，2 次/d，每次 20 min，治疗期间禁服其他中西药。经治3 d，总有效率 97.5%(117/120)。徐东梅等以冰黛糊剂(冰片、白矾、煅石膏、青黛)治疗 50 例乳头皲裂患者，同时与湿润烧伤膏组(50 例)对照，两组均配合电磁波照射 10 min，1 次/d。经治 6 d，治疗组与对照组总有效率分别为 96.0%(48/50)、86.0%(43/50)，组间比较，$P<0.05$。治疗组止痛时间、皮损愈合时间分别为(3.12±1.05)d、(3.98±2.16)d；对照组分别为(5.37±1.89)d、(10.93±3.57)d。组间比较，$P<0.05$，$P<0.01$。关若丹等报道，林毅运用"提脓祛腐"综合疗法(火针洞式烙口术、刮匙棉捻排脓祛腐术、燕尾纱块加压绷缚术等手术治疗方法，以及提脓药捻、金黄散、土黄连液等药物疗法)成功治愈肉芽肿性乳腺炎成脓期患者 23 例。

浆细胞性乳腺炎的治疗与研究，乳腺增生病的治疗及实验研究详见专条。有关中医药治疗乳腺癌的临床和实验研究见"肿瘤科"。

4. 肛肠病

集中在对痔疮、肛瘘、肛周脓肿和肛裂、肛门湿疹、脱肛等的临床报道。

何春梅等采用前瞻性、多中心、平行、随机对照的临床研究方法，以凡士林油纱条引流法为对照组(n=58)，药线蘸提脓祛腐药粉(九一丹、八二丹等)作为试验组(n=55)，换药 1 次/d，疗程 30 d，试验组术后 14 d 脓腔愈合率 56.2%(33/58)高于对照组 48.2%(27/55)($P<0.05$)，但组间脓腔愈合时间比较无明显差异，$P>0.05$；试验组术后第 2 d、10 d、14 d，疼痛积分(5.32±2.22、2.07±1.51、1.05±1.09)，均低于对照组(5.82±2.31、2.69±1.80、1.74±1.02)(均$P<0.05$)；术后当天、2 d、7 d 出血程度低于对照组($P<0.05$)；两组均未出现与治疗有关的不良事件。随访至术后 3 个月，两组各复发 1 例($P>0.05$)。杨其良等对 360 例肛周脓肿患者行内口"⊥"处理一次性根治术加中药敛痔散，结果示一次性治愈率 95.0%(342/360)，总有效率 97.5%(351/360)，无肛门失禁，未发生肛门变形和移位；平均住院天数为 16 d，随访 18 个月未见复发。孙光军等用红藤银花煎坐浴(红藤、银花、苦参、黄柏、枯矾、五倍子等，煎取药液 20～30 min，1 次/d)联合旋磁红外(20 min/次，1 次/d)治疗 25 例肛窦炎患者，对照组(n=25)予红藤银花煎坐浴并口服盐酸左氧氟沙星胶囊。经治 21 d，观察组有效率 96.0%(24/25)高于对照组 72.0%(18/25)($P<0.05$)；观察组各相应症状及体征缓解所需时间短于对照组($P<0.05$)。韩晔等将 80 例高位复杂性肛瘘患者随机均分为两组，治疗组采用低位切除结合高位松挂线分次紧线术，对照组采用低位切开高位挂线术，均以 1 次/d 红油膏纱条引流换药至创面愈合。结果两组治愈率分别为 97.5%(39/40)、92.5%(37/40)($P>0.05$)；治疗组平均住院时间(10.23±1.23 d)明显短于对照组(13.45±2.01 d)($P<0.01$)；治疗组平均治愈时间为 31.31±3.80 d，对照组为 33.58±3.72 d($P>0.05$)。随访 4 个月中，治疗组没有复发病例，对照组复发 1 例，扩创后治愈；术后 1 个月、6 个月，治疗组患者的肛门功能明显优于对照组($P<0.05$，$P<0.01$)。曹科等将 80 例血栓外痔患者随机等分为两组，治疗组采用四黄祛毒方坐浴(黄芩、黄柏、黄连、生大黄、苦参、五倍子等)，对照组采用 1∶5 000 高锰酸钾溶液坐浴，均 1 次/d，药液加热至 40 ℃，坐浴 10 min。经治 7 d，治疗组与对照组总有效率分别为 97.5%(39/40)、87.5%(35/40)，组间比较，$P<0.05$；治疗组疼痛完全缓解时间和血栓痔核完全消失时间分别为(2.10±0.59)d、(6.6±1.9)d，对照组分别为(2.77±0.70)d、(8.2±2.0)d(均$P<0.05$)。

混合痔的治疗详见专条。

5. 男性泌尿性疾病

以前列腺炎、前列腺增生和男性不育症的文献为多，也有附睾炎、男性更年期的临床报道。

王志勇对 120 例ⅢA 型前列腺炎气滞血瘀证予乳酸左氧氟沙星分散片和吲哚美辛肠溶片治疗作为对照组，治疗组 120 例加用桃红泽兰汤(桃仁、红花、泽兰、丹参、莪术、䗪虫等)煎服。经治 4 周，治疗组总有效率 87.3%(72/110)明显优于对照组 64.9%(96/111)($P<0.01$)，两组在改善患者疼痛、尿路症状、对生活质量影响和慢性前列腺炎症状总评分(NIH-CPSI)方面与治疗前相比，均$P<0.01$。治疗组和对照组前列腺液中白细胞(WBC)均减少($P<0.05$)，且治疗组更为显著

($P<0.01$)。李海松等采用多中心、随机对照方法,将160例Ⅲ型气滞血瘀型前列腺炎患者等分为丁桂散敷脐联合前列安栓组(A组)、前列安栓组(B组)。栓剂睡前1粒,纳肛,疗程4周。NIH-CPSI疗效:两组总有效率分别为83.8%(62/74)、68.4%(52/76),($P<0.05$);中医证候疗效,两组总有效率分别为78.4%(58/74)、64.5%(49/76),($P<0.05$)。代睿欣等用滋肾通关片(黄柏、知母、肉桂、鳖甲、牡蛎、王不留行)治疗良性前列腺增生症75例,经治1个月,总有效率76.0%(57/75)。治疗后轻、中度患者国际前列腺症状评分(IPSS)、生活质量指数评分(QOL)均明显降低($P<0.01$),重度患者无改善($P>0.05$)。

张建军等采用角叉菜胶直接注射于前列腺的方法制作大鼠慢性非细菌性前列腺炎急性发作模型,将60只Wistar大鼠随机分为空白对照组、模型对照组、前列康组(0.9 g/kg)、分清肾茶片(苦参、肾茶、土茯苓、川牛膝、丹参、延胡索)高(1.32 g/kg)、中(0.66 g/kg)、低(0.33 g/kg)剂量组,灌服7 d后,分清肾茶片能减少大鼠前列腺组织中的WBC数量($P<0.05$),提高卵磷脂小体(SPL)密度($P<0.01$),并能够降低大鼠前列腺组织中肿瘤坏死因子(TNF-α)和前列腺素E_2(PGE_2)的阳性表达($P<0.05$)。孙洁等以去势加皮下注射丙酸睾酮1 mg/300(g·d)30 d复制大鼠BPH模型,48只Wistar大鼠随机分为正常组、模型组、补肾活血方(淫羊藿、枸杞子、穿山甲、丹参、菟丝子)组、坦索罗辛组。去势第一天起,灌胃1次/d,38 d后补肾活血方、坦索罗辛组膀胱胶原Ⅰ、膀胱胶原Ⅲ阳性面积率及总阳性区域面积比(IOD)均明显较模型组低($P<0.01$);膀胱胶原Ⅰ沉积情况与胶原Ⅲ类似。补肾活血方(1.41±1.33)膀胱胶原Ⅰ/胶原Ⅲ总IOD则明显高于模型组(0.28±0.40)($P<0.01$),与空白组(1.30±0.77)相比,$P>0.05$。

男性不育症的治疗及实验研究详见专条。

6. 周围血管疾病

以糖尿病足、下肢深静脉血栓、下肢动脉粥样硬化、臁疮为主,也有静脉炎、动脉炎等的治疗。

谢吟灵等60例老年下肢动脉粥样硬化性疾病患者随机均分为两组,对照组予辛伐他汀口服,治疗组加服培补疏脉方(黄芪、丹参、当归、桑椹子、地龙、泽泻等)。经治12周,治疗组总有效率83.3%(25/30)优于对照组66.7%(20/30);治疗组治疗后IL-4水平明显升高、IFN-γ水平明显下降,均$P<0.05$,对照组治疗前后无明显差别($P>0.05$);治疗组治疗后动脉内—中膜厚度明显下降($P<0.05$),对照组与治疗前无明显差别($P>0.05$)。李广平等选取下肢动脉粥样硬化性疾病寒湿证8例,血瘀证15例,热毒证12例,健康体检者10例为对照,检测血清高敏C反应蛋白(hsCRP)、TNF-α水平。结果与对照组比较,LEAD寒湿证组血清hsCRP、TNF-α水平轻度升高,血瘀证组和热毒证组血清hsCRP、TNF-α水平明显升高($P<0.01$)。

袁东等用大隐静脉高位结扎、小切口分段结扎术治疗39例下肢静脉曲张患者作为对照组,治疗组40例在此基础上加用自拟益气疏筋方(黄芪、白术、党参、红花、丹参、乳香等)。经治45 d,总有效率治疗组与对照组分别为97.5%(39/40)、84.6%(33/39),组间比较,$P<0.05$;治疗组主要症状、体征、舌象及脉象改善均优于对照组(均$P<0.05$)。石传科等将60例下肢静脉曲张辨证为气虚的患者患者随机均分为两组,治疗组口服玉屏风散合芍药甘草汤(黄芪、防风、苍术、水蛭、牛膝、徐长卿等),对照组服爱脉朗。经治1个月,治疗组显效率为53.3%(16/30),对照组为20.0%(6/30),组间比较,$P<0.05$。治疗组在下肢静脉曲张并发症(静脉溃疡)的收缩率以及下肢水肿方面优于对照组($P<0.05$)。

下肢深静脉血栓、糖尿病足的治疗及实验研究详见专条。

7. 其他外科疾病

有关急性胰腺炎、阑尾炎、胆囊炎、胆结石、肠梗阻、烧伤、外伤、脓毒症的临床报道较多,也有蛇咬伤、冻疮、各类术后等报道。实验研究则集中在急性胰腺炎和烧烫伤以及脓毒症。

石传科等对450例急性阑尾术后的中医证候进行聚类研究,结果脾胃实热证243例54.0%(243/450),脾胃湿热证108例24.0%(108/450),脾虚气滞证99例22.0%(99/450)。陈佳骏等将125例因肝内外胆管结石行胆总管切开取石+T管引流术患者随机分为清利防石汤组(金钱草、海金沙、郁金、滑石、石见穿、威灵仙等)(A

组)、胆维他组(B组)及常规围手术期处理对照组(C组),干预3个月后,A、B两组肝功能ALT、AST、TBIL的降低幅度均大于C组($P<0.05$),但组间比较,$P>0.05$;治疗后A、B两组游离胆红素(UCB)、钙离子(Ca^{2+})的降低幅度及、胆汁酸(TBA)升高幅度均大于C组($P<0.05$),但两组比较,$P>0.05$;治疗后,A组胆道内压力降低幅度大于B、C两组($P<0.05$),B、C两组之间胆道压力降幅比较,$P>0.05$;1年后B超随访,A组复发0例,B组复发率2.4%(1/42),C组复发率9.3%(4/43)。A组的复发率低于B、C两组(均$P<0.05$)。

娄彦妮等选取化疗后出现手足痛不良反应者204例,随机分为试验组136例与对照组68例,分别给予温经通络活血法(老鹳草、川乌、桂枝、红花)和安慰剂外用(洗/浸)+温浴(35～40℃),20 min/次,2次/d,连用7 d。结果试验组治疗前后的数字疼痛分级法(NRS)评分分别为(5.51±1.99)和(2.20±2.20)分,对照组分别为(5.57±1.82)和(4.50±2.44)分,两组治疗后比较,均$P<0.01$;两组疼痛缓解有效率分别为88.1%(120/136)、42.7%(29/68),组间比较,$P<0.05$;手足痛分级的疗效总有效率分别为81.3%(110/136)、26.5%(18/68),组间比较,$P<0.01$。

刘云涛等将SD昆明大鼠100只随机等分为5组。正常对照组不作处理,模型组(6 h、12 h组)(MC)1 ml/100 g·d生理盐水灌胃,桃核承气汤组(6 h、12 h组)(TH)1 ml/100 g·d灌胃,7 d后采用盲肠结扎穿孔法复制脓毒症模型。造模成功后6 h、12 h标本采集结果显示,与同时点MC组比较,TH组小肠组织CD_4 mRNA、TLR4mRNA 12 h时间点表达减少($P<0.05$);TH组6 h和12 h血清TNF-α、IL-6和脂多糖均比模型组下降($P<0.05$,$P<0.01$)。郝蕾等通过夹伤肠管约0.5 cm长的方法制作大鼠粘连性肠梗阻模型,将50只SD大鼠随机等分成5组,通腑泻热灌肠合剂(大黄、虎杖、芒硝、栀子、苦地胆、忍冬藤等)高剂量组(10 ml/kg)、低剂量组(5 ml/kg)、生理盐水组、假手术组及正常组。灌肠2周后,检测结果显示:术后各组与假手术组比较,粘连均有增加;高、低剂量组肠粘连均低于生理盐水组($P<0.05$);高、低剂量组及假手术组、正常组所含IL-10水平均高于生理盐水组($P<0.05$);与假手术组比较,高剂量组、低剂量组所含IL-10,$P>0.05$;各组大鼠肠黏膜分泌型免疫球蛋白A(sIgA)比较,正常组、假手术组高、低剂量组所含sIgA浓度高于生理盐水组($P<0.05$,$P<0.01$);与假手术组比较,高、低剂量组所含sIgA浓度高($P<0.05$,$P<0.01$);生理盐水组sIgA浓度低($P<0.01$)。

重症胰腺炎、烧伤的治疗及实验研究详见专条。

(陈红风　廖明娟)

【慢性皮肤溃疡的治疗及实验研究】

尹恒等将257例下肢慢性皮肤溃疡患者随机双盲入实验组(n=127,生肌玉红膏覆盖创面)与对照组(n=130,凡士林纱布),隔日换药。经治4周,实验组创面坏死脓腐组织脱落积分明显低于对照组($P<0.01$);创面渗出液的形质、色泽、气味、性状及渗液量积分改善均优于对照组($P<0.05$,$P<0.01$);实验组创面细菌感染率降低($P<0.05$);治疗结束时,实验组创面愈合了80%左右,对照组愈合了30%。肖秀丽等将48例慢性皮肤溃疡患者随机分为健脾组(黄芪、太子参、白术、茯苓、生地)、健脾化瘀组(黄芪、太子参、白术、茯苓、丹参、水蛭等)、化瘀组(丹参、水蛭、桃仁、当归)、祛腐组(野菊花、黄柏、紫花地丁、蒲公英)4组。经治8周,健脾化瘀组创面愈合率、促进腐肉脱落、创面愈合时间优于其他各对照组,($P<0.05$)。李克盛等将78例下肢慢性静脉性溃疡患者随机分为治疗组40例和对照组38例,均采用半导体激光(英国DIOMED)治疗。治疗组外敷生肌玉红膏(当归、白芷、紫草、甘草),对照组采用常规换药,均1次/d。4周后,治疗组总有效率90.0%(36/40)优于对照组71.1%(27/38)($P<0.05$);治疗组((14.6±4.8 d)愈合时间较对照组(18.9±5.0 d)更短($P<0.05$)。兴伟等将118例下肢静脉性溃疡患者随机等分为两组。治疗组用四联疗法综合治疗:中药(黄柏、蒲公英、苦参、当归、牛膝、五倍子)外洗,微波照射20 min,自拟生肌愈疡方(珍珠、煅龙骨、血竭、乳香、没药、儿茶等)药末撒布创面,弹力绷带加压包扎;对照组用0.1%雷夫努尔纱条覆盖包扎,均1次/d。经治30 d,治疗组治愈率46.7%(28/60)和总有效率93.3%(56/60)均优于对照组20.7%(12/58)和77.6%(45/58)($P<0.05$);治疗后两组经皮氧分压均提高,治疗组优于对照组($P<0.05$)。肖敏等将68例慢性皮肤慢性溃疡患者随机均分

为治疗组和对照组，分别用康复新液湿敷、生肌散换药，1次/d。经治4周，治疗组皮损面积减少（13.05 cm^2 减少至 0.59 cm^2）优于对照组（13.34 cm^2减少至 2.35 cm^2）（$P<0.05$），试验组与对照组治愈率分别为82.4%（28/34）、70.6%（24/34），组间比较，$P<0.05$；治疗后治疗组Smad3蛋白表达水平下降（$P<0.05$）。黄仲海等应用八珍汤加味结合局部处理（局部清创，MEBO油纱条或疮疡贴覆盖创面）治疗74例（90处创面）慢性皮肤溃疡患者，所有病例均用药至创面愈合。结果痊愈62例，显效9例，好转3例。

王乐平等将朱砂、红粉制成不同浓度的中药膏（以下简称药纱条），将70只SD大鼠随机分为7组：溃疡模型组、基质组（凡士林）及5个中药剂量组（A、B、C、D、E含中药分别为27.2、13.6、6.8、3.4、1.7 mg/cm^2）。连续给药7 d，结果基质组及中药D、E组大鼠创面愈合速度较快（$P<0.01$），A、B组创面愈合速度呈减缓趋势；D、E组用药早期较好的体现了提脓祛腐作用，后期创面平整光滑、质地柔软；各中药组肉芽组织中蛋白及羟脯氨酸含量均明显提高（$P<0.01$）。谢延华等通过切除大鼠背部皮肤浅层，创口内注入金黄色葡萄球菌复制大鼠创伤性溃疡模型，120只随机均分为空白对照组、实验对照组和实验组。分别用生理盐水纱块、生长因子纱块和复方落地生根膏（落地生根、龙眼壳、杨梅根、紫草、合欢皮、乳香等）外敷，1次/d。结果与空白对照组（28.5±3.4）相比，实验组（23.2±1.8 d）和对照组（23.4±1.84 d）愈合时间缩短（$P<0.05$）；RT-PCR法检测CTGF基因在第1 d、7 d，实验组的表达水平高于空白组和对照组，（$P<0.05$）；MMP-2在第14 d，实验组的表达水平（0.972±0.633）高于对照组（0.524±0.241）和空白组（0.113±0.160）（$P<0.05$）。张旭辉等将44只SD大鼠随机分为4组：模型组，回阳生肌膏全方组（肉桂、炮姜、人参、黄芪、川芎、当归等），温阳益气拆方组（肉桂、炮姜、人参、黄芪、白芥子）和活血生肌拆方组（川芎、当归、白蔹），采用“激素干预—皮肤缺损—细菌感染”复合因素叠加法制备慢性皮肤溃疡大鼠模型。结果，给药2 d后，温阳益气组和活血生肌组创面愈合率均高于模型组（$P<0.05$）；给药4 d后，全方组创面愈合率高于模型组（$P<0.05$）。给药3 d后，全方组、温阳益气组的白细胞介素-8含量均高于模型组（$P<0.05$）；活血生肌组与模型组比较，$P>0.05$。给药3 d后，全方组、模型组TNF-α含量均高于温阳益气组和活血生肌组（$P<0.05$，$P<0.01$）。王元元等采用2.5 mol/L NaOH外涂建立大鼠皮肤溃疡模型，将80只雄性Wistar大鼠随机等分为8组，模型对照组，京万红软膏组，蜂蜜高、中、低剂量治疗组（蜂蜜生药10.8、5.4、2.7 g/kg）和蜂胶高、中、低剂量治疗组（0.20、0.10、0.05 g/kg）。1次/d，连续14 d，与对照组相比，京万红对照组、蜂蜜高、低剂量组和蜂胶高、低剂量组大鼠创面愈合时间缩短，$P<0.05$或$P<0.01$；酶联免疫法检测京万红对照组、蜂蜜中、低剂量组和蜂胶高、中、低剂量组大鼠血清中超氧化物歧化酶（SOD）含量增加（$P<0.05$或$P<0.01$）；除蜂胶低剂量组，其余各组微血管密度（MDA）含量下降，但与模型对照组比较，$P>0.05$。马拴全等将90只SD大鼠随机分成创愈膏（陕西中医学院附属医院制剂）组、湿润烧伤膏组、凡士林组，每组30只。采用切除大鼠皮肤全层及皮下组织、创口内注入金黄色葡萄球菌液造成热毒证大鼠皮肤溃疡模型。12 h换药1次至创面愈合。病理学检测结果示术后第3 d、7 d创愈膏组成纤维细胞数、炎细胞数、肉芽组织数、新生毛细血管数均明显多于凡士林组（$P<0.01$），与湿润烧伤膏对照组比较，$P>0.05$；术后第14 d，创愈膏组成纤维细胞数、炎细胞数、肉芽组织数、新生毛细血管数明显减少，与凡士林组比较，$P<0.01$，与湿润烧伤膏组比较，$P>0.05$。

（陈红风　邓　樱）

【带状疱疹的治疗与研究】

侯立军用复元活血汤联合超短波治疗带状疱疹后遗神经痛85例。按就诊顺序奇偶数随机分为两组，均予超短波治疗，治疗组加服复元活血汤加减。经治1个月，治疗组总有效率为93.3%（42/45），对照组为67.5%（27/40），组间比较，$P<0.01$。吉朝阳治疗带状疱疹80例，发病初期即用三棱针或毫针点刺，然后加拔火罐，并服公英解毒汤（蒲公英、龙胆草、山栀、延胡索、黄芩、紫草等），治疗7 d，总有效率为97.5%（78/80）。李宁波将带状疱疹患者随机分为两组，对照组服阿昔洛韦片、维生素B_{12}片，局部外涂莫匹罗星软膏；治疗组服龙胆泻肝汤加减，康复新液局部外用，4次/d，每次1～2 h。经治60 d，治疗组总有效率为96.5%（110/114），对照组为84.9%（90/106），组

间比较,$P<0.05$。刘朝钦等将148例带状疱疹后遗疼痛患者随机分为两组,对照组口服维生素B_1+维生素B_{12};治疗组予服清利湿热剂(龙胆草、栀子、黄芩、柴胡、木通、蜈蚣等)。经连续治疗10 d,治疗组总有效率为95.7%(67/70),对照组为60.3%(41/68),$P<0.01$。蒋蓝运用身痛逐瘀汤加减治疗带状疱疹后遗神经痛31例,经治30 d,总有效率为96.8%(30/31)。荀向红等治疗带状疱疹后神经痛154例,予服脉管复康片(丹参、鸡血藤、乳香、没药),结合毫针泻法针刺夹脊穴,叩刺拔罐,起罐后予以消炎膏(细辛、白鲜皮、苏子、白芷、檀香、丹参等)外敷。经治28 d,总有效率为94.2%(147/154)。龙云群用连花清瘟胶囊(连翘、金银花、石膏、板蓝根、大黄、炙麻黄等)治疗带状疱疹26例,同时予以阿昔洛韦注射液加生理盐水静脉滴注,连用5~7 d,总有效率为96.2%(25/26)。李巧芬以口服阿昔洛韦、肌注维生素B_{12}、病毒唑软膏外涂等治疗儿童带状疱疹44例作为对照组,治疗组辨证服用龙胆泻肝汤、除湿胃苓汤、柴胡疏肝散合桃红四物汤,同时外敷玉露膏、青黛散或三棱针刺。结果治疗组总有效率为86.3%(38/44),对照组为63.6%(28/44)。组间比较,$P<0.05$。

田浩等将64例带状疱疹后遗神经痛患者随机分为两组,治疗组局部采用注射针点刺及负压拔罐治疗,隔日1次,治疗8次;对照组口服普瑞巴林,治疗16 d。结果两组治疗后VAS评分及外周血清P物质与治疗前比较均显著降低,而刺血拔罐组降低更明显低($P<0.01$)。陈金生等选择急性带状疱疹患者25例,随机分为药物治疗组和针灸治疗组,选择12例正常人作为对照组。药物治疗组予抗病毒、营养神经和镇痛药物治疗,针灸治疗组在药物治疗组基础上加用针灸治疗。结果两组患者治疗后VAS评分较治疗前均明显减少,组间比较无明显差异($P>0.05$),针灸治疗组皮疹愈合时间短于药物治疗组($P<0.01$);急性带状疱疹患者c-FLIP表达比正常人表达明显降低($P<0.01$),针灸治疗组治疗后较治疗前表达升高($P<0.01$),药物治疗组治疗前、后表达无明显变化($P>0.05$)。

马迎歌总结王丽平治疗带状疱疹后遗神经痛经验:善取安神穴、腹针培元穴组、阿是穴,配合点刺放血以清热,或艾灸以扶阳。杨迎霞总结李秀敏治疗老年带状疱疹的思路,注重从整体去把握本病,局部与整体辨证相结合;在顾护脾胃、扶助正气的基础上,适当加入疏经通络、活血化瘀、抗病毒之类的药物。王丹妮等总结李发枝治疗艾滋病带状疱疹及其后遗神经痛的配伍精要,常用药物为清热燥湿之黄芩,活血化瘀之红花,清热解毒、利尿渗湿之车前子,清肺化痰之全瓜蒌,养血活血之当归,清泄肝胆经湿热之龙胆草。

(薛　亮　李　斌)

【湿疹的治疗及实验研究】

单敬文将60例急性湿疹患者随机分为两组,治疗组龙胆泻肝汤加减,再取药汁湿敷患处,同时口服西替利嗪;对照组口服强的松、西替利嗪,外敷3%硼酸溶液和艾洛松软膏交替。经治2周,治疗组总有效率为93.8%(30/32),对照组82.14%(23/28),组间比较,$P<0.05$。孔智贤用龙牡治湿汤(生龙骨、煅牡蛎、苍术、黄柏、仙鹤草、防风等)治疗湿热型湿疹36例,对照组36例口服龙胆泻肝丸。经治8周,治疗组总有效率为85.7%(31/36),对照组为61.86%(22/36),组间比较,$P<0.05$。随访3个月,治疗组复发率为25.0%(9/36),对照组为33.3%(20/36)。严仲用湿疹汤(荆芥、苦参、淡竹叶、白蒺藜、地肤子、土茯苓等)治疗慢性湿疹90例,以12 d为1个疗程,共治1~3个疗程。结果治愈63例,总有效率为92.3%(87/90)。谢泽初等以复方木尼孜其颗粒及盐酸西替利嗪片口服治疗急性、亚急性、慢性湿疹32例作为观察组,对照组28例仅服盐酸西替利嗪片。结果两组总有效率分别为90.6%(29/32)、67.9%(19/28)($P<0.05$)。邓光烈将100例湿疹患儿随机等分为A、B两组。A组患儿采用中医方法(急性期基本方为当归、生地黄、防风、何首乌、蛇床子、玉竹等;慢性期基本方为浮萍、紫苏叶、青黛、紫草、荷叶、败酱草等)治疗,B组患儿口服扑尔敏。经治1个月,A组总有效率为98.0%(49/50),B组为80.0%(40/50),组间比较,$P<0.05$。乔敏将60例手足慢性湿疹患者随机等分为两组,治疗组服活血祛风汤,配合中药润愈洗剂洗浴,并外用丹皮酚软膏、曲咪新软膏;对照组服润燥止痒胶囊,并外用丹皮酚软膏、曲咪新软膏。经治4周,治疗组总有效率为93.3%(28/30),对照组为73.3%(22/30),组间比较,$P<0.05$。治疗后两组患者外周血CD_4^+、CD_4^+/CD_8^+指标均较治疗前上升。提示活血祛风汤合润愈洗剂可能通过抑制T细胞活化,调节CD_4^+细

胞水平及 CD_4^+/CD_8^+ 的比值来改善机体的免疫功能，而对慢性湿疹具有治疗作用。

实验研究方面，郭晓明分别用 7%、1%的 2,4－二硝基氯苯溶液制作小鼠接触性湿疹的模型，用 0.5%的 4－氨基吡啶制作小鼠皮肤瘙痒的模型，采用中药汤剂湿疹溻渍方进行溻渍洗浴治疗，结果湿疹溻渍方外用对肿胀炎症及瘙痒模型有显著抑制作用，可通过直接升高湿疹小鼠皮损组织中的 IFN－yRa 和 IL－2 而间接降低 IL－4 的表达，可通过直接降低湿疹小鼠外周血中 CD_8－T 和直接升高 CD_4－T 淋巴细胞的百分比而改善湿疹的病情。提示湿疹溻渍方外用对小鼠湿疹模型有显著的抑制作用，其作用机理与抑制炎症反应、止痒、调节细胞因子分泌的紊乱有关。

李玉柱等总结杜锡贤治疗湿疹经验，认为湿疹在临床表现上不外乎“痒”、“湿”、“顽”、“变”，病理因素“本源于湿，再源于热及风，三者互结，郁于肌肤”。湿热内蕴型应湿热当清，凉血为先，方中每取生地、丹皮等凉血活血，芩、连、知、柏苦寒清热，金银花、连翘透热转气，白鲜皮、泽泻、车前子利湿泻浊；风热搏肤型治以疏风清热利湿，方选消风散加减；血虚风燥型治以养血润燥，祛风止痒，方选当归饮子加减，主张要“先安未受邪之地”，方中独取生地一味，济肾之水，泉源不竭。宋瑜等总结马绍尧治疗湿疹经验，认为湿疹因先天禀赋不足，脾胃虚弱，不能运化水谷，以致湿浊内生，与湿毒、热毒相合而发病；辨证重视不同体质及舌苔情况，因老年小儿，脾健情况不同，且脾胃之气大抵可反映于舌苔；治疗原则为治脾以健运为要，强调祛湿为先，重视清热解毒。日常调护强调顾护脾胃，认为“牛肉羊肉火锅酒，芒果荔枝大闸蟹”是湿疹患者的禁忌饮食。

（孙晓颖　李　斌）

【荨麻疹的治疗与研究】

赵一丁等将 36 例慢性荨麻疹患者随机分为两组，试验组予口服中药汤剂(金银花、连翘、生地黄、当归、蝉衣、牛蒡子等)及西替利嗪(逐渐减量)，对照组仅服西替利嗪。经治 8 周，试验组有效率为 80.6%(29/36)，对照组为 46.9%(17/36)，组间比较，$P<0.05$。张禁等应用左西替利嗪联合复方甘草酸苷治疗慢性荨麻疹。将 68 例患者随机分为两组，均予口服左西替利嗪片，治疗组加服复方甘草酸苷片。经治 4 周，治疗组总有效率为 92.7%(63/68)，对照组为 74.6%(41/55)，组间比较，$P<0.05$。黄蕊等将 72 例风热犯表型荨麻疹患者随机分为两组，均予服依巴斯汀片，治疗组加服石蓝草煎剂加减(生石膏、金银花、龙胆草、黄芩、车前子、马齿苋等。咽痛者加板蓝根、北豆根，痒重者加地肤子、蛇床子，发热恶寒者加蝉蜕、牛蒡子，心烦不寐者加龙骨、牡蛎、酸枣仁)。结果治疗组治愈率为 54.8%(23/42)，总有效率为 90.5%(38/42)；对照组分别为 33.3%(10/30)、70.0%(21/30)。组间比较，均 $P<0.05$。崔勇将 240 例丘疹性荨麻疹患者随机分为两组，治疗组将季德胜蛇药片 8 g 加入炉甘石洗剂 100 ml 中，浸泡溶化外用；对照组单用炉甘石洗剂。经治 10 d，两组患者入组时症状和体征的总积分各为 228 分和 216 分；治疗后总积分各为 21 分和 83 分。治疗组起效时间为 1～2 d，对照组为 2～3 d。组间比较，均 $P<0.001$。

实验研究方面，郭静等研究当归饮子加减方对气血两虚模型慢性荨麻疹小鼠全身皮肤瘙痒的影响。方法：将 64 只 KM 小鼠随机分为空白对照组、模型组、氯雷他定组、当归饮子加减方高、中、低剂量组，并对小鼠于给药当天开始，每天于腹侧皮下注射利血平生理盐水溶液，1 次/d，造模 7 d(致气虚)，与此同时，自给药第 1 d、4 d、7 d 皮下注射 2%乙酰苯肼 6 mg/只(致血虚)。并对除空白组外的各组于末次给药 30 min 后，尾静脉注射 0.012 5%低分子右旋糖酐溶液致敏，记录小鼠在尾静脉注射低分子右旋糖酐溶液后 30 min 内的搔抓潜伏期、搔抓次数(全身瘙痒反应：前爪搔抓头部、后抓挠躯干、嘴咬全身各部位为瘙痒指征）和瘙痒持续总时间。结果与模型组比较，当归饮子加减方各剂量组可显著延长小鼠搔抓潜伏期(均 $P<0.01$)；减少小鼠搔抓次数(均 $P<0.01$)；缩短搔抓持续时间(均 $P<0.01$)，并呈量效关系，且当归饮子各剂量组均可降低血清组胺含量。

向国栓等总结艾儒棣治疗慢性荨麻疹经验，在辨证论治的基础上，始终重视中医整体观，不仅在运方遣药上顾护机体平衡，更根据患者个体差异，指导其饮食宜忌，活动起居等，为疾病的治疗及整体健康的维护创造良好的环境。对于“痒”、“痛”等症状的疾患予龙骨、磁石、石决明等镇心安神之品，加之合欢皮解郁安神，能缓解患者瘙痒时的焦躁情绪，从而改善患者生活质量，促使疾病康复，正所谓“诸痛痒疮，皆属于心”。此外，艾氏注重扶正驱邪,诊治中常加用玉屏风散益气固表、祛风散邪。张大萍总结张作舟治疗慢性荨麻疹经验,认为其病因复杂,或感受风寒、风热之邪;或饮食起居失调,使机体正气受损,致使卫外不固,营卫失和,不得疏达而出现疹块。还有先天禀赋不耐,若劳逸失度,或内伤于七情,导致脏腑气机失调,日久必耗伤阴血,以致水不涵木,风从内生,也可发为本病。辨证分为表虚不固、血虚气弱、阴虚内热和湿热内蕴4种类型施治,表虚不固者用固卫御风汤,血气虚弱者予当归补血汤益气养血,阴虚内热者用养阴宁荨汤以养阴清热,湿热内蕴者用加味平胃散。杨蒴等总结陈宝义治疗小儿荨麻疹经验,认为急性荨麻疹可分风热犯表型、风寒束表型、湿热内蕴型3型,治疗当以祛风为主,并予以疏风清热、疏风散寒、疏风祛湿和中,分别以消风散、桂枝汤和藿连保和汤加减;慢性荨麻疹,瘾疹日久,气血耗伤,血虚生风生燥,气血亏虚则藩篱不固,稍有风邪外袭则发病,病儿常伴有面色少华,倦怠乏力等气血不足之证,治疗当以补虚为主,治病求于本,用益气养血,固表和营之法,方用八珍汤加减。

(李可心　李　斌)

【黄褐斑的治疗及实验研究】

林聪用阳和汤加味治疗面部黄褐斑患者86例,结果显效60例,总有效率为93.0%(80/86)。劳瑞平用李可的乌蛇荣皮汤(酒浸生地、当归、桂枝、川芎、桃仁、红花等)治疗黄褐斑患者42例,痊愈35例,显效5例,有效2例,治愈时间最短10 d,最长4个疗程。毛燕予消斑汤(当归、益母草、红花、川芎、荆芥穗、川牛膝等)治疗气滞血瘀型面部黄褐斑42例,对照组38例服维生素C片。经治3个月,治疗组总有效率92.8%(39/42)显著高于对照组73.7%(28/38)($P<0.01$)。周垒将120例女性黄褐斑患者随机等分为两组,观察组加味逍遥散加减治疗,对照组服维生素C加外擦3%氢毓霜或迪维霜于色斑处。观察组患者治疗前后于月经前1周抽取空腹静脉血,检测其血清性激素水平含量变化。结果观察组总有效率93.3%(56/60)显著高于对照组55.0%(33/60)($P<0.05$),且治疗组治疗后血清FSH、LH、E_2明显下降($P<0.01$)。郭雯等将120例黄褐斑患者随机等分为两组,治疗组服化瘀祛斑汤(桃仁、红花、柴胡、菟丝子、益母草、白僵蚕等),同时采用E光进行治疗,每2周治疗1次,连续4次为1个疗程;对照组用E光治疗。经治8周,治疗组总有效率85.0%(51/60),对照组为55.0%(33/60),组间比较,$P<0.01$。付强等将120例黄褐斑患者随机均分为两组,均予糖皮质激素外用治疗,观察组在此基础上加用通便消痤片(西洋参、大黄、芒硝、枳实、生白术、小红参等)。经治3个月,观察组患者皮损MASI评分改善情况总有效率为85.0%(51/60),对照组为63.3%(38/60),组间比较,$P<0.05$。季艳芳将100例女性黄褐斑患者随机均分为两组,均予服维生素C,并以2%氢醌乳膏早晚涂抹于患处;治疗组在此基础上加服红花逍遥片(竹叶、柴胡、当归、红花、皂角刺、薄荷等)。经治12周,治疗组总有效率为84.0%(42/50),对照组为58.0%(29/50),组间比较,$P<0.05$。治疗组患者平均起效时间、显效时间、治愈时间较对照组患者显著缩短(均$P<0.05$),治疗组患者治疗后面部色斑大面积消退,颜色基本消失或明显变淡,较对照组患者明显好转。

翁丽丽等将275例肾虚型黄褐斑患者随机分为两组,治疗组139例予补肾祛斑汤(牡丹皮、泽泻、熟地黄、山茱萸、丹参、何首乌等),对照组136例予维生素C、维生素E口服。经治3个月,治疗组总有效率85.6%(119/139)显著高于对照组50.7%(69/136),且治疗组的血液流变学各指标在治疗后明显下降,MDA较治疗前明显降低,SOD明显升高(均$P<0.05$)。提示补肾祛斑汤治疗黄褐斑的机制可能与改善患者氧化与抗氧化失衡,调节患者性激素水平,改善患者血液流变学有关。廖燕将69例气滞血瘀型黄褐斑患者随机分为两组,治疗组予柴附冲剂(柴胡、香附、制白附子、当归、白薇、僵蚕等),对照组予维生素C、E胶丸。两组治疗前后采用硫代巴比妥酸比色法检测血清MDA及LPO水平,采用黄嘌呤氧化酶法检测SOD,并观察疗效。经治2个月,治疗组总有效率为85.7%(31/35),复发率为6.7%(2/30);对照组分别为53.0%(16/34)、38.9%(7/18)。组间比较,均$P<0.05$。黄褐斑患者血清LPO及MDA水平较健康对照组明显升高,而SOD水平明显降低(均$P<0.01$)。

实验研究方面,李艳等将常用于色素性疾病研究的C57BL/6J小鼠的随机分为空白对照组、祛斑汤(黄芪、泡参、制首乌、当归、川芎、菟丝子等)低剂量(10 g/kg)组、中剂量(20 g/kg)组、高剂量(40 g/kg)组、维生素C组。各组小鼠灌胃给药30 d后皮肤取材。采用免疫组化法观察皮肤

α-MSH表达，并用χ2检验进行统计学分析。结果祛斑汤高剂量组α-MSH阳性表达率低于空白对照组($P<0.01$)。提示高剂量祛斑汤可以通过降低α-MSH表达这一环节来抑制黑素生成，从而治疗黄褐斑。康金森等采用肌注黄体酮及辅助中波UV照射方法建立黄褐斑小鼠模型，将60只雌性昆明种小鼠随机分成对照组、模型组、维生素E、维生素C颗粒组、红玉祛斑胶囊(红景天、柴胡、红花、茯苓、山药、栀子等)200、400、800 mg/kg剂量组。测定各组小鼠肝脏及皮肤组织中的超氧化物歧化酶(SOD)活性、酪氨酸、丙二醛(MDA)以及皮肤脂褐质水平，同时采用免疫组化法观察药物对小鼠皮肤黑色素细胞的影响。结果与维生素E、维生素C颗粒组比较，红玉祛斑胶囊高剂量组黄褐斑小鼠皮肤中黑色素细胞的数目明显降低，且小鼠皮肤中酪氨酸、脂褐质和MDA的含量也显著低于其他观察组，而SOD的活性较高($P<0.01$，$P<0.05$)。提示红玉祛斑胶囊对黄褐斑小鼠模型具有较好的治疗作用，其作机制可能在于抑制黑色素细胞的增殖和酪氨酸的生成，增强机体清除自由基的能力。

李苹等总结了王成荣诊治黄褐斑经验，认为面部黄褐色斑块与肾之气化不足有关。褐色为黑之略浅者。黑乃水之色，而肾主水，如其气化失常，水色上泛则可见面部色斑。据此而以温肾利水为主治疗女性黄褐斑，常用自拟益肾消斑汤(桂枝、仙茅、淫羊藿、白茅根、皂角刺、桃仁等)加减治疗。俞若熙等报道王琦治疗黄褐斑验案3则，认为黄褐斑的发病与体质有关，其患者多为血瘀质，气滞血瘀为黄褐斑的主要病机。治疗从活血化瘀干预血瘀体质的基础上论治黄褐斑，同时多用芳香花类药物，兼顾致瘀诱因加减用药，不但可以起到活血化瘀的作用，而且疏肝理气，同时可引药上行至头面，还有美容的功效。徐庆等总结杨志波经验，认为黄褐斑病因病机为气血瘀滞，不能上荣于面。治疗主要采用活血化瘀，同时兼以疏肝理气、益气养血健脾、滋阴补肾等。肝肾不足者以六味地黄丸加减；肝郁气滞者，逍遥散合桃红四物汤加减；脾虚湿热者，方用除湿胃苓汤加减；气血亏虚证，方用桃仁四物汤合归脾汤加减。

(柴媛媛　李　斌)

【银屑病的治疗及实验研究】

许斌等将48例银屑病患者随机均分为两组，对照组口服甲氨蝶呤、外用卡泊三醇软膏；治疗组口服疏风养血汤(生地黄、当归、川芎、板蓝根、紫草、蛇床子等)、外用卡泊三醇软膏。经治8周，治疗组治疗后PASI积分为(3.71±2.75)分，总有效率为91.7%(22/24)，对照组分别为(6.58±3.83)分、83.3%(20/24)，组间比较，$P<0.05$。高励聪等运用内外兼治的方法治疗银屑病42例，口服自拟方(生地黄、金银花、白鲜皮、白芨、茜草、地肤子等)，外用中药洗剂(黄芩、连翘、苦参、白鲜皮、薄荷、败酱草等)洗浴全身30 min后，外用尿素、止痒润肤乳等。经治30 d，治愈31例，好转11例。刘爱萍将150例银屑病患者随机等分为3组，西医组患者接受单纯西医治疗(口服阿维A胶囊、静脉滴注复方甘草酸苷注射液、涂抹、外擦氢化可的松软膏，中医组患者辨证治疗：① 血热型：黄芩、荆芥穗、蔓荆子、黄柏、知母、藁本等。② 湿热型：当归、熟地黄、川芎、黄连、黄芩、黄柏等。③ 风热型：川芎、羌活、柴胡、薄荷、红花、桔梗等。④ 风寒型：桂枝、芍药、生姜、大枣、甘草等。⑤ 血虚风燥型：当归、生地黄、白芍、川芎、何首乌、荆芥等)。中西医结合组同时用上述两种方式进行治疗。经治30 d，3组总有效率分别为74.0%(37/50)、54.0%(27/50)、86.0%(43/50)。西医组和中医组比较，$P>0.05$；中西医结合组和西医组比较，$P<0.05$；中西医结合组和中医组比较，$P<0.01$。李强将72例寻常型银屑病患者均分为两组，均予外用他克莫司软膏，治疗组加用窄谱中波紫外线治疗。结果治疗组总有效率为97.2%(35/36)，对照组为86.1%(31/36)，组间比较，$P<0.05$。治疗后治疗组的红斑、鳞屑、浸润、瘙痒评分明显少于对照组(均$P<0.05$)。

李轲将64例寻常型银屑病患者等分为两组，对照组口服雷公藤多苷，治疗组在对照组基础上加用复方苦参注射液静脉滴注。经治4周，治疗组总有效率为87.5%(28/32)；对照组为59.4%(19/32)。组间比较，$P<0.05$。李昌吉等将73例寻常性银屑病患者随机分为两组，治疗组用祛风活血方治疗(荆芥、桂枝、当归、红花、川芎、麻黄等)，对照组用复方青黛丸治疗，两组均同时外用凡士林软膏。经治8周，两组治疗后PASI评分均明显下降(均$P<0.005$)；且以治疗组更明显($P<0.05$)。

刘海琴等用酶联免疫吸附竞争法检测40例

寻常性银屑病患者在使用退银汤(生地黄、土茯苓、当归、何首乌、白蒺藜、乌梢蛇等)前后外周血血清胎盘型钙黏蛋(P-cad)水平,并与40例正常对照组进行比较。结果患者血清P-cad水平为(47.04±11.15)ng/ml,正常对照组P-cad水平(10.92±6.78)ng/ml,组间比较,$P<0.01$。经治12周,银屑病患者血清P-cad水平(23.52±5.31)ng/m明显下降($P<0.01$)。

实验研究方面,余靖宏等以心得安(盐酸普萘洛尔)乳剂涂抹豚鼠耳部造成银屑病模型,观察银屑灵优化方(含赤芍药、肿节风、甘草等)对该模型的病理状态影响并用Baker法评分;建立脂多糖诱导的HaCaT细胞增殖模型,用MTT法检测不同浓度和时间下银屑灵优化方对HaCaT细胞的抑制率。结果银屑灵优化方低、高剂量(5.98、11.96 g/kg)能够显著降低银屑病豚鼠的Baker评分;浓度为250、125、62.5 μg/ml银屑灵优化方对共同培养48 h的HaCaT细胞有不同程度抑制作用,各个浓度银屑灵优化方对培养72 h的HaCaT细胞均有抑制作用(均$P<0.01$)。提示银屑灵优化方能够改善豚鼠银屑病病变,抑制HaCaT细胞过度增殖。

范斌等总结秦万章治疗银屑病经验,根据赵炳南先生提出的"内有血热,外受风邪或夹杂燥热之邪;内外合邪,热壅血络"学说,并结合临床经验,归纳出凉血、活血、养血3大法则。提出:新血证论,以血为纲;重视血瘀,活血为先。并拟定验方润肤饮、凉血清热饮,喜用雷公藤。杨素清等总结王玉玺治疗银屑病经验,提出"毒"邪是银屑病致病的关键因素,强调"毒"邪在银屑病发生发展中的重要作用,从"毒"论治。凡素体阳热偏胜,复感六淫之邪,外邪入里,从阳化热;或因情志内伤,气机壅滞,郁久化火,进而化毒,与血气相搏,外发于肌肤,致全身出现红斑;热极生风,胜而化燥,肌肤失养,则于红斑上鳞屑叠起、瘙痒无度;或由肾精亏损,阴寒毒邪外侵,闭塞腠理玄府,阳气不得外达,蕴久化热,寒闭热伏,毒遏肌表,外发皮肤而致病;毒邪不去,新血无养,皮肤失气血之充润,则有血虚血燥,鳞屑迭起;热盛迫血妄行,日久以致血瘀,而成顽疾。临床运用蜈蚣败毒饮等代表方剂辨证施治,疗效较好。

(李　苏　李　斌)

【痤疮的治疗及实验研究】

韩晓丽等将67例痤疮患者随机分组,治疗组35例予"化瘀解毒散结饮"(生地黄、赤芍药、牡丹皮、金银花、蒲公英、三棱等),对照组32例予当归苦参丸。经治4周,治疗组对患者皮损改善效果优于对照组($P<0.05$)。黄毓等将60例男性轻中度面部痤疮患者随机分为两组各30例,西药组单纯用克林霉素、阿达帕林凝胶外涂,联合组在此基础上加用自拟消痤方(枇杷叶、桑白皮、生地黄、黄芩、牡丹皮、白花蛇舌草等)煎服。经治4周,联合组总有效率为93.3%(28/30),西药组为66.7%(20/30)。组间比较,$P<0.05$。李晓帛等将60例寻常型痤疮患者随机分为两组,治疗组应用中药面膜配合玫芦消痤膏治疗,对照组应用阿达帕林凝胶及四环素治疗。结果治疗组总有效率为87.5%(28/32),对照组为67.9%(19/28),组间比较,$P<0.01$。徐斌等将300例轻、中度寻常痤疮患者随机均分为两组,治疗组红蓝光照射后联合胶原贴敷料外敷,每周2次;对照组每晚单用0.1%阿达帕林凝胶外涂。经治6周,治疗组有效率为87.3%(131/150),对照组为57.3%(86/150),组间比较,$P<0.05$。罗继红用知柏地黄汤加减治疗60例阴虚火旺证的痤疮患者,观察治疗前及治疗后4周患者面部各类皮损的数量、形态(丘疹、脓疱、结节、囊肿)颜色及分布情况,以判断其临床疗效。结果临床痊愈37例,有效率为93.3%(56/60)。

实验研究方面,陈略等分别建立煤焦油致兔痤疮模型和丙酸杆菌致大鼠耳郭痤疮炎症模型,设正常对照组、模型组、清热暗疮片组、五味消毒饮低、中、高剂量组,观察兔耳痤疮形成强度及反应强度,计算鼠耳郭肿胀率。结果与正常对照组比较,模型组家兔耳痤疮形成强度、耳痤疮反应强度明显增加(均$P<0.01$)。与模型组家兔的耳痤疮形成强度、耳痤疮反应强度比较,清热暗疮片组和高剂量组均明显下降($P<0.01$,$P<0.05$)。五味消毒饮中剂量组仅耳痤疮反应强度较模型组下降($P<0.01$)。兔耳组织病理学观察结果表明,五味消毒饮给药后对煤焦油引起的兔耳实验性痤疮形成有较好的抑制作用,与空白对照组相比,模型组造模后1~5 d耳郭肿胀度均明显增大(均$P<0.01$);与模型组比较,清热暗疮片组及五味消毒饮高剂量组在造模后1~5 d均能明显降低大鼠耳郭肿胀度($P<0.01$,$P<0.05$);中剂量组在造模后1 d能明显降低大鼠耳郭肿胀度($P<0.05$),低剂量组在造模后1~5 d对大鼠耳郭肿

胀度均未见明显影响(均$P>0.05$)。提示五味消毒饮能明显降低兔耳痤疮形成强度、耳痤疮反应强度,且能降低丙酸杆菌所致的大鼠耳郭肿胀度,具有明显的抗痤疮作用。

彭红华从颜面局部望诊论治痤痤,认为面部为经脉汇聚之处,亦为脏腑气血之外荣,脏腑在颜面部均有对应分布。周峰峰等通过分析痤疮中医辨证治疗的现状,辨证结合辨病的学术思想,参考中医经典古籍与其长期临床经验认为卫气主身之皮毛,从而从卫气观点论治痤疮,并指出痤疮不是只有热证、阳证,也有可能出现阳虚寒凝或由阳转阴的虚寒证,只是局部热象明显,故治疗时不可一味寒凉,当温凉并用。罗璎等阐述金元名家李东垣"火与元气不两立"之论,探讨痤疮发病的内在机理,研究启示痤疮的治疗当须审其病机,以泻热利湿和益气养阴、升阳散火并重。无论何种证型,不可独用寒凉,应同时酌加益气升阳、驱邪透风之品,重视脾胃虚弱和肝肾亏损在痤疮致病中的重要性,脾胃虚损,元气不足,则火自内生。凡痘疹之类,以外透之法为顺。在治疗上加入益气养阴、升阳散火之品对于痤疮日久以及湿热内阻所致痤疮尤为重要。

(陈 娜 李 斌)

【浆细胞性乳腺炎的治疗与研究】

崔进军等将91例浆细胞性乳腺炎患者分为两组,治疗组63例分为脓肿型、瘘管型和肿块型,分别予托里清毒饮(党参、白芷、蒲公英、金银花、王不留行、路路通等)、血府逐瘀汤合逍遥蒌贝散和阳和汤,30 d为1个疗程,治疗期间配合采用WE2012-A型微波治疗机理疗。对照组28例以抗炎及手术治疗。结果,治疗组总治愈率为88.8%(31/35)、有效率为97.1%(34/35)、复发率为6.4%(2/35),平均疗程为75.2 d,对照组分别为82.1%(23/28)、85.2%(24/28)、17.1%(5/28),34.8 d。治疗组复发率低于对照组($P<0.05$)。盛喜霞采用常规方法(抗厌氧菌药、糖皮质激素治疗及手术)治疗30例浆细胞性乳腺炎患者作为对照组,治疗组加服柴芩消痈汤(柴胡、黄芩、郁金、香附、夏枯草、金银花等)半个月,结果治疗组治疗后红肿、脓肿、乳头内陷畸形、乳头溢液较对照组改善显著(均$P<0.05$),瘘口、腋窝淋巴结肿大较对照组显著改善($P<0.01$),总有效率93.5%(30/32),高于对照组66.6%(20/30),($P<0.05$)。倪毅等将90例伴有乳头溢液或乳管开口堵塞的浆细胞乳腺炎患者分为3组,A组中药治疗(急性炎症期予以疏肝理气、清热解毒、活血消肿为法;慢性炎症期以温阳化痰、散寒通滞为主);B组乳管镜介入治疗(乳管镜下用生理盐水冲洗乳管后缓慢注入0.5%甲硝唑和地塞米松溶液,退镜同时注入地塞米松2.5 mg);C组中药联合乳管镜介入治疗。结果A、B、C组有效率依次为63.3%(19/30),56.7%(17/30)、86.7%(26/30),治愈率依次为16.7%(5/30)、23.3%(7/30)、70.0%(21/30),三组平均疗程依次为(8.80±1.50)周、(7.43±1.04)周、(4.95±2.16)周,上述指标C组疗效好,治疗天数少于A组、B组,均$P<0.05$。

胡金辉等采用健康宣教、辨证施治、结合外治的"三步法"治疗浆细胞性乳腺炎53例,其中肝经蕴热者采用乳康柴芩汤(柴胡、黄芩、栀子、皂角刺、蒲公英、莪术等);余毒未清者采用乳康芪苓汤(在乳康柴芩汤的基础上去黄芩、栀子、莪术,加用黄芪、茯苓、白芷、浙贝母),服8周;外治法分为箍围透药法(如意金黄散加矾冰液)、针刺推挤加垫棉法及切开纱条引流法,均1 d/次,10~15 d为1疗程,共治8周,患者乳房肿块、红肿、疼痛、脓肿及瘘管症状的积分改善值治疗后均明显下降(均$P<0.01$)。王月以矾冰纳米乳(明矾、冰片)外敷,结合中药瓜蒌牛蒡汤(瓜蒌皮、牛蒡子、蒲公英、夏枯草、赤芍药、金银花等)煎服治疗36例浆细胞性乳腺炎患者,经治1个月,治愈24例,总有效率为94.4%(34/36)。沈加君等治疗本病内外兼治,内服以阳和汤为主方加减,外治用中药离子导入(内服中药中沉淀的部分作为导入原料,每日或隔日1次,疗程15 d~9个月,平均4.8个月)理疗,共治疗72例,其中54例治愈,余均经手术治愈。赵臣银等使用局部封闭(利多卡因针、头孢呋辛针、曲安奈德配成混合液10 ml于肿块周围六点注射、肿块及胸肌筋膜间注射。每周封闭治疗1次,治疗4次以上无效者停止治疗)结合乳腺Ⅳ号(熟地黄、生地黄、鹿角片、陈皮、青皮、炙麻黄等)治疗浆细胞性乳腺炎12例,治愈8例,显效4例,疗程2~4个月,术后随访3个月~4年无复发。杨毅等根据临床分期对101例浆细胞性乳腺炎患者分别施行乳管切除术、乳腺区段切除术、乳晕部瘘管切除术、全部或大部皮下腺体切除术和乳头矫形术,术后服用疏肝清热、利湿消肿中药(柴胡、黄芩、栀子、虎杖、金银花、蒲公英

等),治疗后101例全部治愈,治疗时间4～33 d,平均12.4 d。柴好等用升阳益胃汤合阳和汤加减配合手术治疗对60例难治性浆细胞性乳腺炎进行临床观察,其中28例单纯中药治愈;余32例经手术和中药治疗全部康复,治疗时间16～58 d,平均32 d,术后随访时间3个月～2年半,无复发病例。

范洪桥认为本病最重要的病机是气机失常,临证需抓住调畅气机这一核心,采用疏泄肝气以通达胃气(香附、郁金、苏梗之属)、清胃气(黄连、蒲公英、瓜蒌等),宣降肺气以佐金制木(百合、苏叶辛润相须,升降结合),多脏调燮着手。程亦勤认为可将本病分成肿块期、脓肿期、成漏期。肿块期当以中药内服内消为上策,而进入脓肿期和成漏期需要手术方能痊愈,其采用中医切开引流或扩创,配合拖线、乳头切开矫形法,辅助药膏贴敷、冲洗、垫棉绑缚、中药熏洗等外治方法治疗本病,获得良好及确切疗效。赵磊等临证时将本病分为四期:溢液期、肿块期、脓肿期和瘘管期,前两期以内治为主,外治为辅;后两期以手术、外治为主,内治为辅。内治用温阳散结法以阳和汤加减,外治法包括敷贴、药捻引流、切开、拖线等。

(陈红风　时百玲)

【乳腺增生病的治疗及实验研究】

陈霞将96例围绝经期乳腺增生症患者随机均分为两组,治疗组予补肾疏肝(淫羊藿、鹿角霜、肉苁蓉、菟丝子、枸杞子、香附等),对照组予乳癖消片口服。经治2个月,治疗组在缓解乳房疼痛及乳房包块方面总有效率95.8%(46/48)优于对照组83.3%(40/48)($P<0.05$),治疗组治疗后雌激素(E_2)和孕激素(P)水平明显下降,围绝经期相关症状缓解率明显低于对照组(均$P<0.01$)。张秀芳将232例乳腺增生病患者随机分为治疗组123例和对照组109例,治疗组予自拟益肾化癖方(淫羊藿、巴戟天、肉苁蓉、鹿角、柴胡、白芍药等)煎服,对照组予乳康片。经治9周,治疗组痊愈98例,总有效率为97.6%(120/123),对照组分别为73例、87.2%(95/109)。组间比较,$P<0.01$。张久清等将243例乳腺增生病患者随机分为枸橼酸他莫昔芬片(TAM)组、乳癖消片组、联合组(TAM合乳癖消)各81例。经治3个月,联合组总有效率95.1%(77/81)优于TAM组79.0%(66/81)和乳癖消组72.8%(59/81)(均$P<0.05$)。治疗后3组E_2、促黄体激素(LH)均较治疗前降低、P均升高($P<0.05$),联合组P水平高于其他两组($P<0.05$)。

张曼丽将108例青春期乳腺增生病患者随机均分为两组,对照组予乳癖消片口服,治疗组予背腧穴(肝俞、脾俞、膈俞)刺络拔罐联合青春消解汤加减(当归、丹参、炒白术、陈皮、橘核、生牡蛎等)。经治8周,治疗组总有效率96.3%(52/54),对照组83.3%(45/54),组间比较,$P<0.05$。两组治疗后中医症状积分均明显下降,且以治疗组为著(均$P<0.05$)。王宏昌将328例乳腺增生病患者随机分为两组,对照组158例服桂枝茯苓胶囊,治疗组170例加用刮痧疗法,3个月后治疗组总有效率98.2%(167/170),对照组82.9%(131/158),组间比较,$P<0.01$。马仲丽等治疗100例气滞血瘀的乳腺增生病患者,予乳癖散结膏外敷,每48 h更换1次,并服消乳散结胶囊。经治60 d,乳房疼痛、乳房肿块明显改善,中医证候积分明显降低(均$P<0.05$)。胡克非等通过问卷调查18岁至绝经前435例乳腺增生病患者已经242例非乳腺增生病患者,经Logisitic回归分析表明:痛经、孕次>2次、人流次>2次、中等偏低家庭收入、人际关系一般、职业以脑力劳动为主、工作压抑焦虑程度较高、被动吸烟为危险因素。体型偏瘦、教育程度偏高、初潮年龄晚、产次>2次、饮食清淡、偶尔饮酒为保护因素。

肖红玲等将40只Wistar雌性未孕大鼠随机分为正常组、模型组、TAM组(1.8 mg/kg灌胃)和针刺组(对第2对乳房以乳头为中心进行围刺,同时配合电针,余组予自制束鼠器抓取固定30 min)。干预1次/d。连续30 d后,放射免疫分析结果示:模型组E_2、E_2/P、泌乳素(PRL)、睾酮水平均高于正常组($P<0.05$),针刺组和TAM组均低于模型组($P<0.05$);模型组P低于正常组($P<0.05$),针刺组和TAM组P均高于模型组($P<0.05$),针刺组和TAM组差异均无显著差别($P>0.05$)。刘茂军等通过肌肉注射苯甲酸雌二醇0.5 mg/(kg·d)25 d+黄体酮4 mg/(kg·d)5 d后制备成大鼠乳腺增生病模型,将50只模型大随机等分为模型组、乳癖消片组(0.96 g/kg)、乳安片高(6 g/kg)、中(3 g/kg)、低(1.5 g/kg)剂量组。灌胃4周后,乳安片高、中、低剂量组乳头直径、长度、乳头体积较模型组减小($P<0.05$或$P<0.01$),且乳腺质量、系数和子宫

卵巢系数均显著减轻($P<0.05$，$P<0.01$)。乳安片各剂量组能降低大鼠血清E_2、PRL和E_2/P含量，增加P含量，与模型组比较，$P<0.05$或$P<0.01$，高剂量组可增加血清中睾酮含量($P<0.05$)。

徐晓萌等认为乳腺增生病具有气滞血瘀、痰凝互结，兼肝郁气滞、脾虚湿盛、冲任失调为基础的病变特点。治疗以调摄冲任为主。吴雪雪等总结姜兆俊经验，认为乳腺增生病的病机以肾虚肝郁为本，气滞、血瘀、痰凝为标。治当以温肾疏肝为主，兼行气活血、化痰散结。范洪桥等总结刘丽芳治疗乳腺增生病经验，倡导疏肝达肺，佐金制木佐以益气健脾以泄木，且综合考虑，参入调摄冲任、化痰散结、活血通络之剂。

（陈红风　马疆青）

【混合痔的治疗】

手术治疗方面，郭修田等将80例环状混合痔患者随机分为两组各40例，观察组予外剥内扎术联合内括约肌侧切术治疗，对照组采用传统外剥内扎术治疗，术后均熏洗换药2次/d。结果观察组创面愈合时间(25.40±5.85 d)与对照组(24.27±5.26 d)相当($P>0.05$)，但观察组术后3 d内肛门疼痛评分及术后3个月时肛管静息压均低于对照组(均$P<0.05$)。高洪娣等用胶圈齿形套扎加断桥缝合术治疗30例环状混合痔患者，与传统的外剥内扎术治疗作对照(30例)，结果治疗组患者术后当日及术后第1 d、2 d肛门疼痛评分低于对照组($P<0.05$)，治疗组术后并发症的发生率降低($P<0.05$)。何涛等将155例Ⅱ、Ⅲ期环形混合痔患者分为两组，治疗组80例用自动痔疮套扎术(RPH)联合外痔切除术治疗，对照组75例用传统外剥内扎术治疗，结果治疗组在改善术后并发症如肛门疼痛、排尿障碍、术后切缘水肿、术后便血等方面均优于对照组(均$P<0.05$)；治疗组患者伤口愈合时间(17.33±2.184 d)小于对照组(20.29±2.634 d)($P<0.05$)。罗励等采用小切口治疗环状混合痔患者40例，并将采用Milligan－Morgan术合并横切术治疗的40例环状混合痔患者作为对照组，结果治疗组在减轻术后肛门疼痛、肛门狭窄、肛缘水肿及缩短愈合时间等方面均优于对照组(均$P<0.05$)，而大便失禁的发生两组无显著差异($P>0.05$)。吴喜华等将60例环状混合痔患者随机均分成两组，试验组用开环式微创痔上黏膜切除吻合术(TST)加外痔切剥术，对照组用外剥内扎术，术后均运用抗炎、止血、中药内服、坐浴、换药及对症治疗。结果试验组手术时间(22.63±2.45 min)较对照组(35.32±4.29 min)有所降低；术中出血量、住院天数两组分别为：(5.03±1.21)ml、(4.45±1.02)d和(9.03±2.34)ml、(7.34±2.04)d；试验组在肛门狭窄、尿潴留的发生及术后疼痛、肛门功能、肛管静息压、肛管收缩功能方面均优于对照组(均$P<0.05$)。

术后并发症治疗方面，彭云花等将80例行内扎外剥术湿热下注型混合痔患者随机均分为两组，术后除常规治疗外，治疗组服用痔痛安方(当归、赤芍药、黄芪、延胡索等)；对照组服用泰勒宁。经治7 d，治疗组抑制术后疼痛的疗效优于对照组(均$P<0.05$)，治疗组在防治术后肛缘水肿及排便困难方面的总有效率分别达为95.0%(38/40)、87.5%(35/40)，均优于对照组47.5%(19/40)、57.5%(23/40)(均$P<0.05$)；治疗组用药后无不良反应，对照组出现胃脘不适、恶心呕吐各1例，头晕3例。邓业巍等把136例混合痔患者均行外剥内扎术后，随机分为两组，治疗组68例用纳米银敷料，对照组68例用凡士林油纱，两组均采用中药外敷(白矾、芒硝、五倍子、花椒、车前子、艾叶等)，VAS视觉疼痛评分法示：与对照组比较，治疗组患者创面第1 d、第2 d、第3 d疼痛明显减轻($P<0.05$)；治疗组平均创面愈合时间较对照组缩短($P<0.05$)。张晓娇等将74例行外剥内扎术的混合痔患者随机均分为两组，均于术后24 h开始换药，治疗组加芒硝晶体湿敷换药，结果治疗组水肿积分(1.03±0.13)低于对照组(1.49±0.18)($P<0.05$)，减轻术后疼痛方面优于对照组($P<0.05$)。黎海龙将160例行外剥内扎术的混合痔患者随机分为两组各80例，术后治疗组在患者伤口常规换药后行迈能治疗仪接触皮肤治疗30 min，2次/d，对照组仅行伤口常规换药。经治7 d，与对照组相比，治疗组术后疼痛及创面水肿情况明显减轻，且创面愈合时间较对照组缩短($P<0.05$)。

保守治疗方面，李华春采用自拟中药熏洗方(芒硝、明矾、硼砂、冰片、黄柏、苦参)熏洗治疗60例混合痔水肿患者，对照组60例混合痔水肿患者采用高锰酸钾溶液(1∶5 000)熏洗治疗。两组均配合使用马应龙麝香痔疮膏及肛门部微波治疗。用药第7 d水肿积分例数比较及用药第15 d疗效比较，治疗组均优于对照组(均$P<0.05$)。

(陈红凤　盛佳钰)

【深静脉血栓的治疗及实验研究】

郑文郁等以溶栓、抗凝、祛聚等治疗下肢深静脉血栓为对照组，治疗组加用散瘀消肿汤(党参、黄芪、当归、泽兰、茜草、地龙等)，经治30 d，治疗组总有效率90.9%(19/21)优于对照组71.4%(16/22)。

李晓绿以经腘静脉置入溶栓，导管药物滴注的介入疗法治疗急性下肢深静脉血栓形成30例为对照组，治疗组36例在此基础上加服祛湿化瘀汤(当归、两头尖、茯苓、水蛭、薏苡仁、红花等)配合冰硝散(冰片、芒硝)外敷。结果治疗组痊愈33例，显效3例；对照组分别为20例、6例，组间比较，$P<0.05$。肖光辉治疗急性下肢深静脉血栓形成82例，自拟祛湿活血通脉汤(苍术、黄柏、薏苡仁、土茯苓、益母草、泽兰等)煎服，静脉滴注血塞通注射液，联合西药抗凝、溶栓治疗，结果临床治愈27例，总有效率为96.3%(79/82)。陈柏楠等将231例急性下肢深静脉血栓形成患者辨证分为两组。160例湿热下注证患者(方案1组)用四妙勇安汤加味煎服，疏血通、血栓通或血塞通静脉滴注，冰硝散(冰片、芒硝)每日外敷，并予溶栓抗凝治疗。71例热瘀络脉证患者(方案2组)用验方1号(牛角片、紫草、益母草、生大黄、玄明粉)，外用将军散(大黄粉、玄明粉、赤小豆粉、茶水或醋调)外敷1～2次/d。经治4周，方案1组的整体疗效89.4%(143/160)、症状疗效98.8%(158/160)明显优于方案2组76.1%(54/71)、78.9%(56/71)(均$P<0.01$)，方案1组静脉再通有效率80.0%(128/160)高于方案2组73.2%(53/71)($P<0.05$)。

李普升等对31例DVT患者采用四黄水密膏外敷联合下腔静脉滤器置入及局部溶栓序贯治疗。治疗后患肢膝上5 cm、膝下5 cm处周径较治疗前缩小($P<0.05$)。王彬等将60例急性下肢深静脉血栓形成患者均分为中西医结合组和西药组，并设30例健康查体者为正常组。西药组给予尿激酶20万U静脉滴注、低分子肝素钙4 100 U皮下注射，1次/d，结合组在西药组用药的基础上口服消栓通脉颗粒(茵陈、金银花、赤小豆、桃仁、黄柏等)，连续用药14 d。采用流式细胞术及ELI-SA法观察DVT患者外周血Th1、Th2细胞比例变化及血浆中TNF-α、IFN-γ、IL-4、IL-10水平。结果结合组、西药组TNF-α/IL-4、IFN-γ/IL-10比值低于治疗前($P<0.05$)，结合组TNF-α/IL-4、IFN-γ/IL-10比值低于西药组($P<0.05$)。结合组治疗后肢围改善优于西药组(均$P<0.05$)。

庞光枢等运用中药(黄芪、牛膝、玄胡索、当归、防己、穿山甲等)预防髋关节置换术后下肢深静脉血栓37例，对照组(n=37)用华法林治疗，术后连续用药14 d，两组治疗前后肢体周径变化无明显差异($P>0.05$)，中药组患者股静脉血流速度优于对照组($P<0.05$)。张建方等运用补阳还五汤加减预防髋关节置换术后下肢深静脉血栓39例，对照组(n=38)应用拜瑞妥，用药，经治两周，治疗组发生下肢深静脉血栓4例，对照组例，组间比较，$P>0.05$。许敏在控制血糖、抗凝及抗感染的基础上采用下肢推拿、穴位按压结合静脉滴注苦碟子注射液预防老年糖尿病患者人工膝关节置换术后下肢深静脉血栓形成26例，对照组(n=26)予常规控制血糖、抗凝及抗感染，术后14 d，观察组的下肢深静脉血栓发生率(1例有，25例无)低于对照组(8例有，18例无)($P<0.05$)。

肖清明等建立创伤性下肢深静脉血栓兔模型(大白兔麻醉后于右侧大腿根部以7.5J能量击打右侧大腿股骨大转子1.5 cm的范围，然后石膏外固定右下肢于屈髋屈膝位，保持1周)，将30只新西兰大白兔随机分为模型对照组(生理盐水灌胃)、消栓饮(灌胃：黄芪、白芍药、桂枝、当归尾、川牛膝、丹参等，14.49 g/kg)组及低分子肝素组(皮下注射，40 IU/kg)，每组10只，连续给药1周后，血液流变学指标(血浆黏度、全血低、高切还原黏度、红细胞)及纤维蛋白酶原数值均升高，均$P<0.05$。造模后3 d、7 d，消栓饮组及低分子肝素组的血液流变学及凝血功能等指标较对照组均改善，均$P<0.05$；与低分子肝素组比较，消栓饮的血液流变学及凝血功能等指标均无显著差异($P>0.05$)。蔡立民通过兔创伤性下肢深静脉血栓模型(复制动物左后肢体股骨近端骨折石膏外固定模型)，将60只新西兰兔随机分为正常对照组、模型对照组、低分子肝素钙组及活血灵片组(每组各15只)，灌胃9 d，低分子肝素钙组全血黏度、红细胞聚集指数、刚性指数降低，与模型组比较，均$P<0.05$；活血灵片组上述指标与模型组比较均明显下降($P<0.05$)。

刘政等总结侯玉芬辨证施治下肢深静脉血栓形成经验，在临床分期(急性期、慢性期)的基础上，强调分期外治。急性期,多属湿热壅盛,适宜药物外敷疗法,药用复方消肿散(红花、芒硝、冰片)、红花散;迁延期,证属血瘀湿阻,适宜药物溻渍疗法,药用活血消肿散(丹参、红花、鸡血藤、苍术、延胡索、木瓜等);后遗症期,局部辨证为主,灵活择用药物(苦参、白鲜皮、白芷、黄柏、马齿苋等)溻渍、掺药掺布于病变处、中药油膏纱布或软膏外敷等。

(陈红风 周 悦)

【糖尿病足的治疗及实验研究】

沈霖等将33例糖尿病足患者(糖尿病足分级标准中0~2级)随机分为两组,在常规治疗基础上,治疗组17例予葫芦巴总皂苷胶囊,对照组16例予安慰剂。经治12周,治疗组总有效率82.4%(14/17),对照组62.5%(10/16),组间比较,$P<0.05$;治疗组空腹血糖、餐后2 h血糖、糖化血红蛋白均较治疗前显著下降($P<0.01$),且较对照组下降更显著($P<0.05$)。丰哲等将85例糖尿病足患者随机分为两组,对照组43例采用降糖、胰岛素外敷换药、抗生素治疗,治疗组42例加用当归拈痛汤加味(当归、防风、升麻、苍术、白术等)。结果治疗组治愈率为81.0%(34/42),愈显率为97.6%(41/42),对照组分别为39.5%(17/43)、67.4%(29/43)(均$P<0.05$)。童越在常规治疗基础上联合西洛他唑治疗30例糖尿病足患者作为对照组,观察组30例加服滋肾消渴方(附子、黄芪、桂枝、当归、桃仁等)。两组均以4周为1个疗程,3个疗程后,观察组疼痛感、麻木感、间歇性跛行及总体症状与对照组相比均有改善($P<0.05$);在踝、肱动脉比方面,观察组治疗后评分(1.03±0.09)优于对照组(0.86±0.10)($P<0.05$)。王军等将全国5家研究中心的190例糖尿病足溃疡Ⅱ~Ⅳ级患者以治疗组∶对照组=2∶1的比例随机分组。两组采用统一的基础治疗,不同的外治方法:治疗1组67例外治药物为生肌橡皮膏、金黄膏、丹黄消炎液等,治疗2组67例外治药物为橡皮生肌膏、如意金黄散等。对照组60例采用清创术,外用碘伏、凡士林纱布条、生理盐水冲洗/湿敷、高渗盐湿敷、贝复济喷剂的方法治疗。经治8周,治疗1组、2组创面临床痊愈率、创面闭合指数均优于对照组(均$P<0.05$);在疾病疗效及证候疗效方面,两治疗组相比,$P>0.05$。金真等按Wagner分级法将符合0级糖尿病足的住院患者随机分成两组各40例,对照组给予基础治疗,治疗组加用涌泉穴穴位贴敷(肉桂、吴茱萸)、穴位注射(参附注射液注射双侧足三里穴)及中药足浴(红参、制附子、干姜、桂枝、北杏仁等)治疗。经治2周,治疗组基本痊愈6例,总有效率为92.5%(37/40),对照组分别为2例、67.5%(27/40),两组比较,$P<0.05$。治疗组的症候积分及症状积分均低于对照组(均$P<0.05$)。

李旗等采用腹腔注射链脲佐菌素(STZ)加足部薄铁片固定法的方法制备糖尿病足(Wagner溃疡2级)Wistat大鼠模型,随机分为均中药组和模型组,分别予生肌玉红膏和生理盐水局部外用,隔天换药1次,30 d后,miRCURYTM芯片检测示:中药组NM-031512等20个基因表达上调,NM-345201等4个基因表达下调。提示生肌玉红膏可调控糖尿病足大鼠的部分差异基因表达。胡祝红等在STZ腹腔注射法建立糖尿病模型的基础上,通过游泳、冰块降温和液氮冷冻,诱导建立糖尿病足大鼠模型,随机分为5组(光动力治疗加阳和汤组、光动力治疗组、莫匹罗星组、糖尿病足模型组、阳和汤组),每组10只。经治5周,光动力治疗加阳和汤组、光动力治疗组及莫匹罗星组均能降低大鼠糖尿病足评分,其中光动力治疗加阳和汤组与光动力治疗组相比,糖尿病足评分明显降低($P<0.01$)。对于大鼠血糖的影响,光动力治疗加阳和汤组及光动力治疗组血糖值有明显下降,其中光动力治疗加阳和汤组血糖降低更为显著($P<0.01$)。提示光动力学联合阳和汤对糖尿病足大鼠的疗效优于其他治疗组,溃疡愈合最明显。徐杰男等采用腹腔注射STZ建立糖尿病大鼠模型33只,随机分为模型组、益气化瘀中药组(生黄芪、太子参、丹参、黄精、桃仁、地龙)、氨基胍组,并取10只健康大鼠作为正常对照组。糖尿病造模当天于造模大鼠背部制造创面,灌胃给药,1次/d。创面造模后第21 d,益气化瘀中药组、氨基胍组大鼠创面愈合率较模型组有所提高($P<0.01$)。益气化瘀中药组、氨基胍组大鼠创面愈合时间分别为(25.67±2.00)d及(26.00±3.24)d,较模型组(31.13±1.96)d有所缩短($P<0.01$)。提示益气化瘀中药能明显改善糖尿病大鼠整体情况,促进糖尿病大鼠生长,明显促进糖尿病大鼠难愈创面修复愈合。郑德松等通过对STZ注射与薄铁片固定法制备的大鼠糖尿病足溃疡模型应用消毒愈肌膏治疗,通过miRCURYTM芯片检测发现,与对照组相比中药组的骨形态发生蛋白-9、转化生长因子β1表

达增高($P<0.05$)。

路颖等介绍了魏佳平采用中西医结合方法治疗0级糖尿病足的经验,认为"瘀"为糖尿病足发病的主要病机,临床选用活血化瘀方(桂枝、制川乌、黄芪、当归、牛膝、鸡血藤等)为基础方进行化裁,灵活辨证用药,同时注意顾护脾胃,后期给予补益肝肾。阙华发主张在全面评估和系统的全身整体治疗基础上,建立内外合治糖尿病性足溃疡创面的综合治疗方案,细化局部创面的辨证,分期将祛腐、祛瘀、补虚、活血生肌等外治诸法综合有序地序贯应用于糖尿病足的局部治疗,注重祛瘀化腐、活血生肌、补虚生肌、煨脓湿润、煨脓祛腐、煨脓生肌、箍围疗法、拖线技术的临床应用。

(陈红风　盛佳钰)

【烧伤的治疗及实验研究】

叶春江等将100例深Ⅱ度烧伤患者等分为两组,均予基础对症治疗,观察组加用大黄粉口服(3 g/次,3次/d),经治10 d,观察组治疗后消化道反应、大便隐血均较对照组为轻($P<0.05$)。刘永萍等将小面积烧伤患者72例(浅Ⅱ度46例,深Ⅱ度22例,Ⅲ度4例),随机分为两组,治疗组42例清创后用瓦楞子膏(冰片、瓦楞子、香油制备)包扎,对照组30例用传统油纱,1次/d或隔日1次换药,直至疮面愈合。结果治疗组改善烧伤临床症状(疼痛、创面渗出、炎性反应、局部水肿)有效率显著优于对照组($P<0.01$);治疗组总有效率95.3%(38/40)明显优于对照组93.3%(28/30)($P<0.01$)。肖宜敏等将86例深Ⅱ°、Ⅲ°烧伤患者随机等分两组,治疗组采用自制祛腐生肌膏(狼毒、穿山甲、大黄、川芎、血竭、轻粉等)外敷,对照组外用磺胺嘧啶银纱布,均1次/d,直至疮面愈合。结果,治疗组疼痛发生率为7.0%(3/43)、感染发生率为4.7%(2/43)、创面愈合时间为(14.2±1.8)d、瘢痕出现率为9.3%(4/43),对照组分别为100.0%、34.9%(15/43)、(27.6±3.5)d、48.8%(21/43),组间比较,$P<0.05$。游杰将127例Ⅱ°烧伤患者随机分成两组,治疗组63例清创后采用自制紫草油纱布覆盖,12 h换药1次,对照组清创后涂2 mm厚湿润烧伤膏湿润暴露疗法,1 d换药3～4次,直至疮面愈合,结果治疗组总有效率95.3%(60/63)略高于对照组92.2%(59/64)($P>0.05$)。刘华新等将128例烧伤后期残余创面的患者,随机分为两组各64例,试验组用复春散1号药粉用等渗盐水调成混悬液,单层纱布覆盖创面,对照组创面以单层碘伏纱布覆盖,1 d换药1～2次。经治7 d,两组创面治愈率、总有效率、细菌检出率分别为59.4%(38/64)、87.5%(56/64)、12.1%(8/64)和28.1%(18/64)、65.6%(42/64)、33.6%(22/64),组间相比,均$P<0.05$。李丽卿将62例Ⅲ°烧伤病人随机等分为两组,治疗组烧伤创面采用祛腐生肌散油纱条(大黄、白芷、苦参、龙骨、轻粉、当归等)加湿润烧伤膏外敷,对照组切开减张法加1% SD-Ag霜外涂,均1 d换药1～2次,直至疮面完全愈合。结果治疗组病人创面愈合时间为(40.3±6.5)d、瘢痕发生率为6.5%(2/31);对照组分别为(53.7±6.3)d、96.8%(30/31)。组间比较,$P<0.05$,$P<0.01$。

邱伟等将76例轻、中度烧伤患者随机分为两组各38例,对照组给予湿润烧伤膏外敷,换药1次/d,观察组在此基础上加用桃红四物汤。经治14 d,观察组患者创面愈合时间为(9.8±2.6)d,对照组为(11.2±3.1)d,组间比较,$P<0.05$;观察组患者的治疗总有效率94.7%(36/38),对照组76.3%(29/38),组间比较,$P<0.05$)。廖春华等将130例面部Ⅱ°烧伤患者等分为两组,均采用重组人表皮生长因子(EGF)凝胶外敷,治疗组混合血竭粉,对照组混合SD-Ag霜,换药1次/d,直至疮面愈合。结果治疗组愈合时间为(10.27±1.72)d,疼痛VAS评分为(5.01±1.89),愈后瘢痕面积为(6.53±1.65),对照组分别为(15.24±1.65)d、(8.13±1.17)、(9.29±2.97),组间比较,均$P<0.05$。

姜云云等将大鼠随机分为模型组(皮肤上涂抹混合燃料燃烧法制成直径约2 cm的深Ⅱ度烧伤模型)、紫黄乳膏(紫草、黄连、地榆、冰片)高(含生药0.3 g/g)、低剂量(含生药0.15 g/g)组和美宝湿润烧伤膏组,每组12只,涂药1次/d,连续给药28 d。结果与模型组和美宝组相比,7 d、14 d、28 d紫黄乳膏高、低剂量组的平均愈合时间明显缩短($P<0.05$或$P<0.01$),且高剂量组较低剂量组更明显;紫黄乳膏高、低剂量组和美宝组大鼠血清中TNF-α和IL-6水平恢复较模型组快($P<0.05$或$P<0.01$),EGF含量也较模型组高($P<0.05$或$P<0.01$)。

尚新志等总结唐乾利经验,提出了烧伤创面应辨证施治的观点,将烧伤创面分为热毒型、寒热错杂型、虚寒型、湿热内蕴型、气滞血瘀型、经络阻隔型、气血虚寒型、经络痹阻型，认为烧伤创面的发展是一个“动”的过程，只有正确把握每个阶段的虚实寒热，对症下药，才能收到好的疗效。庞宗超等认为中医治疗烧伤，根据患者病情发展，早期主要以活血理气、清热解毒方剂为主，中、后期主要以养阴清热、益气养阴、健脾和胃方剂为主。

（陈红凤　贡丽娅）

【重症胰腺炎的治疗及实验研究】

尹广军将64例重症急性胰腺炎患者随机等分为两组，对照组采用西药常规治疗，治疗组加用中药大黄20 g水煎从胃管处注入，夹闭胃管2 h，1次/d，结果治疗组总有效率81.3%(26/32)优于对照组50.0%(16/32)($P<0.05$)。刘林峰将25例西医常规治疗加大黄（大黄20 g，水煎200 ml）的重症急性胰腺炎患者设为对照组，在此基础上加用威灵仙煎水作为治疗组（n=26）（威灵仙15 g，水煎250 ml，加入20 g大黄，煮沸5 min，水煎200 ml），2次/d，经鼻空肠管注入后夹管2 h，两组均持续7 d，结果治疗组治疗后3 d、7 d的急性生理与慢性健康（APACHEII）评分（6.57±1.98、3.35±1.60）和Balthazar CT（多层螺旋CT）评分（4.44±0.67、2.15±0.32）均低于对照组（8.16±2.10、5.14±2.12）、（5.20±1.09、2.87±0.45）（均$P<0.05$）；治疗组的血淀粉酶、血清C-反应蛋白恢复正常时间（6.5±1.4 d、7.0±1.5 d）、重症监护病房停留时间（2.4±1.3 d）均短于对照组（均$P<0.05$）；患者腹痛、腹胀缓解时间、肠鸣音（大于3次/min）出现时间、首次排便时间均较治疗组短（均$P<0.01$）。王晶将80例重症急性胰腺炎患者等分为两组，采用西医常规对照和加用银翘散颗粒剂水冲150 ml胃管注入治疗。经治5 d，治疗组在降低患者血淀粉酶（217±179 U/L）、白细胞（7.36±2.79 * 10^9/L）及维持患者血钙水平（2.16±0.38 mmol/L）方面均优于对照组（462±213 U/L、13.62±3.12 * 10^9/L、1.96±0.12 mmol/L）($P<0.01$)。刘淑艳等对30例重症急性胰腺炎患者采用常规治疗，另30例在此基础上加用大黄附子活血汤（附子、细辛、柴胡、枳实、青皮、法半夏等）保留灌肠作为治疗组。经治14 d，治疗组总有效率90.0%(27/30)优于对照组30.0%(24/80)($P<0.05$)；腹痛缓解时间（2.4±0.4 d），腹胀缓解时间（3.3±0.5 d），通气（3.1±0.6 d）、开放流质饮食（6.4±1.0 d）、发热缓解时间（4.2±0.4 d）均短于对照组（均$P<0.01$）；血淀粉酶（5.2±2.3 d）、尿淀粉酶（4.2±1.5 d）、WBC恢复正常时间（4.5±2.6 d）明显短于对照组（10.6±3.0 d、7.4±2.2 d、8.4±2.2 d）（均$P<0.01$），住院时间（14.4±2.8 d）明显短于对照组（22.0±2.5 d）($P<0.01$)。

周群燕等将重症急性胰腺炎患者分为两组，对照组（n=35）经鼻肠管置管术予肠内营养支持，治疗组（n=33）加用八珍汤加减鼻肠管滴注。经治14 d，2组免疫指标（IgA、IgG、CD_3^+、CD_4^+/CD_8^+）比较，治疗组升高较对照组明显（均$P<0.05$）；2组炎症因子指标（血清肿瘤坏死因子TNF-α、CPR、白介素IL-6、IL-2）均有所下降，且治疗组下降明显（均$P<0.05$）。

周贤等将120例重症急性胰腺炎患者等分为观察组（西医治疗加芒硝外敷：芒硝500 g放置于中上腹部，每天10 h以上持续外敷）和对照组（西医治疗），结果观察组患者WBC（12.99±1.92 * 10^9/L）、血清CPR（42.92±14.50 mg/L）和IL-6含量（21.95±2.87 ug/L）下降明显早于对照组（14.02±2.57 * 10^9/L、49.64±18.18 mg/L、24.74±3.76 ug/L）（均$P<0.05$）；腹部超声显示观察组1～2周胰腺渗出完全吸收占总人数比为50.9%(29/57)，对照组为28.6%(16/56)；且局部并发症（胰腺脓肿和胰腺假性囊肿）的发生率5.3%(3/57)，对照组17.9%(10/56)，组间比较，均$P<0.05$。

陈洁生等以西医常规保守治疗重症急性胰腺炎患者35例，同时在此基础上加用大承气汤鼻饲或灌肠及血必净注射液静脉滴注作为观察组（n=36）。经治7 d，观察组总有效率94.4%(34/36)优于对照组85.7%(30/35)($P<0.05$)，患者腹痛、腹胀缓解和排气、排便时间均短于对照组（均$P<0.05$）；观察组患者治疗后血清TNF-α、IL-6、I-8水平均低于对照组($P<0.05$)。谈晨将36例SAP患者分为对照组和治疗组各18例，前者采用单纯内科综合治疗，后者在此基础上加用中药灌胃（人参、麦冬、党参、栀子、生大黄、芒硝等），芒硝外敷及穴位针刺（足三里、内关、中脘、下脘）治疗。经治14 d，治疗组的总有效率为77.8%(14/18)，对照组为55.6%(10/18)，两组比较，$P<0.05$。

李晓萍等用4%牛磺胆酸钠逆行胆胰管注射建立重症急性胰腺炎大鼠模型，将54只SD大鼠等分为SAP组、姜黄素治疗组(建立模型前2 h腹腔内注射姜黄素溶液200 mg/kg)和对照组。结果,模型组3 h、6 h、12 h各时间点血清中上皮中性粒细胞活化肽78(ENA-78)水平均明显高于对照组及治疗组(均$P<0.01$);模型组及治疗组术后胰腺组织各时间点ENA-78蛋白表达均显著高于对照组,但同时间点比较治疗组表达明显低于模型组(均$P<0.01$)。奉镭等用4%牛磺胆酸钠逆行胆胰管注射建立重症急性胰腺炎大鼠模型,将45只SD大鼠分为对照组、模型组、川芎嗪治疗组(术后10 min予0.6%川芎嗪注射液10 ml/kg尾静脉注射)。结果,与对照组比较,模型组及治疗组血清淀粉酶、血尿素氮、血肌酐水平均升高(均$P<0.05$),抗细胞凋亡蛋白Bcl-2/促细胞凋亡蛋白Bax比值减少(均$P<0.05$);川芎嗪处理后,Bcl-2/Bax比值较模型组12 h、24 h、48 h各点均升高(均$P<0.05$)。蒋莉娅等用4%牛磺胆酸钠逆行胆胰管注射建立重症急性胰腺炎大鼠模型,将40只Wistar大鼠等分为假手术组、模型组、针刺治疗组(于造模0.5 h后行针刺肺、大肠、脾经穴位及其背腧穴)和针刺对照组(于造模0.5 h后行针刺肺、脾经穴位及其背腧穴)。结果,模型组6 h后血清TNF-α、NO及血清巨噬细胞炎症-2(MIP-2)蛋白表达水平及及肺与大肠组织MIP-2 mRNA表达水平均明显高于假手术组(均$P<0.05$),针刺治疗组各指标均低于模型组及针刺对照组(均$P<0.05$);针刺治疗组、模型组及针刺对照组大鼠MIP-2蛋白及mRNA间均呈正相关(均$P<0.05$)。

朱惠萍介绍任光荣经验,认为气滞、湿热为急性胰腺炎的病因,瘀血作为急性胰腺炎发病过程中的病理产物,在病情发展过程中起着重要作用,“留瘀化热,络瘀化毒”是急性胰腺炎变生他证之重要原因。急性胰腺炎的主要病机为:胃肠气滞、热结血瘀,滞、热为因,瘀为果,但在疾病的发展过程中,此三者可相互影响。

(陈红风)

【男性不育症的治疗及实验研究】

郑毅春等选用滋阴清热法(知母、黄柏、生地黄、车前子、熟地黄、山药等)随证加减联合左氧氟沙星片治疗解脲脲原体(UU)感染性不育症者患者60例,经治75 d,治疗组总有效率100%,对照组为75.0%(45/60),组间比较,$P<0.001$。李轩等对78例UU感染性不育患者予知柏地黄丸及多西环素、罗红霉素、左氧氟沙星等治疗90 d,总有效率87.2%(68/78),抗生素对照组66.00%(33/50),且治疗组精子顶体酶活性、活率、活动力及正常形态百分率均较治疗前显著提高(均$P<0.01$)。王旭初等将气滞血瘀型少弱精症患者60例随机分为两组,治疗组30例予益精汤(柴胡、枳壳、桃仁、红花、小茴香、覆盆子等)口服12周,与左卡尼汀口服液对照,治疗组总有效率86.7%(26/30),对照组60.0%(18/30),组间比较,$P<0.05$;3个月后随访,治疗组配偶妊娠率为46.2%(14/30),对照组为25.0%(8/30),组间比较,$P<0.05$。周华等用聚精丸(熟地黄、何首乌、沙苑子、当归、黄精、党参等)治疗少精症6个月,配偶总妊娠率为18.82%(16/85),较对照组5.0%(2/40),组间比较,$P<0.05$。

徐勇用疏肝补肾活血法(当归、白芍药、柴胡、白术、茯苓、薄荷等)联合穴位(天枢、气海、关元、肾俞、志室、三阴交等)注射药物(士的宁)治疗46例早泄患者。经治30 d,治疗组国际勃起功能指数评分问卷(IELT)中的配偶的性交满意度(14.0±1.53分)较治疗前(7.60±1.20分)显著提高($P<0.01$),治疗组(14.0±1.53分)较穴位注射配合口服药物(盐酸舍曲林)对照组(9.5±1.17分)效果好($P<0.05$)。朱政衡等用复方玄驹胶囊(玄驹、淫羊藿、蛇床子、枸杞子等)联合五倍子共煎,于性交前温浸阴茎治疗32例早泄患者4周,治疗组患者阴道内射精潜伏期治疗后(4.40±1.30 min)较治疗前(0.81±0.20 min)显著增加($P<0.01$),IIEF问卷中的患者(12.10±2.30分)和配偶性交满意度评分(11.80±2.10分),均较治疗前(5.80±1.70分,5.90±1.60分)高($P<0.01$),与单纯五倍子温浸对照组比较更为显著(均$P<0.01$)。刘茜等对70例抗精子抗体阳性的湿热内蕴型免疫性不育症患者的HLA-DQB1基因进行分型研究,结果显示HLA-DQB1*0601等位基因频率明显高于正常对照组($P<0.05$)。

王世平等用雷公藤多甙(灌胃)制备弱精子症模型,生精散(熟地黄、鹿茸、鱼鳔、沉香、巴戟天、淫羊藿等)小(0.01 g/kg·d)、中(0.02 g/kg·d)、大剂量(0.03 g/kg·d)连续给药14 d,与正常对照组(2.04±0.77)比较,雷公藤多甙组精子特异性钙通道(Cat Sper1)表达量(1.08±0.48)显著下降($P<0.01$);治疗后中剂量组(2.47±

0.20)和大剂量组(2.86±0.73)Cat Sper1 表达量显著增加($P<0.01$)，大剂量组 CatSper1 由(1.12±0.50)升高至(2.86±0.73)，提高作用更加明显($P<0.05$)。尹静等运用缩窄左肾静脉建立精索静脉曲张模型，予以强精胶囊(淫羊藿、仙茅、菟丝子、枸杞子、熟地黄、当归等)高(2.16 g/kg·d)、中(1.08 g/kg·d)、低(0.54 g/kg·d)剂量 4 周；高剂量组(47.64±4.60%，32.73±4.33＊10^6/ml)、中剂量组(35.51±4.30%，25.97±3.56＊10^6/ml)精子活力与密度较模型组(26.26±5.89%，15.42±3.48＊10^6/ml)明显增高(均$P<0.01$)。王宁等对白消安制备无精子症动物模型连续给药五子衍宗丸两个生精周期(78 d)，通过全基因表达谱芯片检测，治疗组与正常对照组基因表达具有 2 倍以上明显差异的上调基因 355 个(占 1.12%)，表现在细胞黏附功能、周期、细胞因子细胞因子受体作用、信号通路的影响；下调基因 487 个(占 1.54%)，表现对化学信号途径、泛素介导的蛋白水解、核糖体、胞质 DNA 的传感途径、白细胞跨内皮细胞迁移通路等的影响。

贺慧娥介绍谭新华经验，将男性不育症分为肾阳不足、肾阴亏虚、脾肾两虚、气血两虚、瘀血阻滞、肝经湿热、痰湿内蕴、肾虚湿热瘀血等 8 种证型辨证治疗，且以整体观念为指导，五脏调治，尤重脾肾。

（陈红风　张玉柱）

[附]　参考文献

C

蔡立民，桑传兰，谭志超.活血灵片对创伤性肢体深静脉血栓模型兔的影响[J].广东中医药大学学报，2013，30(4)：515

曹科，韩宝，梅荣，等.四黄祛毒方坐浴治疗血栓外痔的临床观察[J].北京中医药，2013，32(5)：326

柴好，卓容，丘萍.升阳益胃汤合阳和汤加减配合手术治疗难治性浆细胞性乳腺炎临床观察[J].中国民族民间医药，2013，22(10)：81

陈柏楠，刘明，姜元顺，等.急性期下肢深静脉血栓形成中西医结合治疗的多中心研究[J].山东中医药大学学报，2013，37(4)：298

陈刚，郭艳幸.郭艳幸教授治疗慢性骨髓炎经验[J].中医临床研究，2013，5(23)：50

陈佳骏，罗运权，张海阳，等.清利防石汤干预胆色素结石术后结石复发机制研究[J].上海中医药杂志，2013，47(8)：51

陈洁生，吴申锋，张宇光，等.大承气汤联合血必净注射液治疗早期重症急性胰腺炎的疗效观察[J].广州中医药大学学报，2013，30(3)：305

陈金生，宫庆娟，黄秋兰，等.针灸对急性带状疱疹患者血液 c-FLIP 表达的影响[J].实用医学杂志，2013，29(15)：2562

陈略，陈志明.五味消毒饮治疗痤疮的实验研究[J].新医学，2013，44(10)：676

陈霞.补肾疏肝法在围绝经期乳腺增生病中的临床研究[J].四川中医，2013，31(1)：71

程亦勤.中医扩创引流术及药物外治在粉刺性乳痈脓肿、瘘管期的应用[J].中医外治杂志，2013，22(1)：3

崔进军，宗林，陈松，等.辨证分型结合理疗治疗浆细胞性乳腺炎 35 例[J].长春中医药大学学报，2013，29(4)：689

崔勇.外用季德胜蛇药片治疗丘疹性荨麻疹 240 例临床疗效观察[J].兵团医学，2013，36(2)：43

D

代睿欣，白遵光，胡萍，等.滋肾通关片治疗良性前列腺增生症的临床研究[J].中华中医药学刊，2013，31(7)：1614

邓光烈.中医治疗小儿湿疹临床疗效观察[J].亚太传统医药，2013，9(10)：79

邓业巍，王华胜，张胜威.中药外敷结合纳米银医用抗菌敷料改善混合痔术后创面的临床研究[J].中医学报，2013，28(8)：1135

F

范斌，王洁，李斌.秦万章辨治银屑病经验[J].上海中医药杂志，2013，47(1)：17

范洪桥，刘丽芳.刘丽芳教授从“肝升肺降”理论论治乳腺增生病经验[J].中医药通报，2013，12(3)：29

范洪桥，刘丽芳.疏肝达胃、佐金制木法治疗浆细胞性乳腺炎[J].吉林中医药，2013，33(10).998

丰哲，林宗汉，李书振，等.当归拈痛汤加味治疗糖尿病足 42 例临床观察[J].新中医，2013，45(1)：39

奉镭，穆小松，刘翼，等.川芎嗪对重症胰腺炎大鼠肾细胞凋亡的影响[J].中国中医急症，2013，22(1)：36

付强.通便消痤片联合糖皮质激素治疗黄褐斑 60 例[J].中国药业，2013，22(18)：92

G

高洪娣，应光耀，熊国华，等. 胶圈齿形套扎加断桥缝合术治疗环状混合痔的安全性临床研究[J]. 成都中医药大学学报，2013，36(2)：51

高励聪，宁晓洪，李春梅. 中药治疗银屑病 42 例临床观察[J]. 中国冶金工业医学杂志，2013，30(1)：55

高尚璞，李咏梅，冯国强，等. 活血补肾合剂治疗女性肝肾阴虚型脱发临床研究[J]. 上海中医药大学学报，2013，27(2)：48

关若丹，司徒红林，林毅. 林毅教授首创提脓祛腐综合疗法巧治肉芽肿性乳腺炎——典型病案、理论渊源及操作规范[J]. 辽宁中医药大学学报，2013，15(1)：9

郭静，艾儒棣，段渠，等. 当归饮子加减方对气血两虚模型慢性荨麻疹小鼠全身皮肤瘙痒影响的实验研究[J]. 辽宁中医杂志，2013，40(5)：1026

郭雯，柳芳，董艳芳，等. 化瘀祛斑汤联合 E 光治疗女性黄褐斑疗效观察[J]. 中医临床研究，2013，5(21)：55

郭晓明. 湿疹溻渍方治疗婴儿湿疹的临床与实验研究[D]. 北京中医药大学，2013

郭修田，陆彩忠，石建才，等. 外剥内扎术联合内括约肌侧切治疗环状混合痔 40 例[J]. 上海中医药大学学报，2013，47(5)：69

H

韩晓丽，鲍身涛. 化瘀解毒散结饮治疗痤疮 67 例临床疗效观察[J]. 北京中医药大学学报(中医临床版)，2013，20(2)：56

韩炎艳，田兵兵，崔洪泉. 如意金黄膏合莫匹罗星治疗褥疮临床研究[J]. 中医学报，2013，28(4)：596

韩晔，陆宏. 低位切除结合高位松挂线分次紧线术治疗高位复杂性肛瘘的临床观察[J]. 上海中医药大学学报，2013，27(3)：54

郝蕾，谢维捷，陈育忠. 通腑泻热灌肠合剂对粘连性肠梗阻大鼠肠黏膜免疫屏障的保护作用[J]. 新中医，2013，45(7)：168

何春梅，梁宏涛，姚一博，等. 药线疗法治疗肛门直肠周围脓肿的临床规范化研究[J]. 上海中医药杂志，2013，47(6)：70

何涛，雒福东. RPH 联合外痔切除术治疗Ⅱ、Ⅲ期混合痔 80 例[J]. 中医外治杂志，2013，22(4)：12

贺慧娥，何清湖，周青，等. 谭新华治疗男性不育症经验[J]. 湖南中医杂志，2013，29(11)：19

侯立军. 复元活血汤联合超短波治疗带状疱疹后遗神经痛 45 例[J]. 陕西中医，2013，34(6)：720

胡金辉，黄艳茹，莫兴群. "三步法"综合疗法治疗浆细胞性乳腺炎 53 例临床观察[J]. 中医药导报，2013，19(4)：36

胡克菲，郭琪，裴晓华，等. 435 例女性乳腺增生症影响因素的临床研究[J]. 中国实验方剂学杂志，2013，19(9)：319

胡祝红，祝亚男，倪海洋. 阳和汤联合光动力学外照射疗法对糖尿病足大鼠的影响[J]. 中华中医药学刊，2013，31(10)：2262

黄蕊，吴景东. 石蓝草煎剂治疗风热犯表型荨麻疹疗效观察[J]. 辽宁中医药大学学报，2013，15(5)：181

黄毓，樊春笋，王一飞. 中药消痤方内服结合西药外用治疗男性轻中度面部痤疮的疗效评价[J]. 实用临床医药杂志，2013，17(23)：184

黄仲海，梁宪章，吴年腾，等. 原位再生技术结合中医辨证治疗慢性皮肤溃疡 74 例的疗效观察[J]. 广西医学，2013，35(4)：466

J

吉朝阳. 公英解毒汤配合针灸治疗带状疱疹 80 例[J]. 陕西中医，2013，34(10)：1370

季艳芳，张玉红. 红花逍遥片联合维生素 C 及 2%氢醌乳膏治疗黄褐斑的疗效观察[J]. 中国药房，2013，24(40)：3784

姜云云，赵海滨，叶光明，等. 复方紫黄乳膏对大鼠深Ⅱ度烧伤创面的愈合作用[J]. 中药药理与临床，2013，29(5)：132

蒋蓝. 身痛逐瘀汤治疗带状疱疹后遗神经痛 31 例[J]. 中外健康文摘，2013，10(21)：201

蒋莉娅，黄继人，赵弘卿，等. 针刺对重症急性胰腺炎早期急性肺损伤大鼠血清 MIP－2 蛋白及肺与大肠组织 MIP－2mRNA 表达的影响[J]. 中国中西医结合杂志，2013，33(7)：958

金真，林明欣，林燕玲. 运用中医外治三联模式治疗 0 级糖尿病足 40 例临床观察[J]. 中华中医药杂志，2013，28(2)：443

K

康金森，王雪飞，刘发，等. 红玉祛斑胶囊对黄褐斑模型小鼠的影响[J]. 中药药理与临床，2013，29(4)：134

孔智贤. 龙牡治湿汤治疗湿热型湿疹的临床研究[D]. 北京中医药大学，2013

L

劳瑞平. 乌蛇荣皮汤治疗黄褐斑 42 例[J]. 四川中医，2013，31(6)：120

黎海龙. 迈能治疗仪在混合痔术后应用的临床观察[J]. 湖北中医杂志，2013，35(7)：59

李昌吉，何风玲. 祛风活血方治疗银屑病疗效观察[J]. 中国医学文摘，2013，30(3)：139

李广平，李大勇. 动脉硬化闭塞症中医证候与血清

hsCRP、TNF－α表达的研究[J]. 中华中医药学刊，2013，31(8)：1619

李海松，王彬，韩亮，等. 脐疗联合栓剂治疗Ⅲ型前列腺炎(气滞血瘀型)80例临床研究[J]. 北京中医药大学学报(中医临床版)，2013，20(2)：19

李华春，王彬彬，尚锦绣. 自拟中药熏洗方治疗混合痔水肿60例临床观察[J]. 中西医结合研究，2013，5(4)：196

李轲. 复方苦参注射液联合雷公藤多甙治疗寻常型银屑病32例[J]. 江西中医药，2013，44(2)：30

李克盛，张志勇. 半导体激光联合中药外敷治疗慢性下肢静脉性溃疡40例临床观察[J]. 中医药导报，2013，19(2)：49

李丽卿. 祛腐生肌散合用湿润烧伤膏治疗Ⅲ°烧伤的疗效观察[J]. 中国卫生产业，2013，(34)：184

李宁波. 龙胆泻肝汤加减联合康复新液外敷治疗带状疱疹疗效观察[J]. 山西中医，2013，29(11)：18

李苹，王辉皪，严春玲，等. 王成荣诊治黄褐斑经验[J]. 辽宁中医药大学学报，2013，15(11)：108

李普升，王立恒，庞博. 四黄水蜜膏外敷联合介入治疗下肢深静脉血栓临床观察[J]. 新中医，2013，45(6)：66

李旗，田福玲，李继安. 生肌玉红膏对大鼠糖尿病足溃疡RNA基因表达的影响[J]. 上海中医药大学学报，2013，27(4)：73

李强. 窄谱中波紫外线治疗寻常型银屑病的疗效分析[J]. 中国社区医师，2013，15(8)：181

李巧芬. 100例儿童带状疱疹中西医结合治疗的临床分析[J]. 中国医药指南，2013，11(3)：268

李晓帛，邱桂荣. 自制中药面膜复方野菊花液配合玫芦消痤膏治疗寻常型痤疮32例[J]. 中医外治杂志，2013，22(1)：17

李晓绿. 中药配合导管溶栓治疗下肢急性深静脉血栓形成临床研究[J]. 中医学报，2013，28(6)：909

李晓萍，张志坚，屈纪富. 姜黄素对大鼠重症胰腺炎的干预效应研究[J]. 第三军医大学学报，2013，35(8)：759

李轩，何清湖，刘朝圣. 知柏地黄丸对解脲脲原体感染性不育患者精子顶体酶影响的临床观察[J]. 中华中医药杂志，2013，28(6)：1731

李艳，艾儒棣，肖桦. 祛斑汤对小鼠皮肤表达影响的研究[J]. 辽宁中医杂志，2013，40(5)：1028

李玉清. 张灿玾教授治疗痈疽经验[J]. 山东中医杂志，2013，32(2)：118

李玉柱，陈子良. 杜锡贤教授治疗湿疹经验[J]. 陕西中医学院学报，2013，36(1)：27

廖春华，严伟宾. 重组人表皮生长因子凝胶联合血竭粉外用外敷对女性面部Ⅱ度烧伤创面影响观察[J]. 中医临床研究，2013，5(4)：71

廖燕. 柴附冲剂治疗气滞血瘀型黄褐斑及对MDA、LPO和SOD水平的影响[J]. 中药药理与临床，2013，29(1)：152

林聪. 阳和汤加味治疗面部黄褐斑86例[J]. 四川中医，2013，31(6)：118

凌文津，丘平. 揉推排乳手法治疗郁滞期急性乳腺炎120例[J]. 华夏医学，2013，26(2)：356

刘爱萍. 中西医结合治疗银屑病50例[J]. 河南中医，2013，33(5)：748

刘朝钦，肖惠霞，王洛. 清利湿热法治疗带状疱疹后遗症疼痛70例[J]. 吉林中医药，2013，33(2)：168

刘海琴，盛国荣. 退银汤对寻常性银屑病患者外周血P－cad水平的影响[J]. 中国皮肤性病学杂志，2013，27(12)：1239

刘华新，何洪雨，于帅. 外用复春散1号治疗烧伤后期残余创面疗效观察[J]. 中国现代药物应用，2013，7(17)：99

刘林峰. 威灵仙辅助大黄治疗重症急性胰腺炎肠屏障功能障碍作用研究[J]. 辽宁中医药大学学报，2013，15(6)：180

刘茂军，冯玥，申秀萍. 乳安片对大鼠乳腺增生及调节激素水平研究[J]. 天津中医药，2013，30(5)：308

刘茜，武松，王望九. HLA－DQBl基因多态性与湿热内蕴型免疫性不育症相关性研究[J]. 辽宁中医药大学学报，2013，15(2)：81

刘淑艳，黄岚，郑秋，等. 大黄附子活血汤保留灌肠治疗重症急性胰腺炎的疗效观察[J]. 中国中医药科技，2013，20(5)：505

刘永萍，蒋建纲. 瓦楞子膏治疗小面积烧伤的临床观察[J]. 时珍国医国药，2013，24(6)：1455

刘云涛，王大伟，杨荣源，等. 通腑活血法对脓毒症大鼠小肠组织的保护作用及机制研究[J]. 中国中医基础医学杂志，2013，19(6)：645

刘政，刘明，程志新. 侯玉芬教授分期外治法治疗下肢深静脉血栓形成的经验[J]. 环球中医药，2013，6(1)：45

龙云群. 连花清瘟胶囊治疗带状疱疹26例临床观察[J]. 浙江中医杂志，2013，48(9)：663

娄彦妮，陈信义，田爱平，等. 中医外治化疗性手足痛的多中心、随机、对照临床研究[J]. 北京中医药，2013，32(4)：261

路颖，秦挣然. 魏佳平中西医结合治疗0级糖尿病足经验[J]. 山东中医药大学学报，2013，37(2)：135

罗继红. 知柏地黄汤治疗阴虚火旺证痤疮临床观察[J]. 中医学报，2013，28(5)：759

罗励，郭晓华，陈棣兰. 小切口治疗环状混合痔的临床研究[J]. 内蒙古中医药，2013，32(1)：29

罗艳，楼丽华，沃兴德，等. 阳和汤对急性乳腺炎患者

的疗效及T淋巴细胞亚群的影响[J]. 中华中医药学刊，2013，31(5)：1069

罗璎，胡冬裴. 李东垣的“火与元气不两立”理论对痤疮治疗的启示[J]. 四川中医，2013，31(8)：29

M

马拴全，常媛. 创愈膏对大鼠体表溃疡创面修复作用的实验研究[J]. 山西中医，2013，29(6)：51

马迎歌. 王丽萍教授治疗带状疱疹后遗神经痛3则思路探析[J]. 四川中医，2013，31(11)：99

马仲丽，李颖. 中医外敷内服综合疗法治疗气滞血瘀证乳腺增生病临床观察[J]. 中医学报，2013，28(1)：103

毛燕，张小健，赵宾彦. 消斑汤治疗气滞血瘀型黄褐斑42例临床观察[J]. 河北中医，2013，35(5)：684

N

倪毅，殷飞，薛博瑜. 中西医结合治疗浆细胞性乳腺炎90例[J]. 南京中医药大学学报，2013，29(3)：220

P

庞光枢，冯太升. 中药预防髋关节置换术后深静脉血栓形成的临床研究[J]. 中医临床研究，2013，5(16)：33

庞宗超，李惠斌. 中医药治疗烧伤的研究进展[J]. 中国现代医药杂志，2013，15(8)：115

彭红华. 颜面局部望诊论治痤疮[J]. 河南中医，2013，33(1)：46

彭勇，李斌，李锋，等. 健脾祛风方治疗特应性皮炎95例临床观察[J]. 上海中医药大学学报，2013，27(3)：45

彭云花，杨巍. 痔痛安方改善混合痔术后疼痛及并发症临床观察[J]. 吉林中医药，2013，33(8)：805

Q

乔敏. 中药内服外洗治疗手足慢性湿疹疗效观察及机理初探[D]. 山东中医药大学，2013

秦前刚. 中医辨证治疗下肢深静脉血栓形成108例的体会[J]. 中国中西医结合外科杂志，2013，19(6)：697

邱伟，潘咏梅. 桃红四物汤加减联合湿润烧伤膏外敷治疗轻中度烧伤的临床疗效观察[J]. 中国医药指南，2013，11(35)：515

阙华发. 糖尿病性足溃疡创面处理的中医外治法[J]. 中医外治杂志，2013，22(1)：58

S

单敬文. 龙胆泻肝汤治疗急性湿疹60例[J]. 光明中医，2013，28(1)：87

尚新志，黄国林，冯婧，等. 唐乾利教授辨治烧伤创面经验撷英[J]. 中医药信息，2013，30(3)：79

沈加君，丁嫦英，孙芸. 温通法治疗浆细胞性乳腺炎72例[J]. 中国中西医结合外科杂志，2013，19(4)：458

沈霖，李静，卢芙蓉，等. 胡芦巴提取物治疗糖尿病足的作用[J]. 中国中医骨伤科杂志，2013，21(2)：8

盛喜霞. 柴芩消痈汤配合西药治疗浆细胞性乳腺炎32例[J]. 陕西中医，2013，34(5)：559

石传科，李伟，徐丹，等. 玉屏风散合芍药甘草汤加味治疗气虚质下肢静脉曲张疗效观察[J]. 山东中医杂志，2013，32(5)：325

石传科，严志登，罗明，等. 急性阑尾炎术后中医证候聚类研究[J]. 成都中医药大学学报，2013，36(1)：91

石世华，周必胜，崔纬，等. 中药溻渍疗法对下肢丹毒的临床疗效观察[J]. 北京中医药，2013，32(7)：509

宋瑜，李咏梅，顾敏婕，等. 马绍尧从脾论治湿疹经验[J]. 上海中医药大学学报，2013，27(3)：1

孙光军，任建平，郑勇. 中药坐浴联合肛门直肠旋磁红外治疗肛窦炎临床观察[J]. 中医临床研究，2013，5(9)：16

孙洁，李秋芬，田代志，等. 补肾活血方对前列腺增生模型大鼠膀胱胶原沉积的影响[J]. 中华中医药学刊，2013，31(2)：315

T

谈晨. 中药灌胃与芒硝外敷结合西药治疗急重症胰腺炎疗效观察[J]. 陕西中医，2013，34(6)：731

田浩，田永静，王兵，等. 刺血拔罐对带状疱疹后遗神经痛患者血清P物质的影响[J]. 中国针灸，2013，33(8)：678

童越，孔德明. 滋肾消渴方治疗糖尿病足的临床效果分析[J]. 中医临床研究，2013，5(10)：69

W

王彬，刘明，郝清智，等. 中药调节Th1/Th2免疫平衡在下肢深静脉血栓形成治疗中的作用[J]. 中国中西医结合外科杂志，2013，19(4)：355

王丹妮，李真，徐立然，等. 李发枝治疗艾滋病带状疱疹及其后遗神经痛的配伍精要[J]. 中国中药杂志，2013，38(8)：2497

王宏昌. 刮痧联合桂枝茯苓胶囊治疗乳腺增生症疗效观察[J]. 中医学报，2013，28(9)：1408

王晶. 银翘散治疗急性重症胰腺炎临床观察[J]. 吉林中医药，2013，33(2)：157

王军，张庚扬，侯玉芬，等. 糖尿病足溃疡期中医综合外治方案规范的多中心临床研究[J]. 北京中医药大学学报(中医临床版)，2013，20(2)：15

王乐平，罗玲，董建勋，等. 朱红膏促进大鼠慢性皮肤溃疡创面愈合量效关系研究[J]. 中华中医药杂志，2013，28(5)：1237

王宁，张树成，陈西华，等. 五子衍宗丸对无精症小鼠

的免疫促进作用基因表达谱分析[J]. 上海中医药大学学报，2013，27(4)：63

王世平，吕魏峰，孙秀斌，等. 生精散对大鼠精子特异性钙通道的影响[J]. 中华中医药杂志，2013，28(6)：1692

王旭初. 益精汤治疗气滞血瘀型少弱精症疗效观察. 辽宁中医药大学学报，2013，15(8)：196

王元元，张德芹，沈丽，等. 蜂蜜、蜂胶对大鼠皮肤溃疡创面愈合的影响[J]. 天津中医药，2013，30(5)：305

王月，刘丽芳，周亮，等. 矾冰纳米乳结合中药内服治疗浆细胞性乳腺炎临床疗效观察[J]. 四川中医，2013，31(5)：80

王志勇，金冠羽，卢太坤，等. 行气活血法联合西药治疗ⅢA型前列腺炎气滞血瘀证患者疗效观察[J]. 中医药通报，2013，12(1)：57

翁丽丽，单敬文，柯岩，等. 补肾祛斑汤治疗黄褐斑的临床研究[J]. 中华中医药杂志，2013，28(4)：1142

吴喜华，魏志军，何日明，等. TST术加外痔切剥治疗嵌顿环状混合痔临床疗效观察[J]. 辽宁中医药大学学报，2013，15(8)：229

吴雪雪，杨毅，时光喜. 姜兆俊从肾虚论治乳腺增生病经验[J]. 实用中医药杂志，2013，29(12)：1056

X

向国栓，王娟，刘旺，等. 艾儒棣教授治疗荨麻疹临证经验及疗效观察[J]. 云南中医中药杂志，2013，34(5)：1

肖光辉，何立刚，时永豪. 中西医结合治疗急性下肢深静脉血栓形成82例[J]. 北方药学，2013，10(8)：29

肖红玲，张拴成，佘延芬，等. 围刺配合电针对乳腺增生大鼠的治疗作用及其机理研究[J]. 时珍国医国药，2013，24(3)：752

肖敏，陈明岭，方明，等. 蜚蠊提取液治疗皮肤慢性溃疡34例临床观察及其对Smad3基因表达水平的影响研究[J]. 四川中医，2013，31(5)：71

肖清明，王勇，谭胜平，等. 消栓饮对兔下肢深静脉血栓形成血液流变学影响实验研究[J]. 辽宁中医药大学学报，2013，15(5)：39

肖秀丽，张海岩，茅闻婧，等. 健脾化瘀法治疗慢性皮肤溃疡疗效观察[J]. 陕西中医，2013，34(11)：1509

肖宜敏，卢玉璟，边泽新，等. 祛腐生肌膏治疗深Ⅱ°、Ⅲ°烧伤43例[J]. 河南中医，2013，33(9)：1492

谢延华，黎惠金，肖智青，等. 复方落地生根膏对大鼠溃疡面肉芽中CTGF、MMP-2表达的影响[J]. 新中医，2013，45(1)：154

谢吟灵，沈融，沈玲，等. 培补疏脉方联合西药治疗老年下肢动脉粥样硬化性疾病临床研究[J]. 上海中医药杂志，2013，47(2)：38

谢泽初，张瑞芳. 复方木尼孜其颗粒治疗湿疹的临床疗效[J]. 华西医学，2013，28(2)：261

兴伟，陈霄，贾利辉. 四联疗法治疗下肢静脉性溃疡60例临床观察[J]. 河北中医，2013，35(2)：182

徐斌，王芳，徐春兴. 红蓝光照射联合胶原贴敷料治疗寻常痤疮150例疗效观察[J]. 当代医学，2013，19(25)：22

徐东梅. 冰黛糊剂治疗乳头皲裂100例观察[J]. 实用中医药杂志，2013，29(8)：683

徐杰男，阙华发，唐汉钧，等. 益气化瘀中药促进糖尿病大鼠难愈创面修复愈合的实验研究[J]. 新中医，2013，45(6)：153

徐庆，杨志波. 杨志波运用活血化瘀法治疗黄褐斑经验[J]. 实用中医药杂志，2013，29(7)：581

徐晓萌，宋爱莉. 从调摄冲任浅析乳腺增生病的治疗[J]. 辽宁中医药大学学报，2013，15(2)：135

徐勇. 疏肝补肾活血法联合穴位注射治疗早泄46例[J]. 河南中医，2013，33(10)：1736

许斌，曾宪玉. 自拟疏风养血汤治疗银屑病24例[J]. 湖南中医杂志，2013，29(1)：56

许敏. 老年糖尿病患者人工全膝关节置换术后深静脉血栓形成的预防[J]. 中医正骨，2013，25(6)：72

荀向红，李小莉. 中医药综合治疗带状疱疹后神经痛154例[J]. 中国城乡企业卫生，2013，10(5)：126

Y

严仲. 慢性湿疹90例中医治疗体会[J]. 现代医药卫生，2013，29(7)：1087

杨其良，曹永清. 内口"⊥"处理加外用敛痔散一次性治疗肛周脓肿360例的临床观察[J]. 世界中医药，2013，8(6)：633

杨蒴，刘虹，付美芳. 陈宝义教授治疗小儿荨麻疹的经验[J]. 浙江中医药大学学报，2013，37(4)：419

杨素清，谭杰军，闫景东，等. 王玉玺教授从"毒"论治银屑病经验介绍[J]. 新中医，2013，45(1)：192

杨毅，宋爱莉，孙贻安，等. 中西医结合治疗浆细胞性乳腺炎101例[J]. 山东中医杂志，2013，32(8)：570

杨迎霞. 李秀敏教授治疗老年带状疱疹的思路[J]. 河北中医，2013，35(11)：1610

叶春江，张元海，刘利平，等. 大黄粉治疗烧伤41例观察[J]. 浙江中医杂志，2013，48(5)：347

尹广军. 中药大黄辅助治疗重症急性胰腺炎的疗效评价[J]. 中医学报，2013，28(1)：123

尹恒，应语，姚昶，等. 生肌玉红膏治疗下肢慢性溃疡祛腐生肌疗效的临床研究[J]. 南京中医药大学学报，2013，29(2)：121

尹静，王超. 强精胶囊对精索静脉曲张大鼠附睾显微结构的影响[J]. 中国中西医结合外科杂志，2013，19(4)：401

游杰. 紫草油治疗Ⅱ°烧烫伤63例疗效观察[J]. 海峡

药学,2013,25(7):158

余靖宏,赵瑞芝,卢传坚.银屑灵优化方对银屑病豚鼠及炎性刺激角质形成细胞增殖的影响[J].中华中医药杂志,2013,28(5):1531

俞若熙,张惠敏,郑燕飞,等.浅谈王琦治疗黄褐斑经验与思路[J].辽宁中医杂志,2013,40(9):1781

袁东,周栋.益气活血法联合外科手术治疗下肢静脉曲张40例临床观察[J].中医临床研究,2013,5(11):67

Z

张大萍.张作舟老中医治疗慢性荨麻疹经验介绍[J].新中医,2013,45(7):200

张建方,金国强,姚航军,等.补阳还五汤加减预防髋关节置换术后深静脉血栓形成的临床研究[J].中医正骨,2013,25(2):19

张建军,杨琦,王淳,等.分清肾茶片对角叉莱胶致大鼠前列腺炎的治疗作用及对肿瘤坏死因子-α、前列腺素 E_2 的影响[J].中华中医药杂志,2013,28(10):2909

张禁,黎超,杨颜龙,等.左西替利嗪联合复方甘草酸苷治疗慢性荨麻疹的疗效观察[J].中国现代医药杂志,2013,15(2):52

张久清,张彦敏,赵三珍.枸橼酸他莫昔芬片联合乳癖消片治疗乳腺增生81例临床观察[J].河北中医,2013,35(10):1514

张曼丽,庄克生,崔东晖,等.刺络疗法联合青春消解汤治疗青春期乳腺增生症疗效观察[J].新中医,2013,45(9):122

张晓娇,刘世茹,何炜,等.芒硝晶体湿敷治疗混合痔外剥内扎术后水肿、疼痛的临床观察[J].黑龙江中医,2013,(2):19

张秀芳.益肾化癖胶囊治疗乳腺增生病123例临床报道[J].中医临床研究,2013,5(8):23

张旭辉,董建勋,李健,等.回阳生肌方药对慢性皮肤溃疡大鼠创面愈合及炎症因子的影响[J].北京中医药大学学报,2013,36(3):170

赵臣银,李亚玲.局部封闭结合乳腺Ⅳ号治疗浆细胞性乳腺炎12例[J].中国中医药科技,2013,20(2):201

赵磊,薛晓红.薛晓红治疗浆细胞性乳腺炎临证经验[J].光明中医,2013,28(10):2018

赵一丁,田凤艳,姚春海,等.中药方剂联合西替利嗪间隔疗法治疗慢性荨麻疹36例临床观察[J].实用皮肤病学杂志,2013,2(1):42

郑德松,李旗,田福玲.消毒愈肌膏对大鼠糖尿病足溃疡组织BMP-9、TGF-β1表达的影响[J].环球中医药,2013,6(7):485

郑文郁,张现峰.中西医结合治疗下肢深静脉血栓形成[J].光明中医,2013,28(6):1215

郑毅春,潘明沃,朱照平.滋阴清热法抑制解脲脲原体感染、提高精子活力的临床观察.中华中医药学刊,2013,31(1):83

周峰峰,顾庆华.顾庆华教授从卫气论治痤疮经验探微[J].中医药通报,2013,12(3):26

周华,孙大林,金保方,等.聚精丸治疗少弱精子症80例.南京中医药大学学报,2013,29(1):92

周垒.加味逍遥散加减治疗黄褐斑的临床观察[J].湖南中医药大学学报,2013,33(4):71

周群燕,王宏星.八珍汤加减辅助早期肠内营养治疗急性重症胰腺炎31例临床研究[J].江苏中医药,2013,45(6):22

周贤,夏国栋,李昌平,等.芒硝腹部外敷对急性重症胰腺炎疗效研究[J].中国实用医药,2013,8(11):15

朱惠萍.任光荣治疗急性胰腺炎的临床经验[J].江苏中医药,2013,45(9):29

朱政衡.复方玄驹胶囊结合外治法治疗早泄32例[J].云南中医中药杂志,2013,34(6):19

(八)骨伤科

【概述】

2013年度,在各种专业期刊上发表有关骨伤科方面的论文有10 700余篇,其中粗隆间骨折约占8.2%,桡骨远端骨折约占4.0%,压缩性骨折约占3.8%,骨关节炎约占10.7%,骨质疏松症约占30.8%,肩周炎约占4.8%,颈椎病约占17.2%,腰肌劳损约占1.1%,腰椎间盘突出症约占19.6%。论文内容涵盖了中西医的研究进展、临床研究、实验研究和专家经验总结等。

1. 临床研究

中医骨伤的临床研究基于中医传统理论、特色疗法,同时遵循西医学的诊断与治疗理念的发展,不断探索各种骨伤科疾病的最佳疗法。如桡骨远端骨折、压缩性骨折、粗隆间骨折、肩关节周围炎、腰椎间盘突出症、骨关节炎、颈椎病、骨质疏松、腰肌劳损的治疗与研究等,本卷设有专条介绍。

方金锋以淫羊藿浸膏片配合阿伦磷酸钠片治疗老年性骨质疏松,治疗后BMD值,单纯服用阿伦磷酸钠片、淫羊藿浸膏片配合阿伦磷酸钠片,与治疗前比较,$P<0.05$。石宝营等在痛点处注射利多卡因、曲安奈德等药物,以针刀松解结合肩关节回转手法治疗肩关节周围炎83例,随访时间最长的2年7个月,治愈率为51.8%(43/83);显效率为33.7%(28/83)例,好转率为12.0%(10/83)。谢延华通过比较手法复位小夹板外固定与交叉克氏针内固定,观察两组骨折愈合时间、肘内翻的发生率比较,均$P>0.05$,但临床疗效比较,$P<0.01$。手法复位不会破坏骨折处血运,不损伤骨骺;小夹板可根据患肢肿胀程度适时调整松紧度,防止骨折再移位;骨折复位后,通过小夹板及内外侧压垫加压作用使骨折桡偏、后侧放置的加压垫,维持肱骨远端的前倾角,克服了内翻及内旋应力作用,从而有效地降低了肘内翻畸形的发生率。郭天旻等对211例颈椎病患者予石氏牛蒡子汤(炒牛蒡子、僵蚕、白蒺藜、独活、秦艽、白芷等)为主方,分风寒痹阻型、痰湿阻络型、痰瘀交阻型3型治疗,总有效率为94.3%(199/211),其中风寒痹阻型痊愈率3.7%(1/27),显效率14.8%(4/27),有效率81.5%(22/27);痰湿阻络型痊愈率5.7%(6/105),显效率22.7%(24/105);痰瘀交阻痊愈率1.3%(12/79),显效率15.2%(12/79)。石氏认为颈椎病的发生多以风寒痰湿互阻、气血脏腑失和而为病。风寒湿为发病之始,为致病之外因;气血失和、脾肾亏虚、痰湿内生为致病之内因;气血失和、脾肾亏虚为本,风寒痰湿瘀互阻为标。治疗上,石氏强调“调治兼邪,独重痰湿”,侧重于豁痰。

2. 实验研究

李宁等通过制备肾虚型膝骨性关节炎大鼠模型,灌服益肾通痹方低、中、高剂量,与模型组、假手术组比较,益肾通痹方各组大鼠血清MDA、NO均降低,T-SOD及E2均增高,与模型组比较,$P<0.01$,$P<0.05$;以中剂量组较为显著($P<0.01$,$P<0.05$)。提示益肾通痹方可降低肾虚型膝骨性关节炎大鼠血清中MDA、NO的含量,增加T-SOD及E2的含量清除氧自由基,降低脂质过氧化程度从而达到保护关节软骨、防治骨关节炎的目的。杨少锋等对10月龄wistar雌性大鼠去势造模后,予金刚健骨片(补骨脂、熟地黄、川牛膝、鹿角胶、菟丝子、肉苁蓉等)治疗,骨密度、整合素αvβ6均较模型组、骨松宝组有明显提高,整合素αvβ6高于阿仑膦酸钠组(均$P<0.05$)。提示金刚对骨质疏松症具有良好的预防和治疗作用,可显著提高成骨细胞上的整合素αvβ6的表达水平、对去卵巢大鼠的骨代谢恢复正态平衡有良好促进作用。杨利学等对48只椎板切除后新西兰兔经硬膜外分别滴加生理盐水、玻璃酸钠、当归注射液。结果当归注射液组硬膜外瘢痕形成较空白组和模型组少,创伤后炎症反应轻,瘢痕组织中bFGF含量及HYP含量较空白组和模型组低,随着时间的延长,当归注射液组瘢痕组织中bFGF含量及HYP含量较玻璃酸钠组高(均$P<0.05$)。提示当归注射液具有预防硬膜外瘢痕粘连的作用,但随着时间的延长,其

作用较现今公认的防粘连物质玻璃酸钠无明显优势;随着时间的延长,当归注射液预防硬膜外粘连的效果呈下降趋势,可能与其吸收快降解快有关,可通过增大药物剂量改变剂型等方面进行改进。

3. 专家经验

对于专家的治疗经验,应在循证医学的基础上,将其学术思想、治疗手段、辨证分析等独特的见解和宝贵经验,进行综合整理、总结,以给后世学习、借鉴。徐世平等报道,龚正丰认为颈型颈椎病是颈椎病早期,患者临床症状较轻,如诊断及时,治疗得当,病症可自愈。据其多年的临床经验,以活血行气,化痰祛湿止痛为治疗大法,创"颈痛汤"为主方随证化裁治疗本病,疗效显著。对于颈椎病病程日久,病情重,单用中药已无法控制症状,而西医对于本病疗效不显著者,以颈痛汤为主联合使用痹琪胶囊等,长期服用,减轻患者疼痛,同时配合抬头望明月,大鹏展翅,耸肩放松等功能锻炼,改善生活质量。

(施　杞　唐德志　笪巍伟)

【桡骨远端骨折的治疗与研究】

关于桡骨远端骨折的临床研究方面,主要集中在小夹板固定、手法整复、中药外敷治疗等方面。

1. 小夹板固定治疗

小夹板外固定治疗桡骨远端骨折的中医药文献约 50 篇。主要包括小夹板单纯外固定治疗、特殊小夹板固定治疗。孙启涛等应用闭合手法复位、小夹板外固定治疗老年桡骨远端骨折,6 个月后,对患者的腕关节活动度,DASH 评分进行随访,患侧的活动度(包括掌屈、背伸、尺偏、桡偏、旋前、旋后)均较健侧明显降低(均$P<0.05$)。王利民等对 60 例桡骨远端骨折并尺骨茎突骨折患者采取手法复位加小夹板外固定治疗法,回顾性分析患者的骨折及关节面复位、愈合情况以及腕关节功能等。结果本组患者桡骨远端骨折均愈合良好,尺骨茎突骨折愈合优良率 73.3%(44/60)。董森等将符合要求的 100 例新鲜闭合性桡骨远端骨折患者随机均分为两组。治疗组经手法复位后先采用超掌指关节夹板固定,2 周后改为超腕关节夹板固定,对照组采用手法复位超腕关节夹板固定。两组患者均固定 8 周,治疗组桡骨茎突高度丢失值和掌倾角丢失值均小于对照组。按照 Dienst 标准评定腕关节功能,总有效率治疗组 92.0%(46/50)、对照组 88.0%(44/50),治疗组腕关节功能优于对照组。

2. 手法整复

手法整复治疗桡骨远端骨折的临床报道约 80 余篇。手法整复是临床治疗桡骨远端骨折的重要治疗方法之一。

龙开娥等研究了龙氏驳骨膏配合手法复位小夹板固定治疗老年稳定型桡骨远端骨折的疗效,将 114 例稳定型桡骨远端骨折患者随机分为两组,治疗组予龙氏驳骨膏配合手法复位小夹板固定,对照组予手法复位小夹板固定。结果显示,治疗组患者骨折愈合时间、腕部功能恢复情况均显著优越于对照组(均$P<0.05$)。李兰山等将手法整复夹板外固定与切开复位钢板内固定治疗伸直型桡骨远端骨折按 Dienst 功能评定标准对治疗效果进行评定。结果显示,平均随访 10 个月,夹板外固定组优良率 95.1%(59/62)、患者满意度 96.8%(60/62),钢板内固定组优良率 97.0%(33/34)、患者满意度 91.1%(31/34)。两组比较,$P>0.05$。两种方法各有优势,应根据患者的骨折类型、骨质疏松程度,手术耐受程度,对腕关节功能恢复的期望值及治疗费用等合理选择治疗方式。邱继明等观察手法复位联合土家药活血接骨膏外敷治疗桡骨远端骨折的疗效,将 200 例桡骨远端骨折患者随机分为两组,手法复位后治疗组 102 例外敷土家药活血接骨膏,对照组 98 例口服接骨七厘片。经治 35 d,治疗组骨折治疗后肿胀消退时间、疼痛缓解时间、骨折临床愈合、骨性愈合、总愈合率及腕关节功能明显优于对照组(均$P<0.05$)。

3. 基础研究

有关桡骨远端骨折后中医药治疗的基础研究相对较少,主要集中在有关小夹板固定的生物力学研究。

秦洪等运用生物力学的研究方法,对比分析牵引式夹板治疗桡骨远端粉碎性骨折时橡皮筋拉伸及应力松弛与效果的关系,将 236 例桡骨远端粉碎性骨折患者按治疗方法分为两组,治疗组实行牵引式夹板治疗,对照组实行单纯手法整复夹板外固定。治疗后定期拍摄X射线片观察骨折愈合情况，腕关节功能采用Dienst评估标准进行评定。采用Instron电子万能材料试验机3367对牵引的橡皮筋进行橡皮筋拉伸和应力松弛实验，测试橡皮筋的最大应力。结果显示，患者随访5～13个月，得到Dienst功能评估：治疗组优良率93.2%(110/118)，对照组优良率52.6%(62/118)，治疗组优良率显著高于对照组($P<0.01$)。橡皮筋拉伸和应力松弛实验结果显示，橡皮筋的最大应力为46.97 N，最终应力保持在20.60 N，能够达到桡骨远端粉骨折复位治疗的牵引作用。

(唐占英　林　婕)

【股骨粗隆间骨折的治疗与研究】

股骨粗隆间骨折也称为股骨转子间骨折，是指从股骨颈基底至小转子水平以上的骨折。患者的平均年龄略高于股骨颈骨折。股骨转子间血运丰富，很少发生骨折不愈合或股骨头坏死。因临床上多见于老年人，长期卧床极易产生并发症，病死率较高，故目前主要以手术结合中医药治疗为主。

1. 临床治疗

杨鹈祥等用手术结合中药治疗高龄股骨粗隆间骨折患者47例，手术内固定方法采用动力髋内固定(DHS)；早期患者不能进食时采用生脉注射液静脉滴注，后期口服补中益气汤等治疗术后发热，对32例随访12～36个月。结果，疗效评价优良率为96.9%(31/32)。汪宝军等用抗旋股骨近端髓内钉PFNA治疗老年股骨粗隆间骨折患者46例，术后2周内服用活血祛瘀、消肿止痛中药汤剂，术后2～4周则重在和营生新、接骨续筋，术后4周重在补益肝肾、强筋壮骨，随访5～18个月，髋关节功能评分优良率91.3%(42/46)。卢致顺等用中医结合锁定钢板治疗老年性股骨粗隆间粉碎性骨折21例，以骨折三期辨证为基础，以动静结合、筋骨并重、内外兼治、医患合作为原则。早期：行气活血、消肿止痛，方用骨折一方或跌打汤加减。中期：活血和营、接骨续筋，方用骨折二方加减。后期：补益肝肾、调养气血，方用骨折二方或八珍汤加减。术后使用神灯外照、骨科治疗仪、针灸等理疗，各种练功疗法。随访时间6～12个月，根据Harris评分评价：总优良率为95.2%(20/21)。陈宇等用外固定器结合中医药治疗高龄股骨粗隆间骨折患者70例，均采用斯氏针固定髋部近端，2枚皮质骨螺纹钉固定骨折远端，术后根据中医骨折三期辨治原则口服中药，初期活血化瘀、消肿止痛，方用桃红四物汤加牛膝、泽兰、泽泻等；中期和筋续骨，方用续骨活血汤(续断、骨碎补、川芎、土鳖虫、白芍药、党参)加减；后期补气养血、滋补肝肾，方用补肾汤(熟地黄、当归、菟丝子、补骨脂、黄芪)加减。此外，进行抗骨质疏松治疗，口服十味骨康口服液(淫羊藿、白芍药、补骨脂等)。随访70例中，12例出现针道周围炎性反应，8例出现针道感染，均无深部感染及骨髓炎；髋部固定针松动10例，但未影响骨折愈合；髋部固定针穿越股骨头8例；髋内翻畸形愈合15例；膝关节活动度较术前下降16例，其中8例明显受限。

2. 临床研究

黎勇等将60例EvansⅣ型股骨粗隆间骨折患者分为动力髋螺钉(DHS)、动力髋螺钉结合大粗隆支持钢板(DHS结合TSP)、人工股骨头置换术(FHR)3组各20例，所有患者顺利完成手术，随访9～36个月。按Harris髋关节功能评分，DHS组优良率为75.0%(15/20)，DHS结合TSP组为80.0%(16/20)，FHR组为90.0%(18/20)；FHR组手术时间、术中出血量、下地时间短于其他2组(均$P<0.05$)，DHS组手术时间短于DHS结合TSP组($P<0.05$)，术中出血量少于DHS结合TSP组($P<0.05$)。吴旭辉回顾性分析60例老年股骨粗隆间骨折的临床资料，其中20例采用双极人工股骨头置换(ABFH)治疗，20例采用动力髋螺钉治疗，20例采用解剖型钢板固定。结果ABFH组下地活动时间显著短于另外两组(均$P<0.01$)。ABFH组Harris评分显著高于其他两组(均$P<0.05$)。秦磊等选取2010年1月～2012年10月老年骨质疏松股骨粗隆间骨折患者112例，随机分为两组，观察组63例采用新型股骨近端髓内钉PFNA内固定治疗，对照组49例采用动力髋螺钉DHS内固定治疗。两组患者的年龄、性别、病情、病程等一般资料比较无显著性差异(均$P>0.05$)。结果，观察组手术时间和骨折愈合时间较对照组更短，术中出血量也更少，依据Harris评分评定疗效，观察组临床疗效远高于对照组(均$P<0.05$)。

(郐学群)

【胸腰椎骨折的治疗】

张绍文等对胸腰椎骨折患者实施闭合复位,中药治疗(局部涂擦消定膏、内服损伤胶囊和消肿止痛合剂)、功能锻炼(垫枕练功)、支具固定等保守治疗,结果470例患者中3例完全性脊髓损伤的胸腰椎骨折患者治疗后2周较治疗前ASIA评分好转1级,9例部分性脊髓损伤的胸腰椎骨折患者治疗后2周较治疗前ASIA评分好转2级以上。提示只要适应证选择得当,中西医结合保守治疗胸腰椎骨折具有住院时间短、并发症少、疗效显著等优点。卢永勇对32例患者采取腰背伸肌功能锻炼、腰背部垫枕复位治疗,同时内服中药(早期复元活血汤加减,中期桃红四物汤加味,后期四逆散加味)、外敷十味散(白芍药、赤芍药、红花、当归尾、落得打、乳香等),并配合针灸治疗,经皮椎体后凸成形术治疗。结果总有效率100%。吴霖贤等将64例患者平分为椎旁肌入路+中药熏洗(当归、红花、独活、威灵仙、续断、骨碎补等)组(A组)和椎旁肌入路组(B组)。经治3个月,A组总体有效率为100%,B组为87.5%(28/32),组间比较,$P<0.05$。

黄献京以内服(早期复元活血汤加减,中期桃红四物汤加味,后期四逆散加味)与外敷十味散(白芍药、赤芍药、红花、当归尾、落得打、乳香等)及针灸治疗单纯性腰椎压缩性骨折32例。结果总有效率100%。王汉龙等对453例患者采用腰椎悬吊牵引、垫枕复位,配合手法整复及腰背肌功能锻炼和中药内服外敷(早期外敷骨散,服膈下逐瘀汤、大成汤或合五苓散;中期服正骨丸或和营止痛汤等;后期服六味地黄丸或益肾骨康丸等),6～8周后带腰背支具下床活动。结果住院时间平均21 d;出院后随访3个月～1年,优良率92.9%(421/453)。高晓珺等将99例患者分为两组,对照组45例予西医治疗(过伸复位,口服乐力钙胶囊,肌注鲑降钙素,早期功能训练),治疗组在此基础上加服中药(葛根、补骨脂、淫羊藿、穿山甲、川续断、山药等),中后期行中药熏蒸结合中频脉冲电治疗。结果两组治疗后Frankel分级均优于治疗前且以治疗组为著(均$P<0.05$);治疗组胸腰椎功能恢复优良率为98.1%(53/54),对照组为84.5%(38/45),组间比较,$P<0.05$。两组伤椎前高压缩比均明显上升,Cobb角及椎管侵占率均明显下降,且以治疗组为著(均$P<0.05$)。蒋卫方以鹿瓜多肽注射液静脉滴注,内服补肾活血中药(杜仲、狗脊、补骨脂、续断、当归、桃仁等)及功能锻炼治疗52例,经治15 d,随访6～12个月,总有效率为96.2%(50/52)。

叶朝辉等将30例老年骨质疏松胸腰椎骨折患者平分为两组,均行椎体成形术,对照组服钙尔奇D片,治疗组加服补肾益气活血汤。经治3个月,治疗组疼痛视觉模拟评分(VSA)明显低于对照组($P<0.05$)。沈俊玲将老年骨质疏松性胸腰椎骨折患者随机分成两组各20例,对照组予经皮穿刺椎体成形术(PVP)治疗,观察组加服中药(黄芪、党参、桃仁、红花、骨碎补、丹参等)。经治14 d,观察组VSA评分明显低于对照组($P<0.05$)。艾尼瓦尔·艾力等将骨质疏松性胸腰椎骨折患者随机分为两组,对照组50例行经皮椎体后凸成形术,治疗组44例在此基础上加服中药(早期用当归、泽兰、木通、川牛膝、生黄芪、蒲公英等;中后期用川断、炒白术、甘杞子、炒穿山甲、络石藤、淮山药等)治疗,疗程平均2.5个月。结果总有效率治疗组为100%、对照组为96.0%(48/50),组间比较,$P<0.05$。樊新甫等以经皮球囊扩张椎体后凸成形术结合口服十七味大活血胶囊(川芎、红花、血竭、乳香、没药、莪术等)治疗老年骨质疏松压缩性骨折患者41例,结果术后VAS明显降低,术后1 d与术前比较,术后1周与术后1 d比较,均$P<0.05$。陈继征等将72例胸腰椎骨折疏松性骨折患者分为两组,对照组单纯PVP,治疗组加用中药内服(熟地黄、泽泻、肉苁蓉、鸡血藤、骨碎补)治疗。经治3个月,两组VAS评分均明显下降且以治疗组为著(均$P<0.05$)。

胡阳广等将86例胸腰椎骨折后腹胀便秘患者平分成A、B两组,均予服清宁胶囊,B组加用复元活血汤加味治疗。结果B组总有效率97.7%(42/43)明显高于A组86.1%(37/43)($P<0.05$)。王小刚等自拟活血通便汤(桃仁、陈皮、当归、大黄、桂枝、牛膝等)治疗屈曲型腰椎压缩性骨折早期腹胀、便秘52例,结果总有效率92.3%(48/52)。刘方予理气活血中药(厚朴、半夏、当归、赤芍药、桃仁、酒大黄等)口服治疗胸腰椎骨折并发腹胀患者67例,对照组予胃肠减压等常规治疗,经治2 d,治疗组总有效率为94.1%(32/34),对照组为42.4%(14/33),组间比较,$P<0.05$。

(邢秋娟)

【腰肌劳损的治疗与研究】

2013年度腰肌劳损相关文献数量较2012年有所增加，多达400余篇，内容以临床研究为主，实验研究相对较少。临床治疗上多见于保守治疗，包括手法、功法、中药、小针刀、神经阻滞、理疗等，多以综合治疗方式进行。实验研究侧重于探讨腰肌劳损的病理机制方面。

1. 临床治疗

(1) 中医传统技术治疗　曾科学等将慢性腰肌劳损患者随机分为两组各30例，治疗组采用太极推拿手法，对照组采用常规推拿疗法。经治2周，通过VAS评分，两组治疗后均明显下降且以治疗组为著(均$P<0.05$)。治疗组治愈率为80.0%(24/30)，对照组为40.0%(12/30)，组间比较，$P<0.05$。

(2) 药物治疗　程嗣鹤将腰肌劳损患者分为两组，治疗组58例予补肾活血祛痹方(独活、桑寄生、秦艽、牛膝、广地龙、细辛等)内服，外用中药末(细辛、桂枝、没药、白芷、红花、透骨草等)敷贴，对照组52例服双氯芬酸钠缓释胶囊。疗程均为2周，共治1～3个疗程。结果两组VAS评分均明显下降且以治疗组为著($P<0.05$，$P<0.01$)。高艳平将急性腰扭伤患者随机分成两组，治疗组41例予止痛活血汤(桃仁、红花、续断、赤芍药、当归、小茴香等)联合针刺治疗，对照组37例服阿司匹林肠溶片、对乙酰氨基酚片。经治4 d，两组总有效率分别为97.6%(40/41)、86.5%(32/37)，组间比较，$P<0.05$。两组治疗后VAS评分、M-JOA腰痛评分均下降，且以治疗组下降更为明显(均$P<0.05$)。蓝仕以独活寄生汤线口服结合壮医点灸(阿是穴、肾俞、大肠俞、委中、环跳等穴)治疗腰肌劳损患者100例，痊愈率为76.0%(76/100)，好转率24.0%(24/100)。柴政将慢性腰肌劳损患者随机分为两组各35例，均给予推拿按摩治疗，以5 d为1个疗程，共治3个疗程，疗程间休息1 d，观察组同时予伤科接骨片(红花、土鳖虫、朱砂、马钱子粉、制乳香、制没药等)口服。结果两组治疗后VAS评分均明显下降且以观察组为著(均$P<0.05$)。罗巨利等将腰肌劳损患者随机分为两组，治疗组33例采用活血安痛酒(红花、桃仁、延胡索、丹参、羌活、桂枝等)经离子定向导入治疗，对照组口服塞来昔布和盐酸乙派立松。经治3个月后，总有效率分别为97.0(32/33)、87.5%(28/32)。

(3) 小针刀，神经阻滞治疗　彭运飞以小针刀配合截血膏(天花粉、生地黄、姜黄、赤芍药、白芷)外敷治疗腰骸关节劳损患者52例，治愈41例，好转11例。

(4) 综合治疗　方铁根等以太极、推拿手法结合火山泥热敷、干涉波等理疗方法治疗腰肌劳损患者62例，均为1次/d，5次为1个疗程，共治2个疗程。治愈率为67.7%(42/62)，其中1个疗程治疗后显效率达87.1%(54/62)。

手法治疗中，分别有人结合牵引，肌肉力量技术，重要浸渍等方法治疗腰肌劳损，取得明显的疗效。楚德升等以手法联合活动牵引治疗劳损性上腰痛，好转率达98.3%(118/120)，此法强调筋骨并重，有利于恢复上腰部的动力平衡与稳定。对于下腰痛，王桂茂等通过手法结合肌肉力量技术并利用VSA评分，腰部功能R-MQ评价，等速肌力测试对腰背伸肌进行力学测试，发现手法配合肌肉力量技术能明显改善运动员下腰痛的功能障碍，改善腰背伸肌的力学性能，并有协同优化作用。

2. 临床研究

庄如杰等探讨了腰椎终板ModicⅠ型面积改变率与慢性下腰痛之间的相关性，通过对26例ModicⅠ型患者检测其腰椎终板面积改变率，统计腰椎终板Modic面积改变率并采用疼痛视觉模拟评分评估慢性下腰痛的程度，结果发现ModicⅠ型腰椎终板面积改变率与疼痛视觉模拟评分呈正相关性，Pearson相关系数$r=0.418$，$P=0.018$，即终板面积改变率越大，患者下腰痛程度越严重，提示两者间具有正相关性。

(胡志俊　林　婕)

【肩关节周围炎的治疗】

1. 中药内服

院建生用当归四逆汤加减治疗肩关节周围炎患者32例，经治20 d，总有效率为96.9%(31/32)。赫军等用柳豆叶合蠲痹汤加味治疗肩关节周围炎30例，对照组服布洛芬缓释片，两组均配合肩关节锻炼。经治30 d，总有效率治疗组为96.7%(29/30)，对照组为85.7%(24/28)。冀沛峰等将80例患者随机均分为两组，治疗组口服复方风湿宁片(两面针、七叶莲、鸡骨香、过岗龙、宽筋藤、威灵仙),对照组口服芬必得。经治 20 d,两组总有效率分别为 92.5%(37/40)、72.5%(29/40),组间比较,$P<0.05$。

2. 中药外用

吴洋等将风寒湿痹型肩周炎患者随机平分为两组,治疗组用寒立消贴敷剂(生川乌、生草乌、桂枝、赤芍药、桃仁、红花等)外贴肩部,对照组用狗皮膏药外贴肩部最明显的压痛点。经治10 d,治疗组总有效率为 92.5%(37/40),对照组为 77.5%(31/40),两组比较,$P<0.05$。章竞峰将 65 例肩周炎患者随机分为两组,观察组 35 例采用消瘀通络熏条(川乌、草乌、樟脑、细辛、白芷、猪牙皂等)灸法治疗,对照组采用中药(与熏条药味相同)蒸汽熏洗治疗。经治 4 周,观察组镇痛疗效愈显率 91.4%(32/35)明显优于对照组的 20.0%(6/30)($P<0.001$);肩部功能活动改善方面,观察组愈显率 94.3%(33/35)亦优于对照组的 26.7%(8/30)($P<0.001$)。

3. 综合治疗

杨林平将 189 例肩关节周围炎患者随机分为两组,对照组 89 例予常规治疗,治疗组应用臂丛神经阻滞手法松解联合中药(麻黄、桂枝、桑枝、杜仲、三棱、莪术等)热敷治疗,经治 7 d,对照组优良率为 50.6%(45/89),治疗组优良率为 92.0%(92/100),两组比较,$P<0.05$。杨杰保应用玻璃酸钠联合肩周方(当归、伸筋草、丹参、羌活、木瓜、川芎等)内服治疗肩关节周围炎 25 例,经治 5 周,治愈率 24.0%(6/25),总有效率 100%。阳煦等将肩周炎患者平分为两组,治疗组用黄芪桂枝五物汤加减水煎服及浸酒服联合按摩手法治疗,对照组予美罗昔康等西药治疗。结果总有效率治疗组和对照组分别为 100%,88.8%(71/80)。杜海峡等将肩周炎患者随机分为两组各 27 例,对照组单纯肩关节周围及关节腔封闭治疗,治疗组加臭氧注射治疗。两组均每周 1 次,3 次为 1 个疗程。随访 6 个月,两组 VAS 评分均明显下降(均$P<0.05$)。

4. 其他

蒋顺琬等观察参附注射液液压扩张治疗本病的临床疗效及其血清 MMP-9 表达,将 85 例患者分为治疗 1 组(参附注射液+2%利多卡因+曲安耐德)、治疗 2 组(参附注射液+生理盐水+2%利多卡因+曲安奈德)、对照组(生理盐水+2%利多卡因+曲安奈德),每组分别为 29 例、28 例、28 例。治疗 3 周后,各组血清 MMP-9 及 Constant-Murley 肩关节功能评分均明显升高,C-反应蛋白、血沉均明显下降(均$P<0.01$)。总有效率治疗 1 组为 93.1%(27/29),治疗 2 组为 89.3%(25/28),对照组为 75.0%(21/28)。冯晓琳等用拔罐疗法干预不同证型肩周炎存在疗效差异,结果风寒外袭型疗效最好,气滞血瘀型疗效次之,气血亏虚型疗效最差。

(莫　文　王国栋)

【骨质疏松的治疗及实验研究】

郑艳等对 127 例慢性萎缩性胃炎伴骨质疏松症患者中医症状、证型和证素分布情况进行回顾性调查研究,发现其基本病因病机为脾肾亏虚,肾虚、气虚、阴虚、阳虚甚或阴阳两虚为主,并认为脾肾双补应是该病的治疗法则。周叶等对1 333位杭州市居民进行骨质疏松知识问卷调查显示,仅 40%的人群坚持经常摄入富含钙的食物,经常晒太阳;骨质疏松性骨折的知晓率低于 50%;运动方式无负重运动为主;仅有 1/3 的人群知道骨质疏松的预防始于青年;提示骨质疏松知识不够普及,人们对骨质疏松知识的认识存在一些误区和盲点,骨质疏松健康教育应加大宣传力度。

高明月等运用描述性研究方法和关联规则方法,对收集到的近 40 年来治疗骨质疏松症的中医现代病案数据进行整理、分析、归纳,探讨从肾论治骨质疏松症的用药规律和证型分布特点:① 骨质疏松症的病机主要以虚为主,兼以瘀、寒和热。肾虚为主要病机,或兼血瘀,以补肾为基础治疗,联系五脏相关性,兼以活血、健脾等他法。② 高频药物大部分入肾经,具有补肾作用;证型分类以肾虚证远超于其他证型,验证了从肾论治骨质疏松症的实际意义。③ 从肾论治骨质疏松症是以肾虚为主要病机,联系五脏气血关系,以补肾为主,配合其他疗法治疗骨质疏松症的论治方法。从肾论治病人所患的多是原发性骨质疏松症。李东涛等探讨以证候为内容的骨质疏松症中医疗效评价方法,并验证其可靠性。以 100 mm 刻度法及综合评价层次分析法为数学工具,以综合集成研讨厅为研讨方式,共取 36 个中医症状量化分值为底层指标，证候定性的各个症状或症状组合为第二层次指标，以精亏、气虚、阴虚、阳虚、血瘀证5个证候定性为第三层次指标，以证候总评价为顶层指标；量化了骨质疏松症36个常见中医症状；确立了精亏证、气虚证、阴虚证、阳虚证、血瘀证各证候及中医证候总评分量化计算公式。临床验证骨质疏松症患者中医证候总评分与骨密度、生存质量均有线性关系。构建的骨质疏松症中医证候疗效评价方法可反映骨质疏松症患者病情轻重程度，临床验证可靠。

许坤等认为，老年痴呆症与骨质疏松症责之于肾虚髓减，而脑、精髓的联系则是从生化因子水平上的联系，其中精髓就是指肾精化生的对骨骼生长发育具有营养作用的一类"髓"物质。并从载脂蛋白E、钙迁移、雌激素、同型半胱氨酸、细胞因子等因素与骨质疏松症和老年性痴呆间的相互关系作了阐述。梁伟东等认为，糖尿病骨质疏松的中医临床证型大致经过气阴两虚—阴虚燥热—阴虚及阳—瘀血阻络，各证型以脾肾不足为根本，代谢组学可用于该病的证型诊断；治疗方面，中药从多靶点、多系统、多代谢通路影响生理病理变化，运用代谢组学技术中核磁氢谱技术，分析患者治疗前后体液及组织代谢产物的变化，结合模式识别等化学计量学和多元统计分析方法，为拓展临床应用提供有力的依据。杨军等用蛋白质组学的方法研究壮骨止痛方治疗骨质疏松的作用机理，建立去卵巢大鼠骨质疏松症模型，分为壮骨止痛方组、模型组和假手术组，13周后提取股骨组织蛋白质，分析各组间差异蛋白质，结合蛋白质生物信息库对各蛋白质初步鉴定。结果发现了2个差异蛋白，X1为糖原磷酸化酶，X2为线粒体ATP合酶β基。提示壮骨止痛方治疗骨质疏松的过程中，X1、X2这两种蛋白发挥着重要的分子调控作用。

李富龙等将骨质疏松症患者随机分为两组，基础治疗组56例予钙剂＋维生素D，联合治疗组55例＋五行健骨操锻炼。经治6个月，两组受试者的计时起立行走测试(TUG)均下降、Berg平衡量表评定(BBS)得分均升高，动态平衡仪各项指标测试均下降，且以联合治疗组为著($P<0.05$，$P<0.01$)。TUG、BBS测试结果与静、动态平衡仪测定结果具有相关性。提示五行健骨操可改善骨质疏松症患者的平衡能力；TUG、BBS测试结果与静、动态平衡仪测定结果相关，量表评测与仪器评测结合可更好地反映骨质疏松症患者的平衡能力。

实验研究方面，任树军等观察了补肾健脾益气法(鹿角胶、龟板、生黄芪、白术、当归、熟地黄等)对酒精性骨质疏松(AOP)大鼠小肠组织内维生素D受体(VDR)mRNA表达的影响，结果显示高浓度白酒灌胃大鼠16周后VDR mRNA表达水平明显下降，补肾健脾益气法可以上调该模型小肠组织内VDR mRNA表达。高峰等利用基因芯片技术探究淫羊藿苷治疗去势大鼠骨质疏松症的分子机制，制作去卵巢大鼠模型，随机分为两组各10只，治疗组予以淫羊藿苷灌胃，13周后应用基因芯片技术检测淫羊藿苷治疗后去势骨质疏松症大鼠与模型骨质疏松症大鼠相关基因的表达，通过Gene Ontology数据库对差异表达基因进行基因信息学分析。结果显示，淫羊藿苷治疗去势大鼠骨质疏松症共有532条基因发生了差异表达，其中有175条基因上调，357条基因下调。提示多种基因差异表达是淫羊藿苷治疗去势大鼠骨质疏松症的可能分子机制。

(李晨光)

【骨性关节炎的治疗及实验研究】

闫立将60例髌股关节炎患者随机分为两组，分别采用六步理筋手法治疗和电针治疗，结合股四头肌功能锻炼，两组均每周3次，10次为1个疗程。结果发现六步手法和电针治疗均能有效缓解髌股关节骨关节炎的症状，治疗后半年随访，两组VAS评分均明显下降，且以手法组为著(均$P<0.01$)。王玉龙等将101例患者随机分为治疗组52例与对照组49例，分别给予旋牵过伸法加展筋乳(天南星、透骨草、威灵仙、白芷、延胡索、没药等)和单纯旋牵过伸法治疗，20次后观察并评价临床疗效。结果发现两组的临床优良率分别为88.5%(46/52)、67.3%(33/49)($P<0.05$)；治疗后3个月的随访优良率分别为86.5%(45/52)、55.1%(27/49)($P<0.01$)。王文岳等采用随机双盲多中心安慰剂平行对照的研究方法，将480例患者随机分为芎灵消增贴(威灵仙、赤芍药、乳香、没药、木鳖子、蓖麻子等)组360例和安慰剂组120例，经治1周，以Lequesne MG指数和VAS作为疗效评价指标。结果基于Lequesne MG指数评估，芎灵消增贴组总有效率为67.5%(243/360)，安

慰剂组为 28.3%(34/120),组间比较,$P<0.05$;芍灵消增贴组及安慰剂组 Lequesne MG 指数总评分及 VAS 疼痛评分均明显下降且以前者为著(均$P<0.05$)。

实验研究方面,杜江等以切除卵巢法建立骨性关节炎(OA)大鼠模型,并给予龟鹿二仙胶方及其拆方干预 2、4、8 周后,采用免疫组化法观察关节软骨中 Bax 与 Bcl-2 的表达。结果发现龟鹿二仙胶、龟甲加鹿角、龟鹿加人参、龟鹿加枸杞子和盐酸氨基葡萄糖均可抑制模型大鼠软骨细胞 Bax 的表达,并促进 Bcl-2 的表达,龟鹿二仙胶与龟鹿加枸杞效果相当,且优于龟甲加鹿角和龟鹿加人参。方策等采用 Hulth 造模法建立 OA 模型,造模后肌注青霉素 1 周,预防感染,4 周后灌胃给予健骨活血丸(三七、血竭、人工虎骨粉、红花、当归、川芎等)治疗,6 周后取关节液和血清,测定 TNF-α 水平。结果发现中药组关节液和血清中 TNF-α 明显低于对照组($P<0.01$)。李宁等以切除卵巢法制备肾虚型膝骨性关节炎大鼠模型,随机分为模型组、假手术组和益肾通痹方(炙黄芪、白芍药、熟地黄、山萸肉、炙龟板、鹿角片等)低、中、高剂量组和盐酸氨基葡萄糖片组,待模型成功后模型组和假手术组灌服生理盐水,给药组灌服相应的药物,灌胃 1 个月后腹主动脉采血,检测各组大鼠血清 MDA、NO、T-SOD 及 E2 的水平。结果显示,与模型组、假手术组比较,益肾通痹方各组、盐酸氨基葡萄糖片组大鼠血清 MDA、NO 均降低、T-SOD、E2 均增高,以中剂量组较为显著。与模型组比较,$P<0.01$,$P<0.05$。

(梁倩倩)

【颈椎病的治疗与研究】

颜大荃等采用定点复位配合牵引治疗神经根型颈椎病 150 例,定点复位采用旋转提推法或定点小角度托抖法,牵引治疗采用卧位牵引,重量从 6 kg 起持续牵引 20 min,重量逐日增加,最高可达 18 kg,牵引时颈部垫小圆枕并调整不同的枕垫位置而达到不同位置的牵引力。牵引上位颈椎把小圆枕垫于颈胸段,牵引下位颈椎小圆枕向头项部靠近。治疗时先牵引后复位,1 次/d,7 次为 1 疗程,治疗 3 个疗程,每个疗程间隔 2~3 d,治疗结束后 3 个月随访并评估疗效。结果总有效率为 93.3%(140/150)。梁允青等采用推拿、牵引(每日 1~2 次,15 d 为 1 个疗程)及运动等综合疗法治疗混合型颈椎病 338 例,总有效率为 98.5%(333/338)。张楷利采用综合疗法治疗神经根型颈椎病 118 例,内服辨证用药,风寒湿型用羌活胜湿汤加减(羌活、独活、蔓荆子、藁本、防风、川芎等),气滞血瘀型用身痛逐瘀汤加减(牛膝、地龙、香附、秦艽、川芎、桃仁等),气血虚弱型用独活寄生汤合黄芪桂枝五物汤加减(独活、桑寄生、秦艽、防风、细辛、川芎等);中药离子导入用羌活、独活、红花、制川乌、制草乌、蜈蚣等;针灸用电针或穴位注射,取穴夹脊、曲池、外关、风池、合谷、阿是穴等,穴位注射用维生素 B_1 或复方当归注射液;颈椎牵引取坐位,头前倾 15 度角,牵引重量为2~5 kg,每次 30 min,1 次/d,7 次为 1 个疗程。结果总有效率为 93.2%(110/118)。董博等用颈痛消胶囊(黄芪、桂枝、天麻、钩藤、葛根、乳香等)治疗神经根型颈椎病 120 例,7 d 为 1 个疗程,平均治疗 32 d。结果总有效率为 91.7%(110/120)。

万小明等将 60 例椎动脉型颈椎病患者随机等分为两组,中医综合治疗组予颈健方(当归、川芎、葛根、桂枝、田三七、红花等)配合热敏灸(灸百会、风池、颈夹脊、百劳、大椎穴)及佩戴颈围,对照组服西比灵。连续治疗 2 周后观察两组患者临床症状改善情况及椎基底动脉经颅多普勒(TCD)血流变化情况以评定疗效。结果有效率治疗组为 96.7%(29/30),对照组为 80.0%(24/30),组间比较,$P<0.05$。孙岩等将颈椎不稳症患者随机分为两组各 50 例,治疗组采用 Triton 牵引器卧位变角间歇性牵引结合颈椎手法治疗,对照组采用传统颈椎牵引器坐位垂直连续牵引结合颈椎手法治疗,两组均 1 次/d,5 d 为 1 个疗程,共 3 个疗程,疗程间隔 1 d。结果总有效率治疗组为 94.0%(47/50),对照组为 72.0%(36/50),组间比较,$P<0.01$。白翠先等将 102 例椎动脉型颈椎病患者随机分为两组,治疗组 52 例服银杏叶片及颈舒颗粒;对照组 50 例仅给予颈舒颗粒,两组均辅助行颈椎牵引,疗程为 1 个月。以症状改善及血流变检查为疗效评价指标,总有效率治疗组为 96.2%(50/52),对照组为 68.0%(34/50),组间比较,$P<0.05$;两组治疗后全血黏度、血浆黏度均明显下降且以治疗组为著($P<0.01$,$P<0.05$)。桂志雄等将寰枢关节半脱位患者随机均分为两组,治疗组用颈椎牵引摇正调整法治疗,对照组常规牵引。1 次/d,10 次为 1 个疗程。结果

总有效率治疗组为 98.0%(49/50),对照组为70.0%(35/50),组间比较,$P<0.01$。赵赫等将痹痛型颈椎病患者随机均分为两组,治疗组服抗骨关节丸(熟地黄、鹿茸、肉苁蓉、淫羊藿、狗脊、续断等),对照组服颈复康颗粒。经治 2 周,总有效率治疗组为 96.7%(58/60),对照组为 83.3%(50/60),组间比较,$P<0.01$。

李泽佳等提出了基于"治未病"思想探讨椎动脉型颈椎病的防治思路,认为对于椎动脉型颈椎病的防治应树立"以预防为主、防治重心前移"的思想导向。邓素玲等对孙树椿的颈椎病防治思想进行了研讨,对孙氏的"动、静力失衡的发病说","从筋入手的'解'结治疗说","动静结合的未病'防结'说"等作了总结。张董喆探讨了张建福的治疗经验,提出采用提牵旋转法配合内服颈痹舒筋汤(葛根、当归、川芎、鸡血藤、川乌、草乌等)与颈椎功能锻炼治疗颈椎病。

(崔学军)

【腰椎间盘突出症的治疗与研究】

陈焕龄等将腰椎间盘突出症寒湿瘀血型患者随机均分成两组,治疗组予腰骨痹痛汤(丹参、当归、蜈蚣、乌梢蛇、木瓜、杜仲等)治疗,对照组以西医常规保守疗法(牵引配合扶他林、腰痛宁、布洛芬口服)。均以 1 个月为 1 个疗程,显效不佳者共治 3 个疗程,观察治疗前后疼痛及功能障碍改善变化。结果总有效率治疗组为 97.7%(130/133),对照组为 75.9%(101/133)。组间比较,$P<0.05$。夏铎等将重型腰椎间盘突出症患者随机分为两组,治疗组用腰痹舒汤(独活、白附子、鸡血藤、蜈蚣、地龙、熟地黄等),服药后散步及做松弛腰部的活动操;对照组采用牵引、按摩法,配合西乐葆口服。经治 15 d,总有效率治疗组为96.7%(233/241),对照组为 87.6%(170/194),组间比较,$P<0.05$。

李选民将 192 名腰椎间盘突出症患者随机分为两组,治疗组采用补肾活血类中药(桑寄生、伸筋草、鸡血藤、巴戟天、地龙、当归等)配合推拿牵引等外治法治疗,对照组采用传统牵引疗法。经治 30 d,总有效率治疗组为 81.3%(78/96),对照组为 50.0%(48/96)。组间比较,$P<0.05$。李华南等将 300 例腰椎间盘突出症患者随机分为恢复期应用组、缓解期应用组、传统推拿组和西药组。恢复期应用组:急性期采用中药熏蒸、湿敷(海桐皮、透骨草、乳香、没药、当归、花椒等)、中药敷贴(消瘀止痛膏)治疗,缓解期采用软组织放松类手法配合牵引治疗,恢复期采用整复类手法配合牵引和功能锻炼操;缓解期应用组:在缓解期应用整复手法治疗;传统推拿组:在急性、缓解、恢复期中均用整复类手法治疗,其余治疗同恢复期应用组;西药组各期均口服萘丁美酮片,并在急性期静脉滴注神经妥乐平,缓解期配合牵引治疗,恢复期配合牵引和功能锻炼操。均以 30 d 为 1 个疗程,疗程结束后 6 个月随访并观察复发率。结果恢复期应用组总有效率为 98.6(71/72),缓解期应用组为 89.2%(66/74),传统推拿组为 77.5%(55/71),西药组为 75.4%(52/69),恢复期应用组与其他 3 组比较,均$P<0.05$;缓解期应用组、传统推拿组和西药组比较,均$P>0.05$。各组治疗后,静脉血 NO、IL-6 水平及症状、肌骨彩超评分均明显下降,表面肌电频率值均明显升高(均$P<0.05$),恢复期应用组、缓解期应有组 NO、IL-6 水平均低于传统推拿组和西药组(均$P<0.05$);恢复期应用组症状评分、肌骨彩超评分均低于其他 3 组,表面肌电频率值均高于其他 3 组(均$P<0.05$)。提示整复手法恢复期应用可以作为治疗腰椎间盘突出症的优选方案。张德元将腰椎间盘突出症患者随机分为两组,治疗组 200 例运用中药专利方剂(杜仲、续断、肉苁蓉、怀牛膝、狗脊、伸筋草等)联合物理疗法(三维慢速牵引、超短波治疗及电脑中频治疗),对照组仅用物理治疗。经治 14 d,总有效率分别为 97.0%(194/200)、92.0%(92/100)。

许金海等运用聚类分析探讨和总结了施杞治疗腰椎间盘突出症的学术思想和临床用药规律。有 272 份医案纳入研究,共计就诊 428 人次;共用药物 173 味,出现的总频次为 9 623,常用中药有白芍药、柴胡、川芎、当归等 27 味;益气活血药、补肾助阳药、祛风解表药、利水渗湿药、化痰通络药和健脾理气和胃药为常用配伍药类;圣愈汤、身痛逐瘀汤、独活寄生汤、苓桂术甘汤等为基本方药。李具宝等总结和分析近 10 年国内医学期刊公开发表的中药内服治疗腰椎间盘突出症文献中特殊中药的应用现状,发现最终有效文献为 654 篇,中药内服治疗腰椎间盘突出症特殊用药前 20 位的药物排序依次为:桃仁、红花、乳香、没药、玄胡、川乌、草乌、蕲蛇、土鳖虫、三七、细辛、附子、马钱子、骨碎补、血竭、蜈蚣、蚤休、乌梢蛇、龟甲、蛰虫;药物功效分类依次为:活血止痛、活血调经、祛风寒湿、活血疗伤、化瘀止血、发散风寒、息风止痉、补阴、温里、破血消癥药。提示瘀血致痛在腰椎间盘突出症的病机中占有重要的地位。

(叶　洁　许金海)

[附] 参考文献

A

艾尼瓦尔·艾力,庞渊,李岩.经皮椎体后凸成形术结合中药治疗骨质疏松性胸腰椎压缩性骨折(附44例报告)[J].新疆中医药,2013,31(2):17

B

白翠先,白建兰.银杏叶联合颈舒颗粒治疗椎动脉型颈椎病的临床研究[J].中国中医骨伤科杂志,2013,21(8):43

C

柴政.伤科接骨片治疗慢性腰肌劳损35例治疗体会[J].内蒙古中医药,2013,32(14):91

陈焕龄,张辉耀,何云贵.腰骨痹痛汤治疗腰椎间盘突出症寒湿瘀血型266例[J].中医临床研究,2013,5(10):12

陈继征,周瑜博,董振宇,等.椎体成形术结合中药内服治疗女性绝经期胸腰椎骨质疏松性骨折的临床疗效分析[J].浙江中医药大学学报,2013,37(7):869

陈宇,韩清民.固定器结合中医药治疗高龄股骨粗隆间骨折70例疗效分析[J].新中医,2013,45(1):69

程嗣鹤.自拟补肾活血祛痹方为主综合治疗腰肌劳损临床观察[J].中医药临床杂志,2013,25(4):323

楚德升,崔改琴,王海燕.手法联合活动牵引治疗劳损性上腰痛120例[J].中医研究,2013,26(5):72

D

邓素玲,李沛.浅论孙氏对颈椎病的防治思想[J].中国中医骨伤科杂志,2013,21(6):63

董博,袁普卫,姚洁,等.颈痛消胶囊治疗神经根型颈椎病120例[J].中国中医骨伤科杂志,2013,21(3):49

董森,陈祖平,李辉.手法复位超掌指关节夹板超腕关节夹板序贯固定治疗桡骨远端骨折[J].中医正骨,2013,25(7):16

杜海峡,肖文庆,程立军,等.局部封闭加臭氧注射治疗肩周炎的疗效观察[J].中国中医骨伤科杂志,2013,21(7):35

杜江,黄远鹏,李奕修,等.龟鹿二仙胶及其拆方对去势骨关节炎大鼠关节软骨中Bax和Bcl-2的影响[J].中国中医骨伤科杂志,2013,21(3):4

F

樊新甫,彭俊宇,杨礼跃.椎体后凸成形术配合中药治疗老年骨质疏松压缩性骨折的临床研究[J].中医药临床杂志,2013,25(5):414

方策,宋德为,刘元禄.健骨活血丸对骨性关节炎模型兔关节液和血清中TNF-α表达的影响[J].中国中医骨伤科杂志,2013,21(5):12

方金锋.中西医结合治疗老年骨质疏松临床疗效观察[J].世界中西医结合杂志,2013,8(8):809

方铁根,熊常初.中医传统特色疗法结合现代仪器综合治疗腰肌劳损的临床研究[J].光明中医,2013,28(3):532

冯晓琳,任晓晓,刘建武.拔罐疗法治疗肩周炎不同证型的临床疗效观察[J].实用中西医结合临床,2013,13(4):6

G

高峰,莫新民,李劲平.淫羊藿苷治疗去势大鼠骨质疏松症基因表达谱分析[J].中国中医药信息杂志,2013,20(2):43

高明月,吕爱平.从肾论治骨质疏松症证治规律的现代病案分析[J].中华中医药学刊,2013,31(7):1567

高晓珺,张子峰,马丹军.补肾健骨汤配合西药治疗老年骨质疏松性胸腰椎压缩性骨折54例[J].陕西中医,2013,34(5):567

高艳平.止痛活血汤联合针刺治疗急性腰扭伤41例临床观察[J].河北中医,2013,35(6):820

桂志雄,万子超,简俊峰,等.颈椎牵引摇正调整法治疗寰枢关节半脱位100例[J].中国中医骨伤科杂志,2013,21(4):40

郭天旻,王拥军,李浩钢,等.石氏牛蒡子汤加减治疗颈椎病211例[J].中国中医药现代远程教育,2013,11(13):20

H

赫军,李丽华,任晓晓,等.柳豆叶合蠲痹汤治疗肩周炎30例临床观察[J].江苏中医药,2013,45(1):44

胡阳广,王才立,田庆显.复元活血汤加味治疗阳虚

型胸腰椎骨折后腹胀便秘临床疗效和安全性[J]. 中华中医药学刊，2013，31(4)：767

黄献京. 中医治疗单纯性腰椎压缩性骨折 32 例[J]. 河南中医，2013，33(7)：1104

J

冀沛峰，钱龙江. 复方风湿宁片治疗肩关节周围炎 40 例[J]. 河南中医，2013，33(9)：1504

蒋顺琬，马笃军，麦庆春，等. 参附注射液液压扩张治疗冻结肩的临床研究及其血清 MMP-9 表达[J]. 内蒙古中医药，2013，32(15)：15

蒋卫方. 鹿瓜多肽注射液配合中药治疗老年胸腰椎压缩性骨折 52 例[J]. 中医药导报，2013，19(6)：94

L

蓝仕. 独活寄生汤加味合壮医药线点灸治疗腰肌劳损 100 例[J]. 内蒙古中医药，2013，32(17)：11

黎勇，张振山. 3 种手术方法治疗 EvansⅣ型股骨粗隆间骨折疗效比较[J]. 现代中西医结合杂志，2013，22(22)：2439

李东涛，李富玉，王剑，等. 骨质疏松症中医证候疗效评价方法研究[J]. 中医杂志，2013，54(13)：1110

李富龙，史晓，施丹，等. 五行健骨操对骨质疏松症患者平衡能力的影响[J]. 上海中医药大学学报，2013，27(3)：58

李华南，王金贵，孙庆，等. 整复手法治疗腰椎间盘突出症最佳应用时机的多中心随机对照研究[J]. 中医杂志，2013，54(13)：1122

李具宝，熊启良，亓峰，等. 近 10 年文献中特殊中药治疗腰椎间盘突出症的用药规律探讨[J]. 中国中医骨伤科杂志，2013，21(6)：27

李宁，王拥军，施杞. 益肾通痹方对肾虚型大鼠膝骨性关节炎血清 MDA、NO、T-SOD、E2 的影响[J]. 中国中医骨伤科杂志，2013，21(2)：1

李兰山，王明喜，孙鲁. 手法整复夹板外固定与切开复位钢板内固定治疗伸直型桡骨远端骨折对比研究[J]. 实用中医药杂志，2013，29(11)：939

李选民. 补肾活血方配合牵引疗法治疗腰椎间盘突出症 96 例[J]. 陕西中医，2013，34(3)：314

李泽佳，宋敏，唐宝明. 基于"治未病"思想探讨椎动脉型颈椎病的防治思路[J]. 中国中医骨伤科杂志，2013，21(3)：64

梁伟东，熊莉华. 从代谢组学角度论糖尿病骨质疏松的中医研究[J]. 中国中医药信息杂志，2013，20(7)：5

梁允青，梁允霞，徐琨. 综合疗法治疗混合型颈椎病 338 例[J]. 中国民间疗法，2013，21(7)：28

刘方. 理气活血法治疗胸腰椎骨折并发腹胀 34 例临床观察[J]. 国医论坛，2013，28(1)：32

刘彦，蒋宜伟，梁恬，等. 宋敏教授骨质疏松症学术经验撷萃[J]. 中国中医骨伤科杂志，2013，21(8)：64

龙开娥，周松成. 龙氏驳骨膏配合手法复位小夹板固定治疗老年稳定型桡骨远端骨折的疗效观察[J]. 中国民族医药杂志，2013，19(9)：10

卢永勇. 中西医结合治疗单纯性腰椎压缩性骨折 32 例[J]. 河南中医，2013，33(9)：1542

卢致顺，张育志，李艳萍，等. 中医结合锁定钢板治疗老年性股骨粗隆间粉碎性骨折[J]. 光明中医，2013，28(1)：146

罗巨利，周长征，郑凤萍. 活血安痛酒经离子定向导入治疗腰肌劳损的临床观察[J]. 中医药导报，2013，19(2)：43

P

彭运飞. 小针刀配合截血膏外敷治疗腰骶关节劳损 52 例[J]. 中国民族民间医药，2013，22(10)：139

Q

秦洪，梁爱军，钱文亮. 牵引夹板治疗骨折时橡皮筋拉伸和应力松弛测试[J]. 中国组织工程研究，2013，17(13)：2352

秦磊，朱一鹏. 老年骨质疏松股骨粗隆间骨折 2 种内固定方法的应用分析[J]. 现代中西医结合杂志，2013，22(21)：2352

邱继明，陈春华. 手法复位联合土家药活血接骨膏外敷治疗桡骨远端骨折[J]. 中国中医急症，2013，22(8)：1306

R

任树军，邢国利，葛明富，等. 补肾健脾益气法对酒精性骨质疏松大鼠小肠中 VDR-mRNA 表达影响的研究[J]. 中医药信息，2013，30(2)：46

S

沈俊玲. 自拟方联合 PVP 治疗老年骨质疏松性胸腰椎骨折临床观察[J]. 新中医，2013，45(2)：66

石宝营，苏艳美. 痛点针刀松解结合肩关节回转手法治疗肩关节周围炎 85 例[J]. 中国中医骨伤科杂志，2013，21(8)：50

孙启涛，孙鲁. 小夹板治疗老年桡骨远端骨折 120 例[J]. 菏泽医学专科学校学报，2013，25(4)：52

孙岩，张莹莹，施锋. Triton 牵引器结合颈椎手法治疗下颈椎不稳症疗效观察[J]. 中国中医骨伤科杂志，2013，21(5)：41

W

万小明，杨阳，刘碧峰，等. 椎动脉型颈椎病中医综合

治疗的临床体会[J]. 中国中医骨伤科杂志,2013,21(2):32

汪宝军,王竹风. PFNA内固定联合中药治疗老年股骨粗隆间骨折疗效观察[J]. 北京中医药,2013,32(5):377

王桂茂,纪清,沈利龙,等. 手法配合肌肉力量技术治疗训练性下腰痛的应用评价[J]. 现代中西医结合杂志,2013,22(22):2407

王汉龙,赖展龙,柯晓斌,等. 中医保守治疗胸腰椎压缩骨折453例[J]. 现代中西医结合杂志,2013,22(1):76

王利民. 小夹板治疗桡骨远端骨折并尺骨茎突骨折60例[J]. 河南外科学杂志,2013,19(5):99

王文岳,谢利民,张跃,等. 芍灵消增贴治疗骨性关节炎(肝肾不足、瘀血阻络证)的疗效及安全性评价[J]. 中国中医骨伤科杂志,2013,21(6):21

王玉龙,王平,刘爱峰,等. 旋牵过伸法配合展筋乳治疗肱骨外上髁炎52例[J]. 中国中医骨伤科杂志,2013,21(7):13

王小刚,张自强,祁文兵,等. 活血通便汤治疗屈曲型腰椎压缩骨折早期并腹胀、便秘体会[J]. 中医临床研究,2013,5(7):73

吴霖贤,陈长青,庄子颖,等. 椎旁肌入路内固定结合中药熏洗治疗胸腰椎骨折的临床疗效分析[J]. 中国中医骨伤科杂志,2013,21(2):39

吴旭辉. 人工股骨头置换、动力髋螺钉、解剖型钢板固定治疗老年股骨粗隆间骨折的疗效分析[J]. 中国现代医药杂志,2013,15(3):42

吴洋,张剑,顾玲丽. 寒立消贴敷剂治疗风寒湿痹型肩周炎的临床研究[J]. 光明中医,2013,28(9):1879

X

夏铎,李晓声,陈铁柱. 腰痹舒汤治疗重型腰椎间盘突出症241例临床观察[J]. 中医药导报,2013,19(4):19

谢延华,蔡国雄,王爱民,等. 两种方法治疗小儿肱骨髁上骨折的疗效比较[J]. 新中医,2013,45(5):145

徐世平,孙书龙,张弘,等. 龚正丰治疗颈型颈椎病经验[J]. 河南中医,2013,33(6):865

许金海,邬学群,叶洁,等. 基于聚类分析的施杞教授治疗腰椎间盘突出症的用药规律研究[J]. 中国中医骨伤科杂志,2013,21(3):20

许坤,张洪. 老年性痴呆与骨质疏松症相关联系[J]. 辽宁中医药大学学报,2013,15(8):165

Y

颜大荃,冯前,梁恒晔. 定点复位配合牵引治疗神经根型颈椎病150例[J]. 中国中医骨伤科杂志,2013,21(1):46

闫立,梁朝,温建民,等. 六步理筋手法治疗早期髌股关节骨性关节炎[J]. 中国中医骨伤科杂志,2013,21(1):28

杨鸫祥,李洪久,姚啸生,等. DHS结合中药治疗高龄股骨粗隆间骨折患者疗效分析[J]. 辽宁中医药大学学报,2013,15(4):170

杨杰保,潘子毅. 玻璃酸钠联合中药综合治疗肩关节周围炎25例[J]. 浙江中西医结合杂志,2013,23(9):761

杨军,张小莉,莫新民. 从蛋白质组学研究壮骨止痛方治疗骨质疏松症作用机理[J]. 辽宁中医药大学学报,2013,15(11):35

杨利学,邵松涛,王官林,等. 当归注射液预防椎板切除术后硬膜外粘连的实验研究[J]. 中国中医骨伤科杂志,2013,21(4):4

杨林平. 臂丛神经阻滞手法松解联合中药治疗肩关节周围炎临床研究[J]. 中医学报,2013,28(1):144

杨少锋,剑锋,陈青,等. 金刚健骨片对骨质疏松症去卵巢大鼠整合素αvβ6受体水平作用的影响[J]. 中国中医骨伤科杂志,2013,21(6):1

阳煦,安嘉懿,孔建,等. 黄芪桂枝五物汤联合按摩手法治疗肩周炎80例[J]. 陕西中医,2013,34(9):1148

叶朝辉,韩军伟,代根奇. 椎体成形术配合中医药辨证治疗老年性椎体压缩性骨折[J]. 中国民族民间医药,2013,22(9):103

院建生. 当归四逆汤加减治疗肩关节周围炎32例[J]. 河南中医,2013,33(8):1220

Z

曾科学,盖娟娟. 曾氏太极推拿治疗慢性腰肌劳损30例临床观察[J]. 云南中医中药杂志,2013,34(2):38

郑艳,孙云松. 127例慢性萎缩性胃炎伴骨质疏松症的中医证候分布回顾性分析[J]. 中国中医药信息杂志,2013,20(9):13

张德元. 中药专利方剂联合物理疗法治疗腰椎间盘突出症200例临床观察[J]. 中医药导报,2013,19(7):21

张董喆. 张建福教授治疗颈椎病的经验[J]. 中医正骨,2013,25(4):71

张楷利. 综合疗法治疗神经根型颈椎病118例疗效观察[J]. 国医论坛,2013,28(1):27

张绍文,李盛华,樊成虎. 中西医结合保守治疗胸腰椎骨折470例临床疗效观察[J]. 西部中医药,2013,26(5):108

章竞峰. 消瘀通络熏条治疗肩周炎的临床疗效观察

[J]. 黑龙江中医药,2013,42(1):10

赵赫,梁玉香. 抗骨关节丸治疗痹痛型颈椎病 120 例[J]. 光明中医,2013,28(5):928

周叶,洪鸣鸣. 1 333 名居民骨质疏松知识调查[J]. 浙江中西医结合杂志,2013,23(4):328

庄汝杰,陈冠军,庄伟. 腰椎终板 ModicⅠ型面积改变率与慢性下腰痛之间的相关性研究[J]. 中医正骨,2013,25(5):17

(九) 五 官 科

【概述】

2013年,公开发表的五官科论文约1 200篇,其中眼科约占41%,主要集中于视网膜病、内眼病、角膜病、视神经病及外眼病的治疗及实验研究;耳科约占10%,多集中于耳聋、梅尼埃病、中耳炎等的治疗及实验研究;鼻科约占21%,多集中于慢性鼻炎、变应性鼻炎、鼻窦炎等的治疗及实验研究;咽喉科约占11%,多集中于慢性咽炎、声带疾病等的治疗及实验研究;口腔科约占17%,多集中于口腔黏膜及舌齿疾病的治疗。

1. 眼科疾病

(1) 视网膜病　李军等将109例视网膜脱离术后视网膜下积液患者随机分为两组,均予常规静滴抗感染药物,局部点复方托吡酰胺滴眼液、妥布霉素地塞米松滴眼液等,治疗组61例加服中药(党参、枸杞子、丹参、赤芍药、白芍药、覆盆子等)。均于术后第1 d始,连续治疗10 d,视网膜下积液吸收总有效率分别为85.2%(52/61)、66.7%(32/48),组间比较,$P<0.05$。

江伟等探讨明睛颗粒(生蒲黄、墨旱莲、女贞子、丹参等)干预实验性脉络膜新生血管(CNV)模型兔的药效及作用机制。研究结果显示,明睛颗粒高、中、低剂量均能减少眼底荧光渗漏的面积($P<0.05$),对眼底组织病变有保护作用,中剂量组效果最明显。巨噬细胞参与了CNV形成,以Ⅰ型为主,明睛颗粒可诱导巨噬细胞向Ⅱ型转化。

田楠楠等、张庆等研究显示,驻景方加减(楮实子、枸杞子、菟丝子、五味子、三七等)通过滋补肝肾活血通络的功效增加眼部血液循环,改善局部缺血缺氧状况,从而抑制氪激光诱导的豚鼠病理性近视CNV模型中血管内皮生长因子(VEGF)的表达,达到抑制CNV形成的作用。临床上对高度近视眼底病变或干性老年黄斑变性等患者予该方剂,可有助于预防CNV的形成。

张花治等研究表明,原花青素(PC)可上调视网膜缺血—再灌注(RIR)损伤后大鼠视网膜中的Bcl-2蛋白表达,并下调Bax蛋白的表达,据此推测PC可能通过抑制视网膜神经节细胞凋亡的启动,对RIR损伤后的视网膜视神经起到保护作用。刘莹等研究表明,PC对大鼠RIR损伤视网膜的超微结构具有很好的防护作用,并可能通过抑制氧自由基的活性而间接抑制核转录因子-κB(NF-κB)的活化,从而阻断了NF-κB所诱导细胞因子表达的反应链,起到保护视网膜的作用。

视网膜静脉阻塞的治疗及实验研究、糖尿病性视网膜病变的治疗及实验研究、年龄相关性黄斑变性的治疗与研究等均已列专条介绍。

(2) 内眼病　解孝锋等将329例葡萄膜炎患者随机分为两组,均予妥布霉素地塞米松滴眼液、普南普灵眼水及散瞳等西药;中西医结合治疗组167例予辨证分型、中成药、院内制剂、中药熏洗、离子透入、中药注射剂、中药眼用凝胶等综合治疗。对重症病例,明显影响视功能时,视病情予泼尼松免疫抑制剂口服。急性期每2周为1个疗程,观察3个月;慢性期1个月为1个疗程,观察6个月。中西医结合组的总体疗效及视力的提高明显优于西药组,总体复发率明显低于西药组。高延娥等将46例52眼慢性前葡萄膜炎患者随机分为两组,均予散瞳、糖皮质激素及非甾体抗炎药局部点眼、热敷,严重者全身用糖皮质激素和非甾体抗炎药,同时对感染性患者予以敏感的抗感染药物治疗,炎症顽固者予以免疫抑制剂治疗,待症状缓解后,逐步减少药物用量;治疗组24例27眼予辨证(湿热内蕴型、虚火上炎型)施治,随访6个月,中西医结合治疗组有效率明显优于对照组。

冯俊等对以唐由之发明的睫状体平坦部滤过术治疗的73例78眼各类青光眼患者眼压变化、视力变化并对术中及术后并发症进行总结,患者视力保持稳定的占88.5%(69/78),患眼眼压较术前明显下降($P<0.01$),一定程度上改善了视功能,特别是对恶性青光眼的手术成功率较高,手术安全性良好。李诺等研究提示,白蒺藜皂苷能有效提高慢性高眼压下兔视网膜中SOD活性,降低MDA含量,从而对持续性高眼压视网膜氧化应激具有保护作用。并能降低高眼压兔的全血黏度和血浆黏度,可能是其发挥青光眼视神经保护作用的途径之一。

(3) 角膜病　关瑞娟等将160例复发性单纯疱疹病毒性角膜炎患者(HSK)平分为两组，均予0.15%更昔洛韦眼用凝胶局部点眼，治疗组加服黄芪桂枝口服液(生黄芪、炒白术、防风、桂枝、蒲公英、金银花等)。患者均检测治疗前后外周血T淋巴细胞亚群比例。经治4周，随访6个月(失访14例)，治疗组与对照组复发眼率分别为9.5%(7/74)、27.8%(20/72)，治疗组患者CD_3^+、CD_4^+ T细胞明显升高($P<0.05$)，CD_8^+ T细胞下降，CD_4^+/CD_8^+比值明显升高($P<0.05$)，IL-18、IFN-γ含量较治疗前明显升高；而对照组T淋巴细胞、白细胞介素(IL)-18、干扰素(IFN)-γ含量较治疗前无明显变化(均$P>0.05$)。

聂爱芹等研究表明，玉屏风散具有提高HSK潜伏期(PI28 d)和复发期(UVB3 d)模型小鼠体内CD_3^+、CD_4^+ T细胞表达，降低CD_8^+ T细胞表达，改善CD_4^+/CD_8^+比值水平，调节机体细胞免疫功能的作用。

(4) 外眼病　宋剑涛等研究表明，高、中、低剂量川椒方(知母、地肤子、川椒、防风等)组均能减轻模型小鼠眼睑和结膜水肿充血。其体征评分均较模型组降低($P<0.01$，$P<0.05$)，与奥洛他定滴眼液组接近($P>0.05$)。川椒方各剂量组及奥洛他定滴眼液组的血清IL-4、JAK激酶1(JAK1)、信号转导和转录激活因子6(STAT6)含量均低于模型组($P<0.01$，$P<0.05$)。提示川椒方能减轻过敏性结膜炎小鼠的眼部体征并可能抑制IL 4-JAK1-STAT6信号通路的激活。

陈美荣等研究表明，视明宝颗粒(补益肝肾类中药)可以改善猫斜视性弱视造成的视皮层17区及21a区的损害，中、高剂量组明显，其机制可能与中药加速基因的复制转录过程，加快蛋白质的合成，增加突触的形成，增强突触的可塑性，促进细胞代谢及损伤神经元的恢复有关。

此外，对视神经萎缩的治疗、干眼症的治疗及实验研究见专条。郭俊国等追踪近年来代谢组学的国内外研究进展，在对代谢组学概述的基础上，就代谢组学在中西医结合眼科研究中的应用与展望进行综述，并认为随着研究方法的不断改进、分析技术的进一步提高，代谢组学朝着整合化、自动化和高通量的方向发展，在疾病诊断方面将会有更大的突破和发展，对眼科疾病的研究，将开启科学性和定量化研究的新水平。

2. 耳科疾病

(1) 耳鸣耳聋　突发性耳聋的治疗与研究已立专条。李胜利等对工业噪声致感音神经性耳聋豚鼠予复聪汤Ⅰ号口服液(桃仁、穿山甲、红花、川芎、黄芪、莱菔子等)口服和复聪剂Ⅱ号滴耳液(冰片、茯苓、桂圆、麝香等)耳浴30 d后，80%的豚鼠ABR反应阈值恢复到30到40 d BSPL，DPOAE幅值有较明显提高；耳蜗铺片和电镜观察显示，耳蜗毛细胞数目有一定恢复，组织结构有修复现象，再生毛细胞仅出现少量纤毛，而未治疗噪声对照组无此种现象；治疗60 d时，耳蜗毛细胞数目明显增多，Corti器的毛细胞区，有大量的增殖细胞出现，扫描电镜可见成小束的新生纤毛出现在毛细胞缺失部位，同时支持细胞大量增殖；到治疗90 d时，再生的静纤毛束已基本形成，尤其是耳蜗基底部位的毛细胞明显增多，听功能已基本正常。茅犁春等研究显示，天麻提取液天麻素对豚鼠噪声性损伤有一定的预防作用，其机制可能是保护细胞膜稳定并增加耳蜗毛细胞琥珀酸脱氢酶活性，从而增加细胞能量供应改善耳蜗微循环。

宣伟军等研究显示，复方健耳剂(黄芪、女贞子、丹参、郁金、绞股蓝、何首乌等)通过提高小鼠耳蜗组织脑源性神经营养因子(BDNF)表达，具有对抗小鼠老年性耳蜗毛细胞、螺旋神经节神经元凋亡及疆孔神经纤维退变作用。其作用机制可能是促进与酪氨酸蛋白激酶B(TrkB)结合，发挥Ras-MAPK信号转导途径生物学效应；促进谷光甘肽过氧化物酶活性，或核酸代谢等；降低半胱氨酸天冬酶-3(caspase-3)的活性而抑制细胞凋亡进程。

贾琳琳等研究显示，刺五加注射液对外源性谷氨酸所致的豚鼠耳毒性具有拮抗作用，其机制可能为通过改变血流变、促进血液微循环、增加红细胞变形能力、加速血流，从而使过量的外源性谷氨酸得以较快的扩散，减轻对内毛细胞和突触后结构毒性作用。

(2) 中耳炎　徐光等临床研究发现，与健康人对照组比较，分泌性中耳炎患者血清及耳积液HA、白介素水平显著升高，且慢性期患者更为明显($P<0.05$)。其可用于疾病的诊断与治疗监测的指标之一。仲崇玉将280例疗化脓性中耳炎患者随机平分为两组，分别予患耳滴入速效耳净灵(麝香、黄柏、龙胆草、珍珠、连翘、金银花等)、氧氟

沙星滴耳液。经治 3 周,治疗组与对照组治愈率分别为 96.4%(135/140)、70.7%(99/140),组间比较,$P<0.01$。余朝阳等临床研究发现,经治疗后的化脓性中耳炎患者血清及耳分泌物总 IgE、IL-6、IL-8 及 MDA 呈现持续降低的趋势,而 IL-2 及 SOD 则呈现持续升高的趋势,表明其炎性状态在持续改善,其免疫及机体健康状态也呈现持续改善。

3. 鼻科疾病

(1) 变应性鼻炎(AR) 邹建东等将 585 例 AR 肺脾气虚证患者分为三组,试验组 351 例服用五龙颗粒(黄芪、党参、白术、五味子、地龙、枸杞子等),对照组 117 例服用辛芩颗粒和五龙颗粒安慰剂,安慰剂组 117 例服用五龙颗粒安慰剂。经治 7 d,试验组和对照组在鼻痒、喷嚏等单项指标计分的变化均优于安慰剂组($P<0.001$)。晏英等探讨"天人相应"理论对 AR 治疗的临床意义。将 60 例常年性 AR(肺气虚寒、卫表不固型) 患者随机平分为两组,均予益气温阳方(生黄芪、党参、干姜、生麻黄、乌梅、紫草等),根据季节的变化添加不同药物。结果表明,在春季,添加升阳药物组优于添加潜阳药物组($P<0.05$);秋季,添加潜阳药物组优于添加升阳药物组($P<0.05$)。对 AR 的临床与实验研究见专条介绍。

(2) 鼻窦炎 李卓等以鼻炎宁颗粒(主要成分为蜜蜂巢脾)治疗急性鼻窦炎,连续服用 20 d,临床治愈率 15.5%,总有效率 86.2%(100/116)。研究病例中未见不良反应。对慢性鼻窦炎的治疗与研究见专条介绍。

4. 咽喉科疾病

(1) 咽炎 李向宇等与王颖等研究表明,陈皮利咽合剂(陈皮、延胡索、夜交藤、女贞子、合欢皮)大、中、小剂量组干预急性咽炎模型大鼠后,其外周血白细胞数均低于模型组($P<0.01$);大鼠咽部黏膜鳞状上皮、黏膜下结缔组织稍有增生和充血现象明显减轻。其中以中剂量组的作用为最佳。陈皮利咽合剂能改善慢性咽炎家兔咽部黏膜炎症,其作用机制可能与降低全血黏度有关。对慢性咽炎的治疗及实验研究见专条介绍。

(2) 急性化脓性扁桃体炎 刘晓华等将 230 例患者随机平分为两组,均予阿洛西林针静滴,观察组加服万应胶囊(胡黄连、黄连、儿茶、冰片、熊胆、牛黄)、克比奇羚羊角胶囊。5 d 为 1 个疗程,观察组与对照组总有效率分别为 90.4%(104/115)、73.9%(85/115),治疗组在退热、咽部充血消失及脓性分泌物消失时间上均明显短于对照组(均$P<0.01$)。冯文华将 80 例患儿随机平分为两组,均予抗生素及对症用药,治疗组加用开喉剑喷雾剂(八爪金龙、山豆根、蝉蜕、薄荷脑)喷入咽喉。在退热、咽痛缓解、脓性分泌物消失及血象恢复正常的时间上比较,治疗组明显优于对照组($P<0.05$)。

5. 口腔科疾病

(1) 口腔黏膜疾病 孙勤国等研究表明,口疡清方(当归、生地黄、黄连、牡丹皮、紫草、藿香等)干预复发性口腔溃疡模型大鼠后,其 CD_3^+、CD_4^+ T 细胞及 IL-2、IL-4 的表达均有所上升,其中口疡清方中剂量组和左旋咪唑组上升明显,与对照组比较,$P<0.05$。提示口疡清方作用的机制可能与增强模型大鼠的免疫功能及 IL-2、IL-4 的表达有关。对口腔扁平苔藓的治疗与研究见专条介绍。

(2) 舌齿疾病 黄浩等对 7 680 例当代名医医案、1 018 例临床病例中紫舌与病性证素的相关性进行研究,用双层频权剪叉算法计算出紫舌对病性证素的诊断权值。血瘀、气滞不仅是在紫舌病例中出现频率最高的病性证素,其出现紫舌的比率亦高于其它病性证素($P<0.01$),紫舌对它们的诊断权值也是最高的。

刘东辉等将 96 例慢性牙周炎患者随机平分为两组,均予服罗红霉素胶囊剂对患牙作基础治疗,观察组加用双花清胃汤(生地黄、牡丹皮、金银花、黄连、知母,黄柏等)含漱及口服。疗程均为 7 d。观察组与对照组的总有效率分别为 91.7%(44/48)、75.0%(36/48),组间比较,$P<0.05$;龈沟出血指数(SBI)、菌斑指数(PLI)、牙龈指数(GI)及牙周袋深度(PD) 评分均低于对照组($P<0.01$);牙齿沟液中肿瘤坏死因子(TNF)-α、前列腺 E_2 (PGE_2) 和 IL-6 水平低于对照组($P<0.01$);牙齿沟液中病原菌伴放线放线杆菌(Aa)、牙龈卟啉单胞菌(Pg)及福赛类杆菌(Tf)检出率低于对照组($P<0.01$)。

(熊大经 张应文)

【视网膜静脉阻塞的治疗及实验研究】

视网膜静脉阻塞(RVO)的文献报道约 30

篇，治疗以活血化瘀为主。冯绍鸿等报道52例，予服龙血竭片(肠溶衣)2.4 g，3次/d。连服3个月后，患者视力较治疗前明显改善($P<0.01$)，眼底检查结果显示总有效率为93.3%(48/52)，其中显效率为76.9%(40/52)。李爱政将116例RVO患者随机平分为两组，治疗组给予活血化瘀法(桃仁、红花、当归、生地黄、川芎、赤芍药等为基本方，随证加减)施治，对照组予服迈之灵。30 d为1个疗程，治疗组与对照组中央静脉阻塞患者总有效率为分别为76.0%(19/25)、53.9%(14/26)，分支静脉阻塞患者总有效率分别为93.9%(31/33)、59.4%(19/32)。组间比较，均$P<0.01$。姜英梅等报道62例，随机分为两组，均予血塞通注射液0.4 g加入0.9%氯化钠注射液中静脉滴注，1 d1次，观察组(38眼)与对照组分别予服迈之灵片、维生素C。经治2个月后，两组患者的临床疗效及治疗前、后对数视力比较，观察组均明显优于对照组($P<0.05$)。李波等将60例气滞血瘀证RVO患者随机平分为两组，分别予服通脉化瘀汤(桃仁、红花、地龙、丹参、牛膝、川芎等)和丹红化瘀口服液(丹参、当归、川芎、桃仁、红花、枳壳等)。经治3个月后，两组患者治疗后视力均有提高，出血范围均缩小，全身症状均有改善。而通脉化瘀汤组的疗效优于丹红化瘀口服液组($P<0.05$)。

陆秉文等将62例非缺血型RVO患者随机分为两组，均予服地巴唑、复方丹参片等常规药物，治疗组32例加用苦碟子注射液20 ml于生理盐水中静脉滴注，1次/d。治疗4个月后，治疗组的总有效率及总显效率与对照组相比，$P<0.05$。治疗组的黄斑区视网膜神经上皮层厚度与治疗前相比明显降低($P<0.05$)；两组的视网膜循环时间均缩短而治疗组显著优于对照组。

实验研究方面，吴烈等探讨凉血止血法及活血化瘀法调节兔RVO凝血因子及微循环的作用机理。研究表明，凉血止血法以极早期(3 d内)促凝及早中期的抗凝和舒张血管作用为主；活血通络法以早中期的抗凝和舒血管及中后期的促凝和收缩血管作用为主；两法合用在各期均以抗凝作用为主，其早期有较强的舒张血管作用，中晚期有收缩血管作用。樊曦等探讨丹参三七混合液口服对光动力学诱导大鼠实验性视网膜分支静脉阻塞的预防作用。研究表明，丹参三七混合液口服可明显降低血小板黏附率，明显抑制血小板聚集，具有预防视网膜血栓形成的作用。

(刘红娣)

【糖尿病性视网膜病变的治疗及实验研究】

糖尿病性视网膜病变(DR)的文献报道较集中。严京等将确诊为气阴两虚的非增殖期糖尿病视网膜病变患者随机分为两组，分别予服密蒙花方(黄芪、女贞子、黄连、肉桂、密蒙花等)与羟苯磺酸钙胶囊。连续用药3个月后，密蒙花方组与对照组远视力改善有效率分别为13.6%(30/220)、6.5%(15/229)，改善眼底病变有效率分别为37.5%(77/205)、9.0%(20/222)，眼底荧光造影检查有效率分别为20.6%(43/209)、6.3%(14/222)。组间比较，均$P<0.01$。朱惠明等将60例DR患者随机平分为观察组(58眼)与对照组(57眼)，分别予服丹红化瘀口服液(丹参、当归、川芎、桃仁、红花等)与羟苯磺酸钙胶囊。经治12周后，两组有效率分别为82.8%(48/58)、66.7%(38/57)，组间比较，$P<0.05$。两组患者视力均有改善，眼底微血管病变程度评分、黄斑水肿程度评分及视网膜总循环时间与血管内皮细胞生长因子(VEGF)、碱性成纤维细胞生长因子(bFGF)水平均明显下降，而观察组均优于对照组(均$P<0.01$)；全血黏度、血浆黏度、纤维蛋白原、红细胞压积及红细胞沉降率等血液流变指标的改善观察组均优于对照组(均$P<0.01$)。殷莉等报道50例DR患者予服复方丹参滴丸和羟苯磺酸钙，并与服羟苯磺酸钙治疗的50例作对照。连续治疗2个月后，两组患者平均视力均明显提高，眼底视网膜微血管瘤数明显减少(均$P<0.05$)，视野灰度值(MD)明显降低($P<0.05$)，而观察组效果明显优于对照组($P<0.05$)。

姜小帆等严格按照量表编制的方法和程序，初步编制出包含49项条目的DR中医证素评定量表。其特点是在中医理论指导下，从文献研究中提取证素，形成理论构想，以前期研究为蓝本，提取出易于自评的有代表性条目，从而保证了量表结构的合理性、内容的完整性、条目的代表性；填表方式，以自评为主，避免了医生判断的主观性；采用标准化计分方式，将被测者的主观信息进行量化评分，易于操作，便于比较。同时，研究严格按照心理测量方法学和相应的5种不同统计学方法对条目进行综合筛选，方法互为补充，相得益彰，保证了量表所含条目具有良好的敏感性、独立性、代表性、内部一致性和稳定性。

实验研究方面,郭健等研究显示,糖尿病大鼠早期视网膜改变主要是神经元细胞和神经胶质细胞等神经组织的线粒体病变和细胞的变性、凋亡。枸杞多糖的干预可以明显减轻线粒体的病理改变,阻止神经细胞凋亡,其机制并非通过降低血糖,控制大鼠糖尿病发挥作用,而有望用于早期糖尿病视网膜神经病变的防治。刘冬恋等研究显示,牛蒡子苷能改善糖尿病大鼠视网膜的形态结构,增加视网膜的内核层细胞数($P<0.05$)和视网膜各层的厚度($P<0.05$, $P<0.01$),对糖尿病大鼠视网膜病变具有一定的治疗作用。

李春深等研究显示,抵当汤(桃仁、水蛭、虻虫、大黄)给药干预对大鼠糖尿病视网膜光镜下结构的影响均较模型对照组有一定程度的改善,降低了糖尿病视网膜细胞间黏附分子-1(ICAM-1)和血管内皮细胞黏附分子-1(VCAM-1)蛋白的表达,而早期干预作用更为显著,其机制可能是通过减少黏附分子表达,对抗炎症反应,从而发挥延缓大鼠DR保护视网膜的作用。高昕媛等研究显示,高糖作用导致视网膜神经节细胞(RGCs)释放NO、活性氧簇(ROS)增多,糖网明(由三七、黄芪等组成)干预能显著地降低NO、ROS水平($P<0.01$),在一定程度上减轻高糖对新生大鼠RGCs的氧化应激损伤,从而发挥其对RGCs的保护作用。吉鹏等研究显示,参葛颗粒(西洋参、葛根、三七、泽兰、水蛭、黄芪)能有效调控糖尿病大鼠血糖水平,改善其视网膜超微结构的病变。

(张应文　刘红娣)

【年龄相关性黄斑变性的治疗及实验研究】

年龄相关性黄斑变性(AMD)的文献报道约20余篇,黄云飞将80例AMD患者随机平分为两组,治疗组予服黄斑祛湿方加减(茯苓、薏苡仁、浙贝母、生牡蛎、昆布、郁金等),对照组予服维生素E、三磷酸腺苷片、肌苷等。经治4周,治疗组与对照组的总有效率分别为75.0%(30/40)、65.0%(26/40)。卓耀等将62例98眼肝肾阴虚型患者随机分为两组,均予维生素C、维生素E、血塞通等常规用药,治疗组(32例52眼)加服启明丸(熟地黄、山茱萸、山药、枸杞子、菊花、黄芪等)。经治30 d,两组有效率分别为76.8%(41/52)、56.5%(26/46),组间比较,$P<0.05$。两组患者的血浆同型半胱氨酸(Hcy)较治疗前均有改善,P-VER的P100波潜伏期均有缩短、振幅均有提高,而治疗组较对照组更明显($P<0.01$)。

胡艳红等以32例渗出型AMD患者、44例萎缩型AMD患者及50例健康人为观察对象,检测外周血T淋巴细胞及嗜酸性粒细胞表面CCR3的表达,对渗出型患者予服凉血化瘀中药(蒲黄、姜黄、旱莲草、女贞子、当归、川芎等),比较治疗前后患者外周血CCR3的表达。结果表明,渗出型患者外周血T淋巴细胞及嗜酸性粒细胞表面CCR3表达均高于健康对照组($P<0.01$),而治疗前后外周血CCR3的表达无显著性差异($P>0.05$)。萎缩型患者外周血CCR3表达与健康对照组无显著性差异($P>0.05$)。提示渗出型AMD脉络膜新生血管(CNV)的形成可能与外周血T淋巴细胞及嗜酸性粒细胞表面CCR3的高表达有关,凉血化瘀法能有效治疗渗出型AMD,而与CCR3表达非相关。廖继波等将58例渗出型AMD患者平分为两组,均予光动力(PDT)疗法,治疗组加服柴苓汤(柴胡、法半夏、泽泻、茯苓、猪苓、白术等)。疗程为3个月。两组患者治疗后矫正视力提高,同期组间比较,$P>0.05$。而柴苓汤联合PDT组的CNV渗漏面积和CNV复合体厚度均明显小于单纯PDT组($P<0.05$)。

黄冰林等研究表明,枸杞提取物可以有效地降低高脂饮食及氢醌诱发的AMD模型小鼠的半胱氨酸组织蛋白酶B、半胱氨酸蛋白酶抑制剂C的高表达,而体外研究显示,其成分叶黄素和玉米黄质可以刺激H202诱导的人视网膜色素上皮(ARPE-19)细胞的基质金属蛋白激酶(MMP)2、金属蛋白激酶组织抑制因子(TIMP)2的增殖,并下调两者蛋白的表达。

(刘红娣)

【视神经萎缩的治疗】

宋秋颖等将74例108眼患者分为两组,治疗组38例52眼予服明目复元汤(熟地黄、茯苓、山茱萸、山药、枸杞子、女贞子等)及患侧太阳穴贴敷(丹参、麝香、冰片等),对照组予服曲克芦丁、肌苷、腺苷钴胺、胞磷胆碱和维生素B_1等。经治3个月,两组视力总有效率分别为75.0%(39/52)、60.7%(34/56),视野平均缺损(MD)总有效率分别为78.8%(41/52)、58.9%(33/56),视觉诱发电位(F-VEP)P100波潜伏期总有效率分别为76.9%(40/52)、58.9%(33/56)。组间比较,均$P<0.05$。

王跃进等将84例109眼患者随机分为两组,

治疗组 42 例 55 眼予服补肾益气健脾方(枸杞子、炙黄芪、党参、密蒙花、丹参、白术等),对照组予能量合剂、维生素等常规西药。经治 3 个月,两组视力总有效率分别为 81.8%(45/55)、53.7%(31/54),两组 MD 总有效率分别为 81.8%(45/55)、55.6%(30/54),组间比较,均$P<0.05$。

于晓红等将 64 例外伤性患者平分为两组,均予复方樟柳碱注射液于浅动脉旁皮下注射,维生素 B_1、B_{12}注射液等肌内注射;研究组加服四物汤配方颗粒。经治 1 个月,研究组与对照组的有效率分别为 90.6%(29/32)、78.1%(25/32),两组患者治疗后视野改善明显,而研究组改善优于对照组($P<0.05$)。

郑伟将 166 例患者随机平分为两组,均予维生素 B_6与维生素 B_{12}进行肌内注射,能量合剂、血管扩张药物等静脉滴注;实验组加服补肝益肾活血汤(山药、熟地黄、枸杞子、黄芪、石菖蒲、山茱萸等)。经治 2 个月,实验组与对照组的总有效率分别为 89.2%(74/83)、71.1%(59/83),组间比较,$P<0.05$。

(张应文　刘红娣)

【干眼症的治疗及实验研究】

江丹等将 200 例 400 眼干眼症患者随机平分为两组,均予 0.5 g/L 环孢素 A 滴眼液点眼,试验组加秦皮滴眼液点眼。经治 4 周,两组患者的自觉症状均有不同程度减轻,或基本消失;试验组与对照组总有效率分别为 78.0%(78/100)、47.0%(47/100),试验组 SchirmerI 试验(SIT)及泪膜破裂时间(BUT)改善情况均优于对照组($P<0.01$)。

李凯等将来自 6 个眼科临床中心的 560 例水样液缺乏性干眼患者随机分为润目灵组(170 例)、润目灵联合针刺综合疗法组(169 例)和西药对照组(221 例),分别予服润目灵颗粒(鬼针草、菊花、枸杞子)、综合疗法(口服润目灵颗粒联合针刺)以及泪然滴眼液点眼。疗程均为 8 周,润目灵组和综合疗法组在症状积分、证候显愈率、总有效率以及对 SIT 和 BUT 两个指标的改善方面明显优于西药对照组($P<0.05$,$P<0.01$);而在证候显愈率、总有效率和症状积分改善方面,综合疗法优于单纯润目灵治疗组($P<0.05$)。

实验研究方面,施炜等研究表明,鬼针草提取物可显著抑制雄激素水平降低后兔干眼症的发生。其作用机制可能与黄酮类物质化学结构与雄激素类似,可起到拟雄激素效应.从而调节泪腺局部炎症反应有关。同时其拟胆碱作用在增加泪液流量、延长 BUT、改善角膜染色及主观症状方面均有一定的作用。从晨阳等研究发现,参麦合剂(鬼针草、玄参、麦冬)干预兔干眼症模型 14 d 后,与对照组相比,SIT 及 BUT 值均明显增加($P<0.01$);结膜细胞印迹学检查,结膜杯状细胞数量明显增多;光镜检查,部分结膜上皮层数增多、杯状细胞增多。表明参麦合剂能明显增加兔干眼症模型泪液分泌、改善泪膜稳定性和眼表细胞结构。

姚小磊等与李海中等研究发现,密蒙花总黄酮具有拟雄激素效应,可改善雄激素下降导致的干眼病大鼠角膜和泪腺组织的病理改变,能够产生同丙酸睾酮治疗干眼病相似的效果。彭清华等研究表明,通过密蒙花提取物以及染料木黄酮的干预,兔泪腺组织中 TGF-β1 表达显著提高,而使 IL-1β 和 TNF-A 显著降低,减轻了泪腺局部的炎症反应,炎性细胞浸润消失,正常泪腺细胞得到保护,受损组织得以修复。对于雄兔来说,这可能与密蒙花提取物中黄酮类物质具有拟雄激素作用有关,黄酮类物质与泪腺组织中雄激素受体结合后,提高泪腺组织中 TGF-B1 的 mRNA 的水平,以及促进 TGF-B1 蛋白的聚集,从而进一步抑制促炎细胞因子 IL-1、TNF-A 等的生成,促进组织修复。

方芳等研究发现,与大鼠模型组比较,杞菊润目贴(枸杞子、野菊花、珍珠等)连续外用能改善实验性干眼症大鼠泪腺组织结构的病理变化,其各剂量组均可显著增加 SIT ($P<0.05$),延长 BUT ($P<0.01$),其中以杞菊润目贴中剂量组减轻泪腺组织损伤程度的作用明显。

(张应文　刘红娣)

【突发性耳聋的治疗及实验研究】

突发性耳聋的临床治疗多为中西医结合。吕忠等将 62 例患者随机分为两组,均予地塞米松、低分子右旋糖苷、ATP 等常规静脉滴注,治疗组 32 例加用银杏叶提取物。经治 14 d 后,比较 4 个频率(0.5、1、2、4 KHz)气导纯音听阈均值(PAT),提高 15 dB 以上者视为有效。总有效率分别为 87.5%(28/32)、63.3%(19//30),组间比较,$P<0.05$。

郝建莹等将 60 例患者随机平分为两组,均予金纳多注射液、三磷酸腺苷及辅酶 A 静脉滴注,治疗组加服通窍活血汤(川芎、桃仁、当归、葛根、丹参、地龙)。经治 14 d,治疗组与对照组总有效率分别为 86.7%(26/30)、63.3%(19/30),组间比较,$P<0.05$。邵长宝等将 62 例患者随机分为两组,均予金纳多注射液静脉滴注,治疗组 32 例加服龙胆泻肝汤。经治 14 d,听力改善总有效率分别为 87.5%(28/32)、63.3%(19//30),组间比较,$P<0.05$。

王聘益将 91 例患者随机分为两组,均予扩血管剂、激素、神经营养剂及高压氧治疗,治疗组 46 例加服活血通窍汤(柴胡、葛根、川芎、香附、丹参、桃仁等)。经治 20 d,总有效率分别为 87.0%(40/46)、68.9%(31/45),组间比较,$P<0.05$。两组中度聋均显有效,而治疗组优于对照组($P<0.05$)。

唐英等将 60 例患者随机平分为两组,均予西药凯时注射液于生理盐水中静脉推注,维生素 B_1、维生素 B_{12} 肌注治疗,观察组加服耳聋 2 号煎剂(川芎、郁金、柴胡、香附、桃仁、石菖蒲等)。经治 14 d,观察组与对照组耳聋症状改善的总有效率分别为 83.3%(25/30)、46.6%(17/30),组间比较,$P<0.05$。

实验研究方面,梁俊薇等与宁云红等以清肝通窍汤(柴胡、龙胆草、钩藤、黄芩、栀子、白芍药等)干预突发性耳聋豚鼠模型,与对照组比较,血浆 5-HT、ET 含量明显下降,血清 NO 含量升高。表明清肝通窍汤可通过调节 5-HT、ET 及 NO 水平起到治疗作用。

(沈龙柱)

【变应性鼻炎的临床与实验研究】

杨皖菁等将 120 例 AR 患者随机平分为两组,均予服西替利嗪片,治疗组加服鼻炎片(苍耳子、黄芪、辛夷、白芷、知母、防风等)。经治 1 个月后,治疗组与对照组总有效率分别为 90.0%(54/60)、76.7%(46/60),组间比较,$P<0.01$。两组患者血清 C-反应蛋白(CRP)、IL-6、IL-4 指标水平较治疗前均明显下降($P<0.01$),而治疗组下降的幅度优于对照组($P<0.01$)。且治疗组患者不良反应的发生率明显低于对照组($P<0.05$)。杨占军等将 91 例肾阳虚型患者随机分为两组,治疗组 41 例予服金匮肾气丸合苍耳子散为主方加减治疗,对照组予服氯雷他定。另设正常健康的受试者 20 例为空白对照组。研究 AR 患者转录因子 T-bet/GATA-3 的表达及温肾补阳法对其作用。经治 4 周后,治疗组患者 IFN-γ、T-bet 水平明显提高($P<0.05$),IL-4、GATA-3 水平明显下降($P<0.05$),与正常对照组比较,$P>0.05$。而对照组治疗前后无明显改善。提示温肾补阳法可通过调节 T-bet/GATA-3 表达,纠正失衡的 Th1/Th2 细胞因子网络,起到治疗作用。

季红健等分析认为,AR 是一种复杂的病理性免疫反应,有多种免疫活性细胞和细胞因子(如 P 物质、IL-4 和 IFN-γ、一氧化氮合酶、嗜酸性粒细胞等)参与,但嗜酸性粒细胞阳离子蛋白(ECP)与 AR 辨证分型的研究几乎空白,提出以血清 ECP 作为对 AR 辨证分型的一个数值(或者是一个数值区域)区间,可以由此区分 AR 的“寒(气虚证)”“热(肺热证)”性质,反应 AR 不同证型的相应特点。

杨清等研究表明,辛芷鼻敏胶囊(白芷、辛夷花、苍耳子、鹅不食草、葱白、黄芪等)可能通过下调鼻黏膜中 STAT6 基因表达,抑制大鼠 AR 发病过程中 IL-5、IL-13 的水平,达到减少嗜酸性粒细胞浸润进而改善 AR 症状的目的。

朱镇华等研究表明,鼻敏片低、高剂量组均能降低 AR 豚鼠血清中细胞黏附分子-1(ICAM-1)、及其配体淋巴细胞相关抗原-1(LFA-1)、血管细胞间黏附分子-1(VCAM-1)及其配体很晚抗原-4(VLA-4)的含量。与开瑞坦组的表达比较无显著性差异。这可能是鼻敏片治疗变态反应性鼻炎的作用机制之一。

陈岩等研究表明,与豚鼠模型组比较,醒鼻凝胶剂(蝉蜕、冰片等)可有效缓解 AR 豚鼠的搔鼻、喷嚏、流涕等过敏症状,显著降低血清类胰蛋白酶含量。其作用强度同药物浓度呈正相关,其机制是通过稳定肥大细胞,抑制其脱颗粒释放炎症因子,而起到治疗作用。

董先红等研究表明,与大鼠模型组相比,芩蒿滴鼻剂(新疆一枝蒿、黄芩、甘草)高、低剂量均能降低血清特异性 IgE(OVR-sIgE)含量,不同程度的改善嗜酸性粒细胞及其他炎症细胞的浸润,减轻鼻黏膜毛细血管的扩张,而对 AR 模型大鼠起到治疗作用。

陈哲等研究表明,与对照组比较,青藤碱治疗组的小鼠鼻黏膜无明显腺体增生及嗜酸粒细胞浸润;血清中特异性抗 OVA-IgE、IL-4 和 IFN-γ 浓度,Th1 细胞的转录因子 T-bet 和

Th2细胞的转录因子CATA3表达水平均降低。提示青藤碱可能通过调节AR小鼠T-bet和CATA3的表达，改变体内Th1、Th2细胞的比例，从而调节Th1/Th2的平衡达到作用。彭顺林等研究表明，摄涕止鼽汤（黄芪、肉桂、黄精、石菖蒲、地龙、鹅不食草等）能显著降低肾阳虚型AR大鼠的血清中IL-5、ECP的含量，且高剂量组与酮替芬组无显著性差异（$P>0.05$）。卢健敏研究表明，温肺止流丹（人参、荆芥、细辛、鱼脑石、诃子、桔梗等）能够抑制、减轻炎症细胞在AR大鼠及肺气虚AR大鼠鼻黏膜浸润，降低大鼠血清IgE、IL-4、ECP水平而发挥治疗作用。黄水仙等研究表明，鼻康片（羊耳菊、鱼腥草、绣线菊、蓟根、漆姑草、路路通等）可显著降低AR模型小鼠血清IgE和IL-4的水平（$P<0.05$），明显增加IFN-γ的水平（$P<0.05$），通过调节Thl/Th2的平衡来发挥抗AR的作用。李道佩等研究表明，高、低剂量复方苍耳子滴鼻剂（苍耳子、西红花、纯麻油）对AR模型豚鼠鼻粘膜上皮化生、腺体增生、血管增生或扩张及炎性细胞浸润等方面均有改善作用。

（张守杰　张应文）

【慢性鼻窦炎的治疗与研究】

慢性鼻窦炎的临床文献报道较集中。沈勤峰等将360例患者随机平分为两组，均予头孢、大环内酯类等抗生素及局部鼻喷类固醇激素，试验组加服鼻渊通窍颗粒（辛夷、苍耳子、麻黄、白芷等）。经治4周，试验组与对照组的总有效率分别为96.1%（173/180）、63.3%（114/180），组间比较，$P<0.05$。黄晓梅将130例患者随机分为两组，治疗组69例予服苍耳散（苍耳子、白芷、辛夷、薄荷、冰片）吹鼻联合取渊汤（柴胡、辛夷、当归、焦山栀、浙贝母、玄参等），对照组予克拉霉素合呋喃西林麻黄素滴鼻液滴鼻及上颌窦穿刺冲洗。经治2周，总有效率分别为97.1%（67/69）、82.0%（50/61），组间比较，$P<0.05$。李晖等将226例患者随机平分为两组，均予辅舒良（丙酸氟替卡松水溶性鼻喷雾剂）喷鼻，治疗组加服香菊胶囊（化香树果序、黄芪、夏枯草、野菊花、防风、辛夷等）。2周为1个疗程。经治2～4个疗程，治疗组与对照组总有效率分别为92.9%（115/113）、86.7%（98/113），组间比较，$P<0.05$。

韦富贵将72例慢性鼻窦炎和鼻息肉患者随机平分为两组，对照组予常规抗生素、类固醇激素类药，观察组予服鼻渊舒（苍耳子、辛夷、薄荷、白芷、黄芩、栀子等）。治疗2周后对患者临床疗效进行检测，6个月后对患者进行多导睡眠检测，分析睡眠结构。观察组与对照组总有效率分别为92%（33/36）、78%（28/36），组间比较，$P<0.05$。两组非快速眼动睡眠各期、快速眼动（REM）睡眠、微觉醒指数、呼吸暂停通气指数（AHI）和体质量指数等指标治疗前后比较均有显著性差异（$P<0.05$）；治疗后AHI和微觉醒指数两组比较有显著性差异（$P<0.05$）。陈新野等将90例慢性鼻窦炎伴鼻息肉患者随机分为两组，均予内镜术后，行常规治疗，同时采用鼻腔灌注抽吸装置进行鼻腔灌洗，治疗组60例采用败丹黄灌洗液（败酱草、黄芪、丹参、白芷、甘草），对照组予庆大霉素加地塞米松。14 d为1个疗程，第1个疗程，1次/3 d，第2个疗程，1次/5 d，第3个疗程及以后，1次/7 d。分别对鼻塞、鼻漏、嗅觉障碍、头面部不适或疼痛4种临床症状进行VAS评分等。治疗组术后1.5、3个月VAS总分，及术后3个月单项评分，术后6个月、1年鼻漏评分均优于于对照组（$P<0.05$）。

周立等将60例慢性鼻窦炎胆腑郁热型患者随机平分为治疗组与对照组，分别予服龙胆泻肝汤水煎剂、中药安慰剂。采用SF-36量表、VAS量表和SNOT-20量表分别评价患者生存质量变化情况。经治2周后，治疗组与对照组治疗前后VAS积分比较，$P<0.05$；治疗组尤其在缓解患者鼻相关症状（如流脓涕、头痛、咳嗽、鼻涕倒流方面）及增强患者活力方面（减轻疲倦）优势明显。

（沈龙柱）

【慢性咽炎的治疗及实验研究】

谭焕仙等将256例患者随机分为两组，治疗组136例予咽炎方（山豆根、板蓝根、胖大海、威灵仙，加水煎后去渣取汁）熏蒸咽部及中药（将熏蒸所用的药液倒至药布垫上，分别置于双侧颌下腺下区部位）离子导入，对照组采用庆大霉素、糜蛋白酶、地塞米松及生理盐水作咽部超声雾化吸入。经治20 d，临床总有效率分别为96.3%（131/136）、76.7%（102/120），组间比较，$P<0.05$。吴韻敏将100例患者随机分为两组，治疗组55例予服潜阳封髓丹（炙龟板、肉桂、射干、焦黄柏、砂仁、桔梗等），对照组予服阿莫西林胶囊。连续治疗14 d为1个疗程。经治3个疗程，总有效率分别

为 92.7%(51/55)、71.1%(32/45),组间比较,$P<0.05$。

郭秀清将 130 例患者分为两组,均予服阿莫西林或罗红霉素及西瓜霜,治疗组 78 例加中药(麦冬、玄参、生地黄、银花、板蓝根、柴胡等)超声雾化吸入。经治 3 个月后,两组总有效率分别为 91.0%(71/78)、55.8%(29/52),组间比较,$P<0.01$。

张宏等将 118 例患者随机分为研究组与对照组,分别予服蓝芩口服液(板蓝根、黄芩、栀子、黄柏、胖大海)及西地碘含片。7 d 为 1 个疗程。经治 2~3 个疗程,两组患者血清 IL-2、TNF-α 水平及免疫细胞亚群均有明显改善,而研究组改善程度优于对照组;对各主要症状的总有效率研究组均高于对照组,其中在咽痛、咳嗽、咽痒、咽部红肿等症状的改善具有显著优势。

陈昫等临床研究发现,各类消化系统疾病(包括胃一食管反流、胃炎或胃窦炎、胃或十二指肠溃疡)的患者约占慢性咽炎总患者的 33.1%。与此同时,脾胃疾病患者也常伴随咽后壁淋巴滤泡增生,故单纯以清肺利咽治疗效果并不十分理想。其从"咽胃相关"角度探讨慢性咽炎的病因病机及其治疗,认为该病病程缠绵、易于复发,病机特点为脾胃受损、津液无从化生或痰湿内蕴至津液输布失调,治疗当以健脾为要,紧扣病机灵活配合养阴清肺或利咽散结之法,并注重调神养志,以达到事半功倍之效。

王良波等建立慢性咽炎中药复方数据库。收集整理了 1 350 首治疗有效的复方,用药频率统计分析,共使用了 630 味中药,用药 13 771次。使用的中药中,以清热药、补虚药、化痰止咳平喘药使用频率和使用比例最高。提示慢性咽炎的治疗以清热补虚为主,辅佐化痰止咳;常用药以清热药、补虚药、化痰止咳平喘药为主。

王颖等研究表明,陈皮利咽合剂(陈皮、延胡索、夜交藤、女贞子、合欢皮)能改善慢性咽炎家兔咽部黏膜炎症,其作用机制可能与降低全血黏度有关。

(张守杰　张应文)

【口腔扁平苔藓的治疗与研究】

刘铁军等报道 30 例口腔扁平苔藓(OLP),予服化湿行瘀清热方(黄柏、佩兰、赤芍药等)治疗 8 周后,总有效率为 93.3%,其中显效(充血、糜烂完全消失,白色条纹无或轻微;无自觉症状,疼痛完全消失)18 例;患者血清及唾液中 IL-6、血管内皮生长因子(VEGF)、可溶性细胞间粘附分子 1(sICAM-1)水平均较治疗前明显降低($P<0.05$)。提示其机制与调节血清和唾液中 IL-6、VEGF 以及 slCAM-1 表达有关。

丁广德等将 60 例 OLP 患者随机平分为两组,治疗组予疏肝解郁和血清热为主中药(当归、白芍药、丹参、黄芩、生地黄、白鲜皮等)煎服,对照组予服雷公藤多苷片。经治 2 周,治疗组与对照组总有效率分别为 96.7%(29/30)、60.0%(18/30),组间比较,$P<0.05$。

胡利杰等将 70 例 OLP 患者随机平分为两组,均予醋酸曲安奈德局部注射及维生素 A、维生素 C 口服等治疗,观察组加用石辛含片(石膏、黄柏、黄芩、细辛、栀子、姜黄等)含服。经治 6 个月后,观察组与对照组总有效率分别为 94.3%(33/35)、74.3%(26/35),组间比较,$P<0.05$。轩俊丽等将 256 例 OLP 患者随机分为两组,均予醋酸曲安奈德局部注射,治疗组 130 例予加服白芍总苷胶囊。治疗 8 周后观察疗效并随访 6 个月,于治疗前及治疗结束 6 个月时检查患者 T 淋巴细胞亚群变化情况。两组的有效率分别为 79.2%(120/130)、60.3%(104/126),组间比较,$P<0.01$;治疗后 6 个月,治疗组患者血清 CD_3^+、CD_4^+ T 细胞升高,CD_8^+ T 细胞降低,与治疗前相比,P 均<0.01;对照组患者血清 CD_3^+、CD_4^+ 及 CD_8^+ T 细胞值与治疗前相比,均$P>0.05$。刘砚芝等将 72 例 OLP 患者随机平分为两组,均予服白芍总苷胶囊,治疗组加用他克莫司软膏局部涂搽。经治 2 个月后,治疗组与对照组总有效率分别为 97.2%(35/36)、75.0%(27/36),组间比较,$P<0.05$。

邢海霞等报道对 110 例 OLP 患者及 34 例正常人对照组舌象特点进行观察,分析舌象变化与 OLP 临床分型的相关性。OLP 患者组舌色淡红、白苔的检出率显著低于对照组;舌色紫瘀、黄苔、舌苔厚、润滑、燥涩、腻苔的检出率均显著高于对照组(均$P<0.05$)。糜烂型 OLP 患者及舌部 OLP 患者花剥苔的检出率显著增加(均$P<0.05$)。提示 OLP 患者的证候与湿、热、瘀有关,其舌象变化一定程度上可以反映病情变化。

(戚清权)

[附] 参考文献

C

陈美荣,郝永龙,王静波,等.视明宝颗粒对斜视性弱视猫视皮层超微结构研究[J].辽宁中医药大学学报,2013,15(9):50

陈新野,张春林,洪海裕,等.败丹黄灌洗液鼻腔灌洗对慢性鼻窦炎伴鼻息肉患者术后的临床疗效影响[J].中国中西医结合杂志,2013,33(2):180

陈晌,胡玲,张婷,等.基于"咽胃相关"探讨慢性咽炎及其治疗[J].广州中医药大学学报,2013,30(4):579

陈岩,黄枚,褚克丹,等.醒鼻凝胶剂对变应性鼻炎模型豚鼠的作用机制[J].福建中医药大学学报,2013,23(3):23

陈哲,陶泽璋,章哪哪,等.青藤碱对变应性鼻炎小鼠的治疗作用及机制研究[J].临床耳鼻咽喉头颈外科杂志,2013,27(2):81

丛晨阳,温莹,毕宏生,等.参麦合剂对兔干眼症模型泪液分泌及眼表结构的影响[J].世界中医药,2013,8(9):1053

D

丁广德,张铁峰.疏肝清热法治疗口腔扁平苔藓30例[J].山东中医杂志,2013,32(9):640

董先红,顾政一,黄华,等.芩蒿滴鼻剂对变应性鼻炎大鼠疗效的实验研究[J].新疆医科大学学报,2013,36(3):320

F

樊曦,周和政.丹参三七混合液预防视网膜分支静脉阻塞的实验研究[J].中国中医眼科杂志,2013,23(2):88

方芳,张硕峰,贾占红,等.杞菊润目贴对实验性大鼠干眼症的作用研究[J].世界科学技术(中医药现代化),2013,15(8):1696

冯俊,唐由之,于静.睫状体平坦部滤过术治疗青光眼的临床研究[J].中国中医眼科杂志,2013,23(2):117

冯绍鸿,祖微,刘冰,等.中药龙血竭片治疗视网膜静脉阻塞52例临床观察[J].世界中西医结合杂志,2013,8(10):1073

冯文华.开喉剑喷雾剂(儿童型)治疗急性化脓性扁桃体炎的疗效观察[J].吉林医学,2013,34(36):7643

G

高昕媛,匡洪宇,邹伟.糖网明含药血清对高糖条件下视网膜神经节细胞NO、ROS水平的影响[J].中国中医药科技,2013,20(4):338

高延娥,崔彦,毕宏生,中西医结合治疗慢性前葡萄膜炎临床观察[J].辽宁中医杂志,2013,40(6):1192

关瑞娟,亢泽峰,李凌,等.益气解毒中药减少单纯疱疹病毒性角膜炎复发的免疫机理研究[J].中国中医眼科杂志,2013,23(1):17

郭健,徐国兴,侯泽江,等.枸杞多糖对糖尿病大鼠视网膜超微结构的影响[J].中国中西医结合杂志,2013,33(10):1404

郭俊国,颜廷芹,毕宏生,等.代谢组学在中西医结合眼科研究中的应用与展望[J].世界中西医结合杂志,2013,8(3):315

郭秀清.中药雾化吸入治疗慢性咽炎78例临床分析[J].中国中西医结合耳鼻咽喉科杂志,2013,21(2):138

H

郝建莹,关洁,李馨,等.金纳多联合通窍活血汤治疗血瘀耳窍型突发性耳聋疗效观察[J].中国民间疗法,2013,21(6):49

胡利杰,杨阳.中西医结合治疗糜烂型口腔扁平苔藓70例临床观察[J].中国中医基础医学杂志,2013,19(7):843

胡艳红,祁明信,陈胜.凉血化瘀法干预老年性黄斑变性CNV与外周血CCR3表达的相关研究[J].国际眼科杂志,2013,13(3):546

黄冰林,丁淑华,杭丽,等.枸杞提取物及其成分叶黄素压米黄质在体内外对年龄相关性黄斑变性防治的影响[J].中国中西医结合杂志,2013,33(4):531

黄浩,唐亚平,戴芳,等.紫舌与病性证素相关性的研究[J].时珍国医国药,2013,24(7):1706

黄水仙,李勇,谢民强,等.鼻康片对变应性鼻炎小鼠模型Thl/Th2平衡和血清总IgE的影响[J].医学研究杂志,2013,42(5):160

黄晓梅.苍耳散外用联合取渊汤口服治疗慢性鼻窦炎69例疗效观察[J].临床合理用药杂志,2013,6(2上):57

黄云飞.祛湿法治疗痰湿蕴结型老年性黄斑变性40例[J].光明中医,2013,28(8):1635

J

吉鹏,霍勤,胡凤丽.参葛颗粒对糖尿病大鼠视网膜超微结构的影响[J].中医学报,2013,28(5):686

季红健,王东方.变应性鼻炎中医辨证分型与ECP的相关性研究[J].西部中医药,2013,26(5):127

贾琳琳,赵晓莲,张建华,等.刺五加注射液对外源性谷氨酸致豚鼠耳蜗复合动作电位和内耳组织形态的影响

[J]. 中成药,2013,35(9): 2008

江丹,刘新泉. 秦皮滴眼液联合环孢素 A 滴眼液治疗干眼症的疗效[J]. 国际眼科杂志,2013,13(10): 2149

江伟,唐由之,梁丽娜,等. 明睛颗粒对 Matrigel 诱导实验性脉络膜新生血管的干预作用[J]. 中华中医药杂志,2013,28(9): 2572

姜小帆,曾进,段俊国. 糖尿病性视网膜病变中医证素评定量表的编制策略及条目筛选[J]. 中华中医药学刊,2013,31(1): 24

姜英梅,韩峰,金日. 迈之灵治疗视网膜静脉阻塞疗效[J]. 中国药物经济学,2013,9(4): 254

L

李爱政. 中医活血化瘀法在视网膜静脉阻塞中的应用[J]. 中医药导报,2013,19(2): 63

李波,魏妙. 通脉化瘀汤治疗气滞血瘀证视网膜静脉阻塞临床观察[J]. 中国中医眼科杂志,2013,23(1): 21

李春深,常柏,苗戎,等. 抵当汤早期干预对糖尿病大鼠视网膜 ICAM-1 和 VCAM-1 表达的影响[J]. 北京中医药,2013,32(2): 129

李道佩,吴又明,戴卫波. 复方苍耳子滴鼻剂对变应性鼻炎动物模型组织形态学的影响[J]. 中国临床药理学杂志,2013,29(12): 936

李海中,彭清华,王芬,等. 密蒙花总黄酮对去势雄鼠干眼病血清睾酮水平的影响[J]. 国际眼科杂志,2013,13(11): 2174

李晖,刘莉,郭筠芳,等. 香菊胶囊治疗儿童慢性鼻窦炎疗效观察[J]. 湖北中医杂志,2013,35(8): 30

李军,乔淑琴,吴国强. 中药辅助治疗视网膜脱离术后视网膜下积液的临床疗效观察[J]. 西部中医药,2013,26(10): 87

李凯,王育良,龚佳怡. 润目灵联合针刺治疗水样液缺乏性干眼的临床研究[J]. 中国中医眼科杂志,2013,23(3): 165

李诺,黄丽娜,曾平. 白蒺藜皂苷对慢性高眼压兔视网膜 SOD 活性和 MDA 含量的影响[J]. 国际眼科杂志,2013,13(5): 854

李诺,黄丽娜,曾平. 蒺藜总皂苷对慢性高眼压兔血液流变学影响的实验研究[J]. 中国中医眼科杂志,2013,23(2): 92

李胜利,朱宏亮,刘全征,等. 复聪汤对工业噪声致聋豚鼠耳蜗毛细胞修复再生的研究[J]. 中华中医药杂志,2013,28(3): 8111

李向宇,王新帅,王颖. 陈皮利咽合剂对急性咽炎模型大鼠白细胞和咽黏膜影响的研究[J]. 新中医,2013,45(9): 145

李卓,皇甫辉. 鼻炎宁颗粒治疗急性鼻窦炎的临床研究[J]. 世界中医药,2013,8(7): 767

梁俊薇,宁云红,刘成云. 情志因素与突发性耳聋[J]. 湖南中医杂志,2013,29(2): 112

廖继波,马威奇,欧波,等. 柴苓汤联合光动力疗法治疗渗出型老年性黄斑变性的临床观察[J]. 中国中医眼科杂志,2013,23(4): 250

刘东辉,曹阳. 双花清胃汤治疗慢性牙周炎 60 例临床研究[J]. 中国实验方剂学杂志,2013,19(24): 310

刘冬恋,马松涛. 牛蒡子苷对糖尿病大鼠视网膜和视神经病变的治疗作用. [J]. 中华中医药杂志,2013,28(12): 3732

刘铁军,赵双玲,刘健,等. 化湿行瘀清热方剂治疗口腔扁平苔藓试验研究[J]. 实用口腔医学杂志,2013,29(7): 3

刘晓华,林子升,赵进. 羚羊角联合万应胶囊治疗急性化脓性扁桃体炎的临床疗效观察[J]. 中华中医药学刊,2013,31(4): 949

刘砚芝,杨续艳. 白芍总苷结合他克莫司软膏治疗糜烂型口腔扁平苔藓的疗效评价[J]. 黑龙江医学,2013,37(2): 90

刘莹,张花治,白丽君,等. 原花青素对视网膜缺血再灌注损伤大鼠视网膜结构及核转录因子-κB 表达的影响[J]. 中国中医药信息杂志,2013,20(5): 32

卢健敏. 温肺止流丹对变应性鼻炎大鼠免疫调节作用机制的研究[J]. 西部中医药,2013,26(7): 26

陆秉文,吴星伟. 苦碟子注射液治疗非缺血型视网膜静脉阻塞临床研究[J]. 中国中医眼科杂志,2013,23(3): 179

吕忠,唐真武,邓立波,等. 银杏叶提取物治疗突发性耳聋疗效观察[J]. 临床合理用药杂志,2013,6(10 中): 15

M

茅犁春,赵荣祥,叶再元. 天麻素对噪声性耳聋听觉脑干诱发电位及耳蜗毛细胞的影响[J]. 医学研究杂志,2013,42(7): 80

N

聂爱芹,席兴华,程芳,等. 玉屏风散对单纯疱疹病毒性角膜炎模型小鼠细胞免疫功能的影响[J]. 眼科新进展,2013,33(4): 319

宁云红,梁俊薇. 清肝通窍汤对突发性耳聋豚鼠 ET、NO 水平影响研究[J]. 辽宁中医药大学学报,2013,15(3): 35

P

彭清华,姚小磊,彭俊,等. 密蒙花提取物对干眼症雄兔泪腺局部炎症反应影响的研究[J]. 中华中医药学刊,2010,28(7): 1351

彭顺林,刘宝,李菁,等. 摄涕止鼽汤对实验性变应性

鼻炎 IL－5、ECP 含量的影响[J]. 辽宁中医杂志，2013，40(5)：838

S

邵长宝，邵腾皓，杨新艳，等. 金纳多联合龙胆泻肝汤治疗突发性耳聋疗效观察[J]. 中国中医急症，2013，22(1)：124

沈勤峰，沈小燕，朱荣强. 鼻通窍治疗 360 例慢性鼻窦炎的临床疗效分析[J]. 吉林医学，2013，34(30)：6271

施炜，张传伟，王育良. 鬼针草提取物对兔泪液分泌影响及对泪腺细胞凋亡相关基因表达的实验研究[J]. 临床眼科杂志，2013，21(4)：365

宋剑涛，沈志华，高健生，等. 川椒方对过敏性结膜炎小鼠 IL4－JAK1－STAT6 信号通路的影响[J]. 中国中医眼科杂志，2013，23(4)：240

宋秋颖，张增雷，卫冬，等. 明目复元汤联合中药穴位贴敷治疗视神经萎缩的疗效观察[J]. 世界中医药，2013，8(11)：1300

孙勤国，江波，张贤梅，等. 口疡清方对复发性口腔溃疡大鼠的治疗作用及其对白细胞介素－2、白细胞介素－4 表达的研究[J]. 中国医院药学杂志，2013，33(18)：1494

T

谭焕仙，李党焕，施燎明. 中药咽炎方熏蒸联合离子导入治疗慢性咽炎的疗效观察[J]. 中医临床研究，2013，5(3)：27

唐英，张茹，汪旻琦，等. 中药耳聋 2 号治疗突发性耳聋的临床疗效观察[J]. 中医药信息，2013，30(1)：102

田楠楠，亢泽峰，张庆，等. 驻景方对病理性近视脉络膜新生血管 VEGF 表达的影响[J]. 国际眼科杂志，2013，13(8)：1525

W

王良波，金震柱. 1 350 首治疗慢性咽炎中药复方用药规律研究[J]. 北方药学，2013，10(6)：37

王聘益. 中西医结合治疗突发性耳聋 46 例临床观察[J]. 中国中医急症，2013，22(7)：1224

王颖，王新帅，李向宇，等. 陈皮利咽合剂对慢性咽炎模型家兔全血黏度和咽黏膜的影响[J]. 中医杂志，2013，54(12)：1051

王跃进，王斐. 自拟补肾益气健脾方治疗视神经萎缩的临床观察[J]. 中医临床研究，2013，5(6)：7

韦富贵. 鼻渊舒治疗鼻窦炎和鼻息肉及其对睡眠结构的影响[J]. 现代中西医结合杂志学，2013，22(15)：1606

吴烈，桑子瑾，唐棠，等. 凉血止血法与活血通络法调节 RVO 兔模型凝血因子及微循环作用机制的研究[J]. 中国中医眼科杂志，2013，23(1)：2

吴韻敏. 潜阳封髓丹治疗慢性咽炎随机平行对照研究[J]. 实用中医内科杂志，2013，27(5 上)：57

X

解孝锋，庄曾渊，毕宏生，等. 中西医结合治疗葡萄膜炎减少复发的研究[J]. 世界中医药，2013，8(8)：903

邢海霞，刘宏伟，杨续艳，等. 口腔扁平苔藓患者 110 例舌象特点初步分析[J]. 现代中西医结合杂志，2013，22(22)：2404

徐光，刘玉萍. 分泌性中耳炎患者血清及耳积液 HA 及白介素的变化观察[J]. 中国医药科学，2013，3(24)：57

轩俊丽，李颖慧，李媛媛. 白芍总苷胶囊治疗口腔扁平苔藓 130 例临床观察[J]. 中国皮肤性病学杂志，2013，27(8)：861

宣伟军，褚汉启，宣毅. 复方健耳剂对国产 DBA/ZJ 小鼠耳蜗组织脑源性神经营养因子表达影响的初步研究[J]. 中华中医药杂志，2013，28(9)：2748

Y

严京，高健生，接传红，等. 密蒙花方对非增殖期糖尿病视网膜眼底病变影响的研究[J]. 世界中西医结合杂志，2013，8(3)：246

晏英，严道南. "天人相应"指导变应性鼻炎治疗 60 例[J]. 辽宁中医杂志，2013，40(2)：272

杨清，马冬均，姜孝芳，等. 辛芷鼻敏胶囊对变应性鼻炎大鼠血清中细胞因子和鼻黏膜组织中相关基因表达的影响[J]. 中草药，2013，44(20)：2889

杨皖菁，周波，张宇，等. 鼻炎片对变应性鼻炎的疗效及血清炎症因子的影响[J]. 中医药导报，2013，19(7)：39

杨占军，阮岩，王慧敏，等. 温肾补阳法对变应性鼻炎患者转录因子 T－bet/GATA－3 表达的影响[J]. 中医临床研究，2012，4(8)：6

姚小磊，彭清华，彭俊，等. 密蒙花总黄酮对去势导致干眼症雄鼠血清 LH 的影响[J]. 湖南中医药大学学报，2013，33(7)：8

殷莉，张德龙，任骞，等. 复方丹参滴丸配合羟苯磺酸钙治疗糖尿病视网膜病效果观察[J]. 现代中西医结合杂志，2013，22(22)：2449

于晓红，李文明，周晓滨，等. 四物汤配方颗粒联合复方樟柳碱治疗外伤性视神经萎缩的临床研究[J]. 中国当代医药，2013，20(7)：95

余朝阳，钱学贞. 化脓性中耳炎患者治疗前后血清及耳分泌物总 IgE、IL－2、IL－6、IL－8 及氧自由基的变化研究[J]. 现代中西医结合杂志，2013，22(21)：2320

Z

张宏. 蓝芩口服液对慢性咽炎患者 IL－2、TNF－α、免疫细胞亚群及临床症状的改善作用研究[J]. 现代中西

医结合杂志,2013,22(2):125

张花治,刘莹,白丽君,等.原花青素对缺血—再灌注损伤后大鼠视网膜 Bcl-2 和 Bax 表达的影响[J].中国中医眼科杂志,2013,23(2):83

张庆,田楠楠,亢泽峰,等.加减驻景方对实验性脉络膜新生血管的作用研究[J].中国中医眼科杂志,2013,23(2):79

郑伟.中西医结合治疗视神经萎缩 83 例[J].河南中医,2013,33(9):1544

仲崇玉.速效耳净灵治疗化脓性中耳炎 140 例[J].山东中医杂志,2013,32(4):244

周立,陶铮,熊大经.龙胆泻肝汤治疗胆腑郁热型慢性鼻—鼻窦炎的生存质量观察[J].四川中医,2013,31(4):75

朱惠明,江玉,李玲,等.丹红化瘀口服液治疗单纯型糖尿病视网膜病变[J].中国实验方剂学杂志,2013,19(17):320

朱镇华,郑义,胡丹瑛,等.鼻敏片对变态反应性鼻炎豚鼠黏附分子的影响[J].新中医,2013,45(11):136

卓耀,彭廷云.启明丸治疗年龄相关性黄斑变性的临床疗效及对血浆 Hcy 水平的影响[J].中国中医眼科杂志,2013,23(1):36

邹建东,陈小宁,刘芳.五龙颗粒治疗变应性鼻炎肺脾气虚证的临床研究[J].世界中医药,2013,8(11):1298

(十)针 灸

【概述】

2013年度，期刊公开发表的针灸学术论文共5 100余篇，其中中文4 600余篇，英文SCI收录500余篇(其中中国作者发表210余篇)，较2012年略有增加。临床研究仍占据主要内容，达到77.1%，另外还包括机理研究、经验介绍、针灸文献、器械研究、思路方法、针灸教学、针灸在国外等。针灸学的动态可以概括为：针灸作用机制研究从中枢、组织、细胞、分子、基因等多层次展开；针灸临床研究的国际影响力正在提高。

1. 经络研究

张永红等基于临床中激痛点(MTrP)的特殊治疗效果，认为经络与现代物理学的电磁波理论密切相关：持续收缩的肌纤维所发出的异常电磁波可以通过影响整个空间经络能量结构，进而引起其他远隔部位能量的变化，形成连锁反应最终影响到整个人体组织包括内脏，阻遏正常物质以及能量的传导。并认为经络的电磁波能量结构理论可以很好地解释经络的各种功能。

王志功等采用多端口网络理论和电信号传递系数测量方法，对电针作用的实时电学效果进行观察，在蟾蜍体内初步验证了从电信号传递特性出发研究电针作用效果和经络轨迹方法的可行性，为进一步探索经络的生理特性提供了科学依据。

吉长福等研究原始管道系统(PVs)与经络的关系，发现PVs的出现与炎症密切相关，其并不参与针刺对胃肠运动的调节效应，认为PVs和经络不存在相关性。

2. 腧穴研究

腧穴研究主要包括腧穴效应的特异性、腧穴的理化特性和腧穴的分子生物特性等方面。

田宇瑛等发现，针刺合谷后，鼻区，左、右脸颊区的血流量逐渐升高，与针前比较差异有显著或极显著的统计学意义，前额区针后即刻显著增加，随后保持不变，嘴区没有明显变化，认为该研究进一步补充说明了“面口合谷收”的取穴规律。

陆欣玲等发现，针刺左侧合谷可激活右侧额内侧回、右侧颞上回、右侧颞中回、右侧岛叶、左侧尾状核，双侧额下回；针刺右侧合谷可激活左侧额内侧回、左侧颞中回、左侧额下回、右侧辅助运动区。提示针刺合谷穴可激活大脑皮质语言运用中枢、面部反应区、听觉皮区，与合谷穴功能基本吻合。

杨宁等利用穴位的电导性，观察井原、俞募4种穴位间的相关性，发现4种穴位 $0<r<1$，提示井原穴和腹募穴呈正相关。

胡昊斌等发现，电针神门、太渊两穴均可显著降低被试者P300波幅($P<0.01$, $P<0.05$)；电针对P300潜伏期无显著性影响，但电针神门穴有前移P300潜伏期的趋势；电针两穴对脑地形图电压强度分布有不同影响，电针神门穴后高电位反应主要集中在枕叶，少量散布于左侧顶叶及右侧颞部，而电针太渊穴后高电位反应主要散见于顶叶及左侧枕叶。认为不同经穴刺激对大脑皮质信息处理加工的影响不同，提示经穴功能存在相对差异性。

董泉声等发现，皮温47℃(或48℃)的灸法对内毒素导致的发热产生有效的拮抗作用，认为灸法退热的腧穴物质基础是对47℃(或48℃)敏感的多觉型感受器(PR)。

3. 刺灸法研究

针刺研究包括针刺器械、针刺方法、腧穴与针刺法等内容。灸法学研究涉及灸材、施灸方法、灸量、艾灸理化特性与安全性等方面。

蔡荣林等认为，人体特殊部位腧穴仿真针刺实践实训平台的应用可以显著提高医学生的实践动手能力和针刺操作技能。

李晓梅等观察发现，提插补法、提插泻法及平补平泻法均可使足三里局部皮肤血流灌注量增加，其中前二者较平补平泻法更为明显，而补法组血流灌注量增加幅度明显高于泻法组。认为针刺手法操作可明显提高健康人足三里皮肤血流灌注量，且补泻手法不同，影响存在差异。

齐丽珍等依据文献资料就古今灸材作比较，发现古今灸疗临床施灸材料以艾占主要地位，其他材料辅之。

窦传字等发现，艾条燃烧生成自由基，其成分主要为醌/半醌自由基、烷基和烷氧自由基以及NO自由基，储存期为3年和5年艾条燃烧生成的上述自由基均少于1年艾条。艾烟中自由基的检测有望成为鉴别艾的新陈和艾灸安全性评价的重要依据。

4. 针灸临床研究

针灸临床研究的中文文献约3 600余篇，与2012年持平。其中传染病约20篇，涉及乙型肝炎、肺结核、艾滋病、流行性腮腺炎、手足口病等。肿瘤类50余篇，多与术后并发症、镇痛、增强机体免疫功能等有关。消化系统疾病280余篇，主要是便秘、功能性消化不良、结肠炎、腹泻型肠易激综合征、胆囊炎、胃炎、胃溃疡、胃下垂、肠梗阻等。呼吸系统疾病120余篇，主要集中于支气管哮喘、咳嗽、感冒、肺炎等。心血管系统疾病100余篇，涉及冠心病、高血压、心衰、心律失常、心肌损伤等。泌尿系统疾病50余篇，主要有尿失禁、尿潴留、尿频、泌尿系结石、尿路感染、肾盂肾炎、肾衰竭等。新陈代谢疾病150余篇，主要有肥胖、糖尿病、高脂血症、单纯性消瘦、痛风等。神经系统疾病900余篇，主要有中风、面瘫、头痛、神经痛、神经炎、癫痫、眩晕、痴呆等。精神疾病120余篇，主要集中于抑郁症、癔症、精神分裂症等。妇产科疾病210余篇，主要涉及月经病、带下病、妊娠病、产后病、围绝经期综合征。儿科疾病120余篇，主要有脑瘫、哮喘、腹泻、厌食、多动症、遗尿等。皮肤科疾病近150篇，主要集中于带状疱疹、荨麻疹、痤疮、黄褐斑、神经性皮炎、脂溢性脱发、扁平疣、银屑病等。骨伤科疾病770余篇，主要集中于腰椎间盘突出症、颈椎病、膝骨关节炎、肩周炎、急性腰扭伤等。外科疾病130余篇，主要集中于术后不良反应、前列腺炎、痔疮、急性乳腺炎等。五官科疾病160余篇，主要涉及过敏性鼻炎、近视、耳聋、耳鸣、慢性咽炎等。此外，针灸对戒毒、康复、结缔组织病的治疗以及针灸安全性等亦有报道。

另外，Web of Science数据库收录的SCI文献有200余篇，其中期刊影响因子(IF)＞5的有10篇，内容涉及脑功能成像、抑郁症、针刺镇痛、上肢淋巴水肿、急性腰痛、控制癌症放化疗副作用、面瘫、过敏性鼻炎等。Xu SB等研究加强刺激在针灸治疗贝尔面瘫中的作用，采用行针手法使病人得气，设对照组不运用行针手法，结果发现得气组病人在面部功能恢复、残疾评估、生活质量均优于对照组，回归分析显示得气组在面部神经功能改善方面具有积极的作用。

5. 针灸机理研究

2013年针灸作用机理研究文献共有530余篇。涉及的动物模型有100余种，病种有阿尔茨海默病(AD)、多囊卵巢综合征(PCOS)、创伤后应激、心律失常、心动过缓、肠易激综合征、克罗恩病等，针灸干预措施有电针、手法针刺、艾灸、刺血、穴位注射、耳针、头针等，技术涉及分子生物学、功能磁共振成像(fMRI)、SPECT、蛋白组学等。

基于分子生物技术探讨针灸作用机理，仍是针灸实验研究的主要方向。Sun J等探讨电针治疗PCOS的作用机制，发现电针治疗后，8/10的PCOS大鼠动情周期恢复正常且卵巢形态学和超微结构改善；外周血雄激素含量降低且雌激素含量增加，同时，P450arom含量增加且P450C17α含量降低。此外，电针还可显著增加PCOS大鼠卵巢颗粒细胞层P450arom蛋白及其mRNA表达，显著下调卵泡膜细胞层P450C17α蛋白及其mRNA表达。Wang XM等从胞外信号调节激酶(ERK)信号通路，探讨艾灸治疗克罗恩病(CD)肠纤维化的机制，发现CD肠纤维化大鼠结肠Ras、Raf-1、MEK-1、ERK-1/2蛋白及其mRNA表达较正常组大鼠显著增加，艾灸(隔药灸、温和灸)天枢和气海穴能降低CD肠纤维化大鼠结肠Ras、Raf-1、MEK-1、ERK-1/2蛋白及其mRNA的异常表达。杜艳军等观察不同针灸预刺激对AD模型大鼠热休克蛋白HSP70、HSP90的影响及其作用机理，发现经预针灸治疗，预艾灸组、预电针组、预针灸组大鼠海马CA1区HSP70、HSP90的平均光密度表达均较模型组显著提高。提示艾灸预刺激、电针预刺激及针灸预刺激能通过诱导脑内HSP70、HSP90的表达来抑制Aβ毒性级联反应，从而起到保护神经元的作用。

常小荣等研究发现，艾灸温通温补效应的作用机制为艾灸激活穴位(局部始动)，推动气血运行，调节神经—内分泌—免疫网络(调节通路)，调节脏腑功能(效应器官响应)。并阐明艾灸温通温补效应之间的关系为"以温促通、以温达补，以通促补、以补促通，通中有补、补中有通、通补互用"。

Jiang Y 等比较手针(MA)、电针(EA)、经皮穴位电刺激仪(TEAS)三种不同刺激即时以及持续性效应的异同。结果，三者在组块试验的第一阶段刺激时均出现相似的运动感觉区的正激活以及默认模式区的负激活，而在第二阶段刺激时，正激活脑区消失，相较于 MA 和 TEAS，EA 出现了更广泛的负激活。此外，静息状态下三者均使大脑本能网络的激活增加。相较于 TEAS，MA 和 EA 产生的默认模式网络的功能连接更为广泛，而 TEAS 产生了更强的感觉运动网络的功能连接，提示 MA，EA，TEAS 三种不同的针灸刺激有着不同的脑中枢整合机制。

Gao YH 等发现，坐骨神经慢性缩窄性损伤(CCI)大鼠受损后肢的热痛阈下降，经电针治疗后恢复正常。电针干预后 CCI 大鼠下丘脑中共有 17 种蛋白表达显著改变，3 个基因本体进行富集；同时，对糖酵解/糖异生/六碳糖代谢通路具有显著调节作用。提示电针可通过调节多种下丘脑蛋白的表达来缓解疼痛，并通过调节下丘脑葡萄糖代谢来发挥维持能量支持和神经递质的动态平衡作用。

6. 针刺镇痛与针刺麻醉研究

针刺镇痛方面的研究侧重于观察针刺镇痛效应及其机制。Fang JQ 等认为，电针可迅速提高大鼠痛阈并且具有持续性镇痛效应。而踝关节肿胀在注射后第 14 d 被抑制。此外，电针可下调大鼠脊髓背角 p－p38 MAPK 和 p－ATF－2 蛋白及其受体阳性细胞的表达，抑制 VR－1 蛋白及其 mRNA 的表达。其抑制脊髓 p38 MAPK/ATF－2/VR－1 信号通路的激活，可能是电针通过中枢信号转导通路来抑制 CFA 大鼠炎性痛的主要机制之一。梁宜等提出电针下调脊髓背角 NR2B 酪氨酸 1742 位点磷酸化，可能是其抗 CFA 诱导的炎性疼痛的又一作用靶点。

阚宇等研究发现，电针"足三里"和"阳陵泉"穴能明显升高 CCI 大鼠的痛阈，该作用可能与其下调海马神经型一氧化氮合酶、细胞内蛋白激酶 G 基因表达水平有关。Ju ZY 等发现，电针和手针"足三里"、"三阴交"穴均能显著改善大鼠机械性痛觉过敏，电针效果更佳。该作用与改善神经功能与激活脊髓背角 EphrinBs/EphBs 信号系统亚单位密切相关。

Weng ZJ、Guo XX 等观察和分析肠易激综合征(IBS)内脏高敏感大鼠脊髓 L6－S3 节段背根神经节神经元中 $P2X_2$、$P2X_3$、$P2X_4$ 受体在电针治疗前后的改变，探讨电针缓解 IBS 大鼠慢性内脏痛敏的效应机制。结果显示，电针"上巨虚"和"天枢"穴可显著降低大鼠腹部撤回反射评分，抑制脊髓 L6－S3 节段背根神经节神经元 $P2X_2$、$P2X_3$、$P2X_4$ 受体的表达。杨帅等观察到，电针"百会"和"足三里"穴能改善大鼠焦虑状态，调节海马和结肠组织中 5－HT 水平。

针刺麻醉方面的研究较少，且侧重于针刺复合麻醉。吴群等观察比较经皮穴位电刺激(TAES)用于开颅手术全麻中丙泊酚用量、苏醒时间及拔管时间的影响。结果显示，观察组术中丙泊酚平均所需量、尼卡地平平均所需量、苏醒时间及拔管时间均较对照组减少($P<0.05$)。陈雪等观察 TAES 对经蝶入路垂体瘤切除术患者围术期血流动力学、麻醉用药及相关并发症的影响。结果，电刺激组(T 组)、假穴位组(S 组)以及对照组(C 组)均能够维持稳定的血流动力学。T 组在插管后 1 min、拔管及定向力恢复时的平均动脉压、术中暴露鞍区和取瘤阶段瑞芬太尼效应室浓度以及术后定向力恢复时异丙酚效应室浓度均较其余两组低(均 $P<0.05$)。术后 24 h 内 C 组 2 例发生恶心呕吐，其余各组均无相关并发症发生。

7. 文献与针灸流派传承研究

针灸的文献研究主要集中在现代针灸研究文献综述、古代针灸医籍及医家学术研究、基于循证医学的系统评价、文献计量分析(详见专条)、针灸治疗疾病选穴特点分析、针灸疾病谱的研究等。

在系统评价方面，Pennick V 等在 Cochrane Database of systematic reviews 上对针灸防治孕妇骨盆和腰背痛的文献进行系统评价，认为针灸或运动，相较于单纯常规治疗，更为显著地减轻夜晚骨盆痛或腰背痛，且针灸在减轻夜晚骨盆痛方面优于运动。Deare JC 等在 Cochrane Database of systematic reviews 上对针灸治疗肌纤维痛的疗效进行了系统评价，认为相较于标准治疗或不治疗，有低到中等证据表明针灸更能缓解疼痛以及改善肌肉僵硬。有中等证据表明针灸在缓解疼痛、乏力、提高睡眠质量或整体状态上与安慰针灸无显著性差异。电针可能比手针在缓解疼痛和僵硬以及提高整体状态、睡眠和乏力方面更具优势。Corbett MS 等在 Osteoarthritis Cartilage 上发表了针灸与其他物理方法治疗膝骨性关节炎疼痛的网络荟萃分析,认为针灸可以视为减轻膝骨性关节炎疼痛在短期内更为有效的物理疗法之一。

寿依夏、洪营东、何冬凤、孙晶等采用数据挖据等技术,分析了古代针灸治疗眩晕、胸痹、癫证、狂证、三叉神经痛等病症的用穴规律和特点。王文琴、高丽美等分析了古代和现代文献中太冲穴的运用规律。张国山、董利平、章海凤等总结和归纳了古代医藉中各医家灸法的运用特色和临证心得(详见专条)。

许吉等检索发现,2007～2011 年 SCI 收录针灸高被引论文共 240 篇,被引频次是 4 460,篇均被引频次为 18.58,第一作者发表论文最多的是美国,以第一作者发文最多的是来自中国的 Bai LJ,麻省总医院为发文最多的机构,ECAM 收录高被引论文最多。张承舜等检索并归纳和分析了 2008～2011 年来国外 SCI 源期刊文献中的针灸文献的数量、类型、语种、出版物来源、学科类别分布、研究机构和基金资助机构。丁然等对近 10 年 SCIE 源期刊文献中国作者发表的针灸论文进行文献计量分析,发现中国 SCIE 针灸论文以北京、上海、香港、台湾等经济较发达地区为主,国际合作方面略显不足。

在老中医经验总结方面,夏有兵、朱安宁等总结了澄江针灸学派情况(详见专条);彭冬青等总结了金伯华应用《金针赋》针刺手法经验。

8. 重要研究成果

2013 年,李振吉等报道,由吴焕淦承担的国内首个灸法国家重点基础研究发展计划("973"计划)项目"灸法作用的基本原理与应用规律研究"完成结题验收。该项目明确了艾灸临床的安全性和有效性,总结了艾灸温通温补效应规律:人体机能状态及疾病性质是决定艾灸温通温补效应的前提条件,适宜灸法、合理灸程与合理灸时是产生温通温补效应的关键;发现了穴位敏化现象,揭示了辨敏选穴,明显优于辨证选穴,消敏灸量是个体化充足灸量的临床应用新规律;揭示了穴位对传统隔物灸的红外辐射共振是艾灸起效的重要机制。

(吴焕淦　窦传字　包春辉　吴璐一)

【针刺手法及进针量化研究】

1. 行针补泻手法的量化研究

李靖等以高精度动作捕捉系统,测量比较 12 名针灸专家和 12 名初学者在仿真皮肤上操作 10 次平补平泻捻转手法时数据的大小及离散程度的差异。结果专家捻转频率离散系数显著低于初学者($P<0.01$),且专家捻转前的操作时间亦显著短于初学者($P<0.01$);专家与初学者捻转幅度、频率及力量的绝对数值相比,$P>0.05$。艾炳蔚应用微小力医用传感针,实时检测针刺提插捻转手法的提插力和捻转扭矩,20 名健康志愿者,取足三里和天枢穴,及足三里和天枢旁开 10 mm 非穴位。予腹部和下肢同一部位穴位与非穴位针刺提插捻转手法后,医生的提插、捻转力比较,$P>0.05$。下肢穴位足三里穴与腹部穴位天枢穴针刺提插捻转手法后,医生的提插、捻转力比较,$P<0.05$。乔红伟等从文献学角度分析针刺开阖补泻法的量效关系,认为开阖补法在一般按压力度均匀的情况下,以按压时间为首要决定因素,开阖泻法受摇动时间、幅度和方向影响,其中又以摇动时间为首。

2. 穴位进针深度的量化研究

程为平应用 MRI 测量 20 名健康青年关元穴针刺深度,结果直刺的危险深度为 29.5 mm,安全深度为 22.1 mm,男性和女性无显著性差异($P>0.05$),危险深度与身高、体重、BMI 指数无相关性($P>0.05$)。程氏等还应用 MRI 测量 20 名健康青年肾俞穴针刺深度,结果直刺危险深度左肾俞男性为 54.9 mm,女性为 47.5 mm,右肾俞分别为 53.3 mm、为 52.7 mm,危险深度与身高、体重、BMI 指数无相关性($P>0.05$)。许宇飞等应用 MRI 测量 20 名健康志愿者乳根穴针刺深度,结果男性组针刺危险深度:左侧 23.65 ± 1.95 mm、右侧 25.31 ± 2.83 mm;安全深度:左侧 17.73 ± 1.47 mm、右侧 18.99 ± 2.12 mm。女性组针刺危险深度:左侧为 25.14 ± 2.46 mm、右侧为 26.42 ± 2.78 mm;安全深度:左侧为 18.85 ± 2.13 mm、右侧为 19.81 ± 2.24 mm。针刺危险深度男女性别差异比较,$P>0.05$;左右侧差异性比较,$P>0.05$。张惠林等应用 CT 对翳风穴治疗贝尔麻痹的进针深度和角度定位，结果当7号腰椎穿刺针与人体矢状面约120°、与人体冠状面约45°、进针深度约35 mm时，穿刺针针尖可达茎乳孔处，即最佳进针深度、角度。李慧等测定66名女大学生三阴交穴最强针感深度，结果最强针感针刺深度为25.0±7.0 mm，但与周径、纵径无线性相关（$P>0.01$）。

（蒯　乐）

【支气管哮喘的针灸治疗及实验研究】

1. 临床研究

李焕新将患者分为两组，均予布地奈德雾化混悬液4 ml加沙丁胺醇雾化吸入治疗，早晚各1次，试验组在此基础上温针灸肺俞、风门、大椎、身柱、天突、膻中等穴位，每次每穴2壮。1次/d。经治10 d，试验组有效率为96.67%（29/30），对照组为80%（24/30），组间比较，$P<0.05$。夏俊等将患者分两组，对照组取双侧肺俞、膏肓、定喘穴。贴敷药物（白芥子、黄芪、甘草、细辛、麻黄、玄胡索等），隔日换药1次，每次3 h；观察组取双侧尺泽、列缺、足三里、丰隆穴，尺泽、列缺穴用平补平泻法，丰隆用泻法，足三里用补法。隔日针1次，针刺结束后，予穴位贴敷。均每周3次，经治10次后，观察组有效率为95%（38/40），对照组为75%（30/40），组间比较，$P<0.05$。观察组治疗后胸围呼吸差较对照组明显提高（$P<0.01$）。项永晶等将支气管哮喘发作期患者分为四组各30例，治疗组予服热咳喘胶囊（马兜铃、麻黄、全瓜蒌、桑白皮、黄芩、青黛等），电针双侧肺俞、定喘、足三里、丰隆、天突穴，刺激频率为15 Hz，每次20 min，1次/d；针刺组仅用针刺治疗，方法同治疗组；中药组服用热咳喘胶囊；西药组予吸沙美特罗替卡松吸入剂。治疗7 d后观察外周血嗜酸性粒细胞、血清免疫球蛋白E(IgE)、一秒用力呼气容积(FEV1)、呼气峰值流速(PEF)等指标变化。结果，治疗组与西药组疗效明显好于中药组、针刺组（$P<0.05$）；西药组与治疗组比较，$P<0.05$。罗胜等将哮喘慢性持续期患者分为两组，均予低剂量CIS或白三烯调节剂或长效胆受体激动剂的一种或一种以上药物治疗，并按需使用短效胆受体激动药，治疗组44例在此基础上取肺、平喘、气管等耳穴加用磁珠压贴，对照组40例贴胶布做空白对照。1次/3 d，经治疗20次，两组肺功能较治疗前均有改善（$P<0.05$）；而治疗组的哮喘控制测试评分、组胺支气管激发试验结果均优于对照组（$P<0.05$）。

鲍鑫宇等将患者分为两组，均予哮喘规范治疗方案，治疗组在此基础上加用督灸治疗，即大椎到腰俞之督脉处撒上肉桂、川芎等药粉，上铺桑皮纸、生姜泥、艾绒后施灸，每次约2 h，每月1次。经治3次，治疗组有效率为93.33%（28/30），对照组为70%（21/30），组间比较，$P<0.05$。

陈利芳等评价夏季卡介苗多糖核酸穴位注射对支气管哮喘的防治作用，将150例患者随机分为两组，穴注组取双侧足三里和定喘穴，每穴0.5 ml，肌注组常规肌肉注射，每次2 ml，隔日1次，共治疗30次。治疗前后、当年12月份和次年3月份对患者行哮喘控制水平评价、哮喘控制测试ACT评分。结果穴注组哮喘控制疗效、ACT评分均优于肌注组（$P<0.05$），而两组治疗前后肺功能指标无明显变化，且组间无差异（$P>0.05$）。李影捷等在抗炎、化痰、解痉等西医常规治疗基础上用喘可治注射液穴位注射方法治疗支气管哮喘，150例患者随机分为3组，取穴按3个疗程分别选取。第1疗程：定喘、肺俞、足三里、曲池、风门穴；第2疗程：定喘、脾俞、丰隆、天突、大杼穴；第3疗程：定喘、肺俞、足三里、肾俞、曲池穴。喘可治注射组及自体血注射组均以肺俞、定喘为主穴进行穴位注射，西医治疗组则不进行穴位注射，治疗60 d后，3组哮喘控制水平、血清特异性总IgE、嗜酸性粒细胞计数和FEV1%预计值都明显改善，$P<0.05$；且喘可治组及自体血组各项指标均优于西医治疗组，$P<0.05$。

谢建文等观察三伏天贴敷治疗虚寒喘证患者时发现疗效与连续贴敷药物治疗的时间成一定的相关，连续贴药3年，总有效率86.8%，连续贴药4年总有效率93.1%，连续贴药5年总有效率98.0%。田海燕等将100例患者分为穴位贴敷加隔姜灸组和电针加隔姜灸组，两组均取大椎、肺俞、天突等穴，治疗时间均为“一九”“二九”“三九”及“初伏”“中伏”“末伏”的第一天，结果发现两组治疗后各症状积分较治疗前均明显改善，穴位贴敷加隔姜灸组在咳嗽、喘息控制、呼吸快慢、胸闷程度、有无哮鸣音的治疗效果均优于电针加隔姜灸组，且显愈率高于电针组（$P<0.05$）。刘鸿将68例患者随机分为两组，治疗组于“三九”“三伏”第一天分别在膏肓穴、定喘穴贴敷中药药膏并口服扶正平喘汤，对照组舒利迭2次/d，治疗30 d

后发现治疗组血浆中内皮素、血栓素 B2 水平低于对照组($P<0.05$),且治疗组症状及肺功能改善优于对照组($P<0.05$)。

2. 实验研究

杨晓溪等将 SD 大鼠随机分为空白组、哮喘模型组、哮喘模型针刺组各 10 只,哮喘模型针刺组针刺“肺俞”、“风门”穴,行平补平泻手法,隔日 1 次,共 7 次。结果显示,哮喘模型组炎症病理改变明显,针刺干预后,炎症反应明显减轻,但未达到正常组水平,哮喘模型组肺组织 p38 丝裂原活化蛋白激酶(p38 MAPK)、原癌基因 c－fos 蛋白表达量增加($P<0.01$),针刺后 p38MAPK、c－fos 蛋白表达量降低($P<0.01$)。顾文等将 30 只雄性豚鼠随机分为正常组、模型组、穴位组、非穴位组、阳性对照组(氨茶碱粉末敷贴),以卵清白蛋白致敏激发法建立哮喘模型,穴位组选择肺俞、膻中、定喘穴,非穴位组选择肺俞、膻中、定喘穴旁开 1 cm 处,1 次/d,连续贴敷 10 d 后,穴位组与非穴位组 IL－4 血清含量、GATA －3mRNA 表达明显低于模型组,IFN－γ 含量、T－bet mRNA 表达明显高于模型组($P<0.01$),非穴位组血清 IL－4、IFN－γ 含量,T－bet mRNA 和 GATA －3 mRNA 的表达与穴位组差异均有统计学意义($P<0.01$)。

(王文倩　杨永清)

【针灸治疗慢性阻塞性肺疾病的研究】

1. 针灸治疗慢性阻塞性肺疾病(COPD)稳定期的研究

樊茂蓉等予穴位(天突穴、膻中穴、双侧肺俞穴,如若上述穴位出现皮肤反应,可用定喘穴、膏肓穴替换)贴敷中药(熟白芥子、细辛、麻黄、玄胡索、肉桂、生姜)治疗 COPD 稳定期 183 例,于夏季三伏天(初伏、中伏、末伏)第 1～3 d 各贴敷 1 次,每次成人为 2～6 h。治疗后 3、6、12 个月,症状发作次数均较治疗前减少($P<0.01$);各种慢性咳喘病(慢性支气管炎、支气管哮喘、慢性阻塞性肺疾病、慢性咳嗽)经穴位贴敷治疗后疾病发作次数均较贴敷前明显减少($P<0.01$)。

郭泳梅等将稳定期 COPD 患者分为两组,均在规范用药和有氧运动训练的前提下,治疗组予治疗针,安慰组予安慰针,针刺取膻中、乳根(双)、膺窗(双)、天枢(双)、中脘、关元穴,根据常见兼证选取配穴,复感外邪加合谷(单,隔次左右交替);痰浊中阻加丰隆(单,隔次左右交替)隔日 1 次。经治 14 次,治疗组治疗前后 6 min 步行距离(6－MWD)、一秒钟用力呼气容积占预计值百分比(FEV1%)、FEV1 与用力肺活量占预计值百分比(FVC%)的比值(FEV1/FVC)、最大分钟通气量(MVV)差值均较安慰组显著改善($P<0.05$ 或 $P<0.01$);两组临床症状总分和主要症状、整体症状评分均显著改善($P<0.05$ 或 $P<0.01$),组间比较,$P>0.05$。治疗组的生存质量总分、日常生活情况、抑郁症状均有显著改善($P<0.05$ 或 $P<0.01$);而安慰组治疗前后生存质量总分和各组评分比较,$P>0.05$。郭氏还观察了针刺配合有氧运动训练对稳定期 COPD 患者生活质量的影响。7 例 COPD 稳定期患者治疗前后的 COPD 生存质量问卷总分、6 min 步行距离差异具有统计学意义($P<0.05$ 或 $P<0.01$),而肺通气功能检查中 FVC 占预计值的百分比、FEV1/FVC、FEV1 占预计值的百分比差异无统计学意义($P>0.05$),但具有上升趋势。

李娜等对 COPD 稳定期患者均予羧甲司坦及常规抗炎、抗感染、祛痰、解痉平喘等治疗,治疗组 42 例再予火龙督脉铺灸疗法(铺灸药物:桂枝、白芍药、干姜、细辛、白芥子、黄芪等粉碎过 80 目筛后将生姜研泥加入和匀,制成药饼备用;取穴:背部督脉经及膀胱经第一侧线上,大椎至肾俞段)。经治 7 d 后,总有效率分别为 92.9%(39/42)、77.0%(30/40),组间比较,$P<0.05$。治疗后肺功能的改善,组间比较,$P<0.05$。

文幸等将 COPD 患者分为两组,均予西药常规治疗,治疗组 53 例配合艾炷灸背俞穴(肺俞、心俞、肝俞、脾俞、肾俞),每次 5 壮,灸后皮肤潮红、微汗、轻痛为佳。1 次/d,每周 5 次。经治 4 周,治疗组在中医证候“咳嗽”“喘促”积分及治疗后 3 个月生活质量评分,减少 COPD 急性发作次数方面优于对照组($P<0.05$)。

2. 针灸治疗 COPD 急性加重期的研究

周雪采用浮针治疗 COPD 急性加重期(AECOPD)20 例。取穴:选取患者肺部听诊啰音(干性或湿性)最为明显处为进针(P)点,通常选取 5 个点,即 P1～P5。若患者两肺散在啰音(干性或湿性)或未闻及啰音(湿性或干性),则选取膻中、定喘、膏肓作为 P 点(P1～P5)。操作:选用一次性使用中号浮针,在距离 P 点 3～5 cm

处(从下向上),针尖指向P点,快速以15°~30°角斜刺透过皮肤,稍退针尖入皮下,针尖向上略翘,向P点处皮下水平推进至软套管没于皮下,将针尖稍退,向左旋转90°入卡槽,拇指与其他4指对持针柄、以拇指为支点,中指、无名指交替用力,使针尖在皮下做水平扫散扇形运动,快速在皮下扫散约3 min。扫散完毕,不锈钢针座向右旋转出槽,将不锈钢针芯完全退出,软套管留置皮下,胶布固定,5 h后取出软套管。1次/d,连续治疗3次后,肺部听诊呼吸音评分、及气喘评分明显下降($P<0.05$)。肺功能测定二氧化碳分压($PaCO_2$)明显下降($P<0.05$),氧分压(PaO_2)无明显变化($P>0.05$);FVC、FEV1、FEV1%、FEV1/FVC明显升高($P<0.05$);治疗前肺功能分级为2.45±0.64,治疗后明显降低至1.98±0.58级($P<0.05$)。

战文翔等将AECOPD患者分为三组各30例,均予常规抗感染、雾化吸入平喘、抗炎、化痰药物及支持、对症治疗;粗针组加用粗针刺膻中穴,进针100 mm,留针3 h;传统毫针组加用传统毫针刺膻中穴,进针100 mm,留针3 h。均治疗10 d,计算BODE及圣乔治问卷(SGRQ)评分,BODE包括体质量指数(BMI)、气流阻塞程度(FEV1%pred)、呼吸困难(MMRC)、运动能力(6MWD,6 min步行距离)。结果治疗后BODE中的6MWD步行距离、圣乔治问卷(SGRQ)评分,粗针组、传统毫针组与对照组比较,均$P>0.05$;粗针组与传统毫针组比较,$P<0.01$。肺功能、BMI与呼吸困难分级没有明显改善,可能与观察时间短有关。

张艳敏等将140例AECOPD患者随机分为A肺俞组、B支沟组、C抑喘方(肺俞+支沟)组及D西药组,前三组均行针刺治疗,所刺穴位对应各组名称,得气后肺俞穴行平补平泻法(行均匀地提插、捻转手法),支沟穴行提插捻转泻法(行捻转角度大,用力重,频率快及重提轻插手法),时间为1 min,留针30 min;留针中间再行手法1次,2次/d。D组用氧疗、抗感染、解痉平喘等常规治疗。经治14 d后,总有效率A组为81.8%(27/33)、B组为81.2%(26/32)、C组为93.3%(28/30)、D组为76.6%(23/30),四组间比较,$P<0.05$。

雷琰等采用穴位针刺加中草药贴敷治疗AECOPD,选膻中、合谷、列缺、肺俞、足三里、丰隆穴,针刺10次,1次/d;中草药(白芥子、细辛各400 g,延胡索、甘遂、麻黄各100 g。)穴位贴敷选天突、膻中、大椎、定喘、肺俞、肾俞穴,每3~7 d1次。共治3次,不分节气,总有效率为100%(120/120)。

张弛等将AECOPD患者分为两组各30例,均予常规抗感染、氧疗、改善通气等治疗;治疗组加用5号注射器抽取黄芪注射液分别刺入双侧足三里穴,得气后,回抽无回血后注射黄芪注射液0.5 ml,1次/d。经治2周后,治疗组CD_3、IgA、IgG、IgM较治疗前和对照组均明显升高($P<0.01$)。

(纪　军)

【糖尿病及其并发症的针灸治疗与实验研究】

1. 治疗糖尿病

周平南等将新发肥胖2型糖尿病患者随机分两组。对照组采用生活方式(饮食、运动)改变,治疗组在对照组基础上加针刺大椎、合谷、足三里、三阴交、膈俞、肝俞等穴,行捻转平补平泻手法,1次/d,20次为1个疗程,针灸先仰卧位,后俯卧位,休息10 d,进行第2个疗程。3个疗程后,治疗组总有效率为97.5%(39/40),对照组为81.5%(29/36)。

赵微将2型糖尿病患者随机平分为两组,均予服中药(党参、黄芪、茯苓、白术、黄连、豆蔻等),治疗组联合针刺海泉、肺俞、肾俞、肝俞、胃俞、脾俞等穴,行平补平泻手法,1次/d。经治3个月后,治疗组总有效率94.7%(18/19),对照组78.9%(15/19)。

2. 治疗糖尿病并发症

杨雪蓉等将糖尿病神经源性膀胱患者分为两组各30例,均予基础治疗(降糖、降压、降脂、改善微循环、营养神经、抗感染)及膀胱排尿功能训练(白天定时排尿同时压迫小腹,听水流声诱导排尿,排尿后饮水300 ml,随后收缩、放松会阴肌肉数次),治疗组加针刺三阴交、关元、中极、气海、膀胱俞、肾俞,用补法,同时艾灸关元、气海,耳穴贴压交感、肺、脾、肾、膀胱、三焦,隔天一换,两耳交替。治疗2周后,治疗组残余尿量、中医证候积分均下降且优于对照组($P<0.05$)。

任红等将糖尿病神经原性膀胱患者随机单盲平分成两组,均予饮食控制、心理护理、适当运动、调整降糖药物等常规治疗,治疗组加黄芪注射液注射穴位(关元、三阴交、膀胱俞、肺俞),1 次/d。经治 1 个月后,治疗组与对照组的中医症状积分分别为(18.47±1.67)分、(23.19±2.82)分,均较治疗前的(29.25±2.12)分、(29.13±1.69)分降低;组间比较,$P<0.05$;治疗组与对照组的膀胱残余尿量分别为(88.47±16.7)ml、(143.19±28.2)ml,均较同组治疗前的(308.90±22.6)ml、(305.90±20.8)ml 减少,组间比较,$P<0.05$;治疗组总有效率为 85.5%(59/69)、对照组为 78.3%(54/69),组间比较,$P<0.05$。

张必萌等将糖尿病胃轻瘫患者随机分为两组,西药组口服多潘立酮,针刺组针刺足三里、内关、中脘,行提插补泻手法,1 次/d,5 次为 1 个疗程。经治 3 周后,针刺组总有效率为 86.73%(85/98),西药组为 75%(72/96),组间总有效率及针刺改善饱胀的疗效比较,$P<0.01$。

赵斌将麻痹性斜视的糖尿病患者分为两组,均予控制血糖,及应用血管扩张剂、维生素 B_1、弥可保口服或肌肉注射。中医治疗组加以针刺睛明、承泣、球后、上明、瞳子髎、丝竹空等穴,平补平泻手法,球周各穴禁止提插或捻转,留针 30~40 min。1 次/d,10~14 次为 1 个疗程,同时配合桃红四物汤。经治 3 个疗程后,中医治疗组总有效率为 94.4%(32/36),西医治疗组总有效率为 75.9%(22/29),组间比较,$P<0.01$。

3. 实验研究

翟煦等将 50 只雄性 SD 大鼠分为空白对照组 10 只、模型组 13 只、耳甲区组 13 只、体针组 14 只,空白对照组普通饲料,其余各组高脂饲料喂养并造模。至第 31 d 时,在每日 15: 00~18: 00治疗 30 min,耳甲区电刺激 15 Hz,体针组取足三里、三阴交穴电刺激 15 Hz。经治 14 d,与模型组比较,两针刺组血糖均下降($P<0.01$),但体针组更低($P<0.05$)。耳甲区组大鼠背部皮肤水分散失(TEWL)、色差值(L. 值、b. 值)及腹部皮肤含水量(SCH)、色差值(L. 值、b. 值)有明显改善($P<0.05$),体针组背部水分散失(TEWL),腹部红斑指数(EI),腹背部皮肤含水量(SCH)、黑色素指数(MI)、色差值(L. 值、a. 值、b. 值)改善明显。

胥冰等将 SD 大鼠 50 只均分为空白组、模型组、针刺治疗组、中药治疗组、针刺+中药组。除空白组外其余组大鼠腹腔注射 STZ 糖尿病造模。针刺治疗组取肺俞、胰俞、脾俞、肾俞穴或关元、中脘、三阴交、足三里穴,两组穴位交替,中药治疗组予白芍甘草汤灌胃,针刺+中药组在针刺同时联合白芍甘草汤灌胃。治疗 7 周后,针刺+中药组血糖降低明显,血胰岛素水平升高,胰腺 bcl-2 表达增强,各指标与模型组比较,$P<0.05$、$P<0.01$。

董勤等将 136 只 SD 雄性大鼠分为空白组 32 只、模型组 32 只、电针组 36 只、穴位注射组 36 只。除空白组外,其余组大鼠腹腔注射 STZ 糖尿病周围神经病变造模。电针组电刺激肾俞、足三里,疏密波 2/15 Hz,穴位注射组同样穴位注射弥可保 0.1 ml,模型组仅固定大鼠,均隔日 1 次。治疗 60 d 后,两治疗组降糖效果明显,且电针组更优($P<0.01$),坐骨神经感觉神经传导速度改善方面穴位注射组为佳($P<0.01$)。两组均可提高神经生长因子(NGF)及其受体 TrkA 的表达,且治疗 60 d 时穴位注射组改善幅度优于电针组($P<0.05$)。

(张航飞　赵　玲)

【针灸治疗胃病的实验研究】

丁乐等将 40 只雌雄各半家兔均分为空白组(A 组)、模型组(B 组)、常规针刺组(C 组)、子午流注戌时取穴结合常规针刺组(D 组)、子午流注辰时取穴结合常规针刺组(E 组)。A 组不作处理;而 B、C、D、E 组造模,于 24 h 后采用电针针刺,以中脘、足三里为基本穴位,埋针 1 个时辰,1 次/d。经治 7 d 后,模型组胃黏膜损伤指数(UI 值)明显高于空白组($P<0.01$);与模型组比较,常规针刺组、戌时组、辰时组的 UI 值均有明显降低($P<0.01$);辰时组 UI 值低于常规针刺组、戌时组($P<0.05$);空白组的褪黑素(MT)、热休克蛋白 70(HSP70)含量均低于其它各组($P<0.01$);与模型组比较,常规针刺组、戌时组、辰时组的 MT、HSP70 含量均明显增高($P<0.01$);辰时组与常规针刺组、戌时组比较,MT、HSP70 均含量增高($P<0.05$)。

羊燕群等采用适度夹尾刺激法复制功能性消化不良(FD)大鼠模型,分别予电针刺激"足三里"穴及对照性西药治疗,测定各组大鼠摄食量、体重、胃残留率、碳末推进率及血清 Motilin 和 Ghrelin 浓度。实验结果:模型组、西药组和针刺组摄食量与空白组比较均显著下降($P<0.05$);

西药组与针刺组胃残留率减少($P<0.05$);西药组和针刺组相应的碳末推进率较空白组显著升高($P<0.05$);模型组大鼠血清 Motilin 浓度显著下降($P<0.05$);模型组大鼠血清 Ghrelin 相对升高,但无统计学意义($P>0.05$)。石君杰等观察经皮穴位电刺激(TEAS)“足三里”穴对运动性疲劳致胃黏膜损伤大鼠胃黏膜的保护作用及机制。采用跑台运动法建立运动性疲劳致胃黏膜损伤模型大鼠随机分为正常组、模型组、TEAS 组各 8 只。予 TEAS“足三里”穴(连续波、频率 2 Hz、强度 5 mA 治疗 30 min,1 次/d)干预 15 d,与正常组比较,模型组大鼠水平运动分数、垂直运动分数、力竭运动时间均明显减少,胃黏膜损伤指数增加,同时胃黏膜 6-酮-前列腺素 1α(6-keto-PGF1α)、血栓素 B_2(TXB_2)含量明显降低,与模型组比较,TEAS 组水平运动分数、垂直运动分数、力竭运动时间均增加,胃黏膜损伤指数降低,胃黏膜 6-keto-PGF1α、TXB_2 含量升高。与正常组比较,模型组胃黏膜出现不同程度的溃疡现象,与模型组比较,TEAS 组胃黏膜损伤指数明显降低。

余芝等将 SD 大鼠随机分为正常组、饥饿组(禁食 24 h)、阿托品组(M 受体拮抗剂,0.1%,0.8 ml/kg,40 μL/min·kg)、乙酰胆碱组(0.1%,20 μL/min·kg)、克伦特罗组(β2 受体激动剂,0.2%,80 μL/min·kg)、心得安组(β 受体拮抗剂,0.4%,1 ml/kg,40 μL/min·kg)和对穴组,每组 30 只。在胃内放置球囊,并连接到压力传感器检测胃内压力。分别在上述 6 种状态下观察电针(2 Hz/15 Hz,2 mA,2 min)“天枢”“曲池”和“上巨虚”对大鼠胃运动的影响,并观察正常状态下电针“天枢”+“上巨虚”、“天枢”+“曲池”和“上巨虚”+“曲池”对大鼠胃运动的影响(均取左侧腧穴)。结果发现电针“天枢”对胃内压和胃运动均产生明显抑制作用,抑制程度为:饥饿>正常,乙酰胆碱>阿托品,克伦特罗>心得安,电针“曲池”和“上巨虚”对胃内压和胃运动均产生明显兴奋作用,“天枢”+“上巨虚”对胃运动以抑制为主,“上巨虚”+“曲池”表现为兴奋作用,而“天枢”+“曲池”的抑制或兴奋作用均不明显。

董莉莉等将雄性 Wistar 大鼠随机分为正常组、模型组、捆绑组、中脘组、足三里组和合募配穴组各 10 只。除正常组外其余各组大鼠利用捆绑加水浸应激法复制胃溃疡大鼠模型后进行针刺治疗。足三里组取双侧“足三里”穴针刺,中脘组取“中脘”穴针刺,合募配穴组取“足三里”加“中脘”穴针刺,采用平补平泻针法,1 次/d,留针 20 min,经治疗 2 d,捆绑组、模型组大鼠同正常组比较,溃疡指数显著升高($P<0.01$);中脘组、足三里组、合募配穴组同模型组比较,溃疡指数明显下降($P<0.05$,$P<0.01$),且以合募配穴效果更佳。捆绑组、模型组大鼠同正常组比较,下丘脑组织 GnRH mRNA 表达显著增加($P<0.05$,$P<0.01$);各针刺组和模型组相比,GnRH mRNA 表达均显著下降($P<0.01$);各针刺组之间的差异无统计学意义($P>0.05$)。捆绑组、模型组和正常组相比,下丘脑组织 SP mRNA 表达的差异无统计学意义($P>0.05$);足三里组、合募配穴组同模型组相比,SP mRNA 表达显著增加($P<0.01$);合募配穴组表达的增加较足三里组更明显($P<0.05$)

(刘堂义)

【肠易激综合征的针灸治疗及实验研究】

1. 临床研究

Ma YX 等将患者随机分为三组,分别采用隔药灸、隔饼灸、口服匹维溴胺。经治疗 4 周后,三组胃肠道症状评估量表积分分别是(1.98±0.303,2.93±0.302,3.73±0.449),8 周后为(2.75±0.306,3.56±0.329,4.39±2.48),各组间无明显差异。然隔药灸组与匹维溴胺组的腹痛积分比较,$P<0.05$;腹胀比较,$P<0.01$。

刘敏等采用针刺与按摩结合的方法治疗 68 例患者,针刺选取天枢、大横、足三里、脾俞、大肠俞为主穴,并随证配穴。针刺结束后进行掌揉患者腹部,以腕关节旋转动为主施以揉法,幅度不宜过大,手掌持久、有力、柔和的带动其下组织逆时针回旋。隔日 1 次,10 次 1 个疗程。2 个疗程后,有效率达 95.6%(37/40)。

赵红波等将脾胃湿阻证腹泻型患者分为两组,治疗组 34 例采用健脾厚肠法(方用参苓白术汤加减)联合针灸疗法,针刺选取中脘、天枢、足三里、太冲、脾俞、胃俞等穴,先俯卧位斜刺脾俞、胃俞各 0.5 寸,大肠俞直刺 0.8 寸,施捻转补法,得气后,留针 15 min;然后直刺天枢、中脘,施平补平泻法,直刺足三里、太冲以提插捻转补法,得气后,留针 30 min;同时予神阙穴隔姜灸法,致皮肤红润为度,1 次/d。对照组 31 例口服双歧杆菌乳杆菌三联活菌片和马来酸曲美布丁片。经治疗4周后,治疗组各项消化道症状积分降低($P<0.05$,$P<0.01$);对照组仅腹痛、腹胀、排便次数积分较治疗前改善($P<0.05$)。治疗组消化道症状积分均低于对照组($P<0.05$)。在SF-36评分方面,治疗组各指标评分改善优于治疗前及对照组($P<0.05$)。总有效率分别为97.06%(33/34)、77.42%(24/31),组间比较,$P<0.05$;随访6月后,复发率分别为14.71%(5/34)、51.61%(16/31),组间比较,均$P<0.05$。

谢振年等将患者均分为两组,治疗组采用穴位强化埋线疗法,穴位选取大肠俞(双)、天枢(双)、足三里(双)、气海透关元透中极穴,每穴同时重复埋线3次,1次为1个疗程,疗效不佳或病情反复,间隔1月重复埋线1次。对照组口服麻仁软胶囊。随访时间6个月。治疗组与对照组总有效率分别为72.1%(75/104)、14.4%(15/104),组间比较,$P<0.05$;治疗组主要症状积分与治疗前比较,均$P<0.05$,标志物残留数目较对照组明显减少($P<0.05$)。

2. 实验研究

朱文莲等将大鼠分为3组各9只,模型组与电针关元组造模后2周后电针,模型组束缚20 min不针刺。电针关元组和电针大肠俞组束缚同时电针刺激20 min,正常组不作任何操作,隔日1次。经治7次后,与模型组比较,电针大肠俞组、电针关元组大鼠腹部抬起容量阈值明显升高($P<0.05$),电针关元组大鼠背部拱起容量阈值明显升高($P<0.05$);与模型组比较,电针关元组大鼠丘脑中NPY含量显著升高($P<0.01$),电针大肠俞组大鼠脊髓中神经肽Y含量显著升高($P<0.05$)。

秦庆广将60只SD大鼠分为3组各20只。冰水灌胃法建立便秘模型大鼠,番泻叶灌胃法建立腹泻模型大鼠。针刺"天枢"穴,捻转行针1 min,平补平泻,120次/min,结果:① 正常大鼠,针刺"天枢"降低空肠收缩的频率和波幅($P<0.01$,$P<0.01$),抑制空肠的收缩;腹泻大鼠模型中,针刺"天枢"降低了空肠运动的频率和波幅($P<0.01$,$P<0.01$)。针刺"天枢"对正常和腹泻状态大鼠的空肠运动有明显的抑制作用。② 正常大鼠,针刺天枢增加远端结肠运动的频率和波幅($P<0.01$,$P<0.05$);便秘模型大鼠,针刺天枢使远端结肠的运动加快,波幅增大($P<0.05$,$P<0.01$)。

(安广青　李　娜)

【针灸治疗肥胖的临床及实验研究】

1. 临床研究

单敬文将患者分成两组,均取中脘、关元、气海、双侧足三里、脾俞、肾俞为主穴,随证配穴。治疗组40例予温针灸(针刺得气后,于主穴处温针灸,每次1壮,约30 min)与走罐治疗(在腹部任脉、脾胃经脉,背腰部督脉、足太阳膀胱经脉上取穴,于针刺起针后视患者肥胖程度选火罐,在罐口和走罐部位分别涂上适量刮痧油,用闪火法将罐迅速吸附于体表,火罐不宜太紧,然后以手握罐底稍倾斜,沿任脉、经脉或督脉、足太阳膀胱经脉缓缓推拉移动数次,至皮肤潮红即可起罐。每次轮取腹部和背腰部经脉走罐,每次10 min)。对照组38例采用电针治疗。结果治疗组腰围、体重、体重指数(BMI)与治疗前比较,$P<0.05$。治疗后两组腰围、BMI分别比较,均$P<0.05$。

孙健等将腹型肥胖患者分为电针、埋线及联合组各50例,联合组采用电针与埋线合治。电针取穴:① 中脘、气海、滑肉门、外陵、府舍、大横穴。② 水分、关元,天枢、水道,腹结、带脉,足三里、丰隆。双侧对称取穴,每次选一组穴位,交替应用,并随证配穴,针刺进针捻转得气后接电针仪,采用疏密波,以患者能耐受为度,留针30 min。埋线取穴同电针。均每周1次。经治8周后,三组患者的腰围、体重、BMI与同组治疗前比较,$P<0.05$,$P<0.01$。联合组治疗后空腹血糖(FPG)、空腹胰岛素(FINS)、胰岛素敏感指数(ISI)、胰岛素抵抗指数(IRI)与同组治疗前比较,$P<0.01$;体重、BMI及ISI、IRI与电针组和埋线组比较,$P<0.05$,$P<0.01$。联合组和电针组治疗后血浆胆固醇(CH)、甘油三酯(TG)、低密度脂蛋白(LDL)、高密度脂蛋白(HDL)与同组治疗前比较,$P<0.05$,$P<0.01$。埋线组治疗后CH、LDL、HDL与同组治疗前比较,$P<0.05$,$P<0.01$。联合组和埋线组治疗后HDL与电针组比较,$P<0.05$,$P<0.01$。

2. 实验研究

郜婕等将SD大鼠随机分为普食组、模型组、

5 mA 电针组、1 mA 电针组各 10 只，后三组喂食高脂饲料造肥胖大鼠模型。电针组针刺双侧“足三里”“三阴交”，1 次/d，15 min/次。经治 2 周，两电针组体质量及 sOCS－3、PPAR－γmRNA 表达较模型组均降低($P<0.01$)，5 mA 电针较 1 mA电针效果更明显($P<0.01$)。

（安广青　翟国华）

【慢性疲劳综合征的治疗】

茅敏等治疗 45 例慢性疲劳综合征(CFS)患者，取穴：① 百会、膻中、气海、神门、足三里、三阴交、太溪。② 心俞、膈俞、肝俞、脾俞、肾俞。每日一组，两组交替，得气后行平补平泻，留针 30 min，每 15 min 行针 1 次，1 次/d，逢周末休息 2 d。经治 4 周，总有效率为 93.3%(42/45)。刘亚丽等将 CFS 患者分为两组，治疗组选取双侧膀胱经大杼、肺俞、心俞、督俞、膈俞、肝俞等穴，对照组取百会、印堂、神门、太溪、太冲、三阴交等穴。不行提插捻转，留针 30 min，10 次为 1 个疗程。治疗 3 个疗程后，两组治疗前疲劳整体症状量表积分比较，$P>0.05$，治疗后组间比较，$P<0.05$；治疗组与治疗前组内比较，$P<0.01$；对照组与治疗前组内比较，$P<0.05$。治疗组与对照组总有效率分别为 90.7%(29/32)、70.9%(22/31)，组间比较，$P<0.05$。两组治疗前疼痛量表积分比较，$P>0.05$，治疗后组间比较，$P<0.05$；治疗组治疗前后组内比较，$P<0.01$，对照组治疗前后组内比较，$P<0.05$。杨丽洁等将患者分为两组，治疗组选百会、关元、足三里、太溪、脾俞、肾俞为主穴，并随症加减。进针得气后，用平补平泻法，留针 30 min，10 min 行针 1 次。留针双侧足三里，余穴取针，任选一侧足三里行烧山火针法。周一、三、五取正面腧穴治疗，周二、四取背面腧穴治疗，10 次为 1 个疗程。对照组取穴及针刺手法同治疗组，但足三里不行烧山火针法。治疗 3 个疗程，治疗组总有效率为 96.7%(29/30)，对照组为 88.9%(24/27)。

文胜等治疗 60 例患者用麦粒灸悬钟和足三里穴，患者取侧卧位，施术时男性先左后右，女性先右后左，先灸足三里，用大蒜汁涂抹在穴位表面，将艾绒捻成麦粒样大小的艾炷，直接放置在穴位上，点燃线香，用线香引燃艾炷，医者用双掌拢住周围，避免风吹，让艾炷慢慢燃烧，当患者感到灼热疼痛时，嘱其忍耐勿动。同时，医者发出口令，患者跟随重复，由“1”慢慢数至“9”为止。患者疼痛会消失，待艾炷慢慢燃尽，掸去艾灰，可见穴位处出现一个向四周扩散、呈放射状之皱纹，用剪好直径为 25 mm 的圆形胶布覆盖，以拇指紧紧按压 30 s。然后，用同法施灸另一侧之穴位。每次每穴灸 1 壮，1 次为 1 个疗程。患者即刻治疗后及治疗后 30 d 各项症状积分与治疗前比较，$P<0.01$。患者治疗后 30 d 各项症状积分与即刻治疗后比较，$P<0.01$，$P<0.05$。患者即刻治疗后总有效率为 73.3%(44/60)，治疗后 30 d 总有效率为 90.0%(54/60)，组间比较，$P<0.05$。

郑盛惠等将脾肾两虚型患者分为两组，对照组采用俞募配穴针灸，主穴取脾俞、章门、肾俞、京门，配穴取太白、足三里、命门、关元，均为双侧穴，施以补法，留针 30 min。1 次/d，5 次/周。治疗组在上述俞募配穴针灸的基础上加用长蛇灸(将生附子打粉过筛，加压蒸制 3 h，经生物发酵酸化处理后，加糊精适量，调成直径 4 cm、厚 1 cm 附子饼备用，将生姜研磨成生姜泥备用，取艾绒适量备用；取大椎穴至腰俞穴铺敷 5 cm 宽、1 cm 厚的生姜泥，在生姜泥上排列放置附子饼，然后将纯艾绒捏紧成长蛇形，置于附子饼中央，将艾绒头尾点燃待其自然燃尽后再继续铺艾绒施灸，每次约 1 h，灸毕将绷带连同生姜泥、附子饼、艾灰一同移去。灸后如皮肤起泡，可用针刺破水泡放出渗液，用消毒棉签揩干，涂以碘伏，覆盖消毒纱布，换药 1 次/d，至结痂脱落)。每周治疗 1 次。经治 4 周，治疗组总有效率 63.3%(19/30)，对照组总有效率 41.4%(12/29)，治疗组 IL－2、IFN－γ、TNF－α 水平均显著升高($P<0.05$ 或$P<0.01$)，对照组 IL－2、IFN－γ 水平显著升高($P<0.05$)，TNF－α 无明显变化($P>0.05$)。

（王　静）

【中风后肩手综合征的针灸治疗】

叶水林等将患者分为两组，均予基础药物治疗，治疗组患者取侧卧位，在距痛点 6～8 cm 处常规消毒，医者以针尖对准痛点，针体与皮肤呈 15°～25°快速刺入皮下进至痛点附近后，针柄做扇形运动数次，时间 3～4 min，直到病人的疼痛不再减轻或完全消失为止拔出。对照组直刺肩髃、肩髎、肩贞、臂臑、手三里、曲池等穴，留针 30 min，得气后接电针仪，选用强度均以患者能耐受为度。每周连续治疗 5 d，休息 2 d。经治 3 周，治疗组与对照组总有效率分别为 97.5%(39/40)、80.0%(32/40)，组间比较，$P<0.05$；神经功

能缺损程度评分、肩手综合征评估量表评分(SHS)、疼痛视觉模拟评分法(VAS)评分等与对照组比较，$P<0.05$。

郑盛惠等将患者随机分为两组，治疗组取肩髃、肩髎、肩贞、曲池、手三里、外关等穴，进针后施赤风迎源针法(直刺进针至腧穴深层，得气后退针至腧穴浅层，待针下得气，针体自摇，再插至腧穴中层，边提插，边捻转。然后用右手拇、食指呈交互状，拇指头向前，食指头向后，将两指弯曲，由根部用拇指肚及食指第一节桡侧由下而上沿针柄呈螺旋式搓摩，两指一搓一放，如凤凰展翅状，使针感向腧穴周围甚至远端传导)，每隔 10 min 行针法 1 次，留针 30 min。对照组采用康复训练治疗，给予患肢各关节各运动方向进行被动活动，多做抗痉挛模式的活动，如肩关节外展、前臂旋后、腕和手指伸展等。1 次/d，5 次/周(周末休息)。连续治疗 4 周，治疗组与对照组总有效率分别为 89.7%(35/39)、68.4%(26/38)，组间比较，$P<0.05$。治疗组各维度积分与治疗前后比较，均 $P<0.01$；对照组治疗前后比较，$P<0.05$；组间比较，$P<0.01$ 或 $P<0.05$。两组治疗前后健康效用值比较，$P<0.01$，$P<0.05$；治疗组优于对照组($P<0.05$)。

张伟等将患者分为两组。均予卒中单元的基础治疗，观察组取双侧肩髃、肩髎、肩贞、曲池、手三里、合谷等穴，补虚泄实，补健侧泄患侧，先针健侧，再针患侧。1 次/d，留针 30 min，中间行针 1 次，治疗 6 d 后休息 1 d。对照组选穴同观察组，采用普通针刺法治疗。经治 4 周，治疗组与对照组总有效率分别为 92.5%(37/40)、87.5%(35/40)，组间比较，$P<0.05$；两组上肢 Fugl-Meyer 运动功能评分较治疗前后比较，均 $P<0.01$，组间比较，$P<0.01$。

黄昌锦等将 70 例患者随机分为两组，治疗组选取肩峰(在肩外侧，当肩峰端)、天谬次(在背部，当肩胛内上角处)、天宗次(在肩背部，正当冈下窝中)、肩内陵次(在肩前部，当肱骨结节间沟中)、肩痛点次(在肩背部，当肩胛骨腋缘上方，肩胛骨外缘中点)、臑会次(在臂外侧，当三角肌后束下方处)、举肩次(在腋前部，当喙肱肌肌腹处)、鱼际次(在手掌侧，当第一掌骨内侧缘，拇对掌肌，拇收肌抵止处)穴，涂上薄层万花油，用细火针在乙醇灯上烧红赤，快速准确针刺选定经筋点，出针后按压针孔。隔日 1 次，10 次为 1 个疗程。对照组采用普通针刺治疗。结果治疗组与对照组治疗前后 VAS 评分、ROM、简化 Fugl-Meyer 评分及水肿评分比较，$P<0.01$；两组 VAS 评分、ROM 及水肿评分比较，，$P<0.01$；两组简化 Fugl-Meyer 评分比较，$P>0.05$。

曾姿霈等将患者分为两组，治疗组予薄智云所创的腹针疗法，选中脘、下脘、商曲(健侧)、气海、关元、滑肉门(双侧)等穴，其中中脘、下脘、气海、关元穴均深刺，商曲、滑肉门穴中刺，上风湿点、上风湿外点浅刺，前 3 次治疗每日 1 次，之后隔天 1 次，留针 30 min；局部穴位(选患侧天宗、肩隅、曲池、手三里、内关，每次选用 1 穴，轮替使用)注射天麻素注射液和维生素 B_1 注射液，3 d1 次。对照组取患侧肩膈、曲池、手三里、内关、外关、合谷等穴，针刺得气后，接治疗仪，电量以患者耐受为度，每次 30 min。1 次/d，6 次/周。经治疗 4 周，治疗组与对照组总有效率分别为 95.6%(43/45)、77.8%(35/45)，组间比较，$P<0.05$。

周莉等将患者分为两组各 30 例，实验组采用麦粒灸结合系统康复训练，选择患侧肢体井穴：少商、商阳、中冲、少冲、关冲、少泽，肩手部位的肩髃、肩髎、曲池、曲泽、手三里、外关等。艾绒置于穴位上，以线香点燃，待燃尽后在穴位表面涂以万花油，每穴灸 1～2 壮，1 次/d，共治疗 3 周。系统康复训练包括良肢位摆放、主动被动活动。对照组常规针刺治疗，两组基础治疗相同。结果实验组改善 SHSAS 患者的肢体功能和日常生活能力疗效均优于对照组($P<0.05$)；实验组综合疗效亦优于对照组($P<0.05$)；Brunnstrom 分期比较，实验组改善肌力的情况优于对照组($P<0.05$)。

(许　吉)

【针刺治疗 Bell's 面瘫】

李艳等将患者随机分为 9 组各 13 例，通过正交设计探索针刺治疗周围性面瘫留针时间及频次的优化组合方案，发现针刺时间和针刺频次两个因素均是影响面神经功能恢复的显著因素，其最优组合为留针 20 min、隔日针刺 1 次。Liu LA 等将 129 例患者随机分为连续波组、疏密波组、断续波组，穴取地仓、颊车、阳白、太阳、下关、合谷等，分别行相应频率的电针治疗，3 组均 1 次/d，5 次为 1 个疗程，疗程间休息 2 d，共治疗 4 个疗程。结果连续波组、疏密波组、断续波组的痊愈率分别为 68.9%(31/45)、60.0%(24/40)、65.9%(29/44)，经秩和检验组间疗效比较，$P>0.05$。王元将 108 例 Bell's 麻痹患者随机平分为两组，对照组取患侧四白、颧髎、颊车、地仓、翳风、牵正等穴，直刺进针，针刺深度 0.3～0.5 cm，面部诸穴行平补平泻手法，曲池及合谷穴行泻法，留针 30 min，1 次/d。治疗组在对照组的基础上从急性期开始加以阳明经筋排刺，针刺患侧面部诸穴深度0.1～0.3 cm，不行手法治疗，拔针后勿按其孔可令其出血，曲池及合谷穴行泻法，留针 15 min，；静止期及恢复期针刺面部诸穴深度为 0.3～0.5 cm，并加用地仓透颊车、颊车透地仓、攒竹透鱼腰，行平补平泻手法，曲池、合谷行泻法，留针 30 min。1 周为 1 个疗程，每周休息 1 d。经治 4 周后，治疗组与对照组愈显率分别为 70.4%(52/54)、48.1%(44/54)，组间比较，$P<0.01$。

邓丽兴将 96 例患者随机分为两组，对照组取风池、下关、颊车、地仓、迎香、太阳等穴，刺法为颊车透地仓、太阳透下关、阳白透鱼腰，余穴平补平泻，合谷穴照神灯；观察组采用闪罐配合甩针挂钩治疗，即在患侧风池下颈部、颊车、颧髎、太阳、阳白穴闪罐 5～7 次至潮红，用 6 寸长针从患侧颊车下方进针，先深后浅，以能看见针在皮下前进、针尖上对口角至唇边为度，然后把针向一个方向旋捻，左手轻压针体部，隔腮看见针尖接近口吻时稍微用力拉针柄，则面皮皱成深纹数条，一拉一松十余次让患者自己捏针柄，照神灯，留针 20 min，起针时手捏针柄用力甩出。1 次/d，5 次为 1 个疗程，每个疗程间隔 2 d。经治 1 个月，观察组与对照组总有效率分别为 97.9%(47/48)、87.5%(42/48)，组间比较，$P<0.05$。倪瑛等将患者分成两组，均予普通针刺，即取地仓、颊车、阳白、攒竹、迎香、翳风等穴；治疗组加用温针灸足三里，平补平泻法。留针 30 min，10 次为 1 个疗程。经治 3 个疗程，治疗组与对照组总有效率分别为 96.8%(30/31)、76.7%(23/30)，组间比较，$P<0.05$。孟宪璞等将患者分为两组，穴位埋线组 121 例于患侧面部每次取 4 个穴位(第 1 次为阳白、太阳、地仓、颊车，第 2 次为攒竹、丝竹空、颧髎、牵正，第 3 次为眉冲、四白、口禾髎、承浆)埋线，半个月治疗 1 次；对照组针刺取承浆、地仓、颊车、阳白等为主穴，初期用捻转泻法，后期用捻转补法，1 次/d，留针 25 min，10 次为 1 个疗程，休息 2 d 进入下 1 个疗程。经治 2 个月后，有效率分别为 95.5%(116/121)、87.3%(103/118)，组间比较，$P<0.05$。

Yang SB 将 120 例患者分为三组，常规针刺组取阳白、四白、迎香、地仓、颊车、颧髎等穴，合谷垂直进针后提插捻转泻法使之得气，阳白平刺针尖由上朝外下方经皮下透刺至丝竹空，四白斜刺 15 mm，向外上方入眶下孔，地仓、颊车相互透刺，颧髎、翳风直刺平补平泻手法使酸胀针感扩散至半侧面部；人迎针刺组取人迎、地仓、颊车、合谷、地仓穴，合谷针刺方法同常规针刺组，人迎穴针刺在喉结旁开 1.5 寸，胸锁乳突肌前缘处以左手拇指、食指向外轻轻推开颈总动脉后，垂直进针，针尖略向内上方呈 5°～10°夹角，深约 10～15 mm，提插捻转补法使之得气，以向面部传导为佳；术针组在人迎穴针刺组治疗基础上行星状神经节阻滞术。1 次/d，每次 30 min，7 d 为 1 个疗程，疗程间停歇 1 d。连续治疗 3 个疗程，三组患者面神经直接刺激诱发电位(ENoG)潜伏期均显著缩短，且 ENoG 波幅显著升高；术针组 ENoG 潜伏期较常规针刺组显著降低($P<0.05$)，人迎针刺组 ENoG 波幅较其他两组升高(均$P<0.05$)；各组治疗后 R1、R2 值显著缩短，人迎针刺组和术针组治疗前后 R1、R2 差值均显著大于常规针刺组(均$P<0.05$)，且术针组 R1 差值显著大于人迎针刺组($P<0.05$)；术针组临床愈显率为 87.5%(35/40)，优于人迎针刺组的 77.5%(31/40)，且显著高于常规针刺组的 65.0%(26/40，$P<0.05$)。

(邓宏勇)

【针刺治疗失眠】

1. 体针法

陈秀华等将睡眠障碍患者分为三组，飞针针刺组予飞针针刺三阴交、安眠、神门等穴，口服维生素 B_1 和背俞穴埋皮内针；舒乐安定组予服舒乐安定及非穴位针刺和背俞穴穴位贴压；非穴位针刺组予非穴位针刺及口服维生素 B_1 和背俞穴穴位贴压。均治疗 2 周，观察疗效和匹兹堡睡眠质量指数(PSQI)变化情况，飞针针刺组总有效率为 84.1%(90/107)，优于舒乐安定组的 59.7%(62/104)和非穴位针刺组的 25.0%(24/96)(均$P<0.05$)。各组随访时 PSQI 各项评分及总评分均较治疗前明显降低(均$P<0.05$)，飞针针刺组较其他两组降低更明显(均$P<0.05$)。

张全爱将患者分为两组。安眠穴组取安眠穴,刺入得气后予滞针术(单向搓转针体2～3转,待针体紧涩有"滞针"感,用食指轻抵针尾固定针身,拇指由下向上刮动针柄),留针30 min;常规针刺组取三阴交、神门、百会穴,行捻转平补平泻法,留针30 min;1次/d。连续治疗2周后,常规针刺组患者的睡眠质量、入睡时间较治疗前改善(均$P<0.01$),睡眠时间、睡眠效率、睡眠紊乱、催眠药物、日间功能障碍改善及PSQI总分与治疗前比较,均$P>0.05$;安眠穴组患者PSQI各因子评分及总分较治疗前明显改善($P<0.01$, $P<0.05$),且均优于常规针刺组($P<0.01$, $P<0.05$)。安眠穴组总有效率为91.2%(62/68),常规针刺组为74.6%(47/63),组间比较,$P<0.05$。王玲姝等将患者平分为两组,治疗组上午予醒脑针法(针刺内关、水沟、三阴交穴)、晚间予安神针法(针刺四神聪及腹部以神阙为中点上下左右各3寸的4个穴位),内关直刺行捻转提插结合泻法1 min,以酸胀为度;水沟向鼻中膈方向斜刺行重雀啄法,至眼球湿润或流泪为度;三阴交沿胫骨内侧缘与皮肤呈45°斜刺用提插补法,使患侧下肢抽动3次为度;四神聪向百会平刺行捻转补法,以酸胀为度;腹部四穴直刺行平补平泻,以出现麻感为度,留针30 min;对照组针刺取四神聪、神门、三阴交为主穴,随症配穴,按虚补实泻,各穴以出现酸胀感为度,留针30 min。均6 d为1个疗程,疗程间休息1 d。经治疗4个疗程,治疗组总有效率为94.3%(33/35),对照组为91.4%(32/35),组间比较,$P>0.05$。治疗组在睡眠质量、睡眠时间、睡眠效率和日间功能方面的改善优于对照组($P<0.05$)。尹建平等将患者分为两组各30例,治疗组取心俞、肝俞、胆俞、脾俞、胃俞、肾俞穴直刺勿施手法,接电针仪,留针20 min后予点穴(大拇指点压以上各穴,每穴3～4 min,应使指力直透深层)、拔罐(在上述穴位上拔罐,留罐10 min)、药熨疗法(桂枝、川芎、艾叶、大腹皮、厚朴、小茴香等用布包隔水蒸热后熨于穴位约20 min,以皮肤发红为准);对照组予服艾司唑仑。1次/d,连续治疗5 d,休息2 d,10次为1个疗程。经治3个疗程后,两组PSQI评分与同组治疗前比较,$P<0.05$。治疗组PSQI评分与对照组比较,$P<0.05$。治疗组愈显率和总有效率分别为70.0%(21/30)和93.3%(28/30),对照组分别为43.3%(13/30)和76.7%(20/30),组间比较,$P<0.05$,$P<0.01$。

2. 耳针及其他疗法

胡晓颖等对120例血液透析患者失眠症予耳穴埋豆法,选神门、皮质下、心、垂前为主穴,分型配穴,将王不留行1粒放入凹区内,用小胶布固定,嘱患者每日按3～5次,每次3～5 min,以局部有酸、痛、麻感,耳郭发热、发胀,以能耐受为度,3～5 d更换1次,双耳交替施治,5次为1疗程。经治2个疗程后,心脾两虚、脾胃不和两型患者效果较为显著,总有效率分别为96.4%(27/28)、92.3%(26/28);肝阳上亢、心肾不交、痰热内扰也有较好疗效。

雷静涵将患者分为三组,治疗组予杵针(所用的工具分别为七耀混元杵、五星三台杵、金刚杵和奎星笔,取百会八阵、风府八阵及河车印脑段、脑椎段、大椎至命门段行手法。① 医者持金刚杵或奎星笔于百会八阵、风府八阵行点叩手法。力量由轻渐重,由外向内,共10 min,以患者舒适愉悦及刺激部位皮肤潮红,局部有温热感为度。② 医者持金刚杵或奎星笔于百会八阵、风府八阵行运转或开阖手法7 min,以患者舒适愉悦及刺激部位皮肤潮红,局部有温热感为度。③ 医者持七耀混元杵或五星三台杵于河车印脑段、脑椎段行升降手法5 min,力量稍轻,以患者舒适愉悦及刺激部位皮肤潮红,局部有温热感为度。④ 医者持七耀混元杵或金刚杵杵柄于河车路大椎至命门段行升降手法8 min,力量稍重,以患者有酸胀感但可耐受及局部有温热感为度)配合耳穴贴压(取心、脾、肾、神门、交感、皮质下穴,每次一穴,王不留行籽每次贴一侧耳,每2～3 d交替,每日揉按贴敷穴位1次,少于1 min,以局部产生酸、麻、胀、痛感及灼热感为佳);对照1组单用纯杵针治疗,对照2组单用耳穴贴压治疗。结果治疗组治疗后PSOI评分与对照1组和对照2组比较,$P<0.01$。治疗组总有效率为96.4%(54/56),对照1组为84.9%(45/53),对照2组为87.7%(50/57),治疗组分别与对照1组、2组比较,$P<0.01$。叶富英等将癌症围化疗期失眠症患者分为两组,治疗组予腕踝针(以两侧上1为主,伴有天柱、肩井压痛及指颤时,针一侧或两侧上5,针刺后予以输液小敷贴固定8～10 h)配合耳穴贴压(取心、神门、肾、皮质下穴,配肝、脾、肾、胰胆、小肠、生殖器等穴,随症选2～3个配穴,对准敏感点压籽,嘱患

者每日自行按压每穴 3 次，每次按压时间不少于 10 min，临睡前再按压 1 次，每次用一侧耳穴，两耳交替）；对照组口服地西泮。结果两组治疗前睡眠状况自评量表评分比较，$P>0.05$。治疗后睡眠状况自评量表评分与同组治疗前比较，$P<0.01$。治疗组治疗后睡眠状况自评量表评分与对照组比较，$P<0.01$。治疗组与对照组总有效率分别为 90.2%（37/41）、57.5%（23/40），组间比较，$P<0.01$。

（魏海燕　赵　玲）

【针刺治疗女性压力性尿失禁】

王静将患者分为两组，对照组盆底肌功能锻炼。治疗组针刺百会、关元、气海、中极、足三里、三阴交穴，得气后行捻转补法，关元、气海、中极分别点燃艾柱，每次每穴灸 2 壮。1 次/d，10 次为 1 个疗程。经治 2 个疗程后，治疗组总有效率为 96.4%（27/28）、对照组为 53.6%（15/28）。

熊书华将 130 例老年患者均分为两组，均予服补中益气丸和缩泉丸，治疗组针刺选百会、关元、太溪、肾俞、三阴交、足三里等穴，关元、足三里、肾俞用补法；百会、三阴交、太溪、次髎平补平泻，留针 30 min，1 次/d；继用灸法，关元、天枢、上髎、下髎施温和灸，隔 1 d，再灸中极、气海、中髎、次髎。经治 2 个疗程后，治疗组总有效率为 96.9%（63/65），对照组为 95.4%（62/65），组间比较，$P<0.01$。两组患者治疗前盆底肌力水平比较，$P>0.05$，治疗后治疗组盆底肌力水平较对照组，$P<0.01$。

高潇等将 100 例患者均分成两组。治疗组采用针刺（取关元、气海、中极、足三里、三阴交、曲骨穴。关元、气海、中极、曲骨穴均向下平刺得气后施捻转补法，足三里、三阴交穴均直刺，均留针 40 min，1 次/d）和穴位中频电刺激综合治疗（将中频治疗仪两个极片贴于患者中极、会阴两穴，选用功能性电刺激处方，刺激量取患者所能耐受最大量，治疗 20 min）。对照组单用传统针刺。连续治疗 30 d 后，治疗组总有效率 86%（43/50），对照组为 54%（27/50），组间比较，$P<0.05$。

赵琳等将 60 例女性压力性尿失禁患者平分为两组，对照组根据阴部神经走向选择骶尾部 4 个针刺点，上两针刺点位于骶骨边缘旁，平第 4 骶后孔水平处（双侧），下两针刺点位于尾骨旁开 0.5 寸（双侧）；患者取俯卧位，上两针刺点直刺，使针感达尿道或肛门，下两针刺点针向外侧（坐骨直肠窝方向）斜刺，使针感达尿道后，每侧针的针柄与电针仪相连，电刺激采用连续波，以患者能耐受且无不适为度，留针 60 min。隔日治疗 1 次，共治疗 10 次。治疗组采用 UrostymTM 电刺激生物反馈仪对首次就诊患者实施电针阴部神经刺激疗法的监控，期间观察其阴道压力变化。电针阴部神经刺激疗法操作、疗程同对照组。两组治疗前临床症状评分比较，$P>0.05$。治疗后临床症状评分与同组治疗前比较，$P<0.01$。治疗组治疗后临床症状评分与对照组比较，$P<0.01$。治疗组总有效率为 83.3%（25/30），对照组为 53.3%（16/30），组间比较，$P<0.01$。

（刘堂义）

【针灸治疗类风湿关节炎的实验研究】

李世民等观察不同组方祛痹镇痛凝胶膏贴敷“身柱”“至阳”“命门”对胶原性关节炎（RA）大鼠的治疗作用，将 96 只 SD 雄性大鼠，随机分出空白对照组，其余大鼠注射牛Ⅱ型胶原诱发胶原性关节炎，再随机分成模型对照组，A 贴膏组（以雷公藤为主药），B 贴膏组（以马钱子为主药），基质对照组（基质对照贴膏），阳性膏对照组（吲哚美辛贴片）。治疗 15 d 后，与模型对照组相比，关节炎指数 A 贴膏组与 B 贴膏组极显著减小（$P<0.01$），足跖平均肿胀度与血清牛Ⅱ胶原抗体 B 贴膏组均极显著降低（$P<0.01$，$P<0.01$），A 贴膏组均无显著性差异。

姚剑等选取 30 只 Wistar 大鼠，随机分为正常组、模型组、艾灸组，后两组采用风、寒、湿环境因素＋生物因子（弗氏完全佐剂）复合 RA 造模，造模后第 3 d 进行治疗，艾灸组取双侧肾俞、足三里悬灸，20 min/次，1 次/d，连续治疗 15 d。于造模前、造模后及治疗第 15 d 分别测量各组大鼠右后足趾容积，Western blot 法检测滑膜组织中 Ras 蛋白、ERK1/2、磷酸化 ERK1/2（p－ERK1/2）及 Raf 蛋白的相对表达量。结果造模后大鼠右后足趾容积较正常组明显增大（$P<0.01$）；经治疗 15 d，艾灸组大鼠的跖围小于模型组（$P<0.01$）；模型组 Ras、Raf、ERK1/2、p－ERK1/2 蛋白表达较其他各组增加（均 $P<0.01$）；艾灸组 Ras、Raf、ERK1/2、p－ERK1/2 蛋白表达明显低于模型组（均 $P<0.01$）。

杨馨等将日本大耳白兔分为对照组、模型组和艾灸组，艾灸组动物采用艾粒施灸两侧“肾俞”穴各 5 壮，1 次/d，6 d 为 1 疗程，共治 3 个疗程。

结果：造模后各个时间点模型组动物的左、右后膝关节周长均较对照组明显增加($P<0.01$)，治疗后艾灸组动物左、右后膝关节周长均较模型组降低($P<0.05$)；模型组与对照组比较，滑膜细胞SOCS1、SOCS3蛋白含量显著升高($P<0.01$)；艾灸组与模型组比较，滑膜细胞SOCS1、SOCS3蛋白含量降低($P<0.01$)。

卢军等将SD大鼠分为5组，正常组、模型组、中药复方组、电针组、电针+中药复方组各10只；除正常组外，其余各组应用完全弗氏佐剂诱导大鼠关节炎；中药复方(太子参、黄芪、丹参、桂枝、当归、白芍等)组2 ml/100 g灌胃给药，正常组、模型组、电针组给予2 ml/100 g蒸馏水1次/d，共计28 d。实验期间，称重1次/d，以调整给药剂量。电针组参照上海科技出版社出版的《实验针灸学》取命门、足三里穴，直刺进针，接电针仪，持续15 min，1次/d，共28 d。电针加中药复方组，先电针刺激，再予中药2 ml/100 g灌胃给药，方法同上。正常组、模型组及中药复方组不进行针灸治疗，每日用自制鼠架固定15 min。结果与模型组比较，各组均能降低大鼠足肿胀体积($P<0.01$)，大鼠血清IL-1、TNF-α水平明显降低，IL-2水平明显升高($P<0.01$)。

张卫东等将40只雌性Wistar大鼠随机分为正常组、模型组、甲氨蝶呤(MTX)组、火针组，每组10只。火针组点刺夹脊穴、足三里和阿是穴，深度5 mm，3 d治疗1次，共8次；MTX组每只大鼠按灌胃量2.0 mg/kg，每7 d给药1次，共4次。观察各组大鼠体质量、足容积肿胀度、关节疼痛评分、多关节炎指数变化，光镜观察大鼠肝脏组织的病理变化。结果模型组大鼠体质量、足容积肿胀度、关节疼痛评分、多关节炎指数较正常组显著升高($P<0.05$，$P<0.01$)，治疗后上述各指标两治疗组较模型组均明显降低(均$P<0.01$)，并且火针组与MTX组相比差异均有统计学意义($P<0.05$，$P<0.01$)；与正常组比较，模型组大鼠肝细胞之间出现呈簇集状分布的炎性细胞，MTX组和火针组肝细胞之间炎性细胞减少，MTX组肝细胞变性水肿、肝细胞核增大变形。

(邓宏勇)

【针灸治疗带状疱疹】

1. 针法

吴辛甜采用一次性浮针作为治疗工具。在带状疱疹病痛区神经远端选2～3点，针尖指向神经出口处，在进针点针体与皮肤呈15°～30°角，快速刺入，然后将针尖提至皮下，沿皮下疏松结缔组织向前推进，力求无酸麻胀痛等感觉，进针完毕后，再以进针点为支点，手握针座左右摇摆，使针体作扇面平扫5 min，抽出针芯，将软套管的针座用输液贴固定于皮肤表面，留置24 h后拔出。隔天1次，5次为1个疗程。并设常规针刺组作对照。经治疗1个疗程后，两组VAS评分均较治疗前明显降低($P<0.05$)，浮针组较常规针刺组降低更明显(均$P<0.05$)；浮针组和常规针刺组总有效率分别为81.8%(18/22)、61.1%(11/18)。

赵博华将患者分为两组，对照组口服利巴韦林片、卡马西平、维生素B_1、甲钴胺、醋酸泼尼松，连续14 d为1个疗程。观察组采用梅花针扣刺、拔火罐治疗。根据患者发病部位选择合适的体位，患处皮肤严格消毒后，用梅花针从患疱疹后疼痛部位的一端沿皮损区边缘取阿是穴向心性均匀轻叩，将病灶包围后稍用力重扣疱疹及疼痛部位，使其刺破呈点状渗血后，随即在扣刺处拔火罐(留罐时间5 min)，将水性分泌物及渗出血液吸出后起罐，消毒局部。隔日治疗1次，7次为1个疗程。经治2个疗程，观察组总有效率为100%(36/36)，对照组为86.11%(31/36)，组间比较，$P<0.01$。

范永桥等将患者分成两组各40例，实验组采用蛇头穴刺络放血治疗，即蛇头穴位于拇指指指关节背面，两尖端静脉怒张处，取穴时先将拇指指指关节上搓揉，然后压紧拇指掌指关节，在指指关节背面两尖端可见两个怒张的小静脉，用5号一次性头皮针刺破该静脉，并进行上下挤压，挤出血约7～8滴，当颜色变为浅红色即可。次日再用同样方法取健侧蛇头穴刺络放血。隔2 d后若病已愈，可停止放血，若未愈，同上法继续施治。对照组口服阿昔洛韦0.4 g/次，4次/日，阿昔洛韦软膏外用涂于患者处，5次/d。结果带状疱疹患者治疗前CD_3、CD_4、CD_4/CD_8、IL-2、IgG水平显著低于正常人组，而CD_8水平与正常人组无显著性差异。实验组治疗后，CD_3水平显著上升，但仍低于正常人组，CD_8水平显著降低，CD_4/CD_8、IL-2、IgG水平显著升高，达正常人水平。对照组治疗后，CD_3水平显著上升，CD_4水平显著高于治疗前，CD_8水平较治疗前显著降低，CD_4/CD_8、IL-2水平显著升高，达正常人水平，IgG水平与治疗前相比无显著性差异。

陆佳宁等将患者分为两组各48例，对照组予服阿昔洛韦、维生素B_1、腺苷钴胺片，外用炉甘石洗剂日数次，治疗组在此基础上选取阿是穴(病变皮损处)常规消毒，将针尖及针体烧至透红，迅速刺入穴位后立即出针，用棉签按压片刻；再对疱疹部位皮肤常规消毒，取毫针用酒精灯将针尖及针体烧至透红，然后快速点刺在丘疹水疱上，深度达到疱疹底部。先刺早发的疱疹，再刺新发的疱疹。火针治疗后，用消毒好的玻璃火罐在点刺部位拔罐，留罐5～10 min，起罐后用干棉签清理组织液和血液。穴位点刺隔日1次，疱疹部位点刺1次/d。经治1周后，治疗组与对照组相比，皮损消退情况，$P>0.05$；疼痛情况，$P<0.01$。

2. 灸法

雷成业将患者分为两组，对照组37例予服阿昔洛韦片，雷火灸组39例在此基础上，选在有皮损周围部位及在支沟、阳陵泉、丘墟穴上方2～3 cm悬燃，以皮肤能感觉到灼热，但不能烫伤，皮肤被艾条烤的发红即可。每次每部位悬灸约5～10 min。1次/d。结果雷火灸组在疱疹止疱时间、结痂时间、脱痂时间、疼痛缓解程度、疼痛开始缓解时间及疼痛持续时间、带状疱疹综合疗效评分都优于对照组，组间比较，$P<0.05$或$P<0.01$。

左甲等将患者分为两组，西药组予常规西药治疗，铺棉灸组予铺棉灸为主针灸治疗，具体为：患者取适当体位，充分暴露阿是穴。将脱脂干棉花撕成约3 cm×3 cm大小、薄如蝉翼的薄棉片，并根据皮损面积决定施灸棉片的数量。用活力碘常规消毒后，将棉片铺在阿是穴上，用火柴点燃棉片一角，令其迅速燃尽，如法施灸3遍为1次，1次/d。铺棉灸后，在距皮损边缘0.2 cm处用活力碘常规消毒，用1～2寸毫针沿皮下向皮损中心围刺，针距约为1～2 cm。每簇针数与皮损范围成正比，若皮损直径3 cm以下，则按周围神经走向，前后各刺1针；若皮损直径3～5 cm，可刺6～8针；若皮损直径5 cm以上，则刺10～16针为宜。留针30 min，1次/d。围针刺同时，在双侧支沟、后溪穴及皮损相应神经节段及其上下各一节段的患侧夹脊穴处用活力碘常规消毒，用1～2寸毫针实施针刺，得气后留针30 min，1次/d。均以10 d为1个疗程观察疗效，并于研究期间20、30、60及90 d对患者进行随访。铺棉灸疗组总有效率为92.9%(92/99)，西药组为91.2%(94/102)，组间比较，$P>0.05$；视觉模拟评分(VAS)方面，两组干预前后及组间比较，$P<0.01$；疼痛持续时间方面，组间比较，$P<0.01$；后遗神经痛发生情况方面，第30 d组间比较，$P<0.01$。

史兴忠等将患者分为两组，治疗组58例采用灯芯草灸，每次治疗先灸疱疹的“蛇头”“蛇尾”，而后根据疱疹所损伤皮肤面积间距4～5 cm选疹泡以行灸法，然后在同侧足三里点灸1次。一般3 d治疗1次，10 d为1个疗程。对照组59例予服阿昔洛韦分散片。10 d后，灯芯草灸治疗在止疱、止痛、结痂时间方面均优于西药治疗，$P<0.05$。

李娟红等将患者分为两组各26例，治疗组在对照组阿昔洛韦治疗的基础上采用夹脊穴直刺配合臭氧穴位注射治疗，注射臭氧浓度25 mg/L，3～4d治疗1次。治疗后1、7、30与60 d，治疗组VAS评分低于同期对照组($P<0.05$)；治疗后30 d及60 d，对照组和治疗组VAS评分与治疗前自身比较，$P<0.05$。治疗组止疱时间和结痂时间分别是(3.23±1.12)d和(4.03±0.96)d，低于对照组的(5.36±1.89)d和(5.63±1.55)d，组间比较，$P<0.05$；治疗组总优良率为76.0%(16/26)，对照组为38%(9/24)，组间比较$P<0.05$。

张艳丽等采用西药联合穴位注射治疗耳带状疱疹。选用注射用维生素B_1 100 mg，腺苷钴胺0.5 mg，2%利多卡因2 ml；取翳风、太阳、听宫、阿是、阳白、地仓等穴，每次选3～5穴，常规进针深度，得气后注药1.0～1.5 ml，1次/d。10次为1个疗程，治疗5次间隔2 d。2周为1个疗程。共观察2个疗程，随访3个月，有效率与单纯西药治疗比较，$P<0.05$；西药联合穴位注射治疗后VAS评分与单纯西药治疗同期比较，$P<0.05$。

(纪　军)

【灸法文献研究】

张国山等总结《备急千金要方》灸法内容特点为：灸理宏富、卓然特立；灸法原则独具匠心；临证施灸严谨灵活。认为该书对施灸选穴、施灸体位、施灸顺序、施灸剂量、施灸禁忌及灸疮的处理都做了详细的描述，对当今灸法的临床应用和发展有重要的指导意义。

谢文娟等概括《扁鹊心书》灸法的运用特点为：明经络、重元阳、脾肾为本；审虚实、重病灸、早灸为宜；灸量大、选穴精、药灸同施；证治广、验案足、防病延年等。并认为其中有关灸法防病延年的论述对灸法“治未病”理论的发展及临床运用有重要的学术参考价值。

章海凤等对《针灸聚英》中的论灸特点进行了总结，指出该书中关于灸法记载十分丰富，对后世针灸临床具有很重要的参考价值。其特点为：施灸精简，艾灸宜忌；定穴精准，灸疮独重；灸法精选，针药并用；崇尚经典，师古不泥等。邹天雨等对《针灸聚英》中癫痫的艾灸治疗方法进行了论述，结合作者的学术思想，分析了治疗痫证的“时相性”理论，可总结为：痫发昼夜，分灸二跷；灸治痫证，从热引热；清心化痰，兼顾神明。

张佳丽等认为《医学入门》集明代以前医学之大成，该书灸法特点为：针药所不及者，灸法从之；灸善温阳补虚，亦可泻热泻实；施循法度，灸有度量；灸法养生，炼脐益寿等。

张国山等对《针灸大成》中关于灸法理论的继承、发展和创新之处进行了论述，认为该书引经据典、溯古求源；从以病论灸法和以穴论灸法两个方面详述灸疗主治；汇集了明以前针灸医籍中灸法的精华，并对此增补完善；尊古尚今、师古不泥；融会贯通，成一家之言。

何亚敏等探析了《红炉点雪》卷四中对痰火灸法及却病秘诀、养生调息等方法的专述。总结其灸法特色有辨证施灸，不拘热证；灸学严谨，法度明晰；不拘于古，知常达变等方面。

黄琴峰等利用《中医针灸信息库》，对1954～2010年有关艾条灸的针灸临床论文进行文献计量分析与评价，归纳出现代艾条灸的疾病谱，其涉及269个病种，适宜病症为面神经麻痹，常用适宜病症为颈椎病、带状疱疹、尿潴留、腹泻等，次常用适宜病症为胎位不正、遗尿、失眠症。

（张馥晴　刘立公）

【澄江学派研究】

承淡安先后编写了《中国针灸治疗学》《中国针灸学讲义》及《中国针灸学》。张建斌等从成书背景、体例、内容，以及针灸学科体系构建的演变过程等方面，对该三书进行了研究。认为承淡安先生以针灸临床疗效为起点，参考西方医学模式，吸收日本近代针灸研究成果，回归传统针灸经典理论，构建了现代针灸学科体系的基本框架。

夏有兵等总结了承淡安先生针灸量学的观点，从疏简针刺取穴数量、规范毫针规格材质、明确把握针刺强度、关注针刺间隔时间，以及强调灸疗需有适宜刺激量并因人而异、规范灸疗刺激量化标准等。夏氏等还认为，承淡安及其弟子于20世纪中叶使针灸在香港逐步发展繁衍起来；由于特殊的地理及时代因素，香港也成为了我国改革开放前澄江针灸学派向海外传播的重要阵地。夏氏等亦回顾了澄江针灸学派在新加坡的发展与传播，介绍了前期代表人物及针灸教育机构，指出方展纶、何敬慈、萧憬我、邓颂如、刘致中等皆为澄江针灸学派传人，耀华针灸学社、中国针灸医学总院等早期针灸教育机构也为该学派传人创办，并认为新加坡针灸的起步及发展与澄江针灸学派密切相关，并对萧憬我父子、符伯华、陈必廉等澄江针灸学派在新加坡的主要代表人物的针灸学术思想进行初步总结。

孟宪军等总结澄江学派传人、承淡安亲传弟子留章杰的针灸学术特色：无痛运针，三度进针，候气得气以调经络、平衡阴阳，采用“平刺手”技术；善用直接灸，认为有灸疮才有疗效；取穴贵在专精，刺激点宜少不宜多，反对做满身是针的“豪猪医生”；针灸中药并用，治疗疑难病。其现代针灸教育思想：带徒与办班并重，乐于育人，使澄江针灸学术得以传承；宗经络，尚《伤寒》，针灸药并施，取穴精简，重视指力，技高一筹，艺传后辈；重视从实治学，实事求是，不讳己过；带动学生重视针灸教育，薪火相传；一生勤勤恳恳，兢兢业业，济世救人，德崇思邈；重视经验传承，著书创刊，亲编教材，为针灸人才培养不遗余力。

朱安宁等总结了澄江学派传人黄宗勖的针灸学术特色，重视经络，辨证论治；重视得气，善用补泻；重视调理脾胃，针药结合，治各科疑难杂症；擅用外治法，且善用透穴；重视养生保健，善出食疗奇方。

张建斌等总结了澄江针灸学派的再传弟子李玉堂的针灸学术特色，兼收中西之长，阐发针灸理论，拓展针灸临床，基于三维网络构架阐释经络理论，结合神经节段理论阐明背俞穴本质，提出三层立体止痛法。

（张馥晴　刘立公）

[附] 参考文献

A

艾炳蔚.不同部位穴位与非穴位针刺提插捻转手法的实时检测[J].中国中医药现代远程教育,2013,11(22):157

B

鲍鑫宇,周庆伟,钱航.督灸联合西医常规治疗肺肾气虚型缓解期哮喘30例[J].中医研究,2013,26(7):66

C

Corbett MS, Rice SJ, Madurasinghe V, et al. Acupuncture and other physical treatments for the relief of pain due to osteoarthritis of the knee: network meta-analysis [J]. Osteoarthritis and Cartilage, 2013, 21(9): 1290

蔡荣林,胡玲,王频,等.人体特殊部位腧穴仿真针刺实践实训平台建设的研究与实践[J].中国针灸,2013,33(1):67

常小荣,刘密,吴焕淦,等.艾灸温通温补效应的作用机制及其规律研究[J].世界中医药,2013,8(8):875

陈利芳,方剑乔,贾玲红,等.夏季卡介苗多糖核酸穴位注射治疗支气管哮喘:随机对照研究[J].中国针灸,2013,33(1):8

陈秀华,李颖,奎瑜,等.飞针针刺为主治疗睡眠障碍:临床随机对照研究[J].中国针灸,2013,33(2):97

陈雪,王保国,李锦,等.经皮穴位电刺激对经蝶垂体瘤切除患者围术期静脉全麻的影响[J].中国针灸,2013,33(8):732

程为平,季超,马振旺,等.应用MRI测量关元穴针刺安全深度和角度的研究[J].针灸临床杂志,2013,29(3):54

程为平,马振旺,季超,等.针刺肾俞穴危险角度和深度研究[J].中医药信息,2013,30(1):75

D

Deare JC, Zheng Z, Xue CC, et al. Acupuncture for treating fibromyalgia [J]. Cochrane Database of Systematic Reviews, 2013,(5): CD007070

邓丽兴.闪罐配合甩针挂钩治疗周围性面瘫疗效观察[J].按摩与康复医学,2013,4(7):80

丁乐,张泓,张娟,等.子午流注结合常规针刺法对胃黏膜损伤家兔褪黑素及HSP70的影响[J].中医药导报,2013,19(3):9

丁然,焦宏官.SCIE近10年中国针灸论文统计分析[J].中医药导报,2013,19(5):1

董莉莉,刘安国,王军燕,等.合募配穴对应激性胃溃疡大鼠下丘脑促性腺激素释放激素和P物质mRNA表达的影响[J].针刺研究,2013,38(4):291

董利平,马丽.《外台秘要》中运用灸法治疗疝气的学术思想及临床应用[J].西部中医药,2013,26(1):43

董勤,曹雯萍,鲁佳,等.电针与穴位注射对糖尿病周围神经病变大鼠神经保护作用的比较研究[J].时珍国医国药,2013,24(4):1001

董泉声,董新民,先茂全,等.揭示灸法作用的穴位物质基础与阐明灸法退热机理的研究[J].四川中医,2013,31(7):151

窦传字,洪宗国,吴焕淦,等.不同储存年份的艾条燃烧生成自由基的ESR波谱研究[J].世界中医药,2013,8(8):852

杜艳军,周华,孔立红,等.热休克蛋白在逆针灸保护AD模型大鼠海马神经元中的作用研究[J].时珍国医国药,2013,24(6):1505

F

Fang JQ, Du JY, Liang Y, et al. Intervention of electroacupuncture on spinal p38 MAPK/ATF-2/VR-1 pathway in treating inflammatory pain induced by CFA in rats[J]. Moleaular Pain, 2013,(9): 13

樊茂蓉,王冰,焦秋粉,等,冬病夏治穴位贴敷治疗慢性咳喘病临床观察[J].北京中医药,2013,32(8):570

范永桥,杨正明,顾进.应用蛇头穴刺络放血疗法治疗带状疱疹的免疫学机制分析[J].中国医药指南,2013,11(32):502

G

Gao YH, Chen S, Xu Q, et al. Proteomic analysis of differential proteins related to anti-nociceptive effect of electroacupuncture in the hypothalamus following neuropathic pain in rats[J]. Neurochemical Research, 2013, 38(7): 1467

Guo XX, Chen JF, Lu Y, et al. Electroacupuncture at He-Mu points reduces P2X4 receptor expression in visceral hypersensitivity [J]. Neural Regeneration Research, 2013, 8(22): 2069

高丽美,任玉兰,郭太品,等.太冲穴及常见配伍运用规律的文献研究[J].时珍国医国药,2013,24(6):1531

高潇,邢艳丽,董施秋,等.针刺配合穴位中频电刺激对女性压力性尿失禁的影响[J].针灸临床杂志,2013,29(8):15

郜婕,唐成林,刘仁建,等.不同强度电针对肥胖大鼠细胞因子信号转导抑制蛋白-3及过氧化物酶体增殖物激活受体-γ mRNA表达的影响[J].针刺研究,2013,38(1):31

顾文,周春祥,燕艳.穴位敷贴对过敏性哮喘豚鼠Th/Th2失衡的免疫调节效应[J].中华中医药杂志,2013,28(6):1689

郭泳梅,童娟,姚红.针刺疗法对稳定期慢性阻塞性肺疾病患者呼吸功能的影响[J].广州中医药大学学报,2013,30(5):658

郭泳梅,童娟,姚红.针刺配合有氧运动训练对稳定期慢性阻塞性肺病患者生活质量的影响[J].针灸临床杂志,2013,29(8):3

H

何冬凤,任玉兰,唐勇,等.古代不同时期针灸治疗胸痹用穴特点的数据挖掘研究[J].辽宁中医杂志,2013,40(6):1209

何亚敏,刘密,李金香,等.《红炉点雪》论灸法[J].国医论坛,2013,28(3):22

洪营东.探索《针灸甲乙经》中针灸治疗癫证的特定穴运用规律[J].中医外治杂志,2013,22(4):19

胡昊斌,胡玲,董朝阳,等.电针神门、太渊对正常人事件相关电位P300影响的比较[J].针刺研究,2013,38(3):186

胡晓颖,张成亮,何立群.耳穴埋豆改善血液透析患者失眠症120例疗效观察[J].中国中西医结合肾病杂志,2013,14(4):345

黄昌锦,黄应杰,吴艳华.火针经筋结点治疗中风后肩手综合征临床观察[J].上海针灸杂志,2013,32(8):627

黄琴峰,刘婕,吴焕淦.基于《中医针灸信息库》评述艾条灸的疾病谱[J].上海针灸杂志,2013,32(7):529

J

Jiang Y, Wang H, Liu Z, et al. Manipulation of and sustained effects on the human brain induced by different modalities of acupuncture: an fMRI study[J]. PLoS One, 2013, 8(6): e66815

Ju ZY, Cui HS, Guo XH, et al. Molecular mechanisms underlying the effects of acupuncture on neuropathic pain [J]. Neural Regeneration Research, 2013, 8(25): 2350

吉长福,王晓宇,石宏,等.原始管道系统(PVs)与针灸经络关系的研究[J].上海针灸杂志,2013,32(10):795

姜荣荣,徐桂华,陈华,等.中国期刊全文数据库2002～2012年刮痧文献评析[J].中国针灸,2013,33(4):381

K

阚宇,淑萍,高永辉,等.海马一氧化氮/蛋白激酶G信号通路参与针刺对慢性痛大鼠产生的累积性镇痛效应[J].针刺研究,2013,38(2):93

L

Liu LA, Zhu YH, Li QH, et al. Comparison of efficacy and the safety evaluation of electroacupuncture with different waveforms for peripheral facial paralysis patients [J]. World Journal of Acupuncture-Moxibustion, 2013, 23(2): 17

雷成业,薛晓芳,叶禹,等.雷火灸治疗带状疱疹39例[J].中国中医药现代远程教育,2013,11(13):56

雷静涵.杵针配合耳穴贴压治疗失眠症疗效观察[J].上海针灸杂志,2013,32(7):548

雷琰,王惠琴,史蕾,等.穴位针刺加中草药贴敷治疗慢性阻塞性肺疾病急性加重期的临床分析[J].当代医学,2013,19(1):155

李焕新.温针配合精心护理治疗支气管哮喘疗效及护理体会[J].吉林医学,2013,34(32):6872

李慧,陈晓燕,秦玮.探讨三阴交穴适宜针刺深度[J].中医临床研究,2013,5(15):46

李靖,Lawrence Grierson,Mary X Wu,等.捻转针刺手法的运动学及动力学特征研究[J].针刺研究,2013,38(5):415

李娟红,李桂英,程斌.夹脊穴直刺配合臭氧穴位注射治疗急性带状疱疹神经痛疗效观察[J].世界中西医结合杂志,2013,8(4):371

李娜,张中新,李双霞.火龙督脉铺灸治疗慢性阻塞性肺疾病稳定期42例[J].西部中医药,2013,26(9):98

李世民,方剑乔,方芳,等.祛痹镇痛凝胶膏穴位敷贴对胶原性关节炎大鼠的治疗作用[J].浙江中医药大学学报,2013,37(4):432

李晓梅,李岩琪,周丹,等.提插补泻对健康人足三里穴皮肤微循环血流灌注量的影响[J].针刺研究,2013,38(4):297

李艳,范兴良.基于正交设计的针刺治疗周围性面瘫的优化方案研究[J].新中医,2013,45(4):121

李影捷,惠萍,宋天云,等.穴位注射治疗支气管哮喘的临床观察[J].湖南中医药大学学报,2013,33(6):72

李振吉,苏钢强,彭以祺.973计划中医理论基础研究专题2009年项目成果集[M].北京:中国中医药出版社,2013:27

梁宜,方剑乔,房军帆,等.电针对CFA大鼠脊髓背角NR2B酪氨酸1472位点磷酸化的影响[J].中国中西医结合杂志,2013,33(10):1372

廖天华,胡联民,余昭胜,等.穴位贴敷联合注射用格

拉司琼防治化疗相关性恶心呕吐 30 例临床观察[J]. 中医药导报，2013，19(2)：76

刘鸿. 穴位贴敷配合扶正平喘汤对过敏性哮喘外周血 ET－1、TXB_2 及肺功能的影响[J]. 中医药导报，2013，19(2)：71

刘敏，徐亚莉. 针刺结合按摩治疗肠易激综合征 68 例[J]. 河南中医，2013，33(1)：116

刘亚丽，杨桂桂，杨丽娟. 针刺背俞穴治疗慢性疲劳综合征的临床疗效及对心理状态的影响[J]. 中华中医药学刊，2013，31(10)：2327

刘振威，邓鑫，莫金花，等. 同伴教育模式下艾灸疗法干预 HIV 感染者 50 例临床观察[J]. 中医杂志，2013，54(13)：1119

卢军，任景，王晓波，等. 中药复方配合针灸对佐剂性关节炎模型大鼠血清 IL－1、IL－2 及 TNF－α 水平的影响[J]. 新疆中医药，2013，31(3)：59

陆佳宁，张小卿，张宇，等. 火针点刺阿是穴(皮损处)及拔罐联合西药治疗带状疱疹随机平行对照研究[J]. 实用中医内科杂志，2013，27(3)：86

陆欣玲，杨烁慧，宣腾，等. 基于 fMRI 的合谷穴功能特异性研究[J]. 上海中医药大学学报，2013，27(3)：63

罗胜，李俊雄，凌孟晖. 耳穴压贴治疗哮喘慢性持续期的临床疗效观察[J]. 中医临床研究，2013，5(7)：43

M

Ma YX，Liu X，Liu CZ，et al. Randomized Clinical Trial：The Clinical Effects of Herb-Partitioned Moxibustion in Patients with Diarrhoea-Predominant Irritable Bowel Syndrome [J]. Evidence-Based Complementary and Alternative Medicine，2013，2013：8

茅敏，牟欣，陈新，等. 针刺治疗慢性疲劳综合征 45 例临床观察[J]. 成都中医药大学学报，2013，36(1)：80

孟宪军，张建斌，朱安宁. 澄江学派传人留章杰先生针灸学术特色[J]. 中华中医药杂志，2013，28(8)：2320

孟宪军，朱安宁，孙孝忠. 澄江学派传人留章杰先生针灸教育思想简介[J]. 中国针灸，2013，33(6)：566

孟宪璞，吴中秋，肖丽梅，等. 从经筋论治周围性面瘫疗效观察[J]. 中国临床医生，2013，41(2)：62

N

倪瑛，黄钰玲，郑焱. 温针灸足三里治疗周围性面瘫的疗效观察[J]. 四川医学，2013，34(2)：230

P

Pennick V，Liddle SD. Interventions for preventing and treating pelvic and back pain in pregnancy [J]. Cochrane Database of Systematic Reviews，2013，(8)：CD001139

彭冬青，高旭，金伯华. 金伯华应用《金针赋》针刺手法经验总结[J]. 北京中医药，2013，32(3)：214

Q

齐丽珍，马晓芃，洪珏. 古今灸材及灸法的比较[J]. 中华中医药学刊，2013，31(11)：2349

乔红伟，尚小红，贺艳婷，等. 针刺开阖补泻的量效关系初探[J]. 辽宁中医药杂志，2013，40(5)：992

秦庆广，王海萍，刘坤，等. 针刺天枢对正常、便秘和腹泻模型大鼠不同肠段运动功能的双向调节效应[J]. 世界中医药，2013，8(3)：245

任红，袁军，郭淑芹. 穴位注射用于糖尿病神经原性膀胱患者的临床研究[J]. 国际中医中药杂志，2013，35(6)：501

S

Sun J，Jin C，Wu H，et al. Effects of electro-acupuncture on ovarian P450arom，P450c17α and mRNA expression induced by letrozole in PCOS rats[J]. PLoS One，2013，8(11)：e79382

单敬文. 温针灸结合走罐治疗脾肾阳虚型单纯性肥胖症临床观察[J]. 新中医，2013，45(3)：128

石君杰，黄玲芬. 经皮穴位电刺激"足三里"对运动性疲劳胃黏膜损伤大鼠胃黏膜 6－酮-前列腺素 1α、血栓素 B2 的影响[J]. 针刺研究，2013，38(3)：181

史兴忠，许建峰. 灯芯草灸治疗带状疱疹的临床观察[J]. 宁夏医学杂志，2013，35(8)：754

寿依夏，任玉兰，唐勇，等. 基于数据挖掘技术分析古代针灸治疗眩晕的经穴特点[J]. 成都中医药大学学报，2013，36(2)：1

孙健，卢秉慧，曾志平，等. 电针配合穴位埋线对腹型肥胖患者糖脂代谢的影响[J]. 上海针灸杂志，2013，32(5)：365

孙晶，方剑乔，陈勤，等. 与三叉神经痛相关病症的古代针灸处方规律分析[J]. 上海针灸杂志，2013，32(1)：66

孙远征，于佳妮. 原络配穴埋线治疗中风后心肾不交型失眠 40 例[J]. 针灸临床杂志，2013，29(1)：33

T

田海燕，胡佳，王琳. 穴位贴敷与电针治疗支气管哮喘疗效对照观察[J]. 中国针灸，2013，33(6)：485

田宇瑛，黄涛，王广军，等. 应用激光散斑技术观察针刺合谷对面部不同区域血流的影响[J]. 中国中医基础医学杂志，2013，19(2)：183

W

Wang XM，Lu Y，Wu L，et al. Moxibustion Inhibits the ERK Signaling Pathway and Intestinal Fibrosis in Rats with Crohn's Disease[J]. Evidence-Based Complementary and Alternative Medicine, 2013, 2013: 198282

Weng ZJ, Wu LY, Lu Y, et al. Electroacupuncture diminishes P2X2 and P2X3 purinergic receptor expression in dorsal root ganglia of rats with visceral hypersensitivity [J]. Neural Regeneration Research, 2013, 8(9): 802

王静. 针刺结合排灸治疗压力性尿失禁 28 例临床观察[J]. 江苏中医药,2013,45(3): 61

王玲姝,赵桂君,张茗. 醒脑安神针法早晚分时针刺治疗失眠症疗效观察[J]. 上海针灸杂志, 2013, 32(4): 280

王文琴,张永臣,贾红玲. 太冲穴古代文献应用分析[J]. 针灸临床杂志,2013,29(7): 73

王元. 分期针刺法治疗 Bell's 面瘫 54 例[J]. 辽宁中医杂志,2013,40(9): 1905

王志功,吕晓迎,王苏阳,等. 基于电气信号传递特性的"经络"轨迹研究[J]. 针刺研究,2013,38(4): 339

文胜,郑智,蔡章健. 保健灸治疗慢性疲劳综合征疗效观察[J]. 上海针灸杂志,2013,32(7): 558

文幸,陈楚云,梁美爱. 艾炷灸背俞穴对慢性阻塞性肺病稳定期患者生活质量的影响[J]. 世界中医药,2013, 8(6): 658

吴群,张明晓,王璐璐,等. 经皮穴位电刺激对开颅术丙泊酚靶控输注全麻效能的影响[J]. 针刺研究,2013, 38(3): 229

吴辛甜. 浮针治疗带状疱疹性神经痛临床疗效观察[J]. 亚太传统医药,2013,9(12): 92

X

Xu SB, Huang B, Zhang CY, et al. Effectiveness of strengthened stimulation during acupuncture for the treatment of Bell palsy: a randomized controlled trial[J]. Canadian Medical Association Journal. 2013, 185(6): 473

夏俊,钱虹仔. 远道刺配合穴位贴敷治疗支气管哮喘临床观察[J]. 中医临床研究,2013,5(10): 56

夏有兵,程洁,穆艳云,等. 浅析承淡安先生对针灸量学的探索[J]. 针刺研究,2013,38(1): 73

夏有兵,贺霆. 澄江针灸学派在香港的繁衍与传播[J]. 中国针灸,2013,33(10): 951

夏有兵,张建斌,林英,等. 澄江针灸学派在新加坡的传播[J]. 中国针灸,2013,33(1): 79

项永晶,袁维真. 热咳喘胶囊结合针刺治疗哮喘发作期临床疗效观察[J]. 中医临床研究,2013,5(3): 5

谢建文,刘羽祥,邓国全. 三伏天穴位贴敷法治疗虚寒喘症的疗效分析[J]. 内蒙古中医药,2013,32(20): 35

谢文娟,刘密,李金香,等.《扁鹊心书》灸法的运用特点[J]. 国医论坛,2013,28(4): 19

谢振年,王芳丽,李东冰,等. 穴位强化埋线疗法治疗慢传输型便秘的临床应用效果分析[J]. 世界中医药, 2013,8(9): 1018

熊书华. 针灸为主治疗老年功能性尿失禁疗效观察[J]. 陕西中医,2013,34(4): 460

胥冰,刘娟,田磊,等. 针灸联合中药通过抑制胰岛细胞的凋亡发挥对糖尿病大鼠的治疗作用[J]. 陕西中医, 2013,34(6): 757

许吉. 2007～2011 年 SCI 收录针灸高被引论文的计量研究[J]. 中国中医药信息杂志,2013,20(6): 17

许宇飞,李晓陵,曹丹娜,等. 应用 MRI 测量乳根穴针刺深度的研究[J]. 针灸临床杂志,2013,29(4): 73

薛平聚,傅立新. 针灸治疗压力性尿失禁的临床研究进展[J]. 针灸临床杂志,2013,29(1): 77

Y

Yang SB, Mei ZB, Cai SJ, et al. Treatment of peripheral facial paralysis with acupuncture at Rényíng (人迎 ST 9) combined with stellate ganglion block: a randomized controlled trial [J]. World Journal of Acupuncture-Moxibustion, 2013, 23(1): 15

Yang SB, Mei ZG, Cai SJ, et al. Treatment of peripheral facial paralysis with acupuncture at Renying (ST 9) mainly cooperated with stellate ganglion block: a randomized controlled trial[J]. Chinese Acupuneture & Moxibustion, 2012, 32(1): 21

羊燕群,侯陈凤,彭丹,等. 针刺足三里对 FD 胃排空及血清 Motilin 和 Ghrelin 的影响[J]. 中华中医药学刊, 2013,31(4): 881

杨斌,鲁玉桂,秦赢,等. 艾灸仪辅助治疗肺结核及对患者免疫功能的影响[J]. 中国针灸,2013,33(4): 299

杨丽洁. 足三里烧山火针法为主治疗脾肾阳虚型慢性疲劳综合征临床疗效研究[J]. 四川中医, 2013, 31(11): 128

杨宁,欧阳育树,原嘉民,等. 人体十二经脉井原穴和俞募穴的相关性研究[J]. 时珍国医国药, 2013, 24(6): 1523

杨帅,任晓暄,赵雅芳,等. 电针"百会""足三里"穴对慢性内脏痛模型大鼠行为及组织中 5-HT 水平的影响[J]. 吉林中医药,2013,33(4): 400

杨晓溪,崔建美,喇孝瑾,等. 针刺对哮喘大鼠肺组织 p38 蛋白激酶及 c-fos 蛋白表达的影响[J]. 时珍国医国药,2013,24(4): 1004

杨馨,刘旭光,王月,等. 艾灸对类风湿性关节炎家兔滑膜细胞 JAK-STAT 通路负反馈调节家族细胞因子信号抑制因子的影响[J]. 针刺研究,2013,38(2): 129

杨雪蓉,黄俊,徐佩英,等. 针灸联合耳穴贴压治疗糖尿病神经源性膀胱 30 例[J]. 陕西中医,2013,34(1): 64

姚剑，胡玲，宋小鸽，等. 艾灸“肾俞”“足三里”穴对类风湿关节炎大鼠滑膜组织中 Ras - MAPK 信号通路的影响[J]. 世界针灸杂志(英文版)，2013，(2)：29，

叶富英，林胜友，蔡亚红，等. 腕踝针配合耳穴贴压治疗围化疗期失眠症疗效观察[J]. 上海针灸杂志，2013，32(3)：207

叶水林，黄怀，古菁，等. 浮针治疗中风后肩手综合征临床观察[J]. 辽宁中医药大学学报，2013，15(11)：223

殷小兰，侯秋科. 子午流注序贯穴位埋线治疗 HBeAg 阴性乙肝病毒携带者外周血 T 细胞亚群变化的临床观察[J]. 中西医结合肝病杂志，2013，23(1)：17

尹建平，李迎真，郝琳慧，等. 针刺背俞穴为主治疗失眠疗效观察[J]. 上海针灸杂志，2013，32(3)：180

余芝，夏有兵，卢明香，等. 电针不同部位单穴/穴组对大鼠胃运动调节效应的特征及影响因素[J]. 针刺研究，2013，38(1)：40

Z

曾姿霈，吴绍汉，曾科学，等. 腹针结合局部穴位注射治疗中风后肩手综合征临床疗效观察[J]. 按摩与康复医学，2013，4(2)：63

翟煦，荣培晶，王宏才，等. 电针刺激对 2 型糖尿病大鼠皮肤屏障及色泽的影响[J]. 针刺研究，2013，38(1)：7

战文翔，王德敬，吴爱芳，等. 粗针透刺膻中穴对急性加重期慢性阻塞性肺疾病 BODE 指数及生活质量的影响[J]. 中国中医基础医学杂志，2013，19(10)：1187

张必萌，胡智海，寿崟，等. 针刺治疗糖尿病性胃轻瘫多中心随机对照研究[J]. 上海中医药杂志，2013，47(3)：31

张承舜，代晓琴，余曙光. 2008～2011 年 SCI 收录的针灸文献特征分析[J]. 中医药导报，2013，19(1)：94

张弛，刘亮，黄建果. 中医穴位注射对慢性阻塞性肺病急性加重期(AECOPD)患者免疫功能的影响[J]. 临床合理用药杂志，2013，6(12)：3

张国山，刘密，章海凤，等.《备急千金要方》论灸法[J]. 国医论坛，2013，28(3)：24

张国山，刘密，章海凤，等.《针灸大成》论灸法[J]. 国医论坛，2013，28(1)：19

张惠林，王玉明. 翳风穴针刺深度及角度 CT 定位探析[J]. 针灸临床杂志，2013，29(8)：24

张佳丽，刘密，娄必丹，等.《医学入门》论灸法[J]. 国医论坛，2013，28(2)：20

张建斌，李开平，李玉堂. 澄江针灸学派传人李玉堂针灸学术特色简析[J]. 江苏中医药，2013，45(7)：58

张建斌，夏有兵，王欣君，等. 现代针灸学科体系构建轨迹的探析——兼评承淡安《针灸学》三部曲[J]. 针刺研究，2013，38(3)：249

张全爱，孙晓慧，林家驹，等. 安眠穴施用滞针术刮法治疗失眠症：随机对照研究[J]. 中国针灸，2013，33(6)：481

张伟，付磊，易宣超，等. 补虚泄实针刺法结合卒中单元模式对脑卒中后肩手综合征患者上肢功能的影响[J]. 辽宁中医药大学学报，2013，15(12)：119

张卫东，王丕敏，韩润霞，等. 火针治疗类风湿关节炎大鼠疗效及安全性评价[J]. 中国针灸，2013，33(4)：334

张艳丽，黄显峰，梁爱芳，等. 药物联合穴位注射治疗耳带状疱疹临床研究[J]. 中医学报，2013，28(5)：769

张艳敏，廖辉. 针刺抑喘方对慢性阻塞性肺疾病急性加重期患者肺功能和体液免疫的影响[J]. 天津中医药大学学报，2013，32(2)：80

张永红，刘初容，黄飞燕. 从激痛点的治疗效果看经络的能量场结构[J]. 中国针灸，2013，33(2)：124

章海凤，雷毅军，常小荣，等.《针灸聚英》论灸法[J]. 国医论坛，2013，28(1)：21

赵斌，翁文庆. 针刺及中药联合治疗糖尿病性麻痹性斜视 36 例[J]. 浙江中医杂志，2013，48(3)：206

赵博华. 梅花针刺络拔罐法治疗带状疱疹急性期临床观察[J]. 北京中医药，2013，32(5)：371

赵崇智，周仙仕. 灯火灸疗法治疗流行性腮腺炎概况[J]. 中医临床研究，2013，5(13)：121

赵红波，范娴娴，吴晓晶，等. 健脾厚肠法联合针灸治疗脾胃湿阻证腹泻型肠易激综合征临床观察[J]. 新中医，2013，45(4)：124

赵琳，汪司右. 不同频次阴部电针神经刺激疗法对女性压力性尿失禁的影响[J]. 国际中医中药杂志，2013，35(5)：391

赵琳，汪司右. 生物反馈监控电针阴部神经刺激疗法治疗女性压力性尿失禁疗效观察[J]. 上海针灸杂志，2013，32(5)：372

赵微. 针药联合治疗 2 型糖尿病 19 例临床观察[J]. 针灸临床杂志，2013，29(7)：27

郑盛惠，吴玉娟，常洁，等. 赤风迎源针法对脑卒中后肩手综合征患者生存质量的影响[J]. 中医药信息，2013，30(5)：89

郑盛惠，郑生智，吴玉娟，等. 长蛇灸治疗脾肾两虚型慢性疲劳综合征临床疗效及对细胞因子的影响[J]. 中华中医药学刊，2013，31(11)：2555

郑盛惠，郑生智，吴玉娟，等. 长蛇灸治疗脾肾两虚型慢性疲劳综合征随机对照研究[J]. 上海针灸杂志，2013，32(10)：824

周莉，施伟. 麦粒灸结合系统康复治疗脑卒中后肩手综合征Ⅰ期临床研究[J]. 中国中医急症，2013，22(11)：1970

周平南，彭鹏鸣，王蓉娣，等. 针灸治疗新发肥胖 2 型糖尿病疗效观察[J]. 针灸临床杂志，2013，29(1)：21

周雪，陆瑾，符仲华，等. 浮针治疗慢性阻塞性肺疾病

急性加重期20例[J].中国针灸,2013,33(6)：527

朱安宁,孟宪军,钱林超,等.澄江学派传人黄宗勖先生针灸学术特色[J].中国针灸,2013,33(4)：373

朱文莲,李滢,杨帅,等.同神经节段不同穴位对肠易激综合征效应机制的比较研究[J].中华中医药杂志,2013,28(11)：3224

邹天雨,程为平,王薇.《针灸聚英》灸治癫痫的探讨[J].针灸临床杂志,2013,29(2)：50

左甲,何佳,杜晨,等.铺棉灸疗法治疗带状疱疹的临床研究[J].南京中医药大学学报,2013,29(3)：211

(十一) 推　　拿

【概述】

2013年在各类杂志上发表的关于推拿的论文有近千篇，广东深圳举行的全国第十四次中医推拿学术年会收到100多篇学术论文，论文仍以临床研究与治疗经验总结者居多，涉及面也较广，兹将它们所反映推拿学术的进展或动态作简要介绍。

1. 基础研究

姚斌彬等发现推拿治疗可以通过提高轴浆运输马达蛋白 kinesin 及 dynein 的表达，促进轴浆运输功能恢复，进而双向影响神经元细胞及神经支配靶组织，并最终改善坐骨神经损伤大鼠的运动及感觉功能。吴凡等发现推拿可以延长机体对热痛刺激的反应时间，在坐骨神经损伤后可以有效地保护脊髓背角感觉神经元，并抑制神经损伤后所出现的神经源性疼痛。豆梦琳等发现，简谐激励改良斜扳法的疗效与频率有关。(详见专条)

2. 临床研究

(1) 骨伤科疾病的治疗　赵保礼等将青少年颈椎病患者分为两组，对照组32例予推拿治疗，治疗组33例在对照组的基础上联合颈椎操锻炼。治疗14 d后观察两组临床疗效，比较治疗前后视觉模拟评分(VAS评分)、临床症状评分。结果，总有效率治疗组与对照组分别为93.9%(31/33)、71.9%(23/32)，组间比较，$P<0.05$。两组治疗后VAS评分、临床症状评分均较本组治疗前降低($P<0.05$)，治疗组更明显($P<0.05$)。杨军雄等将腰椎间盘突出症患者分为两组，综合组取腹气街部穴位，行双手同刺法，配合脊柱调衡治疗；常规组穴取肾俞、大肠俞及患侧环跳、承扶等，采用常规针刺和推拿治疗。结果，综合组与常规组愈显率分别为91.7%(33/36)、77.1%(27/35)，组间比较，$P<0.05$；治疗前10次的镇痛效应综合组明显优于常规组($P<0.05$)；两组治疗后功能障碍指数(Os－westry)功能障碍指数均显著改善(均$P<0.05$)，综合组优于常规组($P<0.05$)；治疗后健康相关生活质量评分(SF－36)总体健康、身体疼痛、生理功能、社会功能、情感职能维度值综合组优于常规组(均$P<0.05$)；治疗15次后综合组血清TNF－α水平较治疗前降低，且明显低于常规组($P<0.05$)，治疗30次后综合组亦低于常规组($P<0.05$)。张建华等运用倒悬牵引配合整脊推拿手法治疗40例轻度青少年脊柱侧弯(特发性脊柱侧弯29例、后天姿态性脊柱侧弯11例)，23例恢复正常，14例明显好转。洪欣等将膝骨性关节炎患者分为两组。观察组57例实施骨盆矫正骨膜压揉法，对照组60例采用传统推拿手法治疗。结果两组患者在对治疗前后疼痛、关节活动度、肿胀或条索结节感等症状的比较，$P<0.01$；而观察组优于对照组($P<0.01$)。覃荣周等将运动性腰肌劳损患者均分为两组，均予常规治疗基础上采用局部推拿及灸法，治疗组同时引入足底反射疗法。结果治疗组与对照组总有效率分别为100.0%、,88.0%(44/50)，组间比较，$P<0.05$。

(2) 内妇科疾病的治疗　孙中明等观察前列排瘀法治疗慢性盆腔疼痛综合征(CPPS)疗效及NIH－CPSI评分。方法：据NIH前列腺炎综合征分类标准，选择CPPS病例719例，根据EPSRt(前列腺液常规)分成Ⅲa和Ⅲb两组。719例均采用示指一指禅功前列排瘀法治疗，1次/3 d，每次3～5 min，10次为1个疗程。排瘀法治疗前、治疗后作EPSRt及NIH－CPSI评分进行疗效评价。3个疗程后，Ⅲa组显效率18.2%(80/439)，有效率66.1%(290/439)；Ⅲb组分别为16.1%(45/280)，69.6%(195/280)。经统计分析，治疗前后差异有统计学意义($P<0.01$)。两组间疗效差异无统计学意义($P>0.05$)，每一疗程结束后，两组NIH－CPSI各类得分均有明显改善($P<0.01$)。结论：前列排瘀法有排瘀散结，通利腺管，最终排出瘀浊的作用。能有效改善或消除盆腔疼痛综合征症状，提高生活质量。房纬等将肝郁气滞型广泛性焦虑症患者分为两组，腹部推拿组给予按腹、揉腹、运腹、推腹、横擦胸胁、捏脊及推拿头项治疗，西药对照组给予盐酸帕罗西汀片

治疗。均1次/d,15 d为1个疗程。2个疗程后,腹部推拿组总有效率为92.5%(37/40),西药对照组为95.0%(38/40),组间比较,$P>0.05$。两组患者血浆5-HT水平、HAMA量表评分均较治疗前下降($P<0.05$),组间比较,$P>0.05$,腹部推拿组患者随访时HAMA量表评分低于西药对照组($P<0.05$)。腹部推拿组患者治疗后TESS量表评分、副反应发生率明显低于西药对照组($P<0.05$)。姚斐等将慢性疲劳综合征(CFS)患者分为推拿组32例和教育组(CBT组)30例,10次为1个疗程。1个疗程后,两组CFS患者匹兹堡睡眠质量指数(PSQI)积分均有降低,睡眠质量改善;但推拿组患者PSQI积分变化更明显,与CBT组相比,$P<0.05$。张军等将120例早期2型糖尿病患者均分为两组。治疗前、治疗后第4周分别检测空腹血糖(FPG)、腰围、体重指数(BMI)、餐后2 h血糖(2 h PG)、糖化血红蛋白(HbA_{1C})、三酰甘油(TG)、总胆固醇(TC)、胰岛素(FINS)水平、胰岛素抵抗指数(HOMA-IR),评价两组临床疗效。结果治疗组临床总有效率为92.8%(56/60),对照组临床总有效率为75.7%(45/60),两组比较,$P<0.05$。治疗组患者治疗后FPG、腰围、BMI、HbA_{1C}、TG、TC、FINS、HOMA-IR与治疗前比较数值降低,$P<0.01$,与对照组治疗后比较,$P<0.01$。

(3) 儿科疾病的治疗　莫金花等将60例缓解期反复呼吸道感染患儿均分为两组,试验组予推拿配合艾灸治疗,对照组予泛福舒胶囊治疗,疗程3个月,观察期1年。两组治疗后上呼吸道感染次数、气管支气管炎发生次数及病种减少,病程缩短,与治疗前相比,$P<0.01$或$P<0.05$。试验组治疗后气管支气管炎发病次数、病程改善优于对照组,$P<0.05$。试验组治疗后CD_3^+、CD_4^+、IgA、IgG水平较治疗前提高,对照组治疗后CD_3^+、CD_4^+、CD_8^+、CD_4^+/CD_8^+、IgA、IgG水平较治疗前提高,差异均有统计学意义($P<0.05$或$P<0.01$)。对照组治疗后CD_3^+、CD_4^+、CD_8^+、CD_4^+/CD_8^+、IgG改善优于试验组,组间比较,$P<0.05$或$P<0.01$。陈团营等将肺炎患儿分为两组,均予消炎、化痰等对症支持治疗,治疗组加推拿配合中药辨证治疗。经治7 d后,治疗组与对照组痊愈率分别为80.0%(32/40)、55.0%(22/40),组间比较,$P<0.05$;且治疗组患儿咳嗽、咳痰、肺部啰音、气喘等症状消失时间为(4.32±2.34)、(6.34±1.36)、(4.34±1.36)、(3.34±2.64)d,均明显少于对照组的(6.12±3.48)、(7.03±1.43)、(6.03±1.85)、(4.23±1.47)d,组间比较,$P<0.05$。徐珊等将小儿急性泄泻伤食证分为两组,试验组76例采用推拿,对照组30例采用思密达和培菲康治疗。经治6 d后,试验组疗效显著优于对照组($P<0.01$),且在主症(大便次数、质地、性状、质量)的恢复正常时间方面显著早于对照组($P<0.01$)。陈治珍等将小儿急性非感染性腹泻患儿分为试验A组37例、试验B组38例及对照组38例,三组均给予基础治疗(包括喂养指导、预防脱水及纠正脱水),试验A组加服固定处方中药汤剂,试验B组在A组的基础上配合虚证推拿法或实证推拿法,对照组在基础治疗的同时口服思密达。三组均于治疗3 d后,全分析集(FAS)和符合方案集(PPT)的分析结果一致,疗效基本相当,组间比较,$P>0.05$,治疗期间三组病例均未见明显不良反应。

3. 功法和推拿教学

胡伟民等按照推拿功法易筋经中定势站桩时长10 s、20 s、30 s设计三种操练方式,85名老年人随机分入三组,观测操练时心率和自觉运动强度分级的变化情况。结果:每种方式操练心率均有增加($P<0.05$),定势站桩30 s组心率和PRE值均较10 s、20 s组高($P<0.05$),操练中目标心率持续时间占比三种方式间差异无统计学意义($P>0.05$)。孙强等选择其学院推拿专科学生,实验组54例,对照组56例,分别进行传统授课方式和改革后授课方式(采取力学训练法:动作发力训练、力量感觉训练、微力训练、相应功法训练、力学评价)的教学,结果:实验组在考核成绩上明显优于对照组($P<0.05$)。

(严隽陶　许　军)

【推拿手法及其机理的实验研究】

姚斌彬等建立大鼠坐骨神经夹持损伤模型,通过腓肠肌湿质量测量、热痛阈实验观察正常组、假手术组、模型组、模型对照组、推拿组大鼠的病理学、行为学变化;通过免疫组织化学染色观察各组大鼠脊髓内kinesin及dynein表达情况,并统计分析各组间的差异。发现坐骨神经损伤后大鼠的感觉及运动功能明显降低的结果,在推拿治疗后,腓肠肌湿质量测量及热痛阈实验评分明显升高,并在治疗20 d后与正常组无显著性差异;模型组、对照组及推拿组 kinesin 及 dynein 免疫组化表达与正常组相比均有显著性提高，推拿组与模型组、对照组相比也具有显著性差异。认为推拿治疗可以通过提高轴浆运输马达蛋白 kinesin 及 dynein 的表达，促进轴浆运输功能恢复，进而双向影响神经元细胞及神经支配靶组织，并最终改善坐骨神经损伤大鼠的运动及感觉功能。梅旭晖等采用神经夹持损伤的方式建立大鼠坐骨神经损伤模型，观察各组大鼠的行为学变化，脊髓内 NGF 及 p75NTR 表达情况。观察到模型组和模型对照组大鼠行为学检测表明坐骨神经损伤后大鼠的运动及感觉功能明显降低($P<0.05$)，推拿治疗后斜板实验及热痛阈实验评分明显升高($P<0.05$)，与正常组无显著性差异；模型组、模型对照组及推拿组 NGF 及 p75NTR 免疫组化表达与正常组相比均有显著性差异($P<0.05$)，其中模型组及模型对照组 NGF 略升高($P<0.05$)，p75NTR 显著性升高($P<0.05$)，推拿组 NGF 显著性升高($P<0.05$)，p75NTR 显著性下降($P<0.05$)。认为推拿治疗可以通过提高机体 NGF 表达，降低 NGF 的低亲和力受体 p75NTR 释放，从而抑制细胞凋亡机制，最终改善坐骨神经损伤大鼠的运动及感觉功能。吴凡等采用 SD 大鼠坐骨神经夹持损伤为模型，以“按摩手法模拟仪”于大鼠手术侧“殷门”“承山”“阳陵泉”穴施以点法、揉法，通过对大鼠甩尾热痛阈的分析，从行为学角度探寻推拿对坐骨神经损伤后的肢体感觉功能恢复的良性促进作用，为揭示推拿促进神经修复的机制提供理论支持。发现经推拿治疗的坐骨神经损伤大鼠的 50℃热水甩尾时间高于假手术组、模型组及模型对照组，且与模型组比较，差异显著。说明推拿可以延长机体对热痛刺激的反应时间，进一步提示，推拿在坐骨神经损伤后可以有效地保护脊髓背角感觉神经元，并抑制神经损伤后所出现的神经源性疼痛。本研究以热痛刺激作为行为学观察指标，检测损伤神经修复后支配情况，结果表明，可延长机体痛敏反应时间。说明推拿对坐骨神经损伤大鼠产生的疼痛感觉具有一定的抑制作用，其机理可能为保护了脊髓背角感觉神经元。林清等采用细胞培养技术，建立人骨骼肌细胞损伤模型后，将正常细胞和损伤细胞各自分为空白对照组、推拿按法组、推拿㨰法＋维拉帕米组、静态压力组和静态压力＋维拉帕米组。分别对各组细胞进行推拿㨰法样刺激或静压刺激，持续时间 10 min。其后对各组细胞的超氧化物歧化酶(SOD)活性、丙二醛(MDA)含量、肌酸激酶(CK)活性进行检测。结果，推拿㨰法可以提高人骨骼肌细胞内 SOD 活性，降低细胞内 MDA 含量以及细胞上清中的 CK 活性；在加入钙离子拮抗剂(维拉帕米)后，各项指标的变化均受到明显的影响。提示推拿㨰法的力学作用主要通过影响人骨骼肌细胞中钙离子的信号通路，从而激发损伤细胞修复的生物学效应。豆梦琳等假设椎骨为刚体，椎间盘及周围韧带等软组织为黏弹性体，建立模拟 L1～5 的 5 自由度振动系统，对基本方程进行解析求解。结果简谐激励改良斜扳法的疗效与频率有关。在频率≤1 的简谐激励改良斜扳法作用下，病变节段最大位移都大于脉冲激励传统斜扳法下的最大位移。随着病变位置下移，简谐激励改良斜扳法的损伤比相比脉冲激励传统斜扳法逐渐下降，安全性增高。说明使用频率≤1 的简谐激励改良斜扳法，治疗效果优于脉冲激励传统斜扳法，且可控制损伤。周楠等选取 10 名腰突症患者两组各 5 例，并设正常志愿者 5 例正常组。理筋组用理筋手法，理调组采用理筋手法加调整手法。应用 ITK 重建软件对三维重建腰椎椎体 CT 进行有限元分析，比较 3 组手法干预前后腰椎椎体三维位移变化情况。结果，3 组腰突症患者推拿手法治疗后 L1～5 各椎体的空间位置发生了一定改变。理调组 L3 在 X 轴角位移为 $(1.77\pm0.46)°$；L4 在 X，Y 轴角位移分别为 $(1.78\pm0.53)°$、$(1.89\pm0.75)°$，显著大于理筋组和正常组($P<0.05$)；理调组 L1～5 在 X 轴三维角位移分别为 $(1.50\pm0.47)°$、$(1.55\pm0.57)°$、$(1.77\pm0.46)°$、$(1.78\pm0.53)°$、$(1.61\pm0.39)°$，均显著大于正常组($P<0.05$)；理调组 L3 在 Y 轴三维位移为 (2.87 ± 0.74)mm，L4 在 X 轴三维位移为 (1.68 ± 0.64)mm，显著大于理筋组和正常组($P<0.05$)；理调组 L1、L4、L5 在 X 轴三维位移分别为 (1.28 ± 0.21)、(1.68 ± 0.64)、(1.30 ± 0.51)mm，L1～3 在 Y 轴维位移分别为 (1.92 ± 0.42)、(2.25 ± 0.61)、(2.87 ± 0.74)mm，均显著大于正常组($P<0.05$)。理筋手法组 L1～5 各节段三维角位移和位移与正常组相比，均呈现大于正常组的趋势。提示理调手法比理筋手法更能调整失稳或退变节段的空间位置，使腰椎椎体产生水平及旋转移位，而非上下移位，对纠正腰椎“骨错缝”产生重要作用。理筋手

法对腰突症患者腰椎结构有一定的影响,但不显著。

(许　军　严隽陶)

【肩周炎的治疗】

欧汉锋等将106个门诊病例分为美洛昔康加肌筋膜牵拉手法组(A组)、肌筋膜牵拉手法组(B组)和常规推拿手法组(C组),三组均进行手法治疗和自主康复训练,C组进行常规推拿手法,A、B组进行肌筋膜牵拉手法,A在手法结束后进行痛点注射美洛昔康;1次/1 d,7 d为1个疗程,每2个疗程间休息2 d,痛点注射1次/周,共4个疗程。根据Constant－Murley score来评价疗效,根据并发症来评价安全性。结果:A组有效率为100%(34/34),B组为93.7%(30/32),C组为70.0%(28/40),组间比较$P<0.05$;A组与B组比较,$P<0.05$。三组均无并发症发生。周瑜博等将瘀滞型患者均分为两组,均予服舒筋汤配合推拿治疗,治疗组加针刀治疗。经治疗结束后4周,治疗组和对照组分别脱落1例和2例;治疗组总有效率94.3%(34/36),对照组为73.5%(27/36),组间比较,$P<0.05$;治疗后两组肩关节功能评分(UCIA)均显著升高($P<0.05$),且治疗组显著高于对照组($P<0.05$)。郭红阳等将患者分为两组各35例,治疗组采用张力下推拿治疗,对照组采用常规推拿治疗,结果,两组疗效比较经秩和检验,$P<0.05$。陆萍将患者分为针推组37例、针刺组35例、推拿组35例,分别采用针刺结合推拿、单纯针刺、单纯推拿治疗,2个疗程后,针推组治疗率为86.5%(32/37),针刺组为42.9%(15/35),推拿组为54.3%(19/35)。针推组与针刺组相比,$X^2=10.105$,$P<0.05$;与推拿组相比,$X^2=9.027$,$P<0.05$。李敏雅等运用中药湿热敷导入和康复手法综合治疗38例患者,结果总有效率为94.7%(36/38),治疗后肩关节关节活动度有显著改善($P<0.01$)。

(许　军　严隽陶)

【推拿治疗小儿便秘】

韩世春等推拿治疗经中医辨证论治后患儿200例。实秘:清大肠100次、泻肺气100次、退下六腑200次、推下七节骨10次、揉龟尾300次、按揉足三里1 min。虚秘:补脾经200次、清大肠100次、推三关100次、按揉胃俞、脾俞、肾俞5 min,捏脊5～10次,按揉足三里1 min。结果,总有效率100%。冯兆才等将32例痉挛型脑瘫特发性便秘患者均分为两组,治疗组分部位采用不同推拿方法:① 腹部局部推拿:患儿取仰卧位,用食、中、无名、小指指面着力于神阙穴,顺时针沿下脘、左天枢、石门、右天枢方向小幅度环转,使着力面在局部做有节奏的环形平移摩擦。用掌根沿任脉或食、中、无名指三指指腹沿任脉两侧少阴肾经、阳明胃经、太阴脾经从巨阙穴至中极穴做单向直线擦拭。以拇指指端着力于巨阙、中脘、下脘、气海、关元、中极等穴位。② 四肢经穴推拿:患儿取仰卧位,用手掌按揉双侧下肢肌群,点按髀关、血海、足三里、丰隆、上巨虚、下巨虚等穴,并配合下肢膝关节屈伸及外旋运动。用手掌按揉双侧上肢肌群,点按曲池、手三里、外关、合谷等穴,并配合肩关节活动类手法。③ 背部经穴推拿:患儿取俯卧位,用手掌或大、小鱼际按揉背部足太阳膀胱经第一、二侧线,自上而下,反复数次。点按肺俞、脾俞、胃俞、肾俞、大肠俞、小肠俞等俞穴。以拇指与食、中二指指面着力,自长强穴至大椎穴,相对用力提捏捻搓,反复数次。以食、中、无名指指端吸定于督脉及膀胱经第一侧线,自上而下反复推揉数次。对照组用开塞露塞肛。同时口服金双歧。1个月后,治疗组有效率为100%,对照组为75.0%(12/16)。王国毅等将105例患者分为两组,均予服双歧杆菌三联活菌胶囊,治疗组51例联合推拿(清脾经,补肾水,清大肠,揉内劳宫,退六腑,运水入土,下推七节骨,揉足三里)疗法,观察治疗后两组的大便性状评分和每周排便次数。结果治疗组14～28 d大便性状评分优于对照组($P<0.05$),每周排便次数多于对照组。谢洁珊等将100例脑性瘫痪便秘患儿分为两组,均予小儿便秘常规护理,推拿组51例加用小儿推拿,取仰卧位,用大拇指点揉中脘、天枢、足三里穴各1 min后,两手掌根部自膻中穴始往下按抚至脐下关元穴,反复操作10次,最后顺时针摩腹5 min。再取俯卧位,用大拇指往下推七节骨500次,揉龟尾1 min,点揉脾俞、大肠俞各1 min。20 d后,推拿组排便质量提高,伴随症状减轻,与对照组比较,$P<0.05$或$P<0.01$。王开萍将患者分为两组,治疗组直刺双侧腑阳池、天枢,行捻转提插手法不留针。同时推拿顺时针摩腹5 min,捏脊5～10次,推下七节骨200次。偏实证加清天河水2 min,退六腑150次,按弦走搓摩2 min;偏气血亏虚,加推三关2 min,按揉足三里各1 min,偏阴虚加指揉肾经1 min,揉上马1 min,对

照组服王氏保赤丸。结果：治疗组总有效率为95.0%(76/80)，对照组为80.0%(64/80)。罗菲采用推拿配合妈咪爱治疗39例功能性便秘患者，实证便秘以清大肠、退六腑、清补脾土、运内八卦、摩腹、按揉足三里及推下七节骨。虚证便秘以补脾经、推肾水、清大肠、推上三关、摩腹、捏脊及按揉足三里。配合口服妈咪爱。结果总有效率100%。袁慎霞等采用推拿(① 虚证便秘：补脾经、推肾水、清大肠、推三关各300次，顺时针摩腹10 min，捏脊5遍。② 实证便秘：摩腹10 min；清大肠、运内八卦各300次，按揉膊阳池500次；推下七节骨3 min；揉足三里2 min：退六腑3 min)联合金双歧片口服。治疗后患者24、48、72 h结肠传输试验钡剂排出率较治疗前明显提高($P<0.05$)。治愈率为64.3%(36/56)。

（何永瑞　郑贤国）

【推拿治疗小儿厌食】

崔璇等将患者分为两组，推拿组给予推拿疗法，药物组口服健胃消食口服液。结果，推拿组有效率为95.7%(45/47)，药物组84.4%(27/32)，组间比较，$P<0.01$。张雪荣等采用扶阳罐配合推拿疗法治疗脾胃气虚型患者，疗程4周。总有效率为95.0%(57/60)，主症食欲和食量，次症腹胀、面色无华、大便不调与治疗前比较，$P<0.05$；次证中腹痛与治疗前比较，$P>0.05$。陈秀珍将脾胃气虚证患者均分为两组，治疗组用推手摩腹捏脊推拿法，对照组口服调脾合剂。7 d为1个疗程。经治4个疗程后，治疗组与对照组总有效率分别为95.0%(38/40)、87.5%(35/40)，组间比较，$P<0.05$。翟瑞军应用将53例患儿辨证分为脾失健运型、脾胃气虚型、脾胃阴虚型进行推拿治疗。10 d为1个疗程。经治1个疗程，治愈21例，占39.6%；显效19例，占35.8%。第2个疗程后全部治愈。谢一民等将患者均分为两组，均予常规药物治疗，治疗组再行推拿按摩疗法。经治30 d后，治疗组与对照组总有效率分别为94.3%(50/53)、84.9%(45/53)，组间比较，$P<0.05$。临床观察中治疗组未发现有不良反应。

（许　军　严隽陶）

［附］ 参考文献

C

陈团营，马庆华，张新建，等. 推拿配合中药辨证治疗小儿肺炎临床观察[J]. 中华医院感染学杂志，2013，23(13)：3180

陈秀珍. 推手摩腹捏脊推拿法治疗小儿厌食症40例观察[J]. 实用中医药杂志，2012，28(1)：36

陈治珍，许华，许双虹，等. 虚实辨证推拿治疗小儿急性非细菌感染性腹泻的临床对照研究[J]. 广州中医药大学学报，2013，30(1)：40

崔璇，李敏. 推拿治疗小儿厌食症47例[J]. 中国中西医结合消化杂志，2012，20(8)：375

D

豆梦琳，方舟，周楠，等. 中医斜扳疗法治疗腰椎间盘突出的生物力学研究[J]. 医用生物力学，2013，28(3)：304

F

房纬，王金贵，孙庆，等. 腹部推拿为主治疗广泛性焦虑症患者40例临床观察[J]. 中医杂志，2013，54(2)：130

冯兆才，马融，李瑞仕. 推拿治疗痉挛型脑瘫患儿特发性便秘临床观察[J]. 辽宁中医杂志，2013，40(1)：158

G

郭红阳，闰博，齐伟. 推拿治疗肩周炎70例疗效分析[J]. 吉林中医药，2013，33(6)：632

H

韩世春，贺思. 推拿手法治疗小儿便秘200例[J]. 中国疗养医学，2013，22(4)：344

洪欣，景明，龚云秀，等. 骨盆矫正骨膜压揉治疗膝骨性关节炎57例临床疗效观察[J]. 云南中医中药杂志，2013，34(2)：13

胡伟民，龚利，钱义明，等. 老年人推拿功法易筋经不同方式锻炼的运动强度研究[J]. 按摩与康复医学，2013，4(5)：53

L

李敏雅，张曦，戴巧君. 康复手法结合中药湿热敷导入治疗肩周炎38例[J]. 浙江中医杂志，2013，48(5)：357

李英. 采用压痛点强刺激推拿治疗肩周炎临床分析[J]. 中国实用医药，2013，8(4)：236

林清，张宏，赵谦，等. 推拿滚法引发人骨骼肌细胞生物学效应的机制探讨[J]. 上海中医药大学学报，2013，

27(2)：81

陆萍. 针推结合治疗肩周炎 37 例疗效观察[J]. 上海医药,2013,34(14)：28

罗菲. 小儿推拿配合妈咪爱治疗婴幼儿功能性便秘 39 例[J]. 陕西中医,2013,34(7)：881

M

梅旭晖,纪倩,姚斌彬,等. 推拿对坐骨神经损伤大鼠神经生长因子及其受体 p75NTR 的影响[J]. 中华中医药杂志,2013,28(7)：1994

莫金花,韦琴,陈似霞,等. 推拿配合艾灸防治反复呼吸道感染的疗效观察[J]. 中华护理杂志,2013,48(4)：343

O

欧汉锋,罗海燕,魏秋实,等. 美洛昔康痛点注射配合肌筋膜牵拉手法治疗肩关节周围炎[J]. 中国中医骨伤科杂志,2013,21(5)：35

S

孙强,孙丹,孙巍巍. 推拿手法学实验课力学训练法的应用研究[J]. 中国中医药现代远程教育,2013,11(13)：85

孙中明,鲍严钟. 前列排瘀法治疗慢性盆腔疼痛综合征临床研究[J]. 中华中医药学刊,2013,31(3)：678

T

覃荣周,雷鸣鸣,程松苗,等. 推拿灸法配合足底反射疗法治疗运动性腰肌劳损的效果研究[J]. 中外医学研究,2013,11(9)：9

W

王国毅,李亚伶,蒲昭霞. 小儿推拿联合益生菌治疗儿童功能性便秘疗效观察[J]. 西南军医,2013,15(2)：123

王开萍. 针推并用治疗小儿功能性便秘 80 例[J]. 内蒙古中医药,2013,32(26)：28

吴凡,张蓓,郑慧敏,等. 推拿治疗坐骨神经损伤大鼠行为学研究[J]. 成都中医药大学学报,2013,36(1)：41

X

谢洁珊,李玉秀,胡克萍. 护理干预结合推拿法治疗脑瘫患儿便秘疗效观察[J]. 中医儿科杂志,2013,9(6)：55

谢一民,周贤刚,杨闯. 推拿按摩配合药物治疗小儿厌食症疗效分析[J]. 实用中医药杂志,2012,28(12)：988

徐珊,汪受传,李江全,等. 基于生存分析的推拿治疗小儿伤食泻临床研究[J]. 中华中医药杂志,2013,28(1)：275

Y

杨军雄,张建平,于建春,等. 气街干预合脊柱调衡治疗腰椎间盘突出症随机对照研究[J]. 中国针灸,2013,33(4)：289

姚斌彬,梅旭晖,吴剑聪,等. 基于马达蛋白探讨推拿对坐骨神经损伤大鼠轴浆运输功能的影响[J]. 南京中医药大学学报,2013,29(4)：338

姚斐,房敏,姜淑云,等. 经穴推拿对慢性疲劳综合征患者睡眠质量影响的临床研究[J]. 中华中医药杂志,2013,28(2)：559

袁慎霞,赵玉忠. 推拿联合金双歧治疗对儿童功能性便秘结肠动力影像学的影响[J]. 中国中西医结合杂志,2012,32(5)：709

Z

翟瑞军. 推拿疗法治疗小儿厌食症 53 例[J]. 中医外治杂志,2013,22(3)：33

张建华,王展. 倒悬牵引配合整脊治疗轻度青少年脊柱侧弯 40 例[J]. 光明中医,2013,28(7)：1408

张军,马笃军,李惠林,等. 推拿手法治疗早期 2 型糖尿病的临床观察研究[J]. 中国医药导报,2013,10(16)：115

张雪荣,刘晓鹰. 扶阳罐配合推拿疗法治疗小儿厌食症(脾胃气虚证)的临床观察[J]. 辽宁中医杂志,2012,39(9)：1838

赵保礼,张立庄,孙建芳. 颈椎操联合推拿治疗青少年颈椎病 33 例临床观察[J]. 河北中医,2013,35(6)：878

周楠,吕强,方舟. 推拿手法对腰椎间盘突出症腰椎结构三维位移的影响[J]. 医用生物力学,2013,28(3)：269

周瑜博,孟庆才. 舒筋汤结合推拿、针刀疗法治疗瘀滞型肩周炎临床观察[J]. 安徽中医学院学报,2013,32(4)：55

(十二) 气　　功

【概述】

2013年气功学术论文较为丰富。通过中国知网、维普、万方等中文数据库的检索,以"气功"为检索词,检出703篇。其中,期刊论文321篇,博硕士论文136篇,会议论文11篇,报纸文章79篇,外文文献47篇,年鉴63篇,专利3项。二次检索,以"健身"为检索词,有344篇;以"医学"为检索词,有180篇;以"导引"为检索词,有81篇;以"吐纳"为检索词,有84篇;以"周天"为检索词,有14篇。

从近5年文献的数量上看,以"气功"为一级检索词,2012年检出804篇,2011年检出589篇,2010年检出596篇,2009年检出484篇。气功文献逐年呈逐年上升的趋势,尤以2012年和2013年的气功文献检出率最高,反映出近两年以气功为研究内容的文献显著高于往年。虽未达到1999年(1 868篇)的50%,但是,论文的质量、研究的科学性和规范性等方面,已经有了显著进步,特别是全国各中医药高等院校和体育院校,出现了许多高水平的硕博士研究生毕业论文,这也成为本年度气功的研究特色。从二次检索的文献情况分析,健身气功检出率达48.93%,为研究的主要内容,而医学气功的检出率为25.60%,明显低于健身气功,这中间又有健身气功关于研究医学问题的混杂,混杂率达80%以上,也就是说,医学气功的实际文献远不足15%,反映出医学气功本年度的文献贡献率相对偏低,这与近年来国家体育总局健身气功中心配套政策的进一步落实和各省市健身气功的广泛推广有非常密切的关系,也就是健身气功从五年前的平均水平上升到目前优势水平的关键所在。从另外一方面说明,医学气功需要在中医药学的框架内,加大管理投入、资金支持和提高学科及人才队伍建设,尽快支持和引导气功的医疗服务融入科研和产业化发展。本年度文献整体水平分析,气功论文理论探讨型、观察型和文献型等偏多,而基础性和应用基础性实验研究文献偏少,其中尤其缺乏实(试)验设计严谨、高引用性文献。

2013年气功研究存在的主要问题有:对照方案的设计不合理、研究纵深度不够、研究的手段和技术相对滞后等。因此,加大与相关学科的交流,引入更加科学、规范的实(试)验方案,加强机制机理的基础研究,对气功的科学发展显得非常重要和迫切。本年度,魏玉龙、夏宇欣等报道,北京中医药大学开展的气功研究具有代表性,而且研究的深入性和切入点(具象思维理论)也非常符合气功研究厚基础的需求。在多年应用EEG、ERP观测气功调心诱发脑功能效应的研究基础上,2013年开展了"意境作业安神解郁作用的分子机制研究",进行了小样本基础性探索研究,发现钙离子信号通路、细胞因子-细胞因子受体信号通路、脂肪酸代谢通路、JAK－STAT信号通路、神经活性配体-受体信号通路等在意境作业训练前后变化显著,推测意境作业训练可能通过调控脂肪酸代谢通路、细胞因子通路、JAK－STAT信号通路、神经活性配体-受体信号通路的基因表达从而发挥其安神解郁的作用。目前该研究正准备扩大样本,进行深入研究,为气功作用效应提供更加充分的分子生物学证据。

(魏玉龙)

【气功机理研究】

通过中国知网、万方和维普数据库,以关键词"气功"检索,检索时间范围为2013年1月至12月,从检索文献中挑选出关于气功三调及临床疗效作用机理的研究文献共6篇,其中硕士学位论文1篇,实验性研究5篇。

林宇峰等研究了健身气功八段锦对19例2型糖尿病患者血液生化指标的影响,研究结果表明健身气功、八段锦可降低空腹血糖,血总胆固醇、甘油三酯、低密度脂蛋白胆固醇、糖化血红蛋白含量均下降,高密度脂蛋白水平升高。焦润艺等将156名无运动习惯的老年人随机均分为不运动组和八段锦组,观察八段锦练习对老年人红细胞功能的影响。结果,八段锦组红细胞压积、红细胞刚性指数、红细胞聚集指数和红细胞膜MDA含量明显低于无运动组($P<0.01$),红细胞膜SOD活性、红细胞CRI表达和CRI黏附活性明显高于无运动组($P<0.01$)。提示八段锦锻炼能

改善红细胞功能，这可能是八段锦抗衰老的机制。汝雷等观察五禽戏练习对老年人血脂水平的影响，结果表明有规律地练习6个月的五禽戏以后，与无运动组比较，受试者血脂甘油三酯及低密度脂蛋白水平均下降，疾病产生因素削弱，高密度脂蛋白含量增加明显，疾病抵抗因素加强。洪邦辉等分析了易筋经对女大学生痛经影响的作用机制，研究结果表明易筋经锻炼后受试者血液流变学中全血低切黏度、全血高切黏度、血浆黏度、红细胞压积及红细胞聚集指数均显著降低，经血前列腺素 PGF_{2a} 含量显著降低，练习者 SCL－90 情绪因子和焦虑因子得分均降低，结果提示易筋经运动可能是通过以上机制而达到减轻大学生原发痛经的疗效。桂翔在其硕士毕业论文龟息功法对血氧饱和度和心肺功能影响的研究中，以30名扬州大学研究生为研究对象，通过12周的龟息功法练习，受试者血氧饱和度明显下降，心率、舒缩和舒张压都下降明显。结果表明龟息功法通过较长时间的闭气呼气，可以提高人体对于氧气的利用率，提高血红蛋白与氧气的结合能力，减少耗能，降低新陈代谢，从而降低心率和血压，增长人体的闭气时间。气功是调身、调息、调心三调合一的心身修炼技能，达到三调合一境界后身心息融为一体，练功者达到身心合一或天人合一的境界。这时气功练习时的思维形式也不是心身割裂的思维形式，而是心身一体的独特思维形式。郭建红等通过不同思维形式时表面肌电特征的实验研究，初步证明具象思维是以心身合一为基本属性的独特思维形式。该实验应用双向设计、关联检测、相互释义的实验研究模式，采集受试者同一思维主题的抽象思维、形象思维和具象思维作业时胫骨前肌表面肌电信号，对导出波幅数据进行统计分析结果表明，具象思维在波幅极差和标准差上与抽象思维、形象思维数据差异较大，与思维作业前安静态相比，抽象思维、形象思维肌电信号在波幅均值、标准差、极差方面均未显示出显著性差异。具象思维与安静态相比，波幅均值无显著性差异，波幅极差值存在显著性差异。实验证明具象思维时心理状态的变化会伴随生理检测指标的改变，而抽象思维没有表现出这种改变，具象思维与抽象、形象思维不同，是心身合一的独特思维形式，气功练习达到三调合一的境界时使用的主要思维形式应是以心身合一为属性的具象思维形式。

以上6篇实验性文章通过实验学的手段，从气功身心作用机制、气功练习后的生理指标及临床效果等多方面对气功练习的机理进行了多方面、多角度的研究，具有较强实用和研究价值。

（郭建红）

【八段锦的临床研究】

付萍萍等认为中度以上的高血压患者，可以在药物治疗的基础上，辅以太极拳或八段锦锻炼，不仅能提高药物疗效，降低用药剂量，减少药物副作用，还能提高患者生活质量，改善原发性高血压危险因素，从而减少其并发症的发生。总结其可能的降压机制为可以改善精神状态，降低患者血脂和血糖水平，抑制C反应蛋白、肿瘤坏死因子α、白介素6等体液调节因子的分泌、并能使血浆NO、ET处于一种平衡状态，改善血液流变性从而降低外周阻力等。张聪等采用队列研究方法，根据是否习练八段锦将受试人群分为八段锦(62人)和对照(67人)2个队列，进行为期6周的观察。结果，比较第6周末与基线的中医症状分值，八段锦队列人员的神疲、健忘等19个症状的分值显著下降($P<0.05$)，占全部观察症状的86.4%；对照队列人员仅有气短懒言、腰膝酸软等4个症状的分值显著下降($P<0.05$)。第6周末，2个队列在神疲、心烦等14个症状分值差值比较上存在显著性差异($P<0.05$)，占全部观察症状的63.6%。

逢辉等将腰椎间盘突出症患者64例随机均分为治疗组和对照组，分别进行八段锦训练和常规运动训练，训练1次/d，治疗8周。结果，两组患者治疗后腰部视觉模拟(VAS)评分和日本骨科协会(JOA)评分较治疗前明显改善($P<0.05$)，并且治疗组JOA和分项日常生活活动(ADL)评分的改善幅度明显优于对照组($P<0.05$)。万婕等将60例颈肩部肌筋膜疼痛综合征患者随机均分为治疗组和对照组，均予手法治疗，治疗组同时习练习八段锦功法，疗程均为35 d，观察临床疗效及疼痛评分(VAS)情感评分(SF－MPQ)变化情况。结果两组总有效率分别为96.7%(29/30)、73.3%(22/30)，组间比较，$P<0.05$。治疗前后两组VAS、SF－MPQ情感评分均明显减少($P<0.05$)，且治疗组优于对照组($P<0.05$)。张铭等将224例中风病患者随机分为两组，均接受基础药物治疗和康复治疗，治疗组111例增加八段锦疗法早、晚各1次/d，每次

20 min，连续6周。结果两组患者治疗后的Berg平衡量表评分均较治疗前有显著差异（$P<0.05$），且治疗组疗效较对照组更加显著（$P<0.05$）。陈群等将60例高血压患者随机均分为八段锦锻炼组和散步锻炼组，在进行常规药物治疗的基础上，八段锦锻炼组进行八段锦锻炼，2次/d，20 min/次，连续3个月。结果两组锻炼后肱动脉内皮功能检测值均较锻炼前提高（$P<0.05$），且八段锦锻炼组检测值较散步锻炼组高，但组间比较，无显著性差异（$P>0.05$）。与健康志愿者相比，差异均有统计学意义（$P<0.05$），表明2组的检测值均未达到健康志愿者水平。李智滨等将216例2型糖尿病患者分为八段锦运动治疗组、一般有氧运动治疗组、太极拳运动治疗组、对照治疗组，试验分为强化治疗时期和自律治疗时期，分析八段锦在2型糖尿病患者运动治疗中的优势。结果，强化治疗阶段，3个运动治疗组均可以改善症状、优化指标，但在运动次数和运动时间上没有差异（$P>0.05$）。自律治疗阶段，八段锦运动治疗组、一般有氧运动治疗组、对照治疗组各项指标保持了强化治疗时的水平，太极拳治疗组一部分指标则有所反复。在保持运动方面，八段锦运动治疗组完成最为出色。

（赵　丹）

【太极拳对人体生理功能影响及机制研究】

温爱玲等探讨24式陈氏太极拳运动对老年人心率变异性（HRV）的影响。结果显示，受试者心率在运动中升高（$P<0.05$），运动后即刻达到最高（约112 bpm），运动后1 min内迅速恢复，运动后10 min基本恢复到运动前水平。全部窦性心搏R－R间期的标准差在运动过程中明显升高（$P<0.05$），运动后即刻、运动后1 min、运动后3 min、运动后10 min均较运动中均有下降（$P<0.05$，$P<0.01$）。受试者相邻R－R间期之差的均方根值随时间变化不明显。低频功率（LF）与高频功率（HF）均在运动中降低，运动后逐渐升高，变化不明显。LF/HF在运动中和运动后即刻相对安静状态有所升高（$P<0.01$），运动后1 min恢复到运动前水平（$P<0.01$），之后基本不变。杜舒婷等将112例慢性阻塞性肺疾病（COPD）稳定期患者随机分为3组，太极拳组（36例）进行24式杨式太极拳锻炼，锻炼组（38例）进行缩唇腹式呼吸和健步走锻炼，对照组（38例）进行平日常规活动，不另加锻炼项目。均接受12周训练，1次/d，1 h/次。太极拳与缩唇呼吸、步行锻炼均能改善COPD稳定期患者BODE指数及SGRQ评分，减轻患者症状，提高生存质量，两种方案相比，太极拳运动对各项指标的改善效果更明显。杨德洪等探讨太极拳运动后白细胞Th_1/Th_2型细胞因子mRNA的表达情况。研究发现，受试者外周血白细胞γ干扰素（INF－γ）mRNA的表达量逐渐降低，3、6月时表达量均与干预前相比存在差异（$P<0.05$）；白细胞介素4（IL－4）mRNA表达量3月时的表达量与干预前相比存在差异（$P<0.05$）；INF－γmRNA/IL－4mRNA逐渐降低，干预6月时和干预前、干预3月存在差异（$P<0.05$）。提示太极拳运动使健康中老年妇女Th_1/Th_2平衡向Th_2极化。

张河水等研究发现，不同架势太极拳练习对老年男性心血管功能、肺功能及运动能力改善具有明显差异性，架势依赖性非常显著。长期低架太极拳练习对老年男性的心肌收缩力量和速度、心脏泵血效率以及血管弹性；肺通气能力和贮备能力；有氧和无氧运动能力提高以及最大运动能力的维持等具有更为有效的改善作用。李春日等对18名体育学院的在校大学生（4年以上太极拳练习经历），采用表面肌电技术检测站立位和无极桩的双侧腹直肌和竖脊肌表面肌电变化，对每组肌肉与所有肌肉积分肌电比值进行对比分析。结果发现，站桩时腹直肌负荷明显大于站立位（$P<0.01$），竖脊肌负荷明显小于站立位（$P<0.01$）。提示，无极站桩初始阶段脊柱负荷向腹侧移动。杨慧馨等将93例中老年女性分为太极拳组（33例）、快走组（30例）和无锻炼组（30例），比较太极拳锻炼与快走锻炼中老年女性静态平衡机能。结果显示，太极拳锻炼组静态平衡能力优于快走锻炼组和无锻炼组，快走锻炼组静态平衡能力显著优于无锻炼组，差异均有统计学意义（$P<0.05$，$P<0.01$）。

（陆　颖）

[附] 参考文献

C

陈群，沈婕，谢晓燕，等. 八段锦对高血压病血管内皮功能影响的超声研究[J]. 广州中医药大学学报，2013，30(3)：299

D

杜舒婷，邢彬，王春霞，等. 太极拳运动对慢性阻塞性肺疾病患者 BODE 指数和 SGRQ 评分的影响[J]. 中国运动医学杂志，2013，32(5)：403

F

逢辉，宋斌，赵鹏，等. 八段锦促进腰椎间盘突出康复的临床研究[J]. 中医学报，2013，28(8)：1241

付萍萍，张洪斌. 八段锦、太极拳治疗原发性高血压及其降压机制的研究进展[J]. 河北中医，2013，35(10)：1585

G

桂翔. 龟息法对血氧饱和度和心肺功能影响的研究[D]. 扬州大学硕士论文集，2013 年

郭建红，陈昌乐，刘冬全，等. 具象思维心身合一属性的肌电表征[J]. 北京中医药大学学报，2013，36(10)：684

H

洪邦辉，姚鑫，陈波，等. 健身气功易筋经对女大学生原发性痛经的影响和作用机制分析[J]. 现代预防医学，2013，40(11)：2040

J

焦润艺，钟国林，潘华山，等. 健身气功八段锦对老年人红细胞功能的影响[J]. 福建体育科技，2013，32(4)：25

L

李春日，任大鹏，白增华等. 太极拳无极站桩初始阶段积分肌电图变化[J]. 实用中医内科杂志，2013，27(4)：13

李智滨，齐丽丽，赵磊，等. 八段锦在 2 型糖尿病患者有氧运动治疗中的优势[J]. 辽宁中医杂志，2013，40(9)：1858

林宇峰，韦军. 健身气功"八段锦"对 T2DM 干预效果研究[J]. 龙岩学院学报，2013，31(2)：59

R

汝雷，张斌. 健身气功五禽戏对老年人血脂及生理机能影响的研究[J]. 甘肃联合大学学报(自然科学版)，2013，27(2)：75

W

万婕，梁贞文，孙克兴，等. 八段锦功法锻炼结合手法治疗颈肩部肌筋膜疼痛综合征临床研究[J]. 上海中医药杂志，2013，47(8)：54

王强. 试析中医思维模式的本质特点和多元复杂性[J]. 中华中医药杂志，2013，28(2)：301

魏玉龙. 调心与治神浅释[J]. 中医学报，2013，28(12)：1818

魏玉龙，夏宇欣，吴晓云，等. 具象思维与具身心智：东西方认知科学的相遇[J]. 北京中医药大学学报，2013，36(11)：732

温爱玲，熊开宇，张猛，等. 24 式陈氏太极拳运动对老年人 HRV 的影响[J]. 吉林体育学院学报，2013，29(1)：69

X

夏宇欣，刘天君. 移空技术之于应激反应调节的访谈研究[A]. 北京师范大学心理学院华人心理学家学术研讨会论文摘要集[C]. 北京师范大学心理学院，2013：1

夏宇欣，吴晓云，刘天君. 移空技术小组活动对慢性应激反应的干预效果[J]. 中国临床心理学杂志，2013，21(3)：450

夏宇欣，吴晓云，刘天君. 移空技术的特点分析及其未来研究展望[J]. 中国临床心理学杂志，2013，21(5)：852

Y

杨德洪，魏勇. 太极拳运动后白细胞 Th1/Th2 型细胞因子 mRNA 的表达[J]. 山东体育学院学报，2013，29(2)：55

杨慧馨，虞定海. 太极拳锻炼与快走锻炼中老年女性静态平衡机能比较[J]. 中国运动医学杂志，2013，32(5)：437

Z

张聪，廖艳，张煜，等. 习练八段锦对疲劳性亚健康人群中医症状改善作用的队列研究[J]. 北京中医药大学学报(中医临床版)，2013，20(6)：6

张河水，段丽梅. 不同架势太极拳练习对老年男性心肺功能和运动能力影响的差异性[J]. 武汉体育学院学报，2013，47(10)：49

张铭，郭健，白艳杰，等. 八段锦联合康复锻炼对中风病患者平衡功能影响的研究[J]. 时珍国医国药，2013，24(10)：2438

（十三）护　理

【概述】

2013年关于护理的研究内容主要集中在理论研究、辨证施护、中医护理技术、情志护理、循证护理、优质护理、中西医结合护理等方面。针对专科专病特点、突出人性化、个性化的护理特色，注重中医护理实践的指导。

1. 基础理论研究

以史为鉴，探讨经典著作中蕴含的护理思想，这一方面的研究文献不多，但却可以从中看出中医护理学的源远流长。如史连和探讨《伤寒论》药后护理法，包括药后饮用热粥法，扶助正气，增加药力；药后勿饮热粥法，分清体质，防止伤正；药后多饮热水法，补充津液，利于祛邪；药后覆盖衣被法，保暖御寒，助药发汗；药后禁食忌口法，治疗护理，相辅相成；药后纠偏救弊法，病情有变，及时处置。张彩娟等探讨《备急千金要方》与《千金翼方》中老年护理细则，提出应首重饮食，生活有节制，外避风寒，内调情志，导引行气、运动保健。还探讨了刘完素《素问病机气宜保命集》的护理思想，认为其提出的"少年宜养，节饮食，适寒暑，防微杜渐；壮年宜治，辨八邪，分劳佚，当减其毒；老年宜保，养精神，调脏腑，内恤外护；耄年宜延，餐精华，处奥庭，以全其真"人生四个阶段的护理思想堪称中医护理学原则。祁海丽等认为《黄帝内经》中体现了情志护理、饮食护理、注重劳逸结合的护理思想，以及顺应阴阳法则，映射个体化护理思想。朱正刚归纳《黄帝内经》中涉及饮食护理的内容，认为保胃气、存津液是其理论基础，适其性是其重要原则，需要饮食调护来补充药物治疗的不足之处以及"四五"养生模式对指导患者健康科学饮食有重要的现实指导意义。

另一方面，将中医的理论思想运用于护理实践中。马梦晖等将中医体质学说应用于痛风性关节炎患者的护理中，认为中医体质学说以中医基础理论为主导，能够通过对不同体质的生理、病理研究，总结出各种体质的发病规律，减轻其疼痛等症状，促进其关节功能的恢复。李萍探讨了中医平衡理论结合高压氧治疗重型颅脑损伤患者的临床疗效和护理措施。在中医平衡理论的指导下实施辨证护理，能够明显降低重型颅脑损伤患者致残率以及并发症，改善生存质量，对于符合治疗指征的患者应尽早采用。

2. 特色技能

陈世萍探讨了中医护理技术的重要地位，认为按摩术、拔罐术、贴药术、熏洗术、耳穴压豆、中药离子导入术、中药保留灌肠术、太极拳等具有操作器具简单、操作方便、适用范围广、疗效快、经济适用、百姓易接受的特点，体现了"安全、高效、低耗、创新、发展"的原则，扩大了中医护理的工作范畴，使中医护理学有更广阔的发展空间。冯进等对81名新进护理人员采取多途径、多形式的中医护理知识与技能培训。使其中医理论、操作考试成绩、工作能力以及住院患者满意度均高于培训前（$P<0.01$，$P<0.05$）。元国芬等将120例胃食管反流病患者随机均分为两组，对照组予常规护理，观察组予情志调摄、饮食调护、耳穴埋豆、养生起居干预。结果观察组总体疗效明显优于对照组，且远期复发率低。朱正刚等调查了200名长沙市社区居民对中医护理适宜技术操作认知情况。发现社区居民对中医护理的需求及了解程度较高，对中医护理技能功效认可度也较高，但了解途径单一，主要以电视媒体为主，且对中医护理操作疗效认知偏颇。

3. 优质护理

覃美玉将60例恶性肿瘤患者随机均分为两组，均予围手术期常规护理，观察组在此基础上采用优质护理服务模式（包括转变工作模式、优化人力资源配置、无缝隙专科护理等）。结果观察组术前30 min的焦虑、抑郁评分、心率、血压、去甲肾上腺素、肾上腺素浓度均显著低于对照组（$P<0.05$），并在躯体功能、心理功能、社会功能、物质生活状态方面的生活质量评分显著高于对照组（$P<0.05$）。薛晓英等对48例前循环动脉瘤患者采取优质护理服务，包括病情观察、基础及生活护理、风险评估、康复指导、健康宣教、心理护理、

专科护理等,对照组 48 例给予常规护理。结果,实验组的护理工作满意度、健康教育知晓率、健康教育覆盖率、责任护士对患者病情掌握程度均优于对照组($P<0.05$)。何英等将 120 例接受手术治疗的老年髋部骨折患者均分为两组,对照组采用常规护理,观察组依据专科特色采用优质护理。结果观察组护理满意度为 96.7%(58/60),对照组为 83.3%(25/30),组间比较,$P<0.05$。观察组术后压疮、肺部感染、泌尿系感染、深静脉血栓发生率及住院时间显著低于对照组(均 $P<0.05$)。安淑银等对 108 例脑卒中后抑郁患者实施优质护理服务(包括制定优质护理计划、丰富患者住院生活、提高患者幸福指数、建立"护士—患者—家属—社会"支持系统等),患者抑郁指数、护理工作满意度、疾病知识认知水平等均有显著改善(均 $P<0.05$)。

4. 情志护理

赵翠萍等介绍了情志疏导法、情志相胜法、陶冶情志法、顺应四时法、气功调神法等在护理中的应用。王艳艳等介绍了中医情志护理在围手术期患者中的应用。术前护理做到因人而异、有的放矢,术中护理做到热情诚恳、照顾周到,术后护理做到消除顾虑、关心体贴。徐艳玲将 126 例膝骨性关节炎伴抑郁患者随机均分为两组。均予服益肾疏肝通络汤(柴胡、甘草、枳壳、芍药、陈皮、川芎等),治疗组在此基础上施以重建认知、社会及家庭支持治疗、娱乐治疗、松弛训练、饮食及生活指导等心理护理。治疗 6 周后,两组总有效率分别为 87.3%(55/63)、73.0%(46/63),组间比较,$P<0.05$。治疗组的抑郁及疼痛评分显著低于对照组($P<0.05$)。顾家琪等将 90 例腹腔镜手术患者随机均分为两组,均予常规护理,观察组在此基础上实施心理护理。结果治疗组在手术治疗中的焦虑程度、术前血压、心率变化及护理满意度等方面均优于对照组($P<0.05$)。

5. 辨证施护

刘子香将 120 例肿瘤患者随机均分为两组,均予过化疗配合常规护理,试验组在此基础上根据患者的胃肠道反应辨证分为胃热呕吐、瘀毒反胃、胃郁结滞、畏寒呕吐、邪毒蕴积等 6 个证型进行护理。结果治疗组效果优于对照组($P<0.05$)。汤仙等将腰痛病患者均分为两组,试验组辨证分为气滞血瘀、寒湿痹阻、湿热痹阻、肝肾亏虚型,给予饮食、用药、情志等护理,对照组予常规护理。干预 15 d 后,试验组总有效率为 90.0%(27/30),不良反应率为 6.7%(2/30),复发率为 16.7%(5/30),对照组分别为 73.0%(22/30)、20.0%(6/30)、33.3%(10/30),组间比较,均 $P<0.05$。高明焕将乳腺癌根治术后患者辨证分为肝郁气滞、冲任失调、肝郁化火、肝肾阴虚、气血两亏 5 个证型,予以不同的情志、饮食、功能锻炼等,疗效显著。

6. 中西医结合护理

曹磊将 106 例急性心肌梗塞恢复期的患者随机均分为两组,对照组予西医护理,实验组予特色的七情、辨证、药膳等中西医结合的护理。干预 14～50 d,试验组与对照组有效率分别为 92.5%(49/53)、73.6%(39/53),组间比较,$P<0.05$。刘漩将 102 例原发性高血压患者随机均分为两组,均予西医常规护理,观察组在此基础上,从生活起居、饮食、情志、用药及辨证等方面进行护理。两组总有效率分别为 85.2%(52/61)、68.3%(28/41),组间比较,$P<0.05$。李丽娟对 42 例雷诺现象患者除常规西医护理外,给予饮食、情志、环境与皮肤、温热疗以及中药护理等。结果 19 例患者的雷诺现象基本消失,23 例患者明显好转,无一例发生皮肤破损及溃疡。患者肢体活动均有改善,生活质量明显提高。李建华等对 183 高血压脑出血围手术期患者采用中西医结合护理,包括术前做好情绪护理,术后做好病情观察、引流管护理、基础护理、并发症护理、中医康复指导等,效果显著。

(张雅丽　董春玲)

【中风的护理】

梁崇南等将 80 例缺血性中风患者随机均分为两组,均予中风的西医二级预防措施,对照组给予常规护理,治疗组在此基础上给予中医时辰护理干预(即加强子、丑、寅、卯时病情观察;重视卯、申时功能锻炼;根据时辰理论与中药性味功效规律择时服药;着重辰、未时饮食指导;强化戌时情志护理;利用申时进行健康宣教)。4 周后发现,两组患者神经功能缺损评分和 SF-36 量表的总体健康积分、生理功能评分均有显著改善(均 $P<0.05$),且治疗组的改善情况优于对照组(均 $P<0.05$)。谭俊英将 284 例中风患者随机分为两组,

均予一般西医常规护理，观察组加用辨证施护和中药泡洗、按摩拔罐等，比较两组患者的平均住院天数、生活满意率和医护满意率。结果，观察组患者平均住院天数明显低于对照组，好转率和医护满意率均明显高于对照组（均$P<0.05$）。钱艳对缺血性中风患者予心理、日常生活、饮食、语言功能训练、健康教育等护理干预外，对肢体的护理强调给予药浴、熏洗（红花、川草乌、当归、川芎、桑枝等），明显减轻了中风后的肩关节疼痛、手部发胀等直接影响运动功能恢复的症状。

梁秀莉对中风患者辨证分为中经络和中脏腑两类施护，中经络又分为风痰入络、风阳上扰、阴虚风动证，中脏腑又分为闭证和脱证。风痰入络证，饮食宜益气、健脾、通络，如山药苡仁粥、黄芪粥、冬瓜、木耳、赤小豆等，忌食辛辣厚味及发物。中药宜饭后温服，可针刺内关、水沟、丰隆、合谷等穴。风阳上扰证，饮食宜清淡甘寒，如绿豆、芹菜、菠菜、梨等，忌食羊肉、鸡肉、狗肉、大蒜、葱等辛香走窜之品，忌甜食。中药宜温凉服。可针刺内关、三阴交、委中、太冲、太溪等穴。阴虚风动型，饮食应清淡富于营养，宜食大豆、藕、香菇、桃、梨等，忌食鸡肉、狗肉等动风之品。中药宜饭后温凉服。可针刺水沟、尺泽、极泉、太溪、风池等穴。闭证，饮食以清热、化痰、润燥为主，如萝卜、绿豆、丝瓜、冬瓜等，忌羊肉、鸡肉、牛肉、辣椒等辛辣刺激、生冷之品。中药宜浓煎，阳闭宜凉服，阴闭宜热服。可针刺水沟、内关、太冲、合谷等穴。脱证，饮食宜升阳固脱为主，宜食参附粥。中药宜浓煎，温度适宜。可灸神阙、气海、关元等穴，用补法针刺肾俞以回阳固脱。

（张雅丽　董春玲）

【骨折的护理】

曾玲等将106例胫骨平台骨折患者随机均分为两组，对照组予常规护理，试验组予中西医结合护理（包括饮食护理、康复训练、加强情志护理、协助家属完成日常生活护理、患者间现身说教等）。干预4周，试验组优质护理合格率为98.3%（58/59），护理服务满意度为96.6%（57/59），对照组分别为89.4%（42/47）、85.1%（40/47），组间比较，均$P<0.05$。王彦斐等将80例骨折手术后患者随机均分为两组，均予常规护理，观察组在此基础上予以情志、饮食、康复（推拿、按摩、针灸镇痛、熏蒸等）护理等。干预14 d，观察组治疗依从性为95.0%（38/40），满意度为97.5%（39/40），住院并发症发生率为2.5%（1/40），对照组分别为75.0%（30/40）、85.0%（34/40）、12.5%（5/40），组间比较，均$P<0.05$。韦武燕从生活起居、情志、饮食、用药护理及功能锻炼5个方面对256例骨折患儿进行辨证施护。注重顾护脾胃功能，提出“忌口”、“慎口”、“不可令饥”等观点，强调饮食有节、定时定量，合理膳食、不可偏嗜，注意卫生、注重禁忌。结果256例患儿均治愈出院。吴肖红探讨骨盆骨折患者的围手术期护理方法。术前进行心理护理、基础护理帮助患者做好手术准备；术后观察切口情况，进行膳食指导、疼痛护理、胃肠胀气护理（顺时针腹部按摩、便秘患者使用缓泻剂等）、预防并发症、康复功能锻炼等。出院后随访2～24个月，所有患者均未出现肺部感染、压疮和尿路感染等并发症。袁华丽将老年骨质疏松性胸腰椎骨折患者分期辨证施护，初期以促进活血、通腑排气为目的。多鼓励指导病人主动翻身，宜饮清淡可口，易消化，含纤维丰富的食物。中期除继续做翻身防压疮和皮肤护理外，重点功能锻炼，增加胸部活动和肺功能锻炼。减少并发症和骨折后慢性腰背痛及骨质疏松的发生。后期嘱患者离床练习站立及行走，加强床上功能锻炼，下床后做胸腰肌功能康复操。以食补为原则，多吃高营养及含钙、锰、镁等微量元素的食物以促进骨折愈合。

（张雅丽　董春玲）

【消化性溃疡的护理】

李园园将120例脾虚湿热型溃疡性结肠炎（UC）患者随机均分为两组，予中药保留灌肠，观察组配合情志护理。治疗30 d后，两组总有效率分别为95.0%（57/60）、78.3%（47/60），组间比较，$P<0.05$。两组患者肠镜积分较治疗前均有明显改善，但组间比较，$P>0.05$。谢杏文等对慢性UC患者予食荷花粥（鲜荷花200 g，薏苡仁100 g，绿豆50 g，糯米100 g）。辨证为湿热内蕴型患者饮食以素流质或素半流质为宜，忌食辛辣、肥甘荤腥，生冷瓜果及硬固难化之食物。气滞血瘀型患者若有腹胀腹痛者，可行针灸、热敷，并指导患者做自我按摩。脾气虚弱型，不食过冷过热、辛辣、油腻、油煎食物，宜食营养丰富、易消化饮食；饮食适量，不宜过饥过饱。刘俊敏等在中药保留灌肠治疗慢性非特异性溃疡性结肠炎的基础上应用中医护理（包括情志护理、保留灌肠护理、饮食护理、生活起居护理、腹泻护理、药物护理、预防感染、出院健康指导),并与常规护理对照观察。结果观察组的总有效率为94.3%(50/53),对照组为84.2%(48/57),组间比较,$P<0.05$。冷冰对48例UC患者采用药物保留灌肠的同时进行心理护理、饮食护理、中药保留灌肠护理等,总有效率为93.8%(45/48)。弭艳旭等将80例UC患者随机均分为两组,均予一般护理、饮食护理、音乐治疗、心理护理,观察组在此基础上加中药(苍术、茯苓、黄芪、白头、三七粉、白及等)灌肠护理(如出现不耐受,应立即停止灌肠),行腹部按摩、热敷,至腹痛消失。经治4周,观察组与对照组的症状改善总有效率分别为87.5%(35/40)、67.5%(24/40),组间比较,$P<0.05$。张慧等将124例UC患者随机分为两组,均予中药(白术、茯苓、芍药、黄芪、当归、黄连等)内服加中药(五倍子、蒲黄、白头翁、地榆、黄连、夏枯草等)灌肠,观察组66例加以相应的护理干预。经治1个月,观察组总有效率为95.5%(63/66)、复发率为7.14%(2/28),对照组分别为74.1%(43/58)、40.0%(6/15)。

尚云青等将76例胃溃疡患者随机均分为两组,予辨证分型施治,实验组配合食疗辅助。治疗6周后,治疗组总有效率为94.7%(36/38)、治愈率为60.5%(23/38),对照组分别为84.2%(32/38)、36.8%(14/38),组间比较,均$P<0.05$。颜红等将60例重症食道溃疡患者随机均分为两组,对照组予常规护理,观察组予中西医结合护理(包括情志护理、饮食规律、排便护理、提高抵抗力、生活起居规律、坚持腹部顺时针按摩等)。经治3周,观察组与对照组的改善症状总有效率分别为100.0%、86.7%(26/30),组间比较,$P<0.05$。

(张雅丽　董春玲)

[附]　参 考 文 献

A

安淑银,张军,陈晓丽,等.优质护理服务在贫困地区脑卒中后抑郁患者中的应用及效果观察[J].现代中西医结合杂志,2013,22(19):2156

C

曹磊.急性心肌梗塞恢复期的中西医结合护理体会[J].时珍国医国药,2013,24(4):961

陈世萍.中医特色护理在中医院的作用与意义[J].贵阳中医学院学报,2013,35(4):204

F

冯进,张月娟,廖若夷.对新进护理人员进行中医护理知识与技能规范化培训的探讨[J].中医药导报,2013,19(7):114

G

高明焕.乳腺癌根治术后的辨证施护[J].河北中医,2013,35(7):1082

顾家琪,冯钟煦,周秀莲,等.心理护理在腹腔镜手术患者中的应用[J].贵阳中医学院学报,2013,35(3):229

H

何英,刘晓艳,李玲利.优质护理在老年髋部骨折围术期的应用效果观察[J].现代中西医结合杂志,2013,22(14):1580

L

冷冰.中药保留灌肠治疗溃疡性结肠炎护理体会[J].中国民族民间医药,2013,22(9):145

李建华,杨小英,周小香,等.高血压脑出血患者围手术期的中西医结合护理[J].河北中医,2013,35(4):606

李丽娟.雷诺现象的中西医结合护理[J].现代中西医结合杂志,2013,22(4):442

李萍.中医平衡理论结合高压氧对重型颅脑损伤患者的治疗和护理[J].中医药导报,2013,19(8):96

李园园.保留灌肠配合心理护理治疗溃疡性结肠炎(络瘀证)60例[J].中国中医药现代远程教育,2013,11(2):17

梁崇南,潘林平.传统时辰观在缺血性中风患者护理中的运用效果研究[J].广州中医药大学学报,2013,30(5):640

梁秀莉.中风辨证施护[J].辽宁中医杂志,2013,40(5):1005

刘俊敏,贾艳秋.中药保留灌肠治疗慢性非特异性溃疡性结肠炎的临床观察及护理体会[J].河北中医,2013,35(8):1240

刘漩.原发性高血压的中西医结合护理体会[J].河北中医,2013,35(2):288

刘子香.肿瘤化疗患者呕吐的辨证护理体会[J].中医药导报,2013,19(5):115

M

马梦晖，史临平，马坚，等. 中医体质学说在痛风性关节炎护理中的应用[J]. 中医正骨，2013，25(7)：79

弭艳旭，周凤娟. 中药保留灌肠治疗慢性非特异性溃疡性结肠炎的疗效观察及护理体会[J]. 河北中医，2013，35(9)：1400

Q

祁海丽，孙安兵. 从《黄帝内经》管窥现代中医护理理念[J]. 光明中医，2013，28(8)：1547

钱艳. 中医护理干预对缺血性中风患者 Barthel 指数的影响[J]. 中国中医药现代远程教育，2013，11(17)：141

S

尚云青，吴灿东，曹军，等. 中医食疗辅助中医药治疗胃溃疡疗效观察[J]. 新中医，2013，45(2)：15

史连和.《伤寒论》药后护理法临床意义初探[J]. 新中医，2013，45(8)：214

T

覃美玉. 优质护理服务模式在肿瘤内科的应用研究[J]. 现代中西医结合杂志，2013，22(24)：2728

谭俊英. 中风病人施行中西医结合健康教育护理方法[J]. 辽宁中医药大学学报，2013，15(7)：251

汤仙，冯进，张月娟，等. 辨证施护在腰痛病临床运用中的体会[J]. 湖南中医药大学学报，2013，33(3)：95

W

王彦斐，王彩文，白会玲. 中医护理在骨折术后临床护理中的应用[J]. 西部中医药，2013，26(6)：115

王艳艳，李玉香. 中医情志护理在围手术期患者中的应用[J]. 河北中医，2013，35(8)：1250..

韦武燕. 浅谈小儿骨折的中医护理[J]. 光明中医，2013，28(5)：1037

吴肖红. 骨盆骨折患者的围手术期护理[J]. 中医正骨，2013，25(6)：79

X

谢杏文，陈梦玲. 中西医结合治疗护理慢性溃疡性结肠炎[J]. 湖北中医杂志，2013，35(8)：55

徐艳玲. 心理护理对膝骨性关节炎伴抑郁患者整体疗效影响的研究[J]. 时珍国医国药，2013，24(4)：955

薛晓英，黄行芝，张慧. 优质护理服务用于前循环动脉瘤患者的护理效果[J]. 现代中西医结合杂志，2013，22(5)：541

Y

颜红. 中西医结合护理重症食道溃疡随机平行对照研究[J]. 实用中医内科杂志，2013，27(3)：147

元国芬，邱菊萍，江君. 中医护理干预在中虚气逆证胃食管反流病中应用的临床研究[J]. 江苏中医药，2013，45(2)：68

袁华丽. 老年骨质疏松性胸腰椎骨折的中医分期辨证施护[J]. 中国中医骨伤科杂志，2013，21(2)：61

Z

曾玲，陈晓虹，蔡海颜. 中西医结合护理模式指导下的护理干预措施对锁定钢板治疗胫骨平台骨折患者的影响[J]. 时珍国医国药，2013，24(2)：511

张彩娟，余莉萍，甘盼盼，等. 从《备急千金要方》与《千金翼方》探讨中医学老年护理细则[J]. 新中医，2013，45(4)：220

张彩娟，余莉萍，甘盼盼，等. 刘完素养、治、保、延的护理思想探讨[J]. 新中医，2013，45(2)：6

张慧，陈欢笑. 中药内服加灌肠对溃疡性结肠炎的护理研究[J]. 辽宁中医杂志，2013，40(9)：1913

赵翠萍，王京菊. 中医情志护理初探[J]. 中医药导报，2013，19(3)：121

朱正刚，陈燕，蒋新军，等. 长沙市社区居民对中医护理操作认知现状调查[J]. 中医药导报，2013，19(2)：121

朱正刚，陈燕，潘晓彦，等.《黄帝内经》中的饮食护理特点浅析[J]. 中医药导报，2013，19(1)：116

三、中　　药

(一) 中药资源

【概述】

2013年,中药资源高新技术及基础理论的微观研究不断增多,分子生物学已成为中药资源研究的重点。在分子生物学领域中,除物种遗传多样性及基源鉴定等研究外,功能基因的克隆和生物信息学等已成为资源研究的主要内容。

1. 中药材的宏观认识

梁飞等报道,道地药材以强调产地为其特点,其理念在秦汉之际已有,约在明清两代最终确立,并兴盛发展。同时指出中医的实践检验与理论指导是道地药材形成的理论基础,生态环境与药材种质的差异则是其本质原因。许多道地药材的产地,自古以来都没有发生过改变,但也有为数众多的道地药材历经沧桑发生了巨变。药材产地变迁的原因主要与自然环境的改变和人类社会的发展有关。

2. 分子生物学的应用

(1) 分子生物学技术分析生物遗传多样性　侯茜等用随机扩增多态性DNA标记(RAPD)技术对甘肃、陕西、宁夏、四川及青海5个主产地秦艽的11个种群、90个个体基因组DNA的遗传多样性进行分析,将秦艽的11个种群聚为两类:四川和陕西省4个种群聚为一类,甘肃、宁夏和青海省7个种群聚为一类。结果表明,甘肃省环县种群、子午岭种群和华亭种群应作为秦艽的重要种群而优先重点保护。艾强等运用序列相关扩增多态性(SRAP)分子标记方法将川黔境内14个居群川续断的遗传多样性聚为3类,表明川续断居群的遗传多样性水平丰富,遗传变异主要存在居群内,地理位置(海拔)、气候及地理隔离是川续断居群间遗传多样性较高的因素。吴志刚等对8个山药栽培居群中的21个山药品种进行SRAP分析。结果表明,山药品种呈现较高遗传多样性,薯蓣、参薯、褐苞薯蓣、山薯4种基源山药种间遗传差异较大。郝东等采用简单序列重复间(ISSR)标记技术从100条引物中筛选出14条多态性明显、反应稳定的引物,在23份牻牛儿苗供试材料DNA中共扩增出185条谱带,其中多态性条带142条,占76.8%。聚类分析可将所有供试材料区分,并聚为6组,其结果与牻牛儿苗的地理位置、形态性状存在显著的相关性。朱田田等应用ISSR分子标记技术对甘肃10个不同产地的中麻黄样品进行遗传多样性和亲缘关系分析。聚类结果表明,来自不同地区的野生种和栽培种各自聚成一类,地理距离较近的野生种聚为一类。张祎楠等采用ISSR分子技术标记四川主产地川牛膝遗传多样性,结果居群间遗传多样性较小,遗传变异主要由异花授粉造成。阳翠等采用ISSR分子标记技术,对产自宁夏、甘肃、青海、新疆和内蒙古的22个苦豆子居群遗传多样性进行非加权平均距离法聚类和主成分分析(PCA),结果居群间具有较高的遗传多样性,但遗传距离与地理距离没有明显关系。张维瑞等利用目标起始密码子多态性分子标记(SCoT)对河南伏牛、太行、大别和桐柏4大山脉的8个益母草居群、共计66个样品进行遗传多样性分析,居群间的亲缘关系与它们之间的地理距离有着明显的相关性。徐旭栋等采用SCoT技术和非加权平均距离法对20份不同来源的人工栽培铁皮石斛样品进行遗传多样性分析。结果表明,铁皮石斛人工栽培种存在较大的遗传差异。

(2) 功能基因的克隆及生物信息学分析　尚洁等对宁夏枸杞类黄酮/异黄酮生物合成途径中的关键酶-查耳酮合成酶克隆和分析,该家族的cDNA片段长为1 148 bp,编码382个氨基酸,蛋白相对分子质量为4.168×10^{4},等电点为6.22。

程琪庆等获得的 SmHDR 全长基因由 1 647 个核苷酸组成，编码 463 个氨基酸，SmHDR 基因可能参与丹参酮类成分的生物合成。汪孟曦等对沉香原植物白木香的查尔酮合酶基因 AsCHS1 编码区进行克隆，AsCHS1 基因编码区开放阅读框长为 1 194 bp，编码 397 个氨基酸残基。郭溆等利用 RT－PCR 方法获得灵芝 GLCYP450 和 GLNADPH 基因的全长 cDNA 序列，并在序列两端引入相应的限制性内切酶位点，通过酶切及连接反应将 GLCYP450 和 GLNADPH 重组到酵母表达载体 pESC－URA 中，成功构建了酵母表达载体质粒。王亚君等根据丹参毛状根 cDNA 文库中筛选到 NAC EST 序列，克隆了丹参 SmNAC1 的 cDNA 全长序列，该基因的开放阅读框 591 bp，编码 166 个氨基酸，推测其参与了丹参毛状根对 YE＋Ag^{+} 的胁迫应答调节活动。常凯等克隆了大花红景天尿苷二磷酸葡萄糖基转移酶基因组 DNA。结果，该基因的 DNA 序列 2 977 bp，其中包含 1 499 bp 的编码区域（包括 82 bp的内含子序列）和 1 500 bp 的编码区 5′上游侧翼域序列（包括启动子区域）。该基因结构完整，具有典型的功能结合位点，为红景天分子生物学与代谢工程研究提供了参考。张岗等分离到两个铁皮石斛钙依赖蛋白激酶基因 DoCPK2 和 DoCPK3，全长为 2 119 bp 和 2 418 bp，各编码一条由 541 个和 536 个氨基酸组成的肽链，相对分子质量分别为 60.46×10^{3} 和 60.30×10^{3}，前者在根和原球茎中表达量较高，后者在茎和种子中的表达量较低，表明了其在植物生长发育和逆境胁迫等过程中的生物学功能。吴文燕等对克隆的丹参 SmERF1 在不同诱导子处理后不同时间的表达情况进行聚类分析。结果表明，该基因是一个 AP2/ERF 转录因子，属于 AP2/ERF 家族第Ⅶ亚族，其表达受脱落酸、水杨酸、茉莉酸甲酯等激素调节控制。余晓丹等根据 cDNA 文库提供的基因片段设计特异性引物，从红白忍冬中克隆获得 rLjSABATHMT 基因 cDNA 序列及基因组序列，基因 cDNA 序列全长为 1 251 bp，具有完整编码框，编码 365 个氨基酸。SABATHMT 同源基因主要在花中表达，为金银花活性成分调控机制研究提供了基础。鲁增辉等研究表明，冬虫夏草菌侵染贡嘎蝠蛾后枯草杆菌蛋白酶 Pr1 基因表达量显著上升，侵染后的 Pr1 基因表达量是侵染前的 2～3 倍，Pr1 基因在冬虫夏草菌侵染贡嘎蝠蛾的过程中可能起重要作用，为筛选高致病力的冬虫夏草菌奠定了基础。范丙友等从芍药中克隆了肌动蛋白 Actin 基因，半定量 RT－PCR 表达分析。结果表明，Actin 基因在芍药根、茎、叶、花组织中的表达量保持恒定，适合作为芍药功能基因表达分析的内标基因。赵明明等采用抑制差减杂交技术，分别以接菌及未接菌培养 5 周的铁皮石斛种子 cDNA 作为检测子与驱赶子，建立铁皮石斛种子接菌共生萌发抑制性消减 cDNA 文库。结果，得到 100 个具有植物同源性的表达序列标签。随机挑选 5 个目标基因，实时荧光定量 PCR 分析方法，发现这 5 个基因在共生萌发的种子中均上调表达，表明铁皮石斛种子接菌共生萌发涉及多种途径相关基因表达调控。

（3）分子生物学技术在中药鉴定中的应用 易骏等分析了不同种质来源孩儿参 ITS 序列。结果，整个 ITS 区共有 17 个变异位点，不同种质来源孩儿参均有若干个特异性的单核苷酸变异位点，各样品的序列同源性均在 99.9％以上。表明可利用 ITS 区序列差异，鉴别不同种质来源的孩儿参。夏至等对药用菊花和野菊及其近缘易混种 ITS 序列进行 PCR 扩增和测序，通过遗传距离分析，可鉴定出中药材菊花和野菊与其近缘种。曹亮等研究了白术、苍术鉴别 SNP 位点，并设计特异性引物。结果表明，构建的多重 PCR 鉴别体系，通过一个 PCR 反应，能扩增出苍术、白术约 643 bp 的 ITS DNA 质控条带，扩增出白术172 bp 的特异性鉴别条带，有效鉴别了白术、苍术种子。廖婧等收集了常见 23 种药用蛇类的 44 个样品，并进行 COI 条形码序列测定，对实验中各药用蛇类物种进行了准确的鉴定。陈仕江等研究了芫菁科 7 种斑蝥，分析其线粒体 COI 基因序列。结果，种间遗传距离较大，介于 0.10～0.23 之间；系统进化树显示不同属各自聚为一支，同属不同物种的个体也形成各自独立的分支。表明以 COI 基因作为 DNA 条形码进行芫菁科物种鉴定的可行性。刘晓帆等利用 COI 基因对收集的 8 种龟甲正品及其混伪品的 22 份样品进行鉴定。结果，龟甲的正品来源乌龟与其混伪品种间存在较多变异位点，同属聚在一起，且各物种又形成相对独立的支；采用同样方法也可以很好地鉴定水蛭、蚂蟥、柳叶蚂蟥及其混伪品。

3. 中药资源生理生态学研究

田方等应用四格表卡方检验法和相关分析法

研究药用植物地理分布及海拔与中药功效的相关性。结果表明,清热药在青藏高原、行气药在华中地区、解表药在蒙新荒漠地带比例较高,具有显著性差异;清热药等与海拔呈正相关、温里药等与海拔呈负相关。刘红昌等通过实地生境调查,田间定期观察和定株取样分析,表明何首乌在光照充足、雨量充沛、热量丰富、土壤肥沃的区域生长旺盛;随纬度降低,营养生长期延长,生殖生长期延迟。王海等对川芎内生真菌多样性进行研究。结果,川芎的内生真菌群落结构存在不同个体、不同产区间的差异,同产区不同个体内生真菌的相似程度较高,不同产区间的相似程度较低;道地产区都江堰市石羊镇川芎的内生真菌群落结构较其他4个产区丰富,同时与其他产区相似度均很低,并且存在其他产区未见的特有种。杨舒婷等采用指标成分(白术内酯Ⅰ)含量比较和HPTLC指纹图谱法结合相似度分析(夹角余弦值、Pearson相关系数)与PCA,表明白术药材质量主要受产地环境的影响,种内遗传变异对整体化学相似性没有明显作用,但对白术内酯Ⅰ的含量仍有显著影响。杨贤松研究表明银杏叶片光抑制情况下PSⅡ反应中心供体侧和受体侧功能都受到暂时抑制,PSⅡ反应中心发生可逆失活,光合机构并未受到不可逆损伤。

4. 中药资源再生技术研究

杨先国等对丹参太空育种进行了研究。结果,搭载后的太空组丹参具有叶片增大、茎秆较矮,表型差异明显;丹酚酸B与丹参酮Ⅱ$_A$的含量分别提高13%和50%;聚类分析太空组丹参的化学特征与对照丹参具有明显的差异。张海弢等研究不同外植体、菌株、外源激素、侵染时间、预培养时间和共培养时间对王不留行毛状根诱导率的影响。结果,用王不留行叶片作为外植体,外植体预培养60 h,共培养48 h,发根农杆菌R1601侵染10 min,培养基中添加0.1 mg/L吲哚丁酸转化率最高。李晓灿等在白桦悬浮细胞的生长末期添加0.1 mmol/L和1.0 mmol/L的腐胺、精胺和亚精胺,其中1.0 mmol/L腐胺在处理的第2天对细胞干质量和三萜产量的促进效应最大,分别比对照品增加了38.89%和116.35%,并通过羽扇豆醇合酶基因的RT-PCR检测发现多胺对白桦三萜积累具有促进作用。孙乐乐等对白及根腐病的病原物进行研究,经鉴定为尖孢镰刀菌 *Fusarium oxysporum* Schlecht.,并对生长温度、pH值等生物学特性进行研究,为制定有效的防治措施提供依据。

5. 资源调查

杨全等研究表明,广金钱草野生药用植物资源正逐步减少,部分地区很难找到野生资源;人工栽培广金钱草技术不完善、药材质量参差不齐,影响广金钱草进一步的开发和综合利用。赵能武等对药用蕨类植物资源蕴藏量进行了调查。结果表明,雷公山自然保护区共有药用蕨类植物35科75属190种,占贵州药用蕨类植物总数的44%。

6. 其他

何盼等采用基于^{1}H NMR的代谢组学技术对恒山黄芪和川黄芪进行化学分析,共分离出23种成分。其中,恒山黄芪中的天冬氨酸、γ-氨基丁酸、柠檬酸、黄芪甲苷和毛蕊异黄酮葡糖苷含量较高,而川黄芪中的苏氨酸、丙氨酸、乙酸、胆碱、精氨酸、果糖和蔗糖含量较高,几乎检测不到黄芪甲苷;二者的ITS2序列差异较大,共有8处碱基不同。利用化学成分差异和DNA分子遗传技术,都能区分恒山黄芪和川黄芪。

(王喜军)

【药用植物的遗传多样性研究】

1. 基于序列的分析

杨路存等采用叶绿体DNA非编码区直接测序的方法,对青海、甘肃、四川3个省区濒危植物宽叶羌活的遗传多样性和遗传结构进行了研究。14个居群138个个体的序列长度介于509~515 bp,碱基组成A+T含量较高(平均67.6%),根据序列的核苷酸变异共鉴定出31个单倍型。结果表明,大部分遗传变异发生在居群间,居群遗传变异的分布没有明显的地理趋势。提示宽叶羌活居群间高的遗传变异可能是由基因流受阻、遗传漂变、地理隔离造成。

倪梁红等采用居群采样方法,对西藏不同产地17份麻花艽样品的遗传多样性进行比较,以相同产地同属近缘种粗茎秦艽为外类群比对,ITS区序列分析,构建系统树。结果,西藏产麻花艽nrDNA ITS区序列有1个多态性位点,外类群粗茎秦艽6份样品序列完全一致,麻花艽与外类群种间区别明显，17 份不同产地麻花艽被划分为 2 类，为西藏麻花艽药材品质评价及麻花艽核心种质的构建提供了基础资料。

2. AFLP 分析

张薇等用筛选出来的 11 对引物对采自不同产地的 6 份灯盏花种质资源进行 AFLP 遗传多样性分析。结果，共产生 636 条 DNA 片段，其中 604 条为多态性条带，多态位点百分率(PPB)约占 82.40%，在相似系数为 0.706 时，6 份不同地区的灯盏花可聚为 3 类。聚类分析表明，地理来源相同的部分有相对聚合现象或少部分品系出现交差聚类，与其亲缘关系较近有关。

3. SSR 分析

李忠虎等利用磁珠富集法分离党参核基因组微卫星引物，并选取党参 4 个野生居群 48 个样品进行遗传多样性分析。结果，筛选出了 10 个能成功扩增样品的微卫星引物，这些引物扩增产物的等位基因数目为 5～14 个，使用 4 个党参近缘物种进行引物通用性检测，发现有 5 对引物能同时在 4 个物种中成功扩增。表明筛选出的多态性微卫星引物能用于党参的遗传多样性和群体遗传结构研究，同时也能够用于党参属其他近缘物种的群体遗传学研究。

徐敏等应用 SSR 分子标记对秦岭地区野生华中五味子进行遗传多样性分析。结果，9 对 SSR 引物共检测到 61 条带，每对引物扩增出 5～11 条，平均每对引物可扩增出 6.8 条，PPB 为 86.88%。结果显示，秦岭地区华中五味子遗传变异主要存在于居群内，居群间存在一定基因流，洋县居群遗传多样性最高。表明秦岭地区华中五味子遗传多样性丰富，应优先选择陕西汉中、宝鸡和商洛地区华中五味子居群实行就地保护与扩繁，以保证野生华中五味子可持续发展和利用。

4. ISSR 分析

阳翠等采用 ISSR 分子标记，对不同产地的 22 个苦豆子居群的 DNA 进行扩增，对其扩增条带进行遗传多样性分析。结果，51 条 ISSR 引物共检测到 433 个位点，每条引物 5～12 个，平均 8.49 个，PPB 为 93.30%。表明 22 个苦豆子居群间具有较高的遗传多样性。

张祎楠等应用 ISSR 分子标记，对川牛膝主产地 6 个居群、23 份样本进行了植物性状研究及遗传性研究。经过引物筛选试验选出 4 个呈现多态性的引物，总共扩增条带数为 43 条。结果表明，川牛膝的遗传变异在物种水平上，四川主产地川牛膝物种间遗传多样性较大，居群间遗传多样性较小。

王果平等应用 ISSR 分子标记，对新疆贝母属 10 种植物进行遗传多样性分析。结果，扩增总数为 185 条，其中多态性有 181 条，PPB 为 97.84%。遗传差异性分析表明，12 个 ISSR 引物可将新疆贝母不同种之间的遗传差异明显区分，揭示了 10 种贝母种质资源间的遗传多样性与亲缘关系。

5. SRAP 分析

艾强等运用 SRAP 分子标记，对川黔境内川续断的遗传多样性进行分析。10 对引物共检测到 124 个位点，其中 102 个位点具有多态性，PPB 为 82.26%，基于遗传相似度，14 个居群可聚为 3 类。提示川续断居群的遗传多样性水平丰富，遗传变异主要存在居群内。

蔡顺顺等采用 SRAP 分子标记，对来自四川、重庆的 10 份紫苏材料进行遗传多样性分析。结果，用 26 对 SRAP 引物组合扩增出 167 条带，PPB 为 51.57%，四川和重庆地区的平均 PPB 为 27.25%，在两个地区间，SRAP 标记的平均 H 值分别为 0.149 6 和 0.232 8。表明 SRAP 分子标记适用于紫苏材料的遗传多样性分析。

6. SCAR 分析

周涛等通过 RAPD 随机引物筛选，获得头花蓼特异的 RAPD 分子标记片段，经克隆、测序，重新设计特异性引物转化形成稳定的 SCAR 标记，获得 2 条稳定扩增的头花蓼特异片段 Z300、Z1100，根据该特异片段序列设计 4 对特异引物，分别对头花蓼与尼泊尔蓼药材 DNA 进行扩增，其中引物 Z1－2 可从头花蓼药材中扩增获得约 300 bp 的片段，而尼泊尔蓼药材则未扩增出该片段。引物 Z1－2 成功将 Z300 片段转化为 SCAR 分子标记，可作为头花蓼与近缘种尼泊尔蓼药材分子鉴定的依据。

7. SCoT 分析

张维瑞等利用 SCoT 分子标记，对位于河南

4大山脉的8个益母草居群66个样品进行遗传多样性分析。10对引物共扩增出240条带，其中多态性有238条，PPB为99.17%，结果表明，河南野生益母草种群具有较高的遗传多样性，其遗传距离与地理距离存在明显的相关性。

陈大霞等采用SCoT分子标记，对45个来源于6个野生居群桃儿七进行遗传多态性检测。结果，筛选出的27条引物，共检测到350个位点，其中284个为多态位点，平均每条引物扩增所得多态有10.52条，在物种水平上；桃儿七6个野生居群的遗传多样性较为丰富，在居群水平上；遗传多样性水平较低，相同地理来源或相似生境的材料具有聚为一类的倾向。

（倪梁红）

【道地药材形成及其产区变迁的影响】

1. “道地药材”名称由来及其内涵

(1) “道地药材”名称由来　据梁飞等考证，“道地”一词，源于古代行政区划单位，强调了特定地区所产物品的优良品质；中医典籍中，最早应用“道地”一词是在明代《本草品汇精要》；而“道地药材”现存最早出处为明末《牡丹亭》。

(2) “道地药材”的内涵　道地药材之优，全在于其显著的临床疗效。如明代《景岳全书》言苍术：“惟茅山者，其质坚小，其味甘醇，补益功多，大胜他术。”指出茅山苍术最佳，因其性味甘醇，补益之功效非常显著，优于他处所产。表明内在的品质不同往往导致外观的差异。当临床实践证明某地所产药材质优效佳之后，医药学家从药材的形色气味入手，直观而详细地论述优质药材与非优质药材的表象区别，著录于本草书及其他医书中。如陶弘景论当归，以多肉少枝气香为优，以多根枝而细、色白气味薄者为劣。《唐本草》云“黄连，蜀道者粗大节平，味极浓苦，疗渴为最”，指出四川黄连药效极佳，以粗大节平、味极苦为其特点。表明直观的比较，逐渐发展为后世的药材鉴别，成为判断药材性能的主要方式。

2. 道地药材形成原因

梁氏等论述了“道地药材”的形成原因，在秦汉时期就有“道地药材”的理念；而道地药材的最终确立与兴盛发展，约在明清两代，其间经历了千余年的发展。

(1) 中医的实践检验与理论指导是道地药材形成的理论基础　① 从实践的检验而言，道地药材最初的认识来源于中医的临床实践。② 从理论总结而言，我国古代医药学家在实践中不断总结，对于道地药材的认识由浅入深，逐渐形成了较为丰富的理论体系，大致可归纳为3个阶段：道地的“朴素生境观”、“小环境观”、“整体观”。

(2) 生态环境与药材种质的差异是道地药材形成的本质原因　① 从自然环境的差异而论，我国地跨寒温带、温带、亚热带、热带，地形复杂，温度、日照、水分、土壤、海拔等环境条件相差悬殊，自然地理环境复杂多样。不同的地域，适合不同的中药材生长。② 从药材种质的因素而论，不同产地的药材既有可能是属于同种生物的不同品种，也有可能是属于不同种的生物，种质的差别导致其内质、性征、临床功效的巨大差异。

(3) 明清时期的社会发展是道地药材形成的无形推动力　① 受益于政治文化的影响与本草研究的深入。② 得益于经济活动的繁荣与药材交易的兴盛。③ 依托于生产技术的提高与药材栽培炮制的发展。

3. 道地药材产区变迁及其影响因素

(1) 自然生态环境的改变，必定会影响到物种的变迁、兴衰、存亡　梁氏等以大量史料为基础，表明自然环境的改变，一方面直接造成了药材的生长环境出现有利或有害的改变，另一方面也间接刺激了药材自身的基原变异，从而最终导致了某些道地药材产区的消亡或兴起。彭华胜等以泽泻等为例，论述了气候变化对道地药材产区变迁的影响。近2 000年来，泽泻道地产区受气候较大幅度的波动，明清时期由北向南发生了转移。

(2) 人类社会的发展对道地药材变迁的影响　① 新的认识和发现促进道地药材产区变迁：当人们新发现药材比原先所认为的“道地药材”更为质优效佳时，就往往著录新的道地产区。② 人工引种导致新兴产区：有计划地进行野生变家种或从国外、其他地区引进种植，若条件适宜，往往形成新的主产区。③ 政权区划的变革：政权之间的战争，也会导致药材道地产区变迁。④ 过度开采致使道地产区变迁。

4. 道地药材形成机制研究

基于药材道地性内涵及生物学特征及其分子

机制研究，探讨道地药材形成的分子机制已取得一定进展。席培宇等将3个不同产地甘草的β-香树酯醇合成酶基因作为研究对象，通过比较其在不同产地甘草中的序列多态性及其表达差异，从基因层面探索了甘草道地性的形成机制。结果表明，在序列多态性实验中，9个样品的β-AS序列经比对分析共发现108处变异位点，内含子变异位点数高于外显子变异位点数两倍。在表达差异实验中内蒙组、甘肃组和宁夏组的甘草β-AS基因平均相对表达量有显著性差异。表明不同产地甘草β-AS基因多态性的差异以及表达量的差异，可能是导致甘草道地性形成的原因之一。

5. 道地药材的优选模式

道地药材生物的生长、发育与生态环境密切相关，因光照、温度、湿度和空气等不同生态因子的影响而产生不同分布。王德群应用植物分类、植物生态及中药地理等多学科知识，并根据地理分布将中药材生物的分布分为同纬异经、同经异纬、异纬异经、特殊需求4种基本类型，确定同药单向优选、同药双向或多向优选、异药双向或多向优选、同药多选及随机点状优选等5种优选模式。基于中药材生物分布的4种类型和5种优选模式，通过人工调节环境还可扩展地道药材栽培产区。生物性药材经人工驯化、栽培，通过调节环境、温度、水分、海拔高度等多种措施，不仅可使植物药栽培的范围得到扩展，还可在提高产量的同时，提高质量，逐渐形成新的稳定的道地药材。如耐阴植物药太子参、延胡索、半夏、贝母等人工栽培后，改阴性为阳性，增加了光合效应，提高了产量。又如太子参繁殖的块根凉贮越夏，不仅使其生长环境由阴变阳，还可使其分布南移至福建和贵州等地。再如川芎、附子、当归高海拔育苗，低海拔栽培可获高产。通过对药材优选模式的建立，为道地药材的优选开辟了一条新的探索途径。

（陈建伟）

【采收期对中药材含量的影响】

中药材的采收期对中药药效成分具有较大的影响，确定合理的采收期是保证中药的质量和临床疗效的重要环节。

1. 黄连

曾烨等采用UV和HPTLC测定黄连的有效成分。结果，黄连2～3龄阶段为黄连生长最旺盛的时期，酪氨酸、总生物碱、小檗碱、黄连碱、巴马汀和小檗碱的含量增长速度最快。

2. 橘皮

韦正等采用HPTLC测定四川蒲江、眉山夹江及重庆璧山共45批、不同采收期橘皮中的辛弗林含量。结果表明，同一植株不同的采收期对陈皮、青皮中辛弗林成分的影响较大，橘皮未成熟的果实中辛弗林的含量最高，不同生长期橘皮中辛弗林含量随着果实成熟度增加而降低。

3. 苦玄参

丘琴等采用HPTLC分析测定同一产地不同生长期的苦玄参不同药用部位苦玄参苷I_A的含量。结果苦玄参不同药用部位的苦玄参苷I_A在七八月份的含量最高。

4. 当归

肖宇奇等采用HPTLC对当归中阿魏酸、Z-藁本内酯、正丁烯基苯酞等成分的含量变化进行研究。结果，当归在第2年10～11月份时（传统采收期），其生物产量最大，阿魏酸含量较高，而Z-藁本内酯、正丁烯基苯酞含量不高。

5. 人参

姜先刚应用UV法对人参总糖还原糖和可溶性多糖含量进行测定。结果表明，参根中总糖和还原糖含量在果后参根生长初期达到最大值，可溶性多糖含量在果后参根生长后期达到最大值；参茎和参叶中的总糖还原糖和可溶性多糖含量在人参整个生长时期无显著性变化。

6. 枳壳

李正红等采用RP-HPTLC测定不同采收期的江西新干和樟树两个道地产区枳壳药材中活性成分的含量。结果表明，枳壳药材中主要活性成分的含量随采收期的推延总体呈下降趋势，江枳壳在大暑前后采收最佳。

7. 苦参

陈静等采用HPTLC分析不同年限苦参药材不同部位中5种指标性生物碱的含量。结果表明，随着生长年限的增加，各指标性生物碱成分含量随之增加，第4年有效成分增加幅度较小。

8. 连翘

姜红等用分光光度法测定5、8、10月份所采收连翘叶中总黄酮的含量,HPTLC测定其芦丁的含量。结果表明,河北石家庄井陉县洞阳坡连翘叶的最佳采收期为8月份。

9. 杜仲

宣志红等采用HPTLC测定不同时期杜仲叶中绿原酸、京尼平苷酸、京尼平苷的含量。结果表明,绿原酸在7月上旬含量最高,京尼平苷酸在7月下旬含量最高,京尼平苷在6月上旬含量最高。

10. 山绿茶

郑锡任等研究不同采收期山绿茶药材中绿原酸和芦丁的含量。结果表明,1月份采收的山绿茶中含量均较高,7月份采收的山绿茶中含量均较低,山绿茶的合理采收时间可定为1月。

另外,南敏伦等对金莲花、聂浩鸿等对南板蓝根、冯燕燕等对布渣叶不同采收期对药材中所含成分含量的影响也进行了报道。

（陈德兴）

【硫黄熏蒸对中药材有效成分的影响】

硫黄熏蒸作为传统的中药材加工养护方法已有上百年的历史,适量且规范的硫黄熏蒸可以达到防腐、防虫的目的,但滥用或过度使用则会对中药材及饮片质量产生影响。目前,二氧化硫残留限量已实行分级管理,标准已收入《中国药典》(2010年版)第二增补本,标准为:中药材及饮片中亚硫酸盐残留量(以二氧化硫计)不得超过150 mg/kg,山药、牛膝、粉葛、天冬、天麻、天花粉、白及、白芍药、白术、党参10种中药材及其饮片中亚硫酸盐残留量(以二氧化硫计)不得超过400 mg/kg。

1. 硫黄熏蒸对中药材有效成分的影响

(1) 当归　李芸等采用GC-MS分析了当归熏硫前后挥发油的含量,未熏硫、0.20%熏硫、1.00%熏硫、5.00%熏硫分别为0.19%、0.31%、0.19%、0.25%。结果表明,熏硫加工后,挥发油的含量有所增加,但其主要成分占总挥发油的比例有所下降;采用低剂量的硫黄进行熏蒸,对当归挥发油的影响不大;而高剂量熏硫对当归挥发油影响较大。李成义等认为当归熏硫不仅影响药材的外观性状,还影响药材的内在质量。熏硫后当归不同药用部位阿魏酸的含量明显下降,含量高低为归尾>归身>归头,但当归商品等级与阿魏酸的含量变化无明显的相关性。

(2) 白芍药　蔡皓等对硫黄熏蒸前后白芍药HPTLC-UV图谱进行比较研究。结果经硫黄熏蒸后,白芍药成分发生了比较明显的变化,某些共有成分的含量也有不同程度的改变,表明硫黄熏蒸对白芍药的质量影响较大。

(3) 白芷　蒋运斌等报道,熏硫加工白芷后,氧化前胡素、水合氧化前胡内酯、佛手内酯、白当归脑4个化合物在熏硫前后指纹图谱中变化较为明显,自然晒干的白芷样品氧化前胡素和欧前胡素均高于其他经过硫黄熏蒸的样品。表明白芷随着硫黄用量和熏蒸时间的增加,氧化前胡素和欧前胡素的含量下降。

(4) 金银花　邢志霞、孙曙光等通过硫熏金银花后发现绿原酸含量明显增加,不同产地之间的含量差异也较大,其中郑州产金银花中绿原酸含量较低,封丘、山东两地含量较高。刘伟等研究表明,硫熏后金银花中绿原酸含量明显升高,但木犀草苷含量基本无影响,且不同产地两种成分含量相差较大。

2. 中药材中二氧化硫残留量的检测

对二氧化硫残留量的检测,多采用《中国药典》(2010年版)的酸蒸馏碘滴定法。

杨欣等对河南、山东、广西产山药,甘肃兰州、湖南长沙、湖南龙山产百合及湖南邵东产玉竹进行了二氧化硫残留量的测定。结果表明,二氧化硫含量在200～500 μg/g的样品有4个批次,在501～1 000 μg/g的样品有2个批次,其中超过国际食品法典委员会规定的1 000 μg/g限度的有2个批次,最高可达1 466.9 μg/g。卢晓琳等测定了经硫黄熏蒸处理过的药材或饮片中亚硫酸盐(以二氧化硫计)的残留量。结果,自然晒干的白芷样品中二氧化硫残留量低于其他经过硫黄熏蒸的样品;随着硫黄用量和熏蒸时间的增加,二氧化硫残留量升高。李成义等将不同水分党参经过不同时间熏硫后,发现党参水分含量分别控制在15%、25%、35%时,熏硫时间分别控制在21 h、18 h、15 h以内,二氧化硫残留量低于400 mg/kg;水分含量在65.00%左右或趁鲜熏蒸后,二氧化硫残留量超过 400 mg/kg。结果表明，二氧化硫残留量与熏硫时药材水分及熏硫时间有相关性，药材水分越高，熏硫时间越长，二氧化硫残留量越大。张倩等测定了 80 个批次的常用中药饮片中二氧化硫残留量，共计 10 种中药饮片，每种 8 个批次。结果 8 种、18 个批次的中药饮片中二氧化硫残留量均超出拟定的限量，党参和当归的二氧化硫残留量不合格率超过 50.0%。张丹等通过测定发现，未用硫黄熏制的黄芪二氧化硫残留量为25.6 mg/kg，熏制后残留量明显升高，硫黄用量对二氧化硫残留量影响极显著，药材含水量和熏制时间影响不显著。张义生等测定了不同熏蒸法工艺山药中二氧化硫的含量，其中熏蒸次数、硫黄用量对二氧化硫残留量影响较大。陈睿等检测了 13 种、140 批中药饮片。结果，36 批次未检出二氧化硫，占样品总批次的 25.70%；49 批次低于 10 mg/kg；38 批次超出目前推荐的限量（山药、白芍药、党参 ≤ 400 mg/kg，其他 ≤ 150 mg/kg），占总批次的 27%，最高残留达 2 550 mg/kg。王世伟等通过测定 20 种中药饮片的二氧化硫残留量，按照规定标准合格率只有 43%，含量最高的为菊花(5 722 ppm)，其次为牛膝(4 064 ppm)、党参(3 580 ppm)、百合(2 440 ppm)、桔梗(2 410 ppm)。

另外，彭月等用衍生化反应，建立了荧光分光光度法测定中药中二氧化硫的残留量。并对 20 批中药材进行检测，建立了中药材二氧化硫的快速检测方法。朱雪妍等采用离子色谱法，进行中药材的二氧化硫含量测定。钟虹敏等采用有机元素分析法，通过对已知中药材含硫量的数据分析，进行中药材品质的快速鉴定。吉琅等根据活泼金属单质锌在稀盐酸中能还原亚硫酸或亚硫酸盐生成硫化氢，而硫化氢能使乙酸铅试纸变黑的原理，用于中药材中二氧化硫残留量的检测。

（刘学湘　陈建伟）

【产地加工对中药材有效成分的影响】

1. 水洗对有效成分的影响

水洗的目的是借助水的浮力，除去新鲜药材泥沙杂质和分离非药用部位。谭秋生等在研究不同产地加工方式对白芷的影响时，分别采取刷除和水洗方式对药材进行表面除沙。结果，白芷经过水洗后，总灰分和欧前胡素的含量大幅降低，表明白芷在产地加工过程中应避免水洗。

2. 药材“发汗”对有效成分的影响

（1）“发汗”的由来及方法演化　药材“发汗”一词最早来源于中药炮制学专著《雷公炮炙论》。段金廒等对近现代本草著作进行研究，将药材“发汗”归为普通发汗和加温发汗两大类。普通发汗法：将鲜药材或一定程度失水药材进行堆置，必要时需进行覆盖，促其发热、“回潮”，以使其内部水分向外扩散，形成“发汗”的征象，如玄参、地黄、丹参、板蓝根、大黄、续断等。加温发汗法：将鲜药材或一定程度失水药材实施增温措施后，进行密闭堆积使之“发汗”，如皮类药材厚朴、杜仲用沸水烫淋数遍加热，然后堆积发汗，称“发水汗”。云南及其周边地区在茯苓的产地加工过程中，先将柴草烧热，相间铺放茯苓，再盖草密闭促其“发汗”，称“发火汗”。

（2）药材“发汗”的目的　段氏等将药材“发汗”的目的归纳为 4 点：① 促使药材内部水分重新分布，以实现药材内外干燥一致，加快干燥速度。② 有利于生物组织内部的微生物和功能酶系促发资源性化学物质的生物转化与化学转化。③ 有利于改善药材性状，使之外观更为油润、光泽，质地更加致密、硬实，药香气味更为浓郁、醇厚。④ 有助于增强或平抑原药材的某一偏性，以达到改变或缓和药性的目的。

（3）药材“发汗”过程的生物化学转化影响药材品质的形成　段氏等认为药材初加工环节中的“发汗”方法是部分根及根茎类、皮类、菌核等药材在干燥加工过程中采用的独特处理方法，既有利于药用部位内部水分向外分布易于干燥，同时又调节和促进着生物组织中的酶系统与微生物群落活力，启动或加速了初生/次生代谢产物的生物转化与化学转化过程，直接影响着药材品质的形成。其主要酶活性变化特性及其化学转化间的关系为：① 多酚氧化酶(PPO)与化学成分转化：玄参、地黄等的鲜根“发汗”处理的共同机制是药材中所含丰富的酚性物质(如地黄中含有的咖啡酰葡萄糖苷等)在 PPO 催化作用下形成对应的醌类产物，呈色的醌式结构分子进一步聚合或与其他芳香化物结合形成更大的共轭体系，变成黑色或褐色，从而导致药材品质的改变。② 过氧化物酶(POD)与化学成分转化：POD 可促使药用植物中所含的某些碳水化合物转化成木质素，以增加木质化程度。鲜药材“发汗”过程中，由于在一定范围的温度升高和适宜的水分条件下，促使 POD 酶活力升高，可催化过氧化氢氧化酚类和胺类化合物，且具有消除过氧化氢和酚类、胺类毒性的双重作用。③ 水解酶与化学成分转化：在药材“发汗”过程中，组织细胞受损或解离，温度和水分激活了水解酶(如糖苷水解酶、蛋白水解酶、淀粉水解酶等)的功能，促发、加速一系列的水解反应。续断药材堆置“发汗”过程中，由于水解酶的作用使其中糖苷类物质发生酶解，导致药材中总皂苷和续断皂苷 VI 量降低。薄荷、荆芥等芳香全草类药材在“发汗”过程中，促进了萜烯糖苷类成分水解，释放出芳樟醇、香叶醇、己烯醇等游离态香气物质。

3. 干燥方法对有效成分的影响

干燥的目的是除去新鲜药材中大量水分，保证药材质量，利于贮藏。周铜水研究表明，丹参的主要水溶性活性成分丹酚酸 B 是在干燥过程中大量形成的，在新鲜药材中含量甚微，即丹酚酸 B 实际上是一个采后干燥胁迫诱导产物。其他丹酚酸类成分也都是在干燥过程中伴随着丹酚酸 B 的形成而产生的。丹参酮 II_A 和隐丹参酮等丹参酮类成分在新鲜根中有较大含量的积累，但在干燥过程中也增加近一倍以上。这些成分在干燥过程中都呈现倒“V”字形的变化趋势，增长曲线中丹酚酸 B 等成分的含量与样品水分呈明显负相关。黄芩中黄芩苷等黄酮类成分在干燥过程中也呈现类似的变化曲线。表明采后干燥早期过程对于丹参、黄芩这样的宿根类药材，可能会诱导活性成分的大量形成和升高。

(1) 烘干法　宣志红等研究不同干燥加工方式对杜仲叶中主要成分含量的影响。结果，新鲜杜仲叶采用烘干处理后，药材京尼平苷酸和京尼平苷的含量均较高，绿原酸的含量略有降低；而阴干的温度较低，易发生变质现象。表明杜仲叶更适于采用烘干方式进行干燥。王小平等研究表明，40～80℃烘干对丹参药材中丹参酮 II_A 影响不明显，当温度高于 60℃时，对丹酚酸 B 造成明显损失，而当干燥温度高于 70℃时，丹参的表面和断面颜色会受到影响。所以从活性成分的含量、药材外观色泽等方面综合考虑，丹参药材的加工应 40～60℃烘干为宜。聂慧等研究不同干燥方法对百合质量的影响，分别采用 60℃、80℃及 100℃烘干，测定样品中酚性甘油酯类、核苷、氨基酸及多糖等成分的含量。结果表明，在 60～80℃条件下烘干百合较好，温度过高或过低均会影响百合的质量。聂浩鸿等对南板蓝根进行了产地干燥处理。结果，南板蓝根经过烘干后，腺苷含量比阴干和晒干的要高很多，而当烘干温度高于 60℃时，有效成分含量有所降低，表明烘干温度的选择十分重要。杜远等研究表明，采用传统加工、砂炒烘干等方法对金钗石斛的鲜茎进行干燥加工，药材的折干率和浸出物含量较高，可作为金钗石斛的产地加工方法。管汉亮等采用 UPLC－TQ－MS 联用技术，研究不同干燥过程中银杏叶化学成分的变化规律，分析银杏叶在自然晒干、阴干及不同温度下烘干过程中儿茶素类、黄酮及其苷类、双黄酮类、内酯类及酚酸类成分含量变化。结果表明，80℃条件下烘干银杏叶能起到“杀青”的作用，其有利于银杏叶中儿茶素类、黄酮及其苷类、银杏内酯类等成分的转化积累，而对双黄酮类成分含量的影响不明显。

(2) 阴干法　蔡佳良等研究了广藿香的最佳产地加工方法，发现采用传统干燥法，药材中百秋李醇含量最低，而采用阴干法进行干燥，药材中百秋李醇含量最高。

(3) 晒干法　杨小艳等分别采用晒干、烘干、减压干燥、真空冷冻干燥、远红外干燥、微波干燥 6 种方法，以外观性状、总生物碱、总酸含量为指标，研究不同干燥方法对半夏质量的影响。结果表明，晒干半夏的外观性状最好；不同干燥方法的生物碱和总酸含量差异不大。

(4) 微波干燥法　蒋赣等比较了热风、红外、微波和低温吸附等 4 种干燥方法对土茯苓品质的影响。结果表明，以 100 W 微波干燥速率较快，经微波干燥后的产品具有较好的复水性，其中的黄酮成分能很大程度地保留，产品的外观亦未受影响。宣氏等研究了不同微波功率干燥处理杜仲叶的方法。结果，新鲜杜仲叶采用 600 W 微波处理 5 min 后，京尼平苷酸含量较阴凉处晾干时增加 17.11%；800 W 微波处理 5 min 后，京尼平苷含量较阴凉处晾干时增加了 32.30%。由于绿原酸遇热易被破坏，经过微波处理后，杜仲叶中绿原酸含量的下降程度不一，其中 800 W 微波 5 min 后与阴凉处晾干时绿原酸含量相差无几，1 000 W 微波干燥时由于功率稍大，绿原酸含量较阴凉处晾干时下降 12.80%。表明杜仲叶用 800 W 微波杀青 5 min 是一种相对较好的干燥加工方法。严瑞娟等分析了不同产地初加工方式处理杜仲叶的 HPTLC 指纹图谱。结果，蒸制和烫，耗能高、操作不方便，效果一般；炒制外观较差，产品质量不易控制；微波制操作简单、效果好、应用容易而便于推广。

4. 切制对有效成分的影响

谭秋生等研究了白芷的切片加工方法与成分含量的变化。结果表明，白芷经过切片后，色泽变暗、多卷缩、品相较差，但欧前胡素含量却相对很高，因此其是否需要切制有待商榷。

5. 贮藏对有效成分的影响

宣氏等研究了在 0～18 个月中应用 4 种不同温度、避光方式贮藏对杜仲叶有效成分的影响。结果① 在室温条件下：随着存放时间的延长，杜仲叶中京尼平苷酸、绿原酸和京尼平苷含量均出现了不同程度的下降。② 在室温避光条件下放置 18 个月：京尼平苷酸的量下降了 5.67%、绿原酸的量下降了 10.69%、京尼平苷的量下降了 17.45%。③ 在室温不避光条件下：京尼平苷酸的量下降了 6.29%、绿原酸的量下降了 12.76%、京尼平苷的量下降了 18.61%。④ 在低温条件下：随着存放时间的延长，杜仲叶中京尼平苷酸、绿原酸和京尼平苷都出现了不同程度的下降。⑤ 在低温避光条件下放置 18 个月：京尼平苷酸的量下降了 4.25%、绿原酸的量下降了 6.40%、京尼平苷的量下降了 11.63%。⑥ 在低温不避光条件下：京尼平苷酸的量下降了 4.46%、绿原酸的量下降了 8.80%、京尼平苷的量下降了 13.96%。表明杜仲叶宜密封、低温、避光保存。

（邱海龙　陈建伟）

【秦艽的生药学研究】

秦艽始载于《神农本草经》，为龙胆科植物秦艽(*Gentiana macrophylla* Pall.)、麻花秦艽(*G. straminea* Maxim.)、粗茎秦艽(*G. crassicaulis* Duthie ex Burk.)或小秦艽(*G. dahurica* Fisch.)的干燥根，是一味常用中药材。主要分布于甘肃、陕西、山西等地。近年来，由于过度采挖及生态环境的改变等原因，致使野生秦艽资源处于濒危状态。为解决秦艽药材临床用药的不断需求，对其研究有较多的报道。

1. 秦艽的栽培

董凯等在研究秦艽小拱棚育苗技术时，总结出最佳栽培条件的技术要点：育苗选地应在土层深厚肥沃、质地疏松的砂质土壤，前茬种植玉米、小麦、马铃薯等均可；苗床宜地平土细，播前可撒施优质农家肥；精选当年种子，并用500 mg/kg 赤霉素溶液处理；播种最适时间为 11 月上旬；翌年 2 月中旬在播种畦上搭小拱棚；田间管理以防治害虫为主。和桂军通过研究秦艽育苗，对大田地膜移栽技术、田间管理和采收进行了筛选，从而得出一套新的秦艽栽培方式，生育期相对缩短。杨小萍等根据秦艽生理要求，从选茬、整地施肥、播种、田间管理和收获等方面介绍了临洮县秦艽栽培技术：直播栽培的秦艽种植后的第 2 年可以产少量的种子，第 3 年为产籽高峰期，第 3～4 年即可收获药根；而育苗移栽的秦艽，栽植后的第 1 年可收获少量种子，第 2～3 年为产籽高峰期，一般在第 3 年即可收获药根。

米永伟等研究了麻花艽种子灌浆充实动态及其发芽特性。结果表明，采收期应在花后 52～55 d，种子含水率在 10.0%左右时，根据成熟情况分批采用布袋或尼龙袋，并选择晴天采收，所得到种子发芽质量最优。彭云霞等以 3 年生秦艽为研究对象，对不同成熟度秦艽种子形态特征及萌发特性进行研究。结果表明，秦艽鲜种子萌发率和发芽势均随种子成熟度的增加表现出低、高、低的趋势，成熟度不同发芽持续期也不同，成熟以后的发芽速率较快，秦艽鲜种子以开花后 21 d 采收萌发率最高。郭江帆等采用生物测定方法对秦艽种子中存在的抑制种子萌发物质进行了研究。结果表明，秦艽种子中确实存在影响种子萌发的抑制物质。

晋玲等对秦艽愈伤组织缓慢生长保存及其生理指标进行研究。结果表明，不同类型和浓度的高渗化合物对秦艽愈伤组织保存效果的影响差异较大，1.0 mg/L ABA，9.00%蔗糖保存秦艽愈伤组织效果最好，可溶性糖、淀粉和可溶性蛋白质 3 个生理指标，可以在一定程度上反映秦艽愈伤组织在延缓保存时的存活情况。

2. 秦艽的质量评价

段宝忠等对野生抚育粗茎秦艽药材的有效成分和化学指纹图谱进行了研究。结果表明，野生抚育模式药材可作为粗茎秦艽主要种植发展模式。周亚兴等对云南怒江兰坪县不同生长年限粗茎秦艽中龙胆苦苷含量进行比较研究，结果在中排乡、西乡和通甸镇采集到生长3～4年的秦艽根中龙胆苦苷含量最高。安方玉等用HPTLC对甘肃秦艽的龙胆苦苷含量进行研究，结果不同产地秦艽的有效成分龙胆苦苷的含量存在一定的差异。林燕等采用索氏提取法、GC－MS法、计算机检索对3种秦艽花脂溶性成分进行分离和鉴定。结果，在西藏秦艽花、麻花艽花和川西秦艽花的脂溶性成分中分别鉴定了38(94.31%)、35(83.09%)、27(80.84%)个化合物。3种秦艽花脂溶性成分存在一定程度的差异，其中川西秦艽花的脂溶性成分与其他2种的区别较大，其药理活性也可能不同。

郝彩琴等比较了不同提取方法对宁夏六盘山栽培秦艽中龙胆苦苷的含量影响。结果，动态热回流提取法提取率最高，为14.50%。郝氏等进一步研究表明，用正交设计法优选动态回流法提取的最佳工艺条件是：溶剂用量为药材的10倍，提取30 min，提取1次。贾建忠等用近红外光谱法收集秦艽中龙胆苦苷样本的近红外图谱，并用HPTLC测定其含量，得出秦艽提取过程中在线检测龙胆苦苷定量模型，预测效果良好。

3. 秦艽的分子鉴定

化文平等研究秦艽香叶醇－10羟化酶(G10H)基因的克隆及序列时，克隆了秦艽G10H基因，并对其基因及编码蛋白序列的特征进行了生物信息学分析。结果表明，秦艽G10H基因包含一个完整的长1 491 bp的ORF框，编码496个氨基酸；GmG10H与长春花、川西樟牙菜等植物G10H蛋白具有很高的同源性，无跨膜结构域、信号肽等结构，可能定位于细胞质中，定量PCR发现GmG10H主要在秦艽的花和根中进行表达。

He T等用ISSR标记法研究麻花艽的胚胎在发生和再生植物的遗传稳定性，以植物生长激素和细胞分裂素为指标，检查对愈伤组织诱导和植株再生的影响。结果表明，诱导胚胎愈伤组织发生的最佳方式是加入2 mg/L的叶橙剂酸和0.5 mg/L 6－苄氨基嘌呤；拥有根系统的再生小植株能够在绿色环境和土壤中成功的生长，再生植株能保持很高的遗传稳定性。Zhao ZJ等研究麻花艽中生物诱导因子对齐墩果酸积累和三萜合成基因表达的影响，通过低温、UV－B辐射、茉莉酮酸甲酯(MeJA)、水杨酸等分别处理。结果表明，MeJA能显著提高齐墩果酸的积累，并能促进三萜类基因的表达。

4. 秦艽在复方中的定性鉴定

张灿等采用薄层色谱法对颈复康颗粒中羌活、秦艽中所含紫花前胡苷、龙胆苦苷进行定性鉴别。此方法能较好地鉴别颈复康颗粒中的羌活和秦艽。

5. 秦艽的药理研究

秦艽化学成分主要为环烯醚萜类，其中龙胆苦苷具有抗感染的药理作用。王钢等研究秦艽醇提物对胶原诱导性关节炎大鼠血清抗-环瓜氨酸肽(CCP)及肿瘤坏死因子(TNF)－α的影响。结果，大叶秦艽醇提物能够在早期抑制胶原诱导性关节炎大鼠血清中抗－CCP抗体及TNF－α水平，减轻关节肿胀程度，改善滑膜炎症状，保护关节。表明在早期治疗类风湿关节炎方面优势明显。刘然等研究表明，秦艽不局限于传统的祛风湿作用，在神经系统疾病、呼吸道感染、肛肠疾病、皮肤疾病等也有特殊作用。

(钱春生　吴靳荣)

[附]　参考文献

A

艾强，周涛，江维克，等．川续断种质资源遗传多样性的SRAP分析[J]．中草药，2013，43(15)：2155

安方玉，刘丽莎，侯茜．甘肃濒危植物秦艽的龙胆苦苷含量和遗传多样性的研究[J]．天然产物研究与开发，2013，25(B12)：31

C

蔡皓，张科卫，刘晓，等．硫黄熏蒸前后白芍HPTLC－UV特征图谱的比较研究[J]．药物分析杂志，2013，33(1)：128

蔡佳良，郭念欣，姬生国．不同干燥方法对广藿香中百秋李醇含量影响的近红外光谱分析[J]．云南中医中药杂志，2013，34(1)：53

蔡顺顺，张兴翠．四川、重庆不同紫苏遗传多样性的SRAP研究[J]．西南师范大学学报（自然科学版），2013，38(3)：101

曹亮，蒋超，彭华胜，等．白术、苍术种子位点特异性PCR鉴别方法研究[J]．中国中药杂志，2013，38(6)：2567

常凯，马丽利，王亚雄，等．大花红景天尿苷二磷酸葡萄糖基转移酶基因组DNA的克隆及分析[J]．中草药，2013，44(6)：736

陈大霞，赵纪峰，刘翔，等．濒危药用植物桃儿七野生居群遗传多样性与遗传结构的SCoT分析[J]．中国中药杂志，2013，38(2)：278

陈静，王淑美，孟江，等．不同生长年限苦参不同部位的生物碱含量[J]．中国实验方剂学杂志，2013，19(7)：80

陈睿，刘惠军，储忠英，等．上海市场13种中药饮片二氧化硫残留情况检测分析[J]．中国药事，2013，27(5)：457

陈仕江，鲁增辉，廖玉凤，等．7种中药材斑蝥COI基因序列的分子系统学研究[J]．西南农业学报，2013，26(5)：1809

程琪庆，何云飞，李耿，等．丹参4-羟基-3-甲基-2-丁烯基焦磷酸还原酶基因的全长克隆与诱导表达分析[J]．药学学报，2013，48(2)：236

D

董凯．秦艽小拱棚育苗技术[J]．甘肃农业科技，2013，(11)：60

杜远，刘文杰，孙志蓉，等．金钗石斛药材初加工方法的比较研究[J]．中药材，2013，36(3)：374

段宝忠，黄林芳，尚飞能，等．云南野生抚育粗茎秦艽药材的品质评价[J]．中国实验方剂学杂志，2013，19(21)：82

段金廒，宿树兰，严辉，等．药材初加工"发汗"过程及其酶促反应与化学转化机制探讨[J]．中草药，2013，44(10)：1219

F

范丙友，李芳，张文婷，等．芍药肌动蛋白基因的克隆及表达分析[J]．中草药，2013，43(15)：2136

冯燕燕，梁秋娴，李小青，等．布渣叶中总黄酮与牡荆苷质量分数的季节动态变化[J]．广东药学院学报，2013，29(1)：35

G

管汉亮，钱大玮，段金廒，等．银杏叶干燥方法的优化及其机制探讨[J]．中国中药杂志，2013，38(13)：2140

郭江帆，孙佳，魏朔南．秦艽种子内源萌发抑制物的初步探究[J]．种子，2013，32(7)：39

郭淑，孙超，宋经元，等．灵芝三萜合成关键元件GLCYP450及其还原酶GLNADPH的基因克隆及共表达载体构建[J]．药学学报，2013，48(2)：206

H

He T, Yang LN, Zhao ZG. Embryogenesis of *Gentiana straminea* and assessment of genetic stability of regenerated plants using inter simple sequence repeat (ISSR) marker[J]. African Journal of Biotechnology, 2011, 10(39): 7604

郝彩琴，郭鸿雁，冷晓红，等．正交优选动态回流法提取秦艽中龙胆苦苷工艺[J]．西北林学院学报，2013，28(1)：123

郝彩琴，冷晓红．不同提取方法对宁夏六盘山栽培秦艽中龙胆苦苷提取率的影响[J]．西北药学杂志，2013，28(1)：13

郝东，尹海波；赵晓雨，等．牻牛儿苗种质资源遗传多样性的ISSR研究[J]．中国实验方剂学杂志，2013，19(15)：147

何盼，李震宇，范圣此，等．基于代谢组学技术和ITS2序列的恒山黄芪与川黄芪差异性研究[J]．药学学报，2013，48(10)：1595

和桂军．秦艽育苗及大田地膜移栽技术[J]．中国园艺文摘，2013，(6)：227

侯茜，雷英，刘丽莎，等．西部地区濒危药用植物秦艽遗传多样性的RAPD分析[J]．中华中医药杂志，2013，28(1)：214

化文平，王喆之．秦艽香叶醇-10羟化酶(G10H)基因的克隆及序列分析[J]．基因组学与应用生物学，2013，32(4)：510

J

吉琅，廖晴，吕维，等．中药材中二氧化硫残留量快速测定方法[J]．中国实验方剂学杂志，2013，19(10)：66

贾建忠，吴春燕，李小安．近红外光谱法在秦艽提取过程中的应用[J]．药物分析杂志，2013，33(9)：1567

姜红，李兰芳，解丽君，等．不同采收时期连翘叶中总黄酮及芦丁的含量测定[J]．河北中医，2013，35(6)：912

姜先刚，刘海龙，张惠，等．不同生长时期人参中总糖、还原糖和可溶性多糖含量变化[J]．中国实验方剂学杂志，2013，19(16)：142

蒋赣，何顺秋，刘淑侦．不同干燥方法对土茯苓品质的影响[J]．广东药学院学报，2013，29(3)：258

蒋运斌，卢晓琳，杨枝中，等．与熏硫加工相关的白芷化学成分研究[J]．中国实验方剂学杂志，2013，19(22)：4

晋玲，张延红，高素芳．秦艽愈伤组织缓慢生长保存及其生理指标研究[J]．中国现代中药，2013，15(2)：118

L

李成义，魏学明，王明伟，等．不同熏硫方式对党参中

二氧化硫残留量的影响[J]. 中国现代中药，2013，15(6)：487

李成义，祝永甲，王明伟，等. 熏硫对商品当归不同药用部位阿魏酸含量的影响[J]. 甘肃中医学院学报，2013，30(3)：20

李晓灿，詹亚光，王晓东，等. 多胺对白桦悬浮细胞生长和三萜积累的影响[J]. 中草药，2013，44(4)：463

李芸，苗小楼，吴平安，等. GC－MS分析当归熏硫前后挥发油的化学成分[J]. 中药材，2013，36(3)：367

李正红，陈海芳，骆利平，等. 江枳壳不同采收期活性成分 HPTLC 含量测定[J]. 中药材，2013，36(1)：28

李忠虎，刘晓东，王小琦，等. 党参微卫星引物筛选及群体遗传多样性研究[J]. 中草药，2013，44(2)：210

梁飞，李健，张卫，等. "道地药材"浅述[J]. 中国中药杂志，2013，38(9)：1455

梁飞，李健，张卫，等. 道地药材产地变迁原因的探讨[J]. 中国中药杂志，2013，38(10)：1649

梁飞，李健，张卫，等. 谈"道地药材"的形成原因[J]. 中国中药杂志，2013，38(3)：466

廖婧，梁镇标，张亮，等. 常见药用蛇类的 DNA 条形码研究[J]. 中国药学杂志，2013，48(15)：1255

林燕，韩贺东，胡海清，等. 3 种藏药秦艽花脂溶性成分的 GC－MS 分析[J]. 中国实验方剂学杂志，2013，19(24)：102

刘红昌，罗春丽，李金玲，等. 何首乌不同种质生境调查及在贵州地域的生物学特性研究[J]. 中药材，2013，36(6)：864

刘然，王承平，何利黎，等. 秦艽的临床新用及思考[J]. 中药与临床，2013，4(5)：34

刘伟，茹凡书，崔永霞，等. 硫熏和烘干金银花中绿原酸木犀草苷含量对比分析[J]. 中国实验方剂学杂志，2013，19(1)：91

刘晓帆，刘春生，杨瑶珺，等. 基于 COI 基因的龟甲及其混伪品的 DNA 条形码研究[J]. 中国中药杂志，2013，38(7)：947

刘晓帆，刘春生，杨瑶珺，等. 基于 COI 基因的水蛭及其混伪品的 DNA 条形码研究[J]. 北京中医药大学学报，2013，36(1)：63

卢晓琳，马逾英，张福卓，等. 不同硫黄熏蒸程度白芷二氧化硫残留量与有效成分含量的相关性[J]. 中国实验方剂学杂志，2013，19(9)：139

鲁增辉，石萍，陈仕江. 侵染昆虫前后冬虫夏草菌类枯草杆菌蛋白酶基因表达研究[J]. 药学学报，2013，48(7)：1164

M

米永伟，陈垣，郭凤霞，等. 麻花艽种子灌浆充实动态及其发芽特性研究[J]. 草业学报，2013，22(6)：129

N

南敏伦，赵昱玮，司学玲，等. 不同采收期金莲花中 3 种碳苷黄酮成分动态变化[J]. 中国实验方剂学杂志，2013，19(4)：118

倪梁红，赵志礼，孟千万，等. 西藏麻花艽种质资源的遗传多样性分析[J]. 中草药，2013，44(22)：3212

聂浩鸿，张丽艳，杨丹，等. 不同采收期、初加工方法和药用部位南板蓝根中腺苷含量对比研究[J]. 辽宁中医药大学学报，2013，15(11)：76

聂慧，严辉，钱大玮，等. 加工方法对百合质量的影响研究[J]. 中国现代中药，2013，15(4)：308

P

彭华胜，郝近大，黄璐琦. 近 2000 年来气候变化对道地药材产区变迁的影响——以泽泻与枳壳为例[J]. 中国中药杂志，2013，38(13)：2218

彭月，陈鸿平，银玲，等. 中药材二氧化硫残留快速检测方法的建立[J]. 中国实验方剂学杂志，2013，19(8)：44

彭月，李雪莲，银玲，等. 荧光衍生法测定中药二氧化硫残留量研究[J]. 中国中药杂志，2013，38(2)：212

彭云霞，王宏霞. 不同成熟度秦艽种子的发芽特性[J]. 浙江农业科学，2013，(8)：956

Q

丘琴，苏春妹，甄汉深，等. 不同生产期苦玄参中苦玄参苷 IA 含量测定[J]. 中国实验方剂学杂志，2013，19(5)：108

S

尚洁，陈阿丽，潘伟志. 宁夏枸杞查耳酮合成酶基因 cDNA 片段的克隆及生物信息学分析[J]. 中草药，2013，44(20)：2898

孙乐乐，杨永红，刘军凯，等. 白及根腐病病原鉴定和生物学特性研究[J]. 中药材，2013，36(3)：341

孙曙光，刘伟，徐倩，等. 不同产地硫熏和烘干金银花中绿原酸含量的高效液相色谱测定[J]. 时珍国医国药，2013，24(3)：669

T

谭秋生，章文伟，李玲，等. 不同加工方法对白芷质量的影响[J]. 中国中医药信息杂志，2013，20(7)：49

田方，焦多礼，陈学林，等. 药用植物地理成分及海拔与中药功效的相关性研究[J]. 时珍国医国药，2013，24(7)：1746

W

汪孟曦，李文兰，张争，等. 白木香查尔酮合酶

(AsCHS1)基因的克隆和生物信息学分析[J]. 中国中药杂志,2013,38(2):149

王德群. 中药生物的地理分布类型与优质、地道药材的优选模式[J]. 安徽中医学院学报,2013,32(1):73

王钢,王丽琴,王佳,等. 秦艽醇提物对胶原诱导性关节炎大鼠血清抗-CCP及TNF-α的影响[J]. 中国实验方剂学杂志,2013,19(19):302

王果平,樊丛照,李晓瑾,等. 基于ISSR的新疆贝母属植物遗传多样性研究[J]. 中草药,2013,44(7):887

王海,严铸云,何冬梅,等. 多产区川芎内生真菌菌群组成的PCR-DGGE分析[J]. 中国中药杂志,2013,38(12):1893

王世伟,刘霞,席啸虎,等. 我院对中药饮片二氧化硫残留量及加重粉检验的方法和经验[J]. 中国医院药学杂志,2013,33(19):1641

王小平,白吉庆,寇文龙,等. 不同加工与贮藏方法对商洛产丹参药材品质的影响[J]. 中草药,2013,44(11):1407

王亚君,蒋超,赵容,等. 丹参SmNAC1基因的克隆和生物信息学分析[J]. 中国中药杂志,2013,38(13):2063

韦正,陈鸿平,杨丽,等. 同一植株不同生长期橘皮中辛弗林含量动态变化规律研究[J]. 中国实验方剂学杂志,2013,19(10):80

吴文燕,蒋喜红,刘春生,等. 丹参ERF转录因子SmERF1基因的表达分析和亚细胞定位[J]. 中国中药杂志,2013,38(7):957

吴志刚,李小侠,范传颖,等. 相关系列扩增多态性分子标记分析部分山药品种遗传多样性[J]. 中国药学杂志,2013,48(9):681

X

席培宇,刘颖,陈宏昊,等. 基于β-AS基因的甘草道地性形成机制研究[J]. 中国实验方剂学杂志,2013,19(8):153

夏至,李家美,张红瑞,等. 中药材菊花和野菊花的DNA条形码鉴定研究[J]. 时珍国医国药,2013,24(8):1902

肖宇奇,萨日娜,孙宇靖,等. 不同生长年限当归化学成分的动态变化分析[J]. 中成药,2013,35(3):588

邢志霞,崔燕兵,刘伟. HPTLC法测定不同产地硫熏和烘干金银花中绿原酸含量[J]. 中国医药导报,2013,10(6):98

徐敏,吴生,刘小霞,等. 秦岭地区华中五味子SSR遗传多样性分析[J]. 中药材,2013,36(8):1215

徐旭栋,蒋瑞彬,蓝小明,等. 人工栽培铁皮石斛种质资源遗传多样性的SCoT分析[J]. 中华中医药杂志,2013,28(7):2123

宣志红,浦锦宝,梁卫青. 不同采收时期杜仲叶中活性成分变化规律的研究[J]. 中华中医药学刊,2013,31(6):1336

宣志红,寿辉,姚琥,等. 不同干燥加工与贮藏方法对杜仲叶药材质量变化的研究[J]. 中草药,2013,44(11):1431

Y

严瑞娟,张水寒,罗跃龙,等. 不同产地初加工方式处理杜仲叶的HPTLC指纹图谱研究[J]. 中草药,2013,44(14):2085

阳翠,刘萍,刘姣蓉,等. 苦豆子ISSR标记的遗传多样性分析[J]. 中草药,2013,44(10):1323

杨路存,周国英,聂学敏. 濒危植物宽叶羌活天然居群cpDNA非编码区多态性分析[J]. 西北植物学报,2013,33(8):1535

杨全,李书渊,程轩轩,等. 广金钱草资源调查与药材质量评价[J]. 中国实验方剂学杂志,2013,19(3):147

杨舒婷,龚华栋,赵云鹏,等. 产地与种源对白术药材质量的影响[J]. 中药材,2013,36(6):890

杨先国,陈斌,刘塔斯,等. 航天搭载丹参的植物学特征、质量评价及化学指纹图谱研究(英文)[J]. 中华中医药杂志,2013,28(10):2932

杨贤松. 银杏叶片生长过程中的叶绿素荧光动力学研究[J]. 中药材,2013,36(1):1

杨小萍. 秦艽丰产栽培技术[J]. 农业科技与信息,2013,(5):23

杨小艳,李敏,卢道会,等. 不同干燥方法对半夏质量的影响[J]. 成都中医药大学学报,2013,36(3):18

杨欣,刘成,金晓飞. 3种大宗中药材中二氧化硫残留量的测定[J]. 江西中医学院学报,2013,25(3):63

易骏,廖芳平,郑伟文. 不同种质来源孩儿参的rDNAITS区序列分析及鉴别[J]. 中草药,2013,44(10):1318.

余晓丹,蒋超,黄璐琦,等. 红白忍冬SABATH甲基转移酶基因克隆及其生物信息学分析[J]. 中国中药杂志,2013,38(16):2556

Z

Zhao ZJ, Song YG, Liu YL, et al. The effect of elicitors on oleanolic acid accumulation and expression of triterpenoid synthesis genes in *Gentiana straminea* [J]. Biologia Plantarum, 2013, 57(1): 139

曾烨,王学奎,薛翔楠,等. 湖北利川黄连不同生长龄期主要生物碱的分布及变化[J]. 中国实验方剂学杂志,2013,19(11):123

张灿,段树卿,李云霞,等. 颈复康颗粒中羌活、秦艽的鉴别研究[J]. 承德医学院学报,2013,30(6):460

张丹,晋小军,赵洁,等. 硫黄熏制对黄芪中二氧化硫残留量的影响[J]. 时珍国医国药,2013,24(9):2146

张岗,赵明明,张大为,等.铁皮石斛钙依赖蛋白激酶基因的分子克隆及特征分析[J].中国药学杂志,2013,48(12):958

张海弢,包京姗,杨世海,等.王不留行毛状根的诱导及培养[J].中国实验方剂学杂志,2013,19(6):141

张倩,朱育凤.常用中药饮片中二氧化硫残留量的测定[J].中国医院用药评价与分析,2013,13(6):541

张薇,王建军,魏翔,等.AFLP标记对灯盏花遗传多样性及选育品系群体一致性的分析[J].中国中药杂志,2013,38(14):2245

张维瑞,韩远记,薛愧玲,等.河南益母草野生居群遗传多样性的SCoT分析[J].中草药,2013,44(8):1022

张祎楠,裴瑾,马云桐,等.四川产栽培川牛膝遗传多样性的ISSR分析[J].中成药,2013,35(8):1724

张义生,张南方,周才新,等.彭银亭炮制山药工艺二氧化硫残留量比较分析[J].中国医院药学杂志,2013,33(17):1455

赵明明,张岗,宋超,等.铁皮石斛种子接菌共生萌发抑制差减杂交文库的构建及序列分析[J].中国药学杂志,2013,48(5):341

赵能武,黄静,杨理明,等.雷公山保护区药用蕨类植物资源调查[J].中国实验方剂学杂志,2013,19(15):156

郑锡任,张龙,陈勇,等.不同采收期山绿茶药材绿原酸和芦丁的含量比较[J].中国实验方剂学杂志,2013,19(18):65

钟虹敏,张华,尚妍.中药材硫黄熏蒸检测方法[J].世界科学技术(中医药现代化),2013,15(4):685

周涛,谢宇,张丽艳,等.基于SCAR分子标记的头花蓼分子鉴定研究[J].中国中药杂志,2013,38(16):2577

周铜水.丹参的主要活性成分丹酚酸B是采后干燥胁迫诱导的产物[J].中国现代中药,2013,15(3):211

周亚兴,查云盛.兰坪县不同生长年限粗茎秦艽龙胆苦苷含量的比较研究[J].中国民族民间医药,2013,22(11):13

朱田田,晋玲,杜弢,等.甘肃不同产地中麻黄遗传关系的ISSR分析[J].中药材,2013,36(9):1397

朱雪妍,罗轶,黄捷,等.离子色谱法测定中药材中二氧化硫的含量[J].中国药师,2013,16(9):1330

(二) 中药质量评价

【概述】

2013年,随着中药化学、药理、分析等学科的不断进步,特别是新型分析仪器和手段的飞速发展,使中药药效物质基础研究、分析方法研究、质量标准研究等取得了长足的进步,中药质量标准控制和评价水平不断提高。

1. 基于药效物质基础的中药质量评价

中药质量控制和标准的制定采用性状、显微、理化鉴别和生物检定等四大鉴定方法进行真伪鉴别,并选择单一或数个指标成分进行含量测定,以达到控制其有效性的目的。随着中药有效成分研究的不断深入,基于药效物质基础的质量评价方法已成为越来越重要的手段。

桑白皮为常用中药,《中国药典》(2010年版)中仅有以桑白皮药材为对照的薄层色谱(TLC)鉴别,难以有效控制其质量。桑白皮主要成分为黄酮和生物碱类化合物。异戊烯基黄酮类成分桑根酮C、D具有明显的降血压、抑菌等作用,1-脱氧野尻霉素是一种多羟基哌啶类生物碱,具有α-葡萄糖苷酶抑制活性和降血糖等作用。段志涛等以桑根酮D为指标成分建立了该药材的TLC鉴别方法,以桑根酮C、D和1-脱氧野尻霉素为指标成分建立了该药材的含量测定方法,使桑白皮药材、饮片的质量控制标准得到提升。

百部为百部科植物直立百部 *Stemona sessilifolia* (Miq.)Miq.、蔓生百部 *Stemona japonica* (Bl.)Miq. 或对叶百部 *Stemona tuberosa* Lour. 的干燥块根。由于三种百部的化学成分种间差别较大,导致百部的质量标准仅有试管反应的控制要求。原百部碱为直立百部中主要的生物碱类成分,具有较强的镇咳活性。宗镇等以原百部碱为指标性成分,建立了含量测定方法,可用于直立百部药材的质量控制。

蓼大青叶具有清热解毒的功效,靛蓝、靛玉红为其药效物质基础成分。徐珊珊等以靛蓝、靛玉红为指标性成分建立了高效薄层色谱(HPTLC)鉴别方法和以靛蓝为指标性成分建立了HPTLC含量测定方法,并用梯度洗脱色谱条件,采用单因素循环法对该含量测定方法进行了耐用性验证。

秋水仙碱是秋水仙中主要药效物质,具有抗痛风、抗肿瘤、抗肝炎等多种药理作用。李岩等以秋水仙碱为指标性成分建立了秋水仙药材的HPTLC含量测定方法,为秋水仙药材的质量控制提供了依据。

齿瓣石斛 *Dendrobium devonianum* Paxt. 的干燥茎经加工制成的枫斗称紫皮枫,是枫斗的主要来源之一,其种植、加工已成为云南龙陵地区的支柱产业,但目前尚无质量标准。甘小娜等在系统的生药学研究基础上,建立了齿瓣石斛的性状、显微、TLC鉴别方法,并采用硫酸-苯酚法测定其多糖的含量。

韭菜子为百合科植物韭菜 *Allium tuberosum* Rottl. ex Spreng. 的干燥成熟种子,具有温补肝肾,壮阳固精作用,临床用于肝肾亏虚,腰膝酸痛,阳痿遗精,遗尿尿频,白浊带下等症。目前,《中国药典》(2010年版)中仅有性状鉴别,难以控制其品质。韭菜子主要含有硫化物、核苷类、黄酮类、生物碱类等化学成分,但是特征性成分硫化物的含量很低,不能达到药材质量控制的最低检测要求;核苷类与黄酮类成分的专属性不强,在种子中的含量也比较低。而亚油酸有抑制肿瘤、调节脂质代谢、抑制脂肪沉积、促进生长发育等多种功能,是韭菜子的温补肝肾作用的药效物质基础之一。徐红等对韭菜子进行了系统的生药学研究,建立了韭菜子性状、显微鉴别方法,并以亚油酸为指标性成分建立了TLC鉴别方法,完善了韭菜子药材的质量标准。

王永丽等发现,艾叶经炒炭法炮制成醋艾炭或艾炭后,生成间羟基安息香酸,艾叶本身不含有此成分。该化合物具有杀菌、防腐作用。文献报道艾叶炮制成艾炭、醋艾炭后,其止血作用增强,可以推测其止血作用可能与产生间羟基安息香酸等物质有关。所以可用间羟基安息香酸为指标性成分,建立了醋艾炭的含量测定方法。

消炎利胆片由穿心莲、苦木和溪黄草3味中药组成,具有清热、祛湿、利胆的功效,临床上广泛应用于肝胆湿热引起的口苦、胁痛、急性胆囊炎、胆管炎等。《中国药典》(2010 年版)仅有以穿心莲对照药材、穿心莲内酯、脱水穿心莲内酯为指标成分的 TLC 定性鉴别,以溪黄草对照药材、苦木对照药材为对照的 TLC 鉴别;含量测定项也仅有以穿心莲内酯、脱水穿心莲内酯为指标成分的 HPTLC 含量测定方法,难以全面反映其内在质量。4-甲氧基-5-羟基-铁屎米酮为苦木药材的主要特征性成分,具有抗菌、抗炎等作用。杨娜等以4-甲氧基-5-羟基-铁屎米酮为指标性成分,建立了消炎利胆片的 TLC 鉴别和 HPTLC 含量测定方法,为苦木药材、饮片和消炎利胆片制剂质量标准的提升奠定了基础。

2. TLC-生物自显影技术在中药质量控制和活性评价中的应用

TLC-生物自显影技术是一种将 TLC 分离技术与活性检测相结合的快速活性筛选和质量控制方法,目前已应用于中药材抗氧化、抗菌、抑制胆碱酯酶等生物活性的筛选与测定。该技术可以弥补一般 TLC 的不足,不仅可以反映样品间的化学成分的差异,更能反映 TLC 上获得分离的成分间活性的强弱,且操作简单、耗费低、灵敏度和专属性高,便于普及。

在《中国药典》(2010 年版)中,已将 TLC-生物自显影技术应用于紫苏子、地黄等药材的鉴别。

谷丽华等基于 TLC-生物自显影技术,建立了一种采用 2,2-氨基-二(3-乙基-苯并噻唑啉-6-磺酸)二铵盐(ABTS)对中药材自由基清除能力的活性进行筛选、评价的方法。并利用该方法筛选了不同来源的肉苁蓉和灯盏花样品清除 ABTS 自由基活性。

韩松林等利用该技术,经薄层扫描获得各抗氧化成分的峰面积,从而对 2 种洋甘菊(母菊和罗马洋甘菊)的挥发油提取物、黄酮提取物进行 DPPH 自由基清除活性分析,以总峰面积大小为指标比较不同提取物的抗氧化能力,并与 2 种洋甘菊黄酮提取物总的抗氧化活性进行比较。结果,母菊黄酮提取物显现芹菜素、芹苷元-7-葡萄糖苷等 7 个淡黄色抗氧化斑点,罗马洋甘菊黄酮提取物显现芹菜素、芹苷元-7-葡萄糖苷等 8 个淡黄色抗氧化斑点,薄层扫描表明罗马洋甘菊黄酮提取物抗氧化斑点峰面积大于母菊黄酮提取物。闫瑞卿等运用 TLC-生物自显影方法,快速筛选 17 个化合物的清除 DPPH 自由基活性,结果显示金丝桃苷、咖啡酸、儿茶酚、绿原酸具有较强的清除 DPPH 自由基的活性。郭金凤等同样利用此方法,初步筛选出榆叶合叶子的黄酮类成分具有抗氧化活性,并发现榆叶合叶子中的绣线菊苷、金丝桃苷、芦丁、槲皮素都具有抗氧化活性。

乙酰胆碱酯酶抑制剂是目前治疗阿尔兹海默症(AD)的一线药物,对轻、中度 AD 具有较好效果。对 TLC-生物自显影技术建立的乙酰胆碱酯酶(AChE)抑制活性的方法已有较多研究,党朵等采用 TLC-生物自显影法,对从秦艽中分离到的 2 个化合物进行了 AChE 抑制活性筛选,结果显示都具有一定抑制活性。张春梅等利用此方法,对从束骨姜黄植物分离到的化合物进行 AChE 抑制活性筛选,发现郁金二酮、花侧柏烯有一定的抑制活性。陈萍等对香薷、益智仁、生地黄和荷叶等 4 种中药的乙醇提取物进行活性筛选,结果显示均有一定的 AChE 的抑制活性。

谢谦等采用 TLC-生物自显影技术筛选抗炭疽病菌中药及其成分,发现白芷的乙酸乙酯提取物表现出较强的抗真菌活性,并从乙酸乙酯部位分离得到了 4 个具有抗真菌活性的香豆素化合物,即 suberosin、bergapten、alloimperatorin 和 xanthotoxol。

3. 中药安全性评价

中药毒副作用较小,但许多中医古代文献中均提到"毒"即"药",认为凡治病之药皆为毒药。如《神农本草经》记载:"神农尝百草,日遇七十二毒,得茶而解之"。《中国药典》(2010 年版)将有毒中药分为大毒、有毒、小毒 3 级。因此,建立"有毒"中药中毒性成分的定性、定量分析方法,制定含量限度,十分必要。

附子中双酯型生物碱(DAs)和单酯型生物碱(MAs)成分都有一定的毒性。温瑞卿等比较两类成分在生附片和不同附子炮制品中含量差异,结果发现 MAs 对大鼠的毒性至少是 DAs 的 1/64～1/180;炮制后 DAs 含量下降至生品的 1/76.5～1/38.3,而 MAs 含量增加 4.6～5.2 倍或与生品基本持平;炮制品的 MAs/DAs 值较生品提高 30～390 倍,说明附子炮制减毒的原理是合理的。唐小龙等研究了干热烘制和湿热蒸制对附子 6 种酯型生物碱含量的影响,发现两种炮制方法均使得毒性双酯型生物碱含量显著降低,相比于直接用水浸泡、煎煮等处理，可避免总生物碱等有效成分的流失。

程丽丽等采用一测多评法同时定量测定乌头类药材中6种乌头类生物碱的含量，以乌头碱为内标，测定其与次乌头碱、新乌头碱、苯甲酰乌头原碱、苯甲酰次乌头原碱、苯甲酰新乌头原碱的相对校正因子，利用乌头碱和相对校正因子对其他5种生物碱成分进行测定。

硫黄熏蒸中药材，对中药材的养护和储藏起到了一定的积极作用，然而也一直有争议。段煜等综述了近20年的文献，认为硫黄熏蒸养护方法不应该完全摒弃，而是要选择性的传承，提出了对硫黄熏蒸药材进行再评价和积极寻找硫黄熏蒸的替代方法等建议。

4. 中药特征指纹图谱技术的应用

中药指纹图谱是基于对中药物质群整体作用的认识，是实现鉴别中药真实性、评价质量一致性和产品稳定性的可行模式，具有信息量大、特征性强、整体性和模糊性等特点。

高新彪等建立了牡丹皮的HPTLC指纹图谱，运用高分辨LC-MS/MS技术，对20个共有峰中的18个色谱峰进行了定性鉴别。马鸿雁等建立了苦参中黄酮类成分HPTLC的指纹图谱，标定了13个共有色谱峰，并采用对照品指认了5个主要色谱峰，4批同属近缘种山豆根与苦参黄酮对照图谱明显不同。王丹等采用HPTLC指纹图谱方法对不同产地及生长条件黄芩中的化学成分进行检测，采用系统聚类分析、主成分分析及成分组峰面积模式对指纹谱数据进行评价，从而阐明道地、非道地黄芩的化学成分差异。研究发现道地药材与非道地药材指纹谱轮廓特征明显不同，道地药材的黄芩样品指纹谱特征明显区别于其他产地。

超高效液相色谱(UPLC)法具有分析速度快、分离度好、所需流动相少等优点。马天成等建立了川芎的UPLC指纹图谱，标定了18个共有峰，结合保留时间和紫外光谱分析，标识了咖啡酸、香草醛、阿魏酸、洋川芎内酯Ⅰ、洋川芎内酯H、丁基苯酞、藁本内酯和丁烯基苯酞的峰位。洪燕等建立了26个产地苍耳子药材UPLC指纹图谱，确定了19个共有峰，标识了9个峰。邓少东等比较了UPLC法与HPTLC法对化橘红总黄酮指纹图谱的效果，结果UPLC法标识出21个共有峰(8 min)，HPTLC法标识出17个共有峰(80 min)，表明UPLC法具有高效、快速、灵敏、节省溶剂等优点。

（胡海军　王峥涛）

【分子鉴定技术在药用植物研究中的应用】

1. 山茱萸

Hou DY等对山茱萸及其混伪品(山荆子、甘肃荚蒾、滇刺枣、酸枣、枣、苦楝果)的ITS序列进行测序及分析。结果，山茱萸药材的ITS序列长度均为659 bp，种内变异较小，平均K2P遗传距离为0.005，远小于其与混伪品的种间平均K2P遗传距离0.357。不同来源的山茱萸药材ITS2序列无变异，长度均为250 bp，与混伪品的种间平均K2P遗传距离为0.571。ITS/ITS2序列的NJ系统聚类树和BLAST比对结果均可明显区分山茱萸药材及其混伪品，表现出良好的单系性。

2. 人参

Chen XC等基于常用DNA条形码序列(ITS2，*matK*和*psbA*-*trnH*)对4种人参属植物(人参、西洋参、竹节参、三七)共377条序列进行比较分析。结果，在ITS2区检测到5个稳定的单核苷酸多态性SNP位点，可用于鉴定人参属药用植物；对于人参和西洋参的混合粉末，可在SNP位点检测到明显的双峰，并根据峰的高度大致确定混合的比例。表明SNP的分子条形码可作为鉴定人参属与近缘物种以及人参、西洋参混合粉末的常规方法。

3. 半夏

郑丹书等对半夏16个主要分布区收集到的43种半夏，及福建泰宁的滴水珠和江苏南京的虎掌半夏2个近缘种，采用PCR法克隆并分析叶片基因组DNA中*psb*K-*psb*I和*atp*F-*atp*H两段序列。结果，半夏*atp*F-*atp*H序列长为337～342 bp，仅含变异位点7个，其中信息位点1个；*psb*K-*psb*I序列长为432～435 bp，变异位点37个，其中信息位点17个；聚类分析均显示出与表型以及地理居群的不一致。表明*psb*K-*psb*I序列较*atp*F-*atp*H在半夏种内具有较丰富的变异位点，能对半夏进行鉴别及遗传多样性分析。

4. 孩儿参

易骏等利用特异性引物进行PCR扩增、克隆和测序，对不同产地孩儿参的ITS区间碱基序列进行测定。结果，9个不同种质来源孩儿参的整个ITS长度为623～624 bp，ITS1、5.8S、ITS2分别为224 bp、155 bp、244～245 bp，整个ITS区共有17个变异位点，ITS1、ITS2和5.8S的变异位点分别为7、7和3个，不同种质来源的孩儿参均有若干个特异性的单核苷酸变异位点，各样品的序列同源性均在99.9%以上。表明不同产地、不同种质的孩儿参变异是不超过1个种范围内的变异，可利用ITS区序列差异，鉴别不同种质来源的孩儿参。

5. 桃仁

林韵涵等对桃仁(桃、山桃)及其近缘种(扁桃、郁李、杏)的ITS2核基因片段进行扩增和双向测序，分析相关数据并构建NJ树。结果，桃仁两基原物种ITS2序列长度为212～213 bp，序列变异较小；两基原物种ITS2序列与近缘种的种间平均K2P遗传距离大于其种内平均K2P遗传距离；由NJ树可知，桃仁的两基原物种聚为一枝，并与其他近缘种明显分开。

6. 紫苏

夏至等对紫苏属白苏及其变种(紫苏、野生紫苏、回回苏和耳齿紫苏)的ITS和*psbA-trnH*序列进行测序及分析。结果，MP系统树显示不同地域的紫苏和白苏样本聚为一单系分支，紫苏与回回苏构成姐妹群分支，野生紫苏和耳齿紫苏构成一单系分支(支持率均大于90%)，白苏、紫苏与其他变种间的ITS和*psbA-trnH*序列遗传距离明显大于白苏与紫苏间遗传距离，大于各变种内遗传距离。表明白苏和紫苏可合并为一个种紫苏，紫苏与回回苏亲缘关系最近，野生紫苏与耳齿紫苏亲缘关系最近。

7. 党参

赵莎等研究了党参药材及其混伪品(脉花党参、轮叶党参、新疆党参、金钱豹、小花金钱豹、防风、迷果芹)的33份药材样本，提取基因组DNA，通过PCR扩增ITS序列，进行序列比对与分析。结果，党参药材3个基原物种(党参、素花党参、川党参)ITS序列长度为654～655 bp，ITS2序列长度均为239 bp，ITS/ITS2序列种内平均K2P遗传距离均远小于其与混伪品的种间平均K2P遗传距离，可成功用于党参药材的鉴别。

8. 悬钩子

蒋明等测定并分析了15种悬钩子属药用植物的ITS序列。结果，其ITS1、ITS2和5.8S的序列长度分别为255～258、208～211和164 bp，5.8 S序列的长度十分保守，但在碱基组成上存在一定的差异；ITS1和ITS2序列长度及碱基组成变异较5.8 S大存在较多的缺失/插入、转换和颠换现象，信息位点丰富，可用于区分15种悬钩子属植物。

9. 盘龙参

李家敏等根据ITS区序列设计引物，对盘龙参样本进行PCR扩增，扩增产物克隆并测序，进行软件分析。结果，扩增得到的rDNA ITS片段总长为667 bp，ITS变异位点比率为17.10%，信息化位点比率为6.56%，通过ITS序列构建系统树进行聚类分析表明，ITS序列在绶草属种内是保守的，可作为中药盘龙参分子鉴定标记。

10. 鼓槌石斛

郑司浩等建立了一种特异性鉴别鼓槌石斛的方法，运用该特异性引物可实现从同源物种中快速、准确地鉴定出鼓槌石斛，具有特异性好、操作简便、高效、准确等优点。具体方法：从GenBank数据库中下载石斛属ITS序列170余条，对所有序列进行同源性比较，找出各变异位点，在非保守区设计1对特异性引物。对35份石斛属植物DNA模板进行特异性引物PCR扩增，将退火温度升至58℃时，鼓槌石斛能被该引物特异性地扩增，而其他石斛属植物均为阴性，且该引物的灵敏度可达到0.69 ng/μl。

(倪梁红)

【电子鼻在中药材品质评价中的应用】

电子鼻又称气味指纹分析仪，是利用气敏传感器阵列的响应图谱来识别气味的电子系统。近年来电子鼻已应用于中药材品质评价研究，通过分析、识别、检测复杂气味和挥发性成分，对中药材真伪、商品等级、产地、采收期、贮藏有效期进行判别，是中药材质量控制的一种新的手段与方法，有气味指纹图谱技术之称。

1. 中药材真伪鉴别

日本学者御影雅幸等较早采用气味传感器，

以水晶振动子检测器(配有 183AK、453AA、151AJ、112AJ、353AN 5 种传感器元件)对第 14 版日本药局方收载的 97 种市售生药进行了质量评价,表明气味传感器可以鉴别白色无臭茯苓、牡蛎、龙骨粉末等。邹慧琴等采用电子鼻对姜科 10 味常用中药(干姜、姜黄、高良姜等)进行气味检测,基于逐步判别分析法和聚类分析结合典型指标筛选法,建立了中药鉴别中电子鼻传感器阵列的优化方法。

2. 中药材等级与产区评价

现行川芎药材商品规格标准分为一、二、三等级及俗称小川芎的芎苓子等外级(作兽药或香料用)。陈林等采用电子鼻,通过 Alpha SOFTTV l2 软件对所获得的川芎 4 个产地 18 个批次药材样品数据进行主成分分析和判别因子分析。结果表明,同一产地不同等级川芎挥发性组分整体性质接近,难以区分;但可以区分同一产地川芎药材与芎苓子等外级和川芎传统产区与新兴产区的商品药材。

3. 中药产地鉴别

由于气候条件的差异,不同产地的同种中药化学成分有一定差异,某些挥发性成分的差异会导致中药气味的变化。伍世元等研究在自然态下采用 PEN3 电子鼻鉴别不同产地的薄荷,结果对其未知样品的识别率可达到 100%。韩邦兴等利用电子鼻技术评价大白菊气味的整体信息,区分不同产地的大白菊。邵雅雯等利用电子鼻对 3 种产地的白术样品进行检测,结果 3 种产地白术可以被正确鉴别,对所测样本的正确识别率达到 97.80%。

4. 中药采收期的研究

药用植物在生长发育不同时期,有效成分含量处于动态变化中,利用电子鼻检测不同采收期中药材样品的挥发性成分动态变化,可为中药材科学采收提供依据。蔡泳等研究不同采收期金樱子气味指纹变化,不同采收期金樱子样品根据挥发性成分聚类,以 10 月下旬采收时间为界,明显聚为两类。伍世元等报道,利用电子鼻检测可区分不同采收期的阳春砂。韩邦兴等采用电子鼻检测开花前后两种前胡样品气味在传感器上的响应值,其气味变化反应灵敏,可以完全区分。

5. 中药贮存有效期的评价

熊吟等探讨了基于电子感官技术的中药贮存有效期评价方法。认为中药贮存有效期的确定一直是中药质量评价研究领域里的难点和盲点,将电子鼻引入中药的“储藏年限”、“有效期”研究是一个很好的切入点,对科学有效地制订中药贮存有效期评价标准是一种新的尝试。邹慧琴等采用 α - FOX3000 电子鼻对不同贮藏时间(1 年和 3 年)西洋参进行气味检测,并结合多层感知器网络识别技术建立判别模型;通过十折交叉验证和外部测试集验证对所建模型进行系统性能的评估。结果表明,该模型对不同贮藏时间西洋参具有较高的回判正确率(均为 100%),优化前后的传感器阵列均能实现对不同贮藏时间西洋参的鉴别。

(陈建伟　李　祥)

[附]　参 考 文 献

C

Chen XC, Liao BS, Song JY, et al. A fast SNP identification and analysis of intraspecific variation in the medicinal *Panax* species based on DNA barcoding[J]. Gene, 2013, 530(1): 39

Cheng Z, Wu T. TLC bioautography: high throughput technique for screening of bioactive natural products [J]. Combinatorial Chemistry & High Throughput screening, 2013, 16(7): 531

蔡泳,王盛,黄孙娟,等.基于金属氧化物传感器阵列电子鼻技术的不同采收期金樱子气味分析[J].中华中医药杂志,2011,26(6):1433

陈林,刘友平,陈鸿平,等.电子鼻在川芎不同产地不同等级评价中的应用[J].中药与临床,2013,4(4):7

陈萍,王培培,邵国华,等.48 种中药材的乙酰胆碱酯酶抑制活性研究(英文)[J]. Journal of Chinese Pharmaceutical Sciences, 2013, 22(1): 106

程丽丽,许妍妍,ERIC N,等.一测多评法测定乌头类药材中生物碱[J].现代药物与临床,2013,28(4):528

D

党朵,杨中铎,梁冀北.秦艽花中乙酰胆碱酯酶抑制

剂的分离及结构鉴定[J]. 中医药学报,2013,41(3)：16

邓少东,王莲婧,林励,等. 化橘红黄酮类成分 UPLC 与 HPTLC 指纹图谱的比较研究[J]. 中草药,2013,44(9)：1195

段煜,秦昆明,邹娜姝,等. 中药材的硫黄熏蒸养护方法——摒弃还是传承[J]. 中国中药杂志,2013,42(19)：3395

段志涛,高英,周刚. 桑白皮药材的质量标准研究[J]. 中药材,2013,36(4)：553

G

甘小娜,徐英,徐红,等. 紫皮石斛的质量标准研究[J]. 中国中药杂志,2013,38(23)：4113

高新彪,孙磊,乔善义,等. 牡丹皮 HPTLC 指纹图谱研究[J]. 中草药,2013,44(7)：900

谷丽华,俞桂新,王峥涛. 基于 ABTS 自由基的薄层色谱—生物自显影新方法的建立及其在中药抗氧化活性评价中的应用[J]. 上海中医药大学学报,2013,27(3)：99

郭金凤,张俊妹,张芳,等. TLC-生物自显影法筛选榆叶合叶子的抗氧化活性[J]. 中国民族民间医药,2013,22(24)：9

H

Hou DY, Song JY, Yao H, et al. Molecular identification of Corni Fructus and its adulterants by ITS/ITS2 sequences[J]. 中国天然药物,2013,11(2)：121

韩邦兴,陈乃富,周晓坤,等. 基于电子鼻技术分析开花对前胡气味的影响[J]. 食品科学,2010,31(4)：132

韩邦兴,赵杨阳,朱志祥,等. 基于电子鼻技术的不同产地大白菊鉴别研究[J]. 现代中药研究与实践,2012,26(1)：16

韩松林,李新霞,勉强辉,等. 薄层生物自显影技术比较新疆 2 种洋甘菊抗氧化活性[J]. 中国中药杂志,2013,38(2)：193

洪燕,韩燕全,夏伦祝,等. 不同产地苍耳子 UPLC 指纹图谱研究[J]. 中国中药杂志,2013,38(11)：1766

J

蒋明,李嵘嵘,管铭,等. 悬钩子属植物 rDNA ITS 序列的克隆与分析[J]. 中草药,2013,44(14)：2143

L

李家敏,喻鹏. 中药盘龙参 ITS 的序列分子鉴定研究[J]. 种子,2013,32(8)：28

李岩,李晓静,程雪梅,等. HPTLC 法测定秋水仙药材中秋水仙碱[J]. 中成药,2013,35(1)：203

林韵涵,刘霞,胡志刚,等. 基于 ITS2 序列鉴定桃仁及其近缘种[J]. 世界科学技术(中医药现代化),2013,15(3)：429

M

马鸿雁,周婉珊,褚夫江,等. 苦参中黄酮类成分的高效液相指纹图谱及 5 种成分的含量测定[J]. 中国中药杂志,2013,38(16)：2690

马天成,崔思娇,张靓琦,等. 川芎的 UPLC 指纹图谱研究[J]. 中国药房,2013,24(15)：1389

S

邵雅雯,骆德汉,武琳,等. 基于最大散度差准则 LDA 的电子鼻中药材鉴别方法[J]. 仪表技术与传感器,2011,(11)：80

T

唐小龙,易进海,夏燕莉,等. 不同炮制方法对附子 6 种酯型生物碱含量的影响[J]. 中国实验方剂学杂志,2013,19(21)：96

W

王丹,张秋燕,杨兴鑫,等. 基于 HPTLC 指纹图谱的黄芩道地药材与非道地药材的鉴别研究[J]. 中国中药杂志,2013,38(12)：1951

王永丽,尉小慧,赵森森,等. HPTLC 测定醋艾炭间羟基安息香酸的含量[J]. 中国实验方剂学杂志,2013,19(18)：78

温瑞卿,李东辉,赵昕,等. 基于化学分析的毒性中药附子炮制方法的合理性研究[J]. 药学学报,2013,48(2)：286

伍世元,骆德汉,邓炳荣,等. 不同产地和采收期的中药材电子鼻鉴别研究[J]. 传感技术学报,2011,24(1)：10

X

夏至,李贺敏,张红瑞,等. 紫苏及其变种的分子鉴定和亲缘关系研究[J]. 中草药,2013,44(8)：1027

谢谦,李顺祥,江星明,等. 生物活性指导下的白芷中抗真菌香豆素的分离[A]. 2013 全国中药与天然药物高峰论坛暨第十三届全国中药和天然药物学术研讨会论文集[C],2013,64

熊吟,赵婷,闫永红,等. 基于电子感官技术的中药贮存有效期评价方法探讨[J]. 现代中药研究与实践,2013,26(1)：69

徐红,董婷霞,林燕靖,等. 韭菜子的生药学研究[J]. 中国药房,2013,24(3)：246

徐珊珊,李清,王新丽,等. 蓼大青叶质量标准的研究(英文)[J]. 中国药学,2013,22(5)：415

Y

闫瑞卿,张晓拢,孙洁,等. 吴茱萸化学成分清除 DPPH

自由基的活性研究[J]. 天津中医药,2013,30(5): 301

杨娜,郑程,郭夫江,等. 消炎利胆片中 4-甲氧基-5-羟基-铁屎米酮的定性定量方法研究[J]. 药物分析杂志,2013,33(12): 2166

易骏,廖芳平,郑伟文. 不同种质来源孩儿参的 rDNA ITS区序列分析及鉴别[J]. 中草药,2013,44(10): 1318

御影雅幸,田邉牧,新村春香,等. 使用气味传感器对生药质量进行评价[J]. Natural Medicines,2005,59(2): 63

Z

张春梅,王继达,张永睿思,等. 束骨姜黄化学成分及其乙酰胆碱酯酶抑制活性[J]. 山东大学学报(理学版),2013,48(7): 20

赵莎,辛天怡,侯典云,等. 党参药材及其混伪品的 ITS/ITS2 条形码鉴定研究[J]. 世界科学技术(中医药现代化),2013,15(3): 421

郑丹书,张君毅,郭巧生. 半夏及近缘种叶绿体非编码区序列分析[J]. 中草药,2013,44(7): 881

郑司浩,黄林芳,陈士林. 鼓槌石斛特异性 PCR 分子鉴定[J]. 中草药,2013,44(6): 744

宗镇,班永生,张亚中,等. 直立百部质量标准研究[J]. 药物分析杂志,2013,33(12): 2188

邹慧琴,李硕,邢姝,等. 电子鼻技术结合 MLP 网络对不同贮藏时间西洋参的鉴别研究[J]. 中华中医药学刊,2013,31(7): 1683

邹慧琴,李硕,闫永红,等. 基于 RBF-RF 级联分类器电子鼻对中药的快速鉴别[J]. 世界科学技术(中医药现代化),2013,15(9): 1876

邹慧琴,刘勇,陶欧,等. 电子鼻 MOS 传感器阵列优化及其在中药材快速鉴别中的应用[J]. 中国中药杂志,2013,38(2): 161

(三)中药化学

【概述】

2013年,国内外主要医药学术期刊中,中国学者共发表有关中药及天然药物化学研究方面的论文1 000多篇。主要报道从常用中草药、民间草药、民族药物、海洋生物以及中药复方中分离得到的30 000多种化学成分,其中新化合物约3 000种。

1. 常用中药的化学成分研究

常用中药的化学成分研究占报道的40%左右,除大量首次发现的化合物外,新化合物、新骨架被不断发现。Yan YM 等从常用中药灵芝 *Ganoderma lucidum* 中分离得到一对具有旋转门式的杂萜类化合物,(+)-Lingzhiol 和(-)-lingzhiol,这一对新的对映体不仅具有新颖的骨架,同时还表现出良好的生理活性。金银花为忍冬科忍冬属植物忍冬 *Lonicera japonica* 的干燥花蕾,金银花的现代研究已有半个多世纪,已分离鉴定了包括绿原酸、裂环环烯醚萜苷、黄酮、皂苷、脑苷和多酚等不同结构类型的100多个化合物。王芳等对金银花水提取物进行了研究,从中发现了一系列强水溶性的裂环高环烯醚萜等新型活性成分。还对水提取后的药渣再用乙醇提取,并对提取物进行研究,从中分离鉴定了48种成分,除30种成分已有报道外,尚有18种化合物为首次从金银花中分离得到。

Kuo WL 等从厚朴 *Magnolia officinalis* 中分离得到 5-allyl-5′-(1″-hydroxyallyloxy) biphenyl-2,2′-diol、5,5′-diallyl-2′-(allyloxy) biphenyl-2-ol、5,5′-diallyl-2′-(3-methylbut-2-enyloxy)biphenyl-2-ol、(*E*)-5-allyl-3′-(prop-1-enyl) biphenyl-2,4′-diol、4-allyl-2-(2′-methylbenzofuran-5′-yl)phenol 等5种新的联苯型新木脂素。Xiang Z 等从西洋参 *Panax quinquefolium* 中分离出 seudo-ginsenoside RT_6、pseudoginsengenin R_1、3*β*, 6*α*, 20*S*-trihydroxy-12*β*,23*R*-epoxy dammar-24-ene6-*O*-[α-L-rhamnosyl(1→2)-*β*-D-glucopyranosyl]-20-*O*-*β*-D-glucopyranoside、3*β*,20*S*-dihydroxy-12*β*,23*R*-epoxydammar-24-ene 3-*O*-[*β*-D-glucopyranosyl(1→2)-*β*-D-glucopyranosyl]-20-*O*-*β*-D-glucopyranoside 4种新的达玛烷型皂苷。Chaudhuri PK 等从莲 *Nelumbo nucifera* 的根茎中分离得到一种新的化合物 2*α*, 24-diacetoxy-3*β*-hydroxyolean-12-en-28-oic acid。

2. 民族药、民间药的化学成分研究

薰鲁香(Mastich),为漆树科植物黏胶乳香树 *Pistacia lentiscus* 的树脂,主产于地中海一带,是维吾尔医临床常用的进口药材,Gao JB 等从薰鲁香中分离得到14种化合物,其中 amauroamoienin 为新化合物。兰科绶草属植物敖朗黑布(绶草) *Spiranthes sinensis* 是一种蒙药,Li CY 等从中分离出一种新的菲二聚体:2,2′-dihydroxy-5,5′,7,7′-tetramethoxy-9,9′,10,10′-tetrahydro-3,3′-biphenanthrene,和一种新的黄酮:5-hydroxy-3,7-dimethoxy-4′-(1-hydroxy-3-methylbut-3-en-2-yloxy)-flavone。

Liu JY 等从蒙药金莲花 *Trollius chinensis* 的花中分离得到12种化合物,其中有两种黄酮C-糖苷为新化合物:6‴-(3-hydroxy-3-methylglutaroyl)-2″-*O*-*β*-D-galactopyranosyl orientin 和 6‴-(3-hydroxy-3-methylglutaroyl)-2″-*O*-*β*-D-galactopyranosyl vitexin。此外,7-methoxyl-2″-*O*-(3‴,4‴-dimethoxybenzoyl) vitexin 和 2″-*O*-(2‴-methylbutyryl) isoswertisin 是首次从金莲花属植物中得到。兰科植物竹叶兰 *Arundina gramnifolia* 是一味用于解毒的傣药,Hu QF 等从竹叶兰中提取到 gramniphenols C~G 等5个新化合物和8个已知化合物,其中化合物 gramniphenols C、F、G 具有抗烟草镶嵌病毒活性,化合物 gramniphenols D、E 具有抗 HIV-1 活性。

3. 中药的提取分离技术

近十余年来,中药化学研究领域中新技术、新

方法被广泛应用，如高速逆流技术、超临界流体萃取技术、膜分离技术、半仿生提取技术、超微粉碎技术、分子印迹技术、离子液体萃取技术，生物转化技术等均有报道。

（1）分子印迹技术　陈方方等报道，分子印迹技术是指以特定的分子为模板，制备对该分子有特殊识别功能和高选择性材料的技术。与传统色谱分离技术相比，具有分子识别性强、性质比较稳定、固定相制备简便、溶剂消耗量小、模板可回收再利用等优点。采用该技术富集、分离纯化中药活性成分已有报道，所分离纯化的成分有黄酮、多元酚、生物碱、甾体、香豆素等多种结构类型化合物，如衣丽娜等报道用分子印迹技术从中药粗提物中定向分离胡黄连苷Ⅱ。

（2）离子液体萃取技术　邵江娟等报道，离子液体萃取技术是指室温离子液体（由有机阳离子和无机或有机阴离子组成而不含电中性分子）的化合物利用色散作用、氢键作用、静电作用等分子间的作用力而实现萃取的技术。采用的方法有离子液体微波辅助萃取分离、离子液体超声强化萃取分离、离子液体双水相萃取分离、离子液体液-液萃取分离等，应用于中药研究领域，可成功分离黄酮类、酚酸类、生物碱类及萜类成分等。

（3）膜分离技术　徐龙泉等报道，膜分离技术是以选择性透过膜为分离介质，以外界能量或化学位差为推动力，对混合物中特定组分实现分离、提纯和浓缩的分离技术，在中药提取过程中除杂、中药有效成分的分离浓缩、中药浸膏、口服液、注射液的制备过程中都有广泛的应用。

（陈咏林　俞桂新）

【344种中草药中的新成分研究】

在中国天然药物、Journal of Asian Natural Products Research、Natural Product Research、Organic Letters、Phytochemistry、Planta Medica、Helvetica Chimica Acta、Journal of Natural Products、Molecules、Phytochemistry Letters 等10种期刊中，研究人员从344种中药和植物药中分离、鉴定了约1 400种新化合物。

344种中草药中的新成分研究

中药及其基源	新成分名称	分子式	报道者
1. 蜜环菌 *Armillaria mellea*	(*R*)-2-(2-(furan-2-yl)-oxoethyl)-octahydropyrrolo[1,2-*α*]pyrazine-1,4-dione	$C_{13}H_{14}N_2O_4$	Wang YC, et al
2. 厦门乌芝 *Amauroderma amoiensis*	amauroamoienin	$C_{46}H_{54}O_7$	Zhang S, et al
3. 樟芝 *Antrodia camphorata*	lucidenate A	$C_{29}H_{42}O_6$	Liaw CC, et al
	ethyl lucidenate F	$C_{29}H_{40}O_6$	
	15-*O*-acetylganolucidate A	$C_{32}H_{46}O_7$	
	3,11,15,23-tetraoxo-27ξ-lanosta-8,16-dien-26-oic acid	$C_{30}H_{40}O_7$	
	5-hydroxy-5-(methoxymethyl)-4-methylfuran-2(5*H*)-one	$C_7H_{10}O_4$	
	3-(4-methoxy-2-oxo-2*H*pyran-6-yl)propanoic acid	$C_9H_{10}O_5$	
	antrocamphin O	$C_{15}H_{16}O_4$	Chen PY, et al
4. 灵芝 *Ganoderma lucidum*	Lucidenates A	$C_{29}H_{42}O_6$	Li P, et al
	(+)-Lingzhiol	$C_{15}H_{14}O_6$	Yan YM, et al
	(−)-Lingzhiol	$C_{15}H_{14}O_6$	
5. 热带灵芝 *Ganoderma tropicum*	3*β*,7*β*,15*β*-trihydroxy-11,23-dioxo-lanost-8,16-dien-26-oic acid	$C_{30}H_{44}O_7$	Hu LL, et al
	3*β*,7*β*,15*β*-trihydroxy-11,23-dioxo-lanost-8,16-dien-26-oic acid methyl ester	$C_{31}H_{46}O_7$	
	3*β*,15*β*-dihydroxy-7,11,23-trioxo-lanost-8,16-dien-26-oic acid methyl ester	$C_{31}H_{44}O_7$	

续 表

中药及其基源	新成分名称	分子式	报道者
6. 海南灵芝 *Ganoderma hainanense*	16α,26 - dihydroxylanosta - 8,24 - dien - 3 - one	$C_{30}H_{48}O_3$	Ma QY, et al
7. 蕨 *Pteridium aquilinum*	2,3 - trans - 3,4 - trans - 5α,6,11α,12 - tetrahydro - 6,7 - dihydroxy -[1]benzopyrano[3,2 - β][1] benzopyran - 1 - carboxylic acid	$C_{22}H_{18}O_7$	Chen ND, et al
8. 笔直石松 *Lycopodium obscurum*	lycobscurines A	$C_{17}H_{25}NO_2$	Pan K, et al
	lycobscurines B	$C_{17}H_{25}NO_3$	
	lycobscurines C	$C_{17}H_{27}NO_2$	
9. 垂穗石松 *Palhinhaea cernua*	isopalhinine A	$C_{16}H_{21}NO_4$	Dong LB, et al
10. 地刷子石松 *Lycopodium complanatum*	lycospidine A	$C_{15}H_{21}NO_2$	Cheng JT, et al
11. 半边旗 *Pteris semipinnata*	6β,11α - dihydroxy - 15 - oxo - ent - kaur - 16 - en - 19 -oic acid	$C_{20}H_{28}O_5$	Bai R, et al
	7α,11α - dihydroxy - 15 - oxo - ent - kaur - 16 - en - 19 -oic acid	$C_{20}H_{28}O_5$	
12. 荚果蕨 *Matteuccia struthiopteris*	(2S)- 5,7 - dihydroxy - 6,8 - dimethyl - 4′- methoxydihydroflavone - 7 - *O*-(6″- *O*- acetyl)- β-D- glucopyranoside	$C_{26}H_{30}O_{11}$	Zhang D, et al
13. 蛇足石杉 *Huperzia serrata*	ceriponol A	$C_{15}H_{27}O_3$	Ying YM, et al
	ceriponol B	$C_{14}H_{23}O_3$	
	ceriponol C	$C_{15}H_{23}O_3$	
	ceriponol D	$C_{15}H_{23}O_3$	
	ceriponol E	$C_{15}H_{23}O_4$	
	ceriponol F	$C_{16}H_{27}O_3$	
	ceriponol G	$C_{16}H_{26}O_3$	
	ceriponol H	$C_{16}H_{25}O_4$	
	ceriponol I	$C_{16}H_{27}O_5$	
	ceriponol J	$C_{16}H_{23}O_5$	
	ceriponol K	$C_{15}H_{23}O_3$	
	3β- acetoxy - 15α - hydroxylanosta - 8,24 - dien - 21 - oic acid	$C_{32}H_{50}O_5$	
	3β- acetoxylanosta - 7,9(11),24 - trien - 21 - oic acid	$C_{32}H_{48}O_4$	
	huaspenones C	$C_{13}H_{17}NO_4$	Xiang JG, et al
	huaspenones D	$C_{15}H_{17}NO_3$	
14. 台湾杉木 *Cunninghamia konishii*	(6α,7β)- 7,8 - epoxy - 6 - hydroxyabieta - 9(11),13 - dien - 12 - one	$C_{20}H_{28}O_3$	Chen YC, et al
	(12*R*)- 12 - hydroxylabda - 8(17),13(16),14 - trien - 19 - oic acid	$C_{20}H_{30}O_3$	
	(12*R*)- 12 - hydroxylabda - 8(17),13(16),14 - trien - 18 - oic acid	$C_{20}H_{30}O_3$	
	konishone	$C_{18}H_{24}O_2$	
	3β- hydroxy - 5,6 - dehydrosugiol	$C_{20}H_{26}O_3$	

续 表

中药及其基源	新成分名称	分子式	报道者
15. 南洋杉 *Araucaria cunninghamii*	4-n-butoxyl-phenylpropanetriol	$C_{13}H_{24}NO_4$	Chen J, et al
16. 本榧树 *Torreya nucifera*	torreyanoxane	$C_{31}H_{52}O_2$	Cao CM, et al
17. 日本扁柏 *Chamaecyparis obtusa*	3-methoxyphenol 1-*O*-α-L-rhamnopyranosyl-(1→6)-*O*-β-D-glucopyranoside	$C_{19}H_{28}O_{11}$	Zhang YM, et al
18. 长叶竹柏 *Podocarpus fleuryi*	fleuryinols A	$C_{20}H_{30}O_3$	Zhang LC, et al
	fleuryinols B	$C_{20}H_{30}O_3$	
	fleuryinols C	$C_{20}H_{30}O_3$	
19. 麻黄 *Ephedra sinica*	ephedrannin D_1	$C_{30}H_{23}O_{13}$	Zang X, et al
	ephedrannin D_3	$C_{30}H_{23}O_{13}$	
	ephedrannin D_4	$C_{30}H_{23}O_{14}$	
	ephedrannin D_6	$C_{30}H_{23}O_{14}$	
	ephedrannin D_7	$C_{30}H_{23}O_{14}$	
	ephedrannin Tr_1	$C_{45}H_{35}O_{21}$	
	ephedrannin Tr_2	$C_{45}H_{35}O_{20}$	
	ephedrannin Te_1	$C_{60}H_{45}O_{28}$	
	ephedrannin Te_2	$C_{60}H_{45}O_{28}$	
	ephedrannin Te_3	$C_{60}H_{45}O_{27}$	
	ephedrannin Te_4	$C_{60}H_{45}O_{27}$	
	ephedrannin Te_5	$C_{60}H_{45}O_{27}$	
20. 翠云草 *Selaginella uncinata*	6-(5-acetyl-2-methoxyphenyl)-apigenin	$C_{24}H_{18}O_7$	Zou H, et al
	Uncinataflavone	$C_{24}H_{18}O_8$	
21. 草珊瑚 *Sarcandra glabra*	Atractylenolide Ⅳ	$C_{15}H_{22}O_4$	Hu XR, et al
22. 柳叶白前 *Cynanchum stauntonii*	glaucogenin E	$C_{21}H_{28}O_7$	Zhang M, et al
23. 核桃 *Juglans regia*	juglanones A	$C_{20}H_{18}O_5$	Li CY, et al
	juglanones B	$C_{20}H_{18}O_6$	
24. 朝鲜垂柳 *Salix pseudolasiogyne*	3′-*O*-acetylsalicin	$C_{15}H_{20}O_8$	Yang H, et al
	2′,6′-*O*-acetylsalicortin	$C_{24}H_{28}O_{12}$	
25. 面包树 *Artocarpus altilis*	10-oxoartogomezianone	$C_{26}H_{27}O_7$	Lan WC, et al
	8-geranyl-3-(hydroxyprenyl)isoetin	$C_{30}H_{33}O_7$	
	hydroxyartoflavone A	$C_{25}H_{23}O_7$	
	isocycloartobiloxanthone	$C_{25}H_{23}O_7$	
	furanocyclocommunin	$C_{25}H_{25}O_7$	
26. 见血封喉树 *Antiaris toxicaria*	toxicarioside N	$C_{35}H_{54}O_{15}$	Zuo WJ, et al
	toxicarioside O	$C_{29}H_{44}O_{11}$	
27. 构树 *Broussonetia papyrifera*	5,7,3′,4′-tetrahydroxy-3-methoxy-8-geranylflavone	$C_{26}H_{28}O_7$	Guo F, et al

续　表

中药及其基源	新成分名称	分子式	报道者
27. 构树 *Broussonetia papyrifera*	5,7,3′,4′- tetrahydroxy - 3 - methoxy - 8,5′- diprenylflavone	$C_{26}H_{28}O_7$	Guo F, et al
28. 杠板归 *Polygonum perfoliatum*	8 - oxo - pinoresinol	$C_{20}H_{20}O_7$	Wang KW, et al
29. 首乌 *Polygonum multiflorum*	(*E*)- 2,3,5,4′- tetrahydroxystilbene - 2 - *O*-(4″- *O*- a -D- glucopyranosyl)- β- D - glucopyranoside	$C_{26}H_{32}O_{14}$	Li SG, et al
	(*E*)- 2,3,5,4′- tetrahydroxystilbene - 2 - *O*-(6″- *O*- β -Dglucopyranosyl)- β- D - glucopyranoside	$C_{26}H_{32}O_{14}$	
	(*E*)- 2,3,5,4′- tetrahydroxystilbene - 2 - *O*- β - Dglucopyranosyl - 4′- *O* - α - D - glucopyranoside	$C_{26}H_{32}O_{14}$	
	(*E*)- 2,3,5,4′- tetrahydroxystilbene - 2 - *O*- β - D- glucopyranosyl - 5 - *O* - α - D - glucopyranoside	$C_{26}H_{32}O_{14}$	
	(*E*)- 2,3,5,4′- tetrahydroxystilbene - 2 - *O*-(2″- *O*- β -D- fructofuranosyl)- β- D - glucopyranoside	$C_{26}H_{32}O_{14}$	
30. 虎杖 *Polygonum cuspidatum*	Polyflavanostilbene A	$C_{42}H_{38}O_{19}$	Li F, et al
31. 拉萨大黄 *Rheum lhasaense*	rheumlhasol A	$C_{42}H_{32}O_9$	Liu WB, et al
	rheumlhasol B	$C_{42}H_{31}O_9$	
32. 无心菜 *Arenaria serpyllifolia*	1 - hydroxy - 5 - methoxyxanthone 6 - *O*- β - D- glucopyranoside	$C_{20}H_{20}O_{10}$	Zhou G, et al
	3 -(β- D- glucopyranosyloxymethyl)- 2 -(4 - hydroxy - 3 - methoxyphenyl)- 5 -(3 - acetoxypropyl)- 7 - methoxy - (2*R*,3*S*)- dihydrobenzofuran	$C_{28}H_{36}O_{12}$	
	japonicumone A 4′- *O*- β - D - glucopyranoside	$C_{22}H_{26}O_9$	
	japonicumone B 3′- *O*- β - D - glucopyranoside	$C_{22}H_{26}O_{10}$	
	japonicumone B 4′- *O*- β - D - glucopyranoside	$C_{22}H_{26}O_{10}$	
33. 青葙子 *Celosia argentea*	celosin Ⅰ	$C_{53}H_{81}O_{24}$	Wu QB, et al
	celosin Ⅱ	$C_{58}H_{91}O_{28}$	
34. 华中五味子 *Schisandra sphenanthera*	schisandlignans A	$C_{21}H_{22}O_7$	Li YF, et al
	schisandlignans B	$C_{21}H_{22}O_7$	
	schisandlignans C	$C_{22}H_{26}O_7$	
	schisandlignan D	$C_{22}H_{28}O_7$	
	7 -(3,4 - Dimethoxyphenyl)- 7′(4 - hydroxy - 3 - methoxyphenyl)- 8,8′(dimethylbutyl) acetate	$C_{23}H_{30}O_6$	Song QY, et al
35. 滇藏五味子 *Schisandra neglecta*	neglschisandrins E	$C_{22}H_{26}O_6$	Chen M, et al
	neglschisandrins F	$C_{28}H_{34}O_7$	
	schicagenins D	$C_{29}H_{36}O_{11}$	Liang CQ, et al
	schicagenins E	$C_{29}H_{36}O_{11}$	
	schicagenins F	$C_{29}H_{36}O_{11}$	
	negleschidilactones A	$C_{29}H_{36}O_{12}$	
	negleschidilactones B	$C_{29}H_{34}O_{12}$	

续 表

中药及其基源	新成分名称	分子式	报道者
36. 五味子 *Schisandra chinensis*	schisdilactone H	$C_{30}H_{38}O_{11}$	Li LF, et al
	schisdilactone I	$C_{30}H_{38}O_{11}$	
37. 菲律宾南五味子 *Kadsura philippinensis*	taiwankadsurins D	$C_{29}H_{32}O_{13}$	Lin YC, et al
	taiwankadsurins E	$C_{29}H_{32}O_{13}$	
	taiwankadsurins F	$C_{29}H_{28}O_{10}$	
	kadsuphilins N	$C_{30}H_{36}O_{12}$	
	kadsuphilins O	$C_{22}H_{22}O_9$	
38. 鹤庆五味子 *Schisandra wilsoniana*	schisanwilsonins K	$C_{28}H_{32}O_9$	Ma W, et al
	schisanwilsonins L	$C_{24}H_{28}O_7$	
	schisanwilsonins M	$C_{28}H_{34}O_8$	
	schisanwilsonins N	$C_{28}H_{34}O_8$	
	schisanwilsonins O	$C_{22}H_{26}O_7$	
	marlignans M	$C_{23}H_{31}O_7$	Yang GY, et al
	marlignans N	$C_{22}H_{29}O_7$	
	marlignans O	$C_{22}H_{27}O_7$	
	marlignans P	$C_{22}H_{25}O_7$	
	marlignans Q	$C_{22}H_{25}O_7$	
	marlignans R	$C_{24}H_{30}O_7$	
	marlignans S	$C_{24}H_{30}O_7$	
	marphenols C	$C_{13}H_{18}O_7$	
	marphenols D	$C_{14}H_{20}O_8$	
	marphenols E	$C_{20}H_{24}O_8$	
	marphenols F	$C_{20}H_{22}O_8$	
39. 金山五味子 *Schisandra glaucescens*	(7*S*,8*R*,7′*R*,8′*R*)-7-(3,4-methylenedioxyphenyl)-8,8′-dimethyl-8′-hydroxyl-7′-methoxyl-7′-(3′,4′-methylenedioxyphenyl)-tetrahydrofuran	$C_{21}H_{22}O_7$	Zhang PP, et al
	2-hydroxy-11,12-dehydrocalamenene	$C_{15}H_{20}O$	
40. 狭叶五味子 *Schisandra lancifolia*	lancolides A	$C_{29}H_{32}O_{11}$	Shi YM, et al
	lancolides B	$C_{29}H_{32}O_{11}$	
	lancolides C	$C_{29}H_{32}O_{10}$	
	lancolides D	$C_{29}H_{32}O_{10}$	
41. 红毒茴 *Illicium lanceolatum*	*p*-mentha-1(7),8-dien-2-*O*-*β*-D-glucoside	$C_{16}H_{26}O_6$	Liu JF, et al
	trans-2,4-dihydroxy-2,4-dimethyl-trans-1-acetic acid *γ*-lactone	$C_{10}H_{17}O_3$	
42. 光叶紫玉盘 *Uvaria boniana*	bonianol A	$C_{21}H_{20}O_7$	Chen Z, et al
	bonianol B	$C_{21}H_{22}O_7$	
43. 皂帽花 *Dasymaschalon trichophorum*	10-amino-3,6-dihydroxy-2,4-dimethoxyphenanthrene-1-carboxylic acid lactam	$C_{17}H_{13}O_5N$	周晓磊,等

续　表

中药及其基源	新成分名称	分子式	报道者
44. 瓜馥木 *Fissistigma oldhamii*	aristololactam GI	$C_{26}H_{22}NO_6$	Ge YW, et al
	aristololactam GII	$C_{16}H_{12}NO_4$	
	fissistigamide A	$C_{19}H_{19}N_2O_4$	
	fissistigamide B	$C_{19}H_{19}N_2O_4$	
	fissistigamide C	$C_{19}H_{19}N_2O_4$	
45. 宽叶依兰 *Cananga latifolia*	(2*E*,6*E*,10*R*)-11-butoxy-10-hydroxy-3,7,11-trimethyldodeca-2,6-dienoic acid methyl ester	$C_{20}H_{37}O_4$	Yang H, et al
	(2*E*,6*E*)-3,7,11-trimethyl-10-oxododeca-2,6-dienoic acid methyl ester	$C_{15}H_{26}O_3$	
	(2*E*)-3-methyl-5-[(1*S*,2*R*,6*R*)-1,2,6-trimethyl-3-oxocyclohexyl]-pent-2-enoic acid methyl ester	$C_{16}H_{26}O_3$	
	1β-Hydroxy-3-oxo-4β,5α,7α-H-eudesmane 11-*O*-α-Lrhamnopyranoside	$C_{21}H_{36}O_7$	
	4-Epi-aubergenone 11-*O*-2′,3′-di-*O*-acetyl-α-L-rhamnopyranoside	$C_{25}H_{38}O_8$	
	4-Epi-aubergenone 11-*O*-2′,4-di-*O*′-acetyl-α-L-rhamnopyranoside	$C_{25}H_{38}O_8$	
46. 番荔枝 *Annona squamosa*	(4α)-19-nor-ent-kaurane-4,16,17-triol	$C_{19}H_{32}O_3$	Zhou CX, et al
	(4α,16α)-17-(acetyloxy)-19-nor-ent-kaurane-4,16-diol	$C_{21}H_{34}O_4$	
	17-hydroxy-ent-kaur-15-en-19-al	$C_{20}H_{30}O_2$	
47. 牛心果 *Annona reticulata*	annonaretin A	$C_{33}H_{56}O_3$	Thang TD, et al
48. 大八角 *Illicium majus*	majusanic acid A	$C_{20}H_{29}O_5$	Fang Z, et al
	majusanic acid B	$C_{20}H_{29}O_4$	
	majusanic acid C	$C_{21}H_{31}O_3$	
	majusanic acid D	$C_{20}H_{27}O_4$	
	majusanol A	$C_{15}H_{23}O_6$	
	majusanol B	$C_{15}H_{25}O_7$	
49. 红茴香 *Illicium henryi*	illihenlactoneoside A	$C_{20}H_{28}O_{10}$	Zhuang PY, et al
	illihenlactoneoside B	$C_{23}H_{34}O_{14}$	
	illihenlactoneoside C	$C_{22}H_{32}O_{13}$	
	illihenlactoneoside D	$C_{21}H_{34}O_9$	
	illihenlactoneoside E	$C_{21}H_{34}O_9$	
	illihenlactoneoside F	$C_{21}H_{30}O_9$	
	illihenlactoneoside G	$C_{21}H_{32}O_{11}$	
	Illihenazulene A	$C_{15}H_{24}O_2$	
	illihenryifunones A	$C_{14}H_{21}O_4$	
	illihenryifunones B	$C_{20}H_{31}O_9$	
	illihenryifunol A	$C_{14}H_{19}O_3$	

续 表

中药及其基源	新成分名称	分子式	报道者
49. 红茴香 *Illicium henryi*	illihenryipyranol A	$C_{15}H_{21}O_4$	Zhuang PY, et al
	illihenryiones A	$C_{15}H_{21}O_5$	
	illihenryiones B	$C_{21}H_{31}O_{10}$	
	illihenryiones C	$C_{15}H_{19}O_4$	
	illihenryiones D	$C_{21}H_{29}O_9$	
	illihenryiones E	$C_{15}H_{18}O_4$	
	illihenryiones F	$C_{21}H_{29}O_9$	
	illihenryiones G	$C_{21}H_{29}O_9$	
	Illihendione A	$C_{28}H_{36}O_8$	
	illihenryifunone C	$C_{15}H_{20}O_4$	
	illihenryipyranone A	$C_{15}H_{20}O_4$	
50. 少药八角 *Illicium oligandrum*	spirooliganones A	$C_{25}H_{34}O_4$	Ma SG, et al
	spirooliganones B	$C_{25}H_{34}O_4$	
51. 匙叶八角 *Illicium spathulatum*	(1β,4β,6α)- gorgonane - 1,4,11 - triol	$C_{15}H_{28}O_3$	Dong XJ, et al
	(1β,4α,6α)- gorgonane - 1,4,11 - triol	$C_{15}H_{28}O_3$	
	(1β,4β,6β)- gorgonane - 1,4,11 - triol	$C_{15}H_{28}O_3$	
	(1β,4α,6β)- gorgonane - 1,4,11 - triol	$C_{15}H_{28}O_3$	
52. 台湾八角 *Illicium arborescens*	illicarborene A	$C_{25}H_{34}O_3$	Liaw CC, et al
53. 大叶楠 *Machilus ichangensis*	machilusmarin	$C_{36}H_{40}O_6$	Cheng F, et al
54. 粗壮润楠 *Machilus robusta*	(—)- nectandrin B - β - D - glucopyranoside	$C_{26}H_{34}O_{10}$	Bu PB, et al
	(—)-(7*R*,7′*R*,8*S*,8′*R*)- 4,4′- dihydroxy - 3,3′- dimethoxy - 7,7′- epoxylignan - 4 - *O* - β - D - glucopyranoside	$C_{26}H_{34}O_{10}$	
	(—)-(7*R*,7′*R*,8*S*,8′*R*)- 4,4′- dihydroxy - 3,3′- dimethoxy - 7,7′- epoxylignan - 4′- *O* - β - D - glucopyranoside	$C_{26}H_{34}O_{10}$	
	(—)-(8*S*,8′*R*)- 4,4′- dihydroxy - 3,3′,5′- trimethoxylignan - 4′- *O* - β - D - glucopyranoside	$C_{27}H_{38}O_{10}$	
	(—)-(7*R*,8*R*)- syringylglycerol - 8 - *O* - β - D - glucopyranoside	$C_{17}H_{27}O_{11}$	
	(—)- 3 - hydroxy - 2 - methyl - 4 - pyrone - 3 - *O* - β - D - xylopyranosyl -(1→6)- *O* - β - D - glucopyranoside	$C_{17}H_{24}O_{12}$	
55. 乌药 *Lindera strychnifolia*	linderolide G	$C_{15}H_{18}O_3$	Liu Q, et al
	linderolide H	$C_{14}H_{17}O_4$	
	linderolide I	$C_{15}H_{19}O_4$	
	linderolide J	$C_{15}H_{17}O_5$	
	linderolide K	$C_{15}H_{21}O_4$	
	linderolide L	$C_{18}H_{23}O_5$	
	linderolide M	$C_{18}H_{25}O_7$	

续　表

中药及其基源	新 成 分 名 称	分 子 式	报 道 者
56. 白背厚壳桂 *Cryptocarya maclurei*	cryptogiones G	$C_{17}H_{17}O_6$	Feng R, et al
	cryptogiones H	$C_{17}H_{17}O_6$	
	cryptogiones I	$C_{19}H_{23}O_5$	
	cryptogiones J	$C_{17}H_{17}O_4$	
	cryptogiones K	$C_{17}H_{17}O_4$	
	cryptomaclurone	$C_{17}H_{16}O_2$	
	cryptobeilic acids A	$C_{22}H_{21}O_3$	
	cryptobeilic acids A	$C_{20}H_{29}O_2$	
	tsangibeilin B	$C_{22}H_{22}O_4$	
57. 肉桂 *Cinnamomum cassia*	cinnacassosides A	$C_{26}H_{36}O_{12}$	Luo Q, et al
	cinnacassosides B	$C_{31}H_{42}O_{15}$	
	cinnacassosides C	$C_{19}H_{28}O_{13}$	
58. 天竺桂 *Cinnamomum tenuifolium*	Isotenuifolide	$C_{32}H_{58}O_3$	Dong HP, et al
59. 香花木姜子 *Litsea panamonja*	panamonon A	$C_{18}H_{24}O_4$	Wang YS, et al
	panamonon B	$C_{18}H_{24}O_4$	
60. 升麻 *Cimicifuga dahurica*	cimigenol-3-*O*-[2′-*O*-(*E*)-2-butenoyl]-α-L-arabinopyranoside	$C_{39}H_{60}O_{10}$	Nian Y, et al
	25-*O*-acetylcimigenol-3-*O*-[4′-*O*-acetyl]-α-L-arabinopyranoside	$C_{39}H_{60}O_{11}$	
	25-*O*-acetylcimigenol-3-*O*-[3′-*O*-acetyl]-α-L-arabinopyranoside	$C_{39}H_{60}O_{11}$	
	12β-hydroxy-7(8)-en-cimigenol	$C_{30}H_{46}O_6$	
	11β-hydroxy-7(8)-en-cimigenol	$C_{30}H_{46}O_6$	
	11β-hydroxy-15-deoxycimigenol-7(8)-en-3-one	$C_{30}H_{44}O_5$	
	cimigenol-7(8)-en-3-one	$C_{30}H_{44}O_5$	
	cimigenol-1(2),7(8)-dien-3-one	$C_{30}H_{42}O_5$	
	9,10-seco-1(10),7(8),9(11)-triencimigenol	$C_{30}H_{46}O_4$	
	24-*O*-acetylisodahurinol	$C_{32}H_{50}O_6$	
	24-*O*-acetyl-7(8)-en-isodahurinol	$C_{32}H_{48}O_6$	
	15,23-*O*-diacetyl-7(8)-en-shengmanol-3-*O*-α-L-arabinopyranoside	$C_{39}H_{58}O_{11}$	
61. 大三叶升麻 *Cimicifuga heracleifolia*	heracleifolinoside A	$C_{41}H_{64}O_{15}$	Liu Y, et al
	heracleifolinoside B	$C_{41}H_{64}O_{14}$	
	heracleifolinoside C	$C_{41}H_{64}O_{15}$	
	heracleifolinoside D	$C_{41}H_{66}O_{15}$	
	heracleifolinoside E	$C_{41}H_{66}O_{15}$	
	heracleifolinoside F	$C_{43}H_{68}O_{16}$	
	norkhelloside	$C_{23}H_{26}O_{14}$	

续 表

中药及其基源	新 成 分 名 称	分 子 式	报 道 者
62. 白头翁 *Pulsatilla chinensis*	23 - hydroxy - 3β-[(*O*-β-D-glucopyranosyl-(1→4)-α-L-arabinopyranosyl)]lup-20(29)-en-28-oic-acid 28-*O*-β-D-glucopyranosyl-(1→6)-β-D-glucopyranosyl ester	$C_{53}H_{86}O_{23}$	Xu Q, et al
	23 - hydroxy - 3β-[(*O*-α-L-rhamnopyranosyl-(1→2)-[β-D-glucopyranosyl-(1→4)]-α-L-arabinopyranosyl)]lup-20(29)-en-28-oic-acid 28-*O*-β-D-glucopyranosyl-(1→6)-β-D-glucopyranosyl ester	$C_{59}H_{96}O_{27}$	
	3β-[(*O*-β-D-glucopyranosyl-(1→3)-α-L-rhamnopyranosyl-(1→2)-α-L-arabinopyranosyl)]lup-20(29)-en-28-oic-acid 28-*O*-β-D-glucopyranosyl-(1→6)-β-D-glucopyranosyl ester	$C_{59}H_{96}O_{26}$	
	3β-[(*O*-β-D-glucopyranosyl-(1→3)-α-L-rhamnopyranosyl-(1→2)-α-L-arabinopyranosyl)]lup-20(29)-en-28-oic-acid 28-*O*-α-L-rhamnopyranosyl-(1→4)-β-D-glucopyranosyl-(1→6)-β-D-glucopyranosyl ester	$C_{65}H_{106}O_{30}$	
	3-*O*-β-D-glucopyranosyl-hederagenin 23-*O*-α-D-ribofuranoside	$C_{41}H_{66}O_{13}$	Shu Z, et al
63. 甘青铁线莲 *Clematis tangutica*	clematangosides A	$C_{59}H_{97}O_{26}$	Zhang W, et al
	clematangosides B	$C_{59}H_{97}O_{26}$	
	clematangosides C	$C_{60}H_{99}O_{28}$	
	clematangosides D	$C_{66}H_{109}O_{32}$	
64. 辣蓼铁线莲 *Clematis mandshurica*	clematomandshurica saponins F	$C_{77}H_{127}O_{39}$	Gong Y, et al
	clematomandshurica saponins G	$C_{82}H_{135}O_{43}$	
	clematomandshurica saponins H	$C_{76}H_{125}O_{39}$	
	clematomandshurica saponins I	$C_{70}H_{115}O_{34}$	
	clematomandshurica saponins J	$C_{74}H_{113}O_{32}$	
	clematomandshurica saponins K	$C_{68}H_{103}O_{27}$	
65. 单叶升麻 *Beesia calthaefolia*	(20*S*＊,24*R*＊)-16bacetoxy-20,24-epoxy-9,19-cyclolanostane-3β,12β,15α,18,25-pentaol-3-*O*-β-D- xylopyranoside	$C_{37}H_{60}O_{12}$	Li HJ, et al
	(20*S*＊,24*R*＊)-16β-acetoxy-20,24-epoxy-9,19-cyclolanostane-3β,15α,18,25-tetraol-3-*O*-β-Dxylopyranoside	$C_{37}H_{60}O_{11}$	
66. 圆锥铁线莲 *Clematis terniflora*	(6-hydroxyl-1H-indol-3-yl) carboxylic acid methyl ester	$C_{16}H_{19}NO_8$	Li WT, et al
67. 金莲花 *Trollius chinensis*	6‴-(3-hydroxy-3-methylglutaroyl)-2″-*O*-β-D-galactopyranosyl orientin	$C_{33}H_{38}O_{20}$	iu JY, et al
	6‴-(3-hydroxy-3-methylglutaroyl)-2″-*O*-β-D-galactopyranosyl vitexin	$C_{33}H_{38}O_{19}$	
68. 青天葵 *Nervilia fordii*	nervilifordins F	$C_{31}H_{36}O_{18}$	Qiu L, et al
	nervilifordins G	$C_{31}H_{36}O_{18}$	
	nervilifordins H	$C_{36}H_{36}O_{17}$	

续 表

中药及其基源	新成分名称	分子式	报道者
68. 青天葵 *Nervilia fordii*	nervilifordins I	$C_{37}H_{38}O_{18}$	Qiu L, et al
	nervilifordins J	$C_{27}H_{30}O_{15}$	
	nervisides D	$C_{36}H_{60}O_{11}$	Wei LB, et al
	nervisides E	$C_{35}H_{58}O_{10}$	
	nervisides F	$C_{36}H_{60}O_{11}$	
	nervisides G	$C_{35}H_{56}O_{10}$	
	nervisides H	$C_{36}H_{58}O_{11}$	
	7-*O*-β-D-glucopyranosylapigenin-8-*C*-β-D-glucopyranosyl-(1→2)-β-D-glucopyranoside	$C_{33}H_{40}O_{20}$	Chen JM, et al
	24(*S*/β)-dihydrocycloeucalenol-3-(*Z*)-p-hydroxycinnamate	$C_{39}H_{58}O_{3}$	
69. 威灵仙 *Clematis chinensis*	clematochinenosides H	$C_{88}H_{144}O_{49}$	Fu Q, et al
	clematochinenosides I	$C_{110}H_{172}O_{62}$	
	clematochinenosides J	$C_{110}H_{172}O_{62}$	
70. 芍药 *Paeonia lactiflora*	2′-*O*-benzoylpaeoniflorin	$C_{30}H_{32}O_{12}$	Fu Q, et al
	albiflorin R_2	$C_{23}H_{28}O_{11}$	
	albiflorin R_3	$C_{30}H_{32}O_{13}$	
71. 甘青乌头 *Aconitum tanguticum*	Quercetin 3-*O*-α-L-rhamnopyranosyl-(1→2)-[β-D-glucopyranosyl-(1→3)-α-L-(4-*O*-trans-p-coumaroylrhamnopyranosyl)-(1→6)]-β-D-galactopyranoside-7-*O*-α-L-rhamnopyranoside	$C_{54}H_{66}O_{31}$	Xu L, et al
	kaempferol 3-*O*-α-L-rhamnopyranosyl-(1→2)-[β-D-glucopyranosyl-(1→3)-α-L-(4-*O*-trans-pcoumaroyl rhamnopyranosyl)-(1→6)]-β-D-galactopyranoside-7-*O*-α-L-rhamnopyranoside	$C_{54}H_{66}O_{30}$	
	(*Z*)-sinapic acid-4-*O*-β-D-allopyranoside	$C_{30}H_{38}O_{15}$	
	3,4-dihydroxyphenethoxy-8-*O*-β-D-[6-*O*-(4-*O*-β-D-glucopyranosyl)-feruloyl]-glucopyranoside	$C_{30}H_{38}O_{16}$	
	4-dihydroxyphenethoxy-8-*O*-β-D-[6-*O*-(4-*O*-β-D-glucopyranosyl)-feruloyl]-glucopyranoside	$C_{30}H_{38}O_{15}$	
	trichocarpidine	$C_{43}H_{58}N_{2}O_{6}$	Zhang ZT, et al
	trichocarpinine A	$C_{47}H_{62}N_{2}O_{7}$	
	trichocarpinine B	$C_{47}H_{62}N_{2}O_{6}$	
	trichocarpinine C	$C_{46}H_{60}N_{2}O_{7}$	
72. 丽江乌头 *Aconitum forrestii*	14-acetoxy-8-*O*-methylsachaconitine	$C_{26}H_{41}NO_{5}$	Xu JJ, et al
	14-acetoxyscaconine	$C_{25}H_{39}NO_{6}$	
	8-*O*-ethylcammaconine	$C_{25}H_{41}NO_{5}$	
73. 猫爪草 *Ranunculus ternatus*	(*R*)-3-[2-(3,4-dihydroxybenzoyl)-4,5-dihydroxyphenyl]-2-hydroxypropanoate	$C_{17}H_{16}O_{8}$	Deng KZ, et al
	n-butyl (*R*)-3-[2-(3,4-dihydroxybenzoyl)-4,5-dihydroxyphenyl]-2-hydroxypropanoate	$C_{20}H_{22}O_{8}$	
	Ternatusine A	$C_{16}H_{21}NO_{8}$	Zhan Z, et al

续 表

中药及其基源	新 成 分 名 称	分 子 式	报 道 者
74. 附子 *Aconitum carmichaelii*	*N*-(2′-b-D-glucopyranosyl-5′-hydroxysalicyl)-4-hydroxy-3-methoxyanthranilic acid methyl ester	$C_{22}H_{25}NO_{12}$	He CJ, et al
	N-(2′-b-D-glucopyranosyl-5′-hydroxysalicyl)-4-hydroxyanthranilic acid methyl ester	$C_{21}H_{23}NO_{11}$	
75. 腺毛黑种草 *Nigella glandulifera*	nigeglapine	$C_{19}H_{21}N_2O_2$	Liu YM, et al
	nigeglaquine	$C_{25}H_{32}N_2O_8$	
76. 朝鲜淫羊藿 *Epimedium koreanum*	epimediphine	$C_{19}H_{17}NO_4$	Zhang X, et al
77. 地不容 *Stephania epigaea*	3-Nor-4-oxocepharanthine	$C_{36}H_{34}N_2O_7$	Lv JJ, et al
	(—)-1,3,4-Dehydrocepharanthine	$C_{36}H_{33}N_2O_6$	
	(+)-1,3,4-Dehydrocepharanthine-2′β-N-oxide	$C_{36}H_{32}N_2O_7$	
	(+)-1-Dehydrocepharanthine-2′β-N-oxide	$C_{36}H_{32}N_2O_7$	
	Cepharanthine-2α-N-oxide	$C_{36}H_{33}N_2O_7$	
	Cepharanthine-2β-Noxide	$C_{36}H_{33}N_2O_7$	
	Cepharanthine-2′α-N-oxide	$C_{36}H_{32}N_2O_7$	
78. 三白草 *Saururus chinensis*	sauchinones B	$C_{20}H_{20}O_7$	Gao X, et al
	sauchinones C	$C_{19}H_{20}O_6$	
	sauchinones D	$C_{19}H_{20}O_6$	
79. 鱼腥草 *Houttuynia cordata*	houttuynoid G	$C_{32}H_{38}O_{14}$	Chen S, et al
	houttuynoid H	$C_{42}H_{56}O_{15}$	
	houttuynoid I	$C_{38}H_{48}O_{18}$	
	houttuynoid J	$C_{38}H_{48}O_{18}$	
80. 假蒟 *Piper sarmentosum*	sarmentosumol A	$C_{16}H_{24}O$	Yang S, et al
	sarmentosumol B	$C_{16}H_{24}O_2$	
	sarmentosumol C	$C_{32}H_{46}O_3$	
	sarmentosumol D	$C_{32}H_{46}O_3$	
	sarmentosumol E	$C_{32}H_{46}O_3$	
	sarmentosumol F	$C_{32}H_{48}O_3$	
81. 石蝉草 *Peperomia dindygulensis*	dindygulerione C	$C_{32}H_{49}NO_5$	Wang X, et al
	dindygulerione D	$C_{26}H_{46}O_3$	
	dindyguleranone	$C_{34}H_{60}O_3$	
82. 豆瓣绿 *Peperomia tetraphylla*	(+)-methyl 3-acetoxy-3-(7-methoxy-1,3-benzodioxol-5-yl) propanoate	$C_{14}H_{16}O_7$	Li YZ, et al
83. 台湾荖藤 *Piper taiwanense*	diallylcatechol	$C_{18}H_{19}O_4$	Chen S, et al
	neotaiwanensols A	$C_{18}H_{19}O_4$	
	neotaiwanensols B	$C_{18}H_{19}O_4$	
	taiwandimerols A	$C_{19}H_{21}O_5$	
	taiwandimerols B	$C_{20}H_{23}O_6$	
	2,3-diacetoxy-1-methoxy-5-allylbenzene	$C_{14}H_{17}O_5$	

续 表

中药及其基源	新成分名称	分子式	报道者
84. 黄花胡椒 *Piper flaviflorum*	flavifloramides A	$C_{37}H_{38}N_2O_{10}$	Wu Y, et al
84. 黄花胡椒 *Piper flaviflorum*	flavifloramides B	$C_{38}H_{40}N_2O_{10}$	Wu Y, et al
85. 裸果胡椒 *Piper nudibaccatum*	nudibaccatumone	$C_{39}H_{56}O_3$	Liu HX, et al
86. 蒌叶 *Piper betle*	2-(γ′-hydroxychavicol)-hydroxychavicol	$C_{18}H_{18}O_4$	Lin CF, et al
86. 蒌叶 *Piper betle*	pipercerebrosides A	$C_{35}H_{67}NO_{10}$	Chen DZ, et al
86. 蒌叶 *Piper betle*	pipercerebrosides B	$C_{46}H_{91}NO_5$	Chen DZ, et al
87. 银线草 *Chloranthus japonicus*	chlojaponilactones B	$C_{17}H_{18}O_4$	Yan H, et al
87. 银线草 *Chloranthus japonicus*	chlojaponilactones C	$C_{17}H_{18}O_5$	Yan H, et al
87. 银线草 *Chloranthus japonicus*	chlojaponilactones D	$C_{15}H_{16}O_3$	Yan H, et al
87. 银线草 *Chloranthus japonicus*	chlojaponilactones E	$C_{17}H_{22}O_4$	Yan H, et al
88. 竹叶兰 *Arundina gramnifolia*	gramniphenols C	$C_{20}H_{20}O_6$	Hu QF, et al
88. 竹叶兰 *Arundina gramnifolia*	gramniphenols D	$C_{19}H_{18}O_6$	Hu QF, et al
88. 竹叶兰 *Arundina gramnifolia*	gramniphenols E	$C_{19}H_{18}O_6$	Hu QF, et al
88. 竹叶兰 *Arundina gramnifolia*	gramniphenols F	$C_{19}H_{16}O_3$	Hu QF, et al
88. 竹叶兰 *Arundina gramnifolia*	gramniphenols G	$C_{20}H_{18}O_3$	Hu QF, et al
89. 多穗金粟兰 *Chloranthus multistachys*	chloramultiol G	$C_{40}H_{41}O_{14}$	Liu HY, et al
89. 多穗金粟兰 *Chloranthus multistachys*	ent-(3*R*)-3-hydroxyatractylenolide Ⅲ	$C_{15}H_{21}O_4$	Liu HY, et al
89. 多穗金粟兰 *Chloranthus multistachys*	multistalactones A	$C_{15}H_{21}O_5$	Liu HY, et al
89. 多穗金粟兰 *Chloranthus multistachys*	multistalactones B	$C_{15}H_{21}O_4$	Liu HY, et al
89. 多穗金粟兰 *Chloranthus multistachys*	multistalactones C	$C_{15}H_{21}O_4$	Liu HY, et al
89. 多穗金粟兰 *Chloranthus multistachys*	(1*R*,4*S*,5*R*,8*S*,10*S*)-zedoalactone A	$C_{15}H_{23}O_4$	Liu HY, et al
89. 多穗金粟兰 *Chloranthus multistachys*	multistalactones D	$C_{15}H_{21}O_3$	Liu HY, et al
89. 多穗金粟兰 *Chloranthus multistachys*	multistalactones E	$C_{15}H_{21}O_3$	Liu HY, et al
89. 多穗金粟兰 *Chloranthus multistachys*	multistalactones F	$C_{15}H_{21}O_4$	Liu HY, et al
90. 通城虎 *Aristolochia fordiana*	(7*R*,8*S*)-3,4-methylenedioxy-3′-methoxy-4′,7-epoxy-8,5′-neolignan-7′[*E*]-ene	$C_{20}H_{20}O_4$	Zhou Z, et al
90. 通城虎 *Aristolochia fordiana*	(7*R*,8*S*)-3,4-methylenedioxy-4′,7-epoxy-8,3′-neolignan-7′[*E*]-ene	$C_{19}H_{18}O_3$	Zhou Z, et al
90. 通城虎 *Aristolochia fordiana*	(7*S*,8*R*)-3,4-methylenedioxy-8′,9′-dinor-4′,7-epoxy-8,3′-neolignan-7′-aldehyde	$C_{17}H_{15}O_4$	Zhou Z, et al
90. 通城虎 *Aristolochia fordiana*	(7*S*,8*R*)-3,4-methylenedioxy-3′-methoxy-8,9′-dinor-4′,7-epoxy-8,5′-neolignan-7′-aldehyde	$C_{18}H_{17}O_5$	Zhou Z, et al
90. 通城虎 *Aristolochia fordiana*	(7*R*,8*S*)-3-methoxy-4-hydroxy-4′,7-epoxy-8,3′-neolignan-7′[*E*]-ene	$C_{19}H_{20}O_3$	Zhou Z, et al
90. 通城虎 *Aristolochia fordiana*	(7*R*,8*R*)-3,4-methylenedioxy-8′,9′-dinor-4′,7-epoxy-8,3′-neolignan-7′-aldehyde	$C_{17}H_{15}O_4$	Zhou Z, et al
91. 云南马兜铃 *Aristolochia yunnanensis*	aristoyunnolins A	$C_{15}H_{21}NO_5$	Cheng ZB, et al
91. 云南马兜铃 *Aristolochia yunnanensis*	aristoyunnolins B	$C_{15}H_{20}O_4$	Cheng ZB, et al
91. 云南马兜铃 *Aristolochia yunnanensis*	aristoyunnolins C	$C_{16}H_{22}O_3$	Cheng ZB, et al

续 表

中药及其基源	新成分名称	分子式	报道者
91. 云南马兜铃 *Aristolochia yunnanensis*	aristoyunnolins D	$C_{16}H_{20}O_3$	Cheng ZB, et al
	aristoyunnolins E	$C_{15}H_{22}O_2$	
	aristoyunnolins F	$C_{17}H_{24}O_3$	
	7-*O*-ethyl madolin W	$C_{17}H_{26}O_2$	
92. 白毛藤 *Solanum lyratum*	solajiangxin D	$C_{15}H_{24}O_4$	Yao F, et al
	solajiangxin E	$C_{18}H_{28}O_3$	
	solajiangxin F	$C_{18}H_{28}O_4$	
93. 长果大头茶 *Gordonia longicarpa*	longicarposides A	$C_{52}H_{83}O_{23}$	Tang J, et al
	longicarposides B	$C_{52}H_{83}O_{23}$	
	longicarposides C	$C_{47}H_{77}O_{18}$	
	longicarposides D	$C_{52}H_{85}O_{22}$	
	longicarposides E	$C_{57}H_{91}O_{24}$	
	longicarposides F	$C_{62}H_{97}O_{26}$	
	longicarposides G	$C_{62}H_{97}O_{26}$	
	longicarposides H	$C_{62}H_{97}O_{27}$	
	longicarposides I	$C_{59}H_{93}O_{27}$	
94. 大头茶 *Gordonia kwangsiensis*	gordonsaponin A	$C_{53}H_{87}O_{23}$	Fu HZ, et al
	gordonsaponin B	$C_{53}H_{87}O_{24}$	
	gordonsaponin C	$C_{53}H_{93}O_{26}$	
	gordonsaponin D	$C_{53}H_{87}O_{23}$	
	gordonsaponin E	$C_{53}H_{87}O_{24}$	
	gordonsaponin F	$C_{55}H_{89}O_{25}$	
	gordonsaponin G	$C_{58}H_{93}O_{25}$	
	gordonsaponin H	$C_{58}H_{93}O_{26}$	
	gordonsaponin I	$C_{60}H_{95}O_{28}$	
	gordonsaponin J	$C_{62}H_{97}O_{29}$	
	gordonsaponin K	$C_{59}H_{93}O_{26}$	
95. 油茶 *Camellia oleifera*	21β,22α-diangeloyloxy-3β,15α,16α,28-tetrahydroxyolean-12-en-23-al	$C_{40}H_{60}O_9$	Wang SL, et al
	21β-angeloyloxy-3β,15α,16α,28-tetrahydroxy-22α-(2-methylbutanoyloxy)olean-12-en-23-al	$C_{40}H_{62}O_9$	
	21β-angeloyloxy-3β,16α,28-trihydroxy-22α-(2-methylbutanoyloxy)olean-12-en-23-al	$C_{40}H_{62}O_8$	
96. 柃木 *Eurya japonica*	8,8′,7,2′-lignans,(+)-ovafolinin B-9′-*O*-β-D-glucopyranoside	$C_{28}H_{35}O_{13}$	Yang Kuo LM, et al
	(−)-ovafolinin B-9′-*O*-β-D-glucopyranoside	$C_{28}H_{35}O_{13}$	
	(+)-ovafolinin E-9′-*O*-β-D-glucopyranoside	$C_{28}H_{33}O_{13}$	
	(−)-ovafolinin E-9′-*O*-β-D-glucopyranoside	$C_{28}H_{33}O_{13}$	
	eusiderin N	$C_{26}H_{34}O_{12}$	

续 表

中药及其基源	新成分名称	分子式	报道者
96. 柃木 *Eurya japonica*	(7*S*,8*R*)-3,5,5′-trimethoxy-4′,7-epoxy-8,3′-neolignan-9,9′-diol-4-*O*-*β*-D-xylopyranoside	$C_{26}H_{34}O_{11}$	Yang Kuo LM, et al
96. 柃木 *Eurya japonica*	5,7-dihydroxy-4*H*-chromen-4-one-3-*O*-*β*-D-glucopyranoside	$C_{15}H_{16}O_{10}$	Yang Kuo LM, et al
96. 柃木 *Eurya japonica*	5,7-dihydroxy-4*H*-chromen-4-one-3-*O*-*β*-D-xylopyranoside	$C_{14}H_{14}O_9$	Yang Kuo LM, et al
97. 茶树 *Camellia sinensis*	13,26-epoxy-3*β*,11*α*-dihydroxyolean-12-one	$C_{30}H_{48}O_4$	Huang YL, et al
97. 茶树 *Camellia sinensis*	3*β*,11*α*,13*β*-trihydroxyolean-12-one	$C_{30}H_{50}O_4$	Huang YL, et al
98. 兴安藜芦 *Veratrum dahuricum*	neoveratrenone	$C_{19}H_{26}O_3$	Cong Y, et al
98. 兴安藜芦 *Veratrum dahuricum*	1-[11-(ferulyloxy)undecanoyl)]glycerol	$C_{24}H_{36}O_8$	Cong Y, et al
99. 藤黄 *Garcinia hanburyi*	22,23-dihydroxydihydrogambogenic acid	$C_{38}H_{48}O_{10}$	Deng Y, et al
99. 藤黄 *Garcinia hanburyi*	12-hydroxygambogefic acid A	$C_{38}H_{46}O_{10}$	Deng Y, et al
99. 藤黄 *Garcinia hanburyi*	hanburixanthone	$C_{33}H_{40}O_6$	Deng Y, et al
100. 清水金丝桃 *Hypericum nakamurai*	hyperinakin	$C_{23}H_{26}O_5$	Cheng YB, et al
101. 山橘子 *Garcinia multiflora*	multiflorabiphenyl A	$C_{22}H_{24}O_3$	Jing WY, et al
101. 山橘子 *Garcinia multiflora*	24-p-*E*-coumaroyl-tetracosanyl (*E*)-ferulate	$C_{43}H_{64}O_7$	Jing WY, et al
102. 加纳 *Griffonia simplicifolia*	griffonine	$C_{21}H_{13}N_3O_5$	王欣之,等
103. 金丝李 *Garcinia paucinervis*	paucinervin E	$C_{19}H_{18}O_9$	Wu YP, et al
103. 金丝李 *Garcinia paucinervis*	paucinervin F	$C_{20}H_{20}O_9$	Wu YP, et al
103. 金丝李 *Garcinia paucinervis*	paucinervin G	$C_{20}H_{20}O_9$	Wu YP, et al
104. 单花山竹子 *Garcinia oligantha*	oliganthin E	$C_{19}H_{20}O_8$	Wu YP, et al
104. 单花山竹子 *Garcinia oligantha*	oliganthin F	$C_{19}H_{20}O_8$	Wu YP, et al
104. 单花山竹子 *Garcinia oligantha*	oliganthin G	$C_{20}H_{18}O_8$	Wu YP, et al
104. 单花山竹子 *Garcinia oligantha*	oliganthone A	$C_{30}H_{34}O_7$	Gao XM, et al
105. 英桐 *Platanus*×*acerifolia*	platachromone A	$C_{22}H_{20}O_5$	Yang CH, et al
105. 英桐 *Platanus*×*acerifolia*	platachromone B	$C_{22}H_{20}O_5$	Yang CH, et al
105. 英桐 *Platanus*×*acerifolia*	platachromone C	$C_{22}H_{20}O_6$	Yang CH, et al
105. 英桐 *Platanus*×*acerifolia*	platachromone D	$C_{22}H_{20}O_6$	Yang CH, et al
106. 枫香 *Liquidambar formosana*	(2*S*)-5,7,4′-trihydroxyflavan-7-*O*-*β*-D-glucopyranoside	$C_{21}H_{24}O_9$	Zhong RJ, et al
106. 枫香 *Liquidambar formosana*	(2*S*)-5,7,4′-trihydroxyflavan-5-*O*-*β*-D-glucopyranoside	$C_{21}H_{24}O_9$	Zhong RJ, et al
107. 洋吊钟 *Kalanchoe tubiflora*	kalantubolide A	$C_{25}H_{32}O_7$	Huang H, et al
107. 洋吊钟 *Kalanchoe tubiflora*	kalantubolide B	$C_{25}H_{32}O_7$	Huang H, et al
107. 洋吊钟 *Kalanchoe tubiflora*	kalantuboside A	$C_{32}H_{42}O_{12}$	Huang H, et al
107. 洋吊钟 *Kalanchoe tubiflora*	kalantuboside B	$C_{30}H_{40}O_{11}$	Huang H, et al
107. 洋吊钟 *Kalanchoe tubiflora*	(6*S*,7*R*,8*R*,9*S*)-6-oxaspiro-7,8-dihydroxymegastigman-4-en-3-one	$C_{13}H_{21}O_4$	Huang HC, et al

续 表

中药及其基源	新 成 分 名 称	分 子 式	报 道 者
108. 石莲 *Sinocrassula indica*	sinocrassosides A_{13}	$C_{29}H_{32}O_{16}$	Xie HH, et al
	sinocrassosides B_6	$C_{29}H_{32}O_{17}$	
	sinocrassosides B_7	$C_{29}H_{32}O_{17}$	
	sinocrassosides D_4	$C_{32}H_{38}O_{18}$	
109. 多茎委陵菜 *Potentilla multicaulis*	2α,3β,19α,23,30 - pentahydroxyurs - 12 - en - 28 - oic acid - 28 - *O* - β - D - glucopyranosyl ester	$C_{36}H_{48}O_5$	Jia L, et al
	N - hydroxyl - hexahydroazepin - 2,4 - diones	$C_6H_9O_3N$	
110. 山刺玫 *Rosa davurica*	Quercetin 3″- *O* -(2 - *O* - galloyl)- β - D - glucuronide 6″- methyl ester	$C_{29}H_{24}O_{17}$	Ma F, et al
111. 湖北海棠 *Malus hupehensis*	P - phloridzin -(Ⅰ - 5, Ⅱ - 3′)- phloretin - 4 - *O* - glucoside	$C_{42}H_{47}O_{21}$	Wang SQ, et al
	M - phloridzin -(Ⅰ - 5, Ⅱ - 3′)- phloretin - 4 - *O* - glucoside	$C_{42}H_{47}O_{21}$	
	Phloridzin -(Ⅰ - 4,*O*, Ⅱ - 2)- luteolin - 5 - *O* - glucoside	$C_{42}H_{42}O_{21}$	
112. 窄叶鲜卑花 *Sibiraea angustata*	sibiraglucoside A	$C_{27}H_{34}O_{11}$	Wang Z, et al
	sibiraglucoside B	$C_{27}H_{34}O_{11}$	
	sibiraglucoside C	$C_{26}H_{32}O_{11}$	
	sibiraglucoside D	$C_{26}H_{32}O_{11}$	
	sibiraglucoside E	$C_{25}H_{30}O_{10}$	
	sibiraglucoside F	$C_{25}H_{30}O_{10}$	
	sibiraglucoside G	$C_{25}H_{30}O_{10}$	
	sibiraglucoside H	$C_{25}H_{30}O_{10}$	
113. 皱皮木瓜 *Chaenomeles speciosa*	specpolyphenol A	$C_{34}H_{27}O_{15}$	Huang GH, et al
	specpolyphenol B	$C_{16}H_{23}O_9$	
114. 非洲紫檀 *Pterocarpus soyauxii*	pterosonins A	$C_{17}H_{15}O_7$	Su Z, et al
	pterosonins B	$C_{18}H_{17}O_7$	
	pterosonins C	$C_{18}H_{17}O_7$	
	pterosonins D	$C_{17}H_{15}O_6$	
	pterosonins E	$C_{16}H_{13}O_5$	
	pterosonins F	$C_{17}H_{15}O_6$	
115. 刺果苏木 *Caesalpinia crista*	1α - acetoxy - 5α,7β - dihydroxycassa - 11,13(15)- diene - 16,12 - lactone	$C_{22}H_{30}O_6$	Tian QJ, et al
116. 黄花棘豆 *Oxytropis ochrocephala*	3 - *O* - rhamnocitrin - 6 - *O* - benzoyl - β - D - glucopyranoside	$C_{29}H_{26}O_{12}$	Li X, et al
117. 苦石莲 *Caesalpinia minax*	caesalpinolide F	$C_{23}H_{32}O_7$	Sun ZC, et al
	caesalpinolide G	$C_{22}H_{32}O_7$	
	caesalpines A	$C_{23}H_{32}O_7$	Zhao P, et al
	caesalpines B	$C_{23}H_{30}O_7$	
	caesalpines C	$C_{23}H_{30}O_8$	
	caesalpines D	$C_{26}H_{32}O_9$	

续　表

中药及其基源	新 成 分 名 称	分 子 式	报 道 者
118. 胡芦巴 *Common Fenugreek*	graecumoside A	$C_{27}H_{38}O_{11}$	Pang X, et al
	graecumoside B	$C_{33}H_{48}O_{15}$	
119. 千斤拔 *Flemingia philippinensis*	flemicoumarin A	$C_{19}H_{16}O_{8}$	Fu M, et al
120. 新疆沙冬青 *Ammopiptanthus nanus*	ammopiptanosides A	$C_{28}H_{32}O_{15}$	Ji TF, et al
	ammopiptanosides B	$C_{34}H_{42}O_{19}$	
121. 补骨脂 *Psoralea corylifolia*	corylifols D	$C_{20}H_{18}O_{5}$	Song P, et al
	corylifols E	$C_{20}H_{18}O_{5}$	
122. 野番豆 *Uraria clarkei*	(2*R*)- 4′- hydroxy - 2′,5,7 - trimethoxyflavane	$C_{18}H_{20}O_{5}$	Jiang ZY, et al
	(2*R*,4*R*)- 2′,4′- dihydroxy - 5,7 - dimethoxyflavan - 4 - ol	$C_{17}H_{18}O_{6}$	
123. 甘葛藤 *Pueraria thomsonii*	kakkasaponin Ⅱ	$C_{42}H_{66}O_{13}$	Lu J, et al
	kakkasaponin Ⅲ	$C_{47}H_{74}O_{16}$	
124. 眼镜豆 *Entada phaseoloides*	phaseoloideside A	$C_{70}H_{113}NO_{34}$	Xiong H, et al
	phaseoloideside B	$C_{65}H_{105}NO_{32}$	
	phaseoloideside C	$C_{70}H_{113}NO_{36}$	
	phaseoloideside D	$C_{72}H_{115}NO_{37}$	
	butyl 2,5 - dihydroxyphenyl acetate	$C_{12}H_{16}O_{4}$	Chen L, et al
	butyl	$C_{18}H_{26}O_{9}$	
	2 - *O*-*β* - D - glucopyranosyloxy - 5 - dihydroxyphenyl acetate	$C_{18}H_{26}O_{9}$	
125. 阿勃勒 *Cassia fistula*	fistulaflavonoids B	$C_{17}H_{14}O_{6}$	Zhao W, et al
	fistulaflavonoids C	$C_{18}H_{16}O_{6}$	
	[1,2 - *β*]furan,2,9 - dihydroxy - 7 - methoxy - 4 - methylnaphtha[1,2 - *β*]furan - 3(2*H*)- one	$C_{14}H_{12}O_{5}$	Wang LQ, et al
126. 长柄山蚂蟥 *Podocarpium podocarpum*	podocarnone	$C_{30}H_{22}NO_{10}$	Ma XQ, et al
127. 茸毛木蓝 *Indigofera stachyodes*	2*α*,3*α* - epoxyflavan - 5,7,3′,4′- tetraol -(4*β*→8)- flavan - 5″,7″,4‴- triol	$C_{30}H_{24}O_{11}$	Qiu L, et al
	3 - *O*-(3 - nitropropanoyl)- 2,3 - cis - 5,7,3′,4′- tetrahydroxyflavan	$C_{18}H_{17}NO_{9}$	
128. 响铃豆 *Crotalaria albida*	neocroalbidine	$C_{18}H_{29}NO_{6}$	Sun QH, et al
	neocroalbidinone	$C_{18}H_{27}NO_{7}$	
129. 显脉棋子豆 *Cylindrokelupha dalatensis*	cylindroside A	$C_{96}H_{152}O_{44}$	Zhou WB, et al
130. 蒺藜 *Tribulus terrestris*	26 - *O*-*β* - D - glucopyranosyl -(25*R*)- 5*α* - furostane - 12 - one - 3*β*,22*α*,26 - triol - 3 - *O*-*β* - Dglucopyranosyl(1→4)- *β* - D - galactopyranoside	$C_{45}H_{74}O_{20}$	Chen G, et al
	26 - *O*-*β* - D - glucopyranosyl - 25(*R*)- 5*α* - furostan - 12 - one - 3*β*,22*α*,26 - triol - 3 - *O*-*α* - L - rhamnopyranosyl -(1→2)- *O*-[*β* - D - glucopyranosyl - (1→4)]- *β* - D - galactopyranoside	$C_{51}H_{84}O_{24}$	

续 表

中药及其基源	新成分名称	分子式	报道者
131. 云南土沉香 *Excoecaria acerifolia*	acerifolin A	$C_{32}H_{42}O_{10}$	Wu XD, et al
	acerifolin B	$C_{20}H_{32}O_3$	
	excoecarins F	$C_{20}H_{30}O_3$	Huang SZ, et al
	excoecarins G	$C_{20}H_{32}O_3$	
	excoecarins H	$C_{20}H_{28}O_4$	
132. 叶下珠 *Phyllanthus urinaria*	3-*O*-α-L-(2,4-di-*O*-acetyl) rhamnopyranoside-7-*O*-α-L-rhamnopyranoside	$C_{31}H_{34}O_{17}$	Wu C, et al
	Quercetin 3-*O*-α-L-(3,4-di-*O*-acetyl) rhamnopyranoside-7-*O*-α-L-rhamnopyranoside	$C_{31}H_{34}O_{17}$	
133. 异叶三宝木 *Trigonostemon lii*	trigolins A	$C_{38}H_{45}O_{12}$	Li SF, et al
	trigolins B	$C_{38}H_{45}O_{12}$	
	trigolins C	$C_{38}H_{45}O_{12}$	
	trigolins D	$C_{40}H_{47}O_{13}$	
	trigolins E	$C_{40}H_{47}O_{13}$	
	trigolins F	$C_{40}H_{47}O_{13}$	
	trigolins G	$C_{43}H_{47}O_{12}$	
134. 大戟 *Euphorbia pekinensis*	Pekinenin C	$C_{20}H_{31}O_2$	Tao WW, et al
	Pekinenin D	$C_{20}H_{31}O_3$	
	Pekinenin E	$C_{20}H_{31}O_4$	
	Pekinenin F	$C_{20}H_{31}O_2$	
135. 长梗三宝木 *Trigonostemon thyrsoideum*	trigothysoids A	$C_{29}H_{37}O_{10}$	Cheng YY, et al
	trigothysoids B	$C_{38}H_{43}O_{12}$	
	trigothysoids C	$C_{31}H_{39}O_{11}$	
	trigothysoids D	$C_{29}H_{39}O_{10}$	
	trigothysoids E	$C_{31}H_{40}O_{12}$	
	trigothysoids F	$C_{31}H_{40}O_{12}$	
	trigothysoids G	$C_{38}H_{45}O_{12}$	
	trigothysoids H	$C_{39}H_{49}O_{16}$	
	trigothysoids I	$C_{37}H_{47}O_{15}$	
	trigothysoids J	$C_{45}H_{49}O_{13}$	
	trigothysoids K	$C_{38}H_{43}O_{11}$	
	trigothysoids L	$C_{38}H_{43}O_{11}$	
	trigothysoids M	$C_{34}H_{35}O_9$	
	trigothysoids N	$C_{44}H_{59}O_{13}$	
	trigothysoids O	$C_{46}H_{55}O_{12}$	
	trigothysoids P	$C_{44}H_{59}O_{12}$	
136. 麻风树 *Jatropha curcas*	curcusecons A	$C_{20}H_{24}O_5$	Liu JQ, et al
	curcusecons B	$C_{20}H_{25}O_3$	
	curcusecons C	$C_{20}H_{24}O_3$	

续　表

中药及其基源	新　成　分　名　称	分子式	报道者
136. 麻风树 *Jatropha curcas*	curcusecons D	$C_{20}H_{25}O_3$	Liu JQ, et al
	curcusecons E	$C_{20}H_{25}O_3$	
	curcusecons F	$C_{21}H_{28}O_3$	
	curcusecons G	$C_{20}H_{26}O_4$	
	curcusecons H	$C_{20}H_{24}O_3$	
	curcusecons I	$C_{20}H_{27}O_4$	
	curcusecons J	$C_{20}H_{27}O_4$	
	4 - epi - curcusone E	$C_{20}H_{25}O_3$	
	3 - dehydroxy - 2 - epi - caniojane	$C_{20}H_{25}O_4$	
137. 黄花三宝木 *Trigonostemon lutescens*	trigolutesins A	$C_{21}H_{18}N_2O_5$	Ma SS, et al
	trigolutesins B	$C_{23}H_{22}N_2O_6$	
	trigolutes A	$C_{22}H_{20}N_2O_6$	
	trigolutes B	$C_{21}H_{18}N_2O_5$	
	trigolutes C	$C_{23}H_{22}N_2O_6$	
	trigolutes D	$C_{22}H_{22}N_2O_5$	
138. 越南叶下珠 *Phyllanthus cochinchinensis*	phyllanthoid A	$C_{30}H_{38}O_{14}$	Zhao JQ, et al
	phyllanthoid A	$C_{28}H_{38}O_{13}$	
139. 猫眼草 *Euphorbia sieboldiana*	(1β,2α,3β,19β)- 1,2,3,19 - tetrahydroxyolean - 12 - en - 28 - oic acid	$C_{30}H_{48}O_6$	Zhang BB, et al
	(1β,3β,19β)- 1,3,19 - trihydroxyolean - 12 - en - 28 - oic acid	$C_{30}H_{48}O_5$	
	(1β,2α,3β,16β,19β)- 1,2,3,16,19 - pentahydroxyolean - 12 - en - 28 - oic acid	$C_{30}H_{48}O_7$	
	(1β,2α,3β,19β,23)- 1,2,3,19,23 - pentahydroxyolean - 12 - en - 28 - oic acid	$C_{30}H_{48}O_7$	
140. 龙脷叶 *Sauropus spatulifolius*	*N* - hydroxyethyl - 2 - acetylpyrrole	$C_8H_{11}NO_2$	Zou YS, et al
	N -(3 - carboxypropyl)- 2 - acetylpyrrole	$C_{10}H_{13}NO_3$	
	2 -(4 - hydroxy - 2,2,6 - trimethylcyclohexyl) acetic acid	$C_{11}H_{20}O_3$	
141. 黑面神 *Breynia fruticosa*	(7*S*,8*R*,7′*S*)- 9,7′,9′- Trihydroxy - 3,4 - methylenedioxy - 3′- methoxy [7 - *O* - 4′,8 - 5′] neolignan	$C_{20}H_{22}O_7$	Li YP, et al
	(7*S*,8*R*,7′*S*)- 9,9′- Dihydroxy - 3,4 - methylenedioxy - 3′,7′- dimethoxy[7 - *O* - 4′,8 - 5′]neolignan	$C_{21}H_{24}O_7$	
142. 剑叶三宝木 *Trigonostemon xyphophylloides*	trigoxyphins J	$C_{38}H_{58}O_{10}$	Yu L, et al
	trigoxyphins K	$C_{34}H_{34}O_9$	
	3 - *O* - benzoylpluricostatic acid	$C_{37}H_{54}O_5$	
143. 光叶巴豆 *Croton laevigatus*	laevinoid A	$C_{20}H_{22}O_5$	Wang GC, et al
	laevinoid B	$C_{20}H_{23}O_5Cl$	

续 表

中药及其基源	新成分名称	分子式	报道者
144. 巴豆 *Croton tiglium*	12-*O*-(2-Methyl)butyrylphorbol-13-tiglate	$C_{30}H_{42}O_8$	Zhang XL, et al
	12-*O*-Tiglylporbol-13-propionate	$C_{28}H_{38}O_8$	
	13-*O*-Acetylphorbol-20-oleate	$C_{40}H_{62}O_8$	
	13-*O*-Acetyl-4-deoxy-4α-phorbol-20-linoleate	$C_{40}H_{59}O_7$	
	13-*O*-Acetyl-4-deoxy-4α-phorbol-20-oleate	$C_{40}H_{61}O_7$	
	12-*O*-Tiglyl-4-deoxy-4α-phorbol-13-decanoate	$C_{35}H_{52}O_7$	
	12-*O*-Tiglyl-4-deoxy-4α-phorbol-13-phenylacetate	$C_{33}H_{40}O_7$	
	12-*O*-Tiglyl-4-deoxy-4α-phorbol-13-(2-methyl)butyrate	$C_{30}H_{42}O_7$	
145. 黄皮 *Clausena lansium*	(2′*R*)-*N*-(2phenylethyl)-N-methylcinnamamide 2′-*O*-β-D-glucopyranoside	$C_{24}H_{29}NO_7$	Wang GC, et al
	(1*R*),(3*R*)-4-methylene-1-(1-methylethyl)-(1,3)-cyclohexanediol	$C_{10}H_{19}O_2$	
146. 吴茱萸 *Evodia rutaecarpa*	rutaecarpine-10-*O*-β-D-glucopyranoside	$C_{24}H_{23}N_3O_7$	Zhang XL, et al
	evorubodinin	$C_{27}H_{32}O_{10}$	Yang XB, et al
147. 三叉苦 *Melicope pteleifolia*	pteleifolins A	$C_{19}H_{26}O_5$	Yang LJ, et al
	pteleifolins B	$C_{12}H_{12}O_3$	
	pteleifolins C	$C_{18}H_{15}O_3$	
148. 酒饼簕 *Atalantia buxifolia*	buxifoliadine	$C_{16}H_{14}NO_6$	Shan F, et al
	3-methoxy-1,4,5-trihydroxy-10-methylacridone	$C_{15}H_{13}NO_5$	Yang YY, et al
	2,3-dimethoxy-1,4,5-trihydroxy-10-methylacridone	$C_{16}H_{15}NO_6$	
149. 假黄皮 *Clausena excavata*	clauexcavatins A	$C_{19}H_{20}O_5$	Peng WW, et al
	clauexcavatins B	$C_{24}H_{28}O_5$	
150. 鸦胆子 *Brucea javanica*	bruceine M	$C_{21}H_{30}O_9$	Su Z, et al
	brujavanones A	$C_{34}H_{49}O_8$	Dong SH, et al
	brujavanones B	$C_{33}H_{49}O_7$	
	brujavanones C	$C_{32}H_{47}O_6$	
	brujavanones D	$C_{33}H_{51}O_8$	
	brujavanones E	$C_{32}H_{49}O_8$	
	brujavanones F	$C_{34}H_{53}O_8$	
	brujavanones G	$C_{33}H_{49}O_7$	
	brujavanones H	$C_{33}H_{51}O_8$	
	brujavanones I	$C_{33}H_{53}O_7$	
	brujavanones J	$C_{33}H_{53}O_7$	
	brujavanones K	$C_{32}H_{51}O_7$	
	brujavanones L	$C_{32}H_{49}O_6$	
	brujavanones M	$C_{39}H_{63}O_{10}$	
	brujavanones N	$C_{34}H_{55}O_8$	

续　表

中药及其基源	新 成 分 名 称	分 子 式	报 道 者
151. 臭椿 *Ailanthus altissima*	altissimanins A	$C_{30}H_{49}O_3$	Hong ZL, et al
	altissimanins B	$C_{30}H_{49}O_2$	
	altissimanins C	$C_{30}H_{49}O_2$	
	altissimanins D	$C_{60}H_{99}O_7$	
	altissimanins E	$C_{60}H_{99}O_7$	
	altissimacoumarin G	$C_{21}H_{27}O_7$	
152. 楝 *Melia azedarach*	mesendanin K	$C_{20}H_{31}O_{10}$	Yuan C, et al
	mesendanin L	$C_{28}H_{39}O_8$	
	mesendanin M	$C_{27}H_{31}O_{10}$	
	17β,20β-Epoxyergosta-5,24(28)-diene-3β,16β,22α-triol	$C_{28}H_{45}O_4$	
	1α,4α,6β-Trihydroxyeudesmane	$C_{15}H_{29}O_3$	
153. 麻楝 *Chukrasia tabularis* var *velutina*	chukvelutilide G	$C_{47}H_{62}O_{18}$	Luo J, et al
	chukrasine F	$C_{48}H_{48}O_{18}$	
	chukfuransin A	$C_{37}H_{48}O_{14}$	Hu K, et al
	chukfuransin B	$C_{39}H_{50}O_{16}$	
	chukfuransin C	$C_{37}H_{46}O_{13}$	
	chukfuransin D	$C_{38}H_{50}O_{14}$	
154. 大叶山楝 *Aphanamixis grandifolia*	aphanamolide C	$C_{32}H_{40}O_{11}$	Zhang Y, et al
	aphanamolide D	$C_{32}H_{38}O_{12}$	
	aphanamene A	$C_{40}H_{54}O_7$	Zhang HJ, et al
	aphanamene B	$C_{40}H_{52}O_8$	
155. 灰毛浆果楝 *Cipadessa cinerascens*	cipatrijugins G	$C_{27}H_{32}O_9$	Zhang ZG, et al
	cipatrijugins H	$C_{29}H_{36}O_{10}$	
156. 多脉樫木 *Dysoxylum lukii*	(3β)-3,20-dihydroxyergosta-5,24(28)-dien-7-one	$C_{28}H_{44}O_3$	Hu J, et al
	(3β,4β,7α)-ergosta-5,24(28)-diene-3,4,7-triol	$C_{28}H_{46}O_3$	
	(3β,7α)-3,20-dihydroxyergosta-5,24(28)-dien-7-ylacetate	$C_{30}H_{48}O_4$	
157. 非洲桃花心木 *Khaya senegalensis*	khayseneganins A	$C_{27}H_{30}O_9$	Yuan CM, et al
	khayseneganins B	$C_{27}H_{32}O_{10}$	
	khayseneganins C	$C_{29}H_{34}O_{11}$	
	khayseneganins D	$C_{27}H_{34}O_9$	
	khayseneganins E	$C_{27}H_{34}O_{11}$	
	khayseneganins F	$C_{28}H_{36}O_{11}$	
	khayseneganins G	$C_{28}H_{34}O_{11}$	
	khayseneganins H	$C_{30}H_{36}O_{12}$	
	khayseneganin I	$C_{28}H_{36}O_{11}$	Yuan CM, et al
	2α,3α,16β-trihydroxy-20-acetoxy-20(*R*)-pregnane	$C_{23}H_{38}O_5$	

续 表

中药及其基源	新成分名称	分子式	报道者
158. 碧绿米仔兰 *Aglaia perviridis*	perviridisin A	$C_{30}H_{48}O_3$	Pan L, et al
	perviridisin B	$C_{36}H_{42}N_2O_{10}$	
	8b-*O*-Methyl-4′-demethoxy-3′,4′-methylenedioxyrocaglaol	$C_{27}H_{26}O_7$	
	Methyl 8b-*O*-methyl-4′-demethoxy-3′,4′-methylenedioxyrocaglate	$C_{29}H_{28}O_9$	
	perviridisinol A	$C_{30}H_{48}O_3$	
	perviridisinol B	$C_{30}H_{48}O_3$	
	perviridisinol C	$C_{30}H_{50}O_3$	
	(6*R*,9*S*)-9,10-Dihydroxy-4-megastigmen-3-one	$C_{13}H_{22}O_3$	
159. 香椿 *Toona sinensis*	toonins A	$C_{32}H_{40}O_{12}$	Dong XJ, et al
	toonins B	$C_{30}H_{40}O_8$	
160. 米兰 *Aglaia odorata* var *microphyllina*	8αb-methoxy-desmethylrocaglamide	$C_{29}H_{31}O_7N$	Liu S, et al
	3′-hydroxy-8β-methoxy-rocaglamide	$C_{30}H_{33}O_8N$	
161. 川楝 *Melia toosendan*	12α/b-1-*O*-tigloyl-1-*O*-deacetyl-nimbolinin B	$C_{38}H_{50}O_{10}$	Su S, et al
	1-deacetylnimbolinin B	$C_{35}H_{46}O_{10}$	
	nimbolinin B	$C_{37}H_{44}O_{10}$	
	nimbolinin A	$C_{33}H_{44}O_9$	
162. 海木 *Trichilia connaroides*	Secotrichagmalin A	$C_{32}H_{38}O_9$	Wang H, et al
	trichanolide A	$C_{32}H_{38}O_{11}$	
	trichanolide B	$C_{32}H_{39}O_{10}$	
	trichanolide C	$C_{32}H_{39}O_{10}$	
	trichanolide D	$C_{32}H_{41}O_{11}$	
	trichanolide E	$C_{32}H_{41}O_{11}$	
	trijugin I	$C_{28}H_{31}O_{13}$	
	trijugin J	$C_{29}H_{33}O_{13}$	
163. 割舌树 *Walsura robusta*	10β-nitro-isodauc-3-en-15-al	$C_{15}H_{23}NO_3$	侯丽,等
164. 西印度樱桃 *Malpighia emarginata*	norfriedelins A	$C_{29}H_{44}O_4$	Liu JQ, et al
	norfriedelins B	$C_{28}H_{46}O_3$	
	norfriedelins C	$C_{27}H_{44}O_2$	
165. 苦远志 *Polygala sibirica*	polygalins D	$C_{28}H_{32}O_{16}$	Song YL, et al
	polygalins E	$C_{27}H_{30}O_{16}$	
	polygalins F	$C_{27}H_{30}O_{16}$	
	polygalins G	$C_{33}H_{40}O_{21}$	
166. 漆 *Toxicodendron vernicifluum*	Toxicodenanes A	$C_{15}H_{24}O_2$	He JB, et al
	Toxicodenanes B	$C_{15}H_{26}O_3$	
	Toxicodenanes C	$C_{15}H_{24}O_2$	

续　表

中药及其基源	新 成 分 名 称	分 子 式	报 道 者
167. 文冠果 *Xanthoceras sorbifolia*	3 - *O* - β - D - glucopyranosyl(1→6) - β - D - glucopyranosyl - 28 - *O* - α - L - rhamnopyranosyl(1→2)[β - D - glucopyranosyl(1→6)]β - D - glucopyranosyl - 21β,22α - dihydroxylolean - 12,15 - diene	$C_{60}H_{98}O_{28}$	Li YY, et al
	3 - *O* - β - D - glucopyranosyl(1→2) - β - D - glucopyranosyl - 28 - *O* - α - L - rhamnopyranosyl(1→2)[β - D - glucopyranosyl(1→6)]β - D - glucopyranosy - 21β,22α - dihydroxyl - olean - 12 - ene	$C_{60}H_{100}O_{28}$	
168. 加州七叶树 *Aesculus californica*	aesculioside C_1	$C_{55}H_{85}O_{23}$	Yuan W, et al
	aesculioside C_2	$C_{55}H_{87}O_{22}$	
	aesculioside C_3	$C_{55}H_{85}O_{22}$	
	aesculioside C_4	$C_{55}H_{85}O_{22}$	
	aesculioside C_5	$C_{55}H_{87}O_{22}$	
	aesculioside C_6	$C_{55}H_{87}O_{21}$	
	aesculioside C_7	$C_{55}H_{87}O_{21}$	
	aesculioside C_8	$C_{55}H_{87}O_{21}$	
	aesculioside C_9	$C_{66}H_{103}O_{26}$	
	aesculioside C_{10}	$C_{66}H_{103}O_{26}$	
	aesculioside C_{11}	$C_{54}H_{85}O_{20}$	
	aesculioside C_{12}	$C_{66}H_{103}O_{25}$	
	aesculioside C_{13}	$C_{54}H_{85}O_{20}$	
	aesculioside C_{14}	$C_{58}H_{91}O_{21}$	
	aesculioside C_{15}	$C_{54}H_{85}O_{19}$	
169. 毛冬青 *Ilex pubescens*	ilexpublesnin C	$C_{42}H_{64}O_{16}NH_4$	Zhou Y, et al
	ilexpublesnin D	$C_{36}H_{54}O_{11}NH_4$	
	ilexpublesnin E	$C_{53}H_{86}O_{22}NH_4$	
	ilexpublesnin F	$C_{41}H_{64}O_{12}NH_4$	
	ilexpublesnin G	$C_{82}H_{133}O_{28}$	
	ilexpublesnin H	$C_{41}H_{66}O_{16}S$	
	ilexpublesnin I	$C_{41}H_{67}O_{16}S$	
	ilexpublesnin J	$C_{53}H_{86}O_{23}NH_4$	
	ilexpublesnin K	$C_{53}H_{86}O_{23}NH_4$	
	ilexpublesnin L	$C_{36}H_{64}O_{16}NH_4$	
	ilexpublesnin M	$C_{36}H_{54}O_{11}NH_4$	
	ilexoside P	$C_{53}H_{84}O_{23}$	Zhou ZL, et al
170. 称星树 *Ilex asprella*	asprellanosides C	$C_{41}H_{64}O_{15}S$	赵钟祥,等
	asprellanosides D	$C_{41}H_{64}O_{15}S$	
	asprellanosides E	$C_{35}H_{54}O_{10}S$	
	(3β) - 19 - hydroxy - 28 - oxours - 12 - en - 3 - yl β - D-glucopyranosiduronic acid n - butyl ester	$C_{40}H_{64}O_{10}$	

续 表

中药及其基源	新成分名称	分子式	报道者
171. 枸骨 *Ilexcornuta*	oleanolic acid 3β-O-a-L-arabinopyranosyl-(1→2)-b-Dglucuronopyranoside-6-O-butyl ester	$C_{45}H_{72}O_{13}$	Liao L, et al
	oleanolic acid 3β-O-[a-L-arabinopyranosyl-(1→2)-b-Dglucuronopyranoside-6-O-butyl ester]-28-O-b-D-glucopyranoside	$C_{51}H_{82}O_{18}$	
	19α-hydroxy oleanolic acid 3β-O-b-D-glucuronopyranoside-6-O-methyl ester	$C_{37}H_{58}O_{10}$	
	19α-hydroxy urs-12-en-28-oic acid 3β-Oa-L-arabinopyranosyl-(1→)-b-D-glucuronopyranoside-6-O-methyl ester	$C_{42}H_{66}O_{14}$	
	lactone A	$C_{22}H_{16}O_9$	Zhang Y, et al
	rel-[(1R,4S,4αS,7S)-1,2,3,4,4α,5,6,7-Octahydro-4-hydroxy-7-(1-hydroxy-1-methylethyl)-4α-methylnaphthalen-1-yl]methyl 3-Methylbutanoate	$C_{20}H_{34}O_4$	Liu Y, et al
	rel-(3R,5S,5αR,6R,7S,9S,9αS,10R)-10-(Acetyloxy)-5α-[(acetyloxy)methyl]octahydro-9-hydroxy-2,2,9-trimethyl-6-(2-methyl-1-oxobutoxy)-7-(1-oxopropoxy)-2H-3,9α-methano-1-benzoxepin-5-yl Furan-3-carboxylate	$C_{32}H_{44}O_{13}$	
172. 大花卫矛 *Euonymus grandiflorus*	8β-hydroxy-18-nor-4(5),15-isopimaradien-3-one	$C_{19}H_{28}O_2$	Li C, et al
173. 雷公藤 *Tripterygium wilfordii*	triptobenzene R	$C_{20}H_{28}O_2$	Li JY, et al
	triptobenzene S	$C_{20}H_{26}O_3$	
174. 灯油藤 *Celastrus paniculatus*	(1α,2α,8β,9β)-1,8-bis(acetyloxy)-9-(benzoyloxy)-2-hydroxy-β-dihydroagarofuran	$C_{26}H_{34}O_8$	Weng JR, et al
	(1α,2α,8β,9β)-1,8,14-tris(acetyloxy)-2,9-bis(benzoyloxy)-β-dihydroagarofuran	$C_{35}H_{41}O_{11}$	
	(1α,2α,8β,9β)-1,8-bis(acetyloxy)-2,9-bis(benzoyloxy)-14-hydroxy-β-dihydroagarofuran	$C_{33}H_{39}O_{10}$	
175. 山葡萄 *Vitis amurensis*	amurensin O	$C_{28}H_{18}O_8$	Yao CS, et al
176. 咖啡黄葵 *Abelmoschus esculentus*	(3β,21β)-19,21-epoxylup-20(29)-en-3-yl acetate	$C_{32}H_{50}O_3$	Zhou Y, et al
	(3β)-9,18-dihydroxyolean-12-en-3-yl acetate	$C_{32}H_{52}O_4$	
177. 木棉花 *Bombax ceiba*	bombasinol A	$C_{21}H_{24}O_6$	Wang GK, et al
178. 台湾梭罗 *Reevesia formosana*	reevesioside A	$C_{30}H_{43}O_9$	Chang HS, et al
	reevesioside B	$C_{32}H_{45}O_{11}$	
	reevesioside C	$C_{30}H_{45}O_9$	
	reevesioside D	$C_{30}H_{45}O_{10}$	
	reevesioside E	$C_{29}H_{45}O_9$	
	reevesioside F	$C_{30}H_{47}O_8$	

续　表

中药及其基源	新成分名称	分子式	报道者
178. 台湾梭罗 *Reevesia formosana*	reevesioside G	$C_{30}H_{43}O_{10}$	Chang HS, et al
	reevesioside H	$C_{30}H_{43}O_{11}$	
	epi - reevesioside H	$C_{30}H_{43}O_{11}$	
179. 毒鼠子属 *Dichapetalum* sp.	dichapetalins N	$C_{38}H_{46}O_5$	Long C, et al
	dichapetalins O	$C_{38}H_{53}O_5$	
	dichapetalins P	$C_{40}H_{49}O_8$	
	dichapetalins Q	$C_{38}H_{53}O_5$	
	dichapetalins R	$C_{38}H_{55}O_7$	
	dichapetalins S	$C_{38}H_{49}O_6$	
180. 土沉香 *Aquilaria sinensis*	qinanones A	$C_{18}H_{16}O_4$	Yang D, et al
	qinanones B	$C_{18}H_{16}O_4$	
	qinanones C	$C_{18}H_{16}O_4$	
	qinanones D	$C_{17}H_{14}O_3$	
	qinanones E	$C_{17}H_{14}O_3$	
	aquilarabietic acids A	$C_{20}H_{32}O_5$	Yang L, et al
	aquilarabietic acids B	$C_{20}H_{31}O_5$	
	aquilarabietic acids C	$C_{23}H_{35}O_5$	
	aquilarabietic acids D	$C_{20}H_{32}O_5$	
	aquilarabietic acids E	$C_{20}H_{31}O_6$	
	aquilarabietic acids F	$C_{20}H_{29}O_3$	
	aquilarabietic acids G	$C_{20}H_{32}O_5$	
	aquilarabietic acids H	$C_{20}H_{26}O_3$	
	aquilarabietic acids I	$C_{21}H_{30}O_4$	
	aquilarabietic acids J	$C_{22}H_{33}O_3$	
	aquilarabietic acid K	$C_{34}H_{48}O_8$	
181. 柞木 *Xylocarpus moluccensis*	thaixylomolin D	$C_{34}H_{40}O_{11}$	Li J, et al
	thaixylomolin E	$C_{33}H_{40}O_{11}$	
	thaixylomolin F	$C_{38}H_{38}O_{11}$	
182. 天山堇菜 *Viola tianshanica*	tianshanoside A	$C_{32}H_{44}O_{16}$	Qin Y, et al
183. 苦瓜 *Momordica charantia*	(3β,7β,15β,23*E*)- 3,7,15,25 - tetrahydroxycucurbita - 5,23 - dien - 19 - al	$C_{30}H_{48}O_5$	Cheng BH, et al
	(3β,7β)- 3,7,22,23 - tetrahydroxycucurbita - 5,24 - dien - 19 - al	$C_{30}H_{48}O_5$	
	(3β,7β)- 3,7,23,24 - tetrahydroxycucurbita - 5,25 - dien - 19 - al	$C_{30}H_{48}O_5$	
	(3β,7β,23S)- 3,7,23 - trihydroxycucurbita - 5,24 - dien - 19 - al 7 - b - d - glucopyranoside	$C_{36}H_{58}O_9$	
	(3β,7β,23*E*)- cucurbita - 5,23 - diene - 3,7,19,25 - tetrol 7 - b - d - glucopyranoside	$C_{36}H_{60}O_9$	

续 表

中药及其基源	新成分名称	分子式	报道者
183. 苦瓜 *Momordica charantia*	(3β,7β,23*E*)-3,7-dihydroxy-25-methoxycucurbita-5,23-dien-19-al 3-b-d-allopyranoside	$C_{37}H_{60}O_9$	Cheng BH, et al
184. 芫花 *Daphne genkwa*	12-*O*-(2′*E*,4′*E*-decadienoyl)-7-oxo-5-ene-phorbol-13-acetate	$C_{32}H_{42}O_9$	Wang R, et al
	12-*O*-neodecanoyl-7-oxo-5-ene-phorbol-13-acetate	$C_{32}H_{47}O_9$	
185. 中国沙棘 *Hippophae rhamnoides*	hippophin C	$C_{54}H_{64}O_{26}$	Gao W, et al
	hippophin C	$C_{54}H_{64}O_{26}$	
	hippophin D	$C_{53}H_{62}O_{25}$	
	hippophin E	$C_{53}H_{62}O_{25}$	
186. 胡颓子 *Elaeagnus pungens*	3-*O*-β-D-glucopyranosyl-(1→3)-α-L-rhamnopyranosyl-(1→6)-[α-L-rhamnopyranosyl (1→2)]-β-D-galactopyranoside	$C_{39}H_{50}O_{24}$	Ge YB, et al
	3-*O*-β-D-gluco-pyranosyl-(1→3)-α-L-rhamnopyranosyl-(1→6)-β-D-galactopyranoside	$C_{34}H_{42}O_{21}$	
187. 散沫花 *Lawsonia inermis*	lawsochylin A	$C_{17}H_{15}O_2$	Liou JR, et al
	lawsochylin B	$C_{17}H_{15}O_3$	
	lawsochylin C	$C_{18}H_{17}O_3$	
	lawsonaphthoate A	$C_{13}H_{13}O_5$	
	lawsonaphthoate B	$C_{14}H_{15}O_5$	
	lawsonaphthoate C	$C_{14}H_{15}O_6$	
188. 岗松 *Baeckea frutescens*	baeckein E	$C_{38}H_{32}O_{19}$	Jia BX, et al
189. 石榴 *Punica granatum*	7,8-dihydroxy-3-carboxymethylcoumarin-5-carboxylic acid	$C_{12}H_8O_8$	Yuan T, et al
	punicatannin C	$C_{31}H_{32}O_{16}$	
190. 十雄角果木 *Ceriops decandra*	decandrins A	$C_{20}H_{27}O_2$	Wang H, et al
	decandrins B	$C_{20}H_{33}O_3$	
	decandrins C	$C_{20}H_{27}O_3$	
	decandrins D	$C_{20}H_{27}O_2$	
	decandrins E	$C_{20}H_{29}O$	
	decandrins F	$C_{20}H_{31}O_2$	
	decandrins G	$C_{20}H_{29}O_2$	
	decandrins H	$C_{20}H_{31}O_2$	
	decandrins I	$C_{40}H_{57}O_4$	
	decandrins J	$C_{17}H_{25}O_2$	
	decandrins K	$C_{17}H_{25}O_2$	
191. 锁阳 *Cynomorium songaricum*	songarin A	$C_{21}H_{20}O_{10}$	Xie SA, et al
192. 千丈树 *Camptotheca acuminate*	(1*R*,2*E*,4*S*,5*R*)-1-[(2*R*)-5-oxotetrahydrofuran-2-yl]-4,5-dihydroxy-hex-2-en-1-yl(2*E*)-2-methylbut-2-enoate	$C_{15}H_{22}O_6$	Liu Y, et al

续 表

中药及其基源	新成分名称	分子式	报道者
193. 鹅掌柴 *Schefflera heptaphylla*	heptursosides A	$C_{48}H_{76}O_{18}$	Wu C, et al
	heptursosides B	$C_{48}H_{76}O_{18}$	
	heptursosides C	$C_{48}H_{76}O_{19}$	
	heptursosides D	$C_{42}H_{66}O_{15}$	
	heptoleosides A	$C_{48}H_{76}O_{19}$	
	heptoleosides B	$C_{48}H_{76}O_{18}$	
	heptoleosides C	$C_{48}H_{76}O_{18}$	
	heptoleosides D	$C_{42}H_{66}O_{15}$	
	heptdamoside A	$C_{41}H_{68}O_{14}$	
194. 西洋参 *Panax quinquefolium*	3*β*,6*α*,20*S* - trihydroxy - 12*β*,23*R* - epoxydammar -24 - ene 6 - *O* -[*α* - L - rhamnosyl(1→2)- *β* - D - glucopyranosyl]- 20 - *O* - *β* - D - glucopyranoside	$C_{48}H_{80}O_{19}$	Xiang Z, et al
	3*β*,20*S* - dihydroxy - 12*β*,23*R* - epoxydammar - 24 - ene 3 - *O* -[*β* - D - glucopyranosyl(1→2)- *β* - D - glucopyranosyl]- 20 - *O* - *β* - D - glucopyranoside	$C_{48}H_{80}O_{19}$	
	pseudo - ginsenoside RT_6	$C_{36}H_{60}O_{10}$	Liu JP, et al
	pseudoginsengenin R_1	$C_{30}H_{50}O_5$	
195. 人参 *Panax ginseng*	ginsenjilinol	$C_{42}H_{72}O_{15}$	Wang HP, et al
196. 无梗五加 *Acanthopanax sessiliflorus*	(2*E*)- 3,7 - dimethylocta - 2,6 - dienoate - 6 - *O* - *α* - L -arabinopyranosyl -(1→6)- *β* - D - glucopyranoside	$C_{21}H_{34}O_{11}$	Yang CJ, et al
	(3*Z*,6*E*)- 3,7 - dimethyl - 3,6 - octadiene - 1,2,8 - triol	$C_{10}H_{18}O_3$	
197. 辽东楤木 *Aralia elata*	3 - *O* - *β* - D - glucopyranosyl -(1→3)- *β* - D - glucopyranosyl -(1→3)- *β* - Dglucopyranosyl echinocystic acid	$C_{48}H_{78}O_{20}$	Ma ZQ, et al
	3 - *O* - *β* - D - glucopyranosyl -(1→3)- *β* - Dglucopyranosyl -(1→3)- *β* - D - glucopyranosyl oleanolic acid 28 - *O* - *β* - D - glucopyranoside	$C_{54}H_{88}O_{24}$	
198. 三七 *Panax notoginseng*	6 - *O* - *β* - D - glucopyranosyl - 20 - *O* - *β* - D - glucopyranosyl - 20(*S*)- protopanaxadiol - 3 - one	$C_{42}H_{70}O_{14}$	Fu HZ, et al
	20*S* - sanchirhinosides A_1	$C_{40}H_{66}O_{10}$	Zhang Y, et al
	20*S* - sanchirhinosides A_2	$C_{43}H_{72}O_{14}$	
	20*S* - sanchirhinosides A_3	$C_{41}H_{70}O_{13}$	
	20*S* - sanchirhinosides A_4	$C_{41}H_{70}O_{13}$	
	20*S* - sanchirhinosides A_5	$C_{47}H_{80}O_{18}$	
	20*S* - sanchirhinosides A_6	$C_{47}H_{80}O_{18}$	
	sanchirhinoside B	$C_{42}H_{70}O_{13}$	
199. 多伞阿魏 *Ferula ferulaeoides*	8,9 - dihydroxydshamirone	$C_{23}H_{34}O_5$	Liu T, et al
	8,9 - oxoisopropanyldshamirone	$C_{23}H_{34}O_5$	
	ferulaeolactone	$C_{23}H_{34}O_6$	
	ferulaeone A	$C_{25}H_{33}O_5$	Meng H, et al

续 表

中药及其基源	新 成 分 名 称	分 子 式	报 道 者
199. 多伞阿魏 *Ferula ferulaeoides*	ferulaeone B	$C_{25}H_{37}O_6$	Meng H, et al
	ferulaeone C	$C_{23}H_{31}O_3$	
	ferulaeone D	$C_{23}H_{28}O_4$	
	ferulaeone E	$C_{33}H_{48}O_4$	
	ferulaeone F	$C_{33}H_{48}O_4$	
	ferulaeone G	$C_{33}H_{43}O_5$	
	ferulaeone H	$C_{38}H_{55}O_5$	
200. 蛇床花 *Cnidium monnieri*	methylpicraquassioside B	$C_{20}H_{26}O_{11}$	Kim SB, et al
201. 全裂叶阿魏 *Ferula dissecta*	syreiteate A	$C_{23}H_{22}O_6$	Huang J, et al
	syreiteate B	$C_{22}H_{30}O_5$	
202. 川芎 *Ligusticum chuanxiong*	chuanxiongdiolides A	$C_{24}H_{32}O_4$	Huang J, et al
	chuanxiongdiolides B	$C_{24}H_{32}O_5$	
203. 马醉木 *Pieris japonica*	Benzyl 2-hydroxy-4-*O*-β-D-glucopyranosyl-benzoate	$C_{20}H_{22}O_9$	Li YP, et al
204. 羊踯躅 *Rhododendron molle*	2α,10α-epoxy-3β,5β,6β,14β,16α-hexahydroxy-grayanane	$C_{20}H_{32}O_6$	陈绍农,等
	benzyl 2,6-dihydroxybenzoate-6-*O*-α-L-rhamnopyranosyl-(1→3)-β-D-glucopyranoside	$C_{26}H_{32}O_{13}$	
	mollolide A	$C_{20}H_{32}O_8$	Li Y, et al
205. 照山白 *Rhododendron micranthum*	micranthanone A	$C_{20}H_{30}O_4$	Zhang M, et al
	rhodomicranols A	$C_{29}H_{38}O_8$	
	rhodomicranols B	$C_{27}H_{36}O_7$	
206. 走马胎 *Ardisia gigantifolia*	11-*O*-veratroylbergenin	$C_{23}H_{24}O_{12}$	Mu LH, et al
	3-*O*-β-D-glucopyranosyl-(1→3)-β-D-xylopyranosyl-(1→2)-[α-L-rhamnopyranosyl-(1→3)]-β-D-glucopyranosyl-(1→4)-[β-Dglucopyranosyl-(1→2)]-α-L-arabinopyranosyl-3β,16α,28,30-tetrahydroxy-olean-12-ene	$C_{64}H_{106}O_{30}$	
207. 矮桃 *Lysimachia clethroides*	trans-aconitate 5-ethyl ester	$C_8H_{10}O_6$	Liang D, et al
	trans-aconitate 6-ethyl ester	$C_8H_{10}O_6$	
	trans-aconitate 1-ethyl ester	$C_8H_{10}O_6$	
	vanill acid-4-*O*-β-D-(2-*O*-*E*-p-coumaroyl) glucopyranoside	$C_{23}H_{24}O_{11}$	
	protocatechuic acid-3-*O*-β-Dxylopyranoside	$C_{12}H_{14}O_8$	
	(methoxycarbonylmethyl)phenyl-4-*O*-β-D-glucopyranoside	$C_{15}H_{20}O_8$	
208. 过路黄 *Lysimachia christinae*	myricetin 3,3′-di-a-l-rhamnopyranoside	$C_{27}H_{30}O_{16}$	Gao F, et al
	and quercetin 3,3′-di-a-lrhamnopyranoside	$C_{27}H_{30}O_{15}$	
209. 白背枫 *Buddleja asiatica*	asiatoates A	$C_{25}H_{40}O_6$	Ali F, et al
	asiatoates B	$C_{24}H_{38}O_6$	

续　表

中药及其基源	新成分名称	分子式	报道者
210. 钩吻 *Gelsemium elegans*	21-oxokoumine	$C_{20}H_{20}N_2O_2$	Sun M, et al
	furanokoumine	$C_{20}H_{22}N_2O_2$	
211. 三花龙胆 *Gentiana triflora*	gentioxepine	$C_{13}H_{12}O_4$	Wang S, et alI
	(*1S*,*5R*,*9R*)-deglucosyltrifloroside	$C_{29}H_{32}O_{15}$	
	(*1S*,*5R*,*9R*)-scabraside	$C_{40}H_{44}O_{20}$	
212. 贵州獐牙菜 *Dracaena angustifolia*	drangustosides A	$C_{45}H_{72}O_{17}$	Huang HC, et al
	drangustosides B	$C_{39}H_{62}O_{13}$	
213. 大叶匙羹 *Gymnema tingens*	gymnetinosides A	$C_{27}H_{33}O_{16}$	Tian J, et al
	gymnetinosides B	$C_{28}H_{35}O_{17}$	
	gymnetinosides C	$C_{28}H_{37}O_{16}$	
	gymnetinosides D	$C_{27}H_{35}O_{15}$	
	gymnetinosides E	$C_{29}H_{39}O_{17}$	
	gymnetinosides F	$C_{36}H_{43}O_{18}$	
214. 长春花 *Catharanthus roseus*	17-desacetoxyvinblastine N'_b-oxide	$C_{44}H_{56}N_4O_8$	Zhang WK, et al
	20′-desacetoxyvinblastine N'_b-oxide	$C_{46}H_{58}N_4O_9$	
215. 络石藤 *Trachelospermum jasminoides*	3′,7-dimethoxyisoflavanone-4′,5-di-*O*-*β*-D-glucopyranoside	$C_{29}H_{34}O_{16}$	张健,等
216. 岩生羊角棉 *Alstonia rupestris*	scholarisins Ⅰ	$C_{22}H_{24}N_2O_5$	Wang W, et al
	scholarisins Ⅱ	$C_{22}H_{26}N_2O_5$	
	scholarisins Ⅲ	$C_{24}H_{29}N_2O_6$	
	scholarisins Ⅳ	$C_{21}H_{26}N_2O_5$	
	scholarisins Ⅴ	$C_{21}H_{26}N_2O_5$	
	scholarisins Ⅵ	$C_{22}H_{26}N_2O_5$	
	scholarisins Ⅶ	$C_{22}H_{26}N_2O_5$	
217. 玫瑰树 *Ochrosia borbonica*	ochroborines A	$C_{23}H_{26}N_2O_6$	Zhang BJ, et al
	ochroborines B	$C_{23}H_{28}N_2O_7$	
	vallesiachotamine	$C_{21}H_{22}N_2O_4$	
	10-hydroxyisositsirikine	$C_{21}H_{26}N_2O_4$	
	10,11-dimethoxysitsirikine	$C_{21}H_{26}N_2O_4$	
	10-methoxyapoyohimbine	$C_{21}H_{26}N_2O_4$	
	10-hydroxyakuammidine	$C_{21}H_{24}N_2O_4$	
	17-O-b-d-glucoside	$C_{27}H_{34}N_2O_8$	
	15α-hydroxyapparicine	$C_{18}H_{20}N_2O$	
	15α-hydroxy-10-methoxyapparicine	$C_{19}H_{22}N_2O_2$	
218. 九节属 *Psychotria* sp.	psychotrianosides A	$C_{35}H_{59}O_8$	Zhang C, et al
	psychotrianosides B	$C_{46}H_{75}O_{17}$	
	psychotrianosides C	$C_{46}H_{75}O_{16}$	
	psychotrianosides D	$C_{52}H_{87}O_{20}$	

续 表

中药及其基源	新成分名称	分子式	报道者
218. 九节属 *Psychotria* sp.	psychotrianosides E	$C_{52}H_{87}O_{21}$	Zhang C, et al
	psychotrianosides F	$C_{54}H_{89}O_{22}$	
219. 帽柱木 *Mitragyna diversifolia*	mitradiversifoline	$C_{23}H_{29}N_2O_6$	Cao XF, et al
	specionoxeine - *N*(4)- oxide	$C_{23}H_{29}N_2O_6$	
	7 - hydroxyisopaynantheine	$C_{23}H_{29}N_2O_5$	
	3 - dehydropaynantheine	$C_{23}H_{27}N_2O_4$	
	3 - isopaynantheine - *N*(4)- oxide	$C_{23}H_{29}N_2O_5$	
220. 香果树 *Emmenopterys henryi*	3β,19α,23 - trihydroxyurs - 12 - en - 24 - al - 28 - oic acid	$C_{30}H_{46}O_6$	Wu X, et al
	3β,19α,24 - trihydroxy - 23 - norurs - 12 - en - 28 - oic acid	$C_{29}H_{46}O_5$	
	3β,12β- dihydroxy - 5α - pregnane - 14,16 - dien - 20 - one	$C_{21}H_{30}O_3$	
	12β- hydroxy - 5α - pregnane - 14,16 - dien - 3,20 - dione	$C_{21}H_{28}O_3$	
	5 - oxodolichantoside	$C_{28}H_{34}N_2O_{10}$	Wu XD, et al
	deglycocadambine	$C_{21}H_{22}N_2O_5$	
221. 琼岛染木树 *Saprosma merrillii*	3α,6α,30 - trihydroxy - ursan - 28 - oic acid	$C_{30}H_{50}O_5$	Zhang D, et al
	3α,30 - dihydroxy - 6 - oxo - ursan - 28 - oic acid	$C_{30}H_{48}O_5$	
	3α,6α,7α,30 - tetrahydroxy - ursan - 28 - oic acid	$C_{30}H_{50}O_6$	
222. 丁公藤 *Erycibe obtusifolia*	4 - *O*- caffeoyl - 3 - *O*- sinapoylquinic acid methyl ester	$C_{28}H_{29}O_{13}$	Fan L, et al
	5 - *O*- caffeoyl - 4 - *O*- syringoylquinic acid methyl ester	$C_{26}H_{28}O_{13}$	
	4 - *O*- caffeoyl - 3 - *O*- syringoylquinic acid methyl ester	$C_{26}H_{27}O_{13}$	
	7 - *O*-(3 - *O*- sinapoyl - β- D - glucopyranosyl)- 6 - methoxycoumarin	$C_{27}H_{28}O_{13}$	
	7 - *O*-(6 - *O*- sinapoyl - β- D - glucopyranosyl)- 6 - methoxycoumarin	$C_{27}H_{28}O_{13}$	
	7 - *O*-(2 - *O*- sinapoyl - β- D - glucopyranosyl)- 6 - methoxycoumarin	$C_{27}H_{28}O_{13}$	
	7 - *O*-(6 - *O*- syringoyl - β- D - glucopyranosyl)- 6 - methoxycoumarin	$C_{25}H_{26}O_{13}$	
223. 槭叶牵牛 *Ipomoea cairica*	cairicosides A	$C_{70}H_{111}O_{26}$	Yu B, et al
	cairicosides B	$C_{70}H_{111}O_{26}$	
	cairicosides C	$C_{65}H_{101}O_{26}$	
	cairicosides D	$C_{68}H_{108}ClO_{26}$	
	cairicosides E	$C_{61}H_{105}O_{25}$	
	cairicosides F	$C_{63}H_{110}ClO_{25}$	
224. 密脉木 *Myrioneuron faberi*	myriberine A	$C_{18}H_{20}N_2O$	Huang SD, et al

续　表

中药及其基源	新 成 分 名 称	分 子 式	报 道 者
225. 马鞭草 *Verbena officinalis*	4 - epi - barbinervic acid	$C_{30}H_{48}O_5$	Shu JC, et al
226. 黄荆 *Vitex negundo*	2 - methyl pyromeconic acid 3 - *O* - *β* - D - glucopyranoside - 6′-(*O* - 4″- hydroxybenzoate)	$C_{19}H_{20}O_{10}$	Huang J, et al
	6′- *O* - p - hydroxybenzoyl - gardoside	$C_{23}H_{26}O_{12}$	
227. 蔓荆 *Vitex trifolia* var *simplicifolia*	3 - Oxotaraxer - 14 - en - 30 - al	$C_{30}H_{46}O_2$	Huang MY, et al
	vitextrifolins A	$C_{24}H_{40}O_6$	Zheng CJ, et al
	vitextrifolins B	$C_{24}H_{40}O_6$	
	vitextrifolins C	$C_{22}H_{32}O_4$	
	vitextrifolins D	$C_{20}H_{30}O_3$	
	vitextrifolins E	$C_{20}H_{30}O_3$	
	vitextrifolins F	$C_{20}H_{32}O_4$	
	vitextrifolins G	$C_{20}H_{32}O_4$	
228. 云南石梓 *Gmelina arborea*	6 - *O* - a - L -(2″- *O* - trans - cinnamoyl - 3″- Oisovaleryl) rhamnopyranosylcatalpol	$C_{35}H_{46}O_{16}Cl$	Gu W, et al
	6 - *O* - a - L -(2″,3″- di - *O* - trans - phydroxycinnamoyl) rhamnopyranosylcatalpol	$C_{39}H_{43}O_{18}$	
	2 - *O* - trans - cinnamoyl - a - L - rhamnopyranose	$C_{15}H_{18}O_6$	
	3 - *O* - trans - cinnamoyl - a - L - rhamnopyranose	$C_{15}H_{18}O_6$	
	2 - *O* - cis - cinnamoyl - a - L - rhamnopyranose	$C_{15}H_{18}O_6$	
229. 黄毛豆腐柴 *Premna fulva*	premfulvaoside	$C_{45}H_{56}O_{24}$	Niu KY, et al
	actinidicoside	$C_{42}H_{66}O_{15}$	
230. 裸花紫珠 *Callicarpa nudiflora*	methylcallicarpate	$C_{21}H_{30}O_4$	Dong L, et al
	callicarpic acid	$C_{20}H_{28}O_4$	
231. 海州常山 *Clerodendrum trichotomum*	6 - methoxyvillosin C	$C_{21}H_{27}O_6$	Wang WX, et al
	18 - hydroxy - 6 - methoxyvillosin C	$C_{21}H_{27}O_7$	
	(10*R*,16*S*)- 12,16 - epoxy - 11,14 - dihydroxy - 6 - methoxy - 17(15→16)- abeo - abieta - 5,8,11,13 - tetraene - 3,7 - dione	$C_{21}H_{25}O_6$	
	(10*R*,16*S*)- 12,16 - epoxy - 11,14 - dihydroxy - 18 - oxo - 17(15→16),18(4→3)- diabeo - abieta - 3,5,8,11,13 - pentaene - 7 - one	$C_{20}H_{21}O_5$	
	(10*R*,16*R*)- 12,16 - epoxy - 11,14,17 - trihydroxy - 17(15→16),18(4→3)- diabeo - abieta - 3,5,8,11,13 - pentaene - 2,7 - dione	$C_{20}H_{21}O_6$	
	(3S,4*R*,10*R*,16*S*)- 3,4 : 12,16 - diepoxy - 11,14 - dihydroxy - 17(15→16),18(4→3)- diabeo - abieta - 5,8,11,13 - tetraene - 7 - one	$C_{20}H_{23}O_5$	
	12,16 - epoxy - 17(15→16),18(4→3)- diabeo - abieta -3,5,8,11,13 - pentaene - 7,11,14 - trione	$C_{20}H_{19}O_4$	
232. 香青兰 *Dracocephalum moldavica*	acacetin - 7 - *O* -(4″- acetyl)- glucopyranoside	$C_{24}H_{25}O_{11}$	Yang S, et al

续 表

中药及其基源	新 成 分 名 称	分 子 式	报 道 者
233. 细叶香茶菜 *Isodon japonica*	3α,14β,16α - trihydroxy - ent - kaurane	$C_{20}H_{35}O_3$	Liu W, et alI
	glaucocalyxin G	$C_{26}H_{42}O_{10}$	Xiang ZB, et al
234. 活血丹 *Glechoma longituba*	glechomols A	$C_{16}H_{18}O_4$	Zhu QF, et al
	glechomols B	$C_{16}H_{18}O_4$	
	glechomols C	$C_{16}H_{18}O_4$	
235. 荔枝草 *Salvia plebeia*	1α - acetoxy - 8α,9β - dihydroxy - 2 - oxo - eudesman - 3,7(11)- dien - 8,12 - olide	$C_{17}H_{20}O_7$	Cao SY, et al
236. 半枝莲 *Scutellaria barbata*	scutebatas P	$C_{34}H_{38}O_8$	Li YY, et al
	scutebatas Q	$C_{34}H_{38}O_8$	
	scutebatas R	$C_{28}H_{40}O_9$	
237. 地茶 *Thamnolia vermicularis*	Thamnoliadepside C	$C_{18}H_{18}O_6$	Xiang W, et al
	Thamnoliadepside D	$C_{17}H_{18}O_5$	
	Thamnoliadepside E	$C_{17}H_{16}O_7$	
238. 拟缺香茶菜 *Isodon excisoides*	2α,3β - dihydroxy - 11α,12α - epoxy - urs - 28,13bolide	$C_{30}H_{46}O_5$	Jiao K, et al
	2α,3β,24 - trihydroxy - 11α,12α - epoxy - urs - 28, 13β -olide	$C_{30}H_{46}O_6$	
	2α,3α,24 - trihydroxy - 11,20(30)- dien - urs - 28, 13β -olide	$C_{30}H_{44}O_5$	
239. 帚状香茶菜 *Isodon scoparius*	scopariusic Acid	$C_{37}H_{54}O_6$	Zhou M, et al
240. 米团花 *Leucosceptrum canum*	leucosceptroids E	$C_{25}H_{34}O_5$	Luo SH, et al
	leucosceptroids F	$C_{25}H_{34}O_5$	
	leucosceptroids G	$C_{25}H_{36}O_6$	
	leucosceptroids H	$C_{25}H_{36}O_6$	
	leucosceptroids I	$C_{25}H_{36}O_5$	
	leucosceptroids J	$C_{25}H_{36}O_5$	
	leucosceptroids K	$C_{25}H_{34}O_6$	
	leucosceptroids L	$C_{25}H_{32}O_5$	
	leucosceptroids M	$C_{25}H_{32}O_5$	
	leucosceptroids N	$C_{25}H_{36}O_6$	
241. 山藿香 *Teucrium viscidum*	3β - hydroxy - urs - 30 - p - Z - hydroxycinnamoyloxy - 12 - en - 28 - oic - acid	$C_{39}H_{54}O_6$	Hao X, et al
242. 益母草 *Leonurus japonicus*	(—)-(1S*,2S*,3R*)- 3 - ethoxycupar - 5 - ene - 1,2 - diol	$C_{17}H_{30}O_3$	Xiong L, et al
	(—)-(1S*,4S*,9S*)- 1,9 - epoxybisabola - 2,10 - diene - 4 - ol	$C_{15}H_{24}O_2$	
	leonurusoides A	$C_{36}H_{38}O_{19}$	Zhang Y, et al
	leonurusoides B	$C_{36}H_{39}O_{19}$	
	leonurusoides C	$C_{36}H_{38}O_{19}$	
	leonurusoides D	$C_{36}H_{38}O_{19}$	
	leonurusoides E	$C_{36}H_{38}O_{20}$	

续 表

中药及其基源	新成分名称	分子式	报道者
242. 益母草 *Leonurus japonicus*	3-acetoxy-6-hydroxy-15,16-dinorlabd-8(9)-ene-13-yne-7-one	$C_{20}H_{28}O_4$	Peng F, et al
243. 痢止蒿 *Ajuga forrestii*	3α-acetoxy-1α,8β-dihydroxyeudesm-7(11)-en-8,12-olide	$C_{17}H_{24}O_6$	Xiong Y, et al
	3α-acetoxy-1α-hydroxyl-eudesm-8,7(11)-dien-8,12-olide	$C_{17}H_{22}O_5$	
	1α-acetoxy-8α-oxyethyl-2-oxo-eudesman-3,7(11)-dien-8,12-olide	$C_{19}H_{24}O_6$	
	2α,3β,11,12-tetrahydroxy-7β,20-epoxy-8,11,13-abietatriene	$C_{20}H_{28}O_5$	
244. 猫须草 *Orthosiphon aristatus* var *aristatus*	orthoarisins A	$C_{38}H_{44}O_{11}$	Di XX, et al
	orthoarisins B	$C_{36}H_{42}O_{10}$	
	orthoarisins C	$C_{36}H_{40}O_{10}$	
	orthoarisins D	$C_{29}H_{36}O_8$	
	orthoarisins E	$C_{38}H_{46}O_{11}$	
	orthoarisins F	$C_{38}H_{46}O_{11}$	
	orthoarisins G	$C_{38}H_{44}O_{11}$	
	orthoarisins H	$C_{31}H_{40}O_{10}$	
	orthoarisins I	$C_{36}H_{42}O_{11}$	
245. 狮耳花 *Leonotis leonurus*	leoleorin D	$C_{20}H_{37}O_4$	Wu H, et al
	leoleorin E	$C_{20}H_{35}O_4$	
	leoleorin F	$C_{20}H_{35}O_4$	
	16-epi-leoleorin F	$C_{20}H_{35}O_4$	
	leoleorin G	$C_{20}H_{29}O_4$	
	leoleorin H	$C_{20}H_{33}O_4$	
	leoleorin I	$C_{20}H_{33}O_4$	
	leoleorin J	$C_{20}H_{35}O_4$	
246. 地埂鼠尾草 *Salvia scapiformis*	scapiformolactone A	$C_{22}H_{33}O_7$	Lai Y, et al
	scapiformolactone B	$C_{20}H_{29}O_6$	
	scapiformolactone C	$C_{20}H_{29}O_5$	
	scapiformolactone D	$C_{22}H_{35}O_7$	
	scapiformolactone E	$C_{22}H_{35}O_7$	
	scapiformolactone F	$C_{20}H_{33}O_6$	
	scapiformolactone G	$C_{20}H_{33}O_6$	
	scapiformolactone H	$C_{20}H_{33}O_5$	
	scapiformolactone I	$C_{20}H_{31}O_5$	
247. 枸杞 *Lycium chinense*	lyciumin	$C_{12}H_{12}O_4$	Li XN, et al
248. 黄花烟草 *Nicotiana rustica*	rel-2*R*,5*S*,9*S*,10*R*,11*R*,12-trihydroxy-6(7)-spirovetiven-8-one-9-*O*-β-D-glucopyranoside	$C_{21}H_{34}O_9$	Zhou R, et al

续 表

中药及其基源	新成分名称	分子式	报道者
249. 曼陀罗 *Datura stramonium*	(22*R*)-27-hydroxy-7*α*-methoxy-1-oxowitha-3,5,24-trienolide	$C_{20}H_{40}O_5$	Fang ST, et al
	27-*O*-*β*-D-glucopyranoside	$C_{35}H_{50}O_{10}$	
	(22*R*)-27-hydroxy-1-oxowitha-2,5,24-trienolide	$C_{28}H_{38}O_4$	
250. 曼佗罗 *Hyoscyamus niger*	hyoscyamoside G	$C_{40}H_{66}O_{15}$	Zhang W, et al
251. 水茄 *Solanum torvum*	solanolactoside C	$C_{28}H_{44}O_8$	Shu W, et al
	torvoside Q	$C_{38}H_{62}O_{15}$	
	torvpregnanosides A	$C_{33}H_{53}O_{11}$	Lee CL, et al
	torvpregnanosides B	$C_{32}H_{51}O_{11}$	
	torvoside Q	$C_{39}H_{63}O_{13}$	
252. 马铃薯 *Solanum tuberosum*	(3*β*)-14-hydroxysolanid-5-en-3-yl 4-*O*-(6-deoxy-a-l-mannopyranosyl)-b-d-glucopyranoside	$C_{39}H_{63}NO_{11}$	Zhang ZQ, et al
	(3*β*,7*β*)-7-hydroxysolanid-5-en-3-yl 6-deoxy-a-l-mannopyranosyl-(1→2)-[6-deoxy-a-l-mannopyranosyl-(1→4)]-b-d-glucopyranoside	$C_{45}H_{73}NO_{15}$	
	(3*β*)-7-oxosolanid-5-en-3-yl 6-deoxy-a-l-mannopyranosyl-(1→2)-[6-deoxy-a-l-mannopyranosyl-(1→4)]-b-d-glucopyranoside	$C_{45}H_{71}NO_{15}$	
	(3*β*,5*α*,6*β*)-5,6-dihydroxysolanidan-3-yl 6-deoxy-a-l-mannopyranosyl-(1→2)-[6-deoxy-a-l-mannopyranosyl-(1→4)]-b-d-glucopyranoside	$C_{45}H_{75}NO_{16}$	
253. 黄苞大戟 *Datura wrighti*	withawrightolide	$C_{28}H_{38}O_5$	Zhang H, et al
254. 烟草 *Nicotiana tabacum*	6,7-dimethoxy-4′-hydroxy-8-formylflavon	$C_{18}H_{14}O_6$	Chen J, et al
	8-formyl-4′,6,7-trimethoxyflavon	$C_{19}H_{16}O_6$	
	4′,7-dihydroxy-8-formyl-6-methoxyflavon	$C_{17}H_{12}O_6$	
255. 两头毛 *Incarvillea arguta*	(+)-argutoid A	$C_{10}H_{14}O$	Yan YM, et al
	(−)-incarvoid A	$C_{10}H_{14}O$	
	(+)-incarvoid B	$C_{10}H_{18}O_3$	
	incarvoid C	$C_{12}H_{20}O_3$	
256. 石吊兰 *Lysionotus pauciflorus*	3,10-dihydroxyacoronene	$C_{15}H_{24}O_3$	文庆发,等
	(2*R*)-6,8-dihydroxy-a-dunnione	$C_{15}H_{14}O_5$	Zhong YJ, et al
	6,8-dihydroxy-2,7-dimethoxy-3-(1,1-dimethylprop-2-enyl)-1,4-naphthoquinone	$C_{17}H_{18}O_6$	
257. 北美透骨草 *Phryma leptostachya*	Haedoxancoside A	$C_{38}H_{43}O_{19}$	Chen C, et al
	phrymarolin V	$C_{20}H_{18}O_8$	
258. 忍冬 *Lonicera japonica*	(−)-2-hydroxy-5-methoxybenzoic acid 2-*O*-*β*-D-(6-*O*-benzoyl)-glucopyranoside	$C_{21}H_{23}O_{10}$	Wang F, et al
	(−)-4-Hydroxy-3,5-dimethoxybenzoic acid 4-*O*-*β*-D-(6-*O*-benzoyl)-glucopyranoside	$C_{22}H_{25}O_{11}$	

续　表

中药及其基源	新成分名称	分子式	报道者
258. 忍冬 *Lonicera japonica*	(—)-(*E*)-3,5-Dimethoxyphenylpropenoic acid 4-*O*-*β*-D-(6-*O*-benzoyl)-glucopyranoside	$C_{24}H_{27}O_{11}$	Wang F, et al
	(—)-(7*S*,8*R*)-(4-Hydroxyphenylglycerol 9-*O*-*β*-D-[6-*O*-(*E*)-4-hydroxy-3,5-dimethoxyphenyl propenoyl]-glucopyranoside	$C_{26}H_{33}O_{13}$	
	(—)-(7*S*,8*R*)-(4-Hydroxy-3-methoxyphenylglycerol 9-*O*-*β*-D-[6-*O*-(*E*)-4-hydroxy-3,5-dimethoxy phenylpropenoyl]-glucopyranoside	$C_{27}H_{35}O_{14}$	
	(—)-4-Hydroxy-3-methoxyphenol *β*-D-{6-*O*-[4-*O*-(7*S*,8*R*)-(4-hydroxy-3-methoxyphenylglycerol-8-yl)-3-methoxybenzoyl]}-glucopyranoside	$C_{31}H_{37}O_{15}$	
259. 阔叶缬草 *Valeriana fauriei*	isovalerianin A	$C_{17}H_{26}O_{5}$	Liu XG, et al
	valerianin C	$C_{17}H_{24}O_{7}$	
260. 荚迷花 *Viburnum mongolicum*	3*β*,12*β*-dihydroxy-25,26,27-trinordammara-22-en-24,20-olide	$C_{27}H_{42}O_{4}$	Wang X, et al
	3*β*,12*β*-dihydroxy-24*α*-methoxy-25,26,27-trinordammara-20,24-epoxy	$C_{28}H_{48}O_{4}$	
	3*β*-*O*-acetyl-12*β*-hydroxy-23,24,25,26,27-hexanordammarane-20-one	$C_{26}H_{42}O_{4}$	
	12*β*-*O*-acetyl-15*α*-hydoxy-17*β*-methoxy-3-oxo-20,21,22-23,24,25,26,27-octanordammanrane	$C_{25}H_{40}O_{5}$	
	12*β*-*O*-acetyl-15*α*,17*β*-dihydoxy-3-oxo-20,21,22-23,24,25,26,27-octanordammanrane	$C_{25}H_{38}O_{5}$	
	12*β*,15*α*-dihydoxy-3-oxo-17-en-20,21,22-23,24,25,26,27-octanordammanrane	$C_{22}H_{34}O_{3}$	
261. 墓头回 *Patrinia heterophylla*	patriheterdoid B	$C_{15}H_{20}O_{5}$	Yang B, et al
	patriheterdoid C	$C_{25}H_{36}O_{9}$	
262. 缬草 *Valeriana officinalis* var *latiofolia*	volvalerenal F	$C_{16}H_{24}O_{2}$	Chen HW, et al
	volvalerenal G	$C_{15}H_{22}O_{2}$	
	volvalerenic acid D	$C_{17}H_{24}O_{2}$	
263. 蜘蛛香 *Valeriana jatamansi*	jatamanins N	$C_{10}H_{14}O_{6}$	Li YD, et al
	jatamanins O	$C_{17}H_{23}ClO_{7}$	
	jatamanins P	$C_{17}H_{23}ClO_{6}$	Lin S, et al
	chlorovaltrates A	$C_{17}H_{23}ClO_{7}$	
	chlorovaltrates B	$C_{18}H_{26}ClO_{8}$	
	chlorovaltrates C	$C_{19}H_{30}ClO_{9}$	
	chlorovaltrates D	$C_{16}H_{26}ClO_{7}$	
	chlorovaltrates E	$C_{25}H_{40}ClO_{10}$	
	chlorovaltrates F	$C_{22}H_{34}ClO_{9}$	
	chlorovaltrates G	$C_{17}H_{26}ClO_{8}$	

续 表

中药及其基源	新成分名称	分子式	报道者
263. 蜘蛛香 *Valeriana jatamansi*	chlorovaltrates H	$C_{18}H_{27}ClO_8$	Lin S, et al
	chlorovaltrates I	$C_{19}H_{30}ClO_8$	
	chlorovaltrates J	$C_{20}H_{32}ClO_7$	
	chlorovaltrates K	$C_{22}H_{34}ClO_8$	
	chlorovaltrates L	$C_{25}H_{38}ClO_9$	
	chlorovaltrates M	$C_{24}H_{34}ClO_{10}$	
	chlorovaltrates N	$C_{23}H_{34}ClO_8$	
	chlorovaltrates O	$C_{20}H_{30}ClO_7$	
264. 长序缬草 *Valeriana hardwickii*	volvalerenol A	$C_{30}H_{52}O_4$	Wang PC, et al
265. 刺萼参 *Morina nepalensi*	3-*O*-α-L-arabinopyranosyl-(1→3)-[α-Lrhamnopyranosyl-(1→2)]-β-D-xylopyranosyl ursolic acid-28-*O*-β-D-glucopyranosyl-(1→6)-β-D-glucopyranoside	$C_{58}H_{94}O_{25}$	Zhang ZF, et al
	3-*O*-α-L-arabinopyranosyl-(1→3)-[α-L-rhamnopyranosyl-(1→2)]-α-L-arabinopyranosyl ursolic acid-28-*O*-β-D-glucopyranosyl-(1→6)-β-D-glucopyranoside	$C_{58}H_{94}O_{25}$	
266. 羊乳 *Codonopsis lanceolata*	tangshenoside Ⅷ	$C_{46}H_{64}O_{26}$	Ren J, et al
267. 金鸡菊 *Coreopsis lanceolata*	3,2′-dihydroxy-4,3′-dimethoxychalcone-4′-glucoside	$C_{23}H_{26}O_{11}$	Shang Y, et al
	4′-*O*-(2‴-*O*-caffeoyl)2′,3′,3,4-tetrahydroxychalcone	$C_{30}H_{28}O_4$	
	2′,4′,3-trihydroxy-3′,4-dimethoxychalcone	$C_{17}H_{15}O_6$	
268. 苍耳 *Xanthium sibiricum*	pungiolide D	$C_{30}H_{37}O_6$	Wang L, et al
	pungiolide E	$C_{30}H_{37}O_6$	
	8-epi-xanthatin-1α,5α-epoxide	$C_{15}H_{19}O_4$	
	1β-hydroxyl-5α-chloro-8-epi-xanthatin	$C_{15}H_{20}ClO_4$	
	3β-norpinan-2-one 3-*O*-β-D-apiofuranosyl-(1→6)-β-D-glucopyranoside	$C_{20}H_{32}O_{11}$	Jiang H, et al
	(6*Z*)-3-hydroxymethyl-7-methylocta-1,6-dien-3-ol 8-*O*-β-Dglucopyranoside	$C_{16}H_{28}O_8$	
	(6*E*)-3-hydroxymethyl-7-methylocta-1,6-dien-3-ol 8-*O*-β-D-glucopyranoside	$C_{16}H_{28}O_8$	
	7-[(β-D-apiofuranosyl-(1→6)-β-D-glucopyranosyl)oxymethy]-8,8-dimethyl-4,8-dihydrobenzo[1,4]thiazine-3,5-dione	$C_{22}H_{31}NO_{12}S$	
269. 木里木香 *Vladimiria muliensis*	(7*R*,8*S*,7′*R*,8′*S*)-5-methoxyprinsepiol	$C_{21}H_{24}O_9$	Chen J, et al
	(7*R*,8*S*,7′*R*,8′*S*)-5-methoxyprinsepiol-4-*O*-β-D-glucopyranoside	$C_{27}H_{34}O_{14}$	
	(8*S*,7′*R*,8′*S*)-vladinolD-4′-*O*-β-D-glucopyranoside	$C_{26}H_{32}O_{12}$	

续　表

中药及其基源	新 成 分 名 称	分 子 式	报 道 者
270. 阿尔泰狗娃花 *Heteropappus altaicus*	1β-methoxycaryol-9-one	$C_{16}H_{26}O_2$	Huang H, et al
271. 羊耳菊 *Inula cappa*	4-[(6-*O*-(*E*)-caffeoyl)-β-D-glucopyranosyl] vanillic acid	$C_{23}H_{24}O_{12}$	Wu Z, et al
	3-*O*-[β-D-apiofurarnosyl-(1-6)-β-D-glucopyranoxy]-6-hydroxy-p-cymene	$C_{21}H_{32}O_{11}$	
272. 紫背草 *Emilia sonchifolia*	2-{4-hydroxy-7-oxabicyclo [2.2.1]heptanyl}-acetic acid	$C_8H_{12}O_4$	Shen S, et al
	Emiline	$C_{21}H_{23}NO_6$	
273. 加拿大一枝黄花 *Solidago canadensis*	8-dehydroxymethylvisanol	$C_{18}H_{16}O_5$	Huang Y, et al
	9-*O*-[3-*O*-acetyl-β-D-glucopyranosyl]-4-hydroxy-cinnamic acid	$C_{17}H_{20}O_9$	
274. 总状土木香 *Inula racemosa*	8-oxo-tri-nor-eudesm-6-en-5aol	$C_{12}H_{18}O_2$	Zhang T, et al
	tri-nor-eudesm-5-en-7β,8β-diol	$C_{12}H_{20}O_2$	
	racemosalactones A	$C_{15}H_{22}O_3$	Ma YY, et al
	racemosalactones B	$C_{15}H_{21}ClO_4$	
	racemosalactones C	$C_{15}H_{22}O_3$	
	racemosalactones D	$C_{15}H_{22}O_4$	
	racemosalactones E	$C_{15}H_{22}O_3$	
	(4*R*,5*S*,10*S*)-5-hydroxy-11,12,13-trinoreudesm-6-en-8-one	$C_{12}H_{18}O_2$	
	(4*R*,5*R*,10*R*)-4,15-epoxy-11,12,13-trinoreudesman-8-one	$C_{12}H_{18}O_2$	
275. 红花 *Carthamus tinctorius*	saffloquinoside C	$C_{27}H_{30}O_{15}$	Jiang JS, et al
	(−)-4-hydroxybenzoic acid-4-*O*-[6′-*O*-(2″-methylbutyryl)-β-D-glucopyranoside]	$C_{18}H_{24}O_9$	
276. 短葶飞蓬 *Erigeron breviscapus*	erigeronones A	$C_{20}H_{12}O_9$	Li J, et al
	erigeronones B	$C_{14}H_{10}O_7$	
277. 节毛飞廉 *Carduus acanthoides*	syringic acid-4-*O*-β-L-arabinopyranoside	$C_{14}H_{18}O_9$	Liu SK, et al
	kaempferol-3-*O*-α-L-rhamnopyranosyl-7-*O*-β-D-glucuronopyranoside	$C_{27}H_{28}O_{16}$	
278. 小蓟 *Cirsium setosum*	(7*E*,9*R*)-9-hydroxy-5,7-megastigmadien-4-one-9-*O*-α-L-arabinopyranosyl-(1→6)-β-D-glucopyanoside	$C_{24}H_{39}O_{11}$	姜海,等
279. 绢叶旋覆花 *Inula wissmanniana*	(5*R*,7*R*,10*S*)-4,5-Epoxy-4,5-secoeudesma-1,3-dien-12,5-olide	$C_{15}H_{19}O_3$	Cheng XR, et al
	Eudesma-3,11(13)-dien-12,5β-olide	$C_{15}H_{21}O_2$	
	3,4-Dioxo-5α,7α*H*-3,4-secoeudesma-1,11(13)-dien-12-oic acid	$C_{15}H_{21}O_4$	
	(2*R*,4*E*,6*R*,7*S*,9*S*,10*R*)-2-Acetoxy-9-angeloyloxygermacra-4,11(13)-dien-12,6-olide	$C_{22}H_{31}O_6$	
	4*E*-9β-Angeloyloxy-2α-hydroxy-7α,10α*H*-germacra-4,11(13)-dien-12,6α-olide	$C_{20}H_{29}O_5$	

续 表

中药及其基源	新成分名称	分子式	报道者
279. 绢叶旋覆花 *Inula wissmanniana*	(4*E*,6*R*,7*S*,9*S*,10*R*)-9-Angeloyloxygermacra-4,11(13)-dien-12,6-olide	$C_{20}H_{29}O_4$	Cheng XR, et al
	4*E*-9β-Methacryloxy-7α,10α*H*-germacra-4,11(13)-dien-12,6α-olide	$C_{19}H_{27}O_4$	
	4*E*-9β-Hydroxy-7α,10α*H*-germacra-4,11(13)-dien-12,6α-olide	$C_{15}H_{23}O_3$	
	(1*R*,5*S*,7*R*,10*R*)-1-Hydroxy-2-oxoeudesma-3,11(13)-dien-12-oicacid	$C_{15}H_{21}O_4$	
	4β,5α-Dihydroxy-1-oxoeudesma-2,11(13)-dien-12,6β-olide	$C_{15}H_{19}O_5$	
	3-Oxoeudesma-1,4,11(13)-trien-12,6β-olide	$C_{15}H_{17}O_3$	
	(7*R*)-14(10→1)-Abeoeudesma-1,3,5(10),11(13)-tetraen-12-oic acid	$C_{15}H_{19}O_2$	
280. 六棱菊 *Laggera alata*	(3*R*,4*S*,5*R*,6*R*,2′*R*,3′*S*)-3-*O*-(2′,3′-Diacetoxy-2′-methylbutyryl)-cuauhtemone	$C_{24}H_{27}O_8$	Wang GC, et al
	4-*O*-Acetyl-3-*O*-(3′-acetoxy-2′-hydroxy-2′-methylbutyryl)-cuauhtemone	$C_{24}H_{27}O_8$	
	4-*O*-Acetyl-3-*O*-(2′,3′-diacetoxy-2′-hydroxy-2′-methylbutyryl)-cuauhtemone	$C_{26}H_{39}O_9$	
	3-*O*-(3′-Acetoxy-2′-hydroxy-2′-methylbutyryl)-cuauhtemone	$C_{22}H_{35}O_7$	
	4-*O*-Acetyl-3-*O*-(2′,3′-dihydroxy-2′-methylbutyryl)-cuauhtemone	$C_{22}H_{35}O_7$	
	4α-Acetoxy-3α-(3′-acetoxy-2′-methylbutyryloxy)-11-hydroxy-6,7-dehydroeudesman-8-one	$C_{24}H_{37}O_9$	
	3-Oxo-di-nor-eudesma-4-en-11-oic acid	$C_{13}H_{19}O_3$	
	alatoside F	$C_{21}H_{31}O_8$	
	alatoside G	$C_{21}H_{31}O_8$	
	alatoside H	$C_{21}H_{31}O_8$	
281. 准噶尔橐吾 *Ligularia songarica*	songaricalarins A	$C_{28}H_{42}O_9$	Wang Q, et al
	songaricalarins B	$C_{25}H_{36}O_8$	
	songaricalarins C	$C_{31}H_{45}O_9Cl$	
	songaricalarins D	$C_{26}H_{36}O_5$	
	songaricalarins E	$C_{28}H_{40}O_8$	
282. 苣荬菜 *Cichorium endivia*	(3*S*)-1,2,3,4-tetrahydro-β-carboline-3-carboxylic acid	$C_{12}H_{12}N_2O_2$	Wang FX, et al
283. 臭灵丹 *Laggera pterodonta*	(2β)-2-deoxo-2-methoxytessaric acid	$C_{16}H_{24}O_3$	Zhang ZJ, et al
	(3β,10α)-3-methoxyleudesma-4,11(13)-dien-12-oic acid	$C_{16}H_{24}O_3$	
	(3α,4β,8α)-4-(acetyloxy)-3-(2,3-dihydroxy)-2-methyl-1-oxobutoxy-8-hydroxyeudesm-7(11)-eno-12,8-lactone	$C_{22}H_{32}O_9$	

续　表

中药及其基源	新 成 分 名 称	分 子 式	报 道 者
284. 小鱼眼草 *Dichrocephala benthamii*	dichrocephols A	$C_{16}H_{22}O_5$	Tian X, et al
	dichrocephols B	$C_{18}H_{24}O_6$	
	dichrocephols C	$C_{18}H_{24}O_6$	
	dichrocephols D	$C_{22}H_{24}O_6$	
285. 鼠麴草 *Gnaphalium affine*	gnaphaffine A	$C_{25}H_{24}O_{11}$	Li J, et al
	gnaphaffine B	$C_{30}H_{28}O_{13}$	
286. 紫茎泽兰 *Ageratina adenophora*	5 - *O* - trans - o - coumaroylquinic acid methyl ester	$C_{17}H_{20}O_8$	Zhang M, et al
287. 紫菀 *Aster tataricus*	astataricusones A	$C_{30}H_{50}O_2$	Zhou WB, et al
	astataricusones B	$C_{30}H_{50}O_2$	
	astataricusones C	$C_{30}H_{50}O_2$	
	astataricusones D	$C_{30}H_{52}O_3$	
	astataricusol A	$C_{30}H_{52}O_2$	
288. 菊芋 *Helianthus tuberosus*	3 - Hydroxy - 8β - tigloyloxy - 1,10 - dehydroariglovin	$C_{20}H_{22}O_6$	Yuan X, et al
289. 网脉橐吾 *Ligularia dictyoneura*	(4*S*,5*R*,8*R*,10*S*)- 1 - nor - 10 - hydroxy - 8 - methoxyeremophil - 7(11)- en - 12,8 - olide	$C_{15}H_{22}O_4$	Li S, et al
	1β - angeloyloxy - 6α,10β - dihydroxyeremophil - 7(11),8 - dien - 12,8 - olide	$C_{20}H_{26}O_6$	
290. 薇甘菊 *Mikania micrantha*	b - D - glucopyranosyl - 15α -(3 - hydroxyl - 3 - methylbutanoyloxy)- ent - 16 - kauren - 19 - oate	$C_{31}H_{48}O_{10}$	Xu Q, et al
	b - D - glucopyranosyl - 15α - hydroxy - ent - 16 - kauren - 19 - oate	$C_{26}H_{40}O_8$	
291. 吉祥草 *Reineckia carnea*	1α,3α - dihydroxy - 5β - pregn - 16 - en - 20 - one 3 - *O* -α - L - rhamnopyranoside	$C_{27}H_{42}O_7$	Han N, et al
	1β,3β,27 - trihydroxycholest - 16 - en - 22 - one 1,3 - di - *O* - α - L - rhamnoside	$C_{39}H_{64}O_{13}$	
	reinocarnoside A	$C_{33}H_{54}O_{10}$	Wang Q, et al
	reinocarnoside B	$C_{33}H_{54}O_9$	
	reinocarnoside C	$C_{44}H_{72}O_{19}$	
292. 丫蕊花 *Ypsilandra thibetica*	ypsilanogenin	$C_{33}H_{52}O_8$	Xie B, et al
	ypsilanogenin 3 - *O* - β - D - glucopyranoside	$C_{39}H_{61}O_{13}$	
	4′- acetylypsilanogenin 3 - *O* - β - D - glucopyranoside	$C_{41}H_{64}O_{14}$	
293. 开口箭 *Tupistra chinensis*	3 - *O* - β - D - glucopyranosyl -(1→4)- β - D - glucopyranosyl - 5β - furost - 25(27)- en - 1β,3β,22α, 26 - tetraol - 26 - *O* - β - D - glucopyranoside	$C_{45}H_{74}O_{20}$	Liu C, et al
	(25*S*)- 6 - *O* - β - D - glucopyranosyl - 5β - furost - 3β, 6β,22α,26 - tetraol - 26 - *O* - β - D - glucopyranoside	$C_{39}H_{66}O_{15}$	
	(25*S*)- 5β - furost - 1β,2β,3β,4β,5β,22α, 26 -heptaol - 26 - *O* - β - Dglucopyranoside	$C_{33}H_{56}O_{13}$	
294. 黑刺菝葜 *Smilax scobinicaulis*	(25*R*)- 5α - spirostan - 3β,6β - diol 3 - *O* - β - D - glucopyranosyl -(1→4)-[α - L - arabinopyranosyl - (1→6)]- β - D - glucopyranoside	$C_{44}H_{72}O_{18}$	Zhang C, et al

续 表

中药及其基源	新 成 分 名 称	分 子 式	报 道 者
295. 麦冬 *Ophiopogon japonicus*	ophiopogonin P	$C_{56}H_{92}O_{28}$	Guo Y, et al
	ophiopogonin Q	$C_{56}H_{92}O_{28}$	
	ophiopogonins J	$C_{51}H_{82}O_{23}$	Kang ZY, et al
	ophiopogonins K	$C_{56}H_{90}O_{26}$	
	8 - formyl - 7 - hydroxy - 5,4′- dimethoxy - 6 - methylhomoisoflavone	$C_{20}H_{18}O_6$	Zhou CX, et al
	6 - formylisoophiopogonone B	$C_{19}H_{15}O_6$	
	8 - formylophiopogonanone B	$C_{19}H_{18}O_6$	
296. 象脚王兰 *Yucca elephantipes*	elephanosides G	$C_{45}H_{72}O_{18}$	Zhang Y, et al
	elephanosides H	$C_{39}H_{62}O_{14}$	
297. 土茯苓 *Smilax glabra*	smiglabrone A	$C_{26}H_{24}O_{10}$	Xu S, et al
	smiglabrone A	$C_{25}H_{22}O_9$	
	smilachromanone	$C_{18}H_{18}O_6$	
	smiglastilbene	$C_{14}H_{12}O_4$	
	smiglactone	$C_{15}H_{20}O_3$	
	smiglabrol	$C_{15}H_{16}O_5$	
298. 鹿药 *Smilacina henryi*	henryiosides A	$C_{50}H_{80}O_{23}$	Zhang X, et al
	henryiosides B	$C_{50}H_{80}O_{22}$	
	henryiosides C	$C_{50}H_{80}O_{22}$	
	henryiosides D	$C_{50}H_{80}O_{22}$	
	henryiosides E	$C_{50}H_{80}O_{22}$	
299. 卵叶蜘蛛抱蛋 *Aspidistra typica*	typaspidoside A	$C_{56}H_{90}O_{29}$	Cui JM, et al
	25*S* - typaspidoside A	$C_{56}H_{90}O_{29}$	
	tuberostemonoxirine	$C_{22}H_{31}NO_6$	Yue Y, et al
	9*α* - epi - tuberospironine	$C_{18}H_{27}NO_5$	
300. 知母 *Anemarrhena asphodeloides*	anemarnoside A	$C_{45}H_{76}O_{19}$	Liu QB, et al
	anemarnoside B	$C_{45}H_{74}O_{19}$	
	caesanines A	$C_{21}H_{27}NO_3$	Zhang J, et al
	caesanines B	$C_{21}H_{27}NO_3$	
	caesanines C	$C_{22}H_{29}NO_4$	
	caesanines D	$C_{42}H_{56}NO_7$	
301. 平车前 *Plantago depressa*	2 -(3 - hydroxy - 4 - methoxyphenyl)ethanol 1 - *O* - [*α* -L - rhamnopiranosyl -(1→2)- *β* - D - glucopyranoside]	$C_{21}H_{32}O_{12}$	Yu CY, et al
302. 石蒜 *Lycoris radiata*	2*α* - Methoxy - 6 - *O* - ethyloduline	$C_{20}H_{25}NO_5$	黄升殿,等
	(+)- 5,6 - dehydrolycorine	$C_{16}H_{15}NO_4$	Hao B, et al
	(+)- 3*α*,6*β* - diacetyl - bulbispermine	$C_{20}H_{21}NO_7$	
	(+)- 3*α* - hydroxy - 6*β* - acetyl - bulbispermine	$C_{18}H_{19}NO_6$	
	(+)- 8,9 - methylenedioxylhomolycorine - *N* - oxide	$C_{17}H_{17}NO$	
	5,6 - dihydro - 5 - methyl - 2 - hydroxyphenanthridine	$C_{15}H_{13}NO_3$	

续　表

中药及其基源	新　成　分　名　称	分　子　式	报　道　者
303. 德国鸢尾 *Iris germanica*	iriskashmirianin A	$C_{17}H_{12}O_7$	Xie GY, et al
	germanaism H	$C_{22}H_{20}O_{12}$	
304. 灯心草 *Juncus effusus*	juncuenin E	$C_{19}H_{19}NO_2$	Su X, et al
	juncuenin F	$C_{17}H_{16}O_3$	
	juncuenin G	$C_{19}H_{22}O_3$	
	dehydrojuncuenin D	$C_{19}H_{20}O_3$	
	dehydrojuncuenin E	$C_{17}H_{16}O_3$	
	Ethyl 5 - *O* - trans - feruloyl - α - arabinofuranoside	$C_{17}H_{22}O_8$	
305. 白茅 *Imperata cylindrica*	8 - hydroxy - 2 -(2 - phenylethyl) chromone	$C_{17}H_{14}O_3$	刘轩，等
	2 -(2 - phenylethyl) chromone - 8 - *O* - *β* - D - glucopyranoside	$C_{23}H_{24}O_8$	
306. 蒲葵 *Livistona chinensis*	6′- *O* -(2″- hydroxyheptadecanoyl)- b - D - glucosyl - b -sitosterol	$C_{52}H_{92}O_8$	Zeng X, et al
	6′- *O* -(icosa - 9″*Z*,12″*Z* - dienoyl)- b - D - glucosyl - b -sitosterol	$C_{55}H_{94}O_7$	
	Ethyl16 -(dodeca - 4‴*Z*,7‴*Z* - dienyl)- 29 - oxo - 15 -(tetradeca - 5″*Z*,8″*Z*,11″*Z* - trienyl) triacontanoate	$C_{58}H_{104}O_3$	
	Tetracosa - 11*Z*,14*Z*,18*Z* - trienoic acid	$C_{24}H_{42}O_2$	
	16 - Hydroxy - 8 - oxohexadecyl tetradecanoate	$C_{30}H_{58}O_4$	
	10 - Decylnonadecane - 1,19 - diol	$C_{29}H_{60}O_2$	
307. 象头花 *Arisaema franchetianum*	(2*R* *,3*S* *,5*S* *)- *N*,2 - dimethyl - 3 - hydroxy - 5 -(10 - phenyldecyl) pyrrolidine	$C_{22}H_{37}NO$	Su Y, et al
308. 香附子 *Cyperus rotundus*	rotunduside	$C_{33}H_{45}O_{21}$	Zhou Z, et al
309. 温郁金 *Curcuma wenyujin*	(4*S*)- 4 - hydroxy - gweicurculactone	$C_{15}H_{16}O_3$	Yin GP, et al
	zedoalactone G	$C_{15}H_{22}O_4$	
	(1*R*,4*R*,5*S*,10*S*)- zedoalactone B	$C_{15}H_{20}O_5$	
	1*α*,8*α* - epidioxy - 4*α* - hydroxy - 5*αH* - guai - 7(11), 9 -dien - 12,8 - olide	$C_{15}H_{18}O_5$	Dong JY, et al
	8,9 - seco - 4*β*hydroxy - 1*α*,5*βH* - 7(11)- guaen - 8, 10 -olide	$C_{15}H_{24}O_3$	
	8*α* - hydroxy - 1*α*,4*β*,7*βH* - guai - 10(15)- en - 5*β*,8*β* - endoxide	$C_{15}H_{24}O_2$	
	7*β*,8*α* - dihydroxy - 1*α*,4*αH* - guai - 10(15)- en - 5*β*, 8*β*-endoxide	$C_{15}H_{24}O_3$	
	7 - hydroxy - 5(10),6,8 - cadinatriene - 4 - one	$C_{15}H_{20}O_2$	
310. 节鞭山姜 *Alpinia conchigera*	conchignans A	$C_{28}H_{30}O_5$	Xu JJ, et al
	conchignans B	$C_{28}H_{30}O_5$	
	conchignans C	$C_{29}H_{33}O_5$	
311. 益智 *Alpinia oxyphylla*	1 -(3′,5′- dihydroxy - 4′- methoxyphenyl)- 7 -phenyl - 3 - hepta - none	$C_{20}H_{24}O_4$	Bian QY, et al

续 表

中药及其基源	新成分名称	分子式	报道者
311. 益智 *Alpinia oxyphylla*	1-(2,4′-dihydroxy-3′-methoxyphenyl)-7-(4″-methoxyphenyl)-3-heptanone	$C_{21}H_{26}O_5$	Bian QY, et al
	(11*S*)-12-Chloronootkaton-11-ol	$C_{15}H_{24}ClO_2$	Chen P, et al
	(11*R*)-12-Chloronootkaton-11-ol	$C_{15}H_{24}ClO_2$	
312. 山柰 *Kaempferia galanga*	kaempsulfonic acids A	$C_{20}H_{24}O_8S$	王芳林,等
	kaempsulfonic acids B	$C_{20}H_{24}O_8S$	
313. 白豆蔻 *Amomum kravanh*	kravanhol A	$C_{21}H_{26}O_7$	Yin H, et al
	kravanhol B	$C_{21}H_{26}O_6$	
	kravanhins A	$C_{20}H_{29}O_4$	
	kravanhins B	$C_{20}H_{28}O_3$	
	kravanhins C	$C_{20}H_{27}O_4$	
	kravanhins D	$C_{20}H_{32}O_3$	
	(12*Z*,14*R*)-Labda-8(17),12-diene-14,15,16-triol	$C_{20}H_{34}O_3$	
	3β,18-Dihydroxylabda-8(17),13-dien-15,16-olide	$C_{20}H_{30}O_4$	
	(12*E*)-3β,18-Dihydroxylabda-8(17),12-dien-16,15-olide	$C_{20}H_{30}O_4$	
314. 九翅豆蔻 *Amomum maximum*	Amomaxins A	$C_{19}H_{26}O_3$	Yin H, et al
	Amomaxins B	$C_{19}H_{28}O_4$	
315. 见血青 *Liparis nervosa*	{6-*O*-[(4-oxo-4H-pyran-3-yloxy)-*O*-*β*-D-glucopyranosyl]}-4-hydroxy-3,5-bis(3-methyl-2-butenyl)benzoate	$C_{28}H_{34}O_{10}$	Huang S, et al
	{1-*O*-[6-acetyl-*O*-*β*-D-glucopyranosyl]}-4-hydroxy-3,5-bis(3-methyl-2-butenyl)benzoate	$C_{25}H_{34}O_9$	
	3,5-bis(3-methyl-2-butenyl)-4-*O*-(*α*-L-arabinopyranosyl)benzoate	$C_{23}H_{32}O_7$	
	3,5-bis(3-methyl-2-butenyl)-4-*O*-[*β*-D-glucopyranosyl(1→2)-]*α*-L-arabinopyranosyl)benzoate	$C_{29}H_{42}NO_{12}$	
	3,5-bis(3-methyl-2-butenyl)-4-*O*-(*β*-D-glucopyranosyl)benzamide	$C_{23}H_{34}NO_7$	
	3-[(1*E*)-3-hydroxy-3-methyl-1-butenyl-4-*O*-[*β*-D-glucopyranosyl(1→2)-]*α*-L-arabinopyranosyl]]-5-(3-methyl-2-butenyl)benzamide	$C_{28}H_{42}NO_{12}$	
	[(3-hydroxy-3-methylbutyl)4-*O*-(*β*-D-glucopyranosyl)]-5-(3-methyl-2-butenyl)benzamide	$C_{23}H_{36}NO_8$	
	3-(3-hydroxy-3-methylbutyl)-4-*O*-[(*β*-D-glucopyranosyl)-(1→2)-*β*-D-glucopyranosyl]-5-(3-methyl-2-butenyl)benzamide	$C_{29}H_{45}NO_{13}$	
	3-(3-hydroxy-3-methylbutyl)-4-*O*-[(*β*-D-glucopyranosyl)-(1→2)-*α*-L-glucopyranosyl]-5-(3-methyl-2-butenyl)benzamide	$C_{28}H_{43}NO_{12}$	

续　表

中药及其基源	新 成 分 名 称	分 子 式	报 道 者
315. 见血青 *Liparis nervosa*	1 -(ethoxy)- 3 -[(3 - hydroxy - 3 - methylbutyl)- 4 - *O*-[(β- D - glucopyranosyl)-(1→2)- α - L - arabinosyl]- 5 -(3 - methyl - 2 - butenyl) benzoate	$C_{30}H_{46}O_{13}$	Huang S, et al
	nervosine Ⅰ	$C_{30}H_{44}NO_7$	
	nervosine Ⅱ	$C_{30}H_{44}NO_7$	
	nervosine Ⅲ	$C_{37}H_{56}NO_{13}$	
	nervosine Ⅳ	$C_{36}H_{54}NO_{12}$	
	nervosine Ⅴ	$C_{30}H_{46}NO_8$	
	nervosine Ⅵ	$C_{25}H_{34}NO_3$	
316. 绶草 *Spiranthes sinensis*	2,2′- dihydroxy - 5,5′,7,7′- tetramethoxy - 9,9′,10, 10′- tetrahydro - 3,3′- biphenanthrene	$C_{32}H_{30}O_6$	Li CY, et al
	5 - hydroxy - 3,7 - dimethoxy - 4′-(1 - hydroxy - 3 - methylbut - 3 - en - 2 - yloxy)- flavone	$C_{22}H_{22}O_7$	
317. 天麻 *Gastrodia elata*	gastrodin B	$C_{19}H_{22}O_7$	Zhang ZC, et al
	gastrol B	$C_{21}H_{20}O_4$	
318. 杜鹃兰 *Cremastra appendiculata*	1 -(4 - β- D - Glucopyranosyloxybenzyl) 4 - methyl (2*R*)- 2 - isobutylmalate	$C_{22}H_{33}O_{11}$	Wang Y, et al
	1 -(4 - β- D - Glucopyranosyloxybenzyl) 4 - ethyl (2*R*)- 2 - isobutylmalate	$C_{23}H_{35}O_{11}$	
	1 -(4 - β- D - Glucopyranosyloxybenzyl) 4 - methyl (2*R*)- 2 - benzylmalate	$C_{25}H_{31}O_{11}$	
	1,4 - Bis(4 - β- D - glucopyranosyloxybenzyl) (2*R*)- 2 -benzylmalate	$C_{37}H_{45}O_{17}$	
	7 - Hydroxy - 4 - methoxy - 9,10 - dihydrophenanthrene - 2 - *O* - β - Dglucopyranoside	$C_{21}H_{25}O_8$	
	7 - Hydroxy - 5 - methoxy - 9,10 - dihydrophenanthrene - 2 - *O* - β - Dglucopyranoside	$C_{21}H_{25}O_8$	
	4 - Methoxy - 9,10 - dihydrophenanthrene - 2,7 - di - *O* - β - Dglucopyranoside	$C_{27}H_{35}O_{13}$	
	4,4′- Dimethoxy - 9,10 - dyhydro -[6,1′- biphenanthrene]- 2,2′,7,7′- tetraol	$C_{30}H_{24}O_6$	
	(2,3 - trans)- 2 -(4 - Hydroxy - 3 - methoxyphenyl)- 3 - hydroxymethyl - 10 - methoxy - 2,3,4,5 - tetrahydro - phenanthro[2,1 - β]furan - 7 - ol	$C_{25}H_{24}O_6$	
	(2,3 - trans)- 3 -[(2,7 - Dihydroxy - 4 - methoxy - phenanthren - 1 - yl) methyl]- 2 -(4 - hydroxy - 3 - methoxyphenyl)- 10 - methoxy - 2,3,4,5 - tetrahydro - phenanthro[2,1 - β]furan - 7 - ol	$C_{40}H_{33}O_8$	
	(2,3 - trans)- 3 -[2 - Hydroxy - 6 -(3 - hydroxyphenethyl)- 4 - methoxybenzyl]- 2 -(4 - hydroxy - 3 - methoxyphenyl)- 10 - methoxy - 2,3,4, 5 -tetrahydro - phenanthro[2,1 - β]furan - 7 - ol	$C_{40}H_{39}O_8$	

续 表

中药及其基源	新成分名称	分子式	报道者
319. 叠鞘石斛 *Dendrobium denneanum*	2,5-Dihydroxy-4-methoxy-phenanthrene 2-*O*-*β*-Dglucopyranoside	$C_{21}H_{23}O_8$	Lin Y, et al
	2,5-Dihydroxy-4-methoxy-phenanthrene 2-*O*-*β*-Dapiofuranosyl-(1-6)-*β*-D-glucopyranoside	$C_{26}H_{31}O_{12}$	
	2,5-Dihydroxy-4-methoxy-phenanthrene	$C_{27}H_{33}O_{12}$	
	2-*O*-*α*-Lrhamnopyranosyl-(1-6)-*β*-D-glucopyranoside	$C_{15}H_{15}O_5$	
	5-Methoxy-2,4,7,9*S*-tetrahydroxy-9,10-dihydrophenanthrene	$C_{15}H_{15}O_4$	
	4-Methoxy-2,5,7,9*S*-tetrahydroxy-9,10-dihydrophenanthrene	$C_{15}H_{15}O_4$	
	5-Methoxy-4,7,9*S*-trihydroxy-9,10-dihydrophenanthrene	$C_{15}H_{15}O_4$	
	4-Methoxy-2,5,9*R*-trihydroxy-9,10-dihydrophenanthrene 2-*O*-*β*-D-glucopyranoside	$C_{21}H_{25}O_9$	
	1,2,5,9*R*-Tetrahydroxy-9,10-dihydrophenanthrene 5-*O*-*β*-Dglucopyranoside	$C_{21}H_{25}O_9$	
	(—)-(7*S*,8*R*,7′*E*)-4-hydroxy-3,3′,5,5′-tetramethoxy-8,4′-oxyneolign-7′-ene-7,9,9′-triol 7,9′-bis-*O*-*β*-D-glucopyranoside	$C_{34}H_{48}O_{19}$	Xiong L, et al
	denneanoside A	$C_{21}H_{22}O_8$	Li F, et al
	denneanoside B	$C_{27}H_{32}O_{13}$	
	denneanoside C	$C_{27}H_{32}O_{13}$	
	denneanoside D	$C_{27}H_{32}O_{12}$	
	denneanoside E	$C_{26}H_{30}O_{12}$	
	denneanoside F	$C_{21}H_{24}O_9$	
	trochelioid B	$C_{21}H_{32}O_4$	
320. 云南石仙桃 *Pholidota yunnanensis*	1-(4′-hydroxybenzyl)-imbricatin	$C_{23}H_{20}O_5$	Dong FW, et al
	(*E*)-4′-hydroxy-2′,3,3′,5-tetramethoxystilbene	$C_{18}H_{20}O_5$	
	(*E*)-3,4′-dihydroxy-2,6-bis(4-hydroxybenzyl)-2′,3′,5-trimethoxystilbene	$C_{31}H_{30}O_7$	
321. 山蜡梅 *Chimonanthus nitens*	nitensosides A	$C_{21}H_{26}O_{14}$	Li QJ, et al
	nitensosides B	$C_{23}H_{30}O_{15}$	
322. 小叶地不容 *Stephania succifera*	demethylaristofolin C	$C_{18}H_{14}O_6$	Yang DL, et al
323. 栓皮栎 *Quercus variabilis*	3-acetyloxy-epicycloeucalenol-24-one	$C_{31}H_{50}O_3$	Jia LY, et al
324. 白花土元胡 *Corydalis humosa*	1,1-dimethyl-6-methoxy-7-hydroxyl-1,2,3,4-tetrahydroisoquinoline	$C_{12}H_{17}NO_2$	Zheng XK, et al
	(1*R*)-(4-hydroxybenzyl)-7-hydroxyl-8-*O*-*β*-D-glucopyranosyl-1,2,3,4-tetrahydroisoquinoline	$C_{22}H_{27}NO_7$	

续　表

中药及其基源	新 成 分 名 称	分 子 式	报 道 者
325. 暗消藤 *Streptocaulon juventas*	1α,14β-dihydroxy-5β-card-20(22)-enolide 3-*O*-[*O*-β-Dglucopyranosyl-(1→2)-β-D-digitalopyranoside]	$C_{36}H_{57}O_{14}$	Xue R, et al
	Acovenosigenin A	$C_{36}H_{57}O_{14}$	
	16-*O*-acetyl-hydroxyperiplogenin 3-*O*-β-D-digitoxopyranoside	$C_{31}H_{47}O_{10}$	
	Digitoxigenin 3-*O*-[*O*-β-D-glucopyranosyl-(1→6)-*O*-β-Dglucopyranosyl-(1→4)-2-*O*-acetyl-β-D-digitalopyranoside]	$C_{44}H_{70}O_{19}$	
	16-*O*-acetyl-hydroxyacovenosigenin	$C_{25}H_{37}O_7$	
	1β,3β,14β-trihydroxy-5β-card-16,20 (22)-dienolide	$C_{23}H_{33}O_5$	
326. 牛皮消 *Cynanchum auriculatum*	cynauricoside A	$C_{51}H_{74}O_{16}$	Liu S, et al
	cynauricoside B	$C_{63}H_{94}O_{22}$	
	cynauricoside C	$C_{55}H_{96}O_{23}$	
	cynauricoside D	$C_{55}H_{90}O_{22}$	
	cynauricoside E	$C_{58}H_{92}O_{23}$	
	cynauricoside F	$C_{54}H_{88}O_{21}$	
	cynauricoside G	$C_{56}H_{90}O_{22}$	
	cynauricoside H	$C_{47}H_{76}O_{18}$	
	cynauricoside I	$C_{49}H_{78}O_{19}$	
327. 长序虎皮楠 *Daphniphyllum longeracemosum*	hybridaphniphylline A	$C_{37}H_{48}NO_{11}$	Wang F, et al
	hybridaphniphylline B	$C_{37}H_{48}NO_{11}$	
	daphnicyclidin I	$C_{22}H_{27}N_2O_3$	
328. 交让木 *Daphniphyllum macropodum*	macrodumines A	$C_{23}H_{33}NO_5$	Zhang CR, et al
	macrodumines B	$C_{24}H_{35}NO_5$	
	macrodumines C	$C_{24}H_{35}NO_5$	
329. 美丽属海绵 *Callyspongia* sp.	callylactam A	$C_{13}H_{13}NO_2$	Yang B, et al
	callylactam B	$C_{14}H_{16}N_3$	
330. 南海海绵 *Axinella* sp.	2-heptadec-11-enamidoethanesulfonic acid	$C_{19}H_{36}NO_4S$	Huang R, et al
331. 疣状柳珊瑚 *Verrucella umbraculum*	9-acetyl-1,3,7-trimethyl-pyrimidinedione	$C_{11}H_{13}N_3O_3$	Huang R, et al
332. 柳珊瑚 *Anthogorgia caerulea*	caerulsteroid A	$C_{29}H_{48}O_5$	Sun LL, et al
333. 杯形肉质软珊瑚 *Sarcophyton glaucum*	sarglaucol	$C_{20}H_{32}O_2$	Zhang CX, et al
334. 扁小尖柳珊瑚 *Muricella sibogae*	sibogin A	$C_{24}H_{38}O_6$	Li TT, et al
	sibogin B	$C_{23}H_{38}O_5$	
	9,10-secosteroids sibogol A	$C_{29}H_{46}O_2$	
	9,10-secosteroids sibogol B	$C_{29}H_{44}O_2$	
	9,10-secosteroids sibogol C	$C_{29}H_{44}O_2$	

续 表

中药及其基源	新成分名称	分子式	报道者
335. 黄色皮革珊瑚 *Sarcophyton elegans*	sarcophytolides G	$C_{41}H_{64}O_9$	Xi Z, et al
	sarcophytolides H	$C_{41}H_{62}O_7$	
	sarcophytolides I	$C_{42}H_{64}O_8$	
	sarcophytolides J	$C_{41}H_{60}O_7$	
	sarcophytolides K	$C_{41}H_{62}O_{10}$	
	sarcophytolides L	$C_{41}H_{64}O_9$	
336. 蕾二歧灯芯柳珊瑚 *Dichotella gemmacea*	junceellosides E	$C_{35}H_{56}O_8$	Jiang M, et al
	junceellosides F	$C_{34}H_{54}O_8$	
	junceellosides G	$C_{36}H_{58}O_9$	
337. 短指软珊瑚 *Sinularia gaweli*	(22*R*,23*R*,24*R*)-5α,8α-epidioxy-22,23-methylene-24-methylcholest-6,9(11)-dien-3β-ol	$C_{29}H_{44}O_3$	Yen WH, et al
338. 柔指形软珊瑚 *Sinularia flexibilis*	flexibilisquinone	$C_{20}H_{30}O_5$	Lin YF, et al
339. 多棘 *Scolopendra multidens*	5*β*-pregnane-2*α*,6*α*,20(*S*)-triol	$C_{21}H_{36}O_3$	Fu YD, et al
	8-hydroxyl-3-methoxyl138.(Posido-2(1*H*)-quinolone	$C_{10}H_9NO_3$	
340. 埃及伊蚊 *Aedes aegypti*	pipilyasine	$C_{18}H_{33}NO$	Gulzar T, et al
	pipzubedine	$C_{22}H_{41}NO$	
	pipyaqubine	$C_{22}H_{39}NO$	
341. 黑翅土白蚁 *Odontotermes formosanus*	2-ethyl-7-hydroxy-6,7-dihydro-5H-indolizin-3-one	$C_{10}H_{13}NO_2$	Bi SF, et al
342. 中华真地鳖 *Eupolyphaga sinensis*	(*R*)-3-ethyl-6,8-dihydroxy-7-methyl-3,4-dihydroisochromen-1-one	$C_{12}H_{14}O_4$	Jiang W, et al
	(*R*)-6,8-dihydroxy-3,7-dimethyl-3,4-dihydroisochromen-1-one	$C_{11}H_{12}O_4$	
343. 海七鳃鳗 *Petromyzon marinus*	petromyzonin	$C_{15}H_{16}O_5S$	Li K, et al
344. 海燕 *Asterina pectinifera*	pectiniosides H	$C_{33}H_{58}O_{13}S$	Li Z, et al
	pectiniosides I	$C_{31}H_{52}O_{13}S$	
	pectiniosides J	$C_{31}H_{52}O_{13}S$	

（陈咏林　俞桂新）

【62 种中草药中挥发油成分的研究】

1. 根及根茎类

（1）五味藤　周坚等采用 SD 法和 SFE-CO_2法提取五味藤挥发油，并用 GC-MS 法分析鉴定其化学成分。结果，SD 法提取的挥发油分离出 40 个色谱峰，鉴定了 14 种化合物，主要成分是苯甲醛（14.82%）和 α-亚甲基-γ-丁内酯（11.04%）；SFE 法提取的挥发油分离出 25 个色谱峰，鉴定了 13 种化合物，主要成分是 *β*-石竹烯（15.85%）。两种提取方法所得挥发油的化学成分及其含量有较大差异。

（2）温莪术　朱华凤等采用 GC-MS 法对温莪术挥发油和水煎液的乙酸乙酯萃取物化学成分进行分析，通过标准谱库检索结合文献分析。结果，从温莪术挥发油中分离出 49 种化学成分，从温莪术水煎液乙酸乙酯萃取物中分离出 28 种化学成分，其中莪术二酮、斯巴醇和 deoxysericealactone 等

3种成分为二者共有成分。

(3) 黄丝郁金　杨昭武等采用GC－MS分析了12批黄丝郁金挥发油成分,建立了黄丝郁金挥发油GC－MS特征图谱,其中4－熔烯、杜松烯、α－姜黄烯、姜烯、β－倍半水芹烯、芳基姜黄酮、姜黄酮、姜黄新酮为8种主要共有特征峰,占挥发油总量的80%以上。

(4) 新疆藁本　邢珍珍等采用HS－SPME技术和共水蒸馏法提取新疆藁本地下部分的挥发油,并比较其成分的异同。结果,用HS－SPME技术鉴定出22种成分,主要为肉豆蔻醚(75.88%)、乙酸松油酯(9.40%)、香松烯(2.99%)、榄香素(2.76%)、石竹烯(1.29%)等;共水蒸馏法鉴定出13种成分,主要为肉豆蔻醚(87.3%)、乙酸松油酯(3.29%)、α－水芹烯(2.56%)、6－丁基－1,4－环庚二烯(2.81%)、3－蒈烯(1.15%)。

(5) 白术　李滢等采用SD法分别提取生品白术、炒白术挥发油,计算挥发油得率并进行比较。生品白术和炒白术挥发油平均含量($n=3$)分别为1.31%和0.98%;分别检出115个和114个色谱峰,鉴定了其中58种和60种化合物,占相应挥发油总量的93.84%和86.01%。其中绝大多数为单萜或倍半萜类成分。结果表明,白术经炒制后挥发油总含量明显降低,生品白术和炒白术挥发油化学成分基本一致,但各主要成分含量存在明显差异。

(6) 当归　李芸等对当归进行熏硫加工,采用SD法提取挥发油并采用GC－MS进行分析。从其未熏硫、0.20%熏硫、1.00%熏硫、5.00%熏硫当归挥发油中分别鉴定出23、18、25、27种化合物,分别占总挥发油含量的99.84%、100.00%、99.84%、99.63%;当归挥发油的主要成分为α－蒎烯(96.90%)、3,7－二甲基－1,3,6－辛三烯(95.51%)、藁本内酯(86.40%)和正丁烯基藁本内酯(86.97%)。

(7) 三七　李丽明等采用HS－SPME－GC/MS联用技术研究不同规格三七(20头、30头、60头、100头和120头)的挥发性成分。结果,不同规格三七所含的化合物种类、含量有差异,但萜烯类化合物所占比重均较大,其中α－愈创木烯含量最高。

(8) 京大戟　李雪飞等采用SD法从京大戟中提取挥发油成分,利用GC－MS分离出35个峰,鉴定了29种化学成分。主要成分为沉香螺旋醇(49.23%)和四甲基环癸二烯异丙醇(20.66%)。

(9) 知母　钟可等采用GC－MS法对道地知母药材中挥发性成分进行分析和鉴定。从中分离出60个色谱峰,鉴定出其中58种化合物,占挥发油总量的90.22%。挥发油主要为脂肪酸类成分(62.78%),其中亚油酸占总含量的36.43%,棕榈酸占总含量的20.19%。

(10) 秀丽莓　刘慧等采用GC－MS法分离鉴定秀丽莓根经SFE－CO_2法萃取所得精油成分,其得率为3.42%,分离鉴定出39种成分,主要成分为桉叶油二烯－5,11(13)－内酯－8,12(49.09%)、γ－衣兰油烯(1.69%)、β－谷甾醇(6.77%)等。

(11) 川芎　朱立俏等采用SD法提取川芎中挥发油,利用GC－MS分析其挥发油成分,共检测出45个峰,确认其中34种成分,占挥发油总量的75.60%。主要成分为1－(2,5－二甲基苯)哌嗪(35.35%)等。

(12) 华中碎米荠　卢金清等分别采用SD法和HS－SPME法提取华中碎米荠挥发性成分。采用SD－GC－MS法分离出67个色谱峰,鉴别出其中34种化合物,占挥发油总量的94.34%;采用HS－SPME－GC－MS分离出62个色谱峰,鉴别出其中48种化合物,占总挥发性成分的98.29%。共有的挥发性成分为5种,其中含量最高的成分为4－异硫代氰酰基－1－丁烯(65.71%)。

(13) 川白芷　郭耀杰等采用SD法提取挥发油,运用GC－MS技术从川白芷8个不同品种(系)挥发油中共鉴定出78种化合物,主要含醇类和碳烯类化合物;8个品种(系)挥发油中分别鉴定出40、33、36、38、38、42、33、36种组分,共有组分为12种。除B－6品系外,共有组分均占挥发油总量的50.00%以上。说明川白芷不同品种(系)挥发油组分和含量总体一致,但也存在一定差异。

(14) 柳叶白前　田效民等利用SD法提取柳叶白前挥发油,采用GC－MS法分离出37种化学成分,鉴别出其中29种,占挥发油总量的87.28%,其主要成分为己醛(25.73%)、2－正戊基呋喃(15.51%)、1－壬烯－3－醇(4.03%)等。

(15) 射干　杨胜杰等采用SFE－CO_2法萃取

得到射干块茎中的挥发油，并通过 GC－MS 分离、鉴定了 32 种化学成分，占挥发油总量的 93.87%。包含有机酸、烷烃、萜类及衍生物等，主要成分为肉豆蔻酸乙酯（17.38%）、豆蔻酸（14.63%）、棕榈酸乙酯（11.80%）等。

（16）威灵仙　傅瑶等采用 SFE－CO_2法萃取威灵仙挥发油，并通过 GC－MS 分析了 156 种化学成分，占挥发油总含量的 85.03%。主要成分为亚油酸（18.47%）、l－(＋)－抗坏血酸－2，6－二棕榈酸酯（8.83%）、穿贝海绵甾醇（5.48%）。

（17）碰碰香　孔维维等采用 SPME－GC－MS 联用技术对碰碰香不同部位挥发性成分进行分析。从碰碰香的 3 个不同部位共分离出 40 种成分，主要含有酮、烷烃、烯烃、芳香烃、醇和酯等类化合物。根中含量最高的为莰烯（17.42%），茎和叶中含量最高的均为柠檬烯，含量分别为 27.56%和 27.07%。3 个部位中共有成分 5 种。

（18）珊瑚菜　崔海燕等采用 SD 法提取珊瑚菜根、叶与果实挥发油并进行 GC－MS 分析，分别鉴定出 45、48、34 种成分。根部挥发油以萜类、醛酮类和酸类化合物为主，分别占挥发油总量的 36.32%、13.43% 和 13.85%，主要为花侧柏烯（6.35%）、(*E*,*E*)－2，4－癸二烯醛（5.84%）、α－柏木烯（4.39%）等；叶片、果实挥发油以萜类化合物为主，分别占挥发油总量的 46.74%、73.34%，叶片挥发油主要成分为 β－水芹烯（12.72%）、γ－榄香烯（7.04%）、4－(1－甲乙基)－2－环己烯－1－酮（6.58%）等，果实挥发油主要成分为 β－水芹烯（33.44%）、α－水芹烯（12.90%）、3－甲基－2－丁烯－1－醇（8.57%）等。

2. 茎木

（1）竹沥　杨欣等采用干馏法制备 4 种竹沥，用 GC－MS 法进行分析，结果 4 种竹沥中均含有愈创木酚、紫丁香醇和去甲绵马酚等 13 种相同成分。其中愈创木酚为竹沥止咳化痰的活性成分。

（2）桑寄生　李兵等采用 SFE－CO_2法提取桑寄生挥发油，用 GC－MS 法分析鉴定其化学成分。分离鉴定 25 种化合物，占总量的 51.23%，主要成分是甲氧基肉桂酸乙酯（16.5%）、十五烷（5.30%）、香豆素（5.09%）等；从相思树寄生挥发油分离鉴定 11 种化合物，占总量的 53.94%，主要化学成分是 3－(4－甲氧基苯基)－2－丙烯酸乙酯（13.13%）、2，4－二叔丁基苯酚（11.06%）、反式薄荷酮（6.53%）等。

（3）柚寄生　廖彭莹采用 SD 法和 SFE－CO_2法提取柚寄生的挥发性成分，用 GC－MS 进行分析。从 SD 法提取的挥发油中获得 97 个色谱峰，鉴定了其中 49 种成分，已鉴定出成分的相对含量之和占流出峰总面积的 68.44%，含量较高的是樟脑（5.14%）、植酮（4.80%）、植醇（4.60%）等；从 SFE－CO_2 法提取的挥发油中共获得 65 个色谱峰，鉴定了其中 46 种成分，已鉴定出成分的相对含量之和占流出峰总面积的 79.64%，含量较高的是甲氧基肉桂酸乙酯（13.37%）、棕榈酸（8.81%）、亚油酸乙酯（5.66%）等。结果表明，两种提取方法所得到挥发油中成分存在显著差异。

（4）铁皮石斛　杨柳等采用正己烷蒸馏法从铁皮石斛中提取挥发性成分，并用 GC－MS 联用技术，对铁皮石斛茎中的挥发性成分进行测定。共鉴定出 31 种化学成分，其中含量较高的有亚油酸甲酯（5.85%）、二十五烷（10.13%）、22，23－二氢豆甾醇（11.09%）等。

（5）钻叶龙胆　曹雨虹等采用 SD 法提取钻叶龙胆的挥发油，用 GC－MS 技术鉴定出 18 种成分，占挥发油的 98.4%，主要成分为棕榈酸（28.05%）、15－冠醚－5（14.29%）、二十二烷（10.19%）等。

（6）狭叶薰衣草　王强等采集狭叶薰衣草的花、叶及茎，以 SD 法提取挥发油，用 GC－MS 法分析其化学成分。在狭叶薰衣草的花、叶及茎的挥发油中分别检出 80、60 和 16 个色谱峰，分别鉴定出 69、47、15 种化合物，占各部位挥发油组分总色谱峰面积的 94.01%、86.83%、97.35%，所含成分多为萜烯类化合物及其含氧衍生物，3 个部位中共有化合物 15 种。

（7）山绿茶　张龙等采用 SD 法分别提取山绿茶茎和叶的挥发油，通过 GC－MS 法对这两个部位挥发油的成分进行对比研究。从山绿茶茎中鉴定出 24 种成分，占挥发油总量的 94.97%；从叶中鉴定出 33 种成分，占挥发油总量的 98.48%。茎与叶挥发油成分中均含有糠醛、2，4－己二烯、(*Z*)－2，6－二甲基－2，6－辛二烯等化合物。

（8）小花山小橘　马雯芳等分别提取小花山小橘叶、茎的挥发油成分，应用 GC－MS 技术分离和鉴定各化学组分。从小花山小橘叶的挥发油成分中鉴定了 38 种化合物，占总量的 92.28%，以石竹烯含量最高(25.93%)；从其茎挥发油成分中鉴定了 36 种化合物，占总量的 80.57%，亦以石竹烯含量最高(33.15%)。

3. 叶类

(1) 两面针　阿优等采用 SD 法提取两面针叶挥发油，应用 GC 毛细管柱进行分离，采用质谱法检测。结果，不同采收期的两面针叶挥发性主要成分基本相同，均为萜类化合物，其中橙花叔醇含量最高，分别为 9.92%(7 月)、19.59%(8 月)、13.57%(9 月)和 11.13%(10 月)；其次为 α-杜松醇，分别为 8.86%(7 月)、10.62%(8 月)、16.59%(9 月)和 9.97%(10 月)；再次为棕榈酸，分别为 13.07%(7 月)、12.22%(8 月)、8.25%(9 月)和 7.55%(10 月)。

(2) 细叶艾　尤志勉等采用 SD 法从细叶艾中提取挥发油，用 GC-MS 法鉴定出 37 种成分，主要成分为合成右旋龙脑(16.33%)、右旋樟脑(10.11%)、B-瑟林烯(6.63%)等。

(3) 大叶钩藤　王冬梅等采用 SD 法提取大叶钩藤叶的挥发油，经 GC-MS 分析检出 127 个色谱峰，鉴定了其中 85 种成分，约占相对总含量的 96.47%。大叶钩藤叶挥发油主要成分及其相对含量为酯(23.57%)、烯酮类(15.11%)、烷烃类(14.62%)、烯醇类(7.66%)等物质。

(4) 艾叶　靳然等采用 GC-MS 法测定不同产地艾叶中桉油精、侧柏酮、樟脑、龙脑 4 种挥发性成分的含量。结果，各产地艾叶样品均含有桉油精、樟脑、龙脑，部分样品中含有侧柏酮。

(5) 柠檬百里香　吴爽等采用 SD 法从柠檬百里香叶中提取挥发油，利用 GC-MS 法鉴定出 32 种组分，占总出峰面积的 95.44%，主要成分有冰片(28.82%)、百里香酚(14.43%)、3,7-二甲基-1,6-辛二烯-3-醇(8.26%)等。其挥发油对 HepG2 细胞有很强毒性作用，其诱导细胞凋亡机制可能与 NF-κβ65 表达有关。

(6) 喙果皂帽花　宋煌旺等对皂帽花属植物中的挥发油成分进行了研究，利用 SD 法提取喙果皂帽花叶挥发油，并结合 GC-MS 分析，首次从中得到 91 种化合物，鉴定出 73 种。主要成分为双环杜鹃烯(15.63%)、丁子香烯(7.95%)、香叶烯(6.94%)等。

(7) 美人蕉　孔杜林等采用 SD 法提取美人蕉叶的挥发油，运用 GC-MS 分析鉴定出 45 种成分，占总离子流出峰面积的 25.38%。主要有 1,1-二乙氧基乙烷(5.56%)、二甲基氰膦(4.53%)和邻苯二甲酸单(2-乙基己基)酯(3.61%)等。

(8) 鹰爪花　王燕等采用 SD 法制备鹰爪花叶挥发油，并结合 GC-MS 分析，得到 68 种化合物，鉴定出 53 种，主要成分为大根香叶烯 D(16.97%)、榄香醇(8.63%)、α-石竹烯(6.58%)等。

(9) 北美枫香　尚庆文等以 SD 法提取枫香树属植物北美枫香的叶、树皮、心材三个部分的挥发油，以 GC-MS 联用技术对其成分进行分离、鉴定。结果，叶中鉴定出 15 种成分，树皮鉴定出 7 种成分，心材中鉴定出 9 种成分。心材与叶中所含挥发油成分相似，大部分为烷烃类化合物，树皮中则以脂类成分为主。

(10) 佛手　赵静芳等用 SD 法提取佛手叶及果实中的挥发油，采用 GC-MS 分析挥发油组成。结果，金华、杭州两地的佛手叶挥发油含量分别为 0.58%和 0.32%，佛手鲜果挥发油含量为 1.2%；从金佛手叶挥发油中鉴定出 30 种化学成分，从杭佛手叶挥发油中鉴定出 40 种化学成分，挥发油主要成分均为柠檬烯和 α-柠檬醛，金佛手叶中两者含量比杭佛手叶高，并含有一些果实中没有的香气成分。

(11) 香茶菜　许可等用 SD 法提取香茶菜不同部位的挥发油，利用 GC-MS 进行分析。挥发油主要以烷烃、醇、酸、酯为主，从香茶菜茎鉴定出 8 个化合物，香茶菜叶鉴定出 24 种化合物，香茶菜花序鉴定出 17 种化合物，香茶菜根鉴定出 8 种化合物，香茶菜根茎鉴定出 32 种化合物。

(12) 棘茎楤木　陈美航等采用 SD 法，运用 GC-MS 对棘茎楤木叶、根皮和茎皮 3 个部位挥发油的化学成分进行分析和鉴定。从梵净山棘茎楤木 3 个部位挥发油中共鉴定出 95 种化合物，有 8 种共有成分，其主要成分是倍半萜类及其氧化物，其次是烷烃、醛类、酯类和脂肪酸。

4. 花类

(1) 匙羹藤花　丘琴等采用 SD 法提取匙羹藤花挥发性成分，并采用 GC-MS 对其进行分析，分离出 55 种化合物，鉴定了 33 种化合物，占挥发性成分总量的 88.73%。主要为二十一烯(14.64%)、植醇(11.77%)、(*Z*)-2-甲基-2-二十二烷(11.62%)等。

(2) 大纽子　李静晶等采用 SD 法提取大纽子花挥发油,利用 GC-MS 分析检测出 70 种化学成分,鉴定了 64 种,占总提物的 92.73%。其中主要成分为醇类化合物占 33.96%,烯烃类化合物占 14.90%,氧化物占 13.94%,含量最高的为苯乙醇(10.67%)、顺-呋喃型芳樟醇氧化物(6.30%)、香叶醇(4.30%)等。

(3) 蜜本南瓜　张伟等采用 HS-SPME-GC-MS 技术,首次对蜜本南瓜花、茎尖和籽的挥发性成分进行分析。从蜜本南瓜花、茎尖、籽中分别鉴定出 22、20 和 21 种挥发性成分,占总峰面积的 91.89%、89.24%和 96.26%。其中花和茎尖共有 10 种共有成分,花、茎尖和籽有 3 种共有成分。花中 β-波旁烯(17.57%)、二十一烷(11.90%)、二甲基硫醚(9.63%)含量较高;茎尖中癸醛(28.77%)、壬醛(8.97%)、香叶烯 D(7.15%)含量最高;籽中棕榈酸乙酯(29.12%)、2,3-丁二醇(16.90%)和亚油酸乙酯(16.52%)含量较高。

5. 果实

(1) 阿育魏实　刘玲玲以 PDMS、CAR/PDMS、PDMS/DVB 和 DVB/CAR/PDMS 为微萃取纤维头,采用 HS-SPME 方法提取阿育魏实中挥发性成分,采用 GC-MS 进行分离鉴定,其主要成分为 γ-萜品烯(26.21%)、*p*-伞花烃(23.58%)、百里香酚(20.02%)。并与传统的 HD 法提取的挥发性成分进行比较,结果表明主要挥发性物质组分一致,但 HS-SPME-GC-MS 能快速地获得其组成成分,更有利于提取易挥发性化合物,特别是挥发性单萜类和倍半萜类化合物。

(2) 山茱萸　曾富佳等利用 SD 法提取黔产山茱萸挥发油,用 GC-MS 分离出 74 种化学成分,鉴定出 57 种化学成分,其中含量较高的成分为肉桂酸乙酯(21.90%)、1,2-亚甲二氧基-4-甲氧基-5-(-2 烯丙基)-苯(8.53%)、苯二甲酸丁酯(3.63%)等。

(3) 土荆芥　李植飞等采用 SD 法提取挥发油,通过 GC-MS 分析土荆芥果实挥发油的化学成分,共鉴定出 21 种成分,主要为 3-异丙基-6-甲基-7-氧杂双环[4.1.0]庚-2-酮(66.93%)、1-甲基-4-(1-甲基己烯基)环己烯(15.67%)及邻甲基异丙苯(12.96%);其挥发油主要成分为单萜类,具有良好的抗菌作用及抑制 HepG2 细胞增殖作用。

(4) 陈皮　王坚等采用 SD 法提取陈皮挥发油,用 GC-MS 分析与 AMDIS 软件进行解析。从同一植株生长期不同的 4 批陈皮中定性、定量共 72 种化合物,总含量分别为 95.54%、92.14%、98.66%、96.20%。含量最高的化合物是柠檬烯、芳樟醇、γ-萜品烯。

(5) 草果　何俏明等采用 SD 法分别提取草果果仁及果壳的挥发油,并用 GC-MS 法分析鉴定各挥发油的化学成分组成及结构。从 3 个不同批次的草果中共鉴定出 75 种成分。其中从草果仁挥发油样品中分别鉴定出 35、48、42 种组分,分别占挥发油总量的 94.80%、95.60%、93.70%;从果壳挥发油中分别鉴定出 55、70、68 种组分,分别占其挥发油总量的 94.50%、91.50%、91.40%。果仁挥发油共有成分有 33 种,果壳挥发油共有成分有 54 种;果壳与果仁挥发油成分大部分相同,其共有成分主要有 1,8-桉油素、α-蒎烯、β-蒎烯、α-松油醇、橙花叔醇等 29 种成分,分别占果壳和果仁挥发油总成分的 69.27%~77.29%、91.56%~93.88%。草果果壳挥发油的特有成分有 β-桉叶醇、莳醇、反式-松香芹醇、δ-杜松烯、(—)-桃金娘烯醇等 18 种化合物,果仁挥发油中无此类成分。

6. 种子

(1) 天仙子　王秀琴等用 GC-MS 方法分析天仙子中挥发油组成,经毛细管色谱分离并鉴定出 29 个峰。其中含量最高的是棕榈酸(28.30%)、亚油酸(26.85%)、油酸(14.39%)等。并首次采用 GC 对不同炮制品中挥发油成分进行了比较分析。与生品比较,清炒品中多数成分含量均下降,醋制品中多数成分含量大幅度增加,但未见成分组成的质变。

(2) 罗勒子　阿布都许库尔·吐尔逊等用 SD 法提取罗勒子中的挥发油,GC-MS 法分析挥发油的化学成分。共分离出 68 种化合物,鉴定了 64 种成分,占挥发油总成分的 96.82%。主要成分为三十一酸甲酯(18.56%)、对-烯丙基茴香醚(7.04%)、γ-谷甾醇(6.52%)等。

(3) 三尖杉　解修超等采用索氏回流法提取三尖杉种仁的挥发油,用 GC-MS 法分离和鉴定出23种化学成分,主要为油酸(34.53%)、棕榈酸(12.04%)、亚油酸丁酯(9.56%)等。

7. 全草

(1) 鱼腥草　洪佳璇等利用SD法从新鲜鱼腥草中提取挥发油,用GC-MS法鉴定出60种组分,主要为甲基正壬酮(16.97%)、月桂烯(12.95%)、癸酸(7.53%)等。

(2) 茵陈　王玉林等利用SD法提取茵陈挥发油,用GC-MS检测,共有67个色谱峰,鉴定出48种化学成分,占总含量的89.03%。主要组分为正十六烷酸(23.91%)、9,12,15-十八碳三烯酸(19.38%)、镰叶芹醇(11.76%)等。

(3) 柱果绿绒蒿　高昂等采用SD法提取柱果绿绒蒿挥发油,运用GC-MS分析其化学成分。从中鉴定了47种化合物,占其总量的91.87%,主要为十六烷酸(27.65%)、6,10,14-三甲基-2-十五烷酮(16.33%)、叶绿醇(6.81%)等。

(4) 毛大丁草　罗兰等采用SD法提取毛大丁草挥发油,并利用GC-MS技术对挥发油成分进行鉴定。从中检出22个色谱峰,鉴定了17种化合物,占其挥发油总含量的86.18%。其中含量较高的成分有Neryl(*s*)-2-methylbutanoate(35.99%)、4-羟基-3-甲基苯乙酮(8.74%)、棕榈酸(7.48%)等。

(5) 磨盘草　陈勇等采用SD法提取不同产地的磨盘草挥发油,用GC-MS法分析鉴定磨盘草挥发油中主要化学成分,并进行比较。从广西博白、南宁、玉林产的磨盘草挥发油中,共鉴定出6种相同成分,分别是植物醇、棕榈酸,2-十五烷酮-6,10,14-三甲基、油酸酰胺、二十四烷、正二十五烷,但不同产地药材挥发油成分及含量存在差异。

(6) 冬葵　曾富佳等利用有机溶剂-SD法提取冬葵粗粉挥发油,用GC-MS分离并鉴定出20种化学成分,其中含量较高的为已醛(26.70%)、(*E*,*E*)-2,4-癸二烯醛(10.37%)、苯基-1-乙醛(10.19%)等。

(7) 假蒟　王道平等采用HS-SPME-GC-MS技术研究新鲜假蒟全草的挥发性化学成分。共鉴定出48种化合物,按峰面积比占假蒟挥发油化学成分的88.70%,其中β-月桂烯(34.40%)、柠檬烯(8.90%)、芳樟醇(6.00%)等为主要化合物。

(8) 海州香薷和石香薷　李佳等采用HS-SPME-GC-MS技术,从海州香薷和石香薷挥发性成分中分别检出39种和46种成分,分别占挥发性成分总峰面积的70.50%、92.44%。海州香薷挥发性成分中含量较高的为β-石竹烯(34.26%)、1,4,7,-cycloundecatriene,1,5,9,9-tetramethyl-,*Z*,*Z*,*Z*-(9.07%)、α-法尼烯(3.44%);石香薷挥发性成分中含量较高的为β-石竹烯(30.88%)、1,2,3,5,6,8a-六甲基-4,7-二甲基-1-异丙基萘-(1*S*-*cis*)(22.99%)、α-荜澄茄油萜(13.51%)。结果共有成分11种,2种植物所含挥发性成分及含量存在一定差异。

(9) 委陵菜　王小明等选择委陵菜地上部分,采用HS GC-MS分析,鉴定出32种挥发性成分,主要为α-法尼烯(17.68%)、2-乙基呋喃(14.48%)、叶醇(7.96%)等。

(10) 裂叶牵牛　梁娜等采用SFE-CO_2萃取法,得到裂叶牵牛地上部分含有的挥发油,并通过GC-MS分析其化学成分;鉴定出的组分占挥发油总量的91.43%,主要成分有1-碘十八烷(29.71%)、二十九烷(17.02%)、亚麻酸(9.91%)等。

8. 皮

(1) 核桃楸　李金凤等分别采用汽汽萃取法和SD法提取核桃楸皮中挥发油,并通过GC-MS技术对其化学成分进行分析。汽汽萃取法提取的挥发油共鉴定出34种成分,占挥发油总成分97.76%;SD法提取的挥发油共鉴定出19种成分,占挥发油总成分69.06%。2种方法得到的核桃楸皮挥发油组分与含量相差较大,但有5个共有成分,分别为氧化石竹烯、正十六烷、正十九烷,9-十八碳炔和2,3,5,8-四甲基癸烷。

(2) 苦楝　杨烨等采用SD法提取苦楝干皮、枝皮和根皮中的挥发油,并用GC-MS法分离并分析鉴定其成分。从苦楝干皮、枝皮和根皮中分别鉴定出47、62、56种化学成分。苦楝干皮与枝皮的主要成分为棕榈酸,相对含量分别为38.57%、27.18%;苦楝根皮的主要成分为α-可巴烯,相对含量为18.06%。

9. 树脂

多伞阿魏 雷林洁等采用SD法提取多伞阿魏挥发油,并对挥发油成分进行分析。鉴定出44种化合物，主要成分是左旋乙酸冰片酯(17.78%)、愈创木醇(11.44%)、(E)-β-金合欢烯(11.26%)等，未检出多硫化合物。

(谭红胜)

[附] 参考文献

A

Ali F, Khan HU, Afzal M, et al. Two new cholinesterase inhibitors asiatoates A and B from *Buddleja asiatica*[J]. Journal of Asian Natural Products Research, 2013, 15(6): 631

阿布都许库尔.吐尔逊，孙莲，哈及尼沙. GC-MS法分析新疆罗勒子挥发油的化学成分[J].中国民族民间医药，2013，22(6): 21

阿优(Vilaysac kMackhaphonh)，冯洁，李进英，等.不同采收期两面针叶挥发性成分的GC-MS分析[J].时珍国医国药，2013，24(5): 1244

B

Bai R, Zhou Y, Deng S, et al. Two new entkaurane diterpenoids from *Pteris semipinnata* [J]. Journal of Asian Natural Products Research, 2013, 15(10): 1107

Bi SF, Guo ZK, Jiang N, et al. New alkaloid from streptomyces koyangensis residing in *Odontotermes formosanus* [J]. Journal of Asian Natural Products Research, 2013, 15(4): 422

Bian QY, Wang SY, Xu LJ, et al. Two new antioxidant diarylheptanoids from the fruits of *Alpinia oxyphylla* [J]. Journal of Asian Natural Products Research, 2013, 15(10): 1094

Bu PB, Li YR, Jiang M, et al. Glycosides from the bark of *Machilus robusta*[J]. Journal of Asian Natural Products Research, 2013, 15(5): 482

C

Cao CM, Wu YB, Guo RX, et al. Torreyanoxane, a new 3, 4-secoglutinane triterpenoid isolated from the pulp of *Torreya nucifera*[J]. Helvetica Chimica Acta, 2013, 96(3): 375

Cao SY, Ke ZL, Xi LM. A new sesquiterpene lactone from *Salvia plebeia*[J]. Journal of Asian Natural Products Research, 2013, 15(4): 404

Cao XF, Wang JS, Wang XB, et al. Monoterpene indole alkaloids from the stem bark of *Mitragyna diversifolia* and their acetylcholine esterase inhibitory effects[J]. Phytochemistry, 2013, 96: 389

Chang HS, Chiang MY, Hsu HY, et al. Cytotoxic cardenolide glycosides from the root of *Reevesia formosana*[J]. Phytochemistry, 2013, 87: 86

Chaudhuri PK, Singh D. A new triterpenoid from the rhizomes of *Nelumbo nucifera*[J]. Natural product research, 2013, 27(6): 532

Chen C, Zhu H, Zhao D, et al. Two new lignans from *Phryma leptostachya* L. [J]. Helvetica Chimica Acta, 2013, 96(6): 1392

Chen DZ, Xiong HB, Tian K, et al. Two new sphingolipids from the leaves of *Piper betle* L[J]. Molecules, 2013, 18(9): 11241

Chen G, Su L, Feng SG, et al. Furostanol saponins from the fruits of *Tribulus terrestris*[J]. Natural Product Research, 2013, 27(13): 1186

Chen HW, Chen L, Li B, et al. Three new germacrane-type sesquiterpenes with NGF-potentiating activity from *Valeriana officinalis* var. *latiofolia*[J]. Molecules, 2013, 18(11): 14138

Chen J, Leng H, Duan Y, et al. Three new flavonoids from the leaves of oriental tobacco and their cytotoxicity[J]. Phytochemistry Letters, 2013, 6(1): 144

Chen J, Wei H, Xu Y, et al. Antioxidant lignans from the roots of *Vladimiria muliensis* [J]. Planta Medica, 2013, 79(15): 1470

Chen J, Yang ML, Zeng J, et al. Antimicrobial activity of *Araucaria cunninghamii* Sweet and the chemical constituents of its twigs and leaves [J]. Phytochemistry Letters, 2013, 6(1): 41

Chen JM, Wei LB, Lu CL, et al. A flavonoid 8-C-glycoside and a triterpenoid cinnamate from *Nervilia fordii*[J]. Journal of Asian Natural Products Research, 2013, 15(10): 1088

Chen L, Zhang Y, Ding G, et al. Two new derivatives of 2, 5-dihydroxyphenylacetic acid from the kernel of *Entada phaseoloides* [J]. Molecules, 2013, 18(2): 1477

Chen M, Xu X, Xu B, et al. Neglschisandrins E-F: Two new lignans and related cytotoxic lignans from *Schisandra neglecta*[J]. Molecules, 2013, 18(2): 2297

Chen ND, Chen NF, Chen CW, et al. Separation

and structure elucidation of a new homoflavanol derivative from *Pteridium aquilinum* (L.) Kuhn [J]. Natural Product Research, 2013, 27(19): 1764

Chen P, Qu L, Tian L, et al. Two halogenated sesquiterpenoids from the fruits of *Alpinia oxyphylla* [J]. Helvetica Chimica Acta, 2013, 96(6): 1163

Chen PY, Wu JD, Tang KY, et al. Isolation and synthesis of a bioactive benzenoid derivative from the fruiting bodies of *Antrodia camphorata* [J]. Molecules, 2013, 18(7): 7600

Chen S, Huang HY, Cheng MJ, et al. Neolignans and phenylpropanoids from the roots of *Piper taiwanense* and their antiplatelet and antitubercular activities [J]. Phytochemistry, 2013, 93: 203

Chen S, Li T, Yao X, et al. Anti HSV1 flavonoid derivatives tethered with houttuynin from *Houttuynia cordata*[J]. Planta Medica, 2013, 79(18): 1742

Chen YC, Li YC, You BJ, et al. Diterpenoids with antiinflammatory activity from the wood of *Cunninghamia konishii*[J]. Molecules, 2013, 18(1): 682

Chen Z, Liu YL, Xu QM, et al. New polyoxygenated cyclohexene and polyoxygenated secocyclohexene from *Uvaria boniana* [J]. Journal of Asian Natural Products Research, 2013, 15(1): 53

Cheng BH, Chen JC, Liu JQ, et al. Cucurbitane-type triterpenoids from *Momordica charantia* [J]. Helvetica Chimica Acta, 2013, 96(6): 1111

Cheng F, Deng Z, Guo Z, et al. Machilusmarin, a new neuroprotective isocoumarin dimer from the stems of *Machilus ichangensis* Rehd. et Wils[J]. Natural Product Research, 2013, 27(17): 1542

Cheng JT, Liu F, Li XN, et al. Lycospidine A, a new type of lycopodium alkaloid from *Lycopodium complanatum*[J]. Organic Letters, 2013, 15(10): 2438

Cheng XR, Zhang SD, Wang CH, et al. Bioactive eudesmane and germacrane derivatives from *Inula wissmanniana* Hand. Mazz[J]. Phytochemistry, 2013, 96: 214

Cheng YB, Fazary AE, Lin YC, et al. A new antiinflammatory phloroglucinol derivative from *Hypericum nakamurai* [J]. Natural Product Research, 2013, 27(8): 727

Cheng YY, Chen H, He HP, et al. Anti - HIV active daphnane diterpenoids from *Trigonostemon thyrsoideum*[J]. Phytochemistry, 2013, 96: 360

Cheng ZB, Shao WW, Liu YN, et al. Extracellular signal-regulated kinases (ERK) inhibitors from *Aristolochia yunnanensis* [J]. Journal of Natural Products, 2013, 76(4): 664

Cong Y, Guo JG, Liu J. Two new chemical constituents of *Veratrum dahuricum* (Turcz.) Loes. f. [J]. Helvetica Chimica Acta, 2013, 96(2): 345

Cui JM, Kang LP, Yu HS, et al. Two new furostanol saponins from *Aspidistra typica* [J]. Journal of Asian Natural Products Research, 2013, 15(5): 525

曹雨虹,顾健,谭睿,等.钻叶龙胆挥发油化学成分的GC-MS分析[J].中国实验方剂学杂志,2013,19(5): 91

陈方方,师彦平.分子印迹固相萃取技术在天然产物有效成分分离分析中的应用进展[J].色谱,2013,31(7): 626

陈美航,舒华,陈仕学,等.棘茎楤木不同部位挥发油成分的比较[J].中国实验方剂学杂志,2013,19(12): 124

陈绍农,鲍官虎,汪礼权,等.闹羊花中的两个新化合物(英文)[J].中国天然药物,2013,11(5): 525

陈勇,魏后超,农莉,等.气相色谱-质谱联用测定广西不同产地磨盘草的挥发油成分[J].环球中医药,2013,6(8): 572

崔海燕,胡晶红,张永清.珊瑚菜植株不同器官挥发油成分分析[J].山东中医药大学学报,2013,37(1): 61

D

Deng KZ, Xiong Y, Zhou B, et al. Chemical constituents from the roots of *Ranunculus ternatus* and their inhibitory effects on mycobacterium tuberculosis[J]. Molecules, 2013, 18(10): 11859

Deng Y, Guo T, Shao Z, et al. Three new xanthones from the resin of *Garcinia hanburyi*[J]. Planta Medica, 2013, 79(9): 792

Di XX, Wang SQ, Zhang XL, et al. Diterpenoids from the aerial parts of *Orthosiphon aristatus* var. *aristatus*[J]. Phytochemistry Letters, 2013, 6(3): 412

Dong FW, Fan WW, Xu FQ, et al. Inhibitory activities on nitric oxide production of stilbenoids from *Pholidota yunnanensis* [J]. Journal of Asian Natural Products Research, 2013, 15(11): 1256

Dong HP, Wu HM, Chen SJ, et al. The effect of butanolides from *Cinnamomum tenuifolium* on platelet aggregation[J]. Molecules, 2013, 18(10): 11836

Dong JY, Ma XY, Cai XQ, et al. Sesquiterpenoids from *Curcuma wenyujin* with antiinfluenza viral activities [J]. Phytochemistry, 2013, 85: 122

Dong L, Zhang XP, Liu MS, et al. Two new ent-3,4-secolabdane diterpenoids from *Callicarpa nudiflora* [J]. Journal of Asian Natural Products Research, 2013, 15(1): 30

Dong LB, Gao X, Liu F, et al. Isopalhinine A, a

unique pentacyclic lycopodium alkaloid from *Palhinhaea cernua*[J]. Organic Letters, 2013, 15(14): 3570

Dong SH, Liu J, Ge YZ, et al. Chemical constituents from *Brucea javanica*[J]. Phytochemistry, 2013, 85: 175

Dong XJ, Luo SD. Six novel eudesmane-like sesquiterpenes from *Illicium spathulatum*[J]. Helvetica Chimica Acta, 2013, 96(3): 445

Dong XJ, Zhu YF, Bao GH, et al. New limonoids and a dihydrobenzofuran norlignan from the roots of *Toona sinensis*[J]. Molecules, 2013, 18(3): 2840

F

Fan L, Wang Y, Ye W, et al. Chemical constituents from the roots and stems of *Erycibe obtusifolia* and their in vitro antiviral activity[J]. Planta Medica, 2013, 79(16): 1558

Fang ST, Liu X, Kong NN, et al. Two new withanolides from the halophyte *Datura stramonium* L. [J]. Natural Product Research, 2013, 27(21): 1965

Fang Z, Zhang G, Xu S, et al. Diterpenoids and sesquiterpenoids from the twigs and leaves of *Illicium majus*[J]. Planta Medica, 2013, 79(2): 142

Feng R, Wang T, Wei W, et al. Cytotoxic constitutents from *Cryptocarya maclurei* [J]. Phytochemistry, 2013, 90: 147

Fu HZ, Li CJ, Yang JZ, et al. Triterpenoid glycosides from the stems of *Gordonia kwangsiensis*[J]. Phytochemistry, 2013, 85: 167

Fu HZ, Zhong RJ, Zhang DM, et al. A new protopanaxadiol-type ginsenoside from the roots of *Panax notoginseng*[J]. Journal of Asian Natural Products Research, 2013, 15(10): 1139

Fu M, Deng D, Huang R, et al. A new flavanocoumarin from the root of *Flemingia philippinensis* [J]. Natural Product Research, 2013, 27(14): 1237

Fu Q, Wang SB, Zhao SH, et al. Three new monoterpene glycosides from the roots of *Paeonia lactiflora*[J]. Journal of Asian Natural Products Research, 2013, 15(7): 697

Fu Q, Zan K, Zhao MB, et al. Three new triterpene saponins from *Clematis chinensis*[J]. Journal of Asian Natural Products Research, 2013, 15(6): 610

Fu YD, Li ZL, Pu SB, et al. Two new compounds from *Scolopendra multidens* Newport[J]. Journal of Asian Natural Products Research, 2013, 15(4): 363

傅瑶,李颜,霍炎,等. 威灵仙挥发油的超临界萃取工艺优化及 GC-MS 分析[J]. 中国实验方剂学杂志,2013, 19(7): 41

G

Gao F, Zhao D, Deng J. New Flavonoids from *Lysimachia christinae* Hance[J]. Helvetica Chimica Acta, 2013, 96(5): 985

Gao JB, Li GY, Huang J, et al. A new tetracyclic triterpenoid compound from Mastich[J]. Journal of Asian natural products research, 2013, 15(4): 400

Gao W, Chen C, Kong DY. Hippophins C-F, four new flavonoids, acylated with one monoterpenic acid from the seed residue of *Hippophae rhamnoides* subsp. sinensis [J]. Journal of Asian Natural Products Research, 2013, 15(5): 507

Gao X, He J, Zhao Q, et al. Further lignans from *Saururus chinensis*[J]. Planta Medica, 2013, 79(18): 1720

Gao XM, Cui MZ, Yu T, et al. A novel xanthone from *Garcinia oligantha*[J]. Helvetica Chimica Acta, 2013, 96(3): 494

Ge YB, Li MS, Mei ZN, et al. Two new flavonol glycosides from the leaves of *Elaeagnus pungens*[J]. Journal of Asian Natural Products Research, 2013, 15(10): 1073

Ge YW, Zhu S, Shang MY, et al. Aristololactams and aporphines from the stems of *Fissistigma oldhamii* (Annonaceae)[J]. Phytochemistry, 2013, 86: 201

Gong Y, Hua H, Jing Y, et al. Triterpene saponins from *Clematis mandshurica* and their antiproliferative activity[J]. Planta Medica, 2013, 79(11): 987

Gu W, Hao XJ, Liu HX, et al. Acylated iridoid glycosides and acylated rhamnopyranoses from *Gmelina arborea* flowers[J]. Phytochemistry Letters, 2013, 6(4): 681

Guo F, Feng L, Huang C, et al. Prenylflavone derivatives from *Broussonetia papyrifera*, inhibit the growth of breast cancer cells in vitro and in vivo[J]. Phytochemistry Letters, 2013, 6(3): 331

Guo Y, Liu YX, Kang LP, et al. Two novel furostanol saponins from the tubers of *Ophiopogon japonicus*[J]. Journal of Asian Natural Products Research, 2013, 15(5): 459

高昂,赵兵,巩江,等. 柱果绿绒蒿挥发油化学成分及其抗氧化活性的研究[J]. 中国中药杂志,2013, 38(2): 284

郭耀杰,吴卫,李静夜,等. 川白芷不同品种(系)挥发油成分 GC-MS 分析[J]. 中国实验方剂学杂志,2013, 19(8): 110

H

Han N, Chen L, Yin J, et al. Steroidal glycosides from *Reineckia carnea* herba and their antitussive activity [J]. Planta Medica, 2013, 79(9): 788

Hao B, Shen SF, Zhao QJ. Cytotoxic and antimalarial Amaryllidaceae alkaloids from the bulbs of *Lycoris radiata*[J]. Molecules, 2013, 18(3): 2458

Hao X, Zhang J, Xia G, et al. A new triterpenoid from *Teucrium viscidum*[J]. Molecules, 2013, 18(1): 1262

He CJ, Peng C, Xie XF, et al. Two new dianthramide glucosides with cardiomyocytes protective activity from *Aconitum carmichaelii*[J]. Phytochemistry Letters, 2013, 6(2): 299

He JB, Luo J, Zhang L, et al. Sesquiterpenoids with new carbon skeletons from the resin of *Toxicodendron vernicifluum* as new types of extracellular matrix inhibitors[J]. Organic Letters, 2013, 15(14): 3602

Hong ZL, Xiong J, Wu SB, et al. Tetracyclic triterpenoids and terpenylated coumarins from the bark of *Ailanthus altissima* ("Tree of Heaven") [J]. Phytochemistry, 2013, 86: 159

Hu J, Song Y, Shi XD, et al. Ergostane Steroids from *Dysoxylum lukii* [J]. Helvetica Chimica Acta, 2013, 96(12): 2245

Hu K, Liu JQ, Li XN, et al. Chukfuransins A-D, four new phragmalin limonoids with β - furan ring involved in skeleton reconstruction from *Chukrasia tabularis*[J]. Organic Letters, 2013, 15(15): 3902

Hu LL, Ma QY, Huang SZ, et al. Three new lanostanoid triterpenes from the fruiting bodies of *Ganoderma tropicum* [J]. Journal of Asian Natural Products Research, 2013, 15(4): 357

Hu QF, Zhou B, Huang JM, et al. Antiviral phenolic compounds from *Arundina gramnifolia* [J]. Journal of Natural Products, 2013, 76(2): 292

Hu XR, Wu HF, Zhang XP, et al. A new sesquiterpene lactone from *Sarcandra glabra*[J]. Natural Product Research, 2013, 27(13): 1197

Huang GH, Xi ZX, Li JL, et al. Isolation of two new phenolic compounds from the fruit of *Chaenomeles speciosa* (Sweet) Nakai [J]. Phytochemistry Letters, 2013, 6(4): 526

Huang H, Gao XJ, Liu J, et al. A new caryolane sesquiterpene from *Heteropappus altaicus* (Willd.) Novopokr[J]. Natural Product Research, 2013, 27(4-5): 350

Huang H, Lin M, Kuo Y, et al. Cardenolides and bufadienolide glycosides from *Kalanchoe tubiflora* and evaluation of cytotoxicity [J]. Planta Medica, 2013, 79(14): 1362

Huang HC, Huang GJ, Liaw CC, et al. A new megastigmane from *Kalanchoe tubiflora* (Harvey) Hamet [J]. Phytochemistry Letters, 2013, 6(3): 379

Huang HC, Lin MK, Hwang SY, et al. Two antiinflammatory steroidal saponins from *Dracaena angustifolia* Roxb[J]. Molecules, 2013, 18(8): 8752

Huang J, Han HY, Li GY, et al. Two new terpenoid benzoates with antitumor activity from the roots of *Ferula dissecta*[J]. Journal of Asian Natural Products Research, 2013, 15(10): 1100

Huang J, Lu XQ, Lu J, et al. Two new phthalides with BuChE inhibitory activity from *Ligusticum chuanxiong* [J]. Journal of Asian Natural Products Research, 2013, 15(12): 1237

Huang J, Wang GC, Wang CH, et al. Two new glycosides from *Vitex negundo* [J]. Natural Product Research, 2013, 27(20): 1837

Huang MY, Zhong LJ, Xie JM, et al. A new taraxastane-type triterpene from *Vitex trifolia* var. *simplicifolia* [J]. Helvetica Chimica Acta, 2013, 96(11): 2040

Huang R, Peng Y, Zhou X, et al. A new pyrimidinedione derivative from the gorgonian coral *Verrucella umbraculum* [J]. Natural Product Research, 2013, 27(45): 319

Huang R, Peng Y, Zhou X, et al. A new taurine derivative from South China Sea marine sponge *Axinella* sp. [J]. Natural Product Research, 2013, 27(17): 1537

Huang S, Zhou X, Weng J, et al. New nervogenic acid derivatives from *Liparis nervosa*[J]. Planta Medica, 2013, 79(34): 281

Huang SD, Zhang Y, Cao MM, et al. Myriberine A, a new alkaloid with an unprecedented heteropentacyclic skeleton from *Myrioneuron faberi*[J]. Organic Letters, 2013, 15(3): 590

Huang SZ, Ma QY, Fang WW, et al. Three new isopimarane diterpenoids from *Excoecaria acerifolia*[J]. Journal of Asian Natural Products Research, 2013, 15(7): 750

Huang Y, Hao YL, Mai XY. Chemical constituents from *Solidago canadensis* with hypolipidemic effects in HFD - fed hamsters [J]. Journal of Asian Natural Products Research, 2013, 15(4): 319

Huang YL, Nagai S, Tanaka T, et al. Two new

oleanane-type triterpenes isolated from Japanese post-fermented tea produced by anaerobic microbial fermentation[J]. Molecules, 2013, 18(5): 4868

何俏明，覃洁萍，黄艳，等. 草果果仁及果壳挥发油化学成分的 GC－MS 分析[J]. 中国实验方剂学杂志，2013，19(14): 112

洪佳璇，徐淑媛，江丽，等. 鲜品鱼腥草挥发油成分分析[J]. 浙江中医杂志，2013，4(5): 375

侯丽，唐贵华，张于，等. 割舌树中一个新的胡萝卜烷型倍半萜(英文)[J]. 中国天然药物，2013，11(1): 84

黄升殿，张于，何红平，等. 红花石蒜中的一个新石蒜生物碱(英文)[J]. 中国天然药物，2013，11(4): 406

J

Ji TF, Li J, Liang CH. The chemical constituents of the twigs of *Ammopiptanthus nanus*[J]. Journal of Asian Natural Products Research, 2013, 15(4): 332

Jia BX, Ren FX, Jia L, et al. Baeckein E, a new bioactive C － methylated biflavonoid from the roots of *Baeckea frutescens*[J]. Natural Product Research, 2013, 27(22): 2069

Jia L, Wang J, Lv C, et al. Two new compounds from *Potentilla multicaulis* Bunge[J]. Natural Product Research, 2013, 27(15): 1361

Jia LY, Wang J, Lv CN, et al. A new cycloartane nortriterpenoid from stem and leaf of *Quercus variabilis* [J]. Journal of Asian Natural Products Research, 2013, 15(9): 1050

Jiang H, Yang L, Liu C, et al. Four new glycosides from the fruit of *Xanthium sibiricum* Patr[J]. Molecules, 2013, 18(10): 12464

Jiang JS, Chen Z, Yang YN, et al. Two new glycosides from the florets of *Carthamus tinctorius* [J]. Journal of Asian Natural Products Research, 2013, 15(5): 427

Jiang M, Sun P, Tang H, et al. Steroids glycosylated with both dand larabinoses from the South China Sea gorgonian *Dichotella gemmacea*[J]. Journal of Natural Products, 2013, 76(4): 764

Jiang W, Wu X, Wu B. Isolation and identification of two novel attractant compounds from Chinese cockroach (*Eupolyphaga sinensis* Walker) by combination of HSCCC, NMR and CD techniques[J]. Molecules, 2013, 18(9): 11299

Jiang ZY, Bai XS, Liang H, et al. Cytotoxic flavanes from *Uraria clarkei*[J]. Journal of Asian Natural Products Research, 2013, 15(9): 979

Jiao K, Li HY, Zhang P, et al. Three new ursane-type triterpenoids from the aerial parts of *Isodon excisoides* [J]. Journal of Asian Natural Products Research, 2013, 15(9): 962

Jing WY, Jiang C, Ji F, et al. Chemical constituents from the stem barks of *Garcinia multiflora*[J]. Journal of Asian Natural Products Research, 2013, 15(11): 1152

姜海，孟永海，杨柳，等. 小蓟中一个新的大柱香波龙烷苷(英文)[J]. 中国天然药物，2013，11(5): 534

靳然，于密密，赵百孝，等. 气相色谱法测定艾叶 4 个挥发性成分的含量[J]. 药物分析杂志，2013，33(6): 1033

K

Kang ZY, Zhang MJ, Wang JX, et al. Two new furostanol saponins from the fibrous root of *Ophiopogon japonicus* [J]. Journal of Asian Natural Products Research, 2013, 15(12): 1230

Kim SB, Chang BY, Han SB, et al. A new phenolic glycoside from *Cnidium monnieri* fruits [J]. Natural Product Research, 2013, 27(21): 1945

Kuo WL, Chung CY, Hwang TL, et al. Biphenyl-type neolignans from *Magnolia officinalis* and their anti-inflammatory activities [J]. Phytochemistry, 2013, 85: 153

孔杜林，李永辉，范超军，等. 美人蕉叶挥发油的GC－MS 分析[J]. 中国现代中药，2013，15(6): 445

孔维维，吕鼎豪，李华，等. 碰碰香不同部位挥发性成分的分析[J]. 药物分析杂志，2013，33(2): 241

L

Lai YJ, Xue YB, Zhang MK, et al. Scapiformolactones A-I: germacrane sesquiterpenoids with an unusual ＜DELTA＞3 － 15, 6 － lactone moiety from the whole plants of *Salvia scapiformis* [J]. Phytochemistry, 2013, 96: 378

Lan WC, Tzeng CW, Lin CC, et al. Prenylated flavonoids from *Artocarpus altilis*: antioxidant activities and inhibitory effects on melanin production [J]. Phytochemistry, 2013, 89: 78

Lee CL, Hwang TL, He WJ, et al. Antineutrophilic inflammatory steroidal glycosides from *Solanum torvum* [J]. Phytochemistry, 2013, 95: 315

Li C, Li B, Ye J, et al. A new norditerpenoid from *Euonymus grandiflorus* Wall [J]. Natural Product Research, 2013, 27(19): 1716

Li CY, Du HJ, Su XH, et al. Juglanones A and B: two novel tetralone dimers from walnut pericarp (*Juglans regia*)[J]. Helvetica Chimica Acta, 2013, 96(6): 1031

Li CY, Liu J, Su XH, et al. New dimeric

phenanthrene and flavone from *Spiranthes sinensis* [J]. Journal of Asian natural products research, 2013, 15(4): 417

Li F, Pan HM, Liu X, et al. New phenanthrene glycosides from *Dendrobium denneanum* and their cytotoxic activity [J]. Phytochemistry Letters, 2013, 6(4): 640

Li F, Zhan Z, Liu F, et al. Polyflavanostilbene A, a new flavanol-fused stilbene glycoside from *Polygonum cuspidatum* [J]. Organic Letters, 2013, 15(3): 674

Li HJ, Mu LH, Dong XZ, et al. New cycloartane triterpene glycosides from *Beesia calthaefolia* [J]. Natural Product Research, 2013, 27(21): 1987

Li J, Huang D, Chen W, et al. Two new phenolic glycosides from *Gnaphalium affine* D. Don and their anti-complementary activity[J]. Molecules, 2013, 18(7): 7751

Li J, Li MY, Bruhn T, et al. Thaixylomolins AC: limonoids featuring two new motifs from the Thai *Xylocarpus moluccensis* [J]. Organic Letters, 2013, 15(14): 3682

Li J, Yu DQ. Two new constituents from *Erigeron breviscapus* [J]. Journal of Asian Natural Products Research, 2013, 15(9): 969

Li JY, Peng Y, Li L, et al. Two new abietane diterpenoids from the roots of *Tripterygium wilfordii* Hook. f. [J]. Helvetica Chimica Acta, 2013, 96(2): 313

Li K, Brant CO, Huertas M, et al. Petromyzonin, a hexahydrophenanthrene sulfate isolated from the larval sea lamprey (*Petromyzon marinus* L.)[J]. Organic Letters, 2013, 15(23): 5924

Li LF, Liu HQ, Zhang R, et al. Two new schisdilactonetype compounds from *Schisandra chinensis* [J]. Journal of Asian Natural Products Research, 2013, 15(11): 1168

Li P, Deng Y, Wei X, et al. Triterpenoids from *Ganoderma lucidum* and their cytotoxic activities [J]. Natural Product Research, 2013, 27(1): 17

Li QJ, Wang ML, Yang XS, et al. Two new coumarin glycosides from *Chimonanthus nitens* [J]. Journal of Asian Natural Products Research, 2013, 15(3): 270

Li S, Huang H, Liu J, et al. Two new sesquiterpenes from *Ligularia dictyoneura* [J]. Phytochemistry Letters, 2013, 6(3): 315

Li SF, Zhang Y, Huang N, et al. Daphnane diterpenoids from the stems of *Trigonostemon lii* and their anti-HIV-1 activity[J]. Phytochemistry, 2013, 93: 216

Li SG, Chen LL, Huang XJ, et al. Five new stilbene glycosides from the roots of *Polygonum multiflorum* [J]. Journal of Asian Natural Products Research, 2013, 15(11): 1145

Li TT, Tang XL, Chen CL, et al. New eunicellin diterpenes and 9, 10-secosteroids from the gorgonian *Muricella sibogae* [J]. Helvetica Chimica Acta, 2013, 96(6): 1197

Li WT, Yang BX, Zhu W, et al. A new indole alkaloidal glucoside from the aerial parts of *Clematis terniflora* DC [J]. Natural Product Research, 2013, 27(24): 2333

Li X, Zhang SD, Jin HZ, et al. A new flavonol from *Oxytropis ochrocephala* Bunge [J]. Natural Product Research, 2013, 27(6): 554

Li XN, Chu C, Tong SQ, et al. A new furolactonetype lignan from *Lycium chinense* [J]. Natural Product Research, 2013, 27(8): 750

Li Y, Liu YB, Zhang JJ, et al. Mollolide A, a diterpenoid with a new 1, 10 : 2, 3 disecograyanane skeleton from the roots of *Rhododendron molle* [J]. Organic Letters, 2013, 15(12): 3074

Li YD, Wu ZY, Li HM, et al. Iridoids from the roots of *Valeriana jatamansi* [J]. Helvetica Chimica Acta, 2013, 96(3): 424

Li YF, Jiang Y, Huang JF, et al. Four new lignans from *Schisandra sphenanthera* [J]. Journal of Asian Natural Products Research, 2013, 15(9): 934

Li YP, Dong LB, Chen DZ, et al. Two new dihydrobenzofurantype neolignans from *Breynia fruticosa* [J]. Phytochemistry Letters, 2013, 6(2): 281

Li YP, Li YH, Zhong JD, et al. Antioxidant phenolic glycoside and flavonoids from *Pieris japonica* [J]. Journal of Asian Natural Products Research, 2013, 15(8): 875

Li YY, Tang XL, Jiang T, et al. Bioassay-guided isolation of neoclerodane diterpenoids from *Scutellaria barbata* [J]. Journal of Asian Natural Products Research, 2013, 15(9): 941

Li YY, Xiang Z, Cui H, et al. Two new oleananetype saponins from the husks of *Xanthoceras sorbifolia Bunge* [J]. Natural Product Research, 2013, 27(3): 208

Li YZ, Peng DY, Dai M, et al. A new phenylpropanoid from *Peperomia tetraphylla* [J]. Natural Product Research, 2013, 27(9): 837

Li Z, Chen G, Lu X, et al. Three new steroid

glycosides from the starfish *Asterina pectinifera* [J]. Natural Product Research, 2013, 27(20): 1816

Liang CQ, Hu J, Shi YM, et al. Five new nortriterpenoids from the stems of *Schisandra neglecta* [J]. Helvetica Chimica Acta, 2013, 96(6): 1376

Liang D, Hao ZY, Liu YF, et al. Bioactive carboxylic acids from *Lysimachia clethroides*[J]. Journal of Asian Natural Products Research, 2013, 15(1): 59

Liao L, Zhou X, Liu Y, et al. Four new triterpenoidal saponins from *Ilex cornuta* and their cytotoxic activities[J]. Phytochemistry Letters, 2013, 6(3): 429

Liaw CC, Chen YC, Eid Fazary A, et al. A novel prenylated C_6-C_3 compound with estrogenlike activity from the fruits of *Illicium arborescens* [J]. Phytochemistry Letters, 2013, 6(3): 397

Liaw CC, Chen YC, Huang GJ, et al. Antiinflammatory lanostanoids and lactone derivatives from *Antrodia camphorata* [J]. Journal of Natural Products, 2013, 76(4): 489

Lin CF, Hwang TL, Chien CC, et al. A new hydroxychavicol dimer from the roots of *Piper betle*[J]. Molecules, 2013, 18(3): 2563

Lin S, Zhang ZX, Chen T, et al. Characterization of chlorinated valepotriates from *Valeriana jatamansi* [J]. Phytochemistry, 2013, 85: 185

Lin Y, Wang F, Yang LJ, et al. Anti-inflammatory phenanthrene derivatives from stems of *Dendrobium denneanum*[J]. Phytochemistry, 2013, 95: 242

Lin YC, Cheng YB, Liaw CC, et al. New lignans from the leaves and stems of *Kadsura philippinensis*[J]. Molecules, 2013, 18(6): 6573

Lin YF, Kuo CY, Wen ZH, et al. Flexibilisquinone, a new anti-inflammatory quinone from the cultured soft coral *Sinularia flexibilis* [J]. Molecules, 2013, 18(7): 8160

Liou JR, ElShazly M, Du YC, et al. 1, 5-diphenylpent-3-en-1-ynes and methyl naphthalene carboxylates from *Lawsonia inermis* and their anti-inflammatory activity[J]. Phytochemistry, 2013, 88: 67

Liu C, Guo Z, Deng Z, et al. New furostanol saponins from the rhizomes of *Tupistra chinensis* [J]. Natural Product Research, 2013, 27(2): 123

Liu HX, Chen K, Sun QY, et al. Nudibaccatumone, a trimer comprising a phenylpropanoid and two sesquiterpene moieties from *Piper nudibaccatum* [J]. Journal of Natural Products, 2013, 76(4): 732

Liu HY, Ran XH, Gong NB, et al. Sesquiterpenoids from *Chloranthus multistachys* [J]. Phytochemistry, 2013, 88: 112

Liu JF, Li HJ, Wang LX, et al. Two new monoterpenes from the fruits of *Illicium lanceolatum*[J]. Molecules, 2013, 18(10): 11866

Liu JP, Tian X, Liu HY, et al. Two novel dammaranetype compounds from the leaves and stems of *Panax quinquefolium* L[J]. Journal of Asian Natural Products Research, 2013, 15(9): 974

Liu JQ, Peng XR, Li XY, et al. Norfriedelins A-C with acetylcholinesterase inhibitory activity from acerola tree (*Malpighia emarginata*) [J]. Organic Letters, 2013, 15(7): 1580

Liu JQ, Yang YF, Li XY, et al. Cytotoxicity of naturally occurring rhamnofolane diterpenes from *Jatropha curcas*[J]. Phytochemistry, 2013, 96: 265

Liu JY, Li SY, Feng JY, et al. Flavone C-glycosides from the flowers of *Trollius chinensis* and their anticomplementary activity[J]. Journal of Asian Natural Products Research, 2013, 15(4): 325

Liu Q, Ahn JH, Kim SB, et al. Sesquiterpene lactones from the roots of *Lindera strychnifolia* [J]. Phytochemistry, 2013, 87: 112

Liu QB, Peng Y, Li LZ, et al. Steroidal saponins from *Anemarrhena asphodeloides* [J]. Journal of Asian Natural Products Research, 2013, 15(8): 891

Liu SZ, Chen ZH, Wu J, et al. Appetite suppressing pregnane glycosides from the roots of *Cynanchum auriculatum*[J]. Phytochemistry, 2013, 93: 144

Liu S, Wang H, Zuo W, et al. Two new rocaglamide derivatives from twigs of *Aglaia odorata* var. *microphyllina* [J]. Phytochemistry Letters, 2013, 6(1): 5

Liu SK, Que S, Cheng W, et al. Two new glycosides from *Carduus acanthoides* [J]. Journal of Asian Natural Products Research, 2013, 15(11): 1243

Liu T, Osman K, Kaatz G, et al. Antibacterial sesquiterpenoid derivatives from *Ferula ferulaeoides*[J]. Planta Medica, 2013, 79(8): 701

Liu W, Fan BL, Guo HY, et al. Isolation and identification of a new entkaurane diterpenoid from the leaves of *Isodon japonica*[J]. Natural Product Research, 2013, 27(15): 1388

Liu WB, Hu L, Hu Q, et al. New resveratrol oligomer derivatives from the roots of *Rheum lhasaense* [J]. Molecules, 2013, 18(6): 7093

Liu XG, Zhang WC, Gao PY, et al. Two new sesquiterpenes from the roots of *Valeriana fauriei* [J].

Helvetica Chimica Acta, 2013, 96(4): 651

Liu Y, Hu Z, Lin X, et al. A new polyketide from *Diaporthe* sp. SXZ19, an endophytic fungal strain of *Camptotheca acuminate* [J]. Natural Product Research, 2013, 27(22): 2100

Liu Y, Li C, Shi JG, et al. Two new sesquiterpenes from *Euonymus alatus* [J]. Helvetica Chimica Acta, 2013, 92(2): 335

Liu Y, Wu Z, Li C, et al. Heracleifolinosides A-F, new triterpene glycosides from *Cimicifuga heracleifolia*, and their inhibitory activities against hypoxia and reoxygenation[J]. Planta Medica, 2013, 79(34): 301

Liu YM, Jiang YH, Liu QH, et al. Indazoletype alkaloids from the seeds of *Nigella glandulifera* [J]. Phytochemistry Letters, 2013, 6(4): 556

Long C, Aussagues Y, Molinier N, et al. Dichapetalins from *Dichapetalum* species and their cytotoxic properties[J]. Phytochemistry, 2013, 94: 184

Lu J, Sun JH, Tan Y, et al. New triterpenoid saponins from the flowers of *Pueraria thomsonii* [J]. Journal of Asian Natural Products Research, 2013, 15(10): 1065

Luo J, Li Y, Wang JS, et al. Two new C_{15} enolic acyl phragmalintype limonoids from *Chukrasia tabularis* var. velutina [J]. Natural Product Research, 2013, 27(7): 597

Luo Q, Wang SM, Lu Q, et al. Identification of compounds from the water soluble extract of *Cinnamomum cassia* barks and their inhibitory effects against high-glucose-induced mesangial cells [J]. Molecules, 2013, 18(9): 10930

Luo SH, Hua J, Niu XM, et al. Defense sesterterpenoid lactones from *Leucosceptrum canum* [J]. Phytochemistry, 2013, 86: 29

Lv JJ, Xu M, Wang D, et al. Cytotoxic bisbenzylisoquinoline alkaloids from *Stephania epigaea* [J]. Journal of Natural Products, 2013, 76(5): 926

雷林洁,滕亮,赵欣,等.多伞阿魏挥发油提取工艺及化学成分研究[J].中成药,2013,35(6): 1251

李兵,贾年飞,朱小勇,等.二氧化碳超临界萃取法萃取两种不同寄主桑寄生挥发油成分研究[J].时珍国医国药,2013,24(4): 837

李佳,刘红燕,张永清.顶空固相微萃取-气质色谱联用技术分析海州香薷与石香薷中挥发性成分[J].中国实验方剂学杂志,2013,19(16): 118

李金凤,施勃,杜瑞娟,等.不同方法提取核桃楸皮挥发油的气质联用分析[J].中国实验方剂学杂志,2013,19(9): 62

李静晶,王军民,华燕.大纽子花挥发油的化学成分研究[J].中国民族民间医药,2013,22(5): 40

李丽明,任斌,郭洁文,等.不同规格三七挥发性成分研究[J].中药材,2013,36(6): 934

李雪飞,白根本,王如峰,等.京大戟挥发油化学成分分析[J].中药材,2013,36(2): 237

李滢,陶海燕,杨秀伟.生白术和炒白术挥发油成分的GC-MS分析[J].药物分析杂志,2013,33(7): 1210

李芸,苗小楼,吴平安,等.GC-MS分析当归熏硫前后挥发油的化学成分[J].中药材,2013,36(3): 367

李植飞,唐祖年,戴支凯.土荆芥果实挥发油GC-MS分析及其生物活性研究[J].中国实验方剂学杂志,2013,19(5): 265

梁娜,杨胜杰,赵洪菊,等.裂叶牵牛地上部分挥发油化学成分与生物活性研究[J].中成药,2013,35(5): 1023

廖彭莹,卢汝梅,邵敏敏,等.水蒸气蒸馏法和二氧化碳超临界流体萃取法提取柚寄生的挥发性成分[J].时珍国医国药,2013,24(5): 1274

刘慧,热增才旦,刘斌,等.采用GC-MS法分析秀丽莓根精油成分[J].北京中医药大学学报,2013,36(2): 121

刘玲玲,王强,唐军,等.顶空固相微萃取气质联用法分析阿育魏实挥发性成分[J].药物分析杂志,2013,33(4): 607

刘轩,张彬锋,杨莉,等.白茅根中两个新的色原酮和一个新的黄酮苷(英文)[J].中国天然药物,2013,11(1): 77

卢金清,李婷,郭彧,等.SD-HS-SPME-GC-MS分析华中碎米荠挥发性成分[J].中国实验方剂学杂志,2013,19(1): 148

罗兰,邓金梅,廖华卫.GC-MS分析毛大丁草挥发油成分[J].中药材,2013,36(6): 944

M

Ma F, Onoda T, Li W, et al. A new flavonoid glycoside and other chemical constituents from leaves of *Rosa davurica* and their antioxidant activity[J]. Natural Product Research, 2013, 27(23): 2178

Ma QY, Luo Y, Huang SZ, et al. Lanostane triterpenoids with cytotoxic activities from the fruiting bodies of *Ganoderma hainanense* [J]. Journal of Asian Natural Products Research, 2013, 15(11): 1214

Ma SG, Gao RM, Li YH, et al. Antiviral spirooliganones A and B with unprecedented skeletons from the roots of *Illicium oligandrum* [J]. Organic Letters, 2013, 15(17): 4450

Ma SS, Mei WL, Guo ZK, et al. Two new types of bisindole alkaloid from *Trigonostemon lutescens* [J].

Organic Letters, 2013, 15(7): 1492

Ma W, Lu Y, Chen D. Dibenzocyclooctane lignans from the stems of *Schisandra wilsoniana* [J]. Planta Medica, 2013, 79(12): 1051

Ma XQ, Zheng CJ, Zhang Y, et al. Antiosteoporotic flavonoids from *Podocarpium podocarpum* [J]. Phytochemistry Letters, 2013, 6(1): 118

Ma YY, Zhao DG, Gao K. Structural investigation and biological activity of sesquiterpene lactones from the traditional Chinese herb *Inula racemosa* [J]. Journal of Natural Products, 2013, 76(4): 564

Ma YY, Zhao DG, Zhai Y, et al. Trinorsesquiterpenoids from *Inula racemosa* [J]. Phytochemistry Letters, 2013, 6(4): 645

Ma ZQ, Zhang Y, Cai CK, et al. Two new triterpenoid saponins from the leaves of *Aralia elata* [J]. Journal of Asian Natural Products Research, 2013, 15(8): 849

Meng H, Li G, Huang J, et al. Sesquiterpenoid derivatives from *Ferula ferulaeoides* (Steud.) Korov[J]. Phytochemistry, 2013, 86: 151

Mu LH, Feng JQ, Liu P. A new bergenin derivative from the rhizome of *Ardisia gigantifolia* [J]. Natural Product Research, 2013, 27(14): 1242

Mu LH, Huang XW, Guo DH, et al. A new triterpenoid saponin from *Ardisia gigantifolia* [J]. Journal of Asian Natural Products Research, 2013, 15(10): 1123

马雯芳,朱意麟,贾智若,等. 小花山小橘叶、茎挥发油 GC - MS 分析[J]. 中国实验方剂学杂志,2013, 19(1): 95

N

Nian Y, Wang H, Zhou L, et al. Cytotoxic cycloartane triterpenes of the traditional Chinese medicine "Shengma" (*Cimicifuga dahurica*) [J]. Planta Medica, 2013, 79(1): 60

Niu KY, Wang LY, Liu SZ, et al. New iridoid glycoside and triterpenoid glycoside from *Premna fulva* [J]. Journal of Asian Natural Products Research, 2013, 15(1): 1

P

Pan K, Luo JG, Kong LY. Three new Lycopodium alkaloids from *Lycopodium obscurum* [J]. Journal of Asian Natural Products Research, 2013, 15(5): 441

Pan L, Acun a UM, Li J, et al. Bioactive flavaglines and other constituents isolated from *Aglaia perviridis* [J]. Journal of Natural Products, 2013, 76(3): 394

Pang X, Kang LP, Yu HS, et al. New kaurene diterpenoid glycosides from fenugreek seeds[J]. Natural Product Research, 2013, 27(13): 1202

Peng F, Xiong L, Zhao X M. A bicyclic diterpenoid with a new 15, 16 - dinorlabdane carbon skeleton from *Leonurus japonicus* and its coagulant bioactivity [J]. Molecules, 2013, 18(11): 13904

Peng WW, Zheng YQ, Chen YS, et al. Coumarins from roots of *Clausena excavata* [J]. Journal of Asian Natural Products Research, 2013, 15(3): 215

Q

Qin Y, Yin C, Cheng Z. A new tetrahydrofuran lignan diglycoside from *Viola tianshanica* Maxim [J]. Molecules, 2013, 18(11): 13636

Qiu L, Jiao Y, Xie JZ, et al. Five new flavonoid glycosides from *Nervilia fordii* [J]. Journal of Asian Natural Products Research, 2013, 15(6): 589

Qiu L, Liang Y, Tang GH, et al. Two new flavonols, including one flavan dimer, from the roots of *Indigofera stachyodes* [J]. Phytochemistry Letters, 2013, 6(3): 368

丘琴,甄汉深,黄培倩. 匙羹藤花挥发性成分分析[J]. 中药材,2013,36(4): 575

R

Ren J, Lin Z, Yuan Z. Tangshenosides from *Codonopsis lanceolata* roots[J]. Phytochemistry Letters, 2013, 6(4): 567

S

Shan F, Yin YQ, Huang F, et al. A novel acridone akaloid from *Atalantia buxifolia* [J]. Natural Product Research, 2013, 27(21): 1956

Shang Y, Oidovsambuu S, Jeon J, et al. Chalcones from the flowers of *Coreopsis lanceolata* and their in vitro antioxidative activity [J]. Planta Medica, 2013, 79(34): 295

Shen S, Shen L, Zhang J, et al. Emiline, a new alkaloid from the aerial parts of *Emilia sonchifolia* [J]. Phytochemistry Letters, 2013, 6(3): 467

Shi YM, Wang XB, Li XN, et al. Lancolides, antiplatelet aggregation nortriterpenoids with tricyclo [6.3.0.0 (2, 11)] undecane-bridged system from *Schisandra lancifolia* [J]. Organic Letters, 2013, 15(19): 5068

Shu JC, Liu JQ, Chou GX. A new triterpenoid from

Verbena officinalis L[J]. Natural Product Research, 2013, 27(14): 1293

Shu W, Wu C, Zhang Y, et al. Two new steroidal glycosides isolated from the aerial part of *Solanum torvum* Swartz[J]. Natural Product Research, 2013, 27(21): 1982

Shu Z, Chen Z, Liu YL, et al. A new oleananetype triterpenoidal saponin from *Pulsatilla chinensis* [J]. Natural Product Research, 2013, 27(23): 2196

Song P, Yang XZ, Yuan JQ. Cytotoxic constituents from *Psoralea corylifolia*[J]. Journal of Asian Natural Products Research, 2013, 15(6): 624

Song YL, Zhou GS, Zhou SX, et al. Polygalins DG, four new flavonol glycosides from the aerial parts of *Polygala sibirica* L. (Polygalaceae)[J]. Natural Product Research, 2013, 27(13): 1220

Su S, Shen L, Zhang Y, et al. Characterization of tautomeric limonoids from the fruits of *Melia toosendan* [J]. Phytochemistry Letters, 2013, 6(3): 418

Su X, Yuan Z, Liang B, et al. Phenanthrenes from *Juncus effusus*[J]. Planta Medica, 2013, 79(15): 1447

Su Y, Xu JJ, Bi JL, et al. Chemical constituents of *Arisaema franchetianum* tubers[J]. Journal of Asian Natural Products Research, 2013, 15(1): 71

Su Z, Hao J, Xu Z, et al. A new quassinoid from fruits of *Brucea javanica*[J]. Natural Product Research, 2013, 27(21): 2016

Su Z, Wang P, Yuan W, et al. Flavonoids and 3-arylcoumarin from *Pterocarpus soyauxii* [J]. Planta Medica, 2013, 79(6): 487

Sun LL, Shao CL, Hang H, et al. New polyhydroxylated steroid from the South China Sea gorgonian *Anthogorgia caerulea* [J]. Natural Product Research, 2013, 27(13): 1159

Sun M, Hou X, Gao H, et al. Two new koumine-type indole alkaloids from *Gelsemium elegans* Benth[J]. Molecules, 2013, 18(2): 1819

Sun QH, Yang JJ, Wei XH, et al. Two new pyrrolizidine alkaloids from *Crotalaria albida* [J]. Phytochemistry Letters, 2013, 6(3): 449

Sun ZC, Ma GX, Yuan JQ, et al. Two new diterpenes from *Caesalpinia minax* Hance[J]. Natural Product Research, 2013, 27(9): 818

尚庆文,马丽. 北美枫香挥发油化学成分的研究[J]. 内蒙古中医药,2013,32(26): 30

邵江娟,吴昊,赵雅秋,等. 离子液体萃取技术及其在中药领域中的应用[J]. 中草药,2013,44(24): 3561

宋煌旺,宋鑫明,韩长日,等. 喙果皂帽花挥发油 GC-MS分析及活性研究[J]. 中国实验方剂学杂志,2013,19(16): 132

T

Tang J, Yu L, Zhang D, et al. Cytotoxic triterpenoid saponins from the stems of *Gordonia longicarpa*[J]. Planta Medica, 2013, 79(5): 353

Tao WW, Duan JA, Tang YP, et al. Casbane diterpenoids from the roots of *Euphorbia pekinensis*[J]. Phytochemistry, 2013, 94: 249

Thang TD, Kuo PC, Huang GJ, et al. Chemical constituents from the leaves of *Annona reticulata* and their inhibitory effects on NO production[J]. Molecules, 2013, 18(4): 4477

Tian J, Ma Q, Su Y, et al. Hepatoprotective phenolic glycosides from *Gymnema tingens* [J]. Planta Medica, 2013, 79(9): 761

Tian QJ, Ou YH, He XB, et al. One new antitumour cassanetype diterpene from *Caesalpinia crista* [J]. Natural Product Research, 2013, 27(6): 537

Tian X, Ding G, Peng C, et al. Sinapyl alcohol derivatives from the lipo-soluble part of *Dichrocephala benthamii* C. B. Clarke[J]. Molecules, 2013, 18(2): 1720

田效民,李凤,黄顺菊,等. 柳叶白前挥发性成分的GC-MS分析[J]. 中国实验方剂学杂志,2013,19(5): 111

W

Wang F, Jiang YP, Wang XL, et al. Aromatic glycosides from the flower buds of *Lonicera japonica*[J]. Journal of Asian Natural Products Research, 2013, 15(5): 492

Wang F, Mao MF, Wei GZ, et al. Hybridaphniphyllines A and B, Daphniphyllum alkaloid and iridoid hybrids suggestive of DielsAlder cycloaddition in *Daphniphyllum longeracemosum*[J]. Phytochemistry, 2013, 95: 428

Wang FX, Deng AJ, Li M, et al. (3S)-1, 2, 3, 4-Tetrahydro-β-carboline-3-carboxylic acid from *Cichorium endivia*. L induces apoptosis of human colorectal cancer HCT-8 cells[J]. Molecules, 2012, 18(1): 418

Wang GC, Li GQ, Geng HW, et al. Eudesmanetype sesquiterpene derivatives from *Laggera alata* [J]. Phytochemistry, 2013, 96: 201

Wang GC, Li W, Wang Y, et al. A new amide and a new monoterpene from the seeds of *Clausena lansium*[J]. Natural Product Research, 2013, 27(6): 558

Wang GC, Zhang H, Liu HB, et al. Laevinoids A and B: two diterpenoids with an unprecedented backbone from *Croton laevigatus* [J]. Organic Letters, 2013, 15(18): 4880

Wang GK, Lin BB, Rao R, et al. A new lignan with anti-HBV activity from the roots of *Bombax ceiba* [J]. Natural Product Research, 2013, 27(15): 1348

Wang H, Li M, Satyanandamurty T, et al. New diterpenes from a Godavari mangrove, *Ceriops decandra* [J]. Planta Medica, 2013, 79(8): 666

Wang H, Wang J, Kong L, et al. Chemical constituents from *Trichilia connaroides* and their nitric oxide production and αglucosidase inhibitory activities[J]. Planta Medica, 2013, 79(18): 1767

Wang HP, Yang XB, Yang XW, et al. Ginsenjilinol, a new protopanaxatriol-type saponin with inhibitory activity on LPS - activated NO production in macrophage RAW 264.7 cells from the roots and rhizomes of *Panax ginseng*[J]. Journal of Asian Natural Products Research, 2013, 15(5): 579

Wang KW, Zhu JR, Shen LQ. A new lignan with antitumour activity from *Polygonum perfoliatum* L[J]. Natural Product Research, 2013, 27(6): 568

Wang L, Wang J, Wang M, et al. Cytotoxic sesquiterpene lactones from aerial parts of *Xanthium sibiricum*[J]. Planta Medica, 2013, 79(8): 661

Wang LQ, Tang ZR, Mu WH, et al. A new natural naphtho[1, 2b]furan from the leaves of *Cassia fistula* [J]. Journal of Asian Natural Products Research, 2013, 15(11): 1210

Wang PC, Ran XH, Luo HR, et al. Volvalerenol A, a new triterpenoid with a 12 - membered ring from *Valeriana hardwickii* [J]. Organic Letters, 2013, 15(12): 2898

Wang Q, Chen TH, Bastow KF, et al. Songaricalarins A-E, cytotoxic oplopane sesquiterpenes from *Ligularia songarica* [J]. Journal of Natural Products, 2013, 76(3): 305

Wang Q, Hou Q, Guo Z, et al. Three new steroidal glycosides from roots of *Reineckia carnea* [J]. Natural Product Research, 2013, 27(2): 85

Wang R, Li JY, Qi HY, et al. Two new tigliane diterpene esters from the flower buds of *Daphne genkwa* [J]. Journal of Asian Natural Products Research, 2013, 15(5): 502

Wang S, Xu Y, Jiang W, et al. Isolation and identification of constituents with activity of inhibiting nitric oxide production in raw 264.7 macrophages from *Gentiana triflora*[J]. Planta Medica, 2013, 79(8): 680

Wang SL, Chen Z, Tong XJ, et al. Triterpenoids from the roots of *Camellia oleifera* C. Abel and their cytotoxic activities[J]. Helvetica Chimica Acta, 2013, 96(6): 1133

Wang SQ, Zhu XF, Wang XN, et al. Flavonoids from *Malus hupehensis* and their cardioprotective effects against doxorubicin-induced toxicity in H9c2 cells[J]. Phytochemistry, 2013, 87: 119

Wang W, Cheng M H, Wang X H. Monoterpenoid indole alkaloids from *Alstonia rupestris* with cytotoxic, anti-inflammatory and antifungal activities[J]. Molecules, 2013, 18(6): 7309

Wang WX, Xiong J, Tang Y, et al. Rearranged abietane diterpenoids from the roots of *Clerodendrum trichotomum* and their cytotoxicities against human tumor cells[J]. Phytochemistry, 2013, 89: 89

Wang X, Qu W, Liang J. New longchain aliphatic compounds from *Peperomia dindygulensis* [J]. Natural Product Research, 2013, 27(9): 796

Wang X, Wang W. Cytotoxic and radical scavenging nordammarane triterpenoids from *Viburnum mongolicum* [J]. Molecules, 2013, 18(2): 1405

Wang Y, Guan SH, Meng YH, et al. Phenanthrenes, 9, 10 - dihydrophenanthrenes, bibenzyls with their derivatives, and malate or tartrate benzyl ester glucosides from tubers of *Cremastra appendiculata* [J]. Phytochemistry, 2013, 94: 268

Wang YC, Zhang YW, Zheng LH, et al. A new compound from liquid fermentation broth of *Armillaria mellea* and the determination of its absolute configuration [J]. Journal of Asian Natural Products Research, 2013, 15(2): 203

Wang YS, Huang R, Li Y, et al. Panamonon A and B, a pair of novel tetrahydrobenzofuran derivatives from *Litsea panamonja* (Nees) Hook. f[J]. Phytochemistry Letters, 2013, 6(1): 26

Wang Z, Li B, Yu S, et al. Eight new monoterpene acylglucosides from *Sibiraea angustata* [J]. Phytochemistry letters, 2013, 6(3): 461

Wei LB, Yuan HE, Chen JM, et al. Five new cycloartane-type triterpenoid saponins from *Nervilia fordii*[J]. Helvetica Chimica Acta, 2013, 96(1): 150

Weng JR, Yen MH, Lin WY. Cytotoxic constituents from *Celastrus paniculatus* induce apoptosis and autophagy in breast cancer cells[J]. Phytochemistry, 2013, 94: 211

Wu C, Duan Y, Li Y, et al. Triterpenoid saponins

from the stem barks of *Schefflera heptaphylla* [J]. Planta Medica, 2013, 79(14): 1348

Wu C, Wei CS, Yu SF, et al. Two new acetylated flavonoid glycosides from *Phyllanthus urinaria* [J]. Journal of Asian Natural Products Research, 2013, 15(7): 703

Wu H, Li J, Fronczek FR, et al. Labdane diterpenoids from *Leonotis leonurus*[J]. Phytochemistry, 2013, 91: 229

Wu QB, Wang Y, Liang L, et al. Novel triterpenoid saponins from the seeds of *Celosia argentea* L [J]. Natural Product Research, 2013, 27(15): 1353

Wu X, He J, Zhao Q, et al. Triterpenoids and steroids with cytotoxic activity from Emmenopterys henry [J]. Planta Medica, 2013, 79(14): 1356

Wu XD, Wang L, He J, et al. Two new indole alkaloids from *Emmenopterys henryi* [J]. Helvetica Chimica Acta, 2013, 96(12): 2207

Wu XD, Zhang LC, He J, et al. Two new diterpenoids from *Excoecaria acerifolia* [J]. Journal of Asian Natural Products Research, 2013, 15(2): 151

Wu Y, Zheng CJ, Deng XH, et al. Two new bisalkaloids from the aerial part of *Piper flaviflorum* [J]. Helvetica Chimica Acta, 2013, 96(5): 951

Wu YP, Zhao W, Xia ZY, et al. Three new xanthones from the stems of *Garcinia oligantha* and their anti - TMV activity[J]. Phytochemistry Letters, 2013, 6(4): 629

Wu YP, Zhao W, Xia ZY, et al. Three novel xanthones from *Garcinia paucinervis* and their anti - TMV activity[J]. Molecules, 2013, 18(8): 9663

Wu Z, Shen Y, Zhang W. Two new phenolic glycosides from *Inula cappa* DC[J]. Natural Product Research, 2013, 27(8): 719

王道平,危莉,彭小冰,等. 顶空固相微萃取-气质联用法分析新鲜假蒟挥发性化学成分[J]. 中国实验方剂学杂志,2013,19(10): 142

王冬梅,黄林芳. 大叶钩藤叶挥发油成分气相色谱-质谱联用分析[J]. 药物分析杂志,2013,33(2): 234

王芳,蒋跃平,王晓良,等. 金银花的化学成分研究[J]. 中国中药杂志,2013,38(9): 1378

王芳林,罗建光,王小兵,等. 山柰根茎中一对磺酸化的双苯庚烷差向异构体(英文)[J]. 中国天然药物,2013,11(2): 171

王坚,韦正,陈鸿平,等. 源于同一植株陈皮挥发油成分动态变化规律研究[J]. 中国实验方剂学杂志,2013,19(3): 73

王强,施玉格,徐芳,等. 比较研究新疆狭叶薰衣草不同部位挥发油成分[J]. 药物分析杂志,2013,33(3): 404

王小明,蒋海强,吕青涛,等. 顶空静态进样 GC - MS 分析委陵菜中挥发性成分[J]. 广东药学院学报,2013,29(2): 147

王欣之,吴斐华,曲玮,等. 加纳籽中的一个新β-咔啉型生物碱(英文)[J]. 中国天然药物,2013,11(4): 401

王秀琴,王岩,李军,等. GC - MS 分析天仙子及其炮制品中挥发油成分[J]. 中华中医药学刊,2013,31(5): 1044

王燕,陈文豪,陈光英,等. 鹰爪花挥发油 GC - MS 分析及抗肿瘤活性研究[J]. 中国实验方剂学杂志,2013,19(17): 100

王玉林,朱丹晖,冯晓亮,等. GC - MS 和平滑预处理及 SFA 法用于茵陈挥发性成分的分析[J]. 药物分析杂志,2013,33(1): 98

文庆发,钟玉蛟,苏雪会,等. 石吊兰全草中的一个新菖蒲烷类倍半萜(英文)[J]. 中国天然药物,2013,11(2): 185

吴爽,魏凤香,李红枝,等. 柠檬百里香叶挥发油成分分析及对肝癌细胞毒性作用[J]. 中药材,2013,36(5): 756

X

Xi Z, Bie W, Chen W, et al. Sarcophytolides G-L, new biscembranoids from the soft coral *Sarcophyton elegans*[J]. Helvetica Chimica Acta, 2013, 96(12): 2218

Xiang JG, Shan WG, Liang DE, et al. N - bearing furanone derivatives from an endophytic fungus in *Huperzia serrata* [J]. Helvetica Chimica Acta, 2013, 96(5): 997

Xiang WJ, Wang QQ, Ma L, et al. β - orcinol-type depsides from the lichen *Thamnolia vermicularis* [J]. Natural Product Research, 2013, 27(9): 804

Xiang Z, Lv J, Zhou Z, et al. Two new dammarane-type saponins from leaves of *Panax quinquefolium* [J]. Natural product research, 2013, 27(14): 1271

Xiang ZB, Wang GL, Huang LZ, et al. A new entkaurane diterpenoid glycoside from *Isodon japonica* var. glaucocalyx[J]. Journal of Asian Natural Products Research, 2013, 15(5): 574

Xie B, Chen C, Liu H, et al. New 23 - spirocholestane derivatives from *Ypsilandra thibetica*[J]. Planta Medica, 2013, 79(12): 1063

Xie GY, Qin XY, Liu R, et al. New isoflavones with cytotoxic activity from the rhizomes of *Iris germanica* L. [J]. Natural Product Research, 2013, 27(23): 2173

Xie HH, Yoshikawa M. Further acylated flavonol

bisdesmosides from *Sinocrassula indica* [J]. Journal of Asian Natural Products Research, 2013, 15(8): 885

Xie SA, Li GY, Huang J, et al. A new flavanol from *Cynomorium songaricum* [J]. Journal of Asian Natural Products Research, 2013, 15(4): 413

Xiong H, Mei Z, Yang G, et al. Triterpene saponins from *Entada phaseoloides* [J]. Helvetica Chimica Acta, 2013, 96(8): 1579

Xiong L, Cao ZX, Peng C, et al. Phenolic glucosides from *Dendrobium aurantiacum* var. *denneanum* and their bioactivities[J]. Molecules, 2013, 18(6): 6153

Xiong L, Zhou Q M, Peng C, et al. Sesquiterpenoids from the herb of *Leonurus japonicus* [J]. Molecules, 2013, 18(5): 5051

Xiong Y, Qu W, Sun J, et al. Eudesmane sesquiterpenoid lactones and abietane diterpenoids from *Ajuga forrestii* Diels[J]. Phytochemistry Letters, 2013, 6(3): 457

Xu JJ, Zhao DK, Ai HL, et al. Three new C_{19}-diterpenoid alkaloids from *Aconitum forrestii* [J]. Helvetica Chimica Acta, 2013, 96(11): 2155

Xu JJ, Zhao HM, Shen Y, et al. Three unusual sesquineolignans from *Alpinia conchigera* [J]. Journal of Asian Natural Products Research, 2013, 15(8): 833

Xu L, Luo M, Lin LM, et al. Three new phenolic glycosides from the Tibetan medicinal plant *Aconitum tanguticum* [J]. Journal of Asian Natural Products Research, 2013, 15(7): 743

Xu L, Zhang X, Lin LM, et al. Two new flavonol glycosides from the Tibetan medicinal plant *Aconitum tanguticum* [J]. Journal of Asian Natural Products Research, 2013, 15(7): 737

Xu Q, Shu Z, Zhu W, et al. Lupanetype triterpenoidal saponins from *Pulsatilla chinensis* and their anticomplement activities through the classical pathway [J]. Planta Medica, 2013, 79(6): 506

Xu Q, Xie H, Xiao H, et al. Two new entkaurene diterpene glucosides from the roots of *Mikania micrantha* [J]. Phytochemistry Letters, 2013, 6(3): 425

Xu S, Shang MY, Liu GX, et al. Chemical constituents from the rhizomes of *Smilax glabra* and their antimicrobial activity[J]. Molecules, 2013, 18(5): 5265

Xue R, Han N, Sakurai H, et al. Cytotoxic cardiac glycosides from the roots of *Streptocaulon juventas* [J]. Planta Medica, 2013, 79(2): 157

解修超,陈文强,邓百万,等. 三尖杉种仁挥发油的化学成分及生物活性研究[J]. 中国实验方剂学杂志,2013, 19(10): 76

邢珍珍,卢亚玲,孟庆艳,等. 不同方法分析新疆藁本地下部分中的挥发性成分[J]. 药物分析杂志,2013, 33(6): 1076

徐龙泉,彭黔荣,杨敏,等. 膜分离技术在中药生产及研究中的应用进展[J]. 中成药,2013,35(9): 1989

许可,朱冬青,王贤亲,等. 气质联用法分析香茶菜不同部位挥发油的化学成分[J]. 中华中医药学刊,2013, 31(8): 1797

Y

Yan H, Li XH., Zheng XF, et al. Chlojaponilactones B-E, four new lindenane sesquiterpenoid lactones from *Chloranthus japonicus* [J]. Helvetica Chimica Acta, 2013, 96(6): 1386

Yan YM, Ai J, Zhou LL, et al. Lingzhiols, unprecedented rotary door-shaped meroterpenoids as potent and selective inhibitors of p-smad3 from *Ganoderma lucidum* [J]. Organic letters, 2013, 15(21): 5488

Yan YM, Hu M, Yang M, et al. Terpenoids from *Incarvillea arguta* [J]. Journal of Asian Natural Products Research, 2013, 15(1): 9

Yang B, Cheng RB, Wang YQ, et al. Two new cytotoxic iridoid esters from the rhizomes and roots of *Patrinia heterophylla* Bunge [J]. Natural Product Research, 2013, 27(22): 2105

Yang B, Tao H, Zhou X, et al. Two new alkaloids from marine sponge *Callyspongia* sp[J]. Natural Product Research, 2013, 27(45): 433

Yang CH, Yang Y, Liu JH. Platachromone A-D: Cytotoxic 2-styrylchromones from the bark of *Platanus* ×*acerifolia* (Aiton) Willd[J]. Phytochemistry Letters, 2013, 6(3): 387

Yang CJ, Wang ZB, Song PY, et al. Monoterpenoids from *Acanthopanax sessiliflorus* Fruits [J]. Molecules, 2013, 18(3): 3043

Yang D, Mei W, Dai H, et al. 2-(2-phenylethyl) chromone derivatives in Chinese agarwood "Qi-Nan" from *Aquilaria sinensis* [J]. Planta Medica, 2013, 79(14): 1329

Yang DL, Mei WL, Zeng YB, et al. A new antibacterial denitroaristolochic acid from the tubers of *Stephania succifera* [J]. Journal of Asian Natural Products Research, 2013, 15(3): 315

Yang GY, Wang RR, Mu HX, et al. Dibenzocyclooctadiene lignans and norlignans from fruits of *Schisandra wilsoniana* [J]. Journal of Natural Products, 2013, 76(2): 250

Yang H, Kim HS, Jeong EJ, et al. Plant-derived juvenile hormone III analogues and other sesquiterpenes from the stem bark of *Cananga latifolia* [J]. Phytochemistry, 2013, 94: 277

Yang H, Lee S, Sung S, et al. Neuroprotective compounds from *Salix pseudolasiogyne* twigs and their antiamnesic effects on scopolamineinduced memory deficit in mice[J]. Planta Medica, 2013, 79(1): 78

Yang Kuo LM, Zhang LJ, Huang HT, et al. Antioxidant lignans and chromone glycosides from *Eurya japonica*[J]. Journal of Natural Products, 2013, 76(4): 580

Yang L, Qiao L, Ji C, et al. Antidepressant abietane diterpenoids from Chinese eaglewood [J]. Journal of Natural Products, 2013, 76(2): 216

Yang LJ, Jiang K, Tan JJ, et al. Prenylated Benzene Metabolites from *Melicope pteleifolia* [J]. Helvetica Chimica Acta, 2013, 96(1): 119

Yang S, Sun Q, Long C, et al. Sarmentosumols A to F, new monoand dimeric alkenylphenols from *Piper sarmentosum*[J]. Planta Medica, 2013, 79(8): 693

Yang S, Wang L, Guo X, et al. A new flavonoid glycoside and other constituents from *Dracocephalum moldavica*[J]. Natural Product Research, 2013, 27(3): 201

Yang XB, Qian P, Yang XW, et al. Limonoid constituents of *Evodia rutaecarpa* var. bodinieri and their inhibition on NO production in lipopolysaccharide-activated RAW264.7 macrophages[J]. Journal of Asian Natural Products Research, 2013, 15(10): 1130

Yang YY, Yang W, Zuo WJ, et al. Two new acridone alkaloids from the branch of *Atalantia buxifolia* and their biological activity[J]. Journal of Asian Natural Products Research, 2013, 15(8): 899

Yao CS, Huang KS, Lin M, et al. A new stilbene dimer from *Vitis amurensis*[J]. Journal of Asian Natural Products Research, 2013, 15(6): 693

Yao F, Song QL, Zhang L, et al. Three new cytotoxic sesquiterpenoids from *Solanum lyratum* [J]. Phytochemistry Letters, 2013, 6(3): 453

Yen WH, Chen WF, Cheng CH, et al. A new 5α, 8α-epidioxysterol from the soft coral *Sinularia gaweli* [J]. Molecules, 2013, 18(3): 2895

Yin GP, An YW, Hu G, et al. Three new guaiane sesquiterpene lactones from rhizomes of *Curcuma wenyujin* [J]. Journal of Asian Natural Products Research, 2013, 15(7). 723

Yin H, Luo JG, Kong LY. Diarylheptanoids from the fruits of *Amomum kravanh* and their inhibitory activities of nitric oxide production[J]. Phytochemistry Letters, 2013, 6(3): 403

Yin H, Luo JG, Kong LY. Tetracyclic diterpenoids with isomerized isospongian skeleton and labdane diterpenoids from the fruits of *Amomum kravanh* [J]. Journal of Natural Products, 2013, 76(2): 237

Yin H, Luo JG, Shan SM, et al. Amomaxins A and B, two unprecedented rearranged labdane norditerpenoids with a nine-membered ring from *Amomum maximum*[J]. Organic Letters, 2013, 15(7): 1572

Ying YM, Shan WG, Zhang LW, et al. Ceriponols AK, tremulane sesquitepenes from ceriporia lacerate HSZJUTC13A, a fungal endophyte of *Huperzia serrata* [J]. Phytochemistry, 2013, 95: 360

Ying YM, Shan WG, Zhang LW, et al. Lanostane triterpenes from ceriporia lacerate HS - ZJUT - C13A, a fungal endophyte of *Huperzia serrata* [J]. Helvetica Chimica Acta, 2013, 96(11): 2092

Yu B, Luo J, Wang J, et al. Pentasaccharide resin glycosides from *Ipomoea cairica* and their cytotoxic activities[J]. Phytochemistry, 2013, 95: 421

Yu CY, Sun YC, Chen G. A new phenylethanoid glucoside from *Plantago depressa* Willd [J]. Natural Product Research, 2013, 27(7): 609

Yu L, Zuo W, Mei W, et al. Three new terpenoids from *Trigonostemon xyphophylloides* (Croiz.) LK Dai and TL Wu[J]. Phytochemistry Letters, 2013, 6(3): 472

Yuan C, Zhang Y, Hao X, et al. Cytotoxic limonoids from *Melia azedarach* [J]. Planta Medica, 2013, 79(2): 163

Yuan CM, Zhang Y, Tang GH, et al. Khayseneganins AH, limonoids from *Khaya senegalensis* [J]. Journal of Natural Products, 2013, 76(3): 327

Yuan T, Wan C, Ma H, et al. New phenolics from the flowers of *Punica granatum* and their in vitro α-glucosidase inhibitory activities[J]. Planta Medica, 2013, 79(17): 1674

Yuan W, Wang P, Su Z, et al. Cytotoxic triterpenoid saponins from husks of *Aesculus californica* (Spach) Nutt[J]. Phytochemistry, 2013, 90: 95

Yuan X, Cheng M, Gao M, et al. Cytotoxic constituents from the leaves of Jerusalem artichoke (*Helianthus tuberosus* L.) and their structure-activity relationships [J]. Phytochemistry Letters, 2013, 6(1): 21

Yue Y, Deng AJ, Xu DS, et al. Two new stemona

alkaloids from *Stemona tuberosa* Lour[J]. Journal of Asian Natural Products Research, 2013, 15(2): 145

杨柳,刘守金,胡江苗,等. GC-MS法检测铁皮石斛茎中挥发性成分[J]. 中国现代中药,2013,15(5): 362

杨胜杰,刘明川,梁娜,等. 黔产射干挥发油化学成分的GC-MS分析[J]. 中国实验方剂学杂志,2013,19(7): 136

杨欣,金晓飞,李红,等. 不同种类竹沥化学成分的GC-MS比较分析[J]. 江西中医学院学报,2013,25(2): 53

杨烨,王祥培,徐锋,等. 苦楝皮不同部位挥发油化学成分分析[J]. 中国实验方剂学杂志,2013,19(14): 84

杨昭武,李敏,苟寒阳,等. GC/MS内标法建立黄丝郁金挥发油特征图谱研究[J]. 时珍国医国药,2013,24(7): 1652

衣丽娜,李克琴,王秋娟,等. 利用分子印迹技术从中药粗提物中定向分离胡黄连苷 Ⅱ 的研究[J]. 中国中药杂志,2013,38(13): 2136

尤志勉,韩安榜,林崇良. 浙产细叶艾挥发油成分的GC-MS分析[J]. 浙江中医杂志,2013,48(4): 299

Z

Zang X, Shang M, Xu F, et al. A-type proanthocyanidins from the stems of *Ephedra sinica* (Ephedraceae) and their antimicrobial activities[J]. Molecules, 2013, 18(5): 5172

Zeng X, Li CY, Wang H, et al. Unusual lipids and acylglucosylsterols from the roots of *Livistona chinensis* [J]. Phytochemistry Letters, 2013, 6(1): 36

Zhan Z, Feng Z, Yang Y, et al. Ternatusine A, a new pyrrole derivative with an epoxyoxepino ring from *Ranunculus ternatus*[J]. Organic Letters, 2013, 15(8): 1970

Zhang BB, Jiang Q, Liao ZX, et al. New cytotoxic triterpenoids from the aerial parts of *Euphorbia sieboldiana*[J]. Helvetica Chimica Acta, 2013, 96(7): 1281

Zhang BJ, Yan JM, Wu ZK, et al. Alkaloids from *Ochrosia borbonica*[J]. Helvetica Chimica Acta, 2013, 96(12): 2288

Zhang C, Feng S, Zhang L, et al. A new cytotoxic steroidal saponin from the rhizomes and roots of *Smilax scobinicaulis* [J]. Natural Product Research, 2013, 27(14): 1255

Zhang C, Zhang D, Ye W, et al. Antiproliferative triterpenoid saponins from the stem of *Psychotria* sp[J]. Planta Medica, 2013, 79(11): 978

Zhang CR, Liu HB, Dong SH, et al. Alkaloids from the twigs and leaves of *Daphniphyllum macropodum*[J]. Helvetica Chimica Acta, 2013, 96(3): 499

Zhang CX, He XX, Zhang J, et al. New precursor of tetraterpenoids from the soft coral *Sarcophyton glaucum* [J]. Natural Product Research, 2013, 27(9): 782

Zhang D, Chen W, Chen W, et al. Three new ursane-type triterpenoids from the stems of *Saprosma merrillii*[J]. Molecules, 2013, 18(12): 14496

Zhang D, Li SB, Yang L, et al. Two new C methyl flavanones from the rhizomes and frond bases of *Matteuccia struthiopteris*[J]. Journal of Asian Natural Products Research, 2013, 15(11): 1163

Zhang H, Bazzill J, Gallagher RJ, et al. Antiproliferative withanolides from *Datura wrightii*[J]. Journal of Natural Products, 2013, 76(3): 445

Zhang HJ, Luo J, Shan SM, et al. Aphanamenes A and B, two new acyclic diterpene [4+2]- cycloaddition adducts from *Aphanamixis grandifolia* [J]. Organic Letters, 2013, 15(21): 5512

Zhang J, AbdelMageed WM, Liu M, et al. Caesanines A-D, new cassane diterpenes with unprecedented N bridge from *Caesalpinia sappan*[J]. Organic Letters, 2013, 15(18): 4726

Zhang LC, Wu XD, He J, et al. Three new abietane diterpenoids from *Podocarpus fleuryi* [J]. Phytochemistry Letters, 2013, 6(3): 364

Zhang M, Liu WX, Zheng MF, et al. Bioactive quinic acid derivatives from *Ageratina adenophora*[J]. Molecules, 2013, 18(11): 14096

Zhang M, Wang JS, Luo J, et al. Glaucogenin E, a new C_{21} steroid from *Cynanchum stauntonii*[J]. Natural Product Research, 2013, 27(2): 176

Zhang M, Zhu Y, Zhan G, et al. Micranthanone A, a new diterpene with an unprecedented carbon skeleton from *Rhododendron micranthum*[J]. Organic Letters, 2013, 15(12): 3094

Zhang PP, Gao SS, Zhang TT, et al. Two new compounds from *Schisandra glaucescens*[J]. Journal of Asian Natural Products Research, 2013, 15(5): 466

Zhang S, Ma Q, Zhao Y, et al. Chemical constituents from the fungus *Amauroderma amoiensis* and their in vitro acetylcholinesterase inhibitory activities[J]. Planta Medica, 2013, 79(1): 87

Zhang T, Gong T, Chen RY, et al. Two new trinoreudesmanolides from *Inula racemosa*[J]. Journal of Asian Natural Products Research, 2013, 15(4): 368

Zhang W, Yao M, Xi M, et al. Triterpenoid

saponins with antimyocardial ischemia activity from the whole plants of *Clematis tangutica*[J]. Planta Medica, 2013, 79(8): 673

Zhang W, Zhang W, Luo J, et al. A new steroidal glycoside from the seeds of *Hyoscyamus niger*[J]. Natural Product Research, 2013, 27(21): 1971

Zhang WK, Xu JK, Tian HY, et al. Two new vinblastine-type noxide alkaloids from *Catharanthus roseus*[J]. Natural Product Research, 2013, 27(20): 1911

Zhang X, Oh M, Kim S, et al. Epimediphine, a novel alkaloid from *Epimedium koreanum* inhibits acetylcholinesterase[J]. Natural Product Research, 2013, 27(12): 1067

Zhang X, Su YF, Chen L, et al. Steroidal aaponins from the rhizomes of *Smilacina henryi*[J]. Helvetica Chimica Acta, 2013, 96(3): 478

Zhang XL, Sun J, Wu HH, et al. A new indoloquinazoline alkaloidal glucoside from the nearly ripe fruits of *Evodia rutaecarpa*[J]. Natural Product Research, 2013, 27(20): 1917

Zhang XL, Wang L, Li F, et al. Cytotoxic phorbol esters of *Croton tiglium*[J]. Journal of Natural Products, 2013, 76(5): 858

Zhang Y, Deng S, Qu L, et al. Rare syringyl acylated flavonol glycosides from the aerial parts of *Leonurus japonicus* Houtt[J]. Molecules, 2013, 18(3): 2967

Zhang Y, Han LF, Sakah KJ, et al. Bioactive protopanaxatriol type saponins isolated from the roots of *Panax Notoginseng* (Burk.) FH Chen[J]. Molecules, 2013, 18(9): 10352

Zhang Y, Wang JS, Gu YC, et al. Ring A rearranged limonoids from the fruits of *Aphanamixis grandifolia* and their cytotoxicity evaluation[J]. Phytochemistry Letters, 2013, 6(4): 539

Zhang Y, Xiao G, Sun L, et al. A new flavan-3-ol lactone and other constituents from *Euonymus alatus* with inhibitory activities on α-glucosidase and differentiation of 3T3-L1 cells[J]. Natural Product Research, 2013, 27(17): 1513

Zhang Y, Yang CR, Zhang YJ. New steroidal saponins from the leaves of *Yucca elephantipes*[J]. Helvetica Chimica Acta, 2013, 96(9): 1807

Zhang YM, Xu J, Xiao L, et al. A new phenolic glycoside from *Chamaecyparis obtusa* var. brevirameaf. crippsii[J]. Molecules, 2013, 18(1): 1255

Zhang ZC, Su G, Li J, et al. Two new neuroprotective phenolic compounds from *Gastrodia elata*[J]. Journal of Asian Natural Products Research, 2013, 15(6): 619

Zhang ZF, Lu LY, Luo P, et al. Two new ursolic acid saponins from *Morina nepalensis* var. alba Hand-Mazz[J]. Natural Product Research, 2013, 27(24): 2256

Zhang ZG, Cheng YT, Hu GL, et al. Two new trijugin-type limonoids from *Cipadessa cinerascens*[J]. Helvetica Chimica Acta, 2013, 96(12): 2228

Zhang ZJ, He J, Li Y, et al. Three new sesquiterpenes from *Laggera pterodonta*[J]. Helvetica Chimica Acta, 2013, 96(4): 732

Zhang ZQ, Luo JG, Wang JS, et al. Five new steroidal alkaloid glycosides from *Solanum tuberosum*[J]. Helvetica Chimica Acta, 2013, 96(5): 931

Zhang ZT, Chen DL, Chen QH, et al. Bis-diterpenoid alkaloids from *Aconitum tanguticum* var. trichocarpum[J]. Helvetica Chimica Acta, 2013, 96(4): 710

Zhang ZX, Fu Q, Zheng KY. Three new triterpene glycosides from *Ilex asprella*[J]. Journal of Asian Natural Products Research, 2013, 15(5): 453

Zhao JQ, Wang YM, He HP, et al. Two new highly oxygenated and rearranged limonoids from *Phyllanthus cochinchinensis*[J]. Organic Letters, 2013, 15(10): 2414

Zhao P, Chen H, Wang H, et al. Four new cassane diterpenes from the seeds of *Caesalpinia minax*[J]. Phytochemistry Letters, 2013, 6(4): 606

Zhao W, Zeng X, Zhang T, et al. Flavonoids from the bark and stems of *Cassia fistula* and their antitobacco mosaic virus activities[J]. Phytochemistry Letters, 2013, 6(2): 179

Zheng CJ, Zhu JY, Yu W, et al. Labdane-type diterpenoids from the fruits of *Vitex trifolia*[J]. Journal of Natural Products, 2013, 76(2): 287

Zheng XK, Li DD, Yan H, et al. Two new alkaloids from *Corydalis humosa*[J]. Journal of Asian Natural Products Research, 2013, 15(11): 1158

Zhong RJ, Yuan H, Fu HZ, et al. Three new compounds from the leaves of *Liquidambar formosana*[J]. Journal of Asian Natural Products Research, 2013, 15(11): 1249

Zhong YJ, Wen QF, Li CY, et al. Two new naphthoquinone derivatives from *Lysionotus pauciflorus*[J]. Helvetica Chimica Acta, 2013, 96(9): 1750

Zhou CX, Sun LR, Feng F, et al. Cytotoxic diterpenoids from the stem bark of *Annona squamosa* L.

[J]. Helvetica Chimica Acta, 2013, 96(4): 656

Zhou CX, Zou L, Mo JX, et al. Homoisoflavonoids from *Ophiopogon japonicus*[J]. Helvetica Chimica Acta, 2013, 96(7): 1397

Zhou G, Ma X, Zeng K, et al. Inhibitory activity of chemical constituents from *Arenaria serpyllifolia* on nitric oxide production[J]. Planta Medica, 2013, 79(8): 687

Zhou M, Zhang HB, Wang WG, et al. Scopariusic acid, a new meroditerpenoid with a unique cyclobutane ring isolated from *Isodon scoparius*[J]. Organic Letters, 2013, 15(17): 4446

Zhou R, Li DL, Feng GL, et al. A new sesquiterpene glucoside from *Nicotiana rustica* L. [J]. Natural Product Research, 2013, 27(14): 1261

Zhou WB, Liu J, Xing S, et al. Cylindroside A, a new triterpenoid saponin from *Cylindrokelupha dalatensis* and its cytotoxic activity[J]. Journal of Asian Natural Products Research, 2013, 15(12): 1277

Zhou WB, Zeng GZ, Xu HM, et al. Astataricusones A-D and astataricusol A, five new anti-HBV shionane-type triterpenes from *Aster tataricus* L. f[J]. Molecules, 2013, 18(12): 14585

Zhou Y, Chai X, Tu P, et al. Ilexpublesnins C-M, eleven new triterpene saponins from the roots of *Ilex pubescens*[J]. Planta Medica, 2013, 79(1): 70

Zhou Y, Jia X, Shi J, et al. Two new pentacyclic triterpenes from *Abelmoschus esculentus* [J]. Helvetica Chimica Acta, 2013, 96(3): 533

Zhou Z, Luo J, Pan K, et al. Bioactive benzofuran neolignans from *Aristolochia fordiana* [J]. Planta Medica, 2013, 79(18): 1730

Zhou Z, Yin W, Zhang H, et al. A new iridoid glycoside and potential MRB inhibitory activity of isolated compounds from the rhizomes of *Cyperus rotundus* L[J]. Natural Product Research, 2013, 27(19): 1732

Zhou ZL, Feng ZC, Fu CY, et al. A new triterpene saponin from the roots of *Ilex pubescens* [J]. Natural Product Research, 2013, 27(15): 1343

Zhu QF, Wang YY, Jiang W, et al. Three new norlignans from *Glechoma longituba*[J]. Journal of Asian Natural Products Research, 2013, 15(3): 258

Zhuang PY, Zhang GJ, Wang XJ, et al. Prenylated C_6-C_3 compounds from the roots of *Illicium henryi*[J]. Phytochemistry, 2013, 86: 176

Zou H, Xu KP, Zou ZX, et al. A new flavonoid with 6-phenyl substituent from *Selaginella uncinata*[J]. Journal of Asian Natural Products Research, 2013, 15(1): 84

Zou YS, Foubert K, Tuenter E, et al. Antiplasmodial and cytotoxic activities of Striga asiatica and *Sauropus spatulifolius* extracts, and their isolated constituents[J]. Phytochemistry Letters, 2013, 6(1): 53

Zuo WJ, Dong WH, Zhao YX, et al. Two new strophanthidol cardenolides from the seeds of *Antiaris toxicaria*[J]. Phytochemistry Letters, 2013, 6(1): 1

曾富佳,丁丽娜,高玉琼,等.冬葵挥发性成分研究[J].中国民族民间医药,2013,22(14): 19

曾富佳,张珏,高玉琼,等.黔产山茱萸挥发性成分研究[J].中国民族民间医药,2013,22(7): 29

张健,殷志琦,梁敬钰.络石藤地上部分中的一个新异黄酮苷(英文)[J].中国天然药物,2013,11(3): 274

张龙,郑锡任,陈勇,等.山绿茶茎和叶中挥发油成分GC-MS比较分析[J].中国实验方剂学杂志,2013,19(1): 70

张伟,彭涛,卢引,等.HS-SPME-GC-MS分析蜜本南瓜3个部位的挥发性成分[J].世界科学技术(中医药现代化),2013,15(4): 680

赵静芳,蒋立勤,钟晓明.佛手叶挥发性成分的提取鉴定[J].中华中医药学刊,2013,31(8): 1773

赵钟祥,林朝展,祝晨蔯,等.岗梅根中一个新的三萜皂苷(英文)[J].中国天然药物,2013,11(4): 415

钟可,王文全,靳凤云,等.西陵知母药材挥发性成分GC-MS分析[J].中华中医药学刊,2013,31(4): 740

周坚,陈刚,唐维宏.水蒸气蒸馏法与超临界CO_2萃取法提取五味藤挥发油的化学成分比较[J].广西中医药大学学报,2013,16(2): 87

周晓磊,吴久鸿,白皎,等.皂帽花中的一个新生物碱(英文)[J].中国天然药物,2013,11(1): 81

朱华凤,马慧,赵路路,等.GC-MS法比较温莪术挥发油与水煎液中的挥发性成分[J].沈阳药科大学学报,2013,30(7): 532

朱立俏,盛华刚.川芎挥发性成分GC-MS分析[J].山东中医药大学学报,2013,37(2): 164

(四) 中药药剂

【概述】

2013年,有2 000余篇论文报道中药药剂学领域的研究与应用成果,其内容主要涉及中药制药技术的研究、中药新剂型与新制剂的研究。

1. 中药制药技术的研究

在中药制药技术的研究方面,中药粉碎、干燥、提取、分离纯化等内容均有较多的报道。

(1) 粉碎干燥　① 微粉粉碎:李守信等研究表明,生脉散经超微粉碎后,基本无完整细胞存在,粒度均匀;生脉散超微粉中五味子甲素和五味子乙素溶出速率高于细粉,但是180 min后累积溶出量没有明显差异。超微粉碎可使生脉散显微特征变化明显,化学成分的溶出速率加快。贺义恒等研究恒山黄芪粉碎度与黄芪多糖得率之间的关系。结果表明,恒山黄芪粉体粒度≥600目(破壁前),同等粉碎度黄芪多糖的得率CaO法提取优于水法提取,小于800目(破壁后)得率趋于一致。无论是采用水法提取还是CaO法提取,恒山黄芪在粉碎粒度为800目时,选择提取温度80℃,料液比1∶8,黄芪多糖得率达到最高,分别为8.36%和8.49%。王念明等研究黄芩药材不同粒径的粉体学差异,表明随着粒径的减小,粉体粒度、松密度减小,比表面积与孔隙度、接触角增大,休止角先增后减,吸湿性增强;红外光谱与HPTLC指纹图谱显示,在一定时间内,超微粉碎黄芩药材并未引起化学组成成分与分子结构的改变。王春柳等研究表明,七厘散细粉及微粉在高湿环境下含水量均升高,流动性和血竭素含量下降,血竭素溶出无显著变化;在高温环境下2种粉体的含水量均下降,流动性增加,血竭素溶出均降低,细粉中血竭素含量下降,微粉中则无显著变化;光照条件下两种粉体含水量均升高,流动性无显著变化,血竭素含量均下降,细粉中血竭素溶出下降,微粉中则无显著变化。② 喷雾干燥:吕子明等采用正交试验优选黄连浸膏的喷雾干燥工艺,结果为进风口温度180℃,出风口温度80℃,浸膏比重1.15。乌日娜等研究复方沙棘颗粒剂的喷雾干燥工艺,表明浸膏相对密度和进风温度对喷雾干燥工艺影响极显著。最佳工艺为,相对密度1.02(25℃),进风温度100～110℃,进液速度22 ml/min,颗粒成型率32%。严金桥采用正交试验优选丹参-川芎药对的流浸膏喷雾干燥工艺,表明浸膏的相对密度影响显著。最佳工艺为,入塔风温165℃,入塔风压－1 750 Pa,出塔风温70℃,浸膏相对密度为1.18。

(2) 提取　① 煎煮提取:张家成等研究煎药机煎煮旋覆代赭汤时的最佳工艺,结果为煎煮时间50 min,加水量为9倍药材重量。张家成等又运用高压中药煎煮机,研究复方中人参和甘草在高压煎煮时浸泡时间对主要成分溶出的影响。结果,不同浸泡时间对旋覆代赭汤中人参、甘草等主要成分的含量没有显著影响。李毅民等研究了大承气汤常压机器煎煮过程中显著影响有效成分含量的因素,结果最佳工艺为,药材浸泡时间60 min,密闭模式煎煮,煎煮45 min,大黄后下10 min,液料比9∶1。② 微波提取:李石清等采用中心组合设计优选南方红豆杉枝条中多糖的微波提取工艺,结果料液比21.48(V/W),提取时间13.78 min,提取次数3次,微波频率为1 877 MHz。李盈蕾等用效应面法优选青风藤中青藤碱微波提取工艺,结果为20倍量75%乙醇,450 W微波提取2次,每次8.30 min。在此最佳工艺条件下青藤碱得率为0.803%,理论值为0.824%。朱开梅等采用微波辅助提取技术,优选香蕉皮总多酚的最佳提取工艺,结果为加35倍量50%乙醇,380 W微波提取100 s,总多酚提取率2.16%。刘学仁等采用正交试验优化微波辅助提取枳壳的最佳工艺,结果为80%乙醇作溶剂,微波萃取仪功率400 W,时间10 min,温度40℃。李小菊等采用单因素和响应曲面法优选魔芋葡甘露聚糖的最佳提取工艺,结果为提取温度90℃,浸提时间60 min,微波功率700 W,料液比1∶200。魔芋葡甘露聚糖糖提取率为50.3%。③ 超声提取:马瑞丽等采用响应面分析法优选大血藤中总酚超声提取的最佳工艺,结果为含乙醇量56%,提取温度62℃,提取时间34 min,大血藤总酚得率可达10.629%,与理论预测值10.735%的相对误差为

—0.99%。帕丽达·阿布力孜等采用单因素试验和响应曲面法优选牛舌草中总黄酮的提取工艺，结果为加 20 倍量 70% 乙醇，60℃ 超声提取 20 min，总黄酮平均提取率 3.92%。张生等应用响应面法优选超声辅助提取连翘中桦木酸的最佳工艺，结果为乙醇体积分数 80%，提取温度 37℃，液固比 32 ml/g，桦木酸提取率（4.28 ± 0.05）mg/g，与模型预测值（4.30 mg/g）基本一致。黄弦等用响应面分析法优选栀子超声提取的最佳工艺，结果为甲醇体积分数 88.8%，提取温度 72℃，提取时间 36 min，超声强度 70%，液料比 50：1。马合木提·买买提明等采用正交试验优选超声微波协同萃取芜菁籽中总黄酮类物质的最佳提取工艺，结果为提取功率为 400 W，提取液为 65%（v /v）的乙醇溶液，料液比为 1：20（mg/ml），提取时间为 15 min，芜菁籽中总黄酮的得率为 3.03%。④ 超临界 CO_2 流体萃取：林青等采用正交试验优选川芎-香附药对超临界 CO_2 萃取工艺，结果为萃取压力 25 MPa，萃取温度 45℃，萃取时间 2 h，CO_2 流量 20 kg/h。萃取物中 α-香附酮和丁烯基苯酞的平均含量为 3.26%、1.50%。李晓宁等采用正交试验优选超临界 CO_2 流体萃取当归挥发油的工艺，结果为萃取压力 30 MPa，萃取温度 50℃，萃取时间 2 h，CO_2 流量 25 L/h，分离釜Ⅰ压力 8 MPa，温度 50℃，分离釜Ⅱ压力系统尾压，温度 35℃。张建军等采用均匀设计响应曲面分析法优化超临界 CO_2 流体萃取丹参中丹参酮 $Ⅱ_A$ 的最佳萃取工艺，结果为萃取温度 60℃，萃取压力 18 MPa，CO_2 流量 16.50 kg/h，萃取时间 130 min，分离釜压力 12.5 MPa，温度 60℃。王姿媛等采用正交试验优选超临界 CO_2 流体萃取苍术-厚朴药对的最佳工艺，结果为萃取压力 26 MPa，萃取温度 50℃，解析压力 8 MPa，解析温度 35℃，萃取物中和厚朴酚、厚朴酚及苍术素的平均含量为 9.81%、12.52%、7.26%。⑤ 仿生提取：张慧等应用响应面分析法研究复方金钱草中君药（金钱草、路路通、车前子）的半仿生最佳提取工艺，结果为温度 100℃，料液比 1 g：35 ml，提取 3 次，3 次提取液 pH 值分别为 4.0、7.0 和 8.5，总提取 2.5 h，总黄酮质量分数为 9.91 mg/g，总糖质量分数为 62.38 mg/g，浸膏得率为 13.86%。宫春博等采用正交试验优选牡丹皮中丹皮酚的最佳提取工艺，结果为溶剂中同时加酸加盐，氯化钠浓度为 10%，盐酸浓度为 8%，溶媒倍量为 8 倍量，丹皮酚提取率为 95.3%。张德新等采用正交试验优选半仿生提取玉米须中总皂苷的最佳工艺，结果为酸提取时间 90 min，碱提取时间 60 min，超声功率 70 W，料液比为 1：40。⑥ 加压减压提取：王梓等利用 Box-Behnken 设计、响应曲面法建模和优化加速溶剂萃取五味子中 4 个木脂素。结果最佳提取工艺为，溶剂为 87%乙醇，温度 160℃，静态萃取时间 10 min，提取压力 1 500 psi，1 个提取循环，60%冲水量，4 个木脂素的实测值 14.72 mg/g，与模型预测值基本接近。胡德奇等对抱茎苦荬菜进行不同真空度和温度条件下减压提取研究。结果，减压提取工艺明显提高腺苷收率，真空度0.08 MPa，温度 62℃时腺苷收率最高，与常压提取比较相对提高 27.81%，对总黄酮收率影响较小，浸膏收率相对降低。唐梅等采用浸渍-压榨联合提取法，通过 Box-Behnken 设计优选黄芩的最佳提取工艺，结果为 11 倍量水于 60℃浸泡 4 h，压榨，药渣加 2 倍量水洗涤后压榨，重复操作 1 次。总黄酮、黄芩苷提取率分别为 17.630%，9.38%，出膏率 42.7%，与模型预测值非常接近。叶陈丽等采用 Box-Behnken 设计优选黄芩超高压提取工艺条件，结果为乙醇体积分数 72%，提取压力 100 MPa，液固比 100：1，提取时间 10 s，黄芩苷提取率 102.65 mg/g。⑦ 其他方法：侯莉伟等在单因素试验基础上，用 Box-Behnken 响应面设计优选荷叶总黄酮的最佳温浸提取工艺，结果为加 39 倍量 51%乙醇，71℃温浸 2 次，每次62 min，总黄酮提取率 6.21%。陈雪等采用正交试验优选清脂通脉颗粒的醇提取工艺，结果为加 6 倍量 70%乙醇，回流提取 3 次，每次 1.5 h。林小玲等采用星点设计-效应面法优选参芪消岩颗粒的乙醇渗漉提取工艺条件，结果为 16 倍量 80%乙醇，渗漉速度 13 ml/（min·kg），姜黄素提取率 78.82%，干膏得率 8.35%。白永智等采用正交试验优选高压脉冲电场法快速提取黄花乌头中关附甲素的最佳工艺，结果为以 90%乙醇为提取溶剂，电场强度 20 kV/cm，脉冲数为 10，料液比 1：14。黄花乌头中的关附甲素提取率达到 0.391%，浸膏得率为 39.92%。王春民等对二次蒸馏-萃取耦合法和水蒸气蒸馏法提取颈复康制剂挥发油进行比较研究。结果，采用二次蒸馏-萃取耦合法提取颈复康制剂挥发油时，Z-藁本内酯和洋川芎内酯 A 的转移率是水蒸气蒸馏法的

3倍;两种提取方法中苍术素的转移率没有变化。王权等采用正交试验优选苓桂术甘颗粒的最佳水提工艺,结果为加8倍量水,提取3次,每次煎煮1 h。

(3) 分离纯化 ① 絮凝澄清:倪东杰等应用综合评分法-正交设计优选健骨口服液的除杂澄清工艺条件,结果为药液浓度1∶10,ZTC 1+1天然澄清剂2组分,加入顺序为先B组分后A组分,2组分浓度均为1%,用量分别为每100 ml,待处理溶液加入B黏胶液6 ml及A黏胶液3 ml,作用温度为80℃,并搅拌10 min,保温1 h后,固形物去除率为20.03%,淫羊藿苷含量保留率为82.26%。于蓓蓓等采用正交试验优选桑椹补脑膏的最佳絮凝除杂工艺,结果为药液比1∶2,温度50℃,每100 ml药液加1%壳聚糖溶液10 ml,pH4。战兵等采用正交试验优选大黄水提液的壳聚糖絮凝沉降工艺,结果为药液质量浓度0.1 g/ml,壳聚糖加入量10%,药液pH6。壳聚糖沉淀法和乙醇沉淀法均能较好地使水提液沉淀,但两者均会造成蒽醌类成分的损失,前者在降低浸膏率、保留有效成分方面优于后者。孙姣等研究壳聚糖对小儿咳喘灵口服液原药提取液絮凝除杂效果。结果最佳絮凝工艺为,药液温度30℃,加入壳聚糖0.75 g/L,先在搅拌桨叶片顶端线速度为1.31 m/s的条件下快速搅拌120 s,再在0.26 m/s的速度下搅拌15 min,絮凝后的药液在分离因数为1430条件下离心20 min,此时绿原酸的保留率为94.6%,鞣质和蛋白质的去除率分别为44.7%和51.6%,药液浊度为1.1 NTU。药液静置存放90 d后浊度仅为3.5 NTU。与醇沉法相比,壳聚糖对于小儿咳喘灵原药提取液的絮凝除杂效果良好,有效成分绿原酸及多糖的保留率分别提高了6.3%和25.8%,鞣质去除率提高21.6%,药液的浊度仅是醇沉浊度的1/4,放置3个月药液浊度的上升幅度仅为醇沉法的1/5。孙立霞等以人参皂苷含量、总多糖含量、澄明度和稳定性为评价指标,研究KBT-ZTC絮凝澄清法、酶解法、微滤法、酶解-微滤法及絮凝澄清-微滤法对参玉口服液质量的影响。结果表明,最佳澄清处理方法为絮凝澄清-微滤法。② 膜过滤:刘敏彦等研究表明,经过8种不同孔径陶瓷膜过滤后,连花清瘟胶囊水提液均较过滤前明显透明澄清,出膏率也有一定程度的下降。孔径为0.2 μm的陶瓷膜管能保证有效成分转移率和固形物去除率,并有较大的膜通量。李进等研究超滤技术分离纯化板蓝根有效成分的工艺。结果表明,选择截留相对分子量5 000的卷式中空有机超滤膜,在过膜压力0.5 MPa,过膜体积流量30 L/h,超滤3次,体系温度维持室温(22℃)的条件下分离纯化,效果较好。陈伟等研究表明,100 kDa孔径的超滤膜可较好地去除栀子苷药液中热原,对栀子苷成分的影响较小。彭菲等研究不同材质及孔径的超滤膜对有效成分透过率的影响。结果表明,随着膜截留分子量的变大,各人参皂苷类成分的透过率有所提高,且纤维素材质的超滤膜对原人参二醇型皂苷人参皂苷Rb_1、人参皂苷Rb_2、人参皂苷Rb_3、人参皂苷Rc、人参皂苷Rd、人参皂苷Rg_3的透过率明显大于相同截留分子量的聚醚砜膜材质的超滤膜。③ 大孔吸附树脂:朱梦良等优选大孔吸附树脂分离、纯化葛根总黄酮和葛根素的工艺。结果,选用AB-8型大孔吸附树脂,上样液质量浓度1.0 g/ml,葛根与大孔树脂质量比1∶2,径高比1∶6,用2 BV水洗除杂,加2 BV 80%乙醇以2 ml/min洗脱,转移率均>92%,所得葛根总酮纯度达80%,葛根素质量分数25%。浦益琼等研究表明,采用AB-8大孔树脂精制茜草醇提液,以1 g生药/ml茜草浓缩液与等比例去离子水混合后抽滤所得滤液作为上样液,经去离子水洗脱糖分后,再用95%乙醇洗脱有效成分,将所得洗脱液合并,旋转蒸发,减压干燥后,所得提取物中总醌量分别为59.17%、52.25%和54.83%。吴建雄等优选纯化红花中羟基红花黄色素A的工艺,结果为上样液pH4,药材-树脂质量比1∶6,加4 BV水以3 BV/h的流速洗脱除杂,用5%乙醇6 BV以3 BV/h的流速洗脱,收集洗脱液。童婷婷等优化大孔树脂富集纯化大黄地上部位总蒽醌的工艺。结果表明,D101型大孔树脂对大黄地上部位总蒽醌有良好的吸附和解吸性能。最佳上柱工艺为,最大上样量4.54 g/g(生药材/干树脂),pH7,体积流量1 ml/min,药液含生药量2.16 g/ml。加样吸附均匀后,以5倍量树脂柱体积冲洗至流出液几乎无色,改用10%的乙醇再冲洗至流出液无色,用0.4 mol/L NaOH与75%乙醇按体积比1∶5混合,用量为10倍量树脂柱体积,大黄地上部位总蒽醌的质量分数提高到15.25%。陈超等优选AB-8型大孔吸附树脂纯化复方通脉颗粒有效部位的工艺,结果为上样液质量浓度110 g/L,树脂柱径高比1∶10,树脂体积与上样量比2.8∶1(吸附3 h),加2 BV水洗除杂,用6 BV 50%乙醇洗脱,收集洗脱液。

2. 中药新剂型与新制剂的研究

(1) 颗粒剂 李雪玲等采用正交试验优选炎宁无糖颗粒成型工艺,结果为浸膏粉与辅料(糊精)按1∶2混合均匀,以95%乙醇为润湿剂,润湿剂用量为辅料与浸膏总量的30%。王洪珍等研究表明,益髓通经缓释颗粒的最佳成型工艺为,取处方量药材提取物,加入18.75% $HPMC_{K15M}$,以80%乙醇为润湿剂,采用湿法制粒法制备颗粒。颗粒剂中马钱子碱和士的宁的释药行为均符合Higuchi模型,属于扩散释药机制。郭涛等采用均匀设计优选养肝疏胆颗粒处方,结果为干浸膏∶糊精∶乳糖=11∶6∶7。张涛等优化归芪通便颗粒的最佳处方,结果为浸膏粉∶麦芽糊精∶微粉硅胶=5∶3.5∶1.5,用95%乙醇溶液制粒,颗粒的临界相对湿度为74.8%,休止角为34.95°。

(2) 胶囊剂 张恒玉等采用正交试验筛选银杏酮酯自乳化软胶囊的最佳处方,结果为共轭亚油酸乙酯∶吐温85∶乙醇=80∶15∶5,药物含量7%。常温和加速实验3个月内质量稳定。黄巧文等通过舒秘胶囊在^{60}Co辐射前后的性状等变化情况,研究辐射灭菌的效果。结果,经过5 kGy 10 h的^{60}Co辐射,舒秘胶囊性状未改变,微生物限度符合规定,芦荟苷含量与辐射前无明显差异。唐黎等采用研磨法制备大蒜素羟丙基-β-环糊精包合物(HP-β-CD),并制备大蒜素速溶肠溶胶囊。结果最佳工艺为,HP-β-CD 10 g,大蒜素1 g,水4 ml,研磨2 h,真空干燥箱中50℃干燥4 h。

(3) 凝胶膏剂 刘聪敏等采用星点设计-效应面法优选止痛凝胶膏剂基质,结果为NP-700∶铝化合物∶酒石酸∶甘油=1.5∶0.16∶8.8∶0.12,止痛凝胶膏剂中阿魏酸于12 h内累积释放率为(86.31±6.73)%。优选的基质配方载药量高,涂展性、保湿性、黏着力良好,止痛凝胶膏剂中阿魏酸体外释放接近零级方程,具有扩散和溶蚀的双重机制。肖金宝等研究表明,银杏叶提取物温度敏感型鼻用原位凝胶,主要通过扩散而不是溶蚀方式释放,释放曲线符合一级释放方程,有缓释特征。娄杰等采用冷溶法制备眼用温敏型小檗碱白蛋白纳米粒原位凝胶。结果优选的原位凝胶基质的最佳处方为,26%泊洛沙姆407和4%泊洛沙姆188。优化处方在30.9℃为自由流动的液体,经泪液稀释后在34.2℃能够发生相变形成凝胶。国大亮等采用正交试验优选制备黄芩苷鼻用凝胶剂的最佳处方,结果为卡波姆-936用量0.5%,丙三醇用量30%,载药量2%,pH值6.85~7.00,平均黏度1 850~2 350 Pa·s。黄芩苷经猪鼻黏膜扩散符合一级动力学过程,扩散速率约为0.280 6 $\mu g/(mm^2 \cdot h)$。陈小云等正交试验优选辣椒素透皮凝胶的处方,结果为1%羟丙基甲基纤维素-硬脂酸、15%丙二醇、10%甘油。所制备的凝胶为白色半透明胶体,辣椒素12 h累积渗透量为275.45 $\mu g/cm^2$。陈新民等研究丹黄凝胶剂的成型工艺,结果以1.0%卡波姆-940为凝胶基质,2%氮酮为促渗剂,载药量为4.5%制备丹黄凝胶剂。

(4) 巴布剂 祝星等采用均匀设计优选温脐巴布剂的最佳基质配比,结果质量比为,聚丙烯酸钠∶卡波姆∶明胶∶丙二醇∶甘油∶高岭土∶甘羟铝∶柠檬酸=1.8∶0.3∶1.5∶3.0∶14.0∶1.6∶0.16∶0.32。张洪兵等采用单因素试验、星点设计—效应面优化法优选复方止痛巴布剂基质的处方配比,结果质量比为,NP700∶卡波姆940∶甘羟铝∶微粉硅胶∶甘油=5.34∶0.63∶0.2∶6∶30。周福军等优选止痛巴布剂的体外透皮促进剂,结果为3%氮酮+3%丙二醇。N-甲基-2-吡咯烷酮几乎不能增加阿魏酸的透过量,单独加入2%氮酮使阿魏酸透过率增加1.7倍,单独加入3%丙二醇使阿魏酸的透过率增加1.4倍,3%氮酮与3%丙二醇联合使用使阿魏酸的透过率约增加2.2倍。谢友良等研究不同剂量的$^{60}Co-\gamma$射线辐照灭菌对西洋参巴布剂黏附性及主要有效成分含量的影响。结果表明,西洋参巴布剂在不同剂量的$^{60}Co-\gamma$辐照前后其黏附性无明显变化。

(5) 喷雾剂 宋艳丽等采用注入法制备栀子苷醇质体。结果表明,最优处方制备的栀子苷醇质体粒径(173.40±71.02)nm,Zeta电位(−42.50±8.27)mV,包封率(65.80±2.53)%,载药量(5.25±0.15)%。栀子苷醇质体300 min经鼻黏膜单位面积渗透量为23.39 $\mu g/cm^2$,是其脂质体的2.17倍、水溶液的11.03倍。制剂基本无鼻黏膜纤毛毒性。葛克亚等研究表明,万通筋骨喷雾剂样品的透皮速率27.919 $\mu g/(cm^2 \cdot h)$,

6 h 内平均累积透过率 13.53%；绿原酸喷雾剂的透皮速率 6.636 μg/(cm² · h)，6 h 内平均累积透过率 3.78%。刘宏伟等采用改良 Franz 扩散池评价跌打喷雾剂制备工艺的可行性和合理性。结果表明，以大鼠腹部皮肤为用药部位、50%乙醇/生理盐水为接收液，载药量 8%的跌打喷雾剂体外经皮渗透试验效果较好。水杨酸甲酯和丁香酚的体外经皮渗透行为均可较好的拟合零级动力学方程。

(6) 注射剂　缪菊连等通过单因素试验优选三七总皂苷注射液的超滤工艺，结果为三七总皂苷水溶液质量浓度 100 g/L，选用 10 kDa 超滤膜，超滤温度 70℃，洗液体积 1 200 ml，人参皂苷 Rg_1、Rb_1及三七皂苷 R_1各组份透过率均>90%。祝倩倩等研究了注射用芪红脉通制剂工艺超滤前最佳除杂技术。结果最佳工艺为，冷藏 24 h，离心时间 15min，转速 5 000 r/min，活性炭用量 0.3%，温度 40℃，吸附时间 30 min，原药液的 pH 值。徐桂红等通过单因素试验结合正交试验优选注射用活血通络冷冻干燥制剂的成型工艺，结果为 5%甘露醇为填充剂，药液中有效成分质量浓度 30 g/L，预冻速率 30℃/h，制成的冻干粉针剂质量稳定。

(7) 滴丸　符少莲等采用星点设计-效应面法优选脂溶性丹参提取物速释滴丸的处方工艺，结果为以聚乙二醇 2000(PEG2000)：PEG4000＝3.5：6.5 混合作为载体材料制备脂溶性丹参提取物滴丸，滴丸中丹参提取物的含有量为 9%。所制备的滴丸较提取物原料药释药快且完全，在 20 min 与 60 min 的累积溶出率分别达 53%与 83%，分别高出原料药 26%与 43%。吴建雄等采用正交试验优选天舒滴丸的最佳成型工艺，结果以 PEG6000 为基质，二甲基硅油为冷却剂，浸膏：基质＝1：3，药液滴制温度为 75℃。优选的滴制条件为滴距 8 cm，滴速 40～50 滴/min，冷却剂温度为 5～15℃。夏海建等采用固体分散体方法制备雷公藤红素缓释滴丸，并用正交试验优选制备工艺。结果缓释滴丸的最佳处方质量比为，雷公藤红素：单硬脂酸甘油酯：PEG4000＝1：3：7，药料温度 80℃，滴速 20 滴/min，滴距 5 cm，冷凝液温度 15℃。缓释滴丸中药物以非晶形存在，该缓释滴丸 12 h 的最大累积释放率可达 91.2%。王友芳等研究复方天宁滴丸的稳定性并预测有效期。结果，阿魏酸的含量变化符合一级动力学过程，预测有效期为 20.8 个月。李娜等优选丹参酮固体分散体的最佳制备工艺，结果为药辅比 1：5，温度 70℃，PEG4000：PEG6000＝1：1，增溶剂为泊洛沙姆。经差示扫描热分析、X-ray 和红外分析，表明药物以分子状态分散，形成的固体分散体为填充型固态溶液。固体分散体滴丸的最佳制备工艺为，冷凝剂 1 000cs 二甲基硅油，温度 20℃，滴距 4 cm，滴速 30～40 滴/min，制备的丹参酮滴丸平均累积溶出度 85%。

(8) 包合物　李卿等研究消郁安神胶囊中挥发油β-环糊精包合物的热稳定性。结果，挥发油包合物于 40、60、80℃加热 4 h，百秋李醇含量未发生明显变化。张兰等研究软坚消瘿颗粒中挥发油提取及β-环糊精包合工艺研究。结果最佳提取工艺为，用 6 倍量水浸泡药材 2 h，水蒸气蒸馏法提取 6 h。最佳包合工艺为β-CD：软坚消瘿颗粒挥发油＝10：1(g/ml)，包合温度为 40℃，包合时间为 1.5 h。苏秀霞等采用水浴恒温磁力搅拌法制备当归油-HP-β-CD 包合物。结果最佳包合工艺为，当归油 1 ml，HP-β-CD：当归油＝6：1(g/ml)，水：当归油＝15：1(ml/ml)，包合温度为 40℃，包合时间为 4 h。HP-β-CD 与当归油形成了包合物，且在包合过程中未改变当归油的化学成分，提高了当归油的缓释效果。潘娅等用超声波法制备包合物，结果包合工艺为马钱子碱：β-CD＝1：8，包合温度为 50℃，包合时间为 20 min，马钱子碱经包合后溶解度提高了 6.4 倍，其性质在包合前后没有发生改变，稳定性能良好。周秋娜等采用冷冻干燥法，通过正交设计优选黄芩素最佳制备工艺，结果为黄芩素：HP-β-CD＝1：3，温度 45℃，包合时间4 h，包合溶剂水：无水乙醇＝2：3。采用最优包合条件制备的黄芩素-HP-β-CD 包合物得率为 93.97%，包封率为 95.96%，载药率为 5.20%，其粉末经鉴定已形成包合物。齐学洁等采用冷冻干燥法制备白藜芦醇/HP-β-CD 包合物。结果表明，白藜芦醇/HP-β-CD 包合物中，主、客分子的摩尔比为 1：1，白藜芦醇/HP-β-CD 包合物能显著增大药物的溶解度、稳定性和溶出速率。

(9) 固体分散体　刘珊珊等以聚丙烯酸树脂、聚维酮、共聚维酮为亲水性载体材料，采用热熔挤出技术，制备槲皮素固体分散体。结果，制备的槲皮素固体分散体，在人工胃液中 3 min 时槲皮素：聚丙烯酸树脂＝1：9 的药物溶出度可达到 67%，处方槲皮素：木糖醇：聚维酮＝1：3：6的药物溶出度可达到 65%，而在 60 min 时原料药溶出度不足 10%。胡绍英等采用溶剂蒸发法制备雷公藤红素固体分散体。结果表明，雷公藤红素：胶体二氧化硅＝1：12 时制备的固体分散体中，药物可缓慢释放，8 h 时药物的体外释放度达到 90%以上。陈小云等利用硬脂酸对纳米 $CaCO_3$ 进行表面改性，并以该材料为载体制备雷公藤红素缓释固体分散体。结果，药物与改性纳米 $CaCO_3$ 比例为 1：4 时，所制备的固体分散体中雷公藤红素以非晶型分散于载体表面，0.5 h体外释放度为 7.05%，12 h 的释放度达 90.03%，缓释效果良好。刘其媛等以壳聚糖为载体，采用溶剂法制备丹参酮 $Ⅱ_A$ 固体分散体。结果，丹参酮 $Ⅱ_A$-壳聚糖(MW3 000～5 000)按 1：9 比例制备的固体分散体的体外溶出效果最好，60 min时药物的体外累积溶出率达到 90%以上。蒋艳荣等采用喷雾干燥法制备丹参酮 $Ⅱ_A$ 固体分散体。结果，丹参酮 $Ⅱ_A$：共聚维酮＝1：10 制备的固体分散体，丹参酮 $Ⅱ_A$ 以非晶型分散于载体表面，0.5 h体外溶出度可达 100%，吸湿性低于同比例制备的聚维酮固体分散体，经过 3 个月稳定性加速试验后，其药物溶出度和含量未发生显著性变化。

(10) 微丸　严国俊等采用星点设计-效应面法优选流化床侧喷法研究复方垂盆草微丸的制备工艺，结果为喷液速度(泵速)7 r/min，转盘转速 250 r/min，滚圆时间 10 min。赖春花等采用固体分散体增溶技术及流化床上药技术制备载药丸芯，选取丙烯酸树脂- NE30D 对载药丸芯进行包衣。结果优选的包衣工艺为，丙烯酸树脂-NE30D包衣增重 5%，以 20%乳糖为致孔剂，50%滑石粉为抗黏剂，熟化时间 12 h，熟化温度 40℃，包衣微丸呈良好缓释效果，体外释药过程基本符合一级释药模型。赵一洁等采用滴制法制备大黄酸肠溶缓释微丸。结果，自制微丸光滑，圆整度好，且载药均匀，载药率在 96%以上。其在人工胃液中 2 h 的释放度＜5%；在缓冲溶液 pH6.8，释放曲线表明微丸具有明显的缓释特征。沈熊等采用 Box-Behnken 实验设计优选黄芩素微丸的缓释包衣处方为，增塑剂(柠檬酸三乙酯) 11%，丙烯酸树脂聚合物比例 4：1，包衣增重 12%，其在 2、6、12 h 时的释放度预测值分别为 28.34%、58.56%和 95.00%。制得缓释微丸释放度实测值与预测值基本一致。

(11) 微囊　董自亮等采用复凝聚法制备芍药苷微囊，Doehlert 设计优化制备工艺，芍药苷微囊的囊材囊心比、搅拌速率及体系的 pH 值对微囊的包封率与载药量均有显著影响，当囊材囊心比为 4.3：1、搅拌速率为 305 r/min、pH 值为 4 时，制得的芍药苷微囊圆整光滑，无黏连，粒径均匀，包封率可高达 83.81%，载药量为 24.24%，囊径在 200 μm 以下，且有一定的缓释作用。吴素香等以明胶和阿拉伯胶为囊材，采用复凝聚法制备留兰香油微囊。结果，在优化的处方及工艺条件下，所制备的留兰香油微囊圆整，算术平均粒径为 75.17 μm，以柠檬烯和香芹酮计的包封率分别达到 38.9%和 28.9%，载药量分别达到 27.0%和 20.8%。李小玲等采用凝聚法以自制微囊制粒机制备莪术油-壳聚糖缓释微囊。结果，制备的微囊载药量为 44.83%，包封率为 85.22%，体外累计释放度达到 86.45%，微囊大小均匀，成形度好。

(12) 微球　汪洋等采用正交试验优选刺五加提取物缓释微球的最佳制备工艺，结果为海藻酸钠质量分数 3.5%，刺五加提取物与海藻酸钠的质量比 1：1，$CaCl_2$ 质量分数 4.0%，交联时间 2 h，载药量和包封率分别为 10.11%、21.74%。制备的缓释微球粒径约 0.45 mm，12 h 累积释放率达 96.12%。何杨等采用快速膜乳化-溶剂萃取/挥发法制备水飞蓟宾聚乳酸-羟基乙酸共聚物(PLGA)微球。结果，SPG 膜孔径 2.8 μm，过膜压力 1.0 MPa，离心 20 min，固化液为生理盐水。水飞蓟宾 PLGA 微球的最佳制备工艺为，药辅比 1：4，聚乙烯醇(PVA)质量分数 3%，油水相体积比 1：19。制备的微球，平均粒径(2.634±0.35)μm，载药量(14.84±0.76)%，包封率(56.16±3.77)%。贾永艳等采用乳化交联法制备黄连总生物碱明胶微球。结果最佳制备工艺为，明胶质量分数 12%，投药量 1.7%，交联剂用量 15%，水相油相比 1：12。载药微球包封率 63.73%，载药量 6.50%。陈玉玺等采用乳化溶剂挥发法制备 20(S)-原人参 PLGA 微球。结果优选的处方工艺为，油：水相体积比 1：50，PVA 质量分数 0.5%，投药量 20 mg。制备的微球外观圆整，平均粒径约 1.16 μm，收率 35.58%，包封率

41.76%,载药量19.61%,微球在前0.5 h内的释放量18.24%,192 h时累积释放量高达98.99%。

(13) 微乳　王文刚等采用高压匀质法制备注射用紫杉醇亚微乳表明。结果,优化条件下制备的紫杉醇亚微乳粒度分布均匀,平均粒径为(168±22)nm,多分散系数为(0.89±0.05),Zeta电位为-(33.9±0.5)mV,稳定性较好,血管刺激性小。李海燕等研究表明,直肠微乳的最适处方为,穿心莲内酯8 g,吐温-80 300 ml,无水乙醇600 ml,肉豆蔻酸异丙酯30 ml,氮酮30 ml,水适量,pH7,共配成1 L。许日鑫等研究表明,优化的β-细辛醚微乳处方质量比为,β-细辛醚∶肉豆蔻酸异丙酯∶聚氧乙烯蓖麻油∶丙三醇=1∶2∶8∶2。制备的微乳澄清透明,有蓝色乳光,平均粒径为(18.2±0.2)nm,PI为(0.222±0.005),pH值为(6.50±0.01),10 000 r/min离心10 min后和高温灭菌后均无分层现象,平均载药量为(21.5±0.48)mg/ml。

(14) 自微乳　杨鹏飞等采用伪三元相图结合星点设计-效应面法优选银杏内酯B自微乳药物传递系统的处方质量比,辛酸/癸酸三甘油脂∶聚氧乙烯35蓖麻油∶卵磷脂∶乙醇=25.99∶39.47∶9.87∶24.67,载药量(24±1.4)g/L,粒径30~60 nm,并于1周内在常温、高温及低温状态下稳定性良好,通过溶血试验、血管刺激、急性毒性评价给药安全性良好。朱双燕等绘制三元相图筛选鸦胆子油自微乳最佳处方比例,结果为鸦胆子油0.45 g,卵磷脂0.15 g,肉豆蔻酸异内酯0.15 g,聚氧乙烯氢化蓖麻油-40 0.15 g,甘油0.4 g。乳滴粒径为9.2 nm,自乳化时间为20.53 s。在37℃下加入50 ml纯化水形成鸦胆子油自微乳澄清透明,物理稳定性良好。孙丹丹等研究表明,熊果酸自微乳的优化处方为,油相(中链甘油三酸酯)∶乳化剂(聚乙二醇15羟硬脂酸酯)∶助乳化剂(乙醇)=12.5∶62.5∶25。李洪松等筛选苦参碱自微乳最佳处方为,苦参碱∶油酸∶油酸乙酯∶EL40∶异丙醇=0.5∶0.15∶0.15∶0.35∶0.35。制备的苦参碱自微乳为澄明液体,遇水形成O/W型微乳,平均粒径(68.00±0.07)nm,平均载药量为42.689 mg /ml。刘伟星等研究表明,优选葛根素自乳化渗透泵缓控释胶囊的处方,结果为葛根素0.07 g、油酸乙酯0.25 g、聚山梨酯80 0.45 g、PEG400 0.3 g、甘露醇1.07 g、氯化钠1.07 g。通过对制备处方和预测处方在4、8、12 h的释放度的研究,表明该缓控释胶囊符合零级释放模型。朱双燕等研究表明,穿心莲内酯自微乳化最佳处方为,聚山梨酯-80∶油酸乙酯∶甘油=50∶26∶26,乳滴粒径39.5 nm,Zeta电位-15.18 mV,自乳化时间40.53 s。

(15) 纳米粒　陈明霞等优选重组水蛭素-2(rHV2)鼻腔给药纳米粒冻干粉最佳制备工艺,结果是用5%甘露醇∶葡萄糖=1∶1作为冻干保护剂,于-70℃预冻24 h后,置真空冻干箱中冷冻干燥,24 h后取出。该冻干粉中rHV2的含量为1.1 g/mg,光照对rHV2纳米粒冻干粉的外观,再分散性以及包封率影响均较小,而高温对rHV2纳米粒冻干粉的影响较大。rHV2壳聚糖纳米粒具有较高的渗透系数,是生理盐水组的5倍多,冻干粉仍然保持了良好的渗透性。魏颖慧等采用改良的自乳化溶剂扩散法制备壳聚糖修饰雷公藤多苷纳米粒。结果,根据优化条件制备的纳米粒,平均粒径为(207.6±3.4)nm,多分散指数为(0.078±0.009),包封率和载药量分别为(61.83±2.43)%、(10.70±0.37)%,体外释药符合Higuchi方程。李静等制备壳聚糖修饰的雷公藤甲素聚乙二醇-聚乳酸纳米粒。结果,所制备的纳米粒平均粒径、Zeta电位、包封率和载药量分别为(202.62±1.52)nm、(0.17±0.12)mV、(58.20±2.43)%和(1.25±0.13)%。体外释放实验表明,纳米粒体外释放$t_{1/2}$为1.1 h,在10.0 h累积释放率达到74.0%。陈修克等采用改良的自乳化溶剂蒸发法制备雷公藤多苷聚乳酸纳米粒,并用50%脱乙酰度的低分子量壳聚糖对纳米粒进行表面修饰,制备壳聚糖修饰的雷公藤多苷聚乳酸纳米粒。结果,制备的纳米粒平均粒径为(207.6±3.4)nm,多分散系数为(0.078±0.009),包封率为(61.83±2.43)%,载药量为(10.70±0.37)%,在含20%乙醇的pH7.4的PBS缓冲液中体外释药有缓释特征,肾靶向参数为71.97%,是对照组雷公藤多苷聚乳酸纳米粒的3.6倍。曹姗等采用乳化法制备磷脂纳米粒。结果制得纳米粒呈球状,动态光散射法测定其平均粒径(360±8)nm,包封率为(94.6±1.8)%,载药量为(1.13±0.02)%,72 h累计释放80%,加入空白血浆会减慢释放。曾莉等采用自乳化法制备川芎嗪聚乳酸纳米粒。结果以聚乳酸作为载体材料,优化工艺制备的川芎嗪聚乳酸纳米粒包封率为41.78%,渗漏率为4.80%,体外模拟释放表明载药纳米粒具有明显的缓释作用。刘宏盼等采用透析法制备靶向肽修饰的包载紫杉醇的低相对分子质量肝素-全反式维甲酸聚合物纳米粒。结果表明,制得的纳米粒的粒径为(131.7±2.3)nm,Zeta电位为-(27.1±2.3)mV,载药量和包封率分别为(32.03±0.11)%和(84.84±2.63)%。随着孵育时间的延长,纳米粒对B16F10细胞的毒性增加,孵育72 h后对B16F10细胞的半数抑制浓度为(41.6±7.2)ng/ml。体内药效学研究表明,纳米粒的抑瘤率达到75.28%,是混合药物溶液组的1.46倍。朱蓉等研究乳化-溶剂扩散法制备α-常春藤皂苷壳聚糖纳米粒。结果表明,制备的α-常春藤皂苷壳聚糖纳米粒平均粒径88.9 nm,多分散指数值(0.144±0.037),包封率(75.63±4.06)%。

(陶建生 孙晓燕)

【中药闪式提取的研究】

闪式提取法,也称组织破碎提取法,是根据组织破碎原理设计而成的一种新型提取方法,具有提取温度较低、快捷、节约能源的特点,对中药中热敏性和不稳定成分破坏较小。

谢仲德等以芍药苷含量为指标,采用正交试验优选白芍中芍药苷的闪式提取工艺,并与芍药苷乙醇回流法进行比较。结果最优工艺为,70%乙醇:料液=1:12,提取时间1 min。闪式提取法提取的芍药苷的量高于乙醇回流提取法。董自亮等以白芷中欧前胡素、香豆素为质量控制指标,利用闪式提取方法,在单因素试验基础上采用三因素三水平的Box-Behnken设计、响应面分析统计学方法,优化白芷香豆素闪式提取工艺。结果最佳工艺为,乙醇浓度75%,乙醇用量10倍量,提取时间106 s。在此条件下白芷香豆素的提取转移率可达88.754%。时圣明等采用闪式提取法提取三七果中的总皂苷,制备出9个供试品。以人参皂苷Rb_1为对照品,应用HPTLC测定各个供试品中的单体皂苷,优选闪式提取法的最佳工艺。结果表明,闪式提取可得到较高收率的总皂苷,且单体皂苷人参皂苷Rb_1的量较高。孟庆举等以左旋紫草素、羟基萘醌总色素的提取率为评价指标,比较闪式提取、回流提取、超声提取对紫草中有效成分的提取效果,并采用正交设计综合评分法对闪式提取的工艺参数进行优化。结果优选的最佳工艺为,95%乙醇提取3次,每次90 s。在此工艺条件下左旋紫草素、羟基萘醌总色素提取率分别为93.16%、93.89%,出膏率为5.16%。卢岚英等以栀子苷的含量和出膏率作为考察指标,比较闪式与回流提取对栀子提取效果的影响。结果表明,闪式提取所得栀子苷含量和出膏率高于回流法提取。张庆岭以梓醇及干膏的量为评价指标,通过单因素试验及正交试验优选闪式提取的最佳工艺,结果为加3倍量95%乙醇提取1次,提取时间3 min。赵宏等以黄酮提取率为指标,采用正交试验优选银杏叶总黄酮的闪式提取工艺条件。结果表明,当乙醇体积分数为60%,闪式提取时间30 s,料液比1:20时,银杏叶总黄酮的提取率最高,为1.99%。赵宏等以青龙衣提取物中总黄酮含量为指标,采用正交试验优选闪式提取青龙衣总黄酮的最佳工艺。结果表明,当料液比为1:20、闪式提取时间为60 s、乙醇体积分数为70%时,青龙衣总黄酮的提取率最高,为11.73%。曾祖平等以紫草总萘醌和β,β′-二甲基丙烯酰阿卡宁转移率为指标,采用正交试验研究溶剂用量、提取时间、提取电压等对闪式提取紫草中总萘醌提取效率的影响,并与渗漉法进行比较。结果最佳提取工艺为,加14、8倍量95%乙醇,于140 V电压下提取2次,每次2 min。闪式提取法中总萘醌和β,β′-二甲基丙烯酰阿卡宁平均转移率分别为90.72%、70.68%,渗漉法中两者平均转移率分别为79.03%、65.43%。表明闪式提取法优于渗漉法。

(陶建生 孙晓燕)

【中药的酶提取工艺研究】

酶解技术是基于酶的催化具有较高的催化效率、较强的转移性以及温和的催化条件等特性用于中药提取的一项新型技术。

张卉等采用β-葡聚糖酶、果胶酶、提取用酶、纤维素酶以及半仿生-纤维素酶研究甘草酸的半仿生-酶法提取工艺。结果最佳提取工艺为,提取温度80℃,料液比1:18,提取时间为2 h。纪学慧等采用纤维素酶提取法和超声提取法提取中药复方补气升血方药中的有效成分,并通过小鼠酚红排泌实验、炭粒廓清实验、二甲苯致小鼠耳肿胀实验等药效学指标评价探讨两种提取方法提取液的药效学差异。结果表明,纤维素酶提取法的药理作用优于超声提取法。陆世惠等优选酶解预处理后超声提取两面针中氯化两面针碱的工艺。结果最佳工艺为,纤维素酶:果胶酶底物质量比为

1∶250,4 倍量 pH5 缓冲液,室温(30℃)下酶解 30 min,再以 60%乙醇(含 5 g/L 盐酸)超声(250 W)提取 3 次,溶剂量分别为 10、4 和 3 倍量,每次 10 min,氯化两面针碱的提取率可达到 90.26%。年四辉等采用单因素试验,研究淀粉酶法从板蓝根中提取有效成分最佳工艺,结果为酶解温度 65℃、酶解 pH6、酶解时间 30 min、酶用量 40 U/g,使精氨酸、脯氨酸、水杨酸的提取质量分别比未加酶组分别提高 17.45%、18.15%、16.40%。张华采用正交试验,以盐酸小檗碱总浸出物为指标,对酶解提取黄连有效成分工艺参数进行优选。结果最佳酶解条件为,纤维素酶用量 0.15%、酶解时间 120 min、酶解温度 50℃、pH 值 6。验证试验证实该工艺稳定,酶解后进行提取盐酸小檗碱的提取量增加,比《中国药典》(2010 年版)方法增加 18.40%,比优选水提工艺增加 23.70%,纤维素酶可以增加黄连中盐酸小檗碱及其他有效成分的提取率。王勋等采用单因素试验和正交试验,优选复合酶提取天麻多糖的最佳工艺,结果为温度 50℃、加热时间 60 min、酶用量 20 mg、pH 值为 4,天麻多糖得率为 2.48%。杨春静等采用单因素试验筛选酶的种类,并以多糖总提取率为指标,正交设计优选酶法提取墨旱莲多糖的最佳工艺,结果为 pH5,纤维素酶用量 3%,酶解时间3 h,酶解温度 50℃。杨喆茗等采用单因素及正交试验,以柚子皮多糖的提取量为评价指标,优选柚子皮多糖纤维素酶辅助法的最佳提取工艺,结果为料液比 1∶30、反应时间 5.5 h、酶解温度 60℃、pH5.5、酶含量 0.1%。高建德等以苯乙醇苷作为评价指标,采用正交试验优选纤维素酶提取肉苁蓉中苯乙醇苷的最佳工艺,结果为纤维素酶 0.1%,酶解温度 55℃,酶解时间 2.5 h,可提高肉苁蓉有效成分的提取率。杨仙凌等以海藻多糖得率为指标,采用响应面分析法确定纤维素酶法提取海藻多糖的最佳工艺。结果表明,影响多糖得率的因素为,酶解温度>酶解时间>纤维素酶添加量。最佳提取工艺为,纤维素酶添加量 1.2%,酶解温度 46.5℃,酶解时间 100 min。使多糖得率为 4.64%,比传统水提法提高 7.41%。雒馨怡等以总黄酮提取率为指标,在单因素试验基础上采用 Box-Behnken 中心组合设计,用响应面法优化鹿衔草总黄酮的酶联半仿生法得到的提取工艺为,加酶量 1.25 mg/g 料液比 1∶65,酶解时间1 h,提取时间 1.75 h,提取温度 85℃,总黄酮提取率达 5.54%,与预测值 5.68%较为接近。王景翔等采用中性蛋白酶酶解法提取干香菇中的多糖,采用正交试验优选得到最佳提取工艺为,酶与干香菇粉的配比为 1∶30,酶解温度 40℃,酶解 pH7.5,酶解时间 90 min。邵方元等以多糖得率及其含量为指标,结合正交试验和人工神经网络方法,优化胰蛋白酶提取鱼腥草多糖的工艺。结果 BP 神经网络模型优化工艺为,加胰蛋白酶量 2.5%,于 45℃温浸 2.4 h;正交试验优选的工艺条件为,加胰蛋白酶量 2%,于 45℃温浸时间2.5 h;前者的综合评分略高于后者。刘淑蕊等结合正交试验与 BP 神经网络,筛选木瓜蛋白酶提取鱼腥草多糖的最佳工艺。以提取温度、提取时间及酶添加量为输入量,综合评分为输出量。结果由 BP 神经网络得到的最佳提取工艺为,pH7,提取温度 60℃,酶添加量 2.0%,提取时间 2.5 h。经验证,其综合评分高于正交试验的最优组合的得分。

(陶建生　孙晓燕)

【中药片剂制备的研究】

片剂是中药制剂常用的固体形式之一。新型中药片剂的类型包括双层片、骨架片、分散片、漂浮片、泡腾片、渗透泵片、结肠靶向片等,主要涉及处方优化、制备工艺、质量控制、释药特征等方面的研究。

朱肖肖等以片芯崩解时限、溶出度和外观为综合评价指标,采用正交试验优选复方甘草双层片片芯的制备工艺,结果为 5.6%微晶纤维素为填充剂,15.2%羧甲基淀粉钠(CMS－Na)为崩解剂,4.9%滑石粉为润滑剂,5.1%氧化镁为吸收剂。制备的片芯外表光洁,崩解时限(26.4±10)s,溶出度达 99%。郭迎新等采用单因素考察结合正交试验优选银杏黄酮凝胶骨架片的最佳工艺,结果为羟丙甲基纤维素(HPMC)(K4M－K100M 混合)为骨架材料,K4M∶K100M＝4∶1 的用量粘合剂(聚乙烯吡咯烷酮)为 3%,填充剂为乳糖。采用零级、一级、Higuchi 及 Ritger-pappas 模型对药物总黄酮醇苷释放曲线进行拟合,探讨药物释药机制。王建筑等以聚乙二醇 6000(PEG－6000)为载体,制备水飞蓟素固体分散体,采用直接粉末压片制备以魔芋胶为骨架材料的水飞蓟素缓释片。结果表明,制备的水飞蓟素缓释片体外释药规律符合 Ritger-Peppas 动力学模型,可持续释药 12 h。高源等以 HPMC 为骨架材料，乳糖、微晶纤维素（MCC）、淀粉为填充剂，硬脂酸镁为润滑剂制备氢溴酸高乌甲素骨架片。研究各因素对药物释放度的影响，筛选优化处方为，HPMC 40%、MCC 30%、硬脂酸镁0.5%。所制缓释片无突释现象，缓释周期12 h。根据拟合方程，药物释放符合一级释放模型，其释放既有扩散，又有骨架溶蚀。

宋文霞等以均匀设计筛选得到羟基喜树碱/羟丙基-β-环糊精包合物凝胶骨架缓释片制备包合物的最优处方，再以HPMC为凝胶骨架材料，乙醇为黏合剂，湿法制粒压片，制备包合物凝胶骨架缓释片，并进行体外释放实验。结果，包合物的包合率达到80%以上，缓释片的体外释放为一级释放模型，遵循Fick扩散定律。周珊珊等以不同型号的HPMC（K100M、E4M）为骨架材料，采用湿法制粒压片制备葛根素骨架缓释片。以葛根素释放度为指标，优选缓释片的处方，HPMC两种型号K100M和E4M的质量分数分别为片剂总质量的10%、20%；乳糖为填充剂，质量分数为片剂总质量的30%。制备的骨架缓释片具有良好的12 h体外释药特性，其释放规律符合Ritger-Peppas方程曲线，释药过程为药物扩散和骨架溶蚀协同作用。叶端炉等以崩解时间为指标，采用单因素试验优选补肾益脑分散片的处方，交联聚乙烯吡咯烷酮（PVPP）为崩解剂，MCC为填充剂，两种辅料比例为1∶2.7，80%乙醇为黏合剂制备分散片。采用HPTLC测定补肾益脑分散片中补骨脂素、异补骨脂素的总量。结果表明，不同批次补肾益脑分散片中补骨脂素、异补骨脂素的总量及溶出度无明显差异；与其他制剂比较，补肾益脑分散片体外溶出速率较快，且能达到最大溶出率。申雪丽等以崩解时间、混悬系数和抗张强度为指标，采用星点设计-效应面法优化沙棘黄酮提取物分散片的最佳成型处方，结果为PVPP 50.0 mg/片，羟丙基纤维素9.2 mg/片，聚维酮-K30 7.0 mg/片，预测值和测定值非常接近，偏差仅0.32%。高建德等优选平胃分散片的最佳处方工艺，结果为以交联CMC-Na-PVPP-MCC混合物（1∶1∶5）为崩解剂，在4 kg/cm^{2}压力下制备分散片，平均崩解时限为2.5 min。苏占辉等研究表明，金莲花总黄酮分散片的最佳处方为，选择MCC为填充剂148.48 g（37.12%），PEG-6000为润滑剂6.06 g（1.52%），95%乙醇为黏合剂，PVPP为崩解剂，内加34.09 g（8.52%），外加11.36 g（2.84%），金莲花总黄酮干膏粉200 g（50%），制成1 000片。制得的药片崩解时限均小于3 min，片重0.4 g。李琳等研究胃康漂浮缓释片的成型工艺。结果筛选得到辅料及用量分别为，HPMC为45%，羟乙基纤维素为10%，$NaHCO_3$为15%，以10%聚乙烯吡咯烷酮（PVP）的80%醇溶液作为润湿剂，湿法制粒压片，颗粒的临界相对湿度为73.5%。施之琪等采用干粉直接压片制备积雪草总苷胃漂浮片，以漂浮性能和体外释药性能为指标，采用单因素试验及混料设计试验优选胃漂浮片的处方参数。结果最佳处方工艺为，25%积雪草总苷，28.6% HPMC，15.6% $NaHCO_3$，20.8% CMS-Na，10% PEG-20000；制成的片剂起漂时间（3.2±0.2）min，持漂时间>12 h，体外释放符合零级动力学模型。制备的胃漂浮片具有优良的漂浮能力和释药行为，可增加积雪草总苷在胃部的滞留时间，提高对胃溃疡的疗效。吴敏等制备难溶性药物岩白菜素高载药量单室单层渗透泵型控释片。研究以渗透泵片常用辅料为混合载体材料制备固体分散体，利用等渗原理优化片芯处方；以岩白菜素累积释放度为指标，采用星点设计-效应面法优化包衣处方。结果表明，PEG-1500质量分数1.30%，包衣增重9.5%时，制得的岩白菜素高载药量渗透泵片累积释放度接近80%，符合零级释药特征。王立等以碳酸氢钠和柠檬酸为泡腾剂，聚氧乙烯N80为助悬剂制备片芯；以醋酸纤维素为包衣材料，邻苯二甲酸二乙酯为增塑剂，PEG-400为致孔剂制备葛根素泡腾性渗透泵控释片。结果表明，制备的葛根素泡腾性渗透泵控释片，在12 h内呈现零级释放（r>0.9990），药物累积释放度>85%。孙淑萍等采用非水制粒法、固体分散体技术、酸碱分别制粒、再混合压片法工艺制备妇科复方抗菌消炎泡腾片。采用单因素试验优选成型工艺，结果为乳糖和甘露醇为稀释剂，十二烷基硫酸钠、吐温-80加到7%的PVP75%乙醇溶液作为黏合剂，黄连素与$NaHCO_3$一起用PEG-6000进行包裹。汤瑾等采用HPTLC测定白头翁皂苷B_4的含量，按《中国药典》（2010年版）规定的方法，研究复方白头翁结肠靶向片的外观性状、脆碎度、释放度、质量差异，采用经典恒温试验计算制剂的有效期。结果表明，复方白头翁结肠靶向片在室温（25℃）条件下，有效期为2.69年。李艳玲等研究灯盏花素结肠定位片的体外释放性能。结果表明,灯盏花乙素在 pH1.2 稀盐酸溶液 2 h 中未检测到,在 pH6.8 磷酸盐缓冲液中,4 h 累积溶出率均小于 5%,而在 pH7.6 磷酸盐缓冲液中,1 h累积溶出率均达 90%以上。灯盏花素结肠定位片能达到结肠定位释药的目的。易鹏等以肠康宁为模型药物,制得胃溶型的黄芪片和 pH 敏感-酶触发型黄连片,从而制备肠康宁多元释药片。经体外溶出度试验,黄芪片胃溶型在胃部释药,黄连片能较好地达到结肠靶向释药。张娥等研究表明,葛根素包合物膜控控释片的释药行为受衣膜厚度、促渗剂、致孔剂的影响显著,采用最优处方制备的葛根素膜控控释片释放行为符合零级释放特征。

此外,还有许多中药片剂制备研究的相关报道,如杜利月等优选鬼针草总黄酮缓释片的处方工艺、苟美玲等研究白芷总香豆素缓释片的制备及体外释放度、柯仲成等采用星点设计-效应面法优化盐酸小檗碱缓释片处方、袁春玲等研究连钱草总黄酮缓释片的制备工艺及体外释放特性、蔡延渠等将指纹图谱与体外释放度相结合用于研究中药复方制剂喘平缓释片复杂成分体外释放、郑琴等研究大川芎脉冲片的制备工艺及体外释药特性等。

(陶建生　孙晓燕)

【中药脂质体制备的研究】

脂质体是通过磷脂双分子层膜所形成的囊泡包裹药物分子而形成。脂质体具有靶向给药功能,可减低药物毒性,提高药物稳定性,可以同时包裹脂溶性药物和水溶性药物,制备脂质体所用的材料生物相溶性好。

张兰等将大豆卵磷脂∶培化磷脂酰乙醇胺∶紫杉醇=100∶0.5∶5(摩尔比)混合并溶解于氯仿中,采用油水相研磨成乳,然后高压均质的方法制备脂质体。结果,制得的脂质体平均粒径为(140±10)nm,药脂摩尔比在 3%～6%内,包封率均大于 95%。毒性实验表明,紫杉醇脂质体和紫杉醇游离药对 KM 雄性小鼠的最大耐受剂量分别为 64.8 mg/kg 和 29.4 mg/kg。药效实验表明,紫杉醇脂质体剂量依赖性地抑制鼠肝癌 H22 肿瘤生长。紫杉醇脂质体具有较高包封率,与紫杉醇游离药相比可以显著提高治疗指数。王兴慧等采用 pH 梯度结合薄膜分散法制备盐酸小檗碱脂质体,并以包封率为指标,通过正交试验优选盐酸小檗碱脂质体的制备工艺,同时采用透析法研究脂质体的体外释放性质。结果最佳处方工艺为,磷脂胆固醇比 3∶1,药脂比 1∶15,磷脂质量浓度 30 g/L,外水相 pH7。制备的盐酸小檗碱脂质体包封率 89.34%,平均粒径 123.3 nm,Zeta 电位－20.0 mV,24 h 累积释放率 90.46%。郑杭生等研究盐酸青藤碱脂质体的制备工艺。结果表明,最适宜的制备工艺为薄膜分散法,水化液为柠檬酸缓冲液,pH 梯度载药可提高脂质体的包封率,大豆磷脂∶胆固醇=6∶1,一定粒径与处方药量的脂质体包封率大于 80%,成品脂质体的稳定性良好。刘广等采用薄膜分散法制备延胡索乙素柔性脂质体。结果表明,制备的脂质体包封率 82.7%,粒径(112.3±59.2)nm,基本呈正态分布。该制剂 12 h 内累积渗透量 2 121 μg,明显高于对照组酊剂的 1 153 μg,在皮肤内滞留率 53.9%,明显高于酊剂的 11.2%。齐娜等制备熊果酸脂质体并进行体外释放特性的研究。结果表明,优选的处方工艺为,载药量 6 mg,磷脂-胆固醇 2∶1,水和介质摩尔浓度 0.01 mol/L,超声时间 3 min,制备的熊果酸脂质体平均粒径(223.7±68.4)nm,zeta 电位－20.63 mv,包封率(89.85±1.66)%,48 h 体外累计释放率>80%,体外释放符合一级动力学模型。齐滨等采用逆相蒸发法制备西洋参 SOD 脂质体。结果表明,最佳制备工艺为卵磷脂∶胆固醇=4∶1,磷酸盐缓冲液体积 12 ml,西洋参 SOD 加入量 10 mg,制备的西洋参 SOD 脂质体形态均匀,平均粒径480 nm,平均包封率 71.35%。李娜等以包封率为指标,正交试验优选三七总皂苷脂质体冻干粉的处方工艺,采用塑制法制备三七总皂苷脂质体微丸。结果表明,脂质体冻干粉的最佳处方工艺为,大豆磷脂∶胆固醇=6∶1,水相∶有机相=1∶4,药物质量浓度 20 g/L,磷脂用量 150 mg。制备的脂质体微丸溶解后脂质体的平均粒径 220.5 nm,Zeta 电位－71.21 mV,1 h 内溶出度达 81.41%。郑杭生等研究制备全缘千里光碱脂质体、脂质体凝胶剂与普通凝胶剂。结果表明,脂质体凝胶剂与普通凝胶剂的释放行为基本一致,它们的药物释放速率均比脂质体快。将脂质体分散于 Carbopol 凝胶中,对脂质体中全缘千里光碱释放有促进作用。凝胶剂(含脂质体凝胶剂)与单纯脂质体释药机制有差异,前者可能倾向于溶蚀机制释药,后者倾向于扩散机制释药。何超芹等以氢化大豆磷脂和二棕榈酰磷脂酰胆碱为复合磷脂制备马钱子总生物碱复合磷脂脂质体、常规的二棕榈酰磷脂酰胆碱温敏脂质体和常规脂质体,比较三者温敏释放性质。结果表明，马钱子总生物碱复合磷脂脂质体在37℃的释放明显低于温敏脂质体，而在43℃的释放度高于温敏脂质体。常规脂质体由于相变温度很高，在这2种温度下都几乎不释放，复合磷脂脂质体具有更好的温敏释放行为。赵菊香等采用乙醇注入法制备苦参素空间稳定脂质体。结果表明，苦参素空间稳定脂质体平均包封率83.57%，体外释放曲线符合Higuchi方程，具有良好的体外缓释作用。林珈好等以大豆卵磷脂(SPC)和胆固醇(Ch)为膜材，薄膜分散探头超声法制备甘草次酸(GA)-丹参酮Ⅱ$_A$(TanⅡ$_A$)复方脂质体(GT-Lip)。通过单因素试验和正交试验优选最佳处方工艺为，SPC∶Ch质量比6∶1，SPC∶TanⅡ$_A$质量比30∶1，SPC∶GA质量比24∶1，水合温度为30℃，探头超声条件为380 W超声5 min。制备得到的GT-Lip中TanⅡ$_A$、GA的包封率分别为(81.50±0.76)%、(98.63±0.90)%，平均Zeta电位为－(19.00±0.98)mV，平均粒径为(120.5±1.62)nm。牟琳琳等采用离子交换法建立跨膜pH梯度并制备盐酸小檗碱脂质体。结果表明，包封率随外水相pH的升高而增加，最佳pH调节剂为磷酸盐缓冲液，磷脂为氢化大豆卵磷脂时包封率最高，随载药温度的升高和载药时间的增加包封率有提高的趋势，但基本不受加药顺序的影响，最佳药脂比为1∶10。在最优处方工艺下盐酸小檗碱脂质体的包封率为(98.6±0.68)%，平均粒径为124.1 nm。王永利等采用薄膜-超声分散法研究大黄酚脂质体悬混液制备大黄酚冻干脂质体。结果表明，预冻时间为24 h，干燥时间为24 h，以甘露醇∶蔗糖＝1∶1为保护剂，外加法得到的大黄酚冻干脂质体，粒径均匀，复溶性极好，包封率达(61.30±2.2)%。侯甲福等采用薄膜分散-超声法制备穿心莲内酯脂质体。结果最佳制备工艺为，大豆卵磷脂∶胆固醇＝6∶1，大豆卵磷脂∶穿心莲内酯＝4∶1，维生素E 20 mg，超声时间5 min。制备的穿心莲内酯脂质体平均粒径625.8 nm，包封率81.35%。何晓金等采用薄膜超声法制备载药纳米结构脂质载体，利用Box-Behnken效应面设计法筛选载药纳米结构脂质载体的最佳处方。结果表明，最优处方制备的载药纳米结构脂质载体外形呈圆形或椭球形，粒径分布均匀，平均粒径为(58.37±2.60)nm，Zeta电位为－(22.6±0.88)mV，包封率为(93.48±0.86)%，药物以非结晶状分散于纳米结构脂质载体中。

（陶建生　孙晓燕）

[附]　参考文献

B

白永智，李昌禹，赵景辉，等. 高压脉冲电场法快速提取黄花乌头中关附甲素的工艺研究[J]. 中草药，2013，44(10)：1267

C

蔡延渠，陈健，谢吉福，等. 基于指纹图谱喘平缓释片复杂成分均衡释放的评价[J]. 中国中药杂志，2013，38(9)：1360

曹姗，胡凯莉，刘梅，等. 多西紫杉醇口服磷脂纳米粒的制备与处方优化[J]. 中成药，2013，35(9)：1896

陈超，陈国芹，陈阿丽，等. AB-8型大孔吸附树脂纯化复方通脉颗粒有效部位的工艺优选[J]. 中国实验方剂学杂志，2013，19(5)：4

陈明霞，张建宝，于季萍，等. 重组水蛭素-2鼻腔给药纳米粒冻干粉制备工艺及体外渗透特性研究[J]. 中药材，2013，36(6)：999

陈伟，张鹏，彭国平，等. 不同孔径超滤膜对栀子苷热原去除工艺的影响[J]. 中国实验方剂学杂志，2013，19(10)：11

陈小云，张振海，胡琴，等. 辅料羟丙基甲基纤维素-硬脂酸作为辣椒素透皮凝胶基质的研究[J]. 中草药，2013，44(3)：296

陈小云，张振海，胡绍英，等. 基于硬脂酸改性纳米碳酸钙的雷公藤红素缓释固体分散体的研究[J]. 中国药学杂志，2013，48(16)：1380

陈新民，陈丽华，彭稳稳，等. 丹黄凝胶剂成型工艺研究[J]. 中成药，2013，35(5)：944

陈修克，魏颖慧，姚金娜，等. 壳聚糖修饰的雷公藤多苷纳米粒的制备及其肾靶向性研究[J]. 中国中药杂志，2013，38(4)：548

陈雪，田原，于睿，等. 正交试验法优选清脂通脉颗粒醇提工艺[J]. 中国实验方剂学杂志，2013，19(11)：22

陈玉玺，王冰，浦益琼，等. 20(S)-原人参二醇聚乳酸-羟基乙酸缓释微球的制备[J]. 中国实验方剂学杂志，2013，19(6)：4

D

董自亮,卢君蓉,高飞,等. 芍药苷微囊的制备及其体外释药研究[J]. 中草药,2013,44(13):1756

董自亮,徐瑞超. 基于 Box-Behnken 设计-响应面法优化白芷香豆素闪式提取工艺[J]. 中药与临床,2013,4(1):13

杜利月,崔燕兵,郭留城. 鬼针草总黄酮缓释片处方工艺优选[J]. 中国实验方剂学杂志,2013,19(14):67

F

符少莲,冯翠娟,李沙. 星点设计-效应面法优化脂溶性丹参提取物速释滴丸处方工艺[J]. 中成药,2013,35(4):690

G

高建德,金辉,朱书强,等. 平胃分散片工艺研究[J]. 中国中医药信息杂志,2013,20(5):60

高建德,刘雄,魏舒畅,等. 纤维素酶提取肉苁蓉中苯乙醇苷的工艺研究[J]. 中药材,2013,36(2):311

高源,李凤英,刘玲,等. 氢溴酸高乌甲素亲水凝胶骨架片的制备及体外释放[J]. 中国现代应用药学,2013,30(7):740

葛克亚,杜茂波,刘淑芝,等. 万通筋骨喷雾剂的体外经皮渗透效果考察[J]. 中国实验方剂学杂志,2013,19(5):1

宫春博,康怀兴. 加酸加盐水蒸气蒸馏法提取牡丹皮中丹皮酚的工艺研究[J]. 山东中医药大学学报,2013,37(2):162

苟美玲,李玲,孙鹏,等. 白芷总香豆素缓释片的制备及体外释放度的研究[J]. 时珍国医国药,2013,24(1):135

郭涛,庞来祥,程静. 养肝疏胆颗粒成型工艺处方优选[J]. 现代中药研究与实践,2013,26(2):53

郭迎新,李非,赵倩倩,等. 正交设计法优选银杏黄酮凝胶骨架片处方工艺[J]. 中国中药杂志,2013,38(11):1725

国大亮,何新,刘玉璇,等. 黄芩苷鼻用凝胶的制备及其经鼻扩散研究[J]. 中草药,2013,44(10):1253

H

何超芹,胡梦雅,张会,等. 马钱子总生物碱复合磷脂脂质体的制备与温敏释放性质研究[J]. 中国中药杂志,2013,38(9):1366

何晓金,李丹,陈大为,等. Box-Behnken 效应面法优化姜黄素纳米结构脂质载体处方[J]. 沈阳药科大学学报,2013,30(8):583

何杨,刘彬丽,李木子,等. 快速膜乳化-溶剂萃取/挥发法制备水飞蓟宾 PLGA 微球的工艺优选[J]. 中国实验方剂学杂志,2013,19(1):1

贺义恒,张红夏,李亮,等. 恒山黄芪粉碎度与黄芪多糖得率关联度研究[J]. 中草药,2013,44(9):1141

侯甲福,赵玉佳,梁启超,等. 穿心莲内酯脂质体的制备及质量控制[J]. 中国实验方剂学杂志,2013,19(16):35

侯莉伟,杨凤梅,杨明,等. Box-Behnken 设计优化荷叶总黄酮的温浸提取工艺[J]. 中国实验方剂学杂志,2013,19(18):51

胡德奇,华方波,穆春旭. 抱茎苦荬菜(苦碟子)减压提取工艺实验研究[J]. 辽宁中医杂志,2013,40(5):977

胡绍英,张振海,蒋艳荣,等. 雷公藤红素胶体二氧化硅缓释固体分散体研究[J]. 中草药,2013,44(6):692

黄巧文,郭晓芳,张增弟. 舒秘胶囊的辐射灭菌效果研究[J]. 海峡药学,2013,25(3):58

黄弦,左月明,罗光明,等. 多指标评价栀子超声提取工艺[J]. 时珍国医国药,2013,24(7):1568

J

纪学慧,张华. 补气升血方药纤维素酶提取法和超声提取法的药效学比较[J]. 辽宁中医药大学学报,2013,15(7):73

贾永艳,袁玉霞,周宁,等. 黄连总生物碱明胶微球的制备工艺优选[J]. 中国实验方剂学杂志,2013,19(11):11

蒋艳荣,张振海,夏海建,等. 基于共聚维酮的丹参酮 $Ⅱ_A$ 固体分散体的研究[J]. 中国中药杂志,2013,38(2):174

K

柯仲成,程子洋. 星点设计-效应面法优化盐酸小檗碱缓释片处方[J]. 中成药,2013,35(7):1555

L

赖春花,邱天健,郑琴,等. 丹参总酮缓释微丸的制备及处方工艺优化[J]. 中国实验方剂学杂志,2013,19(13):18

李海燕,朱庆文,杜红,等. 穿心莲内酯直肠微乳的 pH 和吸收促进剂用量考察[J]. 中国实验方剂学杂志,2013,19(4):41

李洪松,张学顺,傅春升,等. 苦参碱自微乳化制剂的制备工艺研究[J]. 中草药,2013,44(4):414

李进,王盛,李祥,等. 超滤技术分离纯化板蓝根有效成分的工艺研究[J]. 中成药,2013,35(3):622

李静,周英,徐秀玲,等. 壳聚糖修饰的雷公藤甲素聚乙二醇-聚乳酸纳米粒的制备及质量评价[J]. 中国药学杂志,2013,48(9):700

李琳,陈正君,刘雄,等. 胃康漂浮缓释片的成型工艺

研究[J]. 甘肃中医学院学报，2013，30(3)：31

李娜，崔翰明，李小芳. 三七总皂苷脂质体微丸的制备[J]. 中国实验方剂学杂志，2013，19(18)：35

李娜，崔翰明，吴萍，等. 丹参酮固体分散体滴丸的制备工艺优选[J]. 中国实验方剂学杂志，2013，19(3)：8

李卿，宋国红，秦伟翰，等. 消郁安神胶囊中挥发油β-环糊精包合物的热稳定性考察[J]. 中国实验方剂学杂志，2013，19(14)：17

李石清，徐磊，熊耀康，等. 基于 Box-Behnken 设计优选南方红豆杉多糖微波提取工艺研究[J]. 中华中医药学刊，2013，31(10)：2221

李守信，张则平，邱新建，等. 生脉散超微粉的显微特征和溶出度研究[J]. 现代药物与临床，2013，28(2)：175

李小菊，张越非，钟玲，等. 响应曲面法优化微波辅助提取魔芋葡甘露聚糖的工艺研究[J]. 时珍国医国药，2013，24(3)：525

李小玲，田男，范春雷. 莪术油-壳聚糖缓释微囊的制备及体外释放度研究[J]. 海峡药学，2013，25(4)：6

李晓宁，杨银花，赵博琛，等. 超临界 CO_2 流体技术萃取当归挥发油的工艺优选[J]. 中国实验方剂学杂志，2013，19(14)：27

李雪玲，黄德浩，刘莉，等. 正交设计优选炎宁无糖颗粒成型工艺[J]. 辽宁中医药大学学报，2013，15(1)：58

李艳玲，王锦玉，杨德斌，等. 灯盏花素结肠定位片的制备工艺及体外释放度评价[J]. 中国中药杂志，2013，38(6)：817

李毅民，石志娜，谢瑞芳，等. 大承气汤常压机器煎煮的工艺优化[J]. 中药材，2013，36(4)：657

李盈蕾，陈建华，王寅. 青风藤中青藤碱微波提取工艺的星点设计-效应面法优化[J]. 时珍国医国药，2013，24(3)：659

林珈好，王秀丽，王玉蓉，等. 甘草次酸-丹参酮ⅡA 复方脂质体处方优化及制备工艺研究[J]. 中草药，2013，44(7)：816

林青，李媛，李媚，等. 川芎-香附药对超临界萃取工艺优化及含量测定[J]. 中药材，2013，36(2)：302

林小玲，田成旺，张铁军. 星点设计-效应面法优选参芪消岩颗粒渗漉提取工艺[J]. 中草药，2013，44(4)：430

刘聪敏，白洁，杜守颖，等. 止痛凝胶膏剂的制备及体外释放考察[J]. 中国实验方剂学杂志，2013，19(15)：5

刘广，齐娜，孙考祥，等. 延胡索乙素柔性脂质体的制备与透皮吸收[J]. 中国实验方剂学杂志，2013，19(8)：37

刘宏盼，奚泉，周建平，等. RGD 肽修饰紫杉醇聚合物纳米粒的制备及其药效学研究[J]. 中国药科大学学报，2013，44(3)：228

刘宏伟，朱邻遐，王威，等. 跌打喷雾剂的制备及体外渗透性研究[J]. 现代中药研究与实践，2013，26(2)：46

刘敏彦，张永锋，史东霞，等. 陶瓷膜过滤对连花清瘟胶囊水提液纯化工艺的影响[J]. 中国中医药信息杂志，2013，20(1)：64

刘其媛，张振海，蒋艳荣，等. 基于壳聚糖的丹参酮ⅡA 固体分散体的研究[J]. 中草药，2013，44(4)：420

刘珊珊，赵会英，侯振兴. 热熔挤出法制备槲皮素固体分散体[J]. 中国现代应用药学，2013，30(7)：748

刘淑蕊，薛兴阳，周苏娟，等. 基于 BP 神经网络对木瓜蛋白酶法提取鱼腥草多糖工艺的优化[J]. 广东药学院学报，2013，29(2)：130

刘伟星，李宁，高崇凯. 葛根素自微乳化渗透泵控释胶囊的制备[J]. 中草药，2013，44(12)：1568

刘学仁，蔡品品，姜涛，等. 微波辅助提取枳壳中柚皮苷、新橙皮苷的工艺研究[J]. 中成药，2013，35(2)：420

娄杰，贾运涛，田睿，等. 眼用小檗碱白蛋白纳米粒温敏原位凝胶的制备及性质研究[J]. 中草药，2013，44(3)：277

卢岚英，王萍. 闪式提取与回流法对栀子提取工艺的比较[J]. 陕西中医，2013，34(4)：473

陆世惠，李秀霞. 超声-酶法提取两面针中氯化两面针碱的研究[J]. 中成药，2013，35(4)：841

雒馨怡，陈晓辉，毕开顺，等. 响应面法优化鹿衔草总黄酮的酶联半仿生法提取工艺[J]. 中国实验方剂学杂志，2013，19(12)：19

吕子明，于向红，陈凯，等. 正交试验法优选黄连浸膏的喷雾干燥工艺[J]. 中国实验方剂学杂志，2013，19(1)：10

M

马合木提·买买提明，赛力慢·哈得尔，麦得尼亚提·霍加. 超声-微波协同萃取芜菁籽中总黄酮提取工艺的研究[J]. 中成药，2013，35(2)：417

马瑞丽，张蓉，徐秀泉，等. 响应面分析法优化大血藤中总酚的超声提取工艺[J]. 中成药，2013，35(2)：404

孟庆举，易红，杨华，等. 闪式提取法用于紫草的工艺条件研究[J]. 中国中药杂志，2013，38(14)：2302

缪菊连，黄照昌. 三七总皂苷注射液的超滤工艺考察[J]. 中国实验方剂学杂志，2013，19(2)：35

牟琳琳，徐洋，蒋宫平，等. 改良 pH 梯度法制备盐酸小檗碱脂质体[J]. 中国药学杂志，2013，48(1)：49

N

倪东杰，陆萍. 综合评分法优化健骨口服液的澄清工艺[J]. 解放军药学学报，2013，29(2)：135

年四辉，刘丽敏，张艳华，等. 多指标淀粉酶法提取板蓝根有效成分工艺初步探讨[J]. 中成药，2013，35(3)：625

P

帕丽达·阿布力孜，丛媛媛，米仁沙·牙库甫，等. 响

应面法优化牛舌草总黄酮的超声提取工艺[J]. 中国实验方剂学杂志,2013,19(3):48

潘娅,张燕君,谢昭朐,等. 马钱子碱-β-环糊精包合物的制备及表征[J]. 中成药,2013,35(8):1805

彭菲,叶正良,李德坤,等. 不同材质及不同截留分子量超滤膜对人参皂苷类成分的影响[J]. 中成药,2013,35(5):937

浦益琼,王冰,张彤,等. 大孔树脂柱层析法制备茜草总醌提取物的实验研究[J]. 中成药,2013,35(9):1900

Q

齐滨,刘莉,张楠楠,等. 西洋参SOD脂质体的制备工艺优选和性质评价[J]. 中国实验方剂学杂志,2013,19(18):17

齐娜,刘广,廖迎,等. 熊果酸脂质体的制备及体外释放特性考察[J]. 中国实验方剂学杂志,2013,19(2):28

齐学洁,邱超,姜恒丽,等. 白藜芦醇/羟丙基-β-环糊精包合物的表征及体外溶出研究[J]. 天津中医药,2013,30(8):499

S

邵方元,付腾飞,薛兴阳,等. 正交试验和BP人工神经网络模型优化胰蛋白酶提取鱼腥草多糖的工艺[J]. 中国实验方剂学杂志,2013,19(11):14

申雪丽,袁勇,黄川生,等. 星点设计-效应面法优化沙棘黄酮提取物分散片处方[J]. 中国实验方剂学杂志,2013,19(17):19

沈熊,梁健,黄廼奇,等. Box-Behnken响应面法优化黄芩素微丸的缓释包衣处方[J]. 中成药,2013,35(5):940

施之琪,王洛临,杜建平,等. 积雪草总苷胃漂浮片处方工艺优选[J]. 中国实验方剂学杂志,2013,19(12):15

时圣明,王文倩,袁永兵,等. 三七果中有效成分的闪式提取工艺研究[J]. 药物评价研究,2013,36(2):135

宋文霞,索绪斌,邓妍芳,等. 羟基喜树碱/羟丙基-β-环糊精包合物凝胶骨架缓释片的制备及体外释放[J]. 中成药,2013,35(6):1188

宋艳丽,韩腾飞,李莎莎,等. 栀子苷经鼻给药醇质体喷雾剂的制备及其体外鼻黏膜渗透性研究[J]. 中草药,2013,44(9):1105

苏秀霞,杨玉娜,李凯斌,等. 羟丙基-β-环糊精包合当归油的工艺研究[J]. 中成药,2013,35(2):414

苏占辉,王书君,张滋明,等. 金莲花总黄酮分散片处方工艺优选[J]. 中国实验方剂学杂志,2013,19(6):8

孙丹丹,徐新刚,生立嵩,等. 星点设计-效应面法优化熊果酸自微乳给药系统[J]. 中国实验方剂学杂志,2013,19(8):46

孙姣,秦莉,李桂水,等. 壳聚糖对小儿咳喘灵原药提取液絮凝除杂效果研究[J]. 中草药,2013,44(2):174

孙立霞,常桂娟,李秋萌,等. 参玉口服液澄清工艺优选[J]. 中国实验方剂学杂志,2013,19(17):4

孙淑萍,吴少云,李胜利,等. 妇科复方抗菌消炎泡腾片的成型工艺研究[J]. 中成药,2013,35(2):423

T

汤瑾,刘文,冯果,等. 复方白头翁结肠靶向片的稳定性考察[J]. 中国实验方剂学杂志,2013,19(2):17

唐黎,施璐,陈明,等. 大蒜素速溶肠溶胶囊的研究[J]. 湖北中医药大学学报,2013,15(4):38

唐梅,刘剑云,刘英,等. Box-Behnken设计优化黄芩的浸渍-压榨提取工艺[J]. 中国实验方剂学杂志,2013,19(3):58

童婷婷,谭玉柱,赵高琼,等. 大孔树脂纯化大黄地上部位总蒽醌的工艺研究[J]. 中成药,2013,35(4):848

W

汪洋,焦海胜. 正交试验优选刺五加提取物缓释微球的制备工艺[J]. 中国实验方剂学杂志,2013,19(2):32

王春柳,赵国巍,廖正根,等. 超微粉碎对七厘散稳定性的影响[J]. 中国实验方剂学杂志,2013,19(9):1

王春民,杨冬丽,郑艳春,等. 二次蒸馏-萃取耦合法提取颈复康制剂挥发油的研究[J]. 中成药,2013,35(5):1099

王洪珍,张炜煜. 益髓通经缓释颗粒成型工艺及释药机理的研究[J]. 时珍国医国药,2013,24(5):1117

王建筑,李菲,郝吉福,等. 水飞蓟素骨架型缓释片的制备[J]. 中成药,2013,35(5):1104

王景翔,王娟,赵建录,等. 正交设计优化香菇多糖酶解法提取工艺的研究[J]. 时珍国医国药,2013,24(3):648

王立,张君,王文倩. 葛根素泡腾性渗透泵控释片的制备及其体外评价[J]. 中草药,2013,44(6):686

王念明,张定堃,杨明,等. 超微粉碎对黄芩粉体学性质的影响[J]. 中药材,2013,36(4):640

王权,吴德玲,黄金玲,等. 多指标正交试验优选苓桂术甘颗粒水提工艺[J]. 安徽中医学院学报,2013,32(4):87

王文刚,郭晓华,武向锋. 注射用紫杉醇亚微乳的制备及其性质考察[J]. 解放军药学学报,2013,29(2):112

王兴慧,李俊生,吕佳佳,等. 盐酸小檗碱脂质体的制备工艺优选及体外释放性质考察[J]. 中国实验方剂学杂志,2013,19(18):39

王勋,罗珊珊,蒋嘉烨,等. 酶解法提取天麻多糖的研究[J]. 中药材,2013,36(1):137

王永利,王立华,张江伟,等. 大黄酚冻干脂质体的制备工艺研究[J]. 中草药,2013,44(8):960

王友芳，朱善岚，洪清，等. 复方天宁滴丸稳定性考察[J]. 中国实验方剂学杂志，2013，19(15)：46

王姿媛，何泽民. 苍术-厚朴药对超临界萃取工艺研究及质量控制[J]. 中国实验方剂学杂志，2013，19(4)：155

王梓，李伟，郑毅男. 响应曲面优化加压溶剂提取五味子中4种木脂素[J]. 人参研究，2013，25(1)：27

魏颖慧，赵燕敏，李静，等. 壳聚糖修饰雷公藤多苷纳米粒的制备及其体外释药研究[J]. 中草药，2013，44(5)：541

乌日娜，那生桑，包勒朝鲁. 复方沙棘颗粒剂的喷雾干燥工艺优选[J]. 中国实验方剂学杂志，2013，19(4)：56

吴建雄，秦建平，曹光环，等. 天舒滴丸的成型工艺研究[J]. 现代中药研究与实践，2013，26(4)：49

吴建雄，秦建平，万琴，等. 大孔树脂纯化红花中羟基红花黄色素A的产业化探索[J]. 中国实验方剂学杂志，2013，19(16)：5

吴敏，李德银，谢佳，等. 岩白菜素高载药量渗透泵型控释片的制备[J]. 中国实验方剂学杂志，2013，19(1)：25

吴素香，苏璇，李智慧，等. 复凝聚法制备留兰香油微囊的处方工艺研究[J]. 中成药，2013，35(6)：1193

X

夏海建，张振海，贾晓斌. 雷公藤红素缓释滴丸的研究[J]. 中草药，2013，44(7)：834

肖金宝，李洪斌，刘福强，等. 银杏叶提取物温度敏感型鼻用原位凝胶体外释放研究[J]. 中成药，2013，35(1)：46

谢友良，童玉林，赵学军，等. 辐射灭菌对西洋参巴布剂质量的影响[J]. 中国实验方剂学杂志，2013，19(8)：98

谢仲德，李文烈，方应权，等. 白芍中芍药苷的闪式提取工艺研究[J]. 中成药，2013，35(9)：2037

徐桂红，林夏，曹苗苗，等. 注射用活血通络制剂的冷冻干燥工艺优选[J]. 中国实验方剂学杂志，2013，19(13)：25

许日鑫，石添香，廖娴，等. β-细辛醚微乳的制备及其性质考察[J]. 中草药，2013，44(1)：31

Y

严国俊，蔡宝昌，潘金火，等. 星点设计-效应面法优化复方垂盆草微丸制备工艺[J]. 中药材，2013，36(4)：661

严金桥. 丹参川芎药对流浸膏的喷雾干燥工艺研究[J]. 湖北中医药大学学报，2013，15(2)：37

杨春静，张杰，张华锋，等. 墨旱莲多糖的酶法提取工艺优选[J]. 中国实验方剂学杂志，2013，19(12)：63

杨鹏飞，丁兰萍，蔡晓蕾，等. 银杏内酯B自微乳的处方优选及质量、安全性评价[J]. 中国实验方剂学杂志，2013，19(12)：26

杨仙凌，刘鑫，蒋亚奇. 响应面法优化海藻多糖的酶法提取工艺[J]. 中华中医药学刊，2013，31(8)：1794

杨喆茗，张益铭，许伟民，等. 纤维素酶辅助法提取柚子皮中多糖的工艺研究[J]. 人参研究，2013，25(2)：31

叶陈丽，贺帅，张守尧，等. Box-Behnken 设计优化黄芩超高压提取工艺[J]. 中国实验方剂学杂志，2013，19(3)：40

叶端炉，刘根才，孔晓霞. 补肾益脑分散片的制备及其质量控制研究[J]. 中草药，2013，44(12)：1599

易鹏，李航，文怡静，等. 肠康宁多元释药片剂的制备工艺研究[J]. 中药与临床，2013，4(2)：32

于蓓蓓，闫雪生，郭艳伟，等. 正交试验法优选桑椹补脑膏的壳聚糖絮凝工艺[J]. 中国实验方剂学杂志，2013，19(9)：37

袁春玲，赵亮，王亚娟. 连钱草总黄酮缓释片的制备及体外释放度研究[J]. 中药材，2013，36(1)：127

Z

曾莉，毛春芹，陆兔林，等. 川芎嗪聚乳酸纳米粒的制备和质量研究[J]. 中成药，2013，35(2)：261

曾祖平，钱珊，王宏，等. 紫草总萘醌的闪式提取工艺优选[J]. 中国实验方剂学杂志，2013，19(15)：29

战兵，张超，盛华刚，等. 壳聚糖絮凝沉降法对蒽醌类成分的影响[J]. 中国实验方剂学杂志，2013，19(2)：4

张德新，陈炜，陈松瑞. 半仿生法优化玉米须总皂苷的提取工艺[J]. 湖北中医杂志，2013，35(2)：71

张娥，谭睿，顾健，等. 葛根素包合物膜控控释片的处方优化及体外释药研究[J]. 中国中药杂志，2013，38(1)：49

张恒玉，杨莹，张琳. 银杏酮酯自乳化软胶囊的制备及质量评价[J]. 药学研究，2013，32(1)：29

张洪兵，朱雪瑜，张铁军，等. 星点设计-效应面优化法优选复方止痛巴布剂基质处方[J]. 中草药，2013，44(8)：985

张华. 黄连有效成分酶解法提取工艺研究[J]. 山东中医杂志，2013，32(6)：425

张卉，赵婷婷，戴柳江，等. 半仿生-酶法提取甘草中甘草酸的工艺研究[J]. 中国现代应用药学，2013，30(9)：969

张慧，谭秋龙，黎行山，等. 结合响应面分析法优化复方金钱草中君药的半仿生提取工艺[J]. 广东药学院学报，2013，29(1)：29

张家成，刘峰，张岩，等. 煎药机煎煮加水量与时间对旋覆代赭汤5种有效成分溶出量的影响[J]. 世界中西医结合杂志，2013，8(5)：457

张家成，刘峰，张岩，等. 煎药机煎煮时浸泡时间对旋覆代赭汤5种有效成分溶出量的影响[J]. 环球中医药，

2013,6(2): 88

张建军,全智慧,付建武,等.超临界 CO_2 流体萃取丹参中丹参酮 $Ⅱ_A$ 的工艺研究[J].中成药,2013,35(6): 1329

张兰,韩毅,樊程程,等.软坚消瘿颗粒中挥发油提取及β-环糊精包合工艺研究[J].中华中医药学刊,2013,31(5): 974

张兰,李彦辉,王彩霞,等.紫杉醇脂质体的制备及初步毒性、药效学研究[J].中国药学杂志,2013,48(6): 446

张庆岭.鲜地黄的闪式提取工艺优选[J].中国实验方剂学杂志,2013,19(1): 62

张生,王宇,王少明,等.响应面法优化连翘中桦木酸超声辅助提取工艺[J].中国实验方剂学杂志,2013,19(17): 15

张涛,景明.归芪通便颗粒成型工艺研究[J].甘肃中医学院学报,2013,30(1): 61

赵宏,王宇亮,唐雨薇,等.正交试验法优选青龙衣总黄酮闪式提取工艺[J].辽宁中医杂志,2013,40(7): 1435

赵宏,张宇,王宇亮,等.银杏叶总黄酮闪式提取工艺的正交设计法优化[J].时珍国医国药,2013,24(8): 1852

赵菊香,程怡,吴琼,等.苦参素空间稳定脂质体的包封率测定和体外释放度考察[J].中国实验方剂学杂志,2013,19(3): 4

赵一洁,张丹参,张力,等.大黄酸肠溶缓释微丸的制备及体外释放度考察[J].中成药,2013,35(6): 1199

郑杭生,黄绳武,李范珠,等.盐酸青藤碱脂质体的制备工艺研究[J].中草药,2013,44(4): 408

郑杭生,黄绳武,徐莲英.全缘千里光碱脂质体及其凝胶剂的体外释药比较研究[J].中成药,2013,35(9): 2027

郑琴,周欢,钱佳,等.大川芎脉冲片的制备工艺及体外释药特性研究[J].江西中医学院学报,2013,25(2): 48

周福军,单淇,侯文彬,等.止痛巴布剂的体外透皮促进剂筛选[J].中国实验方剂学杂志,2013,19(15): 20

周秋娜,尉小慧,王峥涛.黄芩素-羟丙基-γ-环糊精包合物制备工艺研究[J].上海中医药杂志,2013,47(8): 82

周珊珊,谭睿,谢彬,等.葛根素骨架缓释片的研制及体外释放评价[J].中国实验方剂学杂志,2013,19(3): 23

朱开梅,顾生玖,骆彩珍,等.微波辅助提取香蕉皮总多酚的工艺优选[J].中国实验方剂学杂志,2013,19(15): 35

朱梦良,招丽君,梁新丽,等.大孔吸附树脂分离纯化葛根总黄酮和葛根素的工艺优选[J].中国实验方剂学杂志,2013,19(4): 23

朱蓉,尹红然,游本刚,等.α-常春藤皂苷壳聚糖纳米粒的制备及其体外评价[J].中成药,2013,35(9): 1906

朱双燕,崔名全,尹蓉莉,等.鸦胆子油自微乳化制剂的处方优化及质量评价[J].中药与临床,2013,4(3): 11

朱双燕,尹蓉莉,崔名全,等.穿心莲内酯自微乳化制剂的处方优化及质量评价[J].中国实验方剂学杂志,2013,19(8): 55

朱肖肖,牟志刚,姚小娟,等.正交试验优选复方甘草双层片片芯的制备工艺[J].中国实验方剂学杂志,2013,19(18): 45

祝倩倩,萧伟,孙永成,等.注射用芪红脉通配液除杂工艺研究[J].中草药,2013,44(6): 696

祝星,富志军,童心,等.温脐巴布剂基质处方的优选[J].解放军药学学报,2013,29(3): 221

(五) 中药炮制

【概述】

2013年，有关中药炮制方面发表的论文约400余篇，除炮制历史沿革、饮片鉴别和贮存等内容外，实验研究的论文约有300余篇。其中以优化炮制工艺研究、炮制前后成分含量的比较研究、炮制前后毒性与药效比较研究和饮片质量标准研究为主。

1. 炮制工艺的研究

（1）简单比较法　黄婷等采用HPTLC法，以补骨脂素、异补骨脂素、补骨脂甲素、补骨脂乙素四种成分为指标，从药汁制（五味子、枸杞、菟丝子、核桃仁）、盐制、水煮3种方法中优选出补骨脂的炮制工艺为药汁制。李凯等比较了不同软化方法对白芍饮片中芍药苷和芍药内酯苷含量的影响，结果闷润法和蒸法均优于减压冷浸法、煮法及浸泡法。

（2）正交试验多指标评价法　刘波等以大黄酸、大黄素、大黄酚、芦荟大黄素和大黄素甲醚为指标，优选小苏打制大黄的最佳炮制工艺，结果为取净大黄饮片，加入浓度为15%、用量为药材重量10%的小苏打溶液拌匀，闷润至液体被吸尽，120℃炒干。王德珍等以小檗碱、表小檗碱、黄连碱和巴马汀碱4种生物碱含量为指标，优选酒黄连、姜黄连、萸黄连的最佳炮制工艺，结果分别为闷润90 min后130℃烘制4 h、闷润60 min后100℃烘制3 h、闷润90 min后160℃烘制2 h。王晓崴等以马钱子碱和士的宁含量为指标，优选醋泡马钱子的最佳炮制工艺，结果为香醋：药液＝3：14(W/V)，醋浸1 d，水漂1 d。黄弦等以水浸出物、醇浸出物及栀子苷质量分数为综合评价指标，优选焦栀子的最佳炮制工艺，结果为180℃炒30 min。仙园园等以总酚酸、总硫苷、刺激性成分（异硫氰酸甲酯、异硫氰酸异丙酯、异硫氰酸丁酯和异硫氰酸异丁酯）的含量为指标，优选刺山柑的最佳炮制工艺，结果为选用过40～50目筛的药材粉末，80℃炒制15 min。

（3）正交试验单指标评价法　汪岩等以可溶性蛋白质质量分数为指标，优选鸡内金最佳机械炒制工艺，结果为每12.5 g鸡内金加砂量500 g，翻炒速度50 r/min，215℃炒制120 s。王航宇等以6-姜酚的含量为指标，优选干姜微波炮制的最佳工艺，结果为微波火力50%，加热3 min。王建科等以甘油三油酸酯含量为指标，优选薏苡仁贵州炮制方法的最佳工艺，结果为取薏苡仁加水浸泡1 h，蒸制15 min，于60℃干燥，再投入6倍量细砂中，于250℃的砂温下翻炒90 s。

（4）效应面法　丁黎艳等以补骨脂素、异补骨脂素、补骨脂甲素、补骨脂乙素的总含量为指标，优选补骨脂盐炙工艺，结果为闷润10.3 h，炒炙12 min，炒炙温度为170℃。周文杰等以哈帕苷、哈帕俄苷、肉桂酸变化率的总评归一值为指标，优选玄参的最佳炮制工艺，结果为浸泡19 min，蒸制1.2 h，切薄片，干燥温度49℃。

（5）其他方法　程亦雄等以淀粉酶、蛋白酶活性为指标，优化神曲的发酵工艺，结果以赛氏曲霉为菌种，150 ml水中加入面粉麦麸12 g和K_2HPO_4 0.15 g，温度28℃，摇床转速180 r/min。陈华国等采用吴茱萸脂溶性及水溶性成分指纹图谱，优选姜制吴茱萸的最佳炮制工艺，结果用量药材：干姜＝100：7，加姜汁闷润时间2 h，150℃炒制8 min。胡娜等以出油量及性状为指标，优选肉豆蔻采用液压榨油机压榨制霜工艺，结果为压榨温度80～90℃，压榨2次，出油率达30.8%。王一硕等以冬瓜皮炭对尿素的吸附力和尿素收率为指标，优选烘箱加热制炭工艺，结果为280℃制炭15 min。包勒朝鲁等以药材的脆性为指标，优化石花微炒的条件，结果为110℃、3 min；烘法的最佳条件为60℃、3 h；炮制品水分应控制在4.1%～5.0%之间。

2. 炮制前后化学成分的比较

（1）图谱定性比较　侯志飞等采用HPTLC指纹图谱，比较生栀子、炒栀子、焦栀子、栀子炭中栀子的各主要成分所占比例发生的变化。结果栀子的主要成分中，环烯醚萜苷类含量呈先降低后升高趋势，有机酸酯类含量呈先升高后降低趋势，西红花苷类含量呈降低趋势。鲁翠香等将炙甘草与甘草的色谱图进行对比研究,结果在 23 min 时两个特征峰消失,在 30 min 时出现了一个新的特征高峰。裘维瀚等建立生、煨葛根的 HPTLC 指纹图谱,确定了生葛根的 14 个特征峰和煨葛根的 19 个特征峰。炮制后葛根素、大豆苷和大豆苷元的量分别增加 1 倍多。朱明贵等研究表明,五味子醋制前后指纹图谱有明显的差异,其中以 5-羟甲基糠醛含量变化最为显著。温慧玲等建立了吴茱萸药材和吴茱萸炮制品(甘草水泡吴茱萸制品、开水泡吴茱萸制品)的指纹图谱。结果吴茱萸炮制后吴茱萸内酯和吴茱萸碱的峰面积均有增加,其中甘草水泡制后峰面积增加更加显著。何晓燕等建立槟榔不同炮制品的 HPTLC 指纹图谱,结果在生槟榔炮制为槟榔炭的过程中新增了 3 个成分峰。

(2) 质谱联用技术的成分鉴定　曾锐等采用超高效液相色谱串联四级杆飞行时间质谱(UPLC-Q-TOF/MS)技术建立橘核及其盐制品的指纹图谱。结果盐制品中圣草枸橼苷、柠檬苦素、诺米林、黄柏酮含量均升高。崔小兵等采用 UFLC/Q-TOF-MS 技术比较白术炮制前后化学成分的变化,白术内酯Ⅰ、白术内酯Ⅱ和正离子模式下 m/z 为 229 的化合物(可能为白术内酯Ⅰ脱氢产物)含量升高,而白术内酯Ⅲ、白术三醇、苍术酮麸炒后含量下降。黄林芳等采用 UPLC-Q-TOF/MS 技术分析了肉苁蓉酒炙前后成分变化。结果,酒炙后松果菊苷、毛蕊花糖苷、β-谷甾醇、胡萝卜苷、蔗糖、次黄嘌呤核苷的量升高,而 8-表马钱酸、丁二酸、京尼平苷的量呈下降趋势。松果菊苷、毛蕊花糖苷、8-表马钱酸、丁二酸可作为区分生品与炮制品的指标性成分。王莉等采用高效液相色谱-电喷雾离子阱质谱(HPTLC-ESI/MS^n)技术,分析荷叶生、炭品总生物碱变化,结果荷叶制炭后荷叶碱、*N*-降荷叶碱、番荔枝碱、甲基莲心碱消失。李红等采用 GC-MS 法分析了干馏 10 min 与 50 min 的竹沥成分差异,分别定性了 38 个和 39 个成分,其中 24 个成分相同,且 50 min 所得成分的平均样品的相对分子质量较大。王秀琴等对天仙子生品和不同炮制品挥发油成分进行研究。结果,清炒品中多数成分含量均下降,醋制品中多数成分含量大幅度增加,未见成分组成的质变。

(3) 成分含量变化的比较　安靖等研究表明,苍耳子炒后羧基苍术苷的含量降低,苍术苷的含量升高。李正红等研究表明,枳壳饮片麸炒后柚皮苷、新橙皮苷、辛弗林、川陈皮素、橘皮素、水合橘皮内酯、橘皮内酯和马尔敏含量均略有下降,而葡萄内酯含量明显上升。吴七十三等研究表明,狼毒经牛奶炮制可降低新狼毒素甲、瑞香素乙、新狼毒素乙的含量。卫昊等研究表明,清蒸大黄与酒蒸大黄中番泻苷 A 和 B 的量随炮制时间的增加而降低,在蒸制 12 h 时已检测不到;(+)-儿茶素、没食子酸、芦荟大黄素、大黄素、大黄酸、大黄酚、大黄素甲醚的量在蒸制 0～6 h 逐渐升高,在蒸制 6～12 h 略有降低。黄鲛等研究表明,细辛炒制可显著降低毒性成分黄樟醚的含量,较好地保留有效成分甲基丁香酚和细辛脂素,起到减毒存效的作用。胡志方等研究 HPTLC-ELSD 测定地黄不同炮制品中单糖含量。结果地黄炮制品中单糖含量远远高于生地黄,建昌帮特色炮制品炆制地黄中单糖含量高于清蒸和酒炖炮制的方法。张焱新等研究表明,浙贝母鲜切饮片的贝母素甲、贝母素乙、浸出物含量比硫熏浙贝母饮片高,石灰蛤粉浙贝母饮片次之,且硫熏浙贝母饮片的硫含量远远高于鲜切浙贝母饮片和石灰蛤粉浙贝母饮片。

3. 炮制前后毒性与药效作用的比较

(1) 药效毒性相结合研究　张乐林等研究表明,京大戟的乙酸乙酯部位既是毒性部位又是药效部位。京大戟醋制后药性缓和,毒性作用显著降低,抗炎作用明显增强。

(2) 毒性、刺激性比较研究　钟凌云等研究表明,厚朴没有毒性,但具有一定刺激性,姜制后可缓和其刺激性作用,樟帮特色姜制法比《中国药典》(2010 年版)姜制法能更好降低生厚朴刺激性作用。梅海霖等研究表明,新疆白喉乌头生品毒性较大,可通过炮制降低毒性,其中以《中国药典》(2010 年版)法和哈萨克族法炮制的毒性较小。王娜等研究表明,马钱子生品、沙烫品及醋煮品的毒力存在差异,以醋煮品的毒性较低。张丽等研究表明,甘遂炮制后可通过影响 LO2 细胞周期与凋亡降低其毒性,且醋制工艺中的炒与醋润在醋制降低甘遂的肝毒性中能够起到协同作用。

(3) 药效作用比较研究　周信等研究生半夏及其炮制品对小鼠主动脉内皮细胞炎性因子分泌的影响。结果,生、清、姜、法半夏均能降低白细胞介素-6、肿瘤坏死因子-α 的分泌,其中清半夏作用最强。覃容贵等研究表明，透骨香用于镇痛抗炎宜采用清炒法炮制。杨毅等研究表明，加工炮制一体化制备的延胡索饮片，其镇痛作用优于传统加工炮制延胡索($P<0.05$)。郭亭亭等研究表明，新疆阿魏及其面粉炒、清炒、醋炙、水煮等炮制品对胃溃疡有一定的治疗效果，其中水煮法的治疗效果更显著。董媛媛等研究表明，杜仲盐制后清除二苯基苦基苯肼自由基活性大于生品。李文兵等研究表明，益智仁石油醚部位具有缩尿作用，盐炙炮制法能增强其作用。王敏江等研究表明，生何首乌及何首乌传统炮制品、发酵炮制品均有显著的降脂作用，其中米根霉发酵制备的发酵品降脂活性更加明显。赵翡翠等研究表明，噶尔乌头生品、《中国药典》(2010年版)炮制品、文献法炮制品浓缩液对体液免疫和细胞免疫可能具有双向调节的作用，而哈萨克族方法炮制品浓缩液对体液免疫和细胞免疫可能具有抑制作用。郑晓珂等研究表明，鲜地黄的雌激素样作用最强、生地黄其次、熟地黄没有雌激素样作用。

(4) 炮制对成分和药效影响的综合研究　覃容贵等研究表明，盐制、醋制、蜜制、姜制、酒制等不同炮制方法对虎耳草中岩白菜素的含量及镇咳、抗炎作用有显著影响，虎耳草止咳宜用醋制品。陈琳等研究表明，商陆醋炙后总皂苷和商陆皂苷甲含量均升高，大鼠排尿量增多，小鼠小肠推动作用减弱。

(5) 其他　张伟等研究表明，补骨脂生品及5种炮制品均有一定的α-葡萄糖苷酶活性抑制作用。成颖等采用多探针技术和 HPTLC-MS/MS 的方法，研究柴胡生品及醋炙品对细胞色素P450酶的影响。结果表明，柴胡生品及醋炙品对CYP2E1、CYP2D6 和 CYP3A4 均产生诱导作用，对 CYP1A2 不产生诱导作用；柴胡生品及醋炙品对 CYP2C9 和 CYP2C19 的影响存在差异，这种差异可能是柴胡经炮制后作用发生变化的原因。崔莉等以超氧化物歧化酶升高量为指标，研究淫羊藿生品及不同炮制品的提取物对小鼠体内药代动力学特征参数的影响。结果表明，药动学特征参数均具有显著性差异，淫羊藿经加热后生物利用度提高，而辅料羊脂油进一步促进其体内吸收。周一帆等研究表明，淫羊藿炮制后能提高淫羊藿苷在大鼠体内的生物利用度。谭鹏等采用 HPTLC 法比较巫山淫羊藿不同炮制品水煎液中朝藿定C、淫羊藿苷、淫羊藿次苷Ⅱ3个黄酮类成分的油水分配系数。结果表明，单体成分与其在饮片中的油水分配系数不同，羊脂油炙后有利于3个黄酮类成分的吸收分布。

4. 炮制品质量控制的研究

(1) 指纹图谱研究　鲍雯雯等建立了牛蒡子及其炮制品的 HPTLC 指纹图谱，用于区分其药材生品和炮制品。温慧玲等建立了樟帮法炮制吴茱萸样品的 HPTLC 指纹图谱。梁永枢等报道，建立并比较4种白术炮制品(白术饮片、麸炒白术、土炒白术、清炒焦白术)的 HPTLC 指纹图谱。赵颖等建立了鼠曲草饮片的 RP-HPTLC 指纹图谱。

(2) 质量控制方法研究　孙佰申等报道，采用 HPTLC-ELSD 建立了同时测定黑参中7个极性和12个非极性皂苷单体含量的方法。周倩等报道，建立了 HPTLC 同时测定艾叶及其炮制品(醋艾叶、艾叶炭、醋艾炭)中棕矢车菊素和异泽兰黄素含量的方法。杜伟锋等用 HPTLC 测定牛蒡苷和牛蒡苷元的含量，采用偏最小二乘法，建立中红外光谱与 HPTLC 法测定值之间的多元校正模型，并预测生品和炮制品中牛蒡苷和牛蒡苷元的含量。徐玉茵等研究表明，吸附力、鞣质含量、pH 值及电导率可作为黄芩标炭炒制的质量控制指标。

(3) 质量标准研究　赵清等建立了蜜麸炒僵蚕的质量标准，确定水分、总灰分、酸不溶性灰分、水溶性浸出物、醇溶性浸出物、草酸铵等的含量。付腾飞等建立牡丹皮炭的质量标准，并建议牡丹皮炭的色素对亚甲基蓝的吸附力不低于7.7 mg/g、鞣质含量不低于0.81 mg/g。韩旭阳等采用 HPTLC 测定吴茱萸内酯、吴茱萸碱、吴茱萸次碱的含量，建立了吴茱萸汁的质量标准。

5. 炮制原理的研究

温瑞卿等比较附子所含双酯型生物碱和单酯型生物碱的毒性大小，以及两类成分在生附片和不同炮制品(无胆制附片和胆制附片)中含量的差异。结果表明，不同炮制方法对两类生物碱和残留无机杂质的影响规律不同，无胆蒸制或炒制工艺的“存性”效果较好。郭啸等研究表明，金礞石炮制后部分八面体结构羟基脱失，八面体结构遭到破坏，使得其阳离子具有了可交换性，进而改善其药性药效。唐力英等研究表明，天南星针晶是产生刺激性毒性的主要成分，其刺激性毒性与针晶的结构形态有关。

（谭 鹏 李 飞）

【基于多指标评价中药炮制工艺的研究】

采用多指标评价中药炮制工艺能够更全面、真实地反映中药饮片的内在质量，为饮片质量标准的制定以及中药饮片的规范化生产提供依据。

安瑜等以重楼皂苷总量、薯蓣皂苷元含量、水分为指标，优选重楼的最佳炮制工艺，结果为润制温度60℃，润制时间30 min，干燥温度65℃，干燥时间45 min。孙笑宇等以金丝桃苷、槲皮素和山奈酚的含量为综合评价指标，优选蒸制菟丝子饼的最佳炮制工艺，结果为20g菟丝子生品加40 ml水闷润10 h，蒸制2 h。龚又明等以总挥发油、吉马酮和姜黄素的含量为指标，优选醋制莪术的最佳微波炮制工艺，结果为莪术饮片加15%米醋闷润45 min，60%微波热力炮制3 min。李群等以传统外观质量和内在质量（总黄酮量、东莨菪内酯量）为评价指标，优选桑白皮的最佳蜜炙工艺，结果为取炼蜜25 g，加入37.5 g沸水稀释，淋入100 g桑白皮中，拌匀，闷润60 min，置炒制容器内，240℃炒制18 min。黄弦等以水浸出物、醇浸出物、栀子苷、西红花苷-Ⅰ及西红花苷-Ⅱ为指标，优选炒栀子的最佳炮制工艺，结果为150℃炒15 min。魏运姣等以甘草酸单铵盐的含量、外观颜色、透心和酥脆度、麻舌感为指标，优选半夏的最佳炮制工艺，结果为甘草煎煮1 h，水煎液浓缩至180 ml，浸泡7 d。韩燕全等综合UPLC指纹图谱相似度和6-姜酚、8-姜酚、10-姜酚的含量及炮制品外观，得到炮姜的最佳工艺为195℃砂烫7 min。赵文龙等以白术内酯Ⅰ、Ⅱ、Ⅲ和苍术酮含量为指标，优选麸炒白术的最佳炮制工艺，结果为170℃炒制2 min，投麸量为10%。王冬梅等兼顾抗氧化活性和多指标成分含量，优化玉竹的酒蒸工艺，结果为酒润2 h，玉竹：黄酒=100：20，酒蒸温度60℃，酒蒸1 h。周倩等采用正交试验，以外观性状、指纹图谱特征峰面积为评价指标，优选黄芪蜜炙的最佳工艺，结果为取黄芪量25%的炼蜜，和水以1：1混合（m：m）后，加入净黄芪片，拌匀，闷润30 min，200～240℃炒至饮片表面温度为100℃。殷放宙等以香豆素、黄酮、酚类等12个成分为指标，采用多指标正交试验法，优选盐制补骨脂的最佳炮制工艺，结果为100 g补骨脂加2 g盐，闷润2 h，150℃炒制10 min。涂瑶生等以川乌中苯甲酰新乌头原碱、苯甲酰次乌头原碱、苯甲酰乌头原碱、新乌头碱、次乌头碱、乌头碱6种生物碱类成分的含量为指标，优选制川乌的最佳炮制工艺，结果为40℃水浸泡24 h，111℃加压蒸制1 h，60℃烘干。肖娟等以松脂醇二葡萄糖苷等6种有效成分、醇溶性浸出物量和损耗率为评价指标，采用权重系数综合评分比较不同辅料炮制对杜仲品质的影响。结果表明，辅料对杜仲炮制品的质量有显著影响，盐炙、清炒、酒炙和糯米炙法所得杜仲成品综合评分高于杜仲原药材，指标成分含量高、损耗少、浸出物得率高。

（蔡宝昌）

【中药炮制品质量控制的研究】

周新惠等以三七生品及不同温度加热炮制品中5种皂苷类成分含量为指标，建立HPTLC法对三七炮制品中皂苷类成分进行含量测定和质量控制。色谱条件：Agilent Zorbax SB-C_{18}（4.6 mm×250 mm，5 μm），乙腈和水梯度洗脱，流速1.0 ml/min，检测波长203 nm，柱温20℃。黄雪丽等以枳实中柚皮苷、橙皮苷、新橙皮苷为指标成分，建立HPTLC法用于枳实药材的质量控制。色谱条件：汉邦Phecda C_{18}色谱柱（4.6 mm×150 mm，5 μm），流动相为2%HAc溶液-甲醇，梯度洗脱，流速1 ml/min，检测波长283 nm，柱温30℃。范连霞等采用HPTLC法同时测定附子饮片（生品和炮制品中）3种双酯型生物碱（乌头碱、新乌头碱和次乌头碱）的含量，对附子质量进行控制。色谱条件：Agilent Extend-C_{18}（4.6 mm×150 mm，5 μm）色谱柱，流动相为乙腈-40 mmol/L乙酸铵（氨水调pH10），梯度洗脱，流速1.0 ml/min，检测波长235 nm，柱温30℃。杨敏等采用HPTLC法测定大黄及炮制品中5种蒽醌（大黄酸、大黄素、大黄酚、大黄素甲醚、芦荟大黄素）的含量，建立大黄炮制品的质量控制方法。色谱条件：Shimadzu C_{18}色谱柱（4.6 mm×250 mm，5 μm），流动相为乙腈-0.1%磷酸，梯度洗脱，流速1.0 ml/min，检测波长254 nm，柱温25℃。侯志飞等采用RP-HPTLC对栀子及其炮制品进行指纹图谱考察，作为定性定量评价栀子不同炮制品质量的依据。色谱条件：CenturySIL C_{18} ODS柱（4.6 mm×250 mm，5 μm），流动相1%乙酸-1%乙腈溶液，低压线性梯度洗脱，流速1.0 ml/min，检测波长265 nm，柱温（30±

0.15)℃。杨彦华等采用HPTLC法建立白术及其麸炒品的指纹图谱，为白术及其炮制品质量评价提供依据。色谱条件：Diamonsil C_{18}(4.6 mm×250 mm，5 μm)色谱柱，流动相为乙腈-水，梯度洗脱，检测波长242 nm，柱温28℃，流速0.8 ml/min。邓广海等采用HPTLC法同时测定草乌及炮制品中乌头碱等6种生物碱的含量，综合评价其安全性和有效性。色谱条件：Dikma kromasil色谱柱(4.6 mm×250 mm，5 μm)，流动相为乙腈：四氢呋喃＝25：15和0.1 mol/L乙酸铵，梯度洗脱，检测波长235 nm，柱温30℃，流速0.8 ml/min。张超建立RP-HPTLC法测定关黄柏及其不同炮制品中黄柏酮、黄柏内酯含量，为控制炮制品的质量提供依据。色谱条件：Kromasil C_{18}色谱柱(4.6 mm×250 mm，5 μm)，流动相为乙腈：水＝50：50，流速1.0 ml/min，柱温25℃，检测波长205 nm。曾颜等建立HPTLC法测定京大戟生品和炮制品中甘遂甾醇、大戟二烯醇和24-亚甲基环阿尔廷醇含量，为京大戟药材及炮制品质量控制提供依据。色谱条件：Agilent XDB-C_8色谱柱(4.6 mm×150 mm，5 μm)，流动相为乙腈：水＝90：10，流速1 ml/min，柱温35℃，检测波长205 nm。刘硕等以巴戟天及不同盐分炮制品中糖分为指标，采用HPTLC-ELSD建立巴戟天及盐巴戟天中糖成分质量控制。色谱条件：Agilent Zorbax Carbohyrate色谱柱(4.6 mm×250 mm，5 μm)，流动相为乙腈-甲醇-水，流速1.2 ml/min，梯度洗脱，柱温35℃，蒸发光检测器检测(漂移管温度105℃，氮气流量2.0 L/min)。

(李伟东)

【13种中药炮制前后化学成分的比较】

1. 斑蝥

王一硕等采用石墨炉、火焰、氢化物发生-冷原子吸收法，测定了斑蝥原药材、生斑蝥、米炒斑蝥及头足翅中Cu、Mn、Zn、Fe、Mg、Ga、K、Pb、Cd、As、汞等微量元素的含量。结果表明，斑蝥各样品中微量元素的含量：K＞Mg＞Fe＞Ca＞Zn＞Mn＞Cu＞Pb＞As＞Hg＞Cd。斑蝥经米炒炮制后Pb、As、Hg、Cd、Fe元素降低，Cu、Mg、Ca元素增高；斑蝥头足翅中Hg、Pb元素的含量比其他部位偏高，内翅As元素的含量最高。斑蝥传统去头足翅和米炒炮制法可有效减毒。

2. 补骨脂

丁黎艳等以抗骨质疏松活性成分(补骨脂素、异补骨脂素、补骨脂甲素、补骨脂乙素)为指标，用HPTLC法测定不同产地生品和盐炙品、雷公炙品、乙醇炙品和微波炙品中4种成分的含量。结果表明，盐炙和微波炙品较生品4种成分总含量降低了10.68%、6.78%，雷公炙品的含量较生品提高48.84%，乙醇炙品的含量降低了24.48%。

3. 苍耳子

朵睿等用HPTLC法研究炒制对苍耳子中羧基苍术苷和苍术苷的影响。结果表明，生品苍耳子中羧基苍术苷含量较高，不含苍术苷；而炒黄后羧基苍术苷的含量降低约90%，转化为苍术苷；炒焦苍耳子中基本不含羧基苍术苷，苍术苷有小幅下降；炒炭后苍术苷显著降低或不能检出。炒制使羧基苍术苷转化为苍术苷，同时进一步降低苍术苷的量，可明显降低苍耳子的毒性。

4. 草乌

杜红等用HPTLC法测定不同类型醋制备的草乌炮制品中3种双醋型生物碱和3种单醋型生物碱的含量差异。结果表明，草乌经过炮制后，双醋型生物碱含量大幅度降低。其中《中国药典》(2010年版)水煮品含量最低，仅为生品的1/10；龙门米醋、玫瑰醋、山西陈醋制品次之，约为生品的1/5；工业乙酸、食用乙酸制品含量最高，超过生品的1/3。单酯型生物碱含量显著增加，其中《中国药典》(2010年版)水煮法含量最高，为生品的5倍；乙酸制品次之，约为生品的3倍；3种食用醋制品为生品的2倍左右。醋制草乌可以达到炮制减毒的目的，食用醋比乙酸的减毒效果更佳。刘帅等用HPTLC法测定诃子汤制、清水制、去鞣诃子汤制草乌中新乌头碱、乌头碱、次乌头碱以及苯甲酰新乌头碱、苯甲酰乌头碱、苯甲酰次乌头碱的含量。结果表明，诃子汤制草乌中单、双酯型生物碱的含量最高、清水制草乌中双酯型生物碱次之、单酯型生物碱最少；去鞣诃子汤制草乌双酯型生物碱含量最少，表明鞣质可抑制生物碱类成分的溶出，达到降低毒性的作用。

5. 附子

唐小龙等用HPTLC法研究干热烘制和湿热

蒸制对附子中所含 6 种酯型生物碱含量的影响。结果表明，附子 200℃干热烘制，双酯型生物碱含量迅速降低，单酯型生物碱先增加后降低，30 min 达到高峰；120℃湿热蒸制，双酯型生物碱迅速消失，单酯型生物碱含量起初显著增加，而后先增后降，60～90 min 达到高峰；105℃高压蒸制，酯型生物碱变化趋势较为缓和，随着蒸制时间增加，双酯型生物碱显著降低，单酯型生物碱显著增加，但明显小于 120℃的蒸制效果。这些炮制方法除湿热蒸制 105℃未达到《中国药典》(2010 年版)要求，其他均符合《中国药典》(2010 年版)规定。

6. 狗脊

徐刚等采用模拟砂烫、升华、水蒸气蒸馏、直接提取挥发油等 4 种方式，从狗脊中收集升华与挥发性成分，并用 UPLC/Q - TOF - MS 法进行定性分析。结果表明，狗脊炮制是一个固体升华和液体挥发的过程。其中狗脊中自身具有的刺激性物质如柠苹酸、6 -姜辣素、月桂酸等通过简单的物理变化受热挥散；且在受热过程中发生化学反应，由糖分解产生糠醛类物质如 5 -羟甲基糠醛等，也具有刺激性。

7. 虎杖

张蕾等用 HPTLC 法研究虎杖生品及不同炮制品中虎杖苷、白藜芦醇和大黄素的含量。结果表明，不同炮制品中虎杖苷含量为：盐制＞醋制＞酒制＞豆汁制；白藜芦醇和大黄素含量为：豆汁制＞酒制＞醋制＞盐制。表明不同的炮制方法对虎杖苷、白藜芦醇和大黄素的含量影响较大，其中豆汁制对 3 种成分的含量影响最大，其虎杖苷含量明显降低，而白藜芦醇和大黄素含量则显著升高。

8. 黄精

曾林燕等用 HPTLC 法比较 3 个品种黄精(滇黄精、黄精和多花黄精)炮制过程中新产生成分及含量的变化。结果表明，与生品比较，3 个品种黄精炮制后新产生 2 种成分，分别为 5 -羟甲基麦芽酚(DDMP)和 5 -羟甲基糠醛(5 - HMF)。多花黄精中 DDMP 的含量随着炮制时间的延长逐渐增加，至炮制 24 h 达到最高，随后开始逐渐降低；5 - HMF 的量随着炮制时间的延长逐渐增加。

9. 卷柏

吴彩霞等用 HPTLC 法研究卷柏及其炮制品中穗花杉双黄酮的含量。结果表明，卷柏生品中穗花杉双黄酮的含量为 0.84％，焦卷柏为 1.07％，卷柏炭为 0.53％。焦卷柏的含量远远高于卷柏生品，而卷柏炭的含量较卷柏生品又有明显降低。

10. 狼毒

庄果等用 HPTLC 法比较狼毒(月腺大戟)生品和不同炮制品(烘干品、水润阴干品、水润烘干品、醋润阴干品、醋润烘干品、乙酸润烘干品)中狼毒乙素、狼毒丙素、岩大戟内酯 B 的含量变化。结果表明，狼毒乙素、狼毒丙素的含量随着温度的升高呈现先上升后下降的趋势，而岩大戟内酯 B 的含量则不断降低。各炮制品中这 3 种成分的含量均以水润烘干品较水润阴干品高，说明适当加热可以增加成分的溶出；对于醋润烘干品和醋润阴干品，虽然烘干使其有效成分含量增加，但岩大戟内酯 B 的含量却大大降低，醋制法较其他方法更能发挥减毒保效的作用，而辅料醋不能用化学试剂乙酸替代。

11. 三七

余河水等采用大孔吸附树脂柱色谱、硅胶柱色谱、Rp - C_{18} 柱色谱、HPTLC 法等分离纯化技术，研究三七炮制品的化学成分变化。结果表明，熟三七《中国药典》(2010 年版)的 70％乙醇提取物中分离得到 23 个单体化合物，其中 20S -人参皂苷 Rg_3、20*R* -人参皂苷 Rg_3、人参皂苷 F_2 和绞股蓝皂苷 XⅦ为首次从三七炮制品中分离得到。三七经过炮制，其中的活性成分三萜皂苷主要发生糖基水解反应和脱水反应。

12. 石斛

欧德明等用 HPTLC 法与苯酚-硫酸法分别比较石斛干品与不同炮制品中石斛碱及多糖含量。结果，石斛碱含量：干品 0.182％、黄酒炙品 0.218％、白酒炙品 0.216％、黄酒润蒸制品 0.225％、白酒润蒸制品 0.283％、蒸制品 0.229％；多糖含量：干品 5.48％、黄酒炙品 5.80％、白酒炙品 7.56％、黄酒润蒸制品 8.31％、白酒润蒸制品 12.5％、蒸制品 8.72％。石斛炮制后石斛碱与多糖含量均有所增高，不同炮制品之间石斛碱和多糖含量也有一定差异。

13. 水蛭

王雨林等采用柱前衍生化 HPTLC 法和凝血酶滴定法测定氨基酸、抗凝血酶活性，比较不同炮制方法对水蛭成分的影响。结果表明，水蛭生品和炮制品中游离氨基酸含量较低，水解氨基酸含量为蚂蟥低于柳叶蚂蟥。蚂蟥和柳叶蚂蟥的抗凝血酶活性差异不大，但高温炮制（砂炒、蜜炙麦麸炒、滑石粉炒）可降低柳叶蚂蟥的抗凝血酶活性。

（张永太）

【11 种中药炮制前后药理作用的比较】

1. 巴豆

陈彦琳等采用家兔血研究加热炮制对巴豆霜溶血效应的影响。结果表明，未经加热或加热时间不足的巴豆，会发生明显的溶血效应，且在较低浓度也能出现相同现象，反应比较灵敏。巴豆粉碎后，应常压蒸制足够时间，再制备巴豆霜，能使巴豆中的巴豆毒蛋白灭活，降低溶血毒性。不同制霜方法中，如果采用淀粉稀释法，不经加热处理，其溶血效应与生巴豆相同；提油返油法有机溶剂可能会残留，导致血细胞凝集变性。故建议不采用生巴豆加淀粉稀释和提油返油法制备巴豆霜。

2. 巴戟天

崔妮等采用腺嘌呤灌胃给药的方法建立小鼠肾阳虚模型，用桂附地黄丸为对照，比较巴戟天不同炮制品补肾壮阳的药理作用。结果表明，各实验组均可以改善肾阳虚小鼠的症状，其中盐巴戟组治疗效果最为显著，其次是制巴戟、巴戟肉、巴戟天。其作用机制可能与改善肾阳虚证小鼠 HPA 轴病理改变和功能抑制状态有关。

3. 北柴胡

赵晶丽等采用 40% CCl_4 制备大鼠慢性肝损伤模型，测定大鼠血清丙氨酸氨基转移酶（ALT）、天门冬氨酸氨基转移酶（AST）、碱性磷酸酶（ALP）、总胆红素（TBiL）、白蛋白（Alb）、总蛋白（TP）水平，并计算白蛋白与球蛋白比值（A/G）；采用胆总管插管术，研究北柴胡不同炮制品对大鼠胆汁流量的影响、不同炮制方法对北柴胡疏肝利胆药效作用的影响。结果表明，北柴胡醋炙组 ALT、AST、ALP、TBiL 含量降低最为显著（$P<0.01$）；蜜炙组次之（$P<0.05$）；生用组和酒炙组对 ALT、AST、ALP 含量有降低作用（$P<0.05$）；醋炙组 TP、Alb、A/G 含量升高最为显著（$P<0.01$ 或 $P<0.05$）；蜜炙组能使 TP、Alb 含量升高（$P<0.01$ 或 $P<0.05$）；生用组和酒炙组仅能使 TP 含量升高（$P<0.05$）。北柴胡醋炙组胆汁流出量增加最为显著（$P<0.05$）。北柴胡醋炙品疏肝利胆作用最强，蜜炙品次之，酒炙品与生柴胡作用相当。

4. 柴胡

王丽娜等研究了柴胡醋制前后的抗炎作用。结果，生柴胡对角叉菜胶所致大鼠足跖肿胀、棉球引起的肉芽增生、二甲苯所致大鼠耳肿胀和毛细血管通透性增加均有拮抗作用（$P<0.05$），醋柴胡对二甲苯所致大鼠耳肿胀有拮抗作用（$P<0.05$）。生柴胡与醋柴胡抗炎作用有差异（$P<0.05$）。表明以肿胀和渗出为指标，生柴胡抗炎作用优于醋柴胡。

5. 大麻药

陈旅翼等研究了大麻药生品和炮制品急性毒性的差异。结果表明，大麻药生品和 3 种炮制品的小鼠口服半数致死量 LD_{50} 为，姜制品＞麸制品＞生品＞酒制品，LD_{50} 值分别为 17.93、16.77、12.11、9.45 g/kg。怠动、腹泻、心跳加速、唾液分泌增加是主要的急毒症状。不同的炮制方法对大麻药的毒性影响较大，其毒性成分与中毒机理尚待进一步研究。

6. 葛根

张丹等采用离体肠张力检测装置，以平均张力为主要指标，研究生、煨葛根对大鼠离体十二指肠平滑肌自发运动的影响，以及氯化钡（$BaCl_2$）、乙酰胆碱（Ach）、去甲肾上腺素（NA）、异丙肾上腺素（ISO）与生、煨葛根对肠肌作用的相互影响。结果表明，生、煨葛根在 2.4～29.1 g/L 范围内能抑制肠肌的自发运动，使平均张力降低且呈剂量依赖性；其低、中、高剂量均能抑制 $BaCl_2$ 引起的痉挛性收缩，对 Ach 引起的肠肌兴奋有拮抗作用，但 Ach 对药液抑制作用后的肠肌未显示出兴奋作用；生、煨葛根对 NA、ISO 引起的肠肌抑制有抑制作用,NA、ISO 对药液引起的肠肌抑制仍能表现出抑制作用。生、煨葛根均能抑制大鼠离体十二指肠平滑肌运动,煨葛根较生葛根作用明显,其作用机制可能是通过阻断 M 受体或直接作用于平滑肌、降低平滑肌细胞内 Ca^{2+} 浓度有关。

7. 何首乌

陈有军等研究了何首乌不同炮制品对大鼠血虚模型的补血作用。结果,何首乌常压豆制 24 h、常压酒豆制 24 h、高压清蒸 4 h 和 8 h、高压豆制 6 h和 8 h 组、高压酒制 6 h 以及高压酒豆制 8 h 组能显著增加血虚大鼠模型的红细胞数量和血红蛋白数量,其中高压豆制何首乌 8 h 组红细胞和血红蛋白数增加效果最佳($P<0.01$)。生何首乌、常压豆制 24 h、酒制 24 h、酒豆制 24 h、高压清蒸 4 h 和 8 h、高压豆制 6 h 和 8 h 以及高压酒制 6 h能够改善血虚大鼠模型的血流变功能紊乱($P<0.05$ 或$P<0.01$)。表明何首乌以黑豆汁或酒为辅料,高压蒸制 6～8 h,补血效果更好。王万根等以体外培养人胚肺二倍体细胞,研究何首乌高压蒸制法、蒸制时间对抗衰老活性的影响。结果表明,3 h 制品何首乌的抗细胞衰减率为 38.04%,其细胞衰亡速率最为缓慢($P<0.001$);生品何首乌、1 h 制品何首乌和正常组细胞间的 SOD 活力无显著性差异($P>0.05$),而 2 h、3 h、4 h 制品何首乌组及传统炮制组均可提高细胞内 SOD 活性。3 h 制品何首乌组细胞内 SOD 含量最高,显著高于对照组细胞内 SOD 酶的活性($P<0.001$)。

8. 黄连

沈晓庆等采用干酵母皮下注射方法制备大鼠发热模型,以阿司匹林作为阳性对照药,研究黄连胆汁炙前后的解热作用。结果表明,生黄连高剂量组解热作用最好,可以持续 12 h,胆汁高剂量组次之,胆黄连组未发现明显解热作用。杨伟鹏等采用巴豆油致小鼠耳肿胀炎症模型,研究吴茱萸汁炮制对黄连抗炎药效及黄连苦寒药性的影响。结果表明,黄连药材和不同炮制品均能减轻小鼠耳肿胀程度,黄连各组给药 14 d 后,大鼠体质量、饮食量、饮水量与对照组比较均有不同程度下降;与对照组比较,疏毛萸连组血黏度升高,白细胞介素 2 降低($P<0.05$),生黄连组促甲状腺素降低($P<0.05$)。不同吴茱萸汁炮制对黄连抗炎药效无明显影响,但可在一定程度上减轻黄连的寒性。

9. 罗仙子

褚夫江等比较传统炮制与现代加工方法对罗仙子抑菌及抗炎作用的影响。结果,经现代加工方法提取、分离获得的罗仙子小分子活性部位的抑菌及抗炎效果明显优于传统炮制方法。在同等剂量的条件下,现代加工法对革兰氏阳性菌及革兰氏阴性菌的最小抑菌浓度及最小杀菌浓度均小于传统法;在抗炎方面,现代加工法优势更为明显,能够显著地改善炎性巨噬细胞的形态,降低炎症因子 TNF-α、IL-6 的表达。表明现代加工方法对罗仙子中抑菌及抗炎物质的活性具有一定的保护作用。

10. 枇杷叶

叶广亿等通过氨水诱发小鼠咳嗽、枸橼酸诱发豚鼠咳嗽、小鼠气管酚红排泌实验、组胺-乙酰胆碱诱发豚鼠哮喘,研究枇杷叶炮制前后不同提取物的止咳化痰平喘作用。结果表明,炙品水提能显著延长小鼠咳嗽潜伏期,减少 4 min 内咳嗽次数,炙品醇提能显著延长咳嗽潜伏期,明显减少咳嗽次数,二者对咳嗽次数的影响有明显差异;生品水提也能有效缓解小鼠咳嗽症状,但作用弱于炙品,与炙品水提比较有明显差异。炙品水提和生品水提能明显延长豚鼠咳嗽潜伏期,各给药组都能明显减少咳嗽次数,炙品水提和炙品醇提延长豚鼠咳嗽潜伏期作用有明显差异。炙品水提能显著增加小鼠气道酚红排泄量,生品水提也能明显增加小鼠气道酚红排泄量,而生品醇提、炙品醇提对小鼠呼吸道酚红排泄量的影响与空白对照组比较无显著性差异。炙品水提和生品水提均能显著延长豚鼠引喘潜伏期,炙品醇提和生品醇提也能明显延长引喘潜伏期,且炙品醇提与炙品水提比较,两者作用有明显差异。

11. 藤黄

窦娟等研究了藤黄不同炮制品对小鼠腹腔炎症与大鼠肠道组织病理学的影响。结果表明,藤黄生品及各炮制品均能导致小鼠腹腔的炎症反应,当藤黄生品给药剂量为 25 mg/kg、给药 3 h 时,其所致炎症反应最强;藤黄经炮制后,其致炎作用有所下降;致炎作用:藤黄生品>藤黄豆腐制品>藤黄清水制品>藤黄高压蒸制品。给药后大鼠的肝脏、肾脏、心脏、胃和食道均未见明显的毒性反应，但十二指肠、空肠有轻度至重度的毒性作用，表现为肠绒毛水肿；3 种藤黄炮制品均会引起给药大鼠肠道的毒性作用，生品藤黄所致的十二指肠和空肠水肿程度最严重，其次是清水制藤黄和藤黄酸；细胞的毒性结果显示，与空白组相比，藤黄生品及炮制品均可明显降低大鼠肠上皮 IEC-6 细胞的活性($P<0.01$)，并使形态变差，且呈一定的剂量相关性，与藤黄生品组相比，藤黄 3 种炮制品组对 IEC-6 细胞的增殖抑制作用($P<0.01$)和形态变差的趋势均显著性降低。

(张永太)

[附] 参考文献

A

安靖，王耀登，盛昌翠，等. 苍耳子炮制前后羧基苍术苷和苍术苷的含量比较[J]. 药物分析杂志，2013，33(11)：1910

安瑜，张文懿，张彩琼，等. 重楼最佳炮制工艺的正交试验优选[J]. 时珍国医国药，2013，24(9)：2140

B

包勒朝鲁，乌兰图雅，那生桑. 石花炮制工艺优化研究[J]. 世界中医药，2013，8(8)：954

鲍雯雯，钟佳丽，丛晓东，等. 不同产地牛蒡子药材炮制前后 HPTLC 指纹图谱研究[J]. 中华中医药学刊，2013，31(2)：258

C

陈华国，马青青，周欣，等. 指纹图谱技术优选姜制吴茱萸的炮制工艺[J]. 中国实验方剂学杂志，2013，19(1)：32

陈琳，吴皓. 商陆醋炙前后化学成分和药效比较[J]. 中国实验方剂学杂志，2013，19(21)：5

陈旅翼，兰洲，林亲雄，等. 大麻药生品和三种炮制品的急性毒性比较[J]. 中南民族大学学报(自然科学版)，2013，32(3)：54

陈彦琳，杜杰，周林，等. 加热炮制对巴豆霜溶血效应影响的初步研究[J]. 中国现代中药，2013，15(3)：219

陈有军，向飞军，金嘉文，等. 何首乌不同炮制品对大鼠血虚模型的补血作用[J]. 世界科学技术(中医药现代化)，2013，15(4)：659

成颖，黄寅，田媛，等. 探针药物法评价柴胡生品及醋炙品对细胞色素 P450 酶的影响(英文)[J]. 中国天然药物，2013，11(3)：302

程亦雄，张婧，戚岑聪，等. 赛氏曲霉深层发酵神曲的工艺优选[J]. 中国实验方剂学杂志，2013，19(19)：42

褚夫江，金小宝，许银叶，等. 传统炮制与现代加工方法对罗仙子抑菌及抗炎作用影响的比较[J]. 中药材，2013，36(6)：893

崔莉，孙娥，钱浅，等. 淫羊藿生品及不同炮制品小鼠药代动力学特征的比较研究[J]. 中国中药杂志，2013，38(10)：1614

崔妮，史辑，贾天柱. 巴戟天不同炮制品补肾壮阳作用的比较研究[J]. 中国中药杂志，2013，38(22)：3898

崔小兵，单晨啸，文红梅，等. 基于 UFLC/Q-TOF-MS 分析麸炒白术的物质基础[J]. 中国中药杂志，2013，38(12)：1929

D

邓广海，林华，龚又明. 草乌及其炮制品中 6 种生物碱类成分的含量测定[J]. 中国实验方剂学杂志，2013，19(7)：35

丁黎艳，郭晏华，黄婷，等. 基于补骨脂抗骨质疏松成分的炮制评价方法研究[J]. 中成药，2013，35(2)：346

丁黎艳，郭晏华，黄婷，等. 星点设计-效应面法优化补骨脂炮制工艺[J]. 中国现代中药，2013，15(1)：56

董媛媛，石智华，邓翀，等. 从抗氧化角度评价杜仲“盐制入肾”的炮制机理[J]. 现代中医药，2013，33(1)：77

窦娟，文红梅，郁红礼，等. 藤黄不同炮制品对小鼠腹腔炎症的影响[J]. 中国药房，2013，24(35)：3268

窦娟，文红梅，郁红礼，等. 藤黄炮制品对大鼠肠道组织病理学研究[J]. 中国实验方剂学杂志，2013，19(5)：279

杜红，刘秋雨，刘晓艳，等. 醋的种类对炮制草乌生物碱类成分的影响[J]. 中华中医药学刊，2013，31(10)：2156

杜伟锋，鲍雯雯，赵耀东，等. 基于中红外光谱的牛蒡子饮片中牛蒡苷和牛蒡苷元快速含量测定方法的建立[J]. 中国新药杂志，2013，22(20)：2431

朵睿，陈燕，刘玉红，等. 苍耳子炒制对羧基苍术苷和苍术苷的影响[J]. 中成药，2013，35(2)：353

F

范连霞，杨会锦，尹华. 中药附子质量控制研究[J]. 海峡药学，2013，25(11)：82

付腾飞，朱琼花，周立艳，等. 牡丹皮炭质量标准研究[J]. 现代医药卫生，2013，29(12)：1761

G

龚又明,邓广海,林华,等.正交试验优选莪术微波炮制工艺[J].中国实验方剂学杂志,2013,19(7):56

郭亭亭,卢军,姜林,等.新疆阿魏及其炮制品对大鼠胃溃疡模型作用的实验研究[J].新疆医科大学学报,2013,36(10):1463

郭啸,王益群,王栋,等.中药金礞石炮制前后红外光谱分析[J].中华中医药杂志,2013,28(3):688

H

韩旭阳,边宝林,李饶饶,等.炮制辅料吴茱萸汁的质量标准[J].中国实验方剂学杂志,2013,19(17):132

韩燕全,洪燕,高家荣,等.基于UPLC特征指纹图谱和指标成分定量测定研究炮姜的炮制工艺[J].中草药,2013,44(1):42

何晓燕,刘玉杰,黄永亮,等.槟榔炒制过程中不同炮制品的指纹图谱分析[J].中国实验方剂学杂志,2013,19(17):44

侯志飞,卢海刚,王刚,等.栀子炮制品的HPTLC指纹图谱[J].中国医药工业杂志,2013,44(7):712

侯志飞,于文国,王刚,等.在线紫外光谱对栀子及其炮制品HPTLC指纹图谱的定性研究[J].中国实验方剂学杂志,2013,19(11):98

胡娜,刘欢,袁子民,等.肉豆蔻制霜新工艺优选及质量评价[J].中国实验方剂学杂志,2013,19(21):10

胡志方,王小平,陈建章.HPTLC-ELSD测定地黄不同炮制品中单糖含量[J].中国实验方剂学杂志,2013,19(13):72

黄鲛,易进海,刘玉红,等.炒制对细辛中黄樟醚、甲基丁香酚和细辛脂素含量的影响[J].中国实验方剂学杂志,2013,19(19):90

黄林芳,李文涛,王冬梅,等.基于UPLC-Q-TOF/MS技术研究酒苁蓉增效的物质基础[J].中草药,2013,44(24):3471

黄婷,郭晏华,丁黎艳,等.药汁制补骨脂对其抗OP化学成分影响[J].辽宁中医药大学学报,2013,15(5):60

黄弦,罗光明,罗扬婧,等.焦栀子的炮制工艺优化及西红花苷类成分含量变化[J].中国实验方剂学杂志,2013,19(14):10

黄弦,罗光明,左月明,等.正交试验法优选炒栀子的炮制工艺[J].中国实验方剂学杂志,2013,19(3):12

黄雪丽,陈玉宇,尧爱珉,等.HPTLC法测定枳实不同炮制品中有效成分的含量[J].广州化工,2013,41(9):141

L

李红,蒋孟良,金晓飞,等.不同干馏时间对竹沥中化学成分的影响[J].中国药房,2013,24(35):3305

李凯,梁勇,刘磐,等.不同软化方法对白芍饮片质量的影响[J].中国实验方剂学杂志,2013,19(3):20

李群,王瑾,张会敏.正交试验法优选桑白皮蜜炙工艺[J].中草药,2013,44(3):286

李文兵,胡昌江,吴珊珊,等.益智仁盐炙对水负荷多尿模型大鼠缩尿作用的研究[J].中国实验方剂学杂志,2013,19(11):261

李正红,夏放高,陈海芳,等.枳壳麸炒前、后主要活性成分的含量变化[J].中国实验方剂学杂志,2013,19(19):18

梁永枢,庄义修,段启,等.白术4种炮制品HPTLC指纹图谱比较[J].中药新药与临床药理,2013,24(3):285

刘波,徐常本.正交试验法优选小苏打制大黄的炮制工艺[J].辽宁中医杂志,2013,40(1):139

刘帅,李飞,侯跃飞,等.诃子中的鞣质成分对诃子汤制草乌的影响-诃子制草乌炮制原理探讨Ⅰ[J].中国实验方剂学杂志,2013,19(5):158

刘硕,马方励,李养学,等.巴戟天及不同盐分炮制品中糖类成分HPTLC-ELSD指纹图谱研究[J].中国实验方剂学杂志,2013,19(4):106

鲁翠香,周萍.高效液相色谱法分析甘草炮制前后化学成分[J].亚太传统医药,2013,9(7):55

M

梅海霖,赵翡翠,李娟,等.新疆白喉乌头及其炮制品对小鼠的急性毒性实验研究[J].新疆医科大学学报,2013,36(7):918

O

欧德明,周一帆,胡昌江,等.不同方法炮制前后石斛中石斛碱及石斛多糖含量测定[J].亚太传统医药,2013,9(8):22

Q

裘维瀚,戴辉,胡泓,等.葛根煨制前后成分的比较研究[J].中成药,2013,35(10):2213

S

沈晓庆,张凡,贾天柱.黄连胆汁炙前后的解热作用研究[J].中药药理与临床,2013,29(2):118

孙佰申,叶光耀,张超超.HPTLC-ELSD同时测定九蒸九曝法炮制的黑参中极性和非极性皂苷[J].药物分析杂志,2013,33(3):388

孙笑宇,程序,贾天柱.正交试验优选蒸制菟丝子饼的炮制工艺[J].中国实验方剂学杂志,2013,19(20):27

T

覃容贵，龙庆德，范菊娣，等. 炮制对虎耳草中岩白菜素及其止咳抗炎作用的影响[J]. 中成药，2013，35(5)：1027

覃容贵，龙庆德，秦拴梅，等. 不同炮制方法对透骨香抗炎镇痛作用及水杨酸甲酯苷含量的影响[J]. 时珍国医国药，2013，24(2)：409

谭鹏，仲玲利，杨蕾，等. 不同炮制方法巫山淫羊藿中3个黄酮类成分油水分配系数的比较[J]. 药物分析杂志，2013，33(8)：1289

唐力英，吴宏伟，王祝举，等. 天南星炮制减毒机制探讨(Ⅱ)[J]. 中国实验方剂学杂志，2013，19(3)：1

唐小龙，易进海，夏燕莉，等. 不同炮制方法对附子6种酯型生物碱含量的影响[J]. 中国实验方剂学杂志，2013，19(21)：96

涂瑶生，全智慧，孙冬梅，等. 川乌炮制工艺优化[J]. 中国实验方剂学杂志，2013，19(5)：13

W

汪岩，翟延君，吕国军，等. 鸡内金机械化炮制工艺优选[J]. 中国实验方剂学杂志，2013，19(4)：65

王德珍，易骏，张翼，等. 酒黄连、姜黄连、萸黄连最佳炮制工艺研究[J]. 中药材，2013，36(1)：35

王冬梅，吕振江，王永红，等. 多指标综合评价玉竹酒蒸炮制工艺[J]. 浙江农林大学学报，2013，30(1)：100

王航宇，李国玉，张珂，等. 正交实验优选干姜微波炮制工艺[J]. 医药导报，2013，32(6)：770

王建科，张永萍，李玮，等. 薏苡仁贵州炮制方法的工艺优化[J]. 贵州农业科学，2013，41(8)：173

王丽娜，汪巍，徐驰，等. 柴胡醋制前后抗炎作用比较研究[J]. 中成药，2013，35(5)：1079

王莉，张学兰，孙玉丽，等. 高效液相色谱-电喷雾离子阱质谱法分析荷叶炮制前后生物碱成分的变化[J]. 中成药，2013，35(4)：780

王敏江，林佩，李云飞，等. 何首乌不同炮制品对肝细胞脂代谢的干预作用研究[J]. 现代药物与临床，2013，28(4)：494

王娜，许海江，孙同文，等. 生品、沙烫品及醋煮品马钱子的急性毒性试验[J]. 中医临床研究，2013，5(4)：25

王万根，张宁华，徐巧红，等. 何首乌高压蒸制法蒸制时间对何首乌抗衰老活性影响的研究[J]. 云南中医学院学报，2013，36(2)：1

王晓崴，易炳学，龚千锋，等. 正交试验法优选醋泡马钱子的炮制工艺[J]. 中国实验方剂学杂志，2013，19(21)：13

王秀琴，王岩，李军，等. GC－MS分析天仙子及其炮制品中挥发油成分[J]. 中华中医药学刊，2013，31(5)：1044

王一硕，张娟，张振凌. 冬瓜皮炭的炮制工艺优选及体外吸附尿毒素活性考察[J]. 中国实验方剂学杂志，2013，19(22)：9

王一硕，赵丽娜，张振凌. 中药斑蝥炮制前后微量元素含量的比较研究[J]. 中药材，2013，36(5)：718

王雨林，王实强，刘玉琴，等. 不同炮制方法对水蛭中氨基酸及抗凝血酶活性的影响[J]. 湖南中医药大学学报，2013，33(11)：42

卫昊，冯改利，郑洁，等. 清蒸和酒蒸对大黄中9种化学成分的影响分析[J]. 中成药，2013，35(4)：777

魏运姣，赵熠，宋红萍，等. 正交设计法研究法半夏的炮制工艺[J]. 中国医院药学杂志，2013，33(2)：134

温慧玲，程齐来，廖梅香，等. 樟帮法炮制吴茱萸样品的指纹图谱[J]. 光谱实验室，2013，30(1)：298

温慧玲，程齐来，吴龙火，等. 基于指纹图谱探讨吴茱萸不同炮制品成分的差异[J]. 中国实验方剂学杂志，2013，19(5)：76

温瑞卿，李东辉，赵昕，等. 基于化学分析的毒性中药附子炮制方法的合理性研究[J]. 药学学报，2013，48(2)：286

吴彩霞，杨宇婷，康文艺. HPTLC法测定卷柏及其炮制品中穗花杉双黄酮的含量[J]. 天然产物研究与开发，2013，25(8)：1089

吴七十三，王青虎，刘瑛，等. 蒙药瑞香狼毒及其奶制品中新狼毒素甲、瑞香素乙、新狼毒素乙的比较研究[J]. 中成药，2013，35(2)：350

X

仙园园，郭小娜，张华，等. 维药刺山柑果实的炮制方法研究[J]. 中草药，2013，44(11)：1420

肖娟，严瑞娟，张水寒，等. 不同炮制方式对杜仲品质的影响[J]. 现代药物与临床，2013，28(6)：874

徐钢，单国顺，鞠成国，等. 狗脊升华与挥发性成分的UPLC/Q－TOF－MS分析[J]. 中草药，2013，43(16)：2308

徐玉茵，朱琼花，孟江. 黄芩炭质量控制标准研究[J]. 中医学报，2013，28(11)：1697

Y

杨敏，许伯慧，汪冬庚，等. 不同炮制方法对大黄中5种蒽醌类化合物含量的影响[J]. 南通大学学报(医学版)，2013，33(5)：385

杨伟鹏，王怡薇，王彦礼，等. 吴茱萸汁炮制对黄连抗炎药效和苦寒药性的影响[J]. 中国中医药信息杂志，2013，20(8)：42

杨彦华，沈晓庆，赵文龙，等. 白术及其麸炒品的HPTLC指纹图谱比较研究[J]. 中国药房，2013，

24(23)：2172

杨毅，孙乙铭，徐建中，等. 延胡索加工炮制一体化饮片与传统炮制饮片镇痛作用比较[J]. 中国现代应用药学，2013，30(10)：1074

叶广亿，李书渊，陈艳芬，等. 枇杷叶不同提取物的止咳化痰平喘作用比较研究[J]. 中药药理与临床，2013，29(2)：100

殷放宙，李林，李伟东，等. 多指标正交法优选盐制补骨脂饮片的炮制工艺[J]. 中国中药杂志，2013，38(3)：346

余河水，张丽娟，宋新波，等. 三七炮制品化学成分研究[J]. 中国中药杂志，2013，38(22)：3910

Z

曾林燕，宋志前，魏征，等. 黄精炮制过程中新产生成分分离及含量变化[J]. 中草药，2013，44(12)：1584

曾锐，付娟，武拉斌，等. UPLC－Q－TOF/MS分析橘核盐制前后成分差异[J]. 中国中药杂志，2013，38(14)：2318

曾颜，侯朋艺，马冰洁，等. HPTLC 同时测定京大戟生品和炮制品中 3 种三萜类成分含量[J]. 中国实验方剂学杂志，2013，19(22)：141

张超. 关黄柏不同炮制品中黄柏酮与黄柏内酯的含量测定[J]. 中药材，2013，36(2)：205

张丹，邢姝丽，李蒙，等. 生、煨葛根对大鼠离体十二指肠平滑肌运动的影响[J]. 上海中医药杂志，2013，47(12)：70

张乐林，葛秀允，孙立立，等. 醋制对京大戟毒性和药效的影响[J]. 中国实验方剂学杂志，2013，19(19)：276

张蕾，郭晏华，黄婷，等. 虎杖生品及不同炮制品中虎杖苷、白藜芦醇和大黄素含量[J]. 辽宁中医药大学学报，2013，15(11)：56

张丽，高兰，颜晓静，等. 不同方法炮制甘遂对 LO2 细胞周期与凋亡的影响[J]. 中国中药杂志，2013，38(6)：825

张伟，尹震花，彭涛，等. 补骨脂生品及炮制品对 α－葡萄糖苷酶抑制活性考察[J]. 中国实验方剂学杂志，2013，19(9)：24

张焱新，杨培培，杜伟锋，等. 浙贝母不同炮制方法质量研究[J]. 中华中医药学刊，2013，31，(12)：2775

赵翡翠，卢军，姜林，等. 新疆准噶尔乌头生品及其炮制品对小鼠免疫功能影响研究[J]. 中华中医药杂志，2013，28(7)：2159

赵晶丽，高红梅. 北柴胡不同炮制品疏肝利胆药效作用初探[J]. 中国实验方剂学杂志，2013，19(16)：235

赵清，秦桂芳，桂雪虹，等. 蜜麸炒僵蚕的质量标准研究[J]. 中国实验方剂学杂志，2013，19(8)：120

赵文龙，吴慧，贾天柱. 麸炒白术的炮制工艺优化[J]. 中国实验方剂学杂志，2013，19(8)：7

赵颖，李文，李鹏，等. 鼠曲草饮片的 RP－HPTLC 指纹图谱研究[J]. 中国药房，2013，24(15)：1391

郑晓珂，刘朝妍，蒋赟，等. 怀地黄雌激素样活性筛选的实验研究[J]. 中国药学杂志，2013，48(21)：1831

钟凌云，兰智慧，祝婧，等. 姜制前后厚朴毒性及刺激性作用研究[J]. 中成药，2013，35(8)：1782

周倩，孙立立，江波，等. RP－HPTLC 法同时测定艾叶及其炮制品中棕矢车菊素和异泽兰黄素的含量[J]. 中国药房，2013，24(47)：4464

周倩，孙立立. 多指标综合评分法优选黄芪最佳蜜炙工艺[J]. 中成药，2013，35(7)：1512

周文杰，傅亚，王云红，等. 中心复合设计-效应面法优化玄参的炮制工艺[J]. 中国实验方剂学杂志，2013，19(4)：10

周新惠，赵荣华，张荣平，等. 三七不同加热炮制品中 5 种皂苷类成分的含量测定[J]. 云南中医学院学报，2013，36(6)：14

周信，张小荣，张秋燕，等. 生半夏及其炮制品对小鼠主动脉内皮细胞炎性因子分泌的影响[J]. 中国实验方剂学杂志，2013，19(10)：261

周一帆，胡昌江，张雪洁，等. 淫羊藿炮制前后在大鼠体内的药代动力学研究[J]. 中成药，2013，35(12)：2717

朱明贵，李丽，肖永庆，等. 五味子醋制前后指纹图谱的分析比较[J]. 中国实验方剂学杂志，2013，19(21)：100

庄果，李俊松，蔡宝昌. 狼毒(月腺大戟)不同炮制品的 HPTLC 图谱及狼毒乙素、狼毒丙素、岩大戟内酯 B 的含量变化研究[J]. 中国中药杂志，2013，38(10)：1526

(六)中药药理

【概述】

2013年,在国内医学刊物上公开发表的中药药理研究报道涉及300余种中药,其中多数为常用药物。热点研究领域仍为中药对心脑血管系统影响及抗肿瘤作用的研究,且大多是对中药有效成分或者有效部位(有效组分)作用机制的研究。

1. 对呼吸系统作用的研究

孙晓芳等报道,三七总皂苷能显著减轻博莱霉素所致小鼠肺纤维化气道上皮细胞凋亡,抑制肺组织中Fas/FasL的过度表达;亦能抑制小鼠肺组织中组织蛋白酶B的过度表达,减轻大鼠肺泡炎和肺纤维化的程度。姜文等报道,茯苓、薏苡仁、冬瓜子能够减轻博莱霉素诱导的肺纤维化,其机制可能与降低转化生长因子-β1(TGF-β1)及肿瘤坏死因子-α(TNF-α)的浓度有关。宫金艳报道,丹参抗肺纤维化的机制在于其抑制结缔组织生长因子在肺组织中的表达。蔡晓璐等报道,穿山龙总皂苷能抑制哮喘小鼠肺组织表达α-平滑肌肌动蛋白(α-SMA),影响平滑肌增厚,改善哮喘小鼠气道重塑状态。康小龙等报道,香青兰总黄酮能够抑制哮喘大鼠TNF-α、白细胞介素-6(IL-6)、IL-13和IL-17等炎性因子的释放,从而缓解哮喘气道炎症。陈晓芳等报道枇杷花醇提物止咳作用的机制可能是通过降低C-纤维释放P物质。

2. 对心血管系统作用的研究

孙娅楠等报道,黄芪注射液可抑制体外培养乳鼠心肌细胞肥大,其机制可能与抑制钙调蛋白激酶途径中钙调蛋白激酶Ⅱ(CaMKⅡ)δ的表达,从而改善心肌收缩功能。毛秉豫等报道,丹参提取物能显著抑制血管紧张素Ⅱ(AngⅡ)诱导的心肌细胞肥大,可能与其对蛋白激酶D1 mRNA的表达调控密切相关。杨光宇等报道,黄芪甲苷对AngⅡ诱导的乳鼠心肌细胞肥大有抑制作用,其机制可能与降低[Ca^{2+}]i及CaMKⅡδB表达有关。吕昕瞳等报道,人参总皂苷对AngⅡ诱导的心肌细胞肥大具有明显抑制作用,其机制可能与抑制钙调神经磷酸酶和细胞外信号调节激酶1信号转导通路有关。何雯等报道,异叶青兰总黄酮能改善高血压大鼠心肌肥厚及心肌纤维化程度,可能与其降IL-1β、TNF-α水平,调节基质金属蛋白酶-9(MMP-9)/基质金属蛋白酶抑制剂-1(TIMP-1)的表达有关。常文静等报道,丹参酮Ⅱ$_A$可抑制压力负荷增加所致大鼠心肌肥厚,减轻心肌纤维化,可能与下调心肌局部心肌结缔组织生长因子和TGF-β1水平有关。刘晓舒等报道,黄芪多糖对高同型半胱氨酸血症大鼠心肌缺血再灌注损伤具有保护作用,其机制在于降低肌酸激酶、乳酸脱氢酶、心肌肌钙蛋白-Ⅰ水平。张莹等报道,黄芪多糖与p38 MAPK阻断剂SB203580联合应用时,可以明显抑制p38通路,下调由其介导的细胞间粘附分子-1(ICAM-1),血管细胞间粘附分子-1(VCAM-1)在内皮细胞质膜上的表达,对抑制大鼠缺血心肌再灌注损伤有协同作用。杨雷等报道,黄芪提取物可明显改善大鼠心肌梗死后异常的血液流变学指标、组织病变及胶原纤维构成比例,其机制可能与下调心肌组织PKD1蛋白的表达相关。陈华文等报道,丹参酮Ⅱ$_A$对脓毒症大鼠心肌凋亡具有保护作用,可能通过降低心脏炎性水平、氧化应激、减轻钙超载,并能部分改善凋亡基因(Bax、Bcl-2、Fas和caspases-3)以及钙调神经磷酸酶的异常表达有关。侯平等报道,麻黄细辛附子汤中的麻黄碱能够增强钙电流峰电流密度,提高细胞内钙离子浓度,因而具有兴奋心肌细胞的作用,此作用与高电压门控性钙通道开放有关;所含β-细辛醚和去甲乌药碱可通过降低细胞内钙离子浓度和轻微阻断钙离子内流而起保护心肌细胞的作用,避免钙超载的损害。汪江涛等报道,一定剂量钩藤碱可使肾性高血压大鼠血压和左心室重量指数(LVMI)回降,血浆AngⅡ含量降低,血浆和心肌中叶素含量升高。付剑江等报道罗布麻叶提取物具有明显的降压作用,其机制可能是激活血管内皮细胞内磷脂酰肌醇3-激酶(PI3K)/蛋白激酶B(Akt)信号转导途径,从而促进内皮型一氧化氮合酶(NOS)磷酸化,提高NOS活性、增加NO。

潘毅等报道,血畅宁(瓜蒌、熟地黄、醋龟甲、丹参、钩藤、三七)可以明显降低自发性高血压大鼠和肾性高血压大鼠的血压,降低LVMI,改善心肌组织结构,增加心肌组织中血管紧张素Ⅱ-2型受体(AT2R)mRNA的表达,同时降低AT1R mRNA的表达。白卫娜等报道,柿叶总黄酮可抑制载脂蛋白E基因敲除小鼠胸腹主动脉粥样硬化(AS)血管内膜血小板选择素、ICAM-1、VCAM-1等粘附分子表达,从而减缓AS病变,但并不依赖于其对血脂的降低作用。王颖超等报道,沙棘黄酮可降低动脉粥样硬化大鼠还原型辅酶Ⅱ氧化酶亚基Nox4及人源氧化低密度脂蛋白的表达,减少ROS生成,防治粥样硬化。卢新华等报道,马齿苋总黄酮可抑制缺氧致血管平滑肌细胞钙超载,调节缺氧条件下血管平滑肌细胞蛋白激酶C活性。王琼等报道,丹参提取物的乙酸乙酯部位对凝血因子Xa和凝血因子Ⅱa均有较好的抑制活性,并且能够浓度依赖性延长凝血酶原时间。叶士勇等报道,淫羊藿苷能够抑制凝血酶、U46619(血栓素A_2类似物)诱导的P-selectin表达和纤维蛋白原的结合,可抑制血小板Akt的磷酸化,可能通过抑制P13K信号通路,降低血小板活化,抑制动脉血栓的形成。

3. 对消化系统作用的研究

刘文东等报道,青蒿琥酯可能通过降低肝组织MMP-2、MMP-9的表达,增加MMP-13的表达,从而发挥抗肝纤维化的作用。郑旭锐等报道,姜黄素抗肝纤维化作用来源于能降低肝星状细胞中JAK2、STAT3蛋白的表达,阻断JAK2-STAT3信号转导。郭洁等报道,葱白提取物对脂肪变性肝细胞有明显的保护作用,其分子机制可能与上调过氧化物酶体增殖物活化受体γ协同刺激因子1α基因的转录活性、增加线粒体琥珀酸脱氢酶活性相关。关翠雯等报道,丹参酮$Ⅱ_A$对雷公藤甲素所致急性肝损伤有保护作用,其机制与激活转录因子NF-E2相关因子/抗氧化反应原件通路有关。张哲等报道,脂多糖可诱导大鼠肝脏Kupffer细胞NF-κB核转位,姜黄素能明显抑制这一效应。朱向东等报道,芍药苷通过下调IL-1β、TNF-α和升高IL-4的表达,调节肠道异常免疫反应、抑制炎症反应,修复溃疡,进而治疗溃疡性结肠炎。李彦龙等报道,薏苡仁水提液通过调节促炎因子与抗炎因子的平衡而发挥其抗炎作用,对溃疡性结肠炎大鼠损伤的肠黏膜有明显的修复作用。杜菲菲等报道,复方儿茶止泻霜可以上调腹泻大鼠结肠水通道蛋白1的表达,减轻结肠黏膜的组织病变。戴关海等报道,胃乐煎能显著增加慢性萎缩性胃炎模型大鼠胃腺体数目、腺体厚度、主细胞数目、壁细胞数目,对血清胃泌素含量有一定的增加作用。段彬等报道,平胃散及其组方药材苍术、厚朴、陈皮水煎液均具有较强的促进大鼠胃排空的作用;厚朴、陈皮挥发油对正常大鼠具有较强的促进胃排空作用,而苍术挥发油无明显促进作用。赵龙等报道,柴芍胃炎颗粒可能通过促进胃泌素、胃动素分泌和增加胃排空率,从而起到改善功能性消化不良模型大鼠胃肠动力障碍的作用。王玉等报道,大黄素对急性放射性肠炎大鼠可明显升高肠组织绒毛高度、黏膜及全层壁厚度,提高肠组织中二胺氧化酶活性,降低细菌移位率,降低肠组织TNF-α表达,减少NO生成。白静等报道,艾叶水提物及其发酵物均能抑制小肠平滑肌收缩,艾叶发酵物作用更强。艾叶水提物作用机制可能与阻断M_3受体相关,艾叶发酵物与阻断M_3受体和H_1受体相关。

4. 对泌尿生殖系统的研究

贾宁等报道,三七总皂苷可升高骨形成蛋白-7、缝隙连接蛋白43的表达水平,同时下调P13K/Akt信号通路及α-SMA阳性细胞百分率,对抗肾间质纤维化。徐浩岑等报道,人参皂苷Rg_1能抑制TGF-β1诱导的大鼠肾小管上皮细胞间充质转分化的作用,可以延缓或抑制肾间质纤维化过程。曾金祥等报道,车前子醇提物能抑制肝脏黄嘌呤氧化酶与腺苷脱氨酶的活性并下调肾脏尿酸转运体mRNA的表达,可能是其降低高尿酸血症小鼠血清尿酸水平的机制。周萍等报道,黄芪、丹参可通过促进肾纤维化抑制因子par-3的表达,减轻肾间质纤维化的进展。苏筠霞等报道,革薢水提物可降低尿酸性肾病模型大鼠肾组织中TNF-α、单核细胞趋化蛋白-1(MCP-1)和ICAM-1的表达及血清MCP-1发挥延缓肾功能损伤的作用。牛彩琴等报道,苦豆子总碱可增强膀胱逼尿肌的收缩作用,机制可能与激活细胞膜上Ca^{2+}通道有关。赵秀军等报道,何首乌饮可升高运动疲劳大鼠血睾酮水平,可能系通过降低睾丸组织细胞色素C氧化酶7α2表达和升高睾酮合成酶的途径。彭娟等建立卵巢颗粒细胞的原代培养体系，发现哈蟆油含药血清能够显著促进卵巢颗粒细胞的增殖。盛磊等报道，人参皂苷 Rh_2 可明显抑制实验性大鼠子宫异位内膜生长，其作用机制可能与降低血清中雌激素、孕激素和抗子宫内膜抗体水平、上调 Bax/Bcl－2 蛋白表达、激活 Caspase－9、Caspase－3 表达有关。

5. 对中枢神经系统作用的研究

马立等报道，三七总皂苷对脑缺血后脑神经损伤有显著保护作用，其机制可能与降低超敏 C 反应蛋白、降低 Hcy 水平、减少线粒体 Ca^{2+} 摄入有关，并能促进血管内皮细胞增殖及体内新生血管生成。张盈等建立大鼠高原低压缺氧模型，研究表明蕨麻乙醇提取物在低压缺氧时可通过促进脑红蛋白的表达，发挥脑保护作用。姚海涛等报道，山茱萸多糖可通过抑制阿尔茨海默病（AD）模型大鼠海马神经元 tau 蛋白在 Ser422 和 Ser396 位点的过度磷酸化，改善 AD 大鼠学习记忆能力。苏亚楠等报道，山茱萸多糖通过抑制 GSK－3β 蛋白过度激活，促进 GSK－3β(Ser9) 蛋白表达途径，防治大鼠 AD 的发生与发展。黄倩等报道，人参皂苷 Rg_1 对慢性温和不可预见性应激诱导的大鼠抑郁行为和额前皮质区突触超微结构的异常有明显的改善作用。栾华梅等报道，人参皂苷 Rb_1 对青霉素诱导的新生大鼠癫痫发作有一定的治疗作用，使海马 CA3 区 Bax 表达相对下降，Bcl－2 表达相对增高。李雪燕等报道，当归多糖具有改善学习记忆能力、延缓衰老的作用，其机制可能与提高 SOD 及端粒酶活性有关。杨宜承等报道，雷公藤内酯可通过上调癫痫模型大鼠海马神经元 Bcl-2、下调 Bax 蛋白表达而抑制大鼠神经元凋亡。赵春霞等报道灵芝孢子粉能有效降低癫痫大鼠海马组织的神经生长因子过度表达，对神经细胞起保护作用。

6. 对骨骼系统作用的研究

董文娟等报道，穿山龙总皂苷可能通过降低滑膜血管内皮生长因子 mRNA、血管生成素－2 及 Tie－2 的表达，抑制滑膜血管新生，发挥治疗类风湿关节炎作用。梁秀军等报道，穿山龙总皂苷治疗类风湿关节炎机制在于明显降低血清 TNF－α、IL－1β 和 IL－6 水平，减轻滑膜组织的病理损伤。汤晓晨等报道，一定浓度的黄芪甲苷能通过抑制人膝骨关节炎退变关节软骨细胞合成 IL－1β，延缓软骨细胞退行性病变。金连峰等报道，骨碎补可通过调控 Bax、Bcl－2 表达来调控软骨细胞异常凋亡，发挥防治膝骨关节炎的作用。徐祥赫等报道，杜仲可通过促进小鼠成骨细胞增殖与分化成熟，并上调骨保护素与 NF－κB 受体活化因子配体的比值，间接抑制破骨细胞的分化和成熟，达到防治骨质疏松症作用。曲雷鸣等报道，淫羊藿含药血清能促进体外培养的 MC3T3－E1 成骨细胞增殖与骨向分化。刘国岩等报道一定浓度骨碎补提取液在体外对骨髓间充质干细胞具有促进其向成骨分化和促进核心结合因子 α1 表达的作用。

7. 抗炎和对免疫系统作用的研究

祁佳等报道，藤茶水提取物具有潜在的清咽抗炎功效，该作用可能与组织中 PGE_2 有关。金国泰等报道六虫骨灵胶囊（含全蝎、穿山甲、蜈蚣等）具有镇痛抗炎作用，抑制 PGE_2 合成是其镇痛作用机制之一。季亢挺等报道，黄芪甲苷对氧化低密度脂蛋白损伤后内皮祖细胞的细胞生物学功能有显著保护作用。褚春民等报道，薯蓣皂苷对胶原性关节炎大鼠具有较强的抗炎作用，机制可能与抑制 NF－κB p65 亚基和环氧酶－2 的表达有关。许博林等报道牦牛活性蛋白能显著增强机体对抗原刺激的应答能力和小鼠淋巴细胞的转化能力，提高吞噬细胞的吞噬能力，并促进小鼠抗体形成细胞生成。韩红彦等报道，通心络胶囊可能通过上调 $CD_4^+CD_{25}^+$ Treg 细胞并抑制 $CD_4^+CD_{28}^-$ T 细胞的过度增殖，进而影响 γ－干扰素（IFN－γ）及基质金属蛋白酶的相应改变，延缓改善动脉粥样硬化的进程。孙宇等报道，黄芪能够有效抑制实验性自身免疫性脑脊髓膜炎小鼠中枢神经系统的炎性反应，与其抑制 $MOG_{35\text{-}55}$ 特异性 T 细胞增殖，减少 Th1、Th17 型细胞因子分泌，促进 Th2 型细胞因子分泌相关。宋占春等报道，大黄素可以降低 IFN－γ 和 IL－17 的水平，对自身免疫性心肌炎大鼠的心肌起到保护作用。尹美珍等报道，一定浓度的艾叶多糖在体外能明显提高小鼠脾细胞分泌的 TNF 和 IL－2 的活性，是其调节免疫功能的部分机制。

8. 防治糖尿病的研究

刘伟等报道，银杏叶提取物可以缓解链脲佐菌素和异丙肾上腺素协同诱导的大鼠糖尿病心肌损害。关悦等报道，羊栖菜多糖可以对抗糖尿病脑缺血大鼠脑组织细胞凋亡，其机制可能与调控survivin基因的表达有关。杨竞等报道，白藜芦醇对大鼠糖尿病肾病的干预作用机制可能与抑制TGF-β1/Smad2信号通路有关。李姝玉等报道，黄芪注射液联用葛根素注射液能减少系膜区肾组织纤黏连蛋白的表达，具有保护肾脏作用。栾海艳等报道，桔梗总皂苷能明显上调2型糖尿病肝病大鼠的BMP-9 mRNA的表达，从而减轻肝损伤。李正红等报道，黄芪对腹膜纤维化具有阻抑作用，其机制可能通过抑制TGF-1，并作用于Smads信号转导通路正、负反馈环路中的Smad2/3、Smad7关键信号蛋白，阻抑腹膜间皮细胞上皮细胞间充质转化的发生。朱德淼等报道，三七三醇皂苷可能通过抑制糖尿病大鼠视网膜神经节细胞内Nogo受体的表达，抑制视网膜氧化应激，保护神经节细胞。金祖汉等报道，黄连降糖片可改善胰岛素抵抗模型动物的胰岛素抵抗，明显降低白内障发生率。

9. 抗肿瘤作用的研究

王艳丽等报道，柴胡皂苷d可以抑制实验大鼠肝癌发生及血管形成，下调AngⅡ和血管内皮细胞生长因子(VEGF)的表达，可能是其抑制肝癌的作用机制之一。郑安红等报道，蝎毒多肽可增强5-氟尿嘧啶(5-Fu)对肝癌H_{22}的抑制作用，其机制可能与抑制癌组织NF-κB通路及MMP-9、VEGF的表达从而抑制新生血管形成有关。陈翔等报道，黄药子醇提物对裸鼠胃癌移植瘤模型有明显的抑瘤作用，其机制可能与下调细胞因子IL-8和可溶性细胞间黏附分子-1的表达有关。马克龙等报道，千金藤碱能抑制结肠癌细胞增殖，增加结肠癌耐药细胞株Lovo/5-FU对5-FU的敏感性，可能与其抑制结肠癌细胞中血红素加氧酶1和醌氧化还原酶1的表达水平有关。车章洪等报道，人参皂苷Rg_3对结肠癌细胞的增殖有抑制作用，机制可能与抑制β-catenin的核转移，进而抑制Wnt/β-catenin信号转导有关。余思云等报道，紫草素能够诱导体外培养的子宫内膜癌Ishikawa细胞凋亡，其机制可能与促进细胞中Bax上调及Bcl-2下调相关。陈立波等报道，苦参碱能有效抑制人宫颈癌Hela细胞的增殖，诱导其凋亡，其机制可能与抑制Survivin基因的表达有关。郭丽华等报道，半枝莲5个黄酮类单体(汉黄芩素、野黄芩苷、芹菜素、木犀草素和黄芩素)均可明显抑制人卵巢癌Skov3细胞增殖，其中汉黄芩素作用最强。金光虎等报道，苦参碱可抑制前列腺癌PC-3M细胞株生长，增加细胞凋亡率，机制与细胞中Bcl-2 mRNA表达水平逐渐下调，Bax mRNA表达水平逐渐上调有关。李顺等报道，氧化苦参碱抑制人膀胱癌细胞Survivin的转录和表达，对caspase-3有上调作用，诱导细胞发生凋亡。周陈姣等报道，苦参碱对人急性红白血病细胞株TF-1 SALL4基因和蛋白表达及Wnt/β-catenin信号通路下游靶基因β-catenin、C-myc、Cyclin DI的抑制，可能在抑制细胞增殖、诱导细胞凋亡过程中起重要作用。王铮华等报道，白杨素可升高人鼻咽癌细胞Cne-2细胞caspase-3的活性，并可诱导细胞周期阻滞。陈俊等报道，苦参碱改构体X在体外可诱导人鼻咽癌Cne-1细胞凋亡，其机制可能是阻滞细胞周期，上调促凋亡蛋白Caspase-3、Caspase-8、Caspase-9、Bax和p53的表达，降低抑制凋亡蛋白Bcl-2的表达。王水英等报道，白山毛桃根提取物能抑制黑色素瘤M21细胞增殖、侵袭迁移能力，其机制可能是下调与肿瘤细胞免疫逃逸密切相关的PD-L1、PD-L2分子基因和蛋白表达。王园园等报道狼毒提取液抗小鼠恶性黑色素瘤B16细胞转移能力可能部分与其下调促转移因子p-Akt，上调抑癌转移因子PTEN的表达有关。曹志友等报道，白附子提取物可抑制人SHG-44脑胶质瘤细胞的增殖及诱导其发生凋亡，其机制与Bcl-2蛋白表达下降和Bax蛋白表达上升有关。陈望昊等报道，汉黄芩素能抑制人胶质瘤细胞株U87细胞的增殖，促进其凋亡，其机制可能与miR-128的上调有密切的相关性。

10. 抗病原微生物作用的研究

刘彬等报道，鱼腥草素钠可增强妥布霉素抗铜绿假单胞菌生物被膜作用。曾春晖等报道，广西藤茶总黄酮可能通过降低金黄色葡萄球菌表面疏水性、增加胞浆膜通透性使细菌形态发生改变，并通过抑制细菌脱氢酶活性发挥抗菌作用。刘蕾等报道，翻白草油在三种作用方式下(直接灭活、病毒复制、病毒吸附阶段)抗呼吸道合胞病毒作用可能与调节Bcl-2蛋白和Bax蛋白的表达有关。苟玲等报道，荆芥、桂枝挥发油含药血清对甲型流感病毒在狗肾传代细胞中的增殖具有显著抑制作用，并具有一定直接杀灭作用，且体内外实验结果一致。

11. 中药药代动力学研究

林建阳等研究了大鼠红景天苷口服及静脉给药的药代动力学，结果红景天苷的绝对生物利用度为41.9%，且吸收迅速。王小兵等报道灯盏花素静脉注射后的药动学过程，在正常大鼠和糖尿病大鼠体内均符合二室模型。灯盏花素在糖尿病大鼠体内的药动学参数与正常大鼠比较，清除率显著性降低。隋忠国等给大鼠分别灌胃一定剂量的五味子酯甲、南五味子提取物后再灌胃他克莫司，结果表明五味子酯甲可明显促进他克莫司在大鼠消化道的吸收。

12. 中药毒理学的研究

王平等报道，山豆根不同组分急性毒性大小顺序依次是醇提组分、水提组分、全组分。曹雨诞等报道，以斑马鱼作为实验动物，甘遂生品的醇提液急性毒性最强，甘遂醋炙品的水提液急性毒性最低。华碧春等报道，黄药子含药血清在体外对肝细胞有毒性作用，与给药剂量及细胞培养时间有关；黄药子与甘草配伍后，对肝细胞的毒性显著降低。陈莹蓉等报道，黄药子醇提物 Caco－2 细胞摄取液对 HL－7702 和 HepG2 细胞有毒性，可部分阐明黄药子肝毒性的物质基础。周思思等报道，在动物急性毒性实验中，人参与附子配伍的减毒作用在一定范围内随着人参剂量的增加而增强。

（仲宗亮　王树荣）

【中药干预血管性痴呆的实验研究】

中药及其有效成分能有效改善血管性痴呆（VD）动物模型的学习记忆和认知功能，药物种类主要涉及活血药、补益药、解表药、开窍药等。

1. 中药抗 VD 与抗氧化作用有关

王莹等研究表明，红景天苷可明显降低 VD 小鼠脑内 NO 含量，并可能通过减少一氧化氮合酶（NOS）的激活，阻止 NO 过量生成，从而提高 VD 小鼠的学习记忆能力。孔德燕研究表明，丹参酮 $Ⅱ_A$ 能够抑制 VD 发生过程中脑组织中 NOS 的活性，使 NO 的生成和释放明显减少，从而减轻其病理损伤，改善 VD 大鼠的学习记忆功能。黄欢等研究表明，白果内酯（BB）对 VD 小鼠具有一定的保护作用，缩短模型小鼠学习反应时间，延长记忆时间，减少错误次数，增加小鼠脑组织 SOD 活性和 MDA 含量，降低乙酰胆碱酯酶（AChE）活性和 NO 含量。罗云等报道，阿魏酸能降低 VD 大鼠大脑海马组织 MDA 含量，提高 SOD 活性，推测抗氧化作用可能是其作用机制之一。潘朝旺等报道，九龙虫能改善 VD 小鼠大脑海马 CA1 区神经元损伤，其机制可能与抑制 VD 小鼠脑内 NOS 活性及降低 NO 含量有关。李炜等研究表明，蛇床子素改善 VD 小鼠的空间学习记忆和探索能力障碍，其机制可能与降低组织 NO 含量和 NOS 活性有关。

2. 中药抗 VD 与调节脑内神经递质或受体功能有关

罗云等研究表明，阿魏酸能显著降低脑内海马组织 AChE 的活性，从而增加脑内 ACh 含量，提高脑内胆碱能系统功能，增强 VD 大鼠学习记忆能力。李君等研究表明，银杏叶提取物可以改善 VD 大鼠空间学习记忆能力，减轻脑缺血再灌注对海马 CA1 区神经元的损伤，可能与上调海马神经元 N－甲基－D－天冬氨酸型离子型谷氨酸受体1型亚单位蛋白及 mRNA 的表达有关。孔德燕研究亦表明，丹参酮 $Ⅱ_A$ 通过增强 VD 大鼠脑组织乙酰胆碱转移酶和 AChE 活性，改善 VD 大鼠的学习记忆功能。胡玉英等研究表明，交泰丸改善 VD 大鼠学习记忆能力的机制可能是通过降低 VD 大鼠脑单胺氧化酶活性，减少单胺类神经递质的氧化分解。刘春丽等研究表明，松果菊苷可以提高 VD 大鼠的学习记忆能力，其机制可能与减轻皮层、海马组织中氧自由基，改善胆碱能神经递质代谢速率有关。

3. 中药抗 VD 与抑制神经细胞凋亡有关

武变瑛等研究表明，银杏叶提取物能明显改善 VD 模型大鼠的认知能力，抑制大鼠海马促细胞凋亡基因 Bax 表达，促进原癌基因 Bcl－2 表达，增加 Bcl－2 和 Bax 比值，推测其抗 VD 与降低神经元对凋亡刺激的敏感性，减少海马神经元的凋亡有关。王丽华等报道三七制剂可减少 VD 大鼠海马神经元的缺血坏死，其机制可能与提高丝裂原活化蛋白激酶表达，抑制神经细胞凋亡有关。王敏等研究表明，竹节参总皂苷可上调慢性脑缺血大鼠海马神经生长相关蛋白的表达，降低海马星形胶质细胞的增生,可能是其提高学习记忆的作用机制。王宇等研究表明,银杏叶提取物明显促进VD大鼠大鼠海马组织PSD－95蛋白表达,抑制海马神经元凋亡,改善大鼠学习记忆能力。蒋青等研究表明,地黄寡糖对VD大鼠有一定的治疗作用,能够显著减少VD大鼠海马CA1区神经元凋亡,其机制可能是与通过调控Bcl－2/bax相关蛋白的表达有关。

4. 中药抗VD的作用与抗炎作用有关

王彩霞等研究表明,独活对VD模型大鼠免疫炎性损伤具有调节作用,可以升高血清中IL－4,降低TNF－α等炎症因子。钟萍等研究表明,小檗碱能改善VD大鼠的行为学症状,可能是通过降低炎症因子IL－1β、IL－8、TNF－α的表达发挥作用。

5. 其他作用

陈连连等研究表明,粉防己碱可改善大鼠脑缺血损伤引起的学习记忆能力障碍,可能与其下调海马齿状回星形胶质细胞S100B蛋白表达,降低大鼠海马细胞内钙离子浓度,对抗钙超载有关。黄新武等研究表明,姜黄素可通过减少海马神经元凋亡,影响Bcl－2及Bax蛋白表达,改善VD模型大鼠学习记忆能力。乔晓鸣等认为沙棘总黄酮能改善全血黏度及血浆黏度,增加脑血流量,改善VD大鼠的行为学,促进缺氧神经细胞功能的恢复,这可能是提高模型大鼠智力的主要机制之一。

(王　欣　胡　爽)

【中药改善神经细胞凋亡的机制研究】

1. 中药改善线粒体途径介导的神经细胞凋亡

Guo DJ等报道,木犀草素对6－羟基多巴胺诱导的大鼠肾上腺嗜铬细胞瘤细胞凋亡具有保护作用,其机制可能是抑制Bax基因的过度表达,抑制Bcl－2基因的下调表达,从而显著降低Bax/Bcl－2的比值。石瑞丽等研究表明,瓜子金皂苷己可以抑制氧糖剥夺/复供所诱导的PC12细胞凋亡,其机制是增加Bcl－2/Bax表达比值,抑制线粒体膜电位水平的降低,稳定线粒体的功能。黄柏胜等研究表明,山楂酸对大鼠大脑皮层神经元氧糖剥夺损伤具有保护作用,可能与凋亡相关蛋白Bax表达降低有关。温旭敏等报道,川芎嗪在过氧化氢诱导PC12细胞凋亡模型中,乳酸脱氢酶释放及细胞活性氧水平显著降低,caspase－3活性降低,Bax/Bcl－2比值降低。刘长安等研究表明,川芎嗪在β淀粉样蛋白($Aβ_{25\text{-}35}$)诱导的体外大鼠海马神经元细胞凋亡模型中通过调节Bax/Bcl－2平衡以抑制神经细胞的凋亡,表明川芎嗪有保护神经细胞的作用。胡微煦等研究表明,白术多糖在一定范围内能有效地抑制神经细胞缺氧性凋亡,其机制是降低凋亡基因及蛋白产生,上调抗凋亡蛋白产生,提高Bcl－2/Bax比例。周本宏等研究表明,天麻多糖对皮质酮损伤的PC12细胞的保护机制可能与抑制细胞内Ca^{2+}浓度超载,调节Bcl－2/Bax比值,及抑制Caspase通路有关。程钢等研究表明,氧化苦参碱对脑缺血损伤有直接的神经保护作用,其机制可能是通过上调Bcl－2及下调Bax、Caspase－3蛋白水平,抑制凋亡发生。

2. 中药改善内质网途径介导的神经细胞凋亡

Li ZY等报道,柴胡总皂苷预处理PC12细胞能够部分剂量依赖性地保护细胞免受皮质酮诱导的毒性损伤,其机制可能是通过下调葡萄糖调节蛋白78、GADD153、人X盒结合蛋白－1的表达以抑制内质网应激反应,起到保护神经细胞作用。王德桂等研究表明,银杏叶提取物金纳多亦能通过降低内质网相关蛋白CHOP的表达及脊髓抑制凋亡,以改善损脊髓神经功能。Wu CX等报道,乔松素能够显著增加缺血再灌注损伤大鼠的GRP78蛋白的表达,减少CHOP/GADD153的表达以及Caspase－12的活化,抑制真核翻译起始因子2α的磷酸化,减少转录激活因子4的表达,减轻因内质网应激造成的凋亡。Ruan L等研究表明,粉防己碱在大脑中动脉闭塞小鼠模型中同样能够抑制GRP78的表达,减轻再灌注损伤。

3. 中药改善死亡受体介导的神经细胞凋亡

Liu DM等研究表明,在氧糖剥夺及复供处理过程中神经细胞Fas－L,Fas相关死亡结构域(FADD)以及TNF－α的蛋白表达显著增加,给予乙酰葛根素组的Fas－L,FADD及TNF－α蛋白含量显著降低,表明乙酰葛根素可以通过下调死亡受体途径的相关基因的表达来抑制神经细胞的凋亡。Zhang S 等报道，金樱子黄酮提取物能够显著地提高脑缺血再灌注损伤大鼠的生存率，减少组织损伤，其与下调 Fas、Fas－L、TNF－α、IL－1β、IL－4 以及 IL－6 等表达有关。陈萌等研究表明，黄芩茎叶总黄酮预处理可减轻脑缺血再灌注损伤大鼠海马组织的病理学改变，使存活的神经元增加，预处理后的海马 Fas、Fas－L 阳性细胞明显减少。其通过下调 Fas、Fas－L 表达和提高大鼠海马组织抗氧化能力起到对损伤海马的保护作用。Liang XY 等研究表明，丹参水提物亦可降低脑缺血再灌注大鼠血清中超敏 C 反应蛋白、IL－8、IL－10、TNF－α 的水平，降低 FADD 及死亡相关蛋白阳性表达水平，从而在脑缺血再灌注大鼠中起到神经保护的作用。

4. 其他

Zhou JJ 等报道，紫红獐牙菜中的有效成分 3－*O*－demethylswertipunicoside 能够抑制 1－甲基－4－苯基吡啶离子诱导的 PC12 细胞的凋亡，其作用机制之一与其抑制凋亡诱导因子（AIF）的核转移有关。Liang JM 等报道，人参皂苷 Rb_1 通过保护线粒体、抑制 AIF 和细胞色素 C 的释放以减轻氧糖剥夺诱导的 SH－SY5Y 细胞的凋亡。Hu GY 等报道，人参皂苷 Rd 通过抑制 PARP－1 的活性，进而阻止 AIF 的核转移，从而减轻局灶性脑缺血大鼠神经损伤。

（申　凯　寇俊萍）

【中药抑制血管生成作用的研究】

1. 抑制血管生长因子及其受体的表达

血管生成依赖于血管生成促进因子和血管生成抑制因子的动态平衡，其中与血管生成关系最为密切的血管生成因子为 VEGF 和碱性成纤维细胞生长因子（bFGF）。郑国灿等研究表明，牛蒡子苷元通过降低 VEGF 的表达水平来调控血管生成因子的平衡，从而抑制肿瘤血管生成。王炎等研究表明，丹参酮 $Ⅱ_A$ 能够抑制裸鼠人肠癌皮下移植瘤的生长和微血管生成，其机制可能与下调 VEGF 和 β－catenin 蛋白表达有关。Yang Y 等报道，紫花前胡素通过抑制血管内皮细胞生长因子受体 2（VEGFR2）活性，达到抑制细胞增殖和血管生成的作用，提示紫花前胡素可能对糖尿病视网膜病的治疗有益。赵春霞等研究表明，青蒿琥酯纳米脂质体与青蒿琥酯原料药能够下调 HepG2 细胞 VEGF 及 VEGFR2 mRNA 表达和蛋白表达，从而抑制肿瘤血管的生成。刘丽丽等报道，益气消癥法中药（党参、川续断、莪术、郁金、白芥子、鳖甲）可明显阻断雌二醇（E_2）对人脐血管内皮细胞株（EA. hy926）细胞增殖的促进作用，降低雌激素受体 α（ERα）与 VEGFR1、VEGFR2 表达，阻断 E_2 对 EA. hy926 细胞凋亡的抑制作用，上调 ERβ 的表达，从而抑制 EA. hy926 细胞的凋亡。龚陈媛等研究表明，石斛联苄类化合物能有效抑制 VEGF 诱导的人脐静脉内皮细胞管腔形成血管新生，其机制主要是阻断了 VEGFR2 及 c－Raf－MEK1/2－ERK1/2 信号级联通路的激活。Yu XB 等报道，二仙汤下调内皮细胞中 VEGFR1 和 VEGFR2 表达，抑制 ERK1/2 和 Akt 的活性，从而抑制血管生成。

2. 促进血管生成抑制因子的表达

血管抑素、内皮抑素是重要的血管生成抑制因子。李斐斐等研究表明，益肺清化颗粒通过降低血管生成促进因子 VEGF 的表达，升高血管生成抑制因子血管抑素和内皮抑素的表达，进而发挥抑瘤作用。

3. 抑制基质金属蛋白酶（MMPs）的活性

姜英等研究表明，木犀草素能有效地抑制乳腺癌 MCF－7 细胞增殖，抑制抑癌基因 Bcl－2 蛋白表达，抑制血管新生和乳腺癌细胞的侵袭，下调星形胶质细胞升高基因－1 和 MMP－2 蛋白表达。邹志坚等研究表明，地锦草通过抑制荷瘤小鼠肿瘤组织的 VEGF、MMP－9 蛋白表达，减少肿瘤血管生成和基质的降解，抑制荷瘤小鼠的肿瘤生长。

4. 抑制血管生成相关细胞的增殖和迁移

曹慧娟等研究表明，黄芩苷在体外对人肺癌 A549 细胞增殖、侵袭、迁移和对脐静脉血管内皮细胞新生血管形成都具有一定的抑制作用。Zhao RP 等报道，麦冬中的一个皂苷单体 DT－13 主要通过下调 p－VEGF2 和 p－Akt 的水平，抑制内皮细胞迁移和血管生成。Zhao B 等报道，没食子酸主要通过下调 EGFR，Akt/pAkt 和 Erk/pErk 通路，显著降低肿瘤细胞增殖和血管的形成。卢碧玉等研究表明，芦荟多糖能够明显抑制人脐静脉内皮细胞 HMEC－1 生长和鸡胚绒毛尿囊膜血管生成。虞迪等研究表明，毛茛有效部位D1通过抑制血管生成拟态相关基因Sema 4D、VE-Cadherin、MMP2和Integrin β5的表达来抑制人胃癌细胞MGC803细胞粘附、细胞迁移和血管生成拟态。

5. 抑制新生血管的成熟

由于VEGF与血管生成素(Ang)为互补和协同的作用关系，Ang-1与Ang-2都可与Tie2受体结合。中药在抑制VEGF表达的同时，一方面可以抑制Ang-1与Ang-2的表达；另一方面从受体的角度可以抑制Ang与Tie2受体结合。邓伟等研究表明，三七可以抑制二乙基亚硝胺诱发大鼠肝癌血管生成，可能是通过抑制Ang-2、Tie-2、HIF-1α及VEGF而发挥预防作用的。崔平等报道，白藜芦醇(Res)可以显著抑制视网膜母细胞瘤细胞生长，且具有剂量和时间依赖性；Res作用后VEGFA、bFGF和Ang-2 mRNA和蛋白表达下降。表明Res具有抗视网膜母细胞瘤血管生成的作用，其机制可能与下调血管生成相关因子VEGFA、bFGF和Ang-2表达有关。

6. 干预细胞内信号转导通路

随着人们对血管生成过程中细胞内信号转导的研究不断深入，干扰信号转导途径中的各种效应物，也是一种很有效的方法。Zeng KW等报道，川麦冬皂苷类代谢成分sprengerinin C抑制VEGFR2介导的PI3K/Akt/mTOR/MMPs和p38 MAPK/MMPs通路，从而抑制血管生成。Zhang L等报道，去甲斑蝥素抑制VEGFR2/MEK/ERK信号通路，从而抑制肿瘤血管的生成。Peng L等研究表明，百里香醌能够抑制NF-κB和下游效应分子，达到抑制肿瘤血管生成和肿瘤生长的作用。Gong CY等报道，穿心莲内酯衍生物主要通过调节细胞内VEGFR2-p38/ERK1/2信号通路抑制血管生成和肿瘤生长。马丽萍等研究表明，合欢皮有效部位能够抑制bFGF诱导的Matrigel种植体内血管生成，此作用与下调pAKT、pERK的表达量有关。

(翟科峰　唐友梅　寇俊萍)

【中药调节内质网应激作用的研究】

内质网是真核细胞内多数蛋白质合成、加工和转运必需的场所。细胞受到刺激后会发生内质网应激反应(ERS)。适度的ERS有助于恢复细胞稳态，维持细胞存活；过度的ERS会引起细胞内蛋白折叠错误，大量Ca^{2+}流入包浆，破坏细胞内稳态。ERS受多种因素的诱发，如缺氧、缺血、能量耗竭、Ca^{2+}紊乱等。

1. 中药调节心血管疾病中ERS的作用

娄利霞等研究表明，丹参Ⅱ$_A$对血管紧张素Ⅱ(AngⅡ)诱导的心肌细胞凋亡具有明显的保护作用，其机制是通过降低ERS分子伴侣葡萄糖调节蛋白78(GRP78)、C/EBP同源蛋白(CHOP) mRNA的表达，继而抑制Caspase-12的转录，减轻了过度的ERS介导的心肌细胞凋亡。付强等研究表明，丹参酮Ⅱ$_A$能上调Bip基因表达，放大ERS信号，诱导兔增殖血管平滑肌细胞(VSMC)凋亡，可能是其抗动脉粥样硬化的机制之一。蔡夏夏等研究表明，槲皮素可能通过抑制ERS相关通路来减轻应激及凋亡，最终改善葡萄糖胺损伤的人脐静脉血管内皮细胞损伤。王琛等、刘蜜等均报道，西洋参茎叶总皂苷能通过抑制过度的ERS介导的细胞凋亡，减轻大鼠心肌缺血/再灌注损伤和大鼠急性心肌梗死后心室重构，显著降低大鼠心肌CHOP、钙网蛋白以及caspase-12蛋白的表达。沈明志等报道，银杏叶提取物可以通过抑制GRP78和CHOP蛋白的表达，对晚期糖基化终产物诱导的心肌细胞损伤发挥保护作用。

2. 中药调节神经系统疾病中ERS的作用

缺血性脑损伤过程中氧气和能量耗竭可激活ERS，引起神经细胞凋亡。Liu D等报道，人参皂苷Rb_1可以通过抑制CHOP通路、氧化应激和线粒体功能紊乱，以对抗高糖诱导的神经细胞损伤。王伟等研究表明，丁苯肽预给药7 d的缺血再灌注大鼠GRP78和CHOP mRNA的表达水平明显降低，脑梗死面积也明显减少，提示丁苯肽可通过调节ERS而起到脑保护的作用。张琰等研究表明，何首乌所含二苯乙烯苷对氧糖剥夺诱导大鼠大脑皮层星形胶质细胞的凋亡具有保护作用，其机制是通过阻断细胞内钙离子介导的ERS或直接抑制ERS特有的凋亡起始因子Caspase-12。Chang XH等报道，茶多酚、茶氨酸、人参皂苷和远志酸(3∶3∶2∶1)混合药物对2型糖尿病引起的认知功能障碍具有改善作用，其机制可能是通过抑制 ERS 过程中 JNK 通路的激活。

3. 中药调节肿瘤细胞 ERS 的作用

药物通过 ERS 途径诱导肿瘤细胞的凋亡，从而达到抑制肿瘤发展的作用。Shen SY 等报道，知母皂苷元的抗肿瘤活性是通过纠正活性氧介导的线粒体功能紊乱和 ERS 导致的细胞坏死。殷文静等研究表明，穿心莲内酯具有抗宫颈癌效应，其机制可能是诱导 ERS，进而促进肿瘤细胞的凋亡。胡庆华等报道，姜黄素对 HeLa 细胞进行干预后，使用 ERS 抑制剂 4－PBA 能够显著降低 HeLa 细胞的凋亡率，同时 HeLa 细胞内 ERS 标志物 GRP78 与凋亡诱导分子 CHOP 的 mRNA 及蛋白表达水平均被显著抑制，表明姜黄素能够通过激活 ERS 相关通路诱导宫颈癌 HeLa 细胞凋亡。Cao AL 等报道，姜黄素还可诱导人胃癌细胞和结肠癌细胞凋亡，这与其影响 ERS 和线粒体功能途径有关。王洁等研究表明，海星中有效成分星皂苷 1 能抑制人胶质瘤 U87 细胞的增殖，其机制是增加 GRP78、GRP94、CHOP 及 Caspase－4 蛋白表达。李玄等研究表明，爵床中分离的新化合物 6′－羟基爵床素 A 能够诱导肝癌细胞 HepG2 细胞内 Ca^{2+} 离子水平升高，激活 ERS 通路，增加 HepG2 细胞的凋亡。

4. 中药调节其他疾病中 ERS 的作用

甘稼夫等研究表明，牛磺酸能够抑制 GRP78 和 CHOP 的表达，显著恢复血管反应性，对大鼠盲肠结扎穿孔脓毒性休克模型具有改善作用。孙升云等研究表明，慢肾康宁对肾间质纤维化大鼠肾脏组织 ERS 中 PERK－eIF2α－ATF4－CHOP 通路过度表达有很好的抑制作用，具有肾脏保护功能。赵珊等研究表明，姜黄素减轻小鼠肺缺血再灌注损伤是通过抑制 ERS 中 JNK 通路过度活化。Wu L 等研究表明，大黄素可以通过抑制 ERS 相关通路，减少胰腺损伤和减轻炎性反应，发挥胰腺炎治疗作用。关翠雯等研究表明，大黄素能够诱导人肾小管上皮 HK－2 细胞凋亡，其作用机制与 ERS 有关。路君等研究表明，棕榈酸酯能够诱导人脐带间充质干细胞凋亡，ERS 可能是细胞凋亡的主要原因。邬姗等研究表明，盐酸小檗碱能够抑制胰岛 β 细胞 ERS 诱导的凋亡，发挥治疗糖尿病的作用。

（周华娜　寇俊萍）

【中药调控小胶质细胞活化的研究】

1. 抑制小胶质细胞炎性因子的释放

Zhang F 等报道，白藜芦醇能显著抑制脂多糖（LPS）刺激导致的小胶质细胞活化，减轻多种促炎因子和毒性因子如肿瘤坏死因子－α（TNF－α）、NO、白细胞介素－1β（IL－1β）的释放。景浩然等研究表明，大黄酚在不影响小胶质细胞细胞活性的情况下，显著抑制 LPS 诱导的小胶质细胞炎性因子 NO、TNF－α 的产生。杨红云等研究表明，羟基红花黄色素能剂量依赖地降低 LPS 活化的小鼠小胶质细胞系 BV2 细胞 NO 的释放，抑制激活诱导细胞死亡。Guo LY 等报道，姜黄素能够抑制人类免疫缺陷病毒Ⅰ型（HIV－1）糖蛋白 gp120 刺激的小鼠小胶质细胞系 N9 释放活性氧（ROS）、TNF－α、单核细胞趋化蛋白－1（MCP－1），减轻小胶质细胞的炎症反应，可能是其发挥神经保护作用的机制之一。王璐等研究表明，姜黄素对弓形虫感染的 BV2 细胞诱导型一氧化氮合酶（NOS）蛋白表达和 NO 的产生有很好的抑制作用，并改善细胞形态。Jiang B 等从益智仁中分得的 3 个新的桉烷倍半萜化合物可明显抑制 LPS 活化的小胶质细胞 NO 和 TNF－α 的释放。景浩然等研究表明，丹红注射液水萃取物中的某些成分以及丹酚酸 A 抑制激活小胶质细胞 NO 的产生，可能是其神经保护的机制之一。马艳等报道，海风藤提取物能抑制 Aβ 寡聚体激活小胶质细胞释放炎性反应因子 IL－1β 和 IL－6。亓珅等研究表明，海风藤提取物对寡聚体和纤丝状 $Aβ_{1-42}$ 激活的小胶质细胞在基因水平上释放炎性因子 IL－1β 和 TNF－α 具有明显的抑制作用。黄金兰等报道，三七总皂苷可明显抑制快速老化痴呆模型小鼠海马小胶质细胞的激活和降低血清 TNF－α、IL－1β、IL－6。

2. 抑制小胶质细胞 NF－κB 通路

Huang C 等报道，何首乌所含二苯乙烯苷通过降低 NF－κB 的结合活性，显著抑制 LPS 激活的小胶质细胞释放的炎症因子 TNF－α、IL－6，使 iNOS 表达下调。Zhang P 等报道，和厚朴酚有潜在的抗炎效应，缘于它能显著抑制 NF－κB 活化从而阻碍抗炎因子的产生。Li J 等报道，羟基红花黄色素 A 可明显抑制 BV2 小胶质细胞的炎症反应，可能是通过抑制 NF－κB 和 p38 磷酸化而发挥的。Teng P 等报道，枸杞多糖能抑制脂多糖活化的 BV2 细胞 NF -κB 和 caspase 3 的激活，从而减少 TNF - α 的释放。

3. 抑制小胶质细胞 Toll 样受体(TLR)激活

涂苑青等研究表明，瑞香素可以抑制 LPS 诱导的小胶质细胞活化产生的炎症因子，其分子机制可能与其调控小胶质细胞 TLR4 信号转导通路有关。朱玉婷等研究表明，槲皮素可明显抑制高糖激活的原代小胶质细胞 TLR4 表达的作用，从而减少 NO 的释放，以及 TNF - α、IL - 1β、NOS mRNA 的表达水平，表明槲皮素发挥抗中枢炎症的作用是通过抑制 TLR4 从而抑制炎症瀑布式级联反应。Hu HX 等报道，瓜蒌桂枝汤能显著降低活化的小胶质细胞中 TLR4 和髓样细胞分化因子 88 的表达，也能抑制 I κB 的磷酸化，阻断 NF -κB 的核转录功能，发挥其抑制炎性因子释放的作用。

4. 抑制小胶质细胞丝裂原活化蛋白激酶(MAPK)通路

Dong XQ 等报道，氧化苦参碱能够抑制 BV2 小胶质细胞炎性介质的释放，是由于其抑制 NF - κB、ERK 1/2、p38 MAPK 和 JNK 通路的激活。Hu HX 等报道，瓜蒌桂枝汤主要是通过 MAPK 通路抑制 LPS 活化的小胶质的迁移，对单核细胞趋化蛋白- 1、巨噬细胞炎症蛋白- 1α 的释放都有一定抑制作用。

5. 其他

Li J 等报道，雪上一枝蒿甲素对高浓度的三磷酸腺苷激活的 BV2 细胞的炎症因子 iNOS，IL -6，IL - 1β mRNA 水平的下调，主要是通过选择性拮抗 P2X7 受体而发挥作用。

(陈红林　寇俊萍)

【中药调节 PI3K/Akt 信号通路的研究】

磷脂酰肌醇 3 -激酶(PI3K)蛋白家族作为对抗凋亡刺激的存活信号，参与细胞增殖、分化、凋亡和葡萄糖转运等多种细胞功能的调节。PI3K/Akt(蛋白激酶 B)信号通路是影响细胞的存活的关键通路之一。

1. 中药通过 PI3K/Akt 通路调节肿瘤凋亡或迁移

Xu HY 等报道，岩大戟内酯 B 对 MCF - 7 乳腺癌细胞具有明显的抑制作用，并诱导肿瘤细胞凋亡。其机制主要是通过下调细胞周期蛋白 D1(cyclinD1)、细胞周期蛋白 E、雷帕霉素的动物靶标(mTOR)、p - PI3K、p - Akt，上调 PTEN 和 p - eIF4E 而发挥作用。Li Y 等报道，异甘草素可以通过下调花生四烯酸代谢网络，使 PI3K/Akt 通路失活，从而引起乳腺癌细胞生长抑制和凋亡。陈菊英等研究表明，紫草素促进乳腺癌 MCF - 7 细胞自噬，其作用机制可能是抑制 PI3K/Akt 通路。朴丽花等研究表明，人参皂苷 Rh_2 通过抑制 PI3K/Akt 信号通路，有效降低 MCF7/Adr 侵袭迁移能力。Sun Y 等报道，绵马素 PB 可抑制肝癌 HepG2 细胞增殖，抑制 PI3K 的表达和 Ser473 Akt、Ser9 GSK3β 的磷酸化，上调 NAG - 1 的表达，发挥促进细胞凋亡的作用。Qiao Y 等报道，草棉黄素对人肝癌细胞 HepG2 具有诱导凋亡作用，与 ROS 介导的线粒体依赖的 PI3K/Akt 失活有关。李一春等研究表明，黄荆子木脂素 3 可抑制 HepG2 细胞的增殖，其机制可能与抑制 Akt、ERK1/2 蛋白磷酸化水平有关。Li QH 等报道，淫羊藿素具有抗急性髓细胞性白血病作用，机制与抑制 MAPK/ERK 和 PI3K/Akt 信号通路和下调 c - myc 有关。Kang XH 等报道，蟾蜍灵通过抑制 Met/PI3K/Akt 通路和诱导死亡信号肽，逆转外源肝细胞生长因子诱导的可逆和不可逆的表皮生长因子受体-酪氨酸激酶抑制剂引起的非小细胞肺癌抵抗。Chen MJ 等报道，麦冬皂苷 B 可引起非小细胞肺癌细胞的自噬，并证实是通过 PI3K/Akt/mTOR 信号通路实现的。毛蜀等研究表明，姜黄素可能通过抑制 PI3K/Akt 信号通路，阻碍髓母细胞瘤 Daoy 细胞的增殖，诱导凋亡。罗发军等研究表明，夜香树花甾体皂苷具有抑制 K562 细胞增殖和促进凋亡的作用，是通过抑制 K562 细胞 PI3K/Akt 信号通路来发挥作用。韩冰冰等研究表明，天花粉蛋白能够抑制小鼠黑色素移植瘤的血管生成拟态，可能与调控 PI3K 的表达有关。

2. 中药通过激活 PI3K/Akt 通路发挥神经保护作用

Chai YS 等报道，小檗碱在脑局部缺血期时下调 p53 和 cyclinD1，上调 p - Bad，减少 caspase3 的分裂，诱导细胞周期阻滞；在灌注期时激活 PI3K/Akt，从而促进细胞存活。小檗碱的神经保护作用是通过诱导细胞周期阻滞和细胞存活以对抗脑缺血损伤。Dong LQ 等报道，厚朴酚通过调节 JNK/线粒体/caspase、PI3K/MEK/ERK 和 PI3K/Akt/FoxO1 通路来抵抗丙烯醛诱导的氧化应激和延长人神经母细胞瘤 SH－SY5Y 细胞的存活。Qi Y 等报道，番红花素通过 PI3K/Akt 通路，对视网膜神经节细胞缺血再灌注损伤起到神经保护的作用。陈亚男等研究表明，红景天苷通过激活 ERK1/2 和 PI3K/Akt/mTOR 信号通路，促进骨髓间充质干细胞向神经细胞定向分化。党惠子等研究表明，姜黄素可能通过调节 Akt 及其磷酸化过程，从而调节 PI3K/Akt 途径的胰岛素信号转导通路，发挥抗阿尔茨海默病作用。

3. 中药通过激活 PI3K/Akt 通路保护肝脏

Zhang YX 等以高脂饲料喂养大鼠制备非酒精性脂肪肝模型以及利用 BRL－3A 和 HepG2 细胞，进行体内和体外试验的研究。结果表明，水飞蓟宾可通过恢复 IRS－1/PI3K/Akt 通路来改善其病理特征，减少脂肪堆积，恢复细胞活力，下调抵抗素的蛋白表达。Liu CM 等通过血清氨基转移酶活性测定和组织病理学分析，表明芝麻素可对抗镍引起的肝毒性，恢复抗氧化酶活性，降低 8-羟基-2-脱氧鸟苷水平，增加 p－PI3K 和 p－PBK/Akt 的水平，抑制肝细胞凋亡。韩淑英等研究表明，荞麦花叶黄酮对糖尿病肝损伤有抑制作用，其机制可能是通过降低血糖、改善胰岛素抵抗，上调 IRS－2、PI3K 蛋白表达及下调 NF－κB 蛋白表达等多途径实现的。

4. 中药通过激活 PI3K/Akt 通路保护心肌

Wang M 等报道，丹参酚酸 B 可有效保护 As_2O_3 诱导的心肌细胞死亡从而起到保护心脏的作用，其机制为激活 PI3K/Akt 通路。Wang Y 等报道，心肌缺血后使用槲皮素处理，通过激活 PI3K/Akt 通路和调节 Bcl－2 及 Bax 蛋白的表达起到保护心肌的作用。李彬彬等研究表明，温阳通脉方具有心肌保护作用，能够减少心肌细胞凋亡，其作用机制可能与 PI3K/Akt 激酶途径激活有关。

5. 其他

Duan XH 等报道，淫羊藿苷可延迟同型半胱氨酸引起的内皮细胞的衰老，可能是通过 PI3K/Akt－eNOS 依赖途径发挥作用。Wang Y 等报道，葛根素对抗顺铂诱导的人成骨细胞 MG－63 的凋亡，并增加细胞的增值与分化，是通过雌激素受体 ERα 和 ERβ，激活 MEK/ERK 和 PI3K/Akt 通路实现的。Zhang Y 等报道，芒果叶提取物可剂量依赖性地减少 KK－Ay 小鼠血糖和甘油三脂，其机制是通过激活 PI3K/Akt 和 AMPK 通路，上调 PI3K，Akt 和 GYS 基因表达，导致血糖下降。

（郑显杰　寇俊萍　余伯阳）

［附］ 参 考 文 献

B

白静，韩婷，胡雷，等. 艾叶水提物及其发酵物对小肠平滑肌收缩性的影响［J］. 时珍国医国药，2013，24(7)：1617

白卫娜，陈英珠，闫静辉，等. 柿叶总黄酮对 apoE－/－小鼠动脉粥样硬化病变中粘附分子表达的影响［J］. 南京中医药大学学报，2013，29(1)：35

C

Cao AL，Li Q，Yin PH，et al. Curcumin induces apoptosis in human gastric carcinoma AGS cells and colon carcinoma HT－29 cells through mitochondrial dysfunction and endoplasmic reticulum stress［J］. Apoptosis，2013，18(11)：1391

Chai YS，Hu J，Lei F，et al. Effect of berberine on cell cycle arrest and cell survival during cerebral ischemia and reperfusion and correlations with p53/cyclin D1 and PI3K/Akt［J］. European Journal of Pharmacology，2013，708(1－3)：44

Chang XH，Lina LN，Zhan LB，et al. The effect of Chinese Jinzhida recipe on the hippocampus in a rat model of diabetes-associated cognitive decline［J］. Complentary Alternative Medicine 2013，13(1)：161

Chen MJ，Du YH，Qui M，et al. Ophiopogonin B－induced autophagy in non-small cell lung cancer cells via inhibition of the PI3K/Akt signaling pathway［J］. Oncology reports，2013，29(2)：430

蔡夏夏，鲍雷，丁叶，等. 槲皮素对葡萄糖胺条件下血管内皮细胞损伤的影响[J]. 食品科学，2013，34(13)：224

蔡晓璐，王真，江立斌. 穿山龙总皂苷对哮喘小鼠气道重塑的影响[J]. 浙江中医药大学学报，2013，37(6)：756

曹慧娟，鄢云彪，戴建业，等. 黄芩苷对人肺腺癌A549细胞的体内外研究[J]. 中国实验方剂学杂志，2013，19(13)：216

曹雨诞，李征军，陈海鹰，等. 甘遂不同炮制品及提取物对斑马鱼的急性毒性研究[J]. 中国现代应用药学，2013，30(2)：140

曹志友，金宏，田晶，等. 白附子提取物对胶质瘤细胞的增殖抑制和诱导凋亡作用及其机制[J]. 吉林大学学报(医学版)，2013，39(4)；649

常文静，赵智明，赵凌杰，等. 丹参酮ⅡA对压力负荷增加大鼠心肌纤维化的改善作用[J]. 微循环学杂志，2013，23(2)：34

车章洪，何百成. 人参皂甙Rg3抑制人结肠癌细胞生长与Wnt/β-catenin信号的关系[J]. 第三军医大学学报，2013，35(13)：1353

陈华文，冯俊，李树生. 丹参酮$Ⅱ_A$对脓毒症大鼠心肌凋亡的保护作用[J]. 中国药学杂志，2013，48(17)：1267

陈菊英，刘朝纯，曾智，等. 紫草素通过PI3K/Akt通路促进人乳腺癌MCF-7细胞自噬[J]. 中国药理学通报，2013，29(2)：194

陈俊，唐安洲，梁钢，等. 苦参碱改构体X调控Caspase-3，Caspase-8和Caspase-9蛋白表达诱导人鼻咽癌CNE1凋亡的研究[J]. 中国药理学通报，2013，29(8)：1136

陈俊，唐安洲，谢貌，等. 苦参碱改构体X对人鼻咽癌CNE1细胞的凋亡诱导作用[J]. 中国实验方剂学杂志，2013，19(17)：266

陈立波. 苦参碱对宫颈癌Hela细胞增殖、凋亡及Survivin基因表达的影响[J]. 中国实验方剂学杂志，2013，19(15)：235

陈连连，陈力学，曾照芳. 粉防己碱对血管性痴呆大鼠齿状回S1000B蛋白表达的研究[J]. 激光杂志，2012，33(1)：72

陈萌，赵淑敏，李涵，等. 黄芩茎叶总黄酮预处理对脑缺血再灌注大鼠海马Fas，FasL的表达和抗氧化能力的影响[J]. 中国实验方剂学杂志，2013，19(4)：228

陈望昊，王慧博，刘宁. 汉黄芩素调节恶性胶质瘤U87细胞增殖和凋亡并影响miR-128的表达[J]. 南京医科大学学报(自然科学版)，2013，33(4)：456

陈翔，吴曙辉，袁杰，等. 黄药子醇提物对人胃癌裸鼠移植瘤的生长和血清IL-8及sICAM-1表达的影响[J]. 湖南中医杂志，2013，29(7). 123

陈晓芳，张倩，吴文倩，等. 枇杷花醇提物止咳化痰作用实验研究[J]. 中成药，2013，35(1)：167

陈亚男，刘辉，赵红斌，等. 红景天苷诱导骨髓间充质干细胞向神经细胞定向分化的机制研究[J]. 药学学报，2013，48(8)：1247

陈莹蓉，王翔，闵丽姗，等. 黄药子醇提物Caco-2细胞摄取液对HL-7702和HepG2细胞毒性研究[J]. 中国现代应用药学，2013，30(4)：368

程钢，秦媛媛，程迪，等. 氧化苦参碱对大鼠局灶性脑缺血损伤的保护作用及其抑制凋亡的作用机制[J]. 中国药理学通报，2013，29(3)：387

褚春民，张洪泉，卜平，等. 薯蓣皂苷对胶原性关节炎模型大鼠环氧合酶2及NF-κB的抑制作用[J]. 中国药理学与毒理学杂志，2013，27(3)：341

崔平，南娜，康洁，等. 白藜芦醇抑制视网膜母细胞瘤株血管生成相关因子VEGFA、bFGF和Ang-2表达的机制[J]. 中国老年学杂志，2013，33(22)：5649

D

Dong LQ, Zhou S, Yang XH, et al. Magnolol Protects Against Oxidative Stress-Mediated Neural Cell Damage by Modulating Mitochondrial Dysfunction and PI3K/Akt Signaling [J]. Journal of Molecular Neuroscience, 2013, 50(3): 469

Dong XQ, Du Q, Yu WH, et al. Anti-inflammatory effects of oxymatrine through inhibition of nuclear factor-kappa B and mitogen-activated protein kinase activation in lipopolysaccharide-induced BV2 microglia cells [J]. Iranian Journal of Pharmaceutical Research, 2013, 12(1): 165

Duan XH, Xu CQ, Huang JH, et al. Icariin delays homocysteine-induced endothelial cellular senescence involving activation of the PI3K/AKT-eNOS signaling pathway[J]. Pharmaceutical Biology, 2013, 51(4): 433

戴关海，童晔玲，张春丽，等. 胃乐煎对慢性萎缩性胃炎模型大鼠作用的实验研究[J]. 中国现代应用药学，2013，30(1)：15

党惠子，李瑞晟，王虹，等. 姜黄素对APP/PS1双转基因小鼠海马CA1区AKT及p-AKT表达的影响[J]. 中国中药杂志，2013，38(19)：3327

邓伟，向清，李宝. 中药三七抑制二乙基亚硝胺诱发大鼠肝癌血管生成的研究[J]. 广西医学，2013，35(11)：1442

董文娟，郭亚春，宋鸿儒. 穿山龙总皂苷对胶原诱导关节炎大鼠滑膜血管内皮生长因子、血管生成素-2及受体Tie-2表达的影响[J]. 中国药学杂志，2013，48(2)：101

杜菲菲，高明，多佳俊，等. 复方儿茶止泻霜对腹泻大鼠结肠黏膜AQP1调节作用[J]. 辽宁中医药大学学报，

2013,15(10): 34

段彬,张建强,陈明,等. 平胃散及其组方药材水煎液对大鼠胃排空的影响[J]. 兰州大学学报(医学版),2013,39(1): 20

F

付剑江,王曦聆,吕红,等. 罗布麻叶提取物的抗高血压作用及其机制研究[J]. 中国实验方剂学杂志,2013,19(7): 159

付强,张妍,沈晓君,等. 丹参酮ⅡA 对血管平滑肌细胞内质网应激相关基因表达的影响[J]. 中国实验方剂学杂志,2013,19(14): 280

G

Gong CY, Xu C, Ji LL, et al. A novel semi-synthetic andrographolide analogue A5 inhibits tumor angiogenesis via blocking the VEGFR2 - p38/ERK1/2 signal pathway[J]. Bioscience Trends, 2013, 7(5): 230

Guo DJ, Li F, Yu PH, et al. Neuroprotective effects of luteolin against apoptosis induced by 6 - hydroxydopamine on rat pheochromocytoma PC12 cells [J]. Pharmaceutical Biology, 2013, 51(2): 190

Guo LY, Xing YY, Pan R, et al. Curcumin protects microglia and primary rat cortical neurons against HIV - 1 gp120 - mediated inflammation and apoptosis[J]. PLoS One, 2013, 8(8): e70565

甘稼夫,胡畔,刘良明. 内质网应激诱导血管反应性降低与线粒体通透性转换孔开放的关系[J]. 中国病理生理杂志,2013,29(2): 231

宫金艳. 丹参对大鼠肺纤维化的影响研究[J]. 湖南中医杂志,2013,29(2): 122

龚陈媛,陆宾,杨莉,等. 石斛联苄类化合物抑制血管新生的机制[J]. 药学学报,2013,48(3): 337

苟玲,何婷,曾南,等. 荆芥、桂枝挥发油含药血清体外抗病毒的实验研究[J]. 时珍国医国药,2013,24(1): 19

关翠雯,金晶,李佳,等. 丹参酮ⅡA 激活 Nrf2/ARE 通路保护雷公藤甲素所致急性肝损伤[J]. 药学学报,2013,48(9): 1397

关翠雯,金晶,朱少华,等. 大黄素诱导人肾上皮HK - 2 细胞凋亡及内质网应激的介导作用[J]. 中草药,2013,44(12): 1501

关悦,李扬,刘佳维. 羊栖菜多糖对糖尿病脑缺血大鼠细胞凋亡的影响[J]. 中国海洋药物,2013,32(2): 63

郭洁,时昭红,张介眉. 葱白提取物对脂肪变性肝细胞 PGC - 1α 表达及线粒体 SDH 活性的影响[J]. 山东医药,2013,53(28): 1

郭丽华,齐聪,杨红,等. 半枝莲黄酮类单体对人卵巢癌 Skov3 细胞增殖的影响[J]. 上海中医药杂志,2013,47(1): 61

H

Hu GY, Wu ZL, Yang F, et al. Ginsenoside Rd blocks AIF mitochondrio-nuclear translocation and NF - κB nuclear accumulation by inhibiting poly(ADP - ribose) polymerase - 1 after focal cerebral ischemia in rats [J]. Neurological Sciences, 2013, 34(12): 2101

Hu HX, Li ZF, Zhu XQ, et al. GuaLou GuiZhi decoction suppresses LPS - induced activation of the TLR4/NF - κB pathway in BV - 2 murine microglial cells [J]. Interntional Journal of Molecular Medicine, 2013, 31(6): 1327

Hu HX, Li ZF, Zhu XQ, et al. GuaLou GuiZhi decoction inhibits LPS - induced microglial cell motility through the MAPK signaling pathway[J]. International Journal of Molecular Medicine, 2013, 32(6): 1281

Huang C, Wang YZ, Wang J, et al. TSG(2,3,4′,5 - tetrahydroxystilbene 2 - *O* - *β* - D - glucoside) suppresses induction of pro-inflammatory factors by attenuating the binding activity of nuclear factor - κB in microglia [J]. Journal of Neuroinflammation, 2013, 10: 129

韩冰冰,李洁. 天花粉蛋白对小鼠黑色素移植瘤血管生成拟态及 PI3K 表达的影响[J]. 中药药理与临床,2013,29(3): 38

韩红彦,贾海珍,潘云红,等. 通心络胶囊对急性冠脉综合征治疗中的免疫调节作用[J]. 辽宁中医药大学学报,2013,15(10): 8

韩淑英,姜妍,王志路,等. 荞麦花叶黄酮对 2 型糖尿病大鼠肝损伤及 IRS - 2、PI3K、NF - κB 表达的影响[J]. 中国药理学通报,2013,29(11): 1582

何雯,郐利娅·伊明,司丽君,等. 异叶青兰总黄酮对高血压大鼠心肌肥厚的影响[J]. 中国药理学通报,2013,29(7): 1008

侯平,杨丽,刘宁,等. 麻黄碱、β-细辛醚和去甲乌药碱对大鼠心肌细胞钙离子浓度和细胞膜钙通道的影响[J]. 中国医科大学学报,2013,42(3): 201

胡庆华,贺建文,赵小军. 姜黄素通过内质网应激途径诱导宫颈癌 Hela 细胞凋亡的实验研究[J]. 陕西医学杂志,2013,42(10): 1279

胡微煦,向勤,文珠,等. 白术多糖抗神经细胞缺氧性凋亡的机制研究[J]. 中药药理与临床,2013,29(4): 84

胡玉英,胡跃强,张青萍,等. 交泰丸对血管性痴呆模型大鼠单胺氧化酶及单胺类神经递质的影响[J]. 中国老年学杂志,2013,33(20): 5028

华碧春,卓实,史道华,等. 甘草减轻黄药子肝毒性的研究[J]. 福建中医药大学学报,2013,23(1): 23

黄柏胜,罗洁,韩仰,等.山楂酸预处理对皮层神经元氧糖剥夺损伤的影响[J].南方医科大学学报,2013,33(3):322

黄欢,曹明成,朱正义,等.白果内酯对血管性痴呆小鼠的保护作用[J].安徽医药,2013,17(3):383

黄金兰,陆璐,黄丹,等.三七总皂苷对快速老化痴呆模型小鼠SAMP8炎症因子及小胶质细胞的影响[J].中国实验方剂学杂志,2013,19(8):171

黄倩,楚世峰,张均田,等.人参皂苷Rg_1的抗抑郁作用及对突触超微结构的影响[J].中国药理学通报,2013,29(8):1124

黄新武,李国春,李华,等.姜黄素对血管性痴呆模型大鼠海马神经元凋亡和蛋白表达的影响[J].中医临床研究,2013,5(15):13

J

Jiang B, Wang WJ, Li MP, et al. New eudesmane sesquiterpenes from Alpinia oxyphylla and determination of their inhibitory effects on microglia[J]. Bioorganic & Medicinal Chemistry Letters, 2013, 23(13): 3879

季亢挺,胡建坚,陈军,等.黄芪甲苷对氧化低密度脂蛋白诱导内皮祖细胞炎症损伤的保护作用[J].中国现代应用药学,2013,30(8):827

贾宁,林琳,朱伟平,等.三七总皂苷对NRK-52E细胞株的BMP-7、connexin43及PI3K/Akt通路的影响[J].时珍国医国药,2013,24(8):1928

姜文,周兆山,胡海波,等.茯苓、薏苡仁与冬瓜子对肺纤维化大鼠血清TGF-β1和TNF-α浓度影响[J].齐鲁医学杂志,2013,28(3):237

姜英,谢鲲鹏,霍洪楠,等.木犀草素下调AEG-1和MMP-2的表达对血管生成和乳腺癌细胞侵袭性的抑制作用[J].生理学报,2013,65(5):513

蒋青,沈明勤,石磊,等.地黄寡糖对血管性痴呆大鼠海马区神经细胞凋亡及相关蛋白表达的影响[J].中国实验方剂学杂志,2013,19(3):192

金光虎,夏海波,李海峰,等.苦参碱对前列腺癌PC-3M细胞生长抑制和凋亡的影响[J].内蒙古医学杂志,2013,45(1):1

金国泰,李博,仲宗亮,等.六虫骨灵胶囊镇痛抗炎作用的实验研究[J].湖南中医杂志,2013,29(7):115

金连峰,韩煜.骨碎补对兔膝骨关节炎关节软骨细胞凋亡相关因子作用实验研究[J].辽宁中医药大学学报,2013,15(11):42

金祖汉,金捷,毛培江,等.黄连降糖片治疗糖尿病的药理作用研究[J].中国现代应用药学,2013,30(8);823

景浩然,胡利民,王少峡,等.丹红注射液及其活性组分对脂多糖诱导的小胶质细胞NO分泌的抑制作用[J].现代药物与临床,2013,28(3):285

景浩然,杨红云,王少峡,等.大黄酚对LPS诱导小胶质细胞炎性因子分泌的影响[J].天津中医药大学学报,2013,32(3):148

K

Kang XH, Xu ZY, Gong YB, et al. Bufalin Reverses HGF-Induced Resistance to EGFR-TKIs in EGFR Mutant Lung Cancer Cells via Blockage of Met/PI3k/Akt Pathway and Induction of Apoptosis [J]. Evidence-based Complementary and Alternative Medicine, 2013, 2013: 243859

康小龙,何承辉,邢建国,等.香青兰总黄酮对哮喘大鼠白细胞介素-6、13、17和肿瘤坏死因子-α的影响[J].中国现代应用药学,2013,30(8):839

孔德燕.丹参酮Ⅱ$_A$对血管性痴呆大鼠脑组织一氧化氮含量、一氧化氮合酶活性及胆碱能系统的影响[J].实用医学杂志,2013,29(17):2797

L

Li J, Ren W, Huang XJ, et al. Bullatine A, a diterpenoid alkaloid of the genus Aconitum, could attenuate ATP-induced BV-2 microglia death/apoptosis via P2X receptor pathways[J]. Brain Research Bulletin, 2013, 97: 81

Li J, Zhang SY, Lu MR, et al. Hydroxysafflor yellow A suppresses inflammatory responses of BV2 microglia after oxygen-glucose deprivation [J]. Neuroscience Letters, 2013, 535: 51

Li QH, Huai L, Zhang CP, et al. Icaritin induces AML cell apoptosis via the MAPK/ERK and PI3K/AKT signal pathways[J]. International Journal of Hematology, 2013, 97(5): 617

Li Y, Zhao HX, Wang YZ, et al. Isoliquiritigenin induces growth inhibition and apoptosis through downregulating arachidonic acid metabolic network and the deactivation of PI3K/Akt in human breast cancer[J]. Toxicology and Applied Pharmacology, 2013, 272(1): 37

Li ZY, Guo Z, Liu YM, et al. Neuroprotective effects of Total Saikosaponins of Bupleurum yinchowense on corticosterone-induced apoptosis in PC12 cells [J]. Journal of Ethnopharmacology, 2013, 148(3): 794

Liang JM, Yu Y, Wang BY, et al. Ginsenoside Rb1 Attenuates oxygen-glucose deprivation-induced apoptosis in SH-SY5Y Cells via protection of mitochondria and inhibition of AIF and cytochrome c release [J]. Molecules, 2013, 18(10): 12777

Liang XY, Li HN, Yang XY, et al. Effect of Danshen aqueous extract on serum hs-CRP, IL-8, IL-

10, TNF-α levels, and IL-10 mRNA, TNF-α mRNA expression levels, cerebral TGF-β1 positive expression level and its neuroprotective mechanisms in CIR rats [J]. Molecular Biology Reports, 2013, 40(4): 3419

Liu CM, Zheng GH, Ming QL, et al. Sesamin protects mouse liver against nickel-induced oxidative DNA damage and apoptosis by the PI3K-Akt pathway[J]. Journal of agricultural food chemistry, 2013, 61(5): 1146

Liu D, Zhang H, Gu WJ, et al. Neuroprotective effects of ginsenoside Rb1 on high glucose-induced neurotoxicity in primary cultured rat hippocampal neurons [J]. PLos One, 2013, 8(11): e79399

Liu DM, Wang ZH, Liu L, et al. Acetylpuerarin increases cell viability and reduces apoptosis in rat hippocampal neurons following oxygen-glucose deprivation/reperfusion[J]. Molecular Medicine Reports, 2013, 8(5): 1453

李彬彬,石月萍.温阳通脉方对大鼠心肌缺血-再灌注损伤的影响及其信号传导途径[J].解放军医学院学报,2013,34(4):386

李斐斐,吴皓,陈璐,等.益肺清化颗粒对 Lewis 肺癌小鼠 VEGF、bFGF、Angiostatin、Endostatin 影响的研究[J].中国中西医结合杂志,2013,33(8):1086

李君,魏涛,张青山,等.银杏叶提取物对血管性痴呆大鼠空间学习记忆和海马 NMDAR1 表达的影响[J].神经解剖学杂志,2012,28(6):621

李姝玉,柴欣楼,吴莹,等.黄芪和葛根素对 2 型糖尿病 KKAy 小鼠的肾脏保护作用及纤黏连蛋白表达的影响[J].北京中医药大学学报,2013,36(2):96

李顺,魏学斌,黄世明,等.氧化苦参碱体外诱导膀胱癌 T24 细胞凋亡[J].第二军医大学学报,2013,34(5):565

李炜,张力,董晓华,等.蛇床子素对痴呆模型小鼠行为学的保护作用[J].神经药理学报,2012,2(2):15

李玄,贺晓丽,童元峰,等.6′-羟基爵床素 A 对 HepG2 细胞内质网应激及胞内 Ca^{2+} 的影响[J].中国实验方剂学杂志,2013,19(13):212

李雪燕,陈开兵,张丽云.当归多糖对衰老模型小鼠行为学、血清和脑 SOD、端粒酶活性的影响[J].现代中医药,2013,33(2):101

李彦龙,伍春,廖志峰,等.薏苡仁水提液对溃疡性结肠炎大鼠血清 IL-6、IL-10 的影响[J].辽宁中医药大学学报,2013,15(9):42

李一春,杨文军,陈艳.黄荆子木脂素 3 对人肝癌 HepG2 细胞增殖的抑制作用及对蛋白激酶 Akt、ERK1/2 信号通路的影响[J].中国药房,2013,24(33):3099

李正红,盛梅笑,张旭,等.黄芪对高糖腹透液诱导大鼠腹膜间皮细胞 EMT 中 TGF-β/Smads 信号通路的影响[J].南京中医药大学学报,2013,29(3):227

梁秀军,孙同友,董文娟,等.穿山龙总皂苷对胶原性关节炎大鼠炎性细胞因子的影响[J].时珍国医国药,2013,24(3):522

林建阳,续晋洁,林秋婕,等.红景天苷在大鼠体内的药物代谢动力学研究[J].山西中医杂志,2013,42(9):971

刘彬,陈逸杰,程惠娟,等.鱼腥草素钠增强妥布霉素抗铜绿假单胞菌生物被膜作用及抗菌协同作用[J].辽宁中医药大学学报,2013,15(11):47

刘春丽,陈虹,姜勇,等.松果菊苷对血管性痴呆大鼠行为学、氧自由基以及胆碱能神经递质代谢速率的影响[J].中国药理学通报,2013,29(7):1035

刘国岩,徐展望,徐琬梨.骨碎补提取物对骨髓间充质干细胞向成骨细胞分化及 Cbfα1 表达的影响[J].山东医药,2013,53(25):10

刘蕾,陈光,王跃新,等.翻白草油对 RSV 感染宿主 HeLa 细胞 Bcl-2 蛋白和 Bax 蛋白表达的影响[J].中国老年学杂志,2013,33(18):4483

刘丽丽,李爽,李海东,等.益气消癥法中药含药血清干预 ER 及 VEGFR 表达抑制 EA.hy926 增殖的研究[J].四川中医,2013,31(7):45

刘蜜,王琛,王晓礽,等.西洋参茎叶总皂苷通过抑制内质网应激相关细胞凋亡减轻大鼠急性心肌梗死后心室重构[J].中国病理生理杂志,2013,29(5):796

刘伟,陈韬,韩洪波,等.银杏叶提取物对 STZ 和 ISO 协同诱发大鼠糖尿病心肌病的治疗作用[J].吉林大学学报(医学版),2013,39(3):503

刘文东,李英娴,娄婷婷,等.青蒿琥酯对肝纤维化大鼠肝组织基质金属蛋白酶表达的影响[J].天津医科大学学报,2013,19(5):362

刘晓舒,孙倩,杨鑫,等.黄芪多糖对 Hhcy 大鼠心肌缺血再灌注的影响[J].辽宁医学杂志,2013,27(1):6

刘长安,朱洁,那莎,等.川芎嗪对 Aβ25-35 诱导体外大鼠海马神经元细胞凋亡的影响[J].天然产物研究与开发,2013,25(5):684

娄利霞,张冬梅,吴爱明,等.丹参酮 $Ⅱ_A$ 对血管紧张素Ⅱ诱导的心肌细胞凋亡的抑制作用[J].中西医结合心脑血管病杂志,2013,11(3):333

卢碧玉,蔡小连.芦荟多糖抑制肿瘤新生血管作用的研究[J].中医药导报,2013,19(1):83

卢新华,王桂霞,何军山.马齿苋总黄酮对缺血缺氧刺激下血管平滑肌细胞蛋白激酶 C 活性的影响[J].中国临床药理学杂志,2013,29(9):685

路君,董会月,林灵婧,等.棕榈酸酯诱导人脐带间充质干细胞内质网应激和细胞凋亡[J].生理学报,2013,65(6):600

栾海艳,张建华,赵晓莲,等.桔梗总皂苷对 2 型糖尿

病肝病大鼠糖脂代谢影响的研究[J]. 中成药，2013，35(6)：1307

栾华梅，于丽丽，刘述磊，等. 人参皂苷对青霉素致癫新生大鼠的影响研究[J]. 时珍国医国药，2013，24(1)：57

罗发军，赵世元，钟振国. 夜香树花甾体皂苷抑制K562细胞增殖及对PI3K/Akt信号通路的调控[J]. 实用癌症杂志，2013，28(6)：583

罗云，赵海平，张婧，等. 阿魏酸对血管性痴呆大鼠学习记忆障碍的改善作用及其机制研究[J]. 药学学报，2012，47(2)：256

吕昕瞳，杨丹莉，邓江，等. 人参总皂苷对血管紧张素Ⅱ所致乳大鼠心肌细胞肥大的抑制作用[J]. 中国药理学与毒理学杂志，2013，27(4)：641

M

马克龙，汪远金，汪天明，等. 千金藤碱对结肠癌细胞5-氟尿嘧啶耐药性的逆转作用和对HO-1和NQO1表达的影响[J]. 江西中医学院学报，2013，25(2)：59

马立，吴明华，梁森，等. 三七总皂苷对脑缺血后神经血管的保护机制[J]. 吉林中医药，2013，33(7)：720

马丽萍，邱丽颖，冯磊，等. 合欢皮有效部位对bFGF诱导小鼠血管生成的影响及其机制[J]. 华西药学杂志，2013，28(6)：583

马艳，邢华医，马学强，等. 海风藤对β淀粉样蛋白寡聚体激活小胶质细胞的影响[J]. 中国神经免疫学和神经病学杂志，2013，20(2)：110

毛秉豫，杨雷，徐国昌，等. 丹参提取物对血管紧张素Ⅱ致培养乳鼠心肌细胞肥大的影响[J]. 中国实验方剂学杂志，2013，19(2)：263

毛蜀，何密斯，刘桂元，等. 姜黄素对髓母细胞瘤PI3K/Akt信号通路的作用[J]. 第三军医大学学报，2013，35(6)：518

N

牛彩琴，张团笑，买文丽. 苦豆子总碱对大鼠膀胱逼尿肌作用机制研究[J]. 辽宁中医药大学学报，2013，15(1)：36

P

Peng L, Liu A, Shen Y, et al. Antitumor and anti-angiogenesis effects of thymoquinone on osteosarcoma through the NF-κB pathway[J]. Oncology Reports, 2013, 29(2): 571

潘朝旺，洪运良，曹宇，等. 九龙虫对血管痴呆型小鼠NO、NOS的影响[J]. 鄂州大学学报，2012，19(5)：15

潘毅，王文靖，阳涛，等. 血畅宁对两种高血压大鼠模型的血压及左室重构的影响[J]. 时珍国医国药，2013，24(6)：1304

彭娟，邓虹珠，马丹丹，等. 哈蟆油对大鼠卵巢颗粒细胞增殖与分泌的影响[J]. 时珍国医国药，2013，24(3)：532

朴丽花，蔡英兰，张默函，等. 人参皂苷Rh2与PI3K/AKT信号通路抑制剂LY294002对乳腺癌细胞转移和侵袭的影响[J]. 中国药房，2013，24(43)：4050

Q

Qi Y, Chen L, Zhang L, et al. Crocin prevents retinal ischemia/reperfusion injury-induced apoptosis in retinal ganglion cells through the PI3K/AKT signalling pathway[J]. Experimental Eye Research, 2013, 107: 44

Qiao Y, Xiang QS, Li Y, et al. Herbacetin induces apoptosis in HepG2 cells: Involvements of ROS and PI3K/Akt pathway[J]. Food and Chemical Toxicology, 2013, 51: 426

亓珅，韩晓娟，王璐，等. 海风藤提取物对激活的小胶质细胞IL-1β和TNF-α表达的影响[J]. 山东大学学报，2013，51(5)：11

祁佳，李莉霞，卜书红，等. 藤茶提取物清咽抗炎作用及其机制的研究[J]. 贵阳中医学院学报，2013，35(1)：19

乔晓鸣，任世存. 沙棘总黄酮对血管性痴呆模型大鼠行为学和血液流变学的影响[J]. 青海医学院学报，2012，33(2)：127

曲雷鸣，龚伟. 淫羊藿含药血清对MC3T3-E1成骨细胞增殖及分化的影响[J]. 中国药房，2013，24(35)：3283

R

Ruan L, Huang HS, Jin WX, et al. Tetrandrine attenuated cerebral ischemia/reperfusion injury and induced differential proteomic changes in a MCAO mice model using 2-D DIGE[J]. Neurochemical Research, 2013, 38(9): 1871

S

Shen SY, Zhang Y, Zhang R, et al. Sarsasapogenin induces apoptosis via the reactive oxygen species-mediated mitochondrial pathway and ER stress pathway in HeLa cells [J]. Biochemical and Biophysical Research Communications, 2013, 441(2): 519

Sun Y, Gao C, Luo M, et al. Aspidin PB, a phloroglucinol derivative, induces apoptosis in human hepatocarcinoma HepG2 cells by modulating PI3K/Akt/GSK3β pathway [J]. Chemico-Biological Interactions, 2013, 201(1-3): 1

沈明志，徐勇，李榕彬，等. 银杏叶提取物对AGEs诱导心肌细胞内质网应激的影响[J]. 现代生物医学进展，2013，13(14)：2633

盛磊，郝树芳，周洁芸，等. 人参皂苷 Rh2 抑制实验性大鼠子宫异位内膜增殖及其作用机制探讨[J]. 中国药理学通报，2013，29(5)：718

石瑞丽，胡金凤，孔令雷，等. 瓜子金皂苷已对连二亚硫酸钠致氧糖剥夺/复供诱导 PC12 细胞凋亡的抑制作用[J]. 中国药理学通报，2013，29(3)：333

宋占春，王占胜，白静慧，等. 大黄素对实验性自身免疫性心肌炎大鼠 IFN－γ 及 IL－17 水平的影响[J]. 中国医科大学学报，2013，42(8)：737

苏筠霞，李建华，刘天喜，等. 革薢水提物对尿酸性肾病大鼠 TNF－α、MCP－1 和 ICAM－1 表达的影响[J]. 中成药，2013，35(5)：1088

苏亚楠，陈立强，张晓波，等. 山茱萸多糖对阿尔茨海默病模型大鼠 GSK－3β 和磷酸化 GSK－3β 的影响[J]. 中国老年学杂志，2013，33(9)：2092

隋忠国，徐文，柳艳平，等. 五味子酯甲对他克莫司在大鼠体内吸收的促进作用研究[J]. 中国药房，2013，24(35)：3280

孙升云，金鑫，黄少君，等. 慢肾康宁对肾间质纤维化大鼠内质网应激 PERK－ATF－4 通路的影响[J]. 中医杂志，2013，54(3)：236

孙晓芳，段斐，刘佳琳，等. 三七总皂苷对肺纤维化小鼠组织蛋白酶 B 表达的影响[J]. 时珍国医国药，2013，24(5)：1134

孙晓芳，段斐，牛建昭. 三七总皂苷对肺纤维化小鼠肺组织 Fas/FasL 表达的影响[J]. 时珍国医国药，2013，24(1)：95

孙娅楠，农一兵，崔晓云，等. 黄芪对乳鼠肥大心肌细胞钙瞬变及钙调蛋白激酶Ⅱ的影响[J]. 中国中医基础医学杂志，2013，19(1)：44

孙宇，王水英，黄梦汶，等. 黄芪对实验性自身免疫性脑脊髓膜炎小鼠的治疗作用及机制研究[J]. 上海中医药大学学报，2013，27(4)：58

T

Teng P, Li YH, Cheng WJ, et al. Neuroprotective effects of Lycium barbarum polysaccharides in lipopolysaccharide-induced BV2 microglial cells [J]. Molecular Medicine Reports, 2013, 7(6): 1977

汤晓晨，俞峰，孙书龙，等. 黄芪甲苷对人膝骨关节炎退变关节软骨 IL－1β 表达的影响[J]. 南京中医药大学学报，2013，29(1)：48

涂苑青，黄丰，朱苗苗，等. 瑞香素对脂多糖诱导的小鼠小胶质细胞炎症反应的保护作用[J]. 时珍国医国药，2013，24(5)：1169

W

Wang M, Sun GB, Sun X, et al. Cardioprotective effect of salvianolic acid B against arsenic trioxide-induced injury in cardiac H9c2 cells via the PI3K/Akt signal pathway[J]. Toxicology Letters, 2013, 216(2－3): 100

Wang Y, Wang WL, Xie WL, et al. Puerarin stimulates proliferation and differentiation and protects against cell death in human osteoblastic MG－63 cells via ER－dependent MEK/ERK and PI3K/Akt activation[J]. Phytomedicine, 2013, 20(10): 787

Wang Y, Zhang ZZ, Wu Y, et al. Quercetin postconditioning attenuates myocardial ischemia/reperfusion injury in rats through the PI3K/Akt pathway [J]. Brazilian Journal of Medical and Biological Research, 2013, 46(10): 861

Wu CX, Liu R, Gao M, et al. Pinocembrin protects brain against ischemia/reperfusion injury by attenuating endoplasmic reticulum stress induced apoptosis [J]. Neuroscience letters, 2013, 546: 57

Wu L, Cai BC, Zheng SZ, et al. Effect of emodin on endoplasmic reticulum stress in rats with severe acute pancreatitis[J]. Inflammation, 2013, 36(5): 1020

汪江涛，丁伯平，柏松，等. 钩藤碱对肾性高血压大鼠血浆 AngⅡ、IMD 及心肌 IMD 含量的影响[J]. 基础医学与临床，2013，33(5)：623

王彩霞，崔家鹏，朱曼迪，等. 中药独活对 AD 和 VD 模型大鼠 IL－4，TNF－α 调节作用的实验研究[J]. 辽宁中医杂志，2011，38(9)：1701

王琛，刘蜜，孙胜，等. 西洋参茎叶总皂苷通过抑制过度内质网应激减轻大鼠心肌缺血/再灌注损伤[J]. 中国病理生理杂志，2013，29(1)：20

王德桂，马泽民，吕国华，等. 金纳多对大鼠急性脊髓损伤内质网应激蛋白 GADD153/CHOP 表达的影响[J]. 海南医学，2013，24(14)：2032

王洁，高振辉，刘文博，等. 海星皂甙 1 对人胶质瘤 U87 细胞抗增殖作用的研究[J]. 现代生物医学进展，2013，13(19)：3658

王丽华，王国辉，金玉玲，等. 三七制剂对血管性痴呆大鼠海马神经元 ERK 的影响[J]. 黑龙江医药科学，2012，35(6)：97

王璐，张义华，孔兰婷，等. 姜黄素对弓形虫感染小胶质细胞 NO 的产生及 iNOS 表达的影响[J]. 中国人兽共患病学报，2013，29(4)：375

王敏，张秋霞，邹海艳，等. 竹节参总皂苷对慢性脑缺血大鼠海马 GFAP、GAP－43 表达的影响[J]. 世界中医药，2013，8(2)：183

王平，吴熙，李俊鹏，等. 山豆根急性毒性实验研究[J]. 时珍国医国药，2013，24(4)：771

王琼，蒋骊龙，肖同书，等. 丹参抑制凝血因子Ⅹa 和Ⅱa 的活性部位研究[J]. 时珍国医国药，2013，

24(5)：1153

王水英，孙宇，金惠，等. 白山毛桃根提取物抑制黑色素瘤M21细胞增殖作用及其机制研究[J]. 辽宁中医杂志，2013，40(10)：2101

王伟，孔维，陈萌，等. 丁苯酞预处理对脑缺血再灌注大鼠内质网应激的影响[J]. 临床神经病学杂志，2013，26(2)：122

王小兵，张帆，赵雪茹，等. 茄灯盏花素在正常大鼠和糖尿病大鼠体内的药动学差异[J]. 兰州大学学报(医学版)，2013，39(2)：41

王炎，刘宣，周利红，等. 丹参酮Ⅱ$_A$对裸鼠人肠癌血管新生的抑制作用[J]. 中国实验方剂学杂志，2013，19(3)：167

王艳丽，宋涛，胡雅楠，等. 柴胡皂甙d对实验性大鼠肝癌Ang-2及VEGF表达的影响[J]. 西安交通大学学报(医学版)，2013，34(5)：664

王莹，刘玉刚，陈占法. 红景天苷对血管性痴呆小鼠学习记忆行为的影响[J]. 河北医药，2013，35(16)：2416

王颖超，柳茵，刘维军，等. 沙棘黄酮对粥样硬化大鼠NADPH氧化酶亚基Nox4及ox-LDL的影响[J]. 云南中医学院学报，2013，36(5)：7

王宇，张明艳，王燕，等. 银杏叶提取物对血管性痴呆大鼠模型学习记忆及PSD-95表达的影响[J]. 中国老年学杂志，2012，32(7)：1428

王玉，周冬枝，夏欣欣，等. 大黄素对急性放射性肠炎肠黏膜屏障的保护作用[J]. 西安交通大学学报(医学版)，2013，34(2)：248

王园园，王义善，杨桂青，等. 狼毒提取液对小鼠恶性黑色素瘤B16细胞体内转移能力的影响[J]. 中国实验方剂学杂志，2013，19(1)：195

王铮华，梁统，李涛，等. 白杨素对人鼻咽癌细胞CNE-2增殖的抑制作用[J]. 中国药科大学学报，2013，44(1)：93

温旭敏，魏涛，白利萍，等. 川芎嗪对H_2O_2诱导PC12细胞凋亡的保护作用研究[J]. 中国药物与临床，2013，13(1)：25

邬姗，陆付耳，董慧，等. 盐酸小檗碱对胰岛β细胞内质网应激相关凋亡的影响[J]. 中国糖尿病杂志，2013，21(6)：544

武变瑛，李利平，张新颖，等. 杏花雨对血管性痴呆大鼠行为及其海马Bcl-2、Bax蛋白表达的影响[J]. 河北大学学报(自然科学版)，2012，32(4)：382

X

Xu HY，Chen ZW，Hou JC，et al. Jolkinolide B induces apoptosis in MCT-7 cells through inhibition of the PI3K/Akt/mTOR signaling pathway[J]. Oncology Reports，2013，29(1)：212

徐浩岑，唐雪骁，刘光陵，等. 人参皂苷R_{g1}抑制TGF-β1诱导肾小管上皮细胞转分化实验研究[J]. 辽宁中医药大学学报，2013，15(2)：34

徐祥赫，刘钊，王虹，等. 杜仲对MC3T3-E1成骨细胞及OPG/RANKL比值的影响[J]. 天津医科大学学报，2013，19(3)：203

许博林，姚星辰，铁军，等. 牦牛活性蛋白对小鼠免疫功能的调节作用[J]. 青海医学院学报，2013，34(1)：54

Y

Yang Y，Yang K，Li YP，et al. Decursin inhibited proliferation and angiogenesis of endothelial cells to suppress diabetic retinopathy via VEGFR2[J]. Molecular and Cellular Endocrinology，2013，378(1-2)：46

Yu XB，Tong Y，Huang WH，et al. Erxian Decoction，a traditional Chinese herbal formula，inhibits angiogenesis in human umbilical vein endothelial cells[J]. Biological & Pharmaceutical Bulletin，2013，36(5)：754

杨光宇，王洪新，赵素玲，等. 黄芪甲苷对血管紧张素Ⅱ诱导大鼠心肌细胞肥大的抑制作用[J]. 中药药理与临床，2013，29(3)：28

杨红云，景浩然，王旭梅，等. 羟基红花黄色素A对小胶质细胞炎性激活的抑制作用[J]. 湖北中医杂志，2013，35(10)：22

杨竞，徐洋，金涛，等. 白藜芦醇通过抑制TGF-β1/Smad2信号通路抗糖尿病肾病[J]. 中国新药与临床杂志，2013，32(4)：307

杨雷，毛秉豫，徐国昌，等. 黄芪提取物对大鼠心肌梗死后心肌组织PKD1蛋白表达的影响[J]. 中国药理学通报，2013，29(4)：535

杨宜承，曾常茜，向彬，等. 雷公藤内酯对癫痫模型大鼠海马神经元凋亡的保护作用研究[J]. 中国药房，2013，24(27)：2516

姚海涛，马金丽，张晓波，等. 山茱萸多糖对阿尔茨海默病模型大鼠tau蛋白的影响[J]. 中国老年学杂志，2013，33(12)：2838

叶士勇，曾春来，向贻佳，等. 淫羊藿苷对血小板活化的影响及其分子机制的研究[J]. 浙江中医杂志，2013，48(8)：609

殷文静，赵君，陈文芬，等. 穿心莲内酯诱导宫颈癌HeLa细胞凋亡的作用及其机制[J]. 中国妇幼保健，2013，28(25)：4220

尹美珍，胡岗，苏振宏，等. 艾叶多糖对小鼠免疫细胞分泌细胞因子及其活性的影响[J]. 时珍国医国药，2013，24(7)：1610

余思云，李运延，胡国华. 紫草素诱导子宫内膜癌Ishikawa细胞凋亡及其机制的研究[J]. 辽宁中医杂志，2013，40(9)：1930

虞迪,朱峰妍,曹志飞,等. 毛茛有效部位 D1 对人胃癌细胞 MGC803 血管生成拟态的作用及其机制[J]. 中国药理学通报,2013,29(2): 261

Z

Zeng KW, Li N, Dong X, et al. Sprengerinin C exerts anti-tumorigenic effects in hepatocellular carcinoma via inhibition of proliferation and angiogenesis and induction of apoptosis [J]. European Journal of Pharmacology, 2013, 714(1-3): 261

Zhang F, Wang H, Wu Q, et al. Resveratrol Protects Cortical Neurons against Microglia-mediated Neuroinflammation[J]. Phytotherapy Research, 2013, 27(3): 344

Zhang L, Ji Q, Liu X, et al. Norcantharidin inhibits tumor angiogenesis via blocking VEGFR2/MEK/ERK signaling pathways [J]. Cancer Science, 2013, 104(5): 604

Zhang P, Liu XY, Zhu YJ, et al. Honokiol inhibits the inflammatory reaction during cerebral ischemia reperfusion by suppressing NF-κB activation and cytokine production of glial cells [J]. Neuroscience Letters, 2013, 534: 123

Zhang S, Qi Y, Xu YW, et al. Protective effect of flavonoid-rich extract from Rosa laevigata Michx on cerebral ischemia-reperfusion injury through suppression of apoptosis and inflammation [J]. Neurochemistry International, 2013, 63(5): 522

Zhang Y, Liu XF, Han LF, et al. Regulation of lipid and glucose homeostasis by mango tree leaf extract is mediated by AMPK and PI3K/AKT signaling pathways [J]. Food Chemistry, 2013, 141(3): 2896

Zhang YX, Hai J, Cao M, et al. Silibinin ameliorates steatosis and insulin resistance during non-alcoholic fatty liver disease development partly through targeting IRS-1/PI3K/Akt pathway[J]. Internaltional Immunopharmacology, 2013, 17(3): 714

Zhao B, Hu MC. Gallic acid reduces cell viability, proliferation, invasion and angiogenesis in human cervical cancer cells[J]. Oncology Letters, 2013, 6(6): 1749

Zhao RP, Sun L, Lin SS, et al. The saponin monomer of dwarf lilyturf tuber, DT-13, inhibits angiogenesis under hypoxia and normoxia via multi-targeting activity [J]. Oncology Reports, 2013, 29(4): 1379

Zhou JJ, Sun Y, Zhao X, et al. 3-*O*-demethylswertipunicoside inhibits MPP^{+}-induced oxidative stress and apoptosis in PC12 cells[J]. Brain Research, 2013, 1508: 53

曾春晖,杨柯,徐明光,等. 广西藤茶总黄酮对金黄色葡萄球菌抗菌机制研究[J]. 中国实验方剂学杂志,2013,19(10): 249

曾金祥,魏娟,毕莹,等. 车前子醇提物降低急性高尿酸血症小鼠血尿酸水平及机制研究[J]. 中国实验方剂学杂志,2013,19(9): 173

张琰. 二苯乙烯苷对氧糖剥夺星形胶质细胞凋亡的影响及其机制[J]. 济宁医学院学报,2013,36(4): 245

张盈,李灵芝,杨虎,等. 蕨麻对低压缺氧大鼠脑组织脑红蛋白表达的影响[J]. 天津中医药,2013,30(4): 224

张莹,徐冰,李庆祥,等. 黄芪多糖干预缺血-再灌注损伤大鼠心肌黏附分子 ICAM-1,VCAM-1 及 p38 通路的研究[J]. 中国实验方剂学杂志,2013,19(12): 151

张哲,闻勤生,倪阵,等. 姜黄素对脂多糖诱导大鼠肝脏 Kupffer 细胞 NF-κB 及下游炎症因子的影响[J]. 胃肠病学和肝病学杂志,2013,22(10): 1030

赵春霞,郝冰. 灵芝孢子粉对戊四氮致痫大鼠 NGF 的影响[J]. 牡丹江医学院学报,2013,34(2): 27

赵春霞,沈雪松,金美华,等. 青蒿琥酯纳米脂质体对人肝癌 HepG2 细胞抗血管生成作用的研究[J]. 中国实验方剂学杂志,2013,19(7): 226

赵龙,喻玉,李丽,等. 柴芍胃炎颗粒对功能性消化不良模型大鼠血浆胃动素与胃泌素的影响[J]. 泸州医学院学报,2013,36(5): 447

赵珊,马迎春,刘亚坤,等. 姜黄素通过抑制内质网应激和 JNK 通路过度活化减轻小鼠肺缺血再灌注损伤[J]. 中国病理生理杂志,2013,29(2): 308

赵秀军,郭银,宋庆亮,等. 何首乌饮对运动疲劳大鼠睾丸组织 Cox7a2 表达的影响[J]. 四川大学学报(医学版),2013,44(2): 205

郑安红,张维东,王兆朋,等. 蝎毒多肽增强 5-氟尿嘧啶对 H22 肝癌抑制作用的机制研究[J]. 中草药,2013,44(11): 1465

郑国灿,王兵,黄聪华,等. 牛蒡子苷元对肿瘤血管生成抑制作用的观察[J]. 中华肿瘤防治杂志,2013,20(3): 177

郑旭锐,樊英华,韦永红,等. 姜黄素对肝星状细胞 JAK2-STAT3 信号通路的影响[J]. 陕西中医,2013,34(9): 1255

钟萍,吴丹红,孙京华. 小檗碱对血管性痴呆大鼠海马 IL-1β、IL-8、TNF-α 表达水平的影响[J]. 卒中与神经疾病,2013,20(1): 16

周本宏,梁艺小,沈恒,等. 天麻多糖对皮质酮损伤 PC12 细胞保护机制研究[J]. 中药材,2013,36(4): 630

周陈姣,史丽君,傅雷华,等. 苦参碱对人急性红白血病细胞株 TF-1 SALL4 基因及 Wnt/β-catenin 信号通路下游靶基因表达的影响[J]. 中国生物制品学杂志,

2013,26(10):1449

周萍,李均,阳小敏,等.黄芪丹参“药对”干预肾纤维化抑制因子 par-3 的量效关系研究[J].上海中医药杂志,2013,47(5):77

周思思,马增春,梁乾德,等.人参附子不同比例配伍对小鼠急性毒性的影响[J].天津中医药,2013,30(1):43

朱德森,刘学政.三七三醇皂苷对糖尿病大鼠视网膜神经节细胞的保护作用[J].天津医药,2013,41(11):1110

朱向东,曹燕飞,王燕,等.芍药苷对溃疡性结肠炎模型大鼠结肠组织病理形态及血清抗炎因子和促炎因子平衡的影响[J].辽宁中医杂志,2013,40(9):1927

朱玉婷,邢同岳,毛海芬.槲皮素对高糖诱导的原代小胶质细胞炎性反应的抑制作用[J].中国医院药学杂志,2013,33(21):1787

邹志坚,胡建新,王晓敏,等.地锦草水提液对 H22 荷鼠 VEGF、MMP-9 蛋白表达的影响[J].中国现代医学杂志,2013,23(36):11

(七) 方剂研究

【概述】

2013年,在方剂学的临床应用与实验研究等方面,又有不少新的研究进展,仅在期刊上公开发表的论文有1 000余篇。

1. 临床应用

(1) 经方应用 毛靓瑶用半夏泻心汤加减治疗胆汁反流性胃炎35例,与莫沙比利对照组比较,结果显效率分别为71.4%(25/35)、57.1%(20/35),总有效率分别为91.4%(32/35)、88.6%(31/35),均有显著差异($P<0.05$)。刘强等报道半夏泻心汤加减治疗消化性溃疡100例,与对照组(西药三联)进行比较,结果在溃疡面积修复、嗳气次数、腹胀腹痛等诸项评分,均有显著差异($P<0.05$)。吕伯中报道柴胡桂枝干姜汤加减治疗慢性羊水过多40例,与对照组(低盐饮食,控制饮水)比较,结果总有效率分别为82.5%(33/40)、36.7%(11/30),组间比较$P<0.01$;羊水指数$P<0.05$,提示本方能改善慢性羊水过多患儿临床体征,降低羊水指数。

(2) 时方应用 孔亮等报道半夏白术天麻汤加减治疗椎-基底动脉供血不足性眩晕60例,与对照组(倍他司汀片和胞磷胆碱钠注射液)比较,结果总效率分别为90.0%(54/60)、73.3%(44/60),组间比较$P<0.05$,治疗前后血液流变学各项指标比较也均有显著差异($P<0.01$)。陈文阁等报道桃红四物汤加减治疗结节性红斑狼疮60例,与对照组(抗生素配合激素治疗)比较,结果显效率分别为66.7%(20/30)、50.0%(15/30),总有效率分别为100.0%(30/30)、83.3%(25/30),均有显著差异($P<0.05$)。

(3) 自拟方应用 刘文娥等报道盆炎丸(黄芪、白术、红藤、丹参、莪术)治疗女性生殖道解脲支原体感染气虚血瘀证,与阿奇霉素对照组比较,两组综合疗效分别为91.4%(85/93)、79.3%(69/87),组间比较 $P>0.01$;两组治疗后解脲支原体感染转阴率分别为61.3%(57/93)、48.3%(42/87),组间比较$P>0.05$;两组治疗后随访复发率分别为12.3%(7/57)、54.8%(23/42),组间比较$P<0.05$。表明本方治疗本病属气虚血瘀证者疗效颇佳,与西药阿奇霉素合用治疗效果更优。周绍荣等报道甲瘤方(香附、夏枯草、象贝、莱菔子、白芍、海浮石、元参、僵蚕、白芥子、泽漆)治疗气滞痰凝型良性甲状腺结节,与优甲乐对照组比较,结果总有效率分别为90.0%(36/40)、27.5%(11/40),组间比较$P<0.05$。

2. 实验研究

方剂的实验研究,注重为临床服务。李静等报道沙参麦冬汤可以提高慢性支气管炎大鼠血清中超氧化物歧化酶(SOD)、谷胱甘肽过氧化物酶(GSH-PX)、过氧化氢酶(CAT)活性,从而提高慢性支气管炎大鼠血清的抗氧化能力,减少氧化应激损伤。夏晓莉等报道柴胡疏肝散对代谢综合征(MS)大鼠肝X受体的影响,认为MS大鼠肝组织中存在肝X受体高表达,本方能降低MS模型大鼠肝X受体的表达,其可能是治疗MS的机理之一。王秀珍等报道,四神丸治疗大鼠溃疡性结肠炎(UC)的机理可能通过提高血清白细胞介素2(IL-2)、白细胞介素4(IL-4)抗炎性细胞因子水平与抑制白细胞介素8(IL-8)炎性细胞因子水平而发挥作用。马雅銮等报道高脂血症小鼠服用黄连解毒汤4周后,血脂无明显改善,但肝脏$CD206^+$ M2型巨噬细胞比例较载脂蛋白E高脂组显著提高($P<0.05$),肝脏脂肪肝病理变化显著减轻。表明本方肝脏保护功能可能与M2型巨噬细胞免疫调节、修复损伤组织有关,其免疫调节作用和肝脏保护作用独立于降脂作用。吴锐等报道加味犀角地黄汤与桃花四物汤对细菌脂多糖诱导的兔内毒素血症中的防治作用,研究从分子水平证实活血化瘀治疗内毒素血症的有效性,而犀角地黄汤较桃红四物汤更能有效抑制脂多糖诱导的TNF-a、CD62P、WP及ET-1的过度表达,改善循环在内毒素血症中具有更强的抗炎作用。

此外,一年来在方剂配伍组成的研究方面、药物应用剂型方面、方剂不同剂量的使用,亦有不少报道,均为临床的广泛应用和提高疗效提供了服务。

（王道瑞）

【小柴胡汤的临床应用与药理作用】

1. 临床应用

(1) 甲型 H1N1 流感　孙丽梅等报道,以小柴胡汤为基础方(柴胡用 20 g)加减治疗甲型 H1N1 流感轻症患者 61 例,西药组(口服磷酸奥司他韦胶囊)18 例。结果,中药组发热、咳嗽、咯痰等流感样症状消失时间明显短于西药组($P<0.05$);头痛、咽痛、恶寒等流感样症状消失时间,咽部红肿、扁桃体肿大等体征恢复正常时间,白细胞恢复正常时间、甲型 H1N1 流感病毒核酸转阴时间与西药组比较均无显著性差异($P>0.05$)。表明小柴胡汤加减治疗甲型 H1N1 流感轻症患者疗效与奥司他韦基本相同,在缓解发热、咳嗽等方面具有一定优势。

(2) 眩晕　何容报道,用小柴胡汤加减治疗美尼尔氏综合征所致眩晕 40 例,对照组(银杏达莫注射液 20 ml+0.9%氯化钠 250 ml 静脉滴注)40 例。结果,治疗组、对照组的总有效率分别为 97.5%(39/40)、80%(32/40),$P<0.05$。

(3) 偏头痛　王双玲等报道,用小柴胡汤合血府逐瘀汤加减方治疗偏头痛 30 例,设对照组(服用西比灵)30 例。结果,两组临床症状综合评分、中医症候积分均较治疗前有所改善,治疗组优于对照组($P<0.05$);临床症状改善率和中医症候改善率治疗组亦优于对照组($P<0.05$);两组患者治疗前血清超敏 C 反应蛋白(hs-CRP)水平均高于正常水平,治疗后 hs-CRP 均明显降低($P<0.05$),但治疗组明显优于对照组($P<0.05$)。表明小柴胡汤合血府逐瘀汤加减方可通过降低 hs-CRP 发挥治疗偏头痛的作用。

(4) 慢性丙型肝炎　怀平艾等报道,用小柴胡汤联合聚乙二醇干扰素 α-2a 治疗慢性丙型肝炎,可缓解患者的症状体征,促进 HCV-RNA 阴转。

(5) 胆汁反流性胃炎　党秀芳报道,用小柴胡汤随症加减治疗胆汁反流性胃炎 45 例,总有效率为 93.3%(42/45)。

(6) 痛经　冯海泉报道,用小柴胡汤加减(柴胡、黄芩、党参、香附、甘草、赤芍、当归、川芎、蒲黄、五灵脂、川牛膝等)治疗气滞血瘀型原发性痛经 18 例。月经前开始服,1 剂/d,3 个月经周期为 1 个疗程。对照组 18 例口服布洛芬。结果两组差异明显($P<0.05$)。

2. 药理作用

(1) 对抗环磷酰胺所致免疫抑制作用　王军等报道,用小柴胡汤低、中、高剂量(10、20、40 g/kg)灌胃,连续 7 d,观察该方对环磷酰胺所致小鼠免疫抑制作用的影响。结果,小柴胡汤对环磷酰胺所致免疫抑制小鼠的胸腺指数有明显的提高作用($P<0.01$),并能升高免疫抑制小鼠血清白介素-2(IL-2)、白介素-6(IL-6)及肿瘤坏死因子-α(TNF-α)的水平($P<0.01$ 或 $P<0.05$),其中小柴胡汤中、高剂量组效果更为显著。表明小柴胡汤能够拮抗环磷酰胺的免疫抑制作用。

(2) 抗肝纤维化作用　江山等报道,用 CCl_4 复制 SD 大鼠肝纤维化模型,给予小柴胡汤不同剂量(3.5、1.79、0.358 g/kg)灌胃,2 次/d,共 8 周。结果,与模型组相比,小柴胡汤高、中剂量组 ALT、AST、总胆红素及谷氨酰转移酶等明显降低($P<0.01$),肝功能显著改善;透明质酸(HA)、Ⅲ型前胶原(PCⅢ)及Ⅳ型胶原(Ⅵ-C)明显降低($P<0.01$ 或 $P<0.05$),血清层粘连蛋白(LN)明显升高($P<0.01$);IL-2 明显升高($P<0.05$),IL-6 显著降低($P<0.05$)。高剂量组白蛋白(ALB)明显升高($P<0.05$),转化生长因子 β1(TGFβ1)明显降低($P<0.05$)。肝脏组织病理检查显示,各治疗组肝纤维化程度明显下降。

(3) 对胃肠运动的影响　郁保生等报道,用慢性束缚应激+过度疲劳+饮食失节的方法造成大鼠功能性消化不良(FD)模型,造模结束后给予小柴胡汤灌胃,连续 14 d。观察小柴胡汤对 FD 大鼠血管活性肠肽(VIP)、胃排空及小肠推进率的影响。结果,与模型组相比,小柴胡汤组大鼠血清 VIP 含量及胃内残留率显著降低,小肠推进率明显升高。表明小柴胡汤可降低 FD 模型大鼠血清中 VIP 的含量,加速胃排空及小肠推进率。曹峰等报道,用不同剂量柴胡(13、10、9.1 g/kg)的小柴胡汤灌胃,观察其对正常大鼠胃窦组织胃动素(MTL)、乙酰胆碱酯酶(AChE)、NO 的影响。结果,与正常对照组比较,柴胡剂量最高的小柴胡汤组 MTL、AChE 含量明显升高($P<0.05$),而胃窦组织 NO 含量无统计学差异($P>0.05$);柴胡为中、低剂量的小柴胡汤组的 MTL、AChE、

NO含量均无统计学差异($P>0.05$)。提示高剂量柴胡的小柴胡汤促进胃动力的作用机制,可能与增加胃窦组织MTL、AChE的含量有关。

(4) 对黑素瘤的抑制作用　周密思等报道,将培养至3代的黑素瘤细胞接种于96孔板,孵育24 h后弃上清液,加入小柴胡汤水煎液,设6个浓度(5、10、20、40、80、160 ug/ml),测定细胞活力、酪氨酸酶活性及黑素的含量。结果,40 ug/ml以上的小柴胡汤水煎液可明显抑制黑素瘤细胞和共培养细胞活力($P<0.01$);小柴胡汤水煎液对黑素瘤细胞及共培养细胞中酪氨酸酶活性、黑素合成均呈剂量依赖性抑制作用,各浓度药品组与对照组比较均有显著性差异($P<0.05$或$P<0.01$);小柴胡汤对于黑素瘤细胞中酪氨酸酶活性、黑素生成的抑制作用与其对于共培养细胞中黑素生成及酪氨酸酶活性的抑制作用无差别($P>0.05$)。表明小柴胡汤在黑素瘤细胞及黑素瘤细胞与HaCaT细胞共培养体系中对黑素瘤细胞增殖、酪氨酸酶活性、黑素合成均有较强的抑制作用。

(5) 抑制肝癌HepG-2细胞作用　李然等报道,用大鼠制备小柴胡汤含药血清,以HepG-2肝癌细胞为研究对象,观察5%、10%、20%含药血清对HepG-2细胞的作用。结果,与空白血清组比较,小柴胡汤含药血清能够抑制HepG-2肝癌细胞增殖,10%含药血清抑制细胞增殖具有时间依赖的特点,凋亡率从6.78%上升至19.51%,且细胞线粒体膜电位明显降低。表明小柴胡汤含药血清能够抑制HepG-2肝癌细胞增殖,促进其凋亡,线粒体途径参与了该过程。

(6) 抗抑郁作用　原红霞等报道,用小柴胡汤石油醚萃取物(部位Ⅰ)、乙酸乙酯萃取物(部位Ⅱ)、水饱和正丁醇萃取物(部位Ⅲ)、水层残留物(部位Ⅵ),各自分为9.0、18.0 g/kg 2个剂量组,对雄性昆明种小鼠连续灌胃7 d,采用强迫游泳和悬尾2种行为绝望试验,比较其抗抑郁作用的药效。结果:部位Ⅱ、部位Ⅵ可明显缩短小鼠强迫游泳不动时间、悬尾不动时间($P<0.05$或$P<0.01$)。表明乙酸乙酯萃取物和正丁醇萃取物为小柴胡汤抗抑郁作用的有效部位。

(李　俊　瞿　融)

【茵陈蒿汤的药理研究与临床应用】

1. 药理研究

(1) 保肝　蔡华丹等报道,茵陈蒿汤水提物和醇提物的成分虽存在明显差别,但两者对大鼠均具有肝损伤的保护作用,其中水提物能明显降低模型大鼠AST、ALT、ALP、TG、总胆红素(T-Bil)含量($P<0.05$,$P<0.01$),改善肝脏的炎症病理状态;醇提物对血清AST、ALT、ALP等部分指标有所改善($P<0.05$,$P<0.01$);但水提取物中栀子苷和大黄素的含量均低于醇提取物。表明以药效为指标,茵陈蒿汤水提物和醇提物对D-氨基半乳糖所致大鼠肝损伤皆有保护作用,以水提取工艺为佳。

(2) 抗肝纤维化　周兴华等报道,用急性肝损伤SD大鼠模型灌胃加味茵陈蒿汤(茵陈30 g,栀子30 g,酒大黄15 g,黄连15 g,黄芩20 g,黄芪30 g,赤芍30 g)。结果,与正常组比较,模型组大鼠肝脏组织TLR-4mRNA和TLR-4蛋白均有极显著增加($P<0.01$);与模型组比较,加味茵陈蒿汤可显著下调TLR-4 mRNA及TLR-4蛋白的表达。表明加味茵陈蒿汤可显著下调大鼠肝细胞中TLR4 mRNA及其TLR4蛋白表达,可能是通过调节大鼠肝组织中TLR4蛋白的信号传导通路,避免其过度激活,进而抑制了NF-$_{\kappa}$B的活化,最终减少了炎性因子的释放,减轻了肝细胞炎症,起到一定的抗肝纤维化作用。

(3) 毒理作用　王坤等用栀子(剂量为12 g/kg)及茵陈蒿汤(剂量为茵陈蒿18 g/kg、栀子12 g/kg、大黄6 g/kg)分别每天灌胃大鼠。结果,茵陈蒿汤组与栀子组相比,ALT、ALP、TBA均显著降低;SOD、SOD/MDA极显著升高,GSH-PX无明显差异;大鼠肝组织中;肿瘤坏死因子(TNF-α)的含量无明显差异;凋亡指数显著降低;Bax、Bax、Bax/Bcl-2均没有明显差异。表明栀子肝毒性的机制与氧化应激、炎症反应诱导肝细胞的坏死及凋亡有关,茵陈蒿汤中的其他组方可减轻栀子的肝毒性。

(4) 其他　张慧芹等报道,茵陈蒿汤醇提物高剂量能降低大鼠血清中ALT、AST含量,水提物低剂量组显著降低大鼠血清TG含量,茵陈蒿汤水提物降低TG及T-Bil的活性强于醇提物;茵陈蒿汤水提液的降血脂及降胆红素作用优于醇提物,而醇提物的抗氧化及抗炎活性高于水煎。也有报道,茵陈篙汤能够针对NASH发病的脂代谢紊乱、氧化应激、脂质过氧化,从而显著修复肝细胞损伤。

2. 临床应用

(1) 治疗药源性肝损伤　李保义等报道,用茵陈蒿汤加味治疗药物性肝损伤65例,对照组服用多烯磷脂酰胆碱胶囊。结果,治疗组和对照组的总有效率分别为95.2%(62/65)、63.1%(41/65),两组比较$P<0.05$。表明茵陈蒿汤加味可降低患者ALT、AST、TBIL水平,减轻黄疸、乏力、纳差等临床症状,提高临床治愈率。

(2) 治疗病毒性肝炎　骆稚平报道,用茵陈蒿汤联合西医治疗早中期慢性乙型重型肝炎16例。结果,肝功能指标(ALT、ATS、TBLI、PAT)两组均有改善,治疗组改善优于对照组($P<0.05$)。王继海报道,用加味茵陈蒿汤治疗急性病毒性淤胆型肝炎30例,结果疗效确切,且优于联合思美泰、优思弗的治疗。于晨媛报道,用茵陈蒿汤加味联合西药干扰素、利巴韦林治疗慢性丙型肝炎65例。结果,治疗组和对照组的总有效率分别为92.3%(60/65)、75.4%(49/65),两组比较差异显著($P<0.05$),两组不良反应发生率有统计学意义($P<0.05$)。

(3) 治疗新生儿黄疸　徐国荣等报道,比较不同煎煮方法制备的茵陈蒿汤治疗新生儿黄疸的疗效。结果,总有效率实验组(茵陈先煎)、对照组(三味药同煎)分别为100%(32/32)、93.8%(30/32),两组比较$P<0.05$,表明茵陈先煎比三种药材同煎的临床治疗效果好。李霞等报道,加味茵陈蒿汤治疗新生儿高胆红素血症,疗效确切,无不良反应。

(4) 治疗胆结石　巫资明等报道,用三镜联合茵陈蒿汤治疗梗阻性黄疸170例,包括单纯胆总管结石、单纯胆囊结石、胆总管并胆囊结石、胆总管并肝内胆管结石、胆总管巨大结石、肝内外胆管并胆囊结石症等。结果,治疗组与对照组比较有显著性差异,表明三镜联合茵陈蒿汤治疗梗阻性黄疸具有创伤小、退黄快、预后好、住院时间短、并发症少等优点。

(5) 治疗母儿ABO血型不合　母婴ABO血型不合是因孕妇与胎儿之间血型不合而产生的免疫性疾病。吴梅婷等报道,用茵陈蒿汤联合西药治疗母儿ABO血型不合246例,取得了较好的治疗结果,新生儿溶血率较单独使用西药组具有显著降低($P<0.05$)。刘梅等报道,用茵陈蒿汤治疗新生儿母婴血型不合溶血病126例。结果,能降低孕妇IgG抗体效价,减少新生儿母婴血型不合溶血病的发生。沈燕慧报道,用双黄连粉针合茵陈蒿汤治疗母儿ABO血型不合78例,对照组用静滴维生素C、口服维生素E。结果,治疗组与对照组的总有效率分别为92.3%(36/39)、76.9%(30/39),两组有显著性差异($P<0.05$)。表明双黄连粉针合茵陈蒿汤治疗母儿ABO血型不合有满意疗效。李兴华报道,用加味茵陈蒿汤治疗母儿ABO血型不合40例。结果表明,加味茵陈汤能有效的降低抗体效价,治疗母儿血型不合,预防新生儿黄疸及溶血病的发生。

(6) 治疗妊娠期肝内胆汁淤积症(ICP)　杨艳芳等报道,茵陈蒿汤联合基础治疗ICP治疗妊娠期肝内胆汁淤积症30例。结果,能缓解瘙痒,降低血胆汁酸水平,改善新生儿出生情况,降低羊水污染率。

(7) 治疗寻常痤疮　许光仓等报道,茵陈蒿汤治疗寻常痤疮的疗效及其对血清IL-4的影响,对照组用丹参酮胶囊治疗。结果,治疗组与对照组的显效率分别为49.0%(40/102)、41.0%(32/78),两组$P>0.05$,但治疗后两组的IL-4均有不同程度的降低,与治疗前相比差异有统计学意义($P<0.01$),表明茵陈蒿汤能明显改善寻常痤疮患者的临床症状,降低IL-4水平。

(8) 治疗急性胆源性胰腺炎(ABP)　许卫华等报道,用大柴胡汤合茵陈蒿汤加减配合西药治疗ABP。结果,中西医结合治疗组比西药对照组疗效好,表明大柴胡汤合茵陈蒿汤加减配合西药治疗ABP,可有效改善ABP患者的临床症状,缩短患者恢复时间,安全有效。

(都广礼　陈德兴)

【金匮肾气丸的药理作用与临床应用】

1. 药理作用

(1) 延缓衰老　魏良浩等报道,金匮肾气丸可以通过增加老年性痴呆大鼠额叶皮质内神经营养因子-3(NT-3)阳性神经元的表达数目,抑制NT-3阳性细胞的凋亡,起到延缓神经元衰老死亡的作用,从而对老年性痴呆起到一定的防治作用。程志安等报道,用金匮肾气丸的含药血清(浓度10%)干预大鼠骨髓间充质干细胞来源的前脂肪细胞成骨分化过程,分别于第6、12、18天观察成骨分化相关基因及成脂分化相关基因的表达水平。结果,成骨分化相关基因于第12和18天出现较显著的基因表达上调变化，如 IGF_1、$RUNX_2$、SPP_1mRNA 的表达；成脂分化相关基因则在第 6 天出现基因表达下调变化，以 $FABP_4$ mRNA 表达为显著。表明本方可能通过促进成骨分化、抑制成脂分化作用，延缓骨质衰老疏松化。

（2）改善生殖功能　龙泳伶等报道，全方及拆方（补阳组、补阴组）对氢化可的松所致肾阳虚雌性大鼠卵巢功能的影响，发现全方组能明显提高血清雌二醇、孕酮的含量；增加大鼠体重、子宫指数、卵巢指数；卵巢病理切片发现各级卵泡总数明显增多，病理性囊性卵泡明显减少。而拆方后的补阳组（附子、桂枝、茯苓、泽泻、丹皮）、补阴组（干地黄、山茱萸、山药、茯苓、泽泻、丹皮）虽也能不同程度改善阳虚时受损的卵巢功能，但效果不佳。表明针对肾阳虚证，单纯补阳、补阴效果不明显，阴阳双补可提高疗效，也阐释了肾气丸“阴中求阳”的配伍理论。陈艳秋等报道，金匮肾气丸能够显著增加腺嘌呤诱导的肾阳虚不育雄性大鼠的体质、精子密度与活率，降低睾丸中 TGF－β_1 表达。表明本方对于肾阳虚不育引起的精子发生过程的异常或障碍，具有一定的改善作用。许翠萍等报道，对于“劳倦过度，房事不节”所致肾阳虚小鼠模型，金匮肾气丸能够显著提高小鼠睾丸端粒酶活性，通过改善下丘脑-垂体-性腺轴功能紊乱，提高小鼠生殖力。周仕轶等报道，金匮肾气丸能通过抑制促凋亡基因表达，改善腺嘌呤致肾阳虚伴生精障碍大鼠附睾成熟精子数，增加睾丸曲细精管厚度，从而提高其生精能力；但对于颌下腺切除的唾液缺乏伴生精障碍大鼠以及肾阳虚合并颌下腺切除大鼠的 Baxhe Bcl－2 表达不具调控作用，对其生精能力改善不明显。

（3）改善听力　黄飞等报道，在庆大霉素所致大鼠听力损伤及修复过程中，金匮肾气丸可通过抑制 Notch2/hesl 信号通路保护并促进听力的恢复。王枫等的报道，金匮肾气丸可以通过降低肿瘤坏死因子－α 表达，从而降低庆大霉素的毒性，对损伤进行了对抗性的防治；也可使 Cav1.2 表达增加，从而影响 Ca^{2+} 运行，以改善听觉。

（4）抗恐惧应激损伤　王红艳等报道，模拟地震造成“恐惧”心理应激，建立“恐伤肾”模型，给予金匮肾气丸干预治疗。结果，金匮肾气丸能显著提高孕鼠的孕仔数，增加仔鼠平均体重，提高仔鼠翻身能力，降低仔鼠血清皮质酮（CORT）水平、升高血清多巴胺水平。表明本方可预防恐伤孕鼠肾精不足，同时通过对应激条件下仔鼠血清 CORT、多巴胺水平的调节，有效地改善仔鼠恐惧应激反应，具有良好的抗恐惧应激损伤作用。

（5）抗疲劳　敖新平等报道，金匮肾气丸能明显提高“力竭性游泳运动疲劳”的雄性大鼠血清中超氧化物歧化酶含量，降低丙二醛、尿素氮、肌酐含量；降低肾脏系数、提高睾丸系数。表明本方具有明显的抗疲劳作用。

（6）抗变态反应　李笋等报道，金匮肾气丸能明显改善肾阳虚变应性鼻炎（AR）模型小鼠鼻黏膜的变态反应症状，降低其血清白介素－4（IL－4）水平，升高肿瘤坏死因子－γ（IFN－γ）、白介素－2（IL－2）水平；降低组胺含量。表明本方可通过下调小鼠血清 IL－4，上调 IFN－γ、IL－2 水平，纠正失衡的 Th1/Th2，从而达到治疗肾阳虚 AR 小鼠的作用。

2. 临床应用

王泽军、吴红专报道，用金匮肾气丸联合西药治疗 2 型糖尿病能明显提高治疗总有效率，并且可以改善患者多项糖代谢和血脂指标。刘保兴等报道，金匮肾气丸可减轻良性前列腺增生合并逼尿肌不稳定患者储尿期症状。吴斌等报道，金匮肾气丸可下调系统性红斑狼疮患者的血清单核细胞趋化蛋白－4 及 IL－4 水平，减少蛋白尿，降低病情活动度，改善临床症状，减少不良反应。杨亚勤等报道，用金匮肾气丸合并穴位注射治疗老年支气管哮喘短期能明显改善患者的临床症状，明显提高肺通气功能，长期疗效好，治愈率高。刘桂章等报道，金匮肾气丸联合奥美拉唑治疗老年性反流性食管炎能显著提高临床疗效、胃镜疗效。吴俊伟等报道，金匮肾气丸能明显改善牙周病治疗后 4 周和 12 周的菌斑指数、龈沟出血指数、牙周探诊深度、附着丧失、探诊出血的临床指标，但长期疗效有待观察研究。

（陈少丽　陈德兴）

【四君子汤的药理作用】

1. 耐缺氧、抗疲劳

李艳丽报道，用四君子汤低、中、高剂量组（37.5、25.0、12.5 g/kg）连续予小鼠灌胃 14 d.

结果,各剂量组均能延长小鼠的负重游泳时间和常压耐缺氧存活时间,降低小鼠血中乳酸含量,其中高、中剂量组作用显著。表明本方具有耐缺氧、抗疲劳作用

2. 增强脾虚动物免疫功能

廖乐乐等报道,以大黄水灌胃建立小鼠脾虚模型,用四君子汤低剂量(12.5 g/kg)和高剂量(25 g/kg)灌胃 7 d。结果,各剂量组的体温、体重量增长及脾脏指数、胸腺指数均显著高于模型组;与模型组相比,四君子汤各剂量组小鼠脾脏、胸腺萎缩现象得到改善,脾脏淋巴细胞聚集、中央动脉闭塞明显改善,红髓区巨核细胞明显增多;胸腺淋巴细胞数量亦较脾虚模型组多,以高剂量组更为明显。表明四君子汤能有效促进脾虚模型小鼠的恢复,其机制可能与促进脾脏和胸腺组织 T 淋巴细胞增殖有关。熊斌等报道,用苦寒泻下、破气耗气、饮食失节加劳倦过度法造成大鼠脾虚模型,用四君子汤 2 g/100 g 灌胃治疗 6 周。结果与模型组比,四君子汤治疗组大鼠在海马 CA1 区及下丘脑腹侧核的 Janus 激酶 1(JAK1)、信号转导和转录激活因子 1(STAT1)、STAT1mRNA 的表达水平较低,细胞因子信号抑制分子 1(SOCS1) 的表达水平较高,两组差异显著,而与正常组比较无显著差异。表明四君子汤可通过影响 JAK - STAT 信号通路起到改善脾虚大鼠机体免疫功能的作用。

3. 对肌萎缩侧索硬化症 AR2 小鼠运动功能的影响

潘卫东等报道,用转基因方法制作能够反映肌萎缩侧索硬化症(ALS)发生与进展的 AR2 小鼠模型以及反映 ALS 症状缓解的 $ADAR2^{flox/flox}$ 小鼠模型,以保留部分运动功能的 $ADAR2^{flox/flox}$ 小鼠为对照组(Ⅰ组),将 AR2 小鼠随机分为空白组(Ⅱ组)、中药低剂量组(Ⅲ组)及高剂量组(Ⅳ组)。中药组用加味四君子汤(四君子汤加黄芪、肉苁蓉)灌胃,高剂量为低剂量的 3 倍。1 次/d。结果,各组小鼠第 8 周开始均有不同程度的运动功能减退,Ⅰ组运动功能减退速度缓慢,Ⅱ组从 12 周开始无论活动度、抓握力还是爬滚筒能力均迅速下降,而中药组运动功能降低程度被延缓,且与中药剂量有关;24 周时Ⅱ组 AR 小鼠的体质量、抓握力和爬滚筒能力与其余 3 组比较明显降低,差异有统计学意义。表明加味四君子汤能够延缓 ALS 小鼠运动功能的衰退。

4. 对慢性心衰大鼠心功能的影响

邱俊等报道,取 SD 大鼠用腹主动脉缩窄法 8 周构建慢性左心衰模型,成模后用四君子汤高、低剂量(11.88 g/kg、2.97 g/kg)灌胃给药,连续 4 周。结果,四君子汤高剂量组可明显改善心衰大鼠心功能,光镜下可见四君子汤高剂量组较模型组心肌纤维排列紊乱、肥大状况与间质水肿、充血状况均有改善。表明四君子汤具有改善慢性左心衰模型大鼠心功能的作用。

5. 抗衰老作用

陈红等报道,对 D -半乳糖致亚急性衰老大鼠模型,用四君子汤灌胃给药,6 周后测定大鼠血清、脑组织、肝脏超氧化物歧化酶(SOD)、谷胱甘肽过氧化物酶(GSH - Px)和丙二醛(MDA)的含量。结果,四君子汤可明显提高衰老模型鼠 SOD、GSH - Px 水平,同时使 MDA 含量明显降低。表明该方可增强衰老大鼠机体抗氧化功能,发挥延缓衰老作用。梁华等报道,四君子汤和四物汤(熟地黄、当归、白芍药、川芎)对 D -半乳糖致亚急性衰老模型雌性小鼠免疫因子白介素- 2(IL - 2)水平的影响。结果,四君子汤组雄性小鼠的 IL - 2 水平显著高于四物汤组和模型组的雄性小鼠;四物汤组雌性小鼠的 IL - 2 水平显著高于四君子汤组和模型组的雌性小鼠。提示四君子汤与四物汤对 D -半乳糖致衰老模型雌性、雄性小鼠免疫因子 IL - 2 的影响具有一定的差异性。

6. 抗肿瘤作用

贾建光等报道,选择不同分化程度的人胃癌细胞株 MKN - 28、SGC - 7901 和 BGC - 823,观察四君子汤及其拆方不同剂量、不同浓度含药血清对胃癌细胞 SP 细胞的生长抑制作用。结果,四君子汤及其拆方含药血清对上述 3 株细胞的 SP 细胞增殖均有明显的抑制作用,以 20%高剂量血清组最为明显。黄浏姣等报道,将低、中、高 3 种剂量的四君子汤含药血清与氟尿嘧啶(FU)合用,分别作用于人胃癌细胞 SGC - 7901,另设空白对照组和 FU 单用组,药物作用时间均为 24 h。结果,FU 对 SGC - 7901 细胞具有 G1/S 期阻滞作用;高剂量四君子汤含药血清与 FU 合用具有明显的 S 期阻滞作用。AV/PI 双染色法计

数显示含药血清与FU合用组,细胞凋亡率分别与对照组比较有显著性差异,且较两药单用组的作用显著增强,呈现剂量依赖性。表明四君子汤能增强FU对人胃癌细胞SGC-7901增殖的抑制和诱导凋亡作用。周昕欣等报道,加味四君子汤(四君子汤加半枝莲、浙贝母、莪术)含药血清作用12、24、48 h,能剂量依赖性抑制B16恶性黑色素细胞增殖,作用24 h为最佳作用时间;中、高剂量组(9.22 g/kg、18.44 g/kg)凋亡率分别为(19.70±0.98)%,(25.21±1.03)%,能显著促进B16恶性黑色素瘤细胞的凋亡($P<0.05$)。说明加味四君子汤可能通过抑制B16恶性黑色素瘤细胞增殖和促进其凋亡的途径,发挥治疗恶性黑色素瘤作用。周氏等还报道,加味四君子汤中、高剂量组分别使B16细胞的侵袭能力显著降低,并显著降低MMP2和MMP9蛋白表达水平,且两者呈剂量依赖式降低。表明加味四君子汤含药血清能显著降低B16恶性黑色素瘤细胞侵袭,并能显著降低与B16恶性黑色素瘤细胞侵袭相关的蛋白MMP2和MMP9表达,这可能是其抑制肿瘤侵袭转移中起重要作用的原因。周氏等同时检测了加味四君子汤含药血清对B16恶性黑色素瘤细胞转录因子核因子-κB(NF-κB)p65活性和表达的影响。结果表明,加味四君子汤含药血清作用24 h后,呈剂量依赖性降低NF-κB(p65)的活性和基因蛋白表达水平,这可能是加味四君子汤含药血清抗恶性黑色素瘤的机制之一。

7. 促进外伤创面愈合

王云飞等建立大鼠右下肢难愈性创面模型,将SD大鼠随机分为模型组、四君子加川牛膝组、四君子汤组、川牛膝组。各组分别给予生理盐水及相应中药灌胃处理,观察各组大鼠创面面积、创面愈合率及创面愈合时间。结果,四君子汤组、四君子加川牛膝组与模型组相比,均可明显缩短创面愈合时间,四君子加川牛膝组创面愈合时间明显少于四君子汤组。表明四君子汤、四君子加川牛膝可以促进大鼠下肢难愈性创面愈合,且以四君子加川牛膝效果明显。

另外,徐秋香等报道,四君子汤不同煎煮方法对脾虚模型动物的影响,比较传统煎煮汤剂、常压煎煮汤剂与高压煎煮汤剂的药效学差别。结果,2种脾虚模型动物经四君子汤治疗后,脾虚症状均得到显著改善,3种煎煮工艺所得四君子汤的治疗作用无显著性差异。

(程 茜 瞿 融)

【中药复方防治肺癌作用机制的研究】

近年来以中医理论为基础的中药复方,发挥多环节、多靶点、多层面的抗肺癌作用,取得一定的研究成果。

1. 中药复方调控细胞周期

中药复方主要通过下调肺癌细胞周期蛋白CyclinD1,阻滞肺癌细胞于G0、G1期,抑制细胞信号转导通路等方面实现对细胞周期的调控。黄河清等研究表明,祛毒扶正汤能有效抑制小鼠Lewis肺癌细胞增殖作用,从而抑制Lewis小鼠肺癌肿瘤生长,其抑癌机制可能与降低血清胸苷激酶(TK1)水平及有效地阻滞细胞于G0、G1期,从而减少S期细胞的分布有关。周燕萍等研究了益气类、养阴类、清热解毒类、活血化瘀类及化痰类的中药复方对人肺癌A549细胞的影响,结果发现,5类中药复方对A549细胞株均有不同程度的抑制作用,其中清热解毒类和活血化瘀类相较于其他3组,具有更明显的抑制作用,其作用机制可能是将A549细胞阻滞于G0、G1期,阻滞肿瘤细胞向S期和G2/M期转化。孙叙敏等报道,复方阿胶浆能够在一定程度延长Lewis小鼠肺癌的生存时间,其作用可能与下调肿瘤组织中CyclinD1、粘附分子CD44的表达水平,干预细胞周期、抑制肿瘤的侵袭性有密切关系。张宏方等报道,调衡方含药血清能显著抑制Lewis肺癌细胞增殖,促进其凋亡,其机制可能与下调Stat3、Stat5的基因表达,抑制细胞信号转导通路有关。

2. 中药复方诱导细胞凋亡

中药复方诱导肺癌细胞的凋亡的机制主要通过调控凋亡相关基因p53、Bcl-2和Survivin等的表达,诱导细胞的凋亡。苏建玲等研究表明,肺康饮口服液能抑制人非小细胞肺癌A549增值及生长,其作用机制可能是上调A549细胞凋亡相关基因p53表达及下调Bcl-2基因表达。李义君等报道,通补消积饮对A549细胞有明显的增殖抑制作用,其作用机制是通过下调增殖细胞核抗原和Survivin基因在A549细胞中的表达。方若鸣等报道,益气除痰方激活内质网应激PERK-eIF2α信号通路诱导A549细胞凋亡,从而抑制A549肺癌裸小鼠移植瘤的生长。另外，马科等研究表明，回药爰康方含药血清呈剂量和时间依赖性抑制Lewis肺癌细胞（LLC）增殖，其机制可能是通过诱导LCC凋亡从而发挥作用。

3. 中药复方抑制新生血管形成

中药复方可以抑制肿瘤血管的形成，其机制主要是抑制肺癌细胞中血管内皮生长因子（VEGF）的表达。来雷等研究表明，复方苦参注射液可抑制肺癌H460细胞的生长和转移，其作用机制与降低VEGF、基质金属蛋白酶9（MMP-9）蛋白表达有关。游捷等研究表明，肺积方对Lewis肺癌小鼠移植瘤的生长具有抑制作用，这种作用可能与减少肿瘤组织中功能性血管的数量，从而抑制肿瘤血管新生有关。刘欣燕等报道，复方回生口服液辅助化疗治疗晚期非小细胞肺癌可显著降低血清中转化生长因子β_1（TGF-β_1）、VEGF的表达，降低肿瘤的免疫抑制作用，起到抑瘤、防止复发转移的作用。胡传杏子报道，参苓白术加味汤能有效降低VEGF、MMP-9表达，提高非小细胞肺癌化疗患者的生活质量。

4. 中药复方抑制肿瘤转移

中药复方主要通过抑制肿瘤细胞对细胞外基质（ECM）的破坏以及下调肿瘤细胞粘附分子的表达，抑制肿瘤转移。陈华圣等研究表明，六君祛痰解毒汤及其拆方对Lewis肺癌转移模型小鼠具有抗肿瘤转移作用，其机制可能与抑制肿瘤细胞对ECM的破坏、使其血清中透明质酸及Ⅳ型胶原水平降低，并下调肿瘤细胞粘附分子CD44的表达、降低其与基质的黏附，进而抑制肿瘤细胞的运动、侵袭和转移有关。曹桂山等研究表明，益气养肺方可以有效辅助治疗非小细胞肺癌，提高治疗实体瘤体疗效，此效应可能是通过降低血清MMP9水平而起作用的。丰哲等报道，参苓白术散加味在治疗肺癌骨转移具有临床疗效，其机制可能是通过抑制肺癌骨转移环氧化物酶-2、VEGF表达而起作用。

5. 中药复方调节免疫功能

中药可通过调节免疫状态而发挥抗肿瘤作用，张晓双等报道，复方乌骨藤胶囊对Lewis肺癌小鼠具有抑瘤作用，其机制就是通过增强肿瘤坏死因子-α和自然杀伤细胞活性，提高荷瘤小鼠的免疫功能从而发挥抗肿瘤的作用。

目前中药复方抗肺癌的实验研究已由形态学深入到微观的细胞、分子、基因水平，众多研究从调节细胞的周期与凋亡、抑制肿瘤血管形成、抑制肿瘤转移及调节免疫功能等多方面对中药复方抑制肺癌的生长与转移的机制进行了阐述，为临床中药复方治疗肺癌提供了科学依据。

（余　秀　寇俊萍）

【中药复方改善缺血性脑损伤的作用机制研究】

1. 对免疫炎症反应的调节作用

周赛男等应用大鼠大脑中动脉阻塞模型，采用RT-PCR，免疫组织化学和蛋白印迹技术研究表明，补阳还五汤可以有效抑制脑缺血后TLR4蛋白的表达增加，从而发挥脑保护作用。Jin Y等报道，在体内应用大脑中动脉模型和体外氧糖剥夺模型，对补阳还五汤改善缺血性脑损伤作用研究表明，其机制可能是通过抑制NF-κB的活化，调节炎症反应的进行发挥脑保护作用。陈利平等用双侧颈总动脉结扎的方法制备慢性脑缺血模型，采用ELISA法检测参龙汤对慢性脑缺血大鼠血清IL-6、IL-8、ICAM-1、TNF-α含量的变化，结果大剂量组可显著降低血清中上述炎性因子含量，这可能是参龙汤对脑缺血神经损伤的保护作用机制之一。

另外，复方桂枝茯苓丸（张建荣等报道）、活络效灵丹（金竹青报道）、健脑益智方（曹瑾等报道）、消栓通络胶囊（严亚锋等报道）等中药复方制剂在脑缺血动物模型上均证实具有较好的脑保护作用，其机制可能是通过对免疫炎症反应的调节发挥作用。

2. 对神经细胞凋亡的抑制作用

宫健伟等研究了地黄饮子对脑缺血再灌注大鼠的作用，结果地黄饮子能通过下调Bax蛋白、上调Bcl-2蛋白和下调Caspase-3蛋白表达，抑制脑缺血再灌注损伤后细胞凋亡，从而发挥脑保护作用。郜峦等研究表明，脑络欣通能够保护脑缺血再灌注损伤大鼠脑组织，其作用机制可能与促进神经生长因子（NGF）表达，激活P13K/Akt信号通路并降低Bad蛋白表达，从而抑制神经细胞凋亡有关。

另外，通络化痰胶囊（富苏等报道）、银丹心脑通(徐忠祥等报道)、中风膏(刘志军等报道)、活脉通络汤(刘海兴等报道)等中药复方制剂在体内脑缺血再灌注模型上的研究也证实均具有抗神经细胞凋亡作用。

3. 对自由基清除和抗氧化作用

吴彪飞等研究表明,参丹芎注射液能够明显减少大鼠急性脑缺血再灌注损伤后脑梗死灶面积和 MDA 含量,增加 SOD 和 GSH-Px 活性,表明其通过抗氧化应激途径呈现的保护作用。宫健伟等研究表明,地黄饮子能显著抑制脑缺血再灌注模型大鼠血清脑组织中 SOD,CAT 和 GSH-Px 活力的降低及 MDA 含量的升高,表明其可通过减轻自由基损伤提高脑组织抗氧化能力而发挥作用。

另外,益气解毒方(朱丽等报道)、丹红注射液(李美娇等报道)、安宫牛黄丸(董世芬等报道)、芪丹通脉片(温晓妮等报道)、参归片(石永平等报道)等中药复方制剂也均具有清除自由基等抗氧化作用,以减少脑缺血再灌注损伤。

4. 对血脑屏障的保护作用

郑咏秋等研究表明,华佗再造浸膏可有效恢复脑缺血再灌注造成的脑微血管内皮水肿和血脑屏障超微结构损伤,减少功能性偶联受体激酶 2 表达,并抑制金属基质蛋白酶-2 和金属基质蛋白酶-9 的表达。李跃等研究表明,益脑康胶囊可以减轻大鼠自体血栓栓塞大脑中动脉闭塞模型溶栓后血脑屏障破坏,可能与其上调 ZO-1 蛋白的表达有关。石贺元等研究表明,脑清喷鼻微乳也可以通过调节紧密连接蛋白的表达和血脑屏障的通透性发挥脑保护作用。

另外,脑泰方(廖君等报道)、当归补血汤(陆莹等报道)、参附注射液(任长虹等报道)等中药复方制剂在对脑缺血后血脑屏障通透性影响的研究中,也证实可以通过抑制金属基质蛋白酶-9 的表达和炎症因子的释放降低血脑屏障通透性。

5. 其他

中药复方较好改善缺血性脑损伤的作用机制的报道还有,如生脉注射液(杨浩鹏等报道)可通过调节 NF-κB 通路,抑制组织因子表达减轻小鼠局灶性脑缺血再灌注损伤;维脑康(郑咏秋等报道)可通过作用 MAPK 信号转导通路调节自噬发挥对缺血性脑损伤的保护作用。

(曹国胜 寇俊萍)

【中药复方抗流感作用机理的研究】

1. 体外细胞培养

田连起等将细胞病变效应法与噻唑蓝比色法相结合,研究大青龙汤颗粒剂对甲型 H1N1 流感病毒感染的狗肾细胞的作用机制。结果表明,该方对脂多糖所致大鼠发热的解热作用显著,且药效持续时间长;可直接灭活病毒,在细胞水平表现出一定的抗甲型 H1N1 流感病毒作用,并呈剂量依赖性;但抑制流感病毒生物合成及阻断吸附、穿入细胞的作用不明显。汪玉冠等研究防感煎剂对甲型 H1N1 流感病毒的体外抑制作用。结果表明,该方对甲型 H1N1 流感病毒感染有显著的预防与直接作用,作用机理可能与直接杀灭病毒、抑制病毒吸附及膜融合作用来阻止流感病毒进入宿主体内增殖复制有关。刘禹翔等以狗肾传代细胞(MDCK)为病毒宿主,研究加味银翘方体外抗甲型流感病毒的作用机制。结果表明,该方对甲型流感病毒所致的 MDCK 病变有较好的抑制作用,效果与达菲相近。常洋等对细胞培养甲型 A/Brisban/10/2008(H3N2)流感病毒,采用病毒细胞形态变化 CPE 法、MTT 染色法,对牛黄清感胶囊抗流感病毒作用进行研究。结果表明,该方具有抑制和预防甲型流感病毒的作用。

2. 动物实验研究

张波等研究表明,麻杏石甘汤能明显减轻流感病毒感染小鼠肺部炎症反应,降低肺指数,其机制可能与抑制神经氨酸酶活性,阻止病毒增殖有关;拆方研究表明麻黄在该方中具有重要作用。孙国倩等报道,清肺解毒方治疗流感病毒滴鼻造模病毒性肺炎小鼠,在一定剂量组死亡保护率明显提高,存活时间明显延长,生命延长率明显增加;小鼠的肺指数、肺脏病毒滴度及肺脏病毒载量显著降低。杜德安研究表明,口服清热消炎宁胶囊能减少病毒感染应激小鼠的发病率和死亡率,并显著延长感染动物的平均存活时间;肺组织病理学研究发现该方可减轻肺损伤,减少肺组织中病毒量;机制可能与降低机体对流感的易感性和抗炎作用有关。任亮等研究表明,清营解表合剂对小鼠免疫功能的作用是通过调节流感病毒感染小鼠外周血 Th 型细胞因子的表达水平,恢复机体的抗感染免疫平衡,提高机体免疫功能起到防治流感病毒感染的作用。刘琪等研究表明,疏风宣肺方各剂量和解表清里中剂量能通过调节MyD88依赖的TLR信号传导通路下调NF-κB活性,发挥抗流感病毒的作用,疏风宣肺方效果优于解表清里方;同时通过观察肺指数、肺组织切片病理形态变化,发现两方均能改善流感病毒感染小鼠的肺组织病理损伤,有抗流感病毒的作用。

3. 药物靶点数据库分析

李立等对麻杏石甘汤中的有效化合物以及PubChem数据库中有效成分的靶蛋白构建分子网络及解析生物学通路,应用IPA软件分析,共发现该方靶蛋白186个,甲流相关基因7个,8条生物通路(含4条细胞免疫通路),表明该方可通过干预细胞免疫相关通路中的多个位点起到防治甲流的作用。

(朱靓贤　陈德兴)

【中药复方及其有效成分改善胰岛素抵抗机制的研究】

胰岛素抵抗(IR)是指胰岛素所作用的靶器官和组织对胰岛素生物学效应的反应性降低或丧失而产生的一系列病理和临床表现。Ye J报道,胰岛素抵抗的发病机制涉及到多方面的因素,有肥胖、炎症反应、内质网应激、氧化应激、线粒体功能紊乱、高胰岛素血症、高血脂症、缺氧等。这些因素大多都与肥胖和衰老相关联,两者是诱发胰岛素抵抗的主要危险因素。

1. 调节脂肪组织稳态,抑制炎症反应

脂肪组织不仅参与了能量储存,而且是一个重要的内分泌组织,其分泌的多种脂肪因子,如脂联素、瘦素、单核细胞趋化蛋白-1(MCP-1)等,参与了机体脂类代谢的调节。与肥胖相关联的炎症反应是胰岛素抵抗的重要诱因。

Zheng X等研究表明,白藜芦醇可以保护2型糖尿病大鼠血管功能,降低肿瘤坏死因子-α(TNF-α)、细胞间黏附分子-1(ICAM-1)、MCP-1等多种炎症因子的表达水平,抑制核因子κB(NF-κB)通路的活化,从而减缓血管内壁的炎症损伤,且白藜芦醇可能是通过激活沉默调节蛋白-1,从而抑制了NF-κB的转录活性。另外,血竭总黄酮(Chen F等报道)、金柴降糖胶囊(左文标等报道)、血脂清颗粒(刘德桓等报道)、祛胰抵方(马建等报道),均可以通过抑制炎症反应来改善胰岛素抵抗。Gao Y等通过3T3-L1细胞的体外实验表明,人参皂苷Re可以通过激活氧化物酶体增殖物激活受体(PPAR)-γ通路,上调脂联素、胰岛素受体底物(IRS)-1等因子的表达水平,并降低TNF-α的表达和分泌,起到减缓胰岛素抵抗的效果。同样,糖脂清方剂(Xia JN等报道)、苓桂术甘汤(汪园园等报道),也是通过影响过氧化物酶体增殖物激活受体PPAR-γ的表达水平来改善胰岛素抵抗。Cui WX等报道,海南冬青三萜类提取物可以改善高脂引起的大鼠非酒精性脂肪肝症状,调节脂质代谢,减轻胰岛素抵抗,这种作用可能与调节PPAR-α和细胞色素P450 2E1(CYP2E1)的表达有关。另外,激活腺苷酸活化蛋白激酶(AMPK)通路和胰岛素通路均可介导葡萄糖的摄取,AMPK通路可以改善IR过程中的炎症反应。此外,小檗碱(Chang W等报道),也都可以通过AMPK改善胰岛素抵抗。

2. 调节内质网应激

内质网应激可能是导致胰岛素抵抗的重要因素,并可能发生在炎症反应之前。游离脂肪酸、缺氧、钙离子稳态的变化、内质网蛋白分子伴侣的突变等诸多因素会扰乱内质网的稳态,进而启动内质网的未折叠蛋白反应(UPR)的三条经典信号通路(ATF6、IRE1和PERK)的各个环节会直接或间接地影响胰岛素发挥生物学效应。如IRE1-α可通过激活和核因子κB抑制蛋白(IκB)激酶(IKK)进而影响胰岛素受体底物的磷酸化,抑制胰岛素信号转导;其他影响方式还包括抑制胰岛素受体后PI3K/Akt通路、影响糖脂代谢相关的转录因子的活化、影响胰岛素的生物合成、导致细胞凋亡等。

Shi FH等研究表明,紫甘薯色素可以改善胰岛素抵抗,显著抑制肝脏中活性氧的产生,同时有效抑制了由活性氧诱导的内质网应激蛋白PERK和eIF2α的活化,继而抑制了c-Jun氨基末端激酶(JNK)和NF-κB的活化。Chang XH等研究表明,大精酸(大黄酸和精氨酸的共结晶物)可通过抑制内质网应激和凋亡来保护2型糖尿病大鼠的肝脏,改善胰岛素抵抗。Zhang ZF等报道,中药复方(由绿茶、人参、远志的提取物组成)可以提高2型糖尿病大鼠的认知功能,增强胰岛素信号传导通路,其机制可能与抑制内质网应激下游的重要信号蛋白JNK有关。

3. 抗氧化应激

氧化应激在胰岛素抵抗的发病因素中扮演了重要角色,可能是构成炎症反应和内质网应激等一系列导致胰岛素抵抗因素的病理基础。

Xiong WT等报道,管花肉苁蓉可以显著降低糖尿病小鼠空腹和餐后血糖水平,其改善胰岛素分泌的机制可能与抗氧化应激有关。Lin M等报道,鱼腥草水提取物可以通过减轻由高脂饮食引起的氧化应激和炎症反应来减弱肝脏中脂肪合成酶类的活性,减少肝脏内饱和脂肪的堆积,改善胰岛素抵抗。

4. 改善线粒体功能

Wang Q等研究表明,鸢尾甙可以减轻棕榈酸所致的内皮细胞胰岛素抵抗,调节内皮细胞的功能。其机制可能与抑制活性氧诱发的炎症反应,在一定程度上恢复线粒体膜电位和胰岛素信号传导通路有关。但目前为止,线粒体功能紊乱与胰岛素抵抗的联系还未研究清楚。

5. 改善高胰岛素血症

高胰岛素血症是胰岛素抵抗早期的重要表现。虽然高胰岛素血症是由胰岛素抵抗所导致的,但高胰岛素血症同样可以诱发胰岛素抵抗,这可能源于胰岛素通路存在负反馈调节,这种负反馈调节可以抑制胰岛素导致的应激反应。

Fang ZH等通过对62位被诊断出2型糖尿病伴有血管损伤病人的研究表明,与对照组相比,丹蛭降糖胶囊可以显著降低患者的空腹胰岛素(FINS)水平和胰岛素抵抗指数。另外,Wang ZQ等报道,猪毛蒿提取物可以有效降低肥胖小鼠FINS水平,并升高肝脏组织中IRS-2的含量,增强IRS-1、胰岛素受体-β、Akt以及AMPKα的磷酸化水平。Liu K等通过搜索并整合数据库信息发现,绿茶可以显著降低患者的空腹血糖值,并可降低空腹胰岛素水平。

6. 其他途径

Lu B等报道,菩人丹可降低糖尿病大鼠的血糖水平,其主要是通过调节血管生成因子,改善胰腺血流状况,维持β细胞的功能,从而缓解胰岛素抵抗;且PKC可能是其作用靶点之一。

胰岛素抵抗作为贯穿糖尿病、高血压、高血脂等代谢疾病的病理基础,其机制复杂,中药在改善胰岛素抵抗方面的研究仍有许多深层次的问题有待探索。

(陈 妍 寇俊萍)

[附] 参 考 文 献

A

敖新平,王明镇,王兴友,等.金匮肾气丸抗雄性大鼠力竭性疲劳的研究[J].时珍国医国药,2013,24(3):607

C

Chen F, Xiong H, Wang J, et al. An-t-idiabetic effect of total flavonoids fr-o-m Sanguis draxonis in type 2 diabet-i-c rats[J]. Journal of Ethnopharmacology, 2013, 149(3):729

Chang XH, Liang LN, Zhan LB, et al. The effect of Chinese Jinzhida recipe on the hippocampus in a rat m-odel of diabetes-associated cognitive decline[J]. Complementary & Alternative Medicine, 2013, 13(1):161

Chang W, Zhang M, Li J, et al. Ber-b-erine improves insulin resistance in cardiomyocytes via activation of 5′-ad-e-nosine monophosphate activated prote-i-n kinase[J]. Metabolism, 2013, 62(8):1159

Cui WX, Yang J, Chen XQ, et al. Triterpenoid-rich fraction from *Ilex hainanensis* Merr. attenuates non-alcoholic fatty liver disease induced by high fat diet in rats[J]. The American Journal of Chinese Medicine, 2013, 41(3):487

蔡华丹,张慧芹,续畅,等.茵陈蒿汤水提物和醇提物活性组分的差异及对D-GalN诱导大鼠急性肝损伤预防作用的比较[J].中国实验方剂学杂志,2013,19(10):216

曹峰,唐阿梅.小柴胡汤中柴胡不同剂量对正常大鼠胃窦组织MTL,AChE,NO含量的影响[J].中国实验方剂学杂志,2013,19(15):232

曹桂山,王玉强,乔钦增.中药益气养肺方联合化疗对晚期非小细胞肺癌患者血清基质金属蛋白酶-9影响的研究[J].山西医药杂志,2013,42(3):330

曹瑾，刘素蓉，韩祖成，等. 健脑益智方对脑缺血再灌注损伤后炎性细胞因子 TNF－α，IL－1β的影响[J]. 新中医，2013，45(10)：136

常洋，周有财，段书敏，等. 牛黄清感胶囊对甲型H3N2 流感病毒抑制和预防作用的实验研究[J]. 中国医药科学，2013，3(16)：27

陈红，陈东波. 四君子汤对衰老大鼠抗氧化功能的影响[J]. 江西中医学院学报，2013，25(1)：68

陈华圣，许爱华，沈婷婷，等. 六君祛痰解毒汤及其拆方对 C57BL/6J 小鼠 Lewis 肺癌转移的抑制作用[J]. 中国实验方剂学杂志，2013，19(6)：249

陈利平，王发渭，孙志高，等. 参龙汤对脑缺血大鼠血清炎性因子的影响[J]. 中国中医急症，2013，22(2)：201

陈文阁，王茜. 桃红四物汤加减治疗结节性红斑 60 例临床观察[J]. 中医药学报，2013，41(4)：106

陈艳秋，南亚昀，张玉芬，等. 金匮肾气丸对肾阳虚大鼠睾丸中 TGF－β1 表达、精子数量及活率的影响[J]. 山东中医杂志，2013，32(3)：191

程志安，韩凌，危建安，等. 六味地黄丸、金匮肾气丸及健骨二仙丸含药血清对 BMSCs 成脂、成骨细胞分化相关基因的影响[J]. 中国中西医结合杂志，2013，33(2)：261

D

党秀芳. 小柴胡汤加减治疗胆汁反流性胃炎 45 例疗效观察[J]. 内蒙古中医药，2013，32(27)：17

董世芬，楼黎明，张硕峰，等. 安宫牛黄丸(含天然麝香或人工麝香)对实验性脑缺血的保护作用[J]. 世界科学技术·中医药现代化，2013，15(1)：85

杜德安. 清热消炎宁可减轻流感病毒引起的肺损伤[J]. 中国中医药信息杂志，2013，20(3)：69

F

Fang ZH，Liu Y，Bao TT，et al. E-f-fect of Danzhijiangtang capsule on monocyte chemoattractant protein－1 mRNA expression in newly diagnosed diabetes subclinical vascular lesions [J]. World Journal of Gastroenterology，2013，19(19)：2963

方若鸣，林丽珠，杨文娟，等. 益气除痰方对小鼠 Lewis 肺癌细胞凋亡的影响[J]. 中药新药与临床药理，2013，24(2)：147

丰哲，林宗汉，陈跃平，等. 参苓白术散加味对肺癌骨转移 COX－2、VEGF 表达调控的影响[J]. 时珍国医国药，2013，24(1)：1055

冯海泉. 小柴胡汤加减治疗气滞血瘀型原发性痛经疗效观察[J]. 湖北中医杂志，2013，35(12)：44

富苏，韩经丹，周杰，等. 通络化痰胶囊对脑缺血损伤大鼠神经细胞凋亡及 Bcl－2，Bax 的影响[J]. 中国实验方剂学杂志，2013，19(8)：242

G

Gao Y，Yang M，Su Y，et al. Ginsen-o-s-ide Re reduces insulin resistance thr-o-u-gh activation of PPAR－γ pathway a-nd inhibition of TNF－α production[J]. Journal of Ethnopharmacology，2013，147(2)：509

郜峦，王键，库宇，等. 脑络欣通及其拆方对脑缺血再灌注大鼠 NGF，PI3K，Akt 以及 Bad 蛋白表达的影响[J]. 中成药，2013，35(11)：2311

宫健伟，叶蕾，樊巧玲. 地黄饮子对脑缺血再灌注模型大鼠 Bax，Bcl－2，Caspase－3 蛋白表达的影响[J]. 中国实验方剂学杂志，2013，19(5)：248

宫健伟，叶蕾，张秀丽，等. 地黄饮子对脑缺血再灌注模型大鼠血清、脑组织 SOD，CAT 和 GSH－Px 及 MDA 的影响[J]. 中国实验方剂学杂志，2013，19(14)：247

H

何容. 小柴胡汤加减治疗美尼尔氏综合征所致眩晕临床效果观察[J]. 亚太传统医药，2013，9(10)：149

胡传杏子. 参苓白术加味汤对非小细胞肺癌化疗患者血清血管内皮生长因子、基质金属蛋白酶－9 表达的影响[J]. 中国医药导报，2013，10(29)：72

怀平艾，郝芳. 小柴胡汤联合聚乙二醇干扰素 α－2a 治疗慢性丙型肝炎的临床研究[J]. 世界中西医结合杂志，2013，8(8)：801

黄飞，刘成福，王小琴. 金匮肾气丸对庆大霉素所致大鼠听力变化及 Notch2/hes1 信号通路表达的影响[J]. 时珍国医国药，2013，24(5)：1083

黄飞，刘成福，王小琴. 金匮肾气丸对庆大霉素诱导肾损伤大鼠肾组织 Notch2/hes1 信号通路的影响[J]. 中国中西医结合肾病杂志，2013，14(1)：29

黄河清，王世聪，陆顺意，等. 中药祛毒扶正汤对肺癌小鼠血清 TK1 表达及肺癌细胞周期影响的实验研究[J]. 光明中医，2013，28(8)：1572

黄浏姣，赵刚，毛明. 四君子汤含药血清与氟尿嘧啶合用对胃癌细胞 SGC－7901 增殖抑制作用研究[J]. 时珍国医国药，2013，24(5)：1236

J

Jin Y，Dong L，Wu C，et al. Buyang Huanwu Decoction fraction protects against cerebral ischemia/reperfusion injury by attenuating the inflammatory response and cellular apoptosis[J]. Neural Regeneration Research，2013，8(3)：197

贾建光，马莉，李靖，等. 四君子汤及拆方含药血清对胃癌细胞株侧群细胞的生长抑制研究[J]. 中国临床药理学与治疗学，2013，18(5)：513

江山，李芳. 小柴胡汤对肝纤维化大鼠的抗肝纤维化作用[J]. 中药药理与临床，2013，29(1)：17

金竹青. 活络效灵丹通过抑制脑组织炎症反应对缺血性脑损伤的保护作用[J]. 浙江中医药大学学报，2013，37(9)：1099

K

孔亮，狄美琪，李超生，等. 半夏白术天麻汤加减治疗椎-基底动脉供血不足性眩晕 60 例临床研究[J]. 中医杂志，2013，54(4)：315

L

Lin M, Hsu P, Yin M. Protective eff-e-cts of Houttuynia cordata aqueous e-x-tract in mice consuming a high satu-r-ated fat diet[J]. Food Funct, 2013, 4(2): 322

Liu K, Zhou R, Wang B, et al. Effect of green tea on glucose control and insulin sensitivity: a meta-analysis of 17 randomized controlled trials [J]. American Journal of Clinical Nutrition, 2013, 98(2): 340

Lu B, Bai Y, Du Z, et al. The effect of Chinese medicine pu-ren-dan on pancreatic angiogenesis in high fat die t/streptozotocin-induced diabetic rats [J]. Indian Journal of Pharmacology, 2013, 45(6): 556

来雷，翟昌林，杨林军，等. 复方苦参注射液对肺癌裸鼠移植瘤的抑制作用及其 MMP-9、VEGF 表达的影响[J]. 中国中医药科技，2013，20(1)：21

李保义，吕晓峰，安春棉，等. 茵陈蒿汤加味治疗药物性肝损伤 65 例[J]. 中国实验方剂学杂志，2013，19(20)：285

李静，李彬彬，尹磊，等. 沙参麦冬汤对慢性支气管炎模型大鼠抗氧化能力的影响[J]. 中医杂志，2013，54(17)：1497

李立，赵静，王雪飞，等. 麻杏石甘汤防治甲型 H1N1 流感分子机制的生物信息学分析[J]. 中国实验方剂学杂志，2013，19(13)：346

李美娇，郭虹，刘青青，等. 丹红注射液对脑缺血缺氧损伤的保护作用[J]. 中国实验方剂学杂志，2013，19(17)：221

李然，刘立萍，马骥，等. 小柴胡汤含药血清对肝癌 HepG-2 细胞的影响[J]. 中国实验方剂学杂志，2013，19(5)：217

李笋，王培源，钟萍，等. 金匮肾气丸对肾阳虚变应性鼻炎缓解期小鼠 Th1/Th2 细胞因子的影响[J]. 中药新药与临床药理，2013，24(3)：258

李霞，朱姬莲. 加味茵陈蒿汤治疗新生儿高胆红素血症 30 例[J]. 中医儿科杂志，2013，9(2)：42

李兴华. 加味茵陈蒿汤治疗 ABO 母儿血型不合 40 例[J]. 光明中医，2013，28(7)：1351

李艳丽. 四君子汤对小鼠耐缺氧及抗运动性疲劳作用研究[J]. 亚太传统医药，2013，9(1)：33

李义君，刘建秋，徐涛. 通补消积饮对人肺腺癌 A549 细胞凋亡的影响[J]. 国际中医中药杂志，2013，35(4)：323

李义君，刘建秋. 通补消积饮对人肺腺癌 A549 细胞增殖影响的研究[J]. 中医药信息，2013，30(2)：90

李跃，孙景波，黄燕. 益脑康胶囊对脑梗死大鼠溶栓后血脑屏障的保护作用及对 ZO-1 蛋白表达的影响[J]. 中国实验方剂学杂志，2013，19(11)：268

梁华，孙燕佩，朱明雪. 四君子汤、四物汤对亚急性衰老模型雌性小鼠 IL-2 影响的实验研究[J]. 辽宁中医杂志，2013，40(2)：193

廖君，张薇，夏兴，等. 脑泰方对局灶性脑缺血大鼠脑组织核因子-κB，基质金属蛋白酶 9 及其抑制剂表达的影响[J]. 中国中医药信息杂志，2013，20(9)：28

廖乐乐，罗翱翔，唐干益，等. 四君子汤对大黄脾虚模型小鼠的影响[J]. 广东药学院学报，2013，29(2)：202

刘保兴，陈国宏. 金匮肾气丸治疗良性前列腺增生症合并逼尿肌不稳定 17 例[J]. 中国中西医结合外科杂志，2013，19(2)：179

刘德桓，陈文鑫，叶靖，等. 血脂清联合阿托伐他汀对高血压合并代谢综合征患者血清炎症因子和胰岛素抵抗的影响[J]. 中国医药导报，2013，10(24)：79

刘桂章，陶鸣浩. 金匮肾气丸联合奥美拉唑治疗老年性反流性食管炎 40 例[J]. 河南中医，2013，33(5)：658

刘海兴，刘玉丽，于嵩，等. 活脉通络饮对大鼠脑缺血再灌注脑组织 caspase-3 表达的影响[J]. 解剖科学进展，2013，19(4)：324

刘梅，唐惠英. 茵陈蒿汤治疗新生儿母婴血型不合溶血病 126 例临床观察[J]. 右江医学，2013，41(3)：370

刘琪，顾立刚，卢娜娜，等. 疏风宣肺方、解表清里方药对流感病毒小鼠 TLR7、MyD88、NF-κBmRNA 及蛋白表达的影响[J]. 中国中西医结合杂志，2013，33(9)：1256

刘琪，顾立刚，周旭澎，等. 疏风宣肺及解表清里方药对流感病毒感染小鼠肺损伤的保护研究[J]. 中华中医药杂志，2013，28(7)：2132

刘强，黄鑫华. 半夏泻心汤加减治疗消化性溃疡疗效观察[J]. 新中医，2013，45(2)：13

刘文娥，谈珍瑜，夏如意，等. 盆炎丸治疗女性生殖道解脲支原体感染气虚血瘀证的临床观察[J]. 中国中西医结合杂志，2013，33(5)：590

刘欣燕，戴献利，侯志华，等. 回生口服液对非小细胞肺癌疗效及转化生长因子 β1 和血管内皮生成因子影响的研究[J]. 临床荟萃，2013，28(6)：643

刘禹翔，曲敬来，曾仲意，等. 加味银翘方体外抗甲型流感病毒实验研究[J]. 新中医，2013，45(8)：187

刘志军，杨瑞龙，杨涛，等. 中风膏对大鼠脑缺血再灌注损伤脑梗死体积及细胞凋亡的影响[J]. 中西医结合心脑血管病杂志，2013，11(3)：337

龙泳伶，李政木. 金匮肾气丸及其拆方对肾阳虚雌鼠卵巢功能的影响[J]. 中国中西医结合杂志，2013，33(7)：967

陆莹，罗亚非，范瑞娟. 当归补血汤对大鼠局灶性脑缺血再灌注血-脑屏障和大脑皮质神经元的影响[J]. 神经解剖学杂志，2013，29(3)：301

骆稚平. 茵陈蒿汤联合西医治疗早中期慢性乙型重型肝炎随机平行对照研究[J]. 实用中医内科杂志，2013，27(13)：64

吕伯中. 柴胡桂枝干姜汤加减治疗慢性羊水过多 40 例[J]. 中医杂志，2013，54(15)：1327

M

马建，韩美子，杜丽坤，等. 祛胰抵方对 2 型糖尿病胰岛素抵抗大鼠 TNF－α 的影响[J]. 中国医药信息，2013，30(4)：51

马科，周慧，边静，等. 回药爱康方含药血清抑制 Lewis 肺癌细胞增殖和诱导凋亡的研究[J]. 肿瘤防治研究，2013，40(12)：1114

马雅銮，李彤，王蓓蓓，等. 黄连解毒汤对高脂血症小鼠肝脏保护作用的观察[J]. 中国中西医结合杂志，2013，33(8)：1107

毛靓瑶，邹维，张芳侠，等. 半夏泻心汤加减治疗胆汁反流性胃炎 35 例[J]. 陕西中医，2013，34(9)：1121

P

潘卫东，Shin Kwak，吴春岚，等. 加味四君子汤对肌萎缩侧索硬化症 AR2 小鼠运动功能的影响[J]. 上海中医药大学学报，2013，27(1)：60

Q

邱俊，刘友章，王超，等. 从四君子汤对慢性心衰大鼠心功能的影响探讨“心脾相关”[J]. 时珍国医国药，2013，24(10)：2564

R

任亮，宋素花，姜璐，等. 清营解表合剂对流感病毒感染小鼠外周血 Th1、Th2 型细胞因子动态表达的影响[J]. 中国实验方剂学杂志，2013，19(11)：255

任长虹，杨勇，吴晓丹，等. 参附注射液对缺血性脑卒中大鼠血脑屏障的影响[J]. 中医药学报，2012，40(5)：76

S

Shi FH，Wu Y，Dai DZ，et al. Hepatosteatosis and hepatic insulin resistance are blunted by argirein，an anti-inflammatory agent，through normalizing endoplasmic reticulum stress and apoptosis in diabetic liver[J]. Journal of Pharmacy and Pharmacology，2013，65(6)：916

沈燕慧. 双黄连粉针合茵陈蒿汤治疗母儿 ABO 血型不合 78 例[J]. 内蒙古中医药，2013，32(15)：50

石贺元，宋宛珊，黄燕. 脑清喷鼻微乳对急性脑梗死大鼠血脑屏障通透性影响及其机制[J]. 中国实验方剂学杂志，2013，19(20)：166

石永平，汪汇，王怀新，等. 参归片对脑缺血损伤的保护作用[J]. 中国应用生理学杂志，2013，29(2)：139

苏建玲，孙黎，罗强，等. 肺康饮口服液对肺腺癌 A549 细胞生长及凋亡的影响[J]. 中国医药导报，2013，10(12)：9

孙国倩，杨静，周喆，等. 清肺解毒方对流感病毒感染小鼠的保护作用[J]. 国际药学研究杂志，2013，40(1)：53

孙丽梅，王军，苏海涛，等. 小柴胡汤加减治疗甲型 H1N1 流感 61 例[J]. 山东中医杂志，2013，32(6)：399

孙叙敏，陈信义. 复方阿胶浆对小鼠 Lewis 肺癌 CyclinD1、CD44 表达的影响[J]. 世界中医药，2013，8(3)：318

T

田连起，黄鹤归，叶晓川，等. 大青龙汤颗粒剂体外抗甲型 H1N1 流感病毒实验研究[J]. 中医学报，2013，28(2)：172

W

Wang Q，Cheng XL，Zhang DY，et al. Tectorigenin Attenuates Palmitate-Induced Endothelial Insulin Resistance v-ia Targeting ROS－Associated Inflam-mation and IRS－1 Pathway[J]. PLoS One，2013，8(6)：e66417

Wang ZQ，Zhang XH，Yu Y，et al. Artemisia scoparia extract attenuates non-alcoholic fatty liver disease in di-e-t-induced obesity mice by enhancing hepatic insulin and AMPK signaling independently of FGF21 pathway[J]. Metabolism，2013，62(9)：1239

汪玉冠，宋康，骆仙芳，等. 防感煎剂含药血清体外抑制甲 1 型流感病毒作用的研究[J]. 中华中医药学刊，2013，31(11)：2466

汪园园，金明华，柯斌，等. 苓桂术甘汤联合热量限摄对胰岛素抵抗模型大鼠的影响及机制研究[J]. 中国中西医结合杂志，2013，33(3)：356

王枫，赵乌兰. 金匮肾气丸对耳聋豚鼠 Cav1.2、TNF－α 表达的影响[J]. 新中医，2013，45(5)：175

王红艳，张先庚，刘琴，等. 金匮肾气丸对恐伤肾模型仔鼠多巴胺水平的调节作用研究[J]. 中国全科医学，2013，16(11)：3957

王红艳，张先庚. 金匮肾气丸对“恐伤肾”模型仔鼠皮质酮水平的调节作用[J]. 辽宁中医杂志，2013，40(2)：362

王继海，黄育华. 加味茵陈蒿汤治疗急性病毒性淤胆型肝炎临床观察[J]. 湖北中医杂志，2013，35(8)：3

王军，苏海涛，孙丽梅，等. 小柴胡汤对免疫抑制小鼠细胞因子影响的研究[J]. 中华中医药学刊，2013，31(10)：2242

王坤，金若敏，陈长勋. 茵陈蒿汤与栀子肝毒性的比较研究[J]. 中药药理与临床，2013，29(1)：8

王双玲，岳振东，李雪梅，等. 小柴胡汤合血府逐瘀汤治疗偏头痛 31 例[J]. 陕西中医，2013，34(10)：1307

王秀珍，毛颖，张喆，等. 四神丸对溃疡性结肠炎大鼠血清 IL-2、IL-4、IL-8 影响的实验研究[J]. 中医药学报，2013，41(3)：105

王云飞，阙华发，高丹，等. 四君子加川牛膝方对大鼠下肢难愈性创面愈合的影响[J]. 上海中医药大学学报，2013，27(3)：95

王泽军. 金匮肾气丸对 2 型糖尿病的疗效分析[J]. 中医临床研究，2013，5(7)：66

魏良浩，潘庆，张跃明.《金匮》肾气丸对阿尔茨海默病模型大鼠额叶皮质神经元 NT-3 表达的影响[J]. 中国中医急症，2013，22(2)：211

温晓妮，乔黎焱. 芪丹通脉片对慢性脑缺血大鼠海马 MDA，SOD 表达的影响[J]. 时珍国医国药，2013，24(10)：2343

巫资明，李初谊. 三镜联合茵陈蒿汤治疗梗阻性黄疸 80 例[J]. 西部中医药，2013，26(8)：94

吴斌，黄利，毛世清，等. 金匮肾气丸对系统性红斑狼疮血清单核细胞趋化蛋白-4 和白细胞介素 4 的影响及疗效观察[J]. 实用医学杂志，2013，29(19)：3245

吴红专. 金匮肾气丸对 2 型糖尿病的临床观察[J]. 中药药理与临床，2013，29(3)：191

吴俊伟，丁旭宣，杨磊，等. 金匮肾气丸治疗牙周病的临床疗效观察[J]. 中国医疗前沿，2013，8(15)：73

吴梅婷，陈玲，项双卫. 茵陈蒿汤联合西药治疗母儿 ABO 血型不合疗效分析[J]. 现代生物医学进展，2013，13(2)：312

吴锐，涂俊玲，谢建祥，等. 加味犀角地黄汤在脂多糖诱导的兔内毒素血症中的防治作用[J]. 辽宁中医杂志，2013，40(2)：339

吴唬飞，孙圆媛，金翠英，等. 参丹芎注射液对大鼠急性脑缺血再灌注损伤的保护作用[J]. 中药药理与临床，2013，29(4)：121

X

Xia JN, Zhang DQ, Du J, et al. Regulation effects of TZQ-F on adip-o-cyte differentiation and insulin action [J]. Journal of Ethnopharmacology, 2013, 150(2): 692

Xiong WT, Gu L, Wang C, et al. Anti-hyperglycemic and hypolipidemic effects of Cistanche tubulosa in type 2 diabetic db/db mice[J]. Journal of Ethnopharmacology, 2013, 150(3): 935

夏晓莉，罗思聪，刘淑玲，等. 柴胡疏肝散对代谢综合征大鼠肝 X 受体的影响[J]. 中医杂志，2013，54(16)：1404

熊斌，钱会南. 四君子汤和玉屏风散对脾虚大鼠脑内信号转导和转录激活因子 1mRNA 水平变化的影响[J]. 湖北中医药大学学报，2013，15(1)：3

熊斌，钱会南. 益气健脾方药对脾虚大鼠脑内 JAK1、STAT1、SOCS1 水平变化的影响[J]. 中华中医药学刊，2013，31(7)：1543

徐国荣，王淑梅. 茵陈蒿汤不同煎煮剂治疗新生儿黄疸临床疗效观察[J]. 中国社区医师医学专业，2013，15(7)：201

徐秋香，郁红礼，吴皓，等. 四君子汤传统煎煮和机器煎煮的药效学差异比较[J]. 中国实验方剂学杂志，2013，19(16)：250

徐忠祥，徐平，张骏，等. 银丹心脑通对脑缺血再灌注大鼠海马区神经细胞凋亡及 Caspase-3 表达的影响[J]. 中华神经医学杂志，2013，12(6)：588

许翠萍，朱庆均，宋洁，等. 金匮肾气丸对肾阳虚小鼠睾丸组织端粒酶活性的促进作用[J]. 中国中西医结合杂志，2013，33(2)：252

许光仑，孔瑞龙. 茵陈蒿汤治疗寻常痤疮的疗效观察及其对血清 IL-4 的影响[J]. 光明中医，2013，28(9)：1830

许卫华，王微，吕冉，等. 大柴胡汤合茵陈蒿汤加减配合西药治疗急性胆源性胰腺炎的临床研究[J]. 环球中医药，2013，6(4)：249

Y

Ye J. Mechanisms of insulin resistance in obesity[J]. Frontiers of Medicine, 2013, 7(1): 14

严亚锋，白海侠. 消栓通络胶囊对急性脑缺血再灌注大鼠脑组织 TNF-α 和 IL-1β 水平的影响[J]. 西部中医药，2013，26(9)：23

杨浩鹏，李龙，柴程芝，等. 生脉注射液对小鼠局灶性脑缺血再灌注损伤后组织因子表达及相关信号通路的影响[J]. 中国实验方剂学杂志，2013，19(14)：194

杨亚勤，孙冰，李闯，等. 穴位注射加金匮肾气丸治疗老年支气管哮喘疗效分析[J]. 实用药物与临床，2013，16(7)：631

杨艳芳，刁晓娣，赵蕴芝，等. 茵陈蒿汤治疗妊娠期肝内胆汁淤积症 30 例临床分析[J]. 新中医，2013，45(2)：71

游捷,赵慧,谭翔文,等.肺积方抑制 Lewis 肺癌肿瘤生长及其抗移植瘤血管生成的实验研究[J].上海中医药大学学报,2013,27(2):61

于晨媛.茵陈蒿汤加味联合西药治疗慢性丙型肝炎 65 例[J].西部中医药,2013,26(9):82

郁保生,张国山,石晓理,等.小柴胡汤对功能性消化不良大鼠血管活性肠肽、胃排空及小肠推进率的影响[J].中国实验方剂学杂志,2013,19(8):251

原红霞,郑靖婕,闫艳.小柴胡汤不同萃取部位抗抑郁作用筛选[J].中国实验方剂学杂志,2013,19(15):211

Z

Zheng XY, Zhu SY, Chang SF, et al. Protective effects of chronic resveratrol treatment on vascular inflammatory injury in streptozotocin-induced type 2 diabetic rats: Role of NF - kappa B signaling [J]. European Journal of Pharmacology, 2013, 720 (1—3): 147

Zhang ZF, Lu J, Zheng YL, et al. Purple sweet potato color attenuates hepatic insulin resistance via blocking oxidative stress and endoplasmic reticulum stress in high-fat-diet-treated mice[J]. Journal of Nutritional Biochemistry, 2013, 24(6): 1008

张波,李玲,卢芳国,等.麻杏石甘汤对流感病毒感染小鼠肺部炎症与神经氨酸酶活性影响的研究[J].中华中医药杂志,2013,28(4):1094

张宏方,吴芳,环诚,等.调衡方对 Lewis 肺癌细胞增殖及 JAK - STAT 信号通路的影响[J].辽宁中医药大学学报,2013,15(3):16

张慧芹,蔡华丹,杨美娟,等.茵陈蒿汤水提物和乙醇提物对 D-氨基半乳糖胺诱导大鼠急性肝损伤保护作用的比较研究[J].北京中医药大学学报,2013,36(2):113

张建荣,潘强,柏江锋,等.复方桂枝茯苓丸对脑缺血再灌注损伤大鼠 TNF - α,ET 的影响[J].中国中医急症,2013,22(11):1841

张晓双,孙建宁,宋延平,等.复方乌骨藤胶囊对 Lewis 肺癌小鼠 TNF - α,NK 活性的影响[J].中国实验方剂学杂志,2013,19(6):220

郑咏秋,刘建勋,徐立,等.维脑康及银杏总内酯对局灶性脑缺血再灌注自噬和神经发生作用研究[J].中国中药杂志,2013,38(13):2182

郑咏秋,姚明江,刘建勋,等.华佗再造浸膏对大鼠局灶性脑缺血/再灌注血脑屏障损伤的保护作用及机制研究[J].中国中药杂志,2013,38(4):585

周密思,陈军,黄海,等.小柴胡汤对黑素瘤细胞酪氨酸酶活性及黑素合成的影响[J].时珍国医国药,2013,24(2):402

周赛男,蔺晓源,郭乐,等.补阳还五汤对局灶性脑缺血大鼠 TLR4 表达的影响[J].中药新药与临床药理,2013,24(1):18

周绍荣,薛慈民.甲瘤方治疗气滞痰凝型良性甲状腺结节临床观察[J].辽宁中医杂志,2013,40(11):2255

周仕轶,于军桥,邵继春,等.金匮肾气丸对颌下腺切除大鼠生精调控的作用及机理研究[J].中药新药与临床药理,2013,24(1):21

周昕欣,金龙,吴晓兰.加味四君子汤含药血清对 B16 恶性黑色素瘤细胞 NF - κB(p65)活性和表达的影响[J].中药药理与临床,2013,29(6):121

周昕欣,王彩霞.加味四君子汤含药血清对 B16 恶性黑色素瘤细胞侵袭和 MMP2、MMP9 表达的影响[J].中药药理与临床,2013,29(1):108

周昕欣,王彩霞.加味四君子汤含药血清对 B16 恶性黑色素瘤细胞增殖和凋亡的影响[J].中国实验方剂学杂志,2013,19(10):178

周兴华,钟振东,钟森,等.加味茵陈蒿汤对肝损伤大鼠 TLR4 mRNA 及其蛋白表达的影响[J].中国实验方剂学杂志,2013,19(15):239

周燕萍,杨航,关江峰,等.5 种不同治法中药对人肺癌 A549 细胞增殖的影响[J].成都中医药大学学报,2013,36(3):15

朱丽,高健,吴传鸿,等.益气解毒方对大鼠局灶性脑缺血氧化应激的影响[J].中国实验方剂学杂志,2013,19(6):171

左文标,杜安业,周传礼,等.调肝泻火法对糖尿病颈动脉硬化患者胰岛素抵抗的影响[J].现代中西医结合杂志,2013,22(28):3103

四、养生保健

【概述】

2013年，中医养生与保健的内容主要集中在几个热点问题上，即对传统养生知识的探讨、亚健康的中医证候及临床防治、治未病的探索、药膳食疗以及延缓衰老等。

1. 基础理论的研究

基础理论的研究主要集中在两个方面，一是在对古代名家及古籍养生思想的研究，二是对养生内涵的研究。前者详见“古代医家养生思想研究”专条。

章德林等研究认为，近现代时期，儒、道、佛各家调息静坐养生在日益社会化世俗化的过程中，呈现出三家圆融整合、各自发挥、各取所需的趋势，医家更是开放包容，兼收并蓄，加之日本调息静坐养生的影响，调息静坐养生著作通俗易懂，方法简便实用，适应社会各阶层养生需求。郭岚等对传统养生九大学术流派进行探讨，认为各大流派在顺应、养性、动形、静神、温补、培元、调气、药饵、食养等方面各有所长。龚鹏等从养生学最能体现中医之道、中医养生学有丰富的实践内容以及立道施术、养生活动的医疗化三个方面来探讨中医养生的道与术。孙晓生等对中医养生学与环境医学的异同进行探讨，分析环境与健康的内在关系，旨在促进中医养生学与现代医学的有机结合，促进人类预防疾病，提高人体健康水平。李董男认为中国传统养生以整体论指导养生实践，重视人类与环境生态和谐相处、形体与道德情志的融合、人与社会的适应。其基本原则是顺应自然、形神合一、动静结合、三因制宜。中国传统养生强调“中正平和”，而在宏观层面上的目标是“天人合一”。

2. 亚健康状态的防治

亚健康状态的研究主要包括体质、证候及临床防治等内容，前者详见“亚健康状态的基础研究”专条。防治主要包括临床研究和实验研究两个方面。

崔骥等辨证筛选大学生亚健康状态气虚型、血虚型、阴虚型、气郁型各20例，分别予四君子汤、四物汤、六味地黄汤、柴胡疏肝散干预2周，检测中药干预前后脉图指标变化。结果，气虚组中，中药干预后 h_1、S、As、Ad 值显著增高（$P<0.05$），h_5/h_1 值显著降低（$P<0.05$）；血虚组中，中药干预后 h_1、S、As、Ad 值与中药干预前相比显著增高（$P<0.05$）；阴虚组及气郁组中，中药干预后 h_1、h_5、S、As、Ad 值与中药干预前相比均显著增高（$P<0.05$）。黄璜等对60名亚健康脑疲劳护士随机均分为两组，对照组给予生活方式健康宣教，观察组在此基础上给予宁神益智方（酸枣仁、石菖蒲、益智仁、丹参、百合、人参等）。治疗2周后，观察组总有效率为93.3%(28/30)，对照组为40.0%(12/30)，组间比较，$P<0.01$。干预后观察组亚健康各维度评分均高于对照组（$P<0.01$），脑疲劳评分低于对照组（$P<0.01$）。

刘艳艳等研究发现，疲劳型亚健康状态下小鼠存在免疫功能异常的情况，维康颗粒（熟地黄、淮山药、党参、山萸肉、黄精、陈皮）可通过改善模型小鼠的免疫功能，促进疲劳型亚健康状态向正常状态转化。

3. 治未病的探索

“治未病”一直是中医养生关注的热点，主要集中在理论研究和临床运用两个方面。后者对临床疾病的指导主要体现在未病先防、既病防变和已愈防复三个方面。

李雨彦等对2002～2011年10年国内发表的文献进行计量学分析，结果显示，对“治未病”研究的文献整体逐年增多，其文献量、文献被引频次、文献的研究层次、文献研究所涉及的学科领域以及有关机构对“治未病”研究的支持都有不同程度的提高。但各机构对“治未病”研究的支持力度有待提升。林丽丽等提出阴阳学说在中医“治未病”中的应用主要体现在顺四时阴阳而养生防病和维护阴阳平衡是治未病的关键，五行学说在中医“治未病”中的应用体现在五行生克乘侮与治未病和辨五行归属而推断病情两方面。

倪红梅等探讨治未病思想与中医健康管理模式，提出“多环节切入＋状态调整＋线性干预”的中医健康管理新模式。王文华等从中医学“治未病”理论的国外声誉、中国治未病健康工程的实施现状、中国治未病发展现状、“治未病”健康管理需要信息资源管理及共享平台的支持、中医药学参与健康管理存在的基本问题等五个方面探讨中医治未病健康管理的现状。何福乐等探讨治未病理论对中医养生体系构建及其产业发展的启示。前者包括强调精、气、神的作用、阐明寿夭论和衰老论、重视治未病理念；后者包括顺应天时、饮食调养、生活节制、调节情志、适量运动以及初病调理。

4. 饮食与养生

食疗是养生的重要内容。李应存等将敦煌医学宝藏中部分与养生食疗有关的内容进行释要，以揭示敦煌医学与《千金方》在养生食疗上的联系。马慧玲等通过查阅大量文献资料，发现蒲公英具多种药理活性以及药膳养生堂存在的巨大价值。梁飞等探讨“服食”养生术对中医本草学、方剂学、治疗学、养生学的影响，认为服食养生对于中医养生学最直接的贡献仍然是饮食养生。于少泓打破固有的思维定势，结合老年人的体质，从药膳食疗方面，探讨“以通为补”的养生方式。

段园园等分析中药降血糖保健食品配方特点，发现84.4%的辅助降血糖保健食品配方中含有中药类原料，使用频数在前15位的依次为黄芪、桑叶、葛根、山药、枸杞子、人参、西洋参、玉竹、银杏叶、麦冬、地黄、知母、黄精、女贞子，与中医药理论治疗消渴病的益气滋阴、清热生津指导原则相符。其他原料中蜂胶、苦瓜、吡啶甲酸铬、南瓜、茶叶、苦荞麦应用比例较高，现代药理研究均具有明确的降糖作用。剂型方面，胶囊剂占65.7%，超过总剂型的半数以上，其中硬胶囊占53.4%、软胶囊占12.3%。其次为片剂(占12.9%)，茶剂、口服液、颗粒剂等占有相对较少的比例。

5. 延缓衰老与养生

延缓衰老的研究一直是中医养生学探讨的热点，主要集中在动物实验方面，具体详见“延缓衰老方药的实验研究”。

基础研究方面，王小平探讨《内经》对衰老的认识。《内经》认为衰老是生命的必然过程，主要与先天禀赋、后天调养及生存环境等因素有关。就其发生机制，有精气神虚衰说、阴阳失调说、脏气虚衰说、气血失和说等观点。王罂滢等对敦煌医学抗衰老方剂的文献进行药理、治法、临床价值研究，提出三点不足：① 对方剂的药理与治法在中医学史上的源流演化梳理不够，对其依据、发展与价值还缺乏全面、充分、深入的论证；② 临床价值研究主要集中于敦煌长寿方、敦煌韦慈方、敦煌面脂方、敦煌大宝胶囊等少数几个方剂，全面、系统的研究尚有待进一步展开；③ 对敦煌医学抗衰老方剂的开发应用研究十分薄弱，成果罕见，亟待加强。冀小伟等总结了中医学对衰老的认识和机理，包括肾虚与衰老、脾虚与衰老、精血津液虚与衰老、痰瘀夹杂与衰老等。

（熊　俊）

【古代医家养生思想研究】

王明强认为“啬”是老子修身养性学说的核心词汇，其本义是将谷物收藏于仓库之中，老子则引申指收敛心神，以此获得“长生久视”。而以“啬”养神之道则在于道家所言“虚静”二字，要做到虚静，就要归根、知常、食母，即持守大道，顺道而行。龚钰清等总结《内经》的养生理论在于强调预防胜于治疗，养生重于治病；强调精神对于养生的重要性、“天人相应”以及人体正气的重要性。养生原则为顺应自然，协调阴阳；远离病邪，防病抗衰；养肾调脾，补精益气；形神共养，动静结合。养生的特色方法有饮食养生、针刺养生、药物养生、起居养生、运动养生以及情志养生。陈明霞等从强调养生以不伤为本，重视饮食起居摄生；提出养生应防微杜渐，详述齿、发、面保健；重视因人制宜原则，倡导辨证养生防病三方面探讨《济阳纲目》中体现的武之望的养生保健思想。李应存研究东汉陇上道医封君达的养生思想，包括爱啬精气，注重房室养生；服用黄精，重视药物保健；减少欲望，防止过劳致虚；食饮有节，去肥浓节酸咸；情志畅达，减思虑损喜怒；顺应四时，春夏泻秋冬藏等方面。李尾咕认为朱熹的养生思想兼具儒、佛、道养生之精华。一生追求简朴的生活方式，坚持存理灭欲，与自然、社会和谐相处，尤其对泉石之美亲近无隙，乐而忘忧。在养心上主张静养为主，动静相宜，揭示了养生动静观的真谛。提倡素食养生、食疗养生等科学的生活方式，并主张加强道德修养，达到内外兼修的目的，诠释了生命延续的本然。蔺焕萍总结清代沈金鳌的养生思想，包括养生重在保精，养生方法注重寡欲、节劳、炼精、饮食、情志、药物、气功等的调摄。曲卫玲等从《老老恒言》探讨老年养生之精要，尤以养静、调脾胃为主，认为“养静为摄生要务”，并从睡眠、昼卧、夜坐等方面来说明养静的理论与方法；注重调养脾胃，尤其在“夏至以后，秋分以前，外则暑阳渐炽，内则微阴初生，最当调停脾胃，勿进肥浓”。

王小芸等总结傅山的食疗养生思想为平衡膳食，营养均衡；饮食有节，三因制宜；调整阴阳，顾护中州。薛芳芸等探讨苏轼“安”与“和”的养生观，告诉人们只有保持内心的宁静与安详，顺应外界事物的变化，保持生理心理与自然社会的和谐，才能泰然处世，颐养天年。另外，从《东坡养生集》中探讨苏东坡的饮食养生观。第一，科学合理的饮食养生观。表现在节制饮食，宽胃养气；素食菜梗，利于健康；节俭饮食，惜福延年。第二，简便易行的食疗养生法。如生姜健脾散寒助阳气，蜂蜜滋补润燥且美容，茶叶除烦去腻怡性情。第三，颇有效验的药疗养生法。如茯苓胡麻延年有奇效，枸杞菊花补精又益气，松脂驻颜乌髯又固齿。孙晓生等从饮食物的选择、因时择食、提倡温食、饮食适量、茶酒饮用方法、营造良好进食环境以及饭后养生方法等方面探讨明代吴正伦《养生类要》中的饮食养生思想。

（熊　俊）

【亚健康状态的基础研究】

支英豪等将413例亚健康失眠患者辨证分为心脾两虚和阴虚火旺型，筛选出对区分2类中医证型有显著贡献的10个变量：目赤、口苦、心烦懊恼、耳鸣、口干咽燥、盗汗、神疲体倦、面色少华、腰膝酸软和小便黄。建立亚健康失眠中医证型预测模型的一致率为81.8%。曲淼等研究发现，心系亚健康状态以疲乏、眼睛不适、健忘、烦躁、头脑昏沉、怕冷、早醒、难以入睡、容易出汗表现的程度较重，不同性别、年龄段、学历、职业表现的症状有差异，多表现为心脾两虚证候、心气虚证候及心阳虚证候。万生芳调查发现，男女性亚健康比例分别为70.22%和67.89%，男性41～45岁组亚健康比例最高，女性46～50岁组亚健康比例最高。亚健康人群与总人群比较，平和体质比例显著下降，亚健康人群男性痰湿体质、女性阳虚体质比例较总人群显著升高，其他偏颇体质比例不同程度上升。于春泉等对3 568例亚健康状态证候分析及证候诊断分类，运用多类逐步判别分析模型建立亚健康状态常见证候的判别函数，得出相关疾病的判别模型。常见证候诊断参考标准的判别模型分析，经过数据库的同类拆分，分为心系类、肝系类、脾系类、肾系类及兼证类证候共计8大类，经判别模型分析建立了心气虚证、心肝血虚证、肝气郁结证、肝肾阴虚证、肾阴虚证、脾气虚证、脾肾阳虚证、肺气虚证等24类证候的判别分析模型。郭丽娜研究发现，亚健康阳虚质疲劳状态人群中以18～34岁年龄段、高学历、脑力劳动者为高发人群，而缺乏体育锻炼、上下班交通拥挤、过度劳累是亚健康阳虚质疲劳状态产生的重要诱因，因此在对这一类人群进行健康指导时，应重视生活方式和心理方面。

于冰琰等分析大学生亚健康状态与中医气虚质的关系与体质特征。研究表明，医科院校学生亚健康总体现患率为62.5%，女性现患率高于男性（$P<0.05$）。气虚质的亚健康大学生分布，女生明显高于男生（$P<0.05$）。其除具有气虚质的表现外，还兼夹了血瘀、气郁、痰湿等症状。亚健康大学生在心理、社会症状方面表现比较突出。黄平等研究发现临床科室的一线护士以平和质居多，而亚健康人群和疾病人群以气虚质、气郁质、血瘀质居多，其各种偏颇体质的分布和所占比例基本相同，提示在护理人员群体中，健康人以平和体质为主，在健康人向亚健康转化的过程中，其中医体质发生了转变。胡晓灵等调查乌鲁木齐市亚健康人群分布情况及其中医证候特点。发现在2 550例被调查者中亚健康状态者2 026例（79.45%）。亚健康人群前10种症状为疲倦、目涩、头晕、心悸、咽干、胸闷、气短、失眠多梦、四肢困重、情志抑郁易怒。中医证候分布由高到低为：肝肾阴虚证、心脾两虚证、肝郁化火证、肝气郁结证、肝脾虚证、脾虚湿阻证、肺脾气虚证、痰热内扰证。女性以肝肾阴虚证及肝气郁结证多见，男性以肝肾阴虚证、心脾两虚证为主。汉族以肝肾阴虚、心脾两虚为主，少数民族以肝肾阴虚、脾虚湿阻、痰热内扰为主。肝肾阴虚证多集中在40～49岁。各证型在年龄、性别、民族方面差异均有统计学意义（$P<0.05$）。

薛晓琳等对疲劳性亚健康进行了中医药物和非药物干预研究，在此基础上提出亚健康中医临床干预研究中的几个关键环节。① 研究类型应根据研究目的、研究对象、干预方法及可行性等情况而确定。② 受试对象选择标准主要包括对亚健康状态的判定、对主症"疲劳"进行时间上和程度上的界定以及证候的准确辨识。③ 疗效评价指标体系从确定主要评价指标、次要评价指标、尽可能地避免非干预措施带来的影响以及多个评价时点的设立等方面进行确定。④ 通过保证受试者的知情权、注重随访及与受试者的有效沟通来增强受试人群的依从性。李乃民等探讨"未病"与"亚健康"之间的关系,认为未病学是中国中医学博大精神理论体系在人类健康与疾病观、病证防治观、社会人文观等方面的核心表述,内容丰富,涉及面广,有自身精确的认知检测理论与方法,以及有效的辨证施治手段,而亚健康仅说明在现代医学诊断模式之外还存在着不健康人群。王泓午等提出中医健康状态精辨识理论框架包括精充足辨识和精不足辨识 2 个类别,每个类别含有形象、窍象、神志象、舌象、脉象五个方面内容。

(胡　菲)

【延缓衰老方药的实验研究】

袁淑莘等将 90 只小鼠随机均分为正常组、模型组、阳性对照组、补益营卫高中低剂量组,观察补益营卫方(人参、甘草等)对 D-半乳糖衰老小鼠模型过氧化氢酶(CAT)、谷胱甘肽过氧化物酶(GSH-Px)活性以及白介素-2(IL-2)、干扰素-r(IFN-r)的影响。结果,与模型组相比,补益营卫方能够提升小鼠血清中 CAT、GSH-Px 和匀浆中 CAT 活性,高剂量组提升显著($P<0.05$)。高、低剂量组 IL-2、IFN-r 的水平显著升高(均$P<0.01$)。徐纪平等将 48 只雄性 SD 大鼠随机均分为游泳对照组和杞藿饮(刺五加、枸杞子、淫羊藿、马齿苋、红景天、肉苁蓉等)高、中、低剂量组,观察杞藿饮对力竭游泳大鼠肝细胞衰老及其超微结构的影响。结果表明,高、中、低浓度杞藿饮组血清 NO、谷丙转氨酶(ALT)、谷草转氨酶(AST)水平与游泳对照组比较均明显降低(均$P<0.05$),高、中浓度杞藿饮组血清 NO、ALT、AST 水平与低浓度组比较降低更明显(均$P<0.05$)。3 个杞藿饮组肝细胞 H_2A 磷酸化阳性细胞数均明显少于游泳对照组(均$P<0.05$),肝细胞超微结构表明损伤程度明显轻于游泳对照组,且与浓度增加呈正相关。刘慧兰等将 80 只老化小鼠均分为对照组、模型组、红芪水提液浓缩液(HRCF)组,观察 HRCF 组对快速老化小鼠学习记忆能力的改善作用和对脑组织内单胺类神经递质的影响。结果,模型组快速老化小鼠隐蔽平台的逃避潜伏期明显延长,脑组织中去甲肾上腺素(NE)、多巴胺(DA)、5-羟色胺(5-HT)及 5-羟吲哚乙酸(5-HIAA)含量显著降低($P<0.01$)。与模型组比较,HRCF 组小鼠隐蔽平台的逃避潜伏期明显缩短,脑组织中 NE、DA、5-HT 及 5-HIAA 含量明显增加,$P<0.05$ 或$P<0.01$。宋庆亮等采用 3β-HSD 特异性染色鉴定体外培养的大鼠睾丸 Leydig 细胞,分为正常组、Leydig 细胞衰老损伤组、何首乌饮(何首乌、肉苁蓉、怀牛膝、淫羊藿、丹参、茯苓)预防组和何首乌饮治疗组,观察何首乌饮对 Leydig 细胞衰老模型 β-半乳糖苷酶表达的影响。结果,与正常组比较,衰老组 Leydig 细胞 β-半乳糖苷酶的表达明显升高($P<0.05$)。与衰老组比较,何首乌饮预防组、治疗组 Leydig 细胞 β-半乳糖苷酶的表达明显降低($P<0.05$)。何首乌饮治疗组与预防组 Leydig 细胞 β-半乳糖苷酶的表达比较($P>0.05$)。

王晓宁等研究表明,自然衰老大鼠学习记忆和空间识别能力减弱,还脑益聪颗粒剂(制首乌、人参、石菖蒲、黄连、川芎)可改善自然衰老大鼠 AD 模型的学习记忆功能,可保护脑组织海马结构,提高血清及组织中抗氧化能力和总抗氧化能力的活性,减少 β-淀粉样蛋白的生成。史爱武等研究发现,高浓度补肾抗衰汤(菟丝子、黄精、熟地黄、紫石英、肉苁蓉、巴戟天等)干预可以显著延长 N_2、daf-2、daf-16 型突变体线虫的寿命($P<0.01$),增加 daf-16 型的基因表达并降低 daf-2 的基因表达。谢艳华等研究发现,倒卵叶五加及复方佳蓉片可以上调 D-半乳糖致亚急性衰老大鼠睾丸间质细胞中的 Bcl-2 蛋白的表达和下调 Bax 蛋白的表达,从而抑制睾丸间质细胞的凋亡,对抗D-半乳糖引起组织细胞的衰老。郑世铎等研究表明,抗衰益智胶囊(熟地黄、枸杞子、黄芪、肉苁蓉、胆南星、麝香等)治疗组大鼠脑组织内乙酰胆碱酯酶活性降低,胆碱乙酰转移酶活性升高,NE、DA、5-HT 含量增高,与模型组比较,均$P<0.05$。刘焕兰等研究发现,琼玉口服液能明显提高衰老小鼠脑组织超氧化物歧化酶活性和降低血清丙二醛含量,提高机体防御自由基的损害能力,增强脏器指数,具有抗脂质过氧化物的作用。陈旭研究认为,益气养阴中药复方(白人参、麦冬、枸杞子、茯苓、何首乌、九节菖蒲等)能通过下调衰老细胞 P_{16}基因的表达来延缓细胞衰老,并且具备优于维生素 E 的抗衰老作用。石少慧等研究发现,

六味地黄汤可通过抑制肾脏 Caspase-3 表达及活性，延缓衰老。张明明等研究发现，何首乌饮方剂能延缓衰老大鼠卵巢细胞凋亡的发生，其机制可能是通过干预凋亡相关基因 FOX、SIRTI 及c-Myc 蛋白表达抑制卵巢细胞的凋亡。

（肖梅华）

［附］ 参 考 文 献

C

陈明霞，冷伟. 浅析《济阳纲目》养生保健思想[J]. 陕西中医学院学报，2013，36(2)：19

陈旭. 益气养阴组方对细胞衰老干预作用及其机理的实验研究[J]. 长春中医药大学学报，2013，29(2)：196

崔骥，许家佗，邸智，等. 大学生亚健康状态中药干预前后脉图分析[J]. 中华中医药杂志，2013，28(5)：1564

D

段园园，黄月纯，魏刚，等. 中药降血糖保健食品配方特点分析[J]. 陕西中医学院学报，2013，36(4)：110

G

龚鹏，江岩. 中医养生的道与术[J]. 河南中医，2013，33(4)：546

龚钰清，盛国光. 论《黄帝内经》之养生观[J]. 贵阳中医学院学报，2013，35(2)：1

郭岚，王平. 中华传统养生九大学术流派探析[J]. 中国中医基础医学杂志，2013，19(6)：699

郭丽娜，林淑娴，潘爱娣，等. 亚健康阳虚质疲劳状态人群健康指导探讨[J]. 辽宁中医药大学学报，2013，15(1)：99

H

何富乐，胡美兰. 治未病理论对中医养生体系构建及其产业发展的启示[J]. 中华中医药学刊，2013，31(7)：1598

胡晓灵，付玲，杜少华，等. 乌鲁木齐市亚健康人群 2026 例中医证候分析[J]. 中医杂志，2013，54(3)：231

黄璜，吴敏，王颖，等. 宁神益智方治疗护士亚健康脑疲劳的临床疗效观察[J]. 护理学报，2013，20(11A)：64

黄平，罗仁，谭永法. 临床护士亚健康状态与中医体质关系调查分析[J]. 护士进修杂志，2013，28(6)：507

J

冀小伟，张连城. 中医对衰老的认识[J]. 中医杂志，2013，54(17)：1527

L

李董男. 试论中国传统养生的原则和目标[J]. 北京中医药大学学报，2013，36(4)：227

李乃民，张永丰，刘珊，等. 有关"未病"与"亚健康"关系探析[J]. 亚太传统医药，2013，9(11)：51

李尾咕. 朱熹的养生思想与实践[J]. 湖州师范学院学报，2013，35(1)：58

李应存. 东汉陇上著名道医封君达养生精华探析[J]. 西部中医药，2013，26(4)：34

李应存，柳长华. 敦煌医学卷子中与《千金方》有关的养生食疗内容释要[J]. 西部中医药，2013，26(3)：36

李雨彦，彭立生. "治未病"研究的文献计量学分析[J]. 辽宁中医药大学学报，2013，15(9)：157

梁飞，张瑞贤，李健，等. 谈"服食"养生术对中医学的影响[J]. 中国中医基础医学杂志，2013，19(4)：390

林丽丽，何文彬. 试论阴阳五行学说在中医"治未病"中应用[J]. 辽宁中医药大学学报，2013，15(6)：134

蔺焕萍，马新红.《沈氏尊生书》养生思想浅析[J]. 河南中医，2013，33(9)：1418

刘焕兰，武夏林，曲卫玲，等. 琼玉口服液对衰老小鼠脑组织 SOD 活性及血清中 SOD 和 MDA 含量的影响[J]. 吉林中医药，2013，33(3)：278

刘慧兰，张俊英，卫东锋. 红芪水提浓缩液对快速老化小鼠学习记忆和单胺类神经递质的影响[J]. 中国中医药信息杂志，2013，20(8)：36

刘艳艳，孙晓敏，欧阳明子，等. 维康颗粒对疲劳型亚健康小鼠免疫功能影响的实验研究[J]. 江苏中医药，2013，45(5)：73

M

马慧玲，吴丽雅，张华豪. 建立蒲公英药膳养生堂的探讨[J]. 中国中医药现代远程教育，2013，11(14)：97

N

倪红梅，程羽，郭盈盈，等. 治未病思想与中医健康管理模式研究探索[J]. 南京中医药大学学报(社会科学版)，2013，14(1)：16

Q

曲淼，张明雪，何丽云. 中医心系亚健康状态调查研究[J]. 中国中医基础医学杂志，2013，19(3)：324

曲卫玲，刘焕兰. 从《老老恒言》探讨老年养生之精要[J]. 环球中医药，2013，6(11)：829

S

石少慧,王怀颖,张晶晶,等.六味地黄汤对衰老小鼠肾脏 Caspase-3 表达及活性的影响[J].中国老年学杂志,2013,33(2):349

史爱武,陆勤,侯莉莉,等.补肾抗衰汤影响秀丽隐杆线虫衰老的机制研究[J].辽宁中医杂志,2013,40(1):52

宋庆亮,郭银,周蕾,等.何首乌饮对 Leydig 细胞衰老模型β-半乳糖苷酶表达的影响[J].承德医学院学报,2013,30(2):106

孙晓生,陈晔.中医养生学与环境医学异同的探讨[J].新中医,2013,45(1):201

孙晓生,米菲菲.《养生类要》的饮食养生思想研究[J].新中医,2013,45(4):218

W

万生芳.亚健康状态人群中医体质特点分析[J].中国中医药科技,2013,20(2):106

王泓午,于春泉,陆小左,等.论中医健康状态精辨识理论框架的构建[J].世界中医药,2013,8(1):5

王明强.《老子》"啬"释及其养生意蕴[J].中国中医基础医学杂志,2013,19(4):362

王文华,刘洪宇,张美英,等.中医治未病健康管理的现状[J].天津中医药,2013,30(4):254

王小平.《内经》关于衰老的认识探析[J].山东中医杂志,2013,32(3):75

王小芸,赵怀舟,王象礼.傅山食疗养生思想初探[J].中国中医基础医学杂志,2013,19(4):373

王晓宁,刘剑刚,刘美霞,等.还脑益聪方对老龄认知障碍大鼠氧化应激和抗衰老指标作用的研究[J].北京中医药,2013,32(11):820

王瑿滢,王玉珠.敦煌医学抗衰老方剂研究概况[J].西部中医药,2013,26(4):30

X

谢艳华,杨倩,周暄宣,等.倒卵叶五加及复方佳蓉片对衰老大鼠睾丸间质细胞 Bcl-2、Bax 的作用[J].陕西中医,2013,34(9):1257

徐纪平,刘保海,孙金山,等.杞藿饮对力竭游泳大鼠肝细胞衰老及其超微结构的影响[J].海军医学杂志,2013,34(2):76

薛芳芸.苏轼"安"与"和"养生观的启示[J].北京中医药大学学报,2013,36(2):83

薛芳芸,许鑫.《东坡养生集》中饮食养生观探析[J].时珍国医国药,2013,24(3):704

薛晓琳,王天芳,林殷.亚健康中医干预研究中的几个关键环节[J].北京中医药大学学报(中医临床版),2013,20(6):1

Y

于冰琰,毕建璐,陈晶,等.大学生亚健康状态与气虚质关系的调查分析[J].时珍国医国药,2013,24(8):1966

于春泉,岳振松,孟静岩,等.基于可拓理论建立亚健康的诊断信息智能化处理模型研究[J].天津中医药,2013,30(9):566

于少泓.药膳食疗中"以通为补"的老年人养生方式[J].山东中医杂志,2013,32(9):645

袁淑苹,马生吉,周小平.补益营卫方对 D-半乳糖衰老模型抗氧化酶及免疫因子的影响[J].时珍国医国药,2013,24(2):259

Z

张明明,贾晓梅,王超,等.何首乌饮对衰老大鼠卵巢组织凋亡相关蛋白 FOX、SIRTI 和 c-Myc 的调节作用[J].医学动物防制,2013,29(12):1368

章德林,蒋力生,沈澍农.近现代调息静坐养生传承演变要略[J].江西中医学院学报,2013,25(1):14

郑世铎,徐海荣,段永强,等.抗衰益智胶囊对衰老大鼠脑组织胆碱神经递质及单胺类神经递质的影响[J].中国中医药信息杂志,2013,20(7):33

支英豪,胡万华,陈克龙,等.亚健康失眠中医证型的 Logistic 回归分析及预测模型的建立[J].中华中医药杂志,2013,28(10):2991

五、医史文献

(一) 古籍文献

【概述】

2013年古籍文献方面发表的论文涉及文字训诂、古籍校勘、文献考证等方面，其中有国家中医药管理局“中医药古籍保护与利用能力建设”项目的初步成果。

1. 文字训诂

金栋等考证指出，《素问·生气通天论》“汗出偏沮，使人偏枯”句之“沮”，当为“袒”字之讹，形似传抄致讹。偏沮，当为“偏袒”，即脱掉衣服，露出半身。袒，脱衣袒露。“汗出偏沮（袒），使人偏枯”，指大汗出后若脱衣袒露半身，容易感受风邪，（日久）使人偏枯——半身不遂。《素问》认为，偏枯，为风邪所中，是由于“汗出受风”而罹患，即由于人体正气不足，卫阳不固，汗出则腠理疏松，风邪乘虚而入，侵入人体半身深部，导致经络营卫气血不畅，肢体筋脉失于濡养，发为偏枯。汉唐宋以前医家多遵之，金元以后则多质疑之，而今之中风病，则非中风所致。

沈成等认为，因《素问》“男女对举”行文惯例，由“女子不月”可知“不得隐曲”应特指男性。另外，从文理来看，“隐”通“檃”，“隐曲”即“檃曲”，意为“使曲为直”。而在《素问》的语境中，所谓“使曲为直”，即使下垂的阴茎勃起。有关隐曲的疾病，即为男子性功能障碍——阳痿。

袁开惠等认为，“善溹”描述肝脉外证，语出《难经·十五难》。“善”作多、易解，“溹”言汗出，“善溹”当作“容易汗出”解。医书也见“溹溹”一词。“溹溹”为“溹”之重言，意思也由水洗义引申而来表示杯中水尽，点滴而下。《金匮要略》有“覆杯溹溹”一词描述脾死脉。此语正是对《内经·平人气象论》中“水之流（溜），屋之漏”的提炼与解读。

2. 古籍校勘

严泽等认为，《博物志》中“虽食者，百病妖邪钟焉”之“虽食”当为“杂食”；《备急千金要方》《医心方》及《太平御览》中“食不欲杂，杂则或有所犯”的论述出自西晋名医王叔和；《太平御览》所载《养生论》的作者高湛当为东晋的张湛，《养生论》实为《养生要集》之误。

董立业等提出，宋人在《新校〈备急千金要方〉序》提及，校补《千金要方》时曾参照《素问》《九墟》《灵枢》《甲乙》《外台秘要》及诸家本草、前古脉书等，“凡所派别，无不考理，互相质证，反复稽参，然后遗文疑义，焕然悉明。”从中亦可看出，宋人是以用字的规范化，以内容的完整性、条理化、系统化为原则，对《千金要方》的医论部分进行了全面整理。其中他们对《素问》的补充，并以之填充《千金要方》原书的做法，不仅显示出北宋校正医书局对《素问》理论的完善与发展，而且体现出宋代医学注重求“理”循“道”的特点，这正是宋代理学“重理”的治学观念在医学领域的具体表现。

3. 文献考证

杨继红等介绍了现存古代中医文献的海外分布情况：在日本，古代中医文献主要分布在图书馆、公私文库、古寺庙等地；在美国，中文古籍藏于各大图书馆的东亚图书馆中；在俄罗斯，主要藏于俄罗斯科学院东方研究所的爱尔米塔日博物馆的中国敦煌黑城馆。

李柳骥等考证，《伤寒论句解》作者李文锦，字襄渑，号治庵、淑景堂主人，金陵（今南京）人，家住金陵天印山南的许村。大约生于康熙四十七年（1708），具体卒年不详，约在乾隆朝末期。李氏性豪迈，喜交游，医卜星相，诗词书画皆有涉猎，后专于医，著有《伤寒论句解》和《医家二十四则》。《伤寒论句解》包括《医圣张仲景伤寒杂病论淑景堂亲解》14卷和《思问集》7卷。前书为李氏注释发挥《伤寒论》之作，于1768年成书；后书又包含了《淑景堂改订注释寒热温平药性赋》4卷、《淑景堂奋医杂著》1卷、《医药箴言》1卷、《淑景堂医药集案》1卷，于1765年成书。

王旭光等考察吴崑著作版本，发现《医方考》6卷成于1584年；1594年撰成《素问吴注》24卷；1618年撰成《针方六集》6卷，由程标捐资刊刻。吴崑尚撰有《脉语》2卷，成书年代不详。《医方考》有明刊本、日本及朝鲜刊本、旧抄本、现代版本4类版本。《吴注素问》有明清刊本、日本刊本、旧抄本、影印本、现代版本5类版本。《针方六集》有明刊本、抄本、影印本及现代版本4类版本。《脉语》多与《医方考》合刊，除部分现代版本未附《脉语》之外，《脉语》的版本大致同于《医方考》。

张雪丹等介绍日本江户时期三部医学抄本：伊泽兰轩《兰轩外台方标记》、丹波元胤《药雅》、锦霞卜元学《医方漫录》，其中《兰轩外台方标记》以宋本《外台秘要方》为底本，以《素问》《灵枢》《伤寒论》《肘后方》《千金方》等10余种古籍为参校本，对宋本《外台方》作了详尽地校勘考证。《药雅》以《伤寒论》《金匮要略》中36种具有代表性的药物为主线，对这些药物及含有这些药物的药对、方剂作医理、药理的详细阐述。《医方漫录》采撷《伤寒》《金匮》至清代之名医方剂，不拘古今，不分和汉，兼收并蓄，故以“漫录”为名。方下标注出处，并详述其主治及方剂治法，方便实用。辑录医书70余种，其中日本医书20余种，所辑方剂以汉方为主，和方以私家医方为主。

高程熙等认为，《内经拾遗方论》或为明代刘浴德、朱练撰述《增补内经拾遗方论》时的托名著作，其底本可能是金代刘完素所著《黄帝素问宣明论方》一书前两卷。

王缙等指出，《外科百效全书》又名《新刻秘授外科百效全书》、《图像外科百效全书》，明末龚居中所著，现存版本15种，据卷帙多少分4卷本和6卷本两大系统。4卷本唯致和堂本一种，内容量与6卷本同。是本刻字规范，印刷清晰，部分书页或有缺字，但无阅读障碍。其余皆为6卷本，按版刻形制特点及相互关系，可再分3类：① 锄经园本和发祥本，二者结构、内容相似度极高，版本源流关系密切。② 以宏道堂本为代表之版本，包括宏道堂本、大文堂本、善成堂本等，是最庞杂的一类；但其分卷、卷首分卷语句类、内容缺失的位置且多为木刻，行款也大部分相同。③ 为明刻本与清刻本。明刻本藏于上海中医药大学图书馆，分元、亨、利、贞四册，是存世最早本，但内容缺损严重，且有后人配补现象，不堪作为底本。

李玉清认为，《中国本草全书》收录的《本草发明》，所据影印版本为中国中医科学院图书馆藏明刊本，为残本。除此版本外，《本草发明》另有上海图书馆藏明刊本及日本抄本，均为足本。上海图书馆藏明刊本与中国中医科学院图书馆藏明刊本实为同一版本，仅书中“明《本草》类辨”一文所在位置不同。日本抄本当为据明刊本抄成。

刘鹏发现，上世纪初裘吉生与金月笙分别刊刻发行《吴鞠通先生医案》(收于《续修四库全书》)。裘氏所刻为4卷本，据书中丙辰(1916)二月高汝贤序文所云，是本乃30年前高氏由胡氏处所得，惜未刊行，仅于友人中转相传钞，后裘吉生欲刊行《医药丛书》，高氏遂详加校雠，并付丛书收入以广其传。王妮认为，裘庆元辑编《罗谦甫治验案》所据的《卫生宝鉴》家藏抄本，与现在流行《卫生宝鉴》版本，不是同一系统的版本；薛清录《中国中医古籍总目》所载《罗谦甫治验案》长春抄本，实为巢念修辑编《卫生宝鉴》的另一部书，书名为《罗谦甫医案》；《中国中医古籍总目》记载的《罗谦甫治验案》绍兴医药学报社刻本和《医药丛书十一种》实为同一版本、同一印次书，属同书异名。

邓月娥认为，《孕育玄机》两个古籍版本均为抄本，清康熙乾尧抄本抄于清代康熙五十二年(1713)；清《陶氏贤奕书楼丛书》本约抄录于晚清时期或之后的民国期间。通过仔细对比发现，二者主体内容基本一致，仅前者的自序中内容有圈改，疑为后人所为；后者缮写比前者更加规范。可知2个古籍版本的文献来源相同，不排除“丛书本”抄自“乾抄本”之可能。

王涛等认为，《医宗宝镜》初刻于清嘉庆三年戊午(1798)，由凌云楼梓行，是为“清嘉庆三年戊午(1798)凌云楼刻本”；至清末先由上海蜚英书局据初刻本石印出版发行，之后由上海文瑞楼出版，即“清末上海蜚英书局石印本”、“民国上海锦章书局石印本”。该书是由多部前人医学著作内容组合而成，很可能出自书商或者书坊主之手。

另有新出土文献研究，可见专条。

(张如青　肖梅华)

【《黄帝内经》训诂学研究】

1. 文字训诂

王诚指出“卧出”一词见于汉代文献，意为睡觉、睡着。《素问·五藏生成篇》中"卧出"也是此义。朱鹏举结合《内经》中的描述，参考马王堆汉墓出土医书，认为"瘨疝"、"癞疝"、"颓疝"是同一病名的不同写法，指以男性前阴肿坠为主要表现的疾病，后世习作"癞疝"。"瘨癃"、"癃瘨"虽词序不同，但与"癞癃疝"一样，皆指疝之重症。狄碧云等认为《灵枢·经脉》"胆足少阳之脉……足外反热"，"热"字衍。党思捷等认为《内经》中的"搏"字有三种解释：① 指经脉、脉象及"相搏"，俱当作"搏"。② 指持脉的动作，作"索取"解。③ 作"至"解。傅海燕等分析了《内经》中"咽"类术语的含义，认为"咽"既表示水谷入胃的通道，也指咽部，偶指喉结。表示咽部，可以用"咽"、"嗌"、"咽嗌"、"咽喉"、"喉咽"。表示水谷入胃的通道，可以用"咽"与"咽路"。王宝华考证《灵枢》"守形"，认为将"守形"注为"粗守形者，守刺法也"有待商榷。"守形"其义指医生难以运用望诊及脉诊法，充分精确地了解患者病情，只能依照患者主诉进行局部治疗。陈中等指出《内经》"结络"从生理言是经筋联络，从病理言有经络的联络、络脉聚结、脉络郁结等义。王正山等认为，隋代萧吉《五行大义》乃隋以前研究阴阳五行集大成者，有 9 处《黄帝内经》引文，与今本《黄帝内经》略有不同，如五脏的阴阳属性、肝为罢极之本、脾为仓廪之本等。萧吉对所引《黄帝内经》之文，多从阴阳五行的角度加以解释，与后世注有所不同。律正严等认为《素问·上古天真论》"幼而徇齐"，当释为幼年学习顺应中正的做人道理。

2. 校勘方法

狄碧云等提出研究《灵枢经》异文有助于正讹、训释、揭示医理、校释他书文字，认为目前该研究存在失引、误引、误勘、错误分析类别等问题。符箴认为清儒在《内经》校勘中运用"揭示同源通用"、"单纯系源以加深理解"及"解决依音借用字"三种音训方法以探求词的语源关系，并通过语音线索解决借字造成的阅读障碍。阴小爱等认为，林亿等综合使用了对校、本校、他校、理校等方法，且本校中据原文、注文、文例作校，他校中以同时代医学、文史类文献及其他书作校，理校中据文理、医理作校。王丽考察了《太平御览》引用《素问》文字共 11 条，能确定者 10 条，其中，"地气上为寒"应不是引自《素问》通行本，"又天气下而为雨"亦未见于此，疑《太平御览》所引为《素问》另一版本。

（李海峰）

【中医文献研究方法研究】

张凯等采用频繁集与关联规则对《王仲奇医案》的用药规律进行分析。以"咳血"、"虚劳"以及"湿温"医案为研究对象，通过分析医案信息结构以对医案原文进行数据预处理，构建《王仲奇医案》数据库，并通过整合 Apriori 关联规则算法，设计并实现"新安中医临证指导系统"，完成数据挖掘结果可视化，提供"临床查询应用"功能以及用药规律的关联性分析。张丽颖等将文本挖掘技术引入到中医药科研项目数据管理中，采用文本预处理、文本建模、时序规则发现、关联规则发现、推理规则发现和高频规则发现、文本分类、聚类分析和孤立点分析等方法，对中医药科研项目进行数据管理，对于项目的知识提取、项目管理的效率都有很重大的价值。戴俭宇等将知识发现技术应用于古代医案的整理中。首先对《名医类案》、《续名医类案》进行版本认定、文字校对和名词术语标准化，以从肾论治医案为研究对象，建立医案的纳入、排除标准，理清从肾论治医案，通过数据库知识发现技术，对医案的病名、证名、体质、病因、病机、症状、治则、治法、方剂、中药、针灸、调护等内容分类系统研究，并以上述 12 项内容为变量，进行频数聚类和关联分析，从一个新的视角深刻解读肾藏象理论。

江蓉星等运用计算机技术，按学科和朝代建立了巴蜀中医药古籍医家及书目全文图片数据库，并按病案、方剂、针灸等不同属性分别确立聚类、复杂网络、关联规则数据挖掘模式，建立巴蜀中医药古籍知识库。钱占红等提出建立中医临床基础学科病案数据库，以激发学生学习中医经典的兴趣，使学生熟练掌握运用中医辨证思维方法，提高教师的教学水平。程静则对古医籍文本的数字处理方法进行了探讨。

李彦文等将知识地图的方法用于中医药信息部门的研究中。采用系统分析方法，进行中医药信息部门知识地图的总体框架设计，重点分析基于知识地图集的知识地图功能模块的构建。

（许　吉）

[附] 参考文献

C

陈中,王朝阳,张月,等.《黄帝内经》“结络”本义[J].中华中医药杂志,2013,28(9):2528

程静.论古医籍文本的数字处理[J].中医文献杂志,2013,31(3):29

D

戴俭宇,郑洪新.于KDD技术对《名医类案》、《续名医类案》从肾论治医案的系统研究[J].中华中医药杂志,2013,28(7):2094

党思捷,袁林,王威,等.《黄帝内经》中“搏”字不作“搏击”解的探讨[J].中医文献杂志,2013,31(4):10

邓月娥.《孕育玄机》版本及其源流[J].中华医史杂志,2013,43(1):46

狄碧云,孙兆杰,范登脉.浅谈《灵枢经》的异文研究[J].中医文献杂志,2013,31(3):12

董立业,曾凤.宋人以《素问》校补《千金要方》内容考[J].北京中医药大学学报,2013,36(5):314

F

符箴.清儒《素问》校释三种音训方法之比较[J].凯里学院学报,2013,31(5):91

傅海燕,马丽佳.《黄帝内经》“咽”类术语的辨析及其意义[J].中医文献杂志,2013,31(3):24

G

高程熙,赵博.《内经拾遗方论》小考[J].中医文献杂志,2013,31(3):17

郭强.民国时期广东中医药学校的三种《喉科讲义》[J].中医文献杂志,2013,31(1):8

H

胡真,王华.中医药文化的内涵与外延[J].中医杂志,2013,54(3):192

J

江蓉星,聂佳,许霞,等.蜀中医药古籍数字化建设及数据挖掘模式研究与实践[J].成都中医药大学学报,2013,36(2):97

金栋,金雪宁,李冬梅,等.偏沮小考[J].中医文献杂志,2013,31(2):27

L

李柳骥,张戬,肖红艳,等.《伤寒论句解》作者及成书年代考[J].中华医史杂志,2013,43(1):48

李彦文,赵英凯,崔蒙,等.中医药信息部门知识地图的构建研究[J].中华中医药学刊,2013,31(1):176

李玉清.《本草发明》版本考[J].中华医史杂志,2013,43(2):112

梁杏,兰凤利.中医脉学在西方的译介与传播——以英文译介为中心[J].中华医史杂志,2013,43(5):271

刘鹏.《续修四库全书》所收《吴鞠通先生医案》的版本[J].中华医史杂志,2013,43(2):125

Q

钱占红,韩雪梅,麻春杰,等.中医临床基础学科建立病案数据库探讨[J].河南中医,2013,33(6):906

S

沈成,张亭立,孙文钟.隐曲当作勃起解[J].中华中医药学刊,2013,31(1):30

W

王宝华.“守形”含义辨析[J].北京中医药,2013,32(9):680

王诚.《黄帝内经》“卧出”辩正[J].中医文献杂志,2013,31(1):18

王缙,和中浚.《外科百效全书》存世版本的现状考察和研究[J].中华中医药学刊,2013,31(3):516

王丽.《太平御览》引“黄帝”医药学著作考[J].中医药文化,2013,8(2):37

王妮.《罗谦甫治验案》版本研究[J].长春中医药大学学报,2013,29(3):552

王涛,朱德明.《医宗宝镜》版本源流考辨[J].浙江中医药大学学报,2013,37(8):970

王旭光,陆翔.吴崑著作版本考[J].中华医史杂志,2013,43(2):114

王正山,张其成.《五行大义》引《内经》考[J].中华医史杂志,2013,43(3):226

Y

严泽,舒秀明,林殷,等.“食不欲杂”出处文献考[J].北京中医药大学学报,2013,36(4):235

杨继红,张凡,郝娟.现存古代中医文献的海外分布概况[J].世界中西医结合杂志,2013,8(4):424

阴小爱,张登本.《素问》“新校正”的校勘方法[J].河北中医,2013,35(5):757

袁开惠,陈慧娟,孙文钟.中医古籍词语考释三则[J].北京中医药大学学报,2013,36(6):380

Z

张凯，寿志勤，郭亚光，等. 用频繁集与关联规则挖掘《王仲奇医案》用药规律[J]. 安徽中医学院学报，2013，32(3)：20

张雷.《治百病方》不等于《武威汉代医简》[J]. 中华医史杂志，2013，43(2)：118

张丽颖，马鸣华，金岩. 文本挖掘方法在中医药科研项目数据管理中应用研究[J]. 辽宁中医药大学学报，2013，15(11)：131

张雪丹，张如青. 日本江户时期医家珍稀抄本三种概述[J]. 中医药文化，2013，8(2)：24

朱鹏举.《内经》"㿉(癞、颓)疝""㿉癃""癃㿉""癞癃疝"钩沉[J]. 世界中西医结合杂志，2013，8(4)：330

(二)医 家 学 派

【概述】

2013 年中医学术流派的理论研究主要是对中医学术流派概念内涵、形成因素、特色优势、传承发展规律、经验教训等领域进行了深入研究。

1. 学术流派的理论研究

洪净对中医学术流派传承发展中一些关键性问题进行了研究,提出中医学术流派的概念,对于如何保护、传承与发展中医学术流派等学术研究过程中必须深入思考和认真解决的重大的、规律性问题进行了探讨。认为在共性的传承传播规律中寻找适合流派生存发展的土壤和空间,应立足于"继承",着眼于"创新",充分挖掘流派文化的价值内涵,增强流派文化的凝聚力和吸引力,注重中医学术流派之间相互沟通、融合借鉴、科学整合,在彰显中医学术流派特色的基础上提高临床疗效、扩大影响、吸纳参与者,发展壮大流派。

宋咏梅在分析中医学术流派发展面临两大问题时提出,当代中医学术呈现出流派特色淡化和传承危机两大问题。分析其原因,主要涉及社会历史文化背景的变迁、教育传承模式的嬗变、现行医疗体制及医院管理模式的影响三个方面。所面临的问题,一是领军人物学术特色淡化,二是学术传承出现危机。

王雪茜在分析中医学术流派传承的核心内容与关键要素时提出,应以"道"为本,以德为行,以"法"为干,各依其宗,以"术"传法、以"技"建功。中医药学继承与发展的主要内容和载体是中医文化、中医学术和临证经验。道、法、术的传承保证了中医学术的整体性和连续性。其在分析中医学术流派传承的三大要素时认为,"源"、"流"、"派"即是构成中医学术流派的基础框架,又是流派传承和发展的重要环节。流派加强了中医学术传统特色的传承,推动、促进了中医学的繁荣与发展。

王鹏采用文献研究与专家访谈、问卷调查、实地调研相结合的方法,对当代中医学术流派的研究与传承发展情况进行了总结。其分别从传统学术流派研究、专科性学术流派研究、少数民族医学流派研究、现代中医学术流派研究、中医学术流派现代传承发展情况、存在的主要问题及发展建议等方面报告了研究结果。认为推动新时期中医学术流派的发展,必须从政策层面进一步创造有利于中医学术流派生存壮大的社会环境,逐渐形成新的具有发展潜力和社会影响的学术流派。

张志强认为中医药学学科的发展离不开学派建设,学派促进学科的发展,这是学科发展所经历的一条必由之路。中医药理论的创立、发展及完善,自始至终学派都在发挥关键的作用。但学派意识的欠缺却是目前存在的一个严重问题,它导致学术创新和交流受阻、归属感和凝聚力削弱、新兴学派构建和发展迟滞。其认为中医药学的发展需要学派意识的强化,新兴学派的构建是中医药学发展的标志。

2. 少数民族学术流派的研究

少数民族医学专科学术流派研究是学术流派中不能忽略的研究内容,2013 年发文不多,但系统总结了少数民族医学专科学术流派的传承脉络、诊疗特点等。

莫清莲就壮医学派的发展源流、学术特色、代表医家及其学术贡献等方面做了详细阐述。壮医学派的学术特色是以"阴阳为本,三气同步"的整体观,"三道两路"的生理病观,"毒虚致病"的病因学说,"调气解毒补虚"的治疗原则。文中还介绍了代表医家罗家安、班秀文、覃保霖、龙玉乾、黄瑾明、黄汉儒及其学术贡献。认为要不断发展、壮大壮医学派,应从理论和临床方面对壮医药进行更深入的研究;探讨壮族文化、哲学思想与壮医药的关系;用壮医理论指导疑难病症的临床治疗,使壮医学为维护百姓的健康发挥作用。

庞宇舟从师承教学角度探讨了壮医药传承与发展的影响。认为师承教学在传统医药和壮医药传承中的重要作用,它是包括中医药在内传统医药传承的主要形式,是传承壮医药理论与临床技能的主要载体,是发展壮医药的有效途径。师承教学有利于保持和发展壮医药传统特色,是壮医药院校教学模式的有效补充,对壮医药人才的成长具有多方面积极作用。

(王振国　范　磊)

【近现代伤寒名家学术思想研究】

张仁岗对近代伤寒大家曹颖甫的临床医案汇编《经方实验录》进行分析，指出其在继承仲景学说的同时，又多有发扬，特点包括活用小方治难症，擅用峻剂起沉疴，不被世俗成见所拘泥，重视辨证，用药寒热不拘，个性鲜明。谷建军对清末辽宁地区著名伤寒学派医家庆恕(云阁)的《伤寒论》研究方法进行了总结，从伤寒六经提纲、按证类方论伤寒、伤寒证辨、编纂伤寒歌括四部分归纳其学术特点。张爱民等对岭南伤寒名医陈庆保《伤寒类编》进行研究，指出该书遵从仲景的伤寒有五之说，以六经为纲、五种伤寒为目、因伤寒以聚方的编排体系体现出新的系统性和条理性，使伤寒病证的概念更趋清楚明晰，更贴近临床辨证论治思维，开辟了研究《伤寒论》的新途径，同时其临证用药谨慎稳重，方解精辟简练，体现了经方大家之特色。此外，伤寒学派之外的几位著名医家对伤寒学术思想的阐发亦颇有代表性。如林亭秀等分析了张锡纯《伤寒论讲义》从气化角度重新阐释《伤寒论》，包括用气化揭示六经病的病因病机，阐述经方对人身气化升降出入的调节作用，以及着眼气化解决少阳病传变顺序等疑难问题，拓宽了经方治疗今病的新思路。王杰等通过近代中医针灸大师承淡安所著的《伤寒论新注》一书，对其伤寒学术思想进行了挖掘，归纳其特点主要有针方互参、助药之不及，衷中参西，兼容并蓄，格物致知、侧重功能，错简重订，充实舌脉等几点。

现代伤寒名家学术思想研究方面，燕茹等记述了山西名老中医刘绍武对厥阴病的研究观点，即厥阴病的提纲应为“厥阴之为病，手足逆冷、脉细、恶寒、肢节痹痛”，其性质属表部的阴性病，其主方为当归四逆汤。孙守信等对甘肃伤寒学家刘举俊的部分学术观点进行了整理，如对伤寒温病实质相同的认识，对《金匮要略》中“四季脾旺不受邪”、“缓急”以及越婢加术汤条文的重新理解等。闫军堂等对伤寒名家刘渡舟运用经方的临床经验进行了系统的整理研究，介绍其善用柴胡剂类方治疗肝胆病，及其治疗黄疸八法、肝炎胁痛十法；善用柴胡剂、泻心剂类方治疗脾胃病，及其治疗胃痛十二法；善用柴胡剂、苓桂剂类方治疗头痛，及其治疗头痛十二法；善用柴胡剂、苓桂剂类方治疗呼吸系统疾病，及其治疗咳嗽十法；善用桂枝剂、苓桂剂、瓜蒌薤白剂等类方治疗心系疾病，及其治疗胸痹心痛十法等。通过论述其治疗特色、方证病机、组方用药的独到经验，以及典型病例的治验实录，体现出刘渡舟对仲景学术思想的继承、运用与发挥，对临床治疗颇有启迪。

(张苇航)

【温病治法研究】

郑春素认为，吴鞠通继承并发扬了叶天士用苦辛法治疗温病的理论，创立、规范苦辛温法的方剂。以苦温药和辛温药相合，应用可分为温阳气以通经络，温胃阳以消食滞，化湿浊以畅气机，健脾气以止疼，散寒湿以除顽痹，补脾气以止下痢等。李秀安等则认为，吴鞠通对温病的辨治有独到之处，特别是温病后期，热羁下焦，消灼肾阴，其治以滋肾法为主，并针对病机演变而分别辅以复脉、填精、敛汗、止涩、泻火、清心、降逆、熄风、透邪、利咽、攻下、护阳等诸法，丰富了温病的治法。康风河认为，吴鞠通在温病治疗中重视体质辨治，以保津存阴为主线，探讨体质辨治，强调温病的个体化治疗，体现在辛凉忌汗、甘寒忌苦寒、甘苦忌渗利、甘寒慎攻下、阴阳双治忌滋腻壅滞、瘥后调理忌余邪复发六个方面。

王菊等认为汗法在温病中是可以运用的，温热类温病不可发汗，可选凉药透汗；湿热类温病不可大汗，可选芳化微温的药物微汗；伏气温病选辛凉开达之药，清热宣气；对于无外感症状的伏气温病，张锡纯也主张用寒凉药物因势利导，内蕴之热可化汗而解。马红等讨论养阴生津法在温病治疗中具有补养阴液和祛邪除病双重作用，养阴生津方药之甘寒濡润药性是其祛邪的药学基础，其祛邪作用主要体现在能清热、润下、散瘀、消痰，而作用机理是既有养阴以扶正祛邪之功，又有直接祛邪泻实之效。张健荣等对温病热毒血瘀证分析，从现代研究和临床运用等角度证实除叶天士强调的“凉血散血”外，养阴生津、清热解毒、凉血散瘀、疏理气机、补益元气等法对改善和治疗瘀血或瘀血倾向均有良好作用。

张灿玾等概括治疗温病包括解表法、和解法、化湿法、清热法、攻下法、开窍法、熄风法、滋阴法等 8 种最基本的方法。在临床使用时，又当根据疾病的复杂情况，或单用一法，或二法三法合用。郑春素探讨温疫具有外邪入侵、胃府失和、气机失常、内外生毒、邪郁积阳等病机特点，因此治疗上应重视补正、治胃、衡通、解毒、养阴等方法，注重审因论治。

（胡　蓉）

【盱江医学研究】

盱江流域自古文风鼎盛，人才辈出，更不乏在医学史上产生深远影响的医家医籍。“盱江医学”概念自上世纪八十年代由江西中医学院杨卓寅提出，并得到学界认可。

1. 整体研究

谢强发现早在汉代江西的盱江流域已经有了医家的医事活动和著述，自汉代迄民国，盱江流域16个县市有医家963人、医籍684种，江西古代十大名医中有8位出自盱江流域。并考察了盱江医学2 000余年的发展源流。谢氏等还提出第一个盱江喉科医生为范淑清，后危亦林师从范氏，著《世医得效方》，首设口齿兼咽喉科专卷。盱江喉科对我国喉科的发展、兴盛、创新有着重要的影响。如清代著名新安喉科医家郑梅涧父亲郑于丰、叔父郑于蕃，均曾受业于盱江流域南丰喉科名医黄明生。徐春娟认为，席弘、陈自明、危亦林、龚廷贤、龚居中、李梴、黄宫绣等7位盱江名医重视针灸，并富有经验，各有特点，某些医家特别着重于灸疗，弥补了当时“重针轻灸”的不足。徐氏还认为，危亦林、李梴、龚廷贤等著作在日本、朝鲜、越南等国的翻刻，对日本汉方医学及朝鲜医学的形成、发展产生了一定影响。

2. 医家研究

徐春娟等对龚廷贤著作成书年代、内容宗旨、学术影响、版本流传及国内馆藏情况进行了系统考证。王东坡等认为龚廷贤论治饮食损伤独具特色，不仅继承李东垣饮食分治思想，同时提出脾胃分治、辨因论治理论。其治胃擅用疏通、慎用消导，治脾擅用健运兼以益肾，并创制治饮食损伤诸方；注重饮食养生，提出三宜五不宜；对于脾胃虚弱者强调食疗，创食疗法及糕饼方。这些理论对饮食损伤疾病的预防及治疗具有重要的现实意义。龚氏临床亦重针灸，聂建军等总结了龚廷贤在艾灸熏脐养生、针刺配合放血及艾灸治疗急重症、针灸治疗妇科及儿科疾病的学术思想。陈明霞等通过对龚廷贤主要著作中有关便秘证治原文的研读，从“详论燥结致秘，独重润燥通便”，“重视简便疗法，广收单方验方”，“强调便秘外治，多有发明改进”等三方面探讨龚氏便秘诊治思想，以供临床借鉴。

祛邪反应是疾病治疗过程中必然出现的机体反应，有轻、重、缓、急、顺、逆之区分，谭永东总结了喻嘉言有关祛邪反应的认识及处理方法，并指出喻氏对祛邪反应和误治两者之间的区别所在。

3. 医著研究

何亚敏等对龚居中《红炉点雪》中灸法治痨瘵的内容进行了总结，认为龚氏打破了前人灸法不宜用于热证的禁锢，将灸法运用于阴虚内热证的痨瘵，不仅注重灸材与炎源的选择，而且对于穴位的配伍、灸量的大小、灸治的次序、灸治的禁忌以及灸后的调养等都有所阐发。张佳丽等对危亦林《世医得效方》中的灸法思想及用灸特点进行了分析，认为此书虽不为针灸专书，却在灸法的运用上颇具特色。其一表现在灸法证治广泛涉及临床各科；其二是选穴配伍精当，注重灸治次序；其三是根据病情轻重以定灸量；其四施灸方式多样，灸后调护措施齐全。相宏杰等通过对陈自明《外科精要》中灸法治疗痈疽医案的系统分析，总结了陈氏使用灸法治疗痈疽的诊疗思想，并对其灸法特点、选穴特色、火候的掌握及操作宜忌等作了详细的论述，以期有益于现代临床对该病的诊疗。

舒艳芳等对龚廷贤代表著作《万病回春》对耳聋的辨治进行讨论。龚氏认为“治耳者，以肾为主”，并从部位上分左右，从病机上分虚实、风火等调治，治疗上以补肾、降火、调养气血为主，以虚实为纲，提出辨治耳鸣耳聋的思路，对于指导临床具有重要的意义。左玉静等对《万病回春》中的4则头痛病案进行赏析，分别从肝、脾、肾三脏及其气血方面论述了作者治疗头痛的方法及其用药特点，并于每一个医案后附现代病案，由此举一反三，透过其头痛病案学习中医辨证的思路和方法。徐超等对《医门法律》中咳嗽的论治内容进行分析，认为在病机的认识上重内外合邪，用药上以清轻顾脾胃为原则。相宏杰等通过研究《妇人大全良方》中有关妇人月水不通的方剂，总结陈氏治疗月水不通等特点。病因方面，陈氏认为妇人常由“劳伤血气致令体虚”“受风冷邪气客于胞内”内外两方面因素损伤冲任，使胞络内血绝不通而经闭，病因重视气血亏虚、风冷乘袭；治疗方面，陈氏重视“补通”以调经。通过统计分析陈氏治疗月水不通的34首方剂，发现其用药方面具有重视养血活血，药性偏温平，药味多苦辛甘，善用虫类药攻坚通络，服药方法灵活多样等特点，均体现了“补通”以调经的治疗原则。《种杏仙方》一书久藏清宫大内，系明代赣医龚廷贤所著，是书汇集了龚氏从医期间搜集积累的经验效方，所收方剂大多以物廉、简便、亲验为特点。采撷精要，切于实用，是珍贵的医学文献资料。王大忠对其医药内容及价值进行了探析。艾华等讨论了明代医家龚延贤的《万病回春》中“医家十要”“病家十要”和“医家病家通病”篇中所涉及的医德内涵、病人就诊原则等医学伦理学内容，认为其思想对改善医患关系有建设性意义，对构建和谐医患关系有借鉴意义。龙奉玺基于《喻嘉言医学三书》从创新的思维方法、严谨的治学态度和仁爱的职业道德三个方面探讨喻昌学术精神。秦燕春从社会文化的角度对喻嘉言《寓意草》中的医案进行剖析，认为疾病亦为社会现象，甚至可以是一个时代世风与人性的象征，并从《寓意草》中反映的明末社会风气谈及喻嘉言的生平经历以及其学术思想对现代疾病诊疗的意义。

（李　丛）

【新安医学研究】

1. 文化研究

王键总结新安医学的六大综合特色：一是理论创新活跃，注释经典也多发明，启蒙普及不忘创新，继承与创新有机统合；二是秉持徽学和谐传统，滋阴温补、伤寒温病虽学派林立，但求同包容，学说纷呈与交流融合有机统合；三是世医代代因袭，家族链与学术链融合交织、有机统合；四是徽域儒道佛并兴，医而好儒但不排斥佛道，以儒通医与融合道佛有机统合；五是根植于本土历史地理时空而又不断向外辐射，融入中医药学大循环而又植入“新安学术”基因于其中，“时空新安”与“学术新安”有机统合；六是生发于徽文化的沃土，硬实力与软实力一体两翼，医学科学与徽学文化有机统合，以满足群众医疗养生和精神文化的双向需求。

黄玉燕认为，《老老余编》强调了保养对老人的重要性，当从起居护持、饮食调护、助其养性延年、教其适当锻炼、以平剂疗疾等方面孝养老人。

王旭光认为《素问吴注》是新安理学大背景影响下的产物。吴昆在注解《素问》时，仿效《四书集注》的体例。《素问吴注》对汪昂和张介宾注解《素问》产生了一定影响。

李新军认为新安医家弃儒从医的原因有：① 本人喜爱医学，把治病救人作为志向。② 自己体弱多病及父母亲人患病，转而学医。③ 仕途不顺或对科考失望等原因弃儒从医。④ 对庸医误人的痛恨，勤奋学医。⑤ 家族世代行医的影响。李达等认为可以用“仁、义、礼、智、信”概括新安医家的职业道德。

2. 医家医籍研究

王键认为汪机、徐春甫、孙一奎、吴昆、汪昂、叶桂、程钟龄、吴谦、郑宏纲、程文囿十位医家对新安医学做出巨大贡献，可谓“十大新安医家”。王氏还认为《名医类案》《古今医统大全》《赤水玄珠》《伤寒论条辨》《医方考》《本草备要》《医学心悟》《不居集》《医宗金鉴》《重楼玉钥》《医述》等 11 部医著可作为新安医派的代表著作。

朱为坤认为新安医家洪基系明朝崇祯年间安徽新安人，在新安创办“胞与堂”药店，辑录 80 种效验方成册即《胞与堂丸散谱》，后又增补养生、房中、种子诸法，而成《摄生总要》。还介绍了该书现存版本馆藏情况。

毛逸斐等认为，《本草备要》的附图，并非汪昂本人所附，为后世翻刻时所加。《本草备要》编撰特点有：① 引文丰富，博采众长。② 药性病情，互相阐发；③纠正时弊，嘉惠后学。④ 语言精练，文字流畅。毛氏还认为，《本草备要》所选药物因贴近临床，切于实用被各版高等中医院校《中药学》教材收载，收载数量随时间推移呈增长趋势。

3. 学术思想研究

王键等总结了“新安医学十大学说”，分别为：营卫一气说、动气命门说、错简重订说、元阴元阳说、暑必兼湿说、卫气营血辨证说、医门八法说、外损致虚说、养阴清肺说、燥湿为纲说。王氏等还总结新安固本培元派形成历史及临床特点：明初中期汪机用人参、白术、黄芪和营卫、温补脾胃阳气，到其再传弟子孙一奎以温补下元为重，或合干姜、附子固先后天之本、培脾肾元气并举并治，以汪机门生们为主体的新安固本培元治法学派形成。此后，明清众多的新安名医，包括歙西槐塘—冯塘程系、歙西余系、歙西澄塘吴系、休宁汪系等新安世医家族链医家，在各自的临床实践中不断地丰富和发展温补培元之治，逐渐形成了以固本培元为学术主张，温养气血、培补脾肾元气为治法，临床善用人参、白术、黄芪或合干姜、附子共用。王氏认为,新安医家在治法上除“固本培元”外,在长期临床实践中还形成了“调理脾胃”、“养阴护阴”、“准《伤寒》法”等特色治法。“调理脾胃”法与“固本培元”法一源双流,以“后天元阴元阳不足”论治为分野,从培补“脾胃元气”到“脾胃分治”,从脾虚分阴阳论治到脾胃各分阴阳论治,以吴澄理脾阴、叶天士养胃阴最具特色;“养阴护阴”法从新安固本培元派滋阴以扶阳的考虑出发,由“补水滋阴”到“理脾阴”,由治疫治杂症重“养胃阴”到“养阴清肺”治白喉,再到“养阴润燥”治燥疫,以清代叶天士、郑氏喉科、余国珮等为代表,俨然形成新安养阴清润派;“准《伤寒》法”从“杂病准《伤寒》”到“温病不废《伤寒》”,从分“乱伤寒”、“杂伤寒”到分正伤寒为“述古”、类伤寒为“新法”,最终完成了由“温病属伤寒”到“寒温根叶相连”的进化,丰富和发展了中医治法体系。王氏还认为,新安医家处方用药有“平正轻简”、“轻清灵巧”、“稳准狠猛”三大风格。与固本培元派相对应。“平正轻简”是指处方平和、用药精简、用量轻巧;与养阴清润派相对应,“轻清灵巧”是指处方用药质轻、灵动,药味少,剂量轻。无论是“平正轻简”还是“时方轻灵”,均以轻巧灵验取胜。“稳准狠猛”用药风格与“准《伤寒》法”密切相关,是针对徽州山区急重伤寒热病,早攻、频攻以刈病根,以认证准、用药猛、剂量重、下手狠为特点。

许燕通过病案研究,发现郑重光治疗暑病不概用香薷,亦长于以干姜、桂、附子等辛温药治疗阴暑之证;脱证以参、芪救逆固脱;气虚则习用生脉饮清补之,益气生津而不恋邪,并注意服药时以粥养胃。

程金莲认为,《医宗金鉴·刺灸心法要诀》作为《医宗金鉴》的针灸部分,以歌诀的形式介绍脏腑、经络、腧穴、刺灸法等,全书配有多幅插图,介绍腧穴时分按部和按经两种形式,重点突出,既避免了按部取穴割裂经络理论的弊端,又便于按部取穴。吴谦重视特定穴、重用奇穴的思想在书中也有突出的体现。张昆则认为,《医宗金鉴》中除艾以外,记载的灸材有草纸、药锭、桑枝、蜡。且灸药结合,艾灸方法多样,且灸量受施灸部位、艾炷大小等多种因素影响。

刘昭认为,汪机重视针灸前病证诊断,并且把脉诊作为针灸施治的依据所在,认为微数之脉慎不可灸,夏季和脉浮者不可灸。汪机认为,灸法适用于风寒湿痹、素体阳虚、阳气下陷或阳气欲绝诸虚百损等症候。汪机还在书后附了禁灸穴歌,以使后人在灸法的运用中有所借鉴。姜德友认为,汪机强调外疡由内而生,治病必本于里,时刻注意保护脾胃,禁忌多用寒凉药。同时还指出一些传统说法的可行性或片面性。汪机外治善用灸法,提出借助火烙以及隔蒜灸的火力,使毒气有处可散,脓瘀有处可泄。汪机指出疮疡用针为贵,但应根据肌肉的厚薄,来确定施针的浅深,旨在去脓血以泄其毒。

汪伟认为,吴澄提出“外损致虚”说,认为虚损一证,不单内伤,外感亦可致损。吴澄为外损的治疗提出解托、补托二法,扩展了中医学临床治疗虚损的思路。

沈钦荣认为,程松厓用“八纲”统领脉法,脏腑辨证辨病互补,遵崇仲景。

（丁　晶）

【孟河医派学术思想研究】

1. 整体研究

杜鹃等认为,孟河四家诊疗咽喉疾病各有特色:费伯雄重视火、痰致病,认为咽喉病证多与肝肾肺相关;马培之以寒热、虚实为咽喉疾病辨证要点;对喉痧的治疗尤以丁甘仁研究深入透彻,对其病因病机、传变过程和治则均有相应论述。治疗中孟河四家除常用内服汤剂外,还有丸药、吹药、外贴药、敷药、穴位按摩等方法,药物以轻灵、精巧见长。孙世辉等以《孟河四家医集》总结其湿热(包括痰热)型痹证治疗用药特点:用药首用当归养血;注重顾护胃气,祛风利湿喜用较清淡温和之品;化痰药选用不伤胃气之品;慎用补法,少用活血化瘀虫类破血药;以理气药和缓急止痛药,以甘凉清淡之品顾护肝胃之阴。钟远等认为,孟河医派学术理论来源于《黄帝内经》《伤寒论》等中医经典,发展中师古不泥,无门户之见,融合各家,寒温并用,开创寒温融通的辨证论治体系;临床诊疗中以辨证为宗,治法灵活多变,用药醇正和缓,尽显轻灵、平淡之特色。

2. 各家研究

王鹏总结费伯雄论治中风经验,认为中风总纲为气血损亏,外风乘隙而入,施治着意于调和营卫,使风从卫出;如见痰火内蕴、外风乘客之证,则以清营化痰、熄风理气为主。临证注重从脏腑气血入手辨治，用药长于应用血药，体现出其一贯主张的和缓醇正之风。孙玉英等研究孟河医派费家带下证治法演进与临证运用，费伯雄强调治脾为主，次则固肾，并指出肝木侮土，内热伤阴是病因病机之一。费绳甫强调清肝火养胃阴的运用，兼顾带有五色，分别治之，注意带下证发病的多因性与治法的临证变化。费子彬继承费氏治脾固肾、养阴清肝、五色分治诸法，兼采傅青主、叶天士等名家经验，将费氏治疗带下经验进一步完善。季乔雪等分析费伯雄治咳的重点放在所病的脏腑，而不在肺；治肺咳之虚实当分微甚，治肺寒重在温阳化饮，治肺热重甘凉滋润，用药以和缓为贵，选用性能平和的方药缓慢图治，同时治必兼顾平素嗜好。

王传博等讨论丁甘仁治咳喘医案，丁氏认为咳嗽病因繁杂，多为内外合邪，故审症求因，分述论治，视疾之轻重缓急，而灵活用药；喘之发病，多责痰饮，因脏腑功能失调，加之病邪侵身所致，故治疗当予以调理脏腑祛除病邪。马明越等认为，丁氏辨治湿温病的经验有三大特点：① 将湿温病扩大到六经范畴。② 重视少阳、厥阴经的枢机作用，善用柴胡。③ 经方和时方并用，经方为主，加用芳化、苦燥、淡渗、疏达之品以助化湿。丰亚云认为丁氏将失眠之因大要不外乎心肾，涉及肝、胃，无出于阴阳，其医案可分为七型，治疗上兼顾阴阳，虚实同治，重视心肾，在辨证的基础上加诸多安神之品。蔡芳霓等认为，丁氏治疗脾胃病擅长经方，善用反治，遣药轻灵，注重健脾，以通为补。付先军等以《诊方辑要》为研究对象，采用文本挖掘与关联网络构建方法，总结分析丁甘仁临床用药规律。用药注重量轻力宏，好用健脾化痰药物，讲究炮制，也喜欢使用生、鲜、嫩中药，对中药的道地性十分重视，喜用二陈汤加减，在配伍方面化痰药与泄浊药的配伍堪为效法。

鲍健欣等分析秦伯未膏方调治特色，秦氏认为膏方的滋补功效，主要分为温补、清补、涩补、平补四类，若出现兼症则需随机应变，强调膏方是以驱病为主，不赞同病家视膏方为唯一补品而贸然进服。

（胡　蓉）

【朱丹溪治疗脾胃病学术思想研究】

王礼凤认为，朱丹溪广泛论述了脘腹痛的病因病机，诊断重视问诊，辨证谨遵八纲，强调因人制宜，并提出凡痛必用温通、诸痛不可补气、腹痛多用芍药等，形成其辨治脘腹痛的独特理论。

刘云霞认为，朱丹溪胃病多从痰论治，治痰顺气为先，采用有温、吐、补、清、消、反佐、饮食调养等多种治法，重视因时、因人制宜处方。

杨建猛等研究了朱丹溪对噎膈病的认识，即该病病机与气、血、痰、火有关，分血虚、气虚、有热、有痰等证型，强调治疗应以“养血生津、降火化结”为主，如牛羊乳、韭汁、竹沥、童便、蜜、姜汁、甘蔗汁等是必用之药。

（张志峰）

［附］ 参考文献

A

艾华，蒋一玮，赵建磊，等. 龚延贤《万病回春》对当代医德与医患关系的借鉴[J]. 中国医学伦理学，2013，26(1)：62

B

鲍健欣，袁久林，邸若虹，等. 秦伯未膏方调治特色[J]. 中医文献杂志，2013，31(2)：49

C

蔡芳霓，叶进.《丁甘仁医案》调治脾胃病特色浅析[J]. 上海中医药杂志，2013，47(6)：19

陈明霞，冷伟. 龚廷贤便秘诊治思想浅析[J]. 陕西中医学院学报，2013，36(4)：28

程金莲.《医宗金鉴·刺灸心法要诀》点评与体会[J]. 北京中医药，2013，32(4)：280.

D

杜鹃，王振国. 孟河四家诊疗咽喉疾病特色的研究[J]. 世界中西医结合杂志，2013，8(1)：64

F

丰亚云. 丁甘仁治疗不寐经验总结[J]. 内蒙古中医药，2013，32(34)：58

付先军，王振国，范磊，等. 基于《诊方辑要》文本挖掘与关联网络的丁甘仁临床用药经验挖掘研究[J]. 江苏中医药，2013，45(8)：63

G

谷建军.辽宁医学名家庆云阁伤寒学术思想述略[J].中医文献杂志,2013,31(3):39.

H

何亚敏,刘密,李金香,等.《红炉点雪》论灸法[J].国医论坛,2013,28(3):22

黄玉燕.《老老余编》中的敬老思想[J].吉林中医药,2013,33(3):315.

J

季乔雪,李达,鹿林,等.费伯雄治咳经验浅谈[J].中医药临床杂志,2013,25(4):363

姜德友.《外科理例》学术特点研究[J].中医药信息,2013,30(5):6.

K

康凤河.吴鞠通温病治疗中的体质辨治[J].吉林中医药,2013,33(7):654

L

李达.浅谈新安医家的职业道德[J].中医药临床杂志,2013,25(4):356.

李新军.新安医家弃儒从医的原因探讨[J].郑州航空工业管理学院学报(社会科学版),2013,32(5):36.

李秀安,黎忠民.《温病条辨》滋肾十二法析要[J].国医论坛,2013,28(3):20

林亭秀,乔艳文.试析张锡纯《伤寒论讲义》中的气化观[J].环球中医药,2013,6(7):523.

刘云霞.《丹溪心法》胃病辨治方法浅析[J].浙江中医杂志,2013,48(3):208

刘昭.《针灸问对》论灸法[J].国医论坛,2013,28(4):17

龙奉玺.基于《喻嘉言医学三书》探讨喻昌学术精神[J].医学与哲学,2013,34(2A):90

M

马红,付梓云,杨进.论养阴生津法在温病治疗中的作用[J].南京中医药大学学报,2013,29(5):401

马明越,于文明.丁甘仁运用六经辨治湿温经验探析[J].中医杂志,2013,54(4):352

毛逸斐.《本草备要》研究评述[J].安徽中医学院学报,2013,32(3):17

莫清莲,戴铭,等.壮医学派探析[J].中国中医基础医学杂志,2013,19(5):574

N

聂建军,熊云.龚廷贤的针灸学术思想[J].中国社区医师,2013,15(8):206

P

庞宇舟,黄贵华.师承教学对壮医药传承与发展的影响[J].广西中医学院学报,2005,8(3):153

Q

秦燕春.最是人间留不住——《寓意草》及其他[J].书屋,2013,(8):84

S

沈钦荣.新安医家程松厓学术思想探析[J].中华中医药学刊,2013,31(1):12

舒艳芳,滕磊.《万病回春》辨治耳聋的特点[J].长春中医药大学学报,2013,29(2):5

宋咏梅,王振国,刘更生.中医学术流派发展面临两大问题[N].健康报,2013年5月8日第5版

孙世辉,张苗苗.孟河医家治疗湿热型痹证用药特色[J].河北中医,2013,35(8):1234

孙守信,刘永强.伤寒学家刘举俊学术观点拾零[J].国医论坛,2013,28(5):6

孙玉英,申春悌.孟河医派费家带下证治法演进与临证运用研究[J].长春中医药大学学报,2013,29(2):189

T

谭永东.喻嘉言祛邪反应学术思想探析[J].中国中医基础医学杂志,2013,19(8):863

W

汪伟.吴澄"外损致虚"理论探析[J].江西中医药,2013,44(9):3

王传博,王婕琼,李泽庚.丁甘仁诊治咳喘撷华[J].中医药临床杂志,2013,25(4):365

王大忠.宫藏秘本《种杏仙方》的医药内容及价值探析[J].陕西中医学院学报,2013,36(6):27

王东坡,张惠敏,林燕,等.龚廷贤饮食损伤证治特色研究[J].安徽中医学院学报,2013,32(1):10

王键.新安医学的主要特色[J].中华中医药杂志,2013,28(2):439

王键.十大新安医家[J].中华中医药杂志,2013,28(3):739

王键.十大新安医著[J].中华中医药杂志,2013,28(4):1008

王键.新安医学十大学说(上)[J].中华中医药杂志,2013,28(6):1787

王键.新安医学十大学说(下)[J].中华中医药杂志,2013,28(7):2051

王键.新安固本培元派[J].中华中医药杂志,2013,

28(8)：2341

王键.新安医家治法创新[J].中华中医药杂志，2013，28(10)：2980

王键.新安医家处方用药风格[J].中华中医药杂志，2013，28(11)：3295

王杰，李孝波，贺文彬，等.承澹安《伤寒论新注》学术思想研究[J].中医杂志，2013，54(12)：2158

王菊，杨宇，周士杰，等.浅议温病中的汗法[J].国医论坛，2013，28(5)：10

王礼凤.朱丹溪脘腹痛文献研究[J].天津中医药，2013，30(2)：96

王鹏，王振国，刘更生，等.当代中医学术流派研究与传承发展[J].中医杂志，2013，54(10)：814

王鹏.孟河医家费伯雄论治中风经验探要[J].中医杂志，2013，54(16)：1367

王旭光.《素问吴注》发微[J].安徽中医学院学报，2013，32(6)：17

王雪茜，鲁艺，闫军堂，等.中医学术流派传承的三大要素[J].中医学报，2013，28(11)：1652

王雪茜，闫军堂，赵琰，等.中医学术流派传承的核心内容与关键要素[J].北京中医药大学学报，2013，36(10)：653

X

相宏杰，闫石，刘艳辉，等.陈自明应用灸法治疗痈疽经验探析[J].四川中医，2013，31(9)：30

相宏杰，闫石，刘艳辉，等.陈自明治疗月水不通的用药特点探析[J].世界中西医结合杂志，2013，8(3)：287

谢强，黄冰林.盱江医学发展纪年[J].江西中医学院学报，2013，25(3)：15

谢强，魏小明，杨淑荣.盱江医学喉科喉针流派溯源[J].中国耳鼻喉科学研究杂志，2013，12(1)：18

谢强，周思平.盱江医家医籍及地域分布略考(续一)[J].江西中医药，2013，44(4)：3

谢强，周思平.盱江医家医籍及地域分布略考(续二)[J].江西中医药，2013，44(5)：3

谢强，周思平.盱江医家医籍及地域分布略考[J].江西中医药，2013，44(3)：3

徐超，李映霞.《医门法律》治咳小议[J].江西中医药，2013，44(4)：20

徐春娟，斐丽，陈荣，等.试析盱江医学的国际影响[J].中医杂志，2013，54(4)：273

徐春娟，斐丽.明代医林状元龚廷贤医著考证[J].中医文献杂志，2013，31(1)：29

徐春娟.盱江医家针灸学术思想研究[J].时珍国医国药，2013，24(6)：1435

许燕.《素圃医案》暑证治验浅析[J].浙江中医药大学学报，2013，37(7)：856

Y

闫军堂，刘晓倩，马小娜，等.刘渡舟教授治疗头痛十二法[J].辽宁中医药大学学报，2013，15(8)：68

闫军堂，刘晓倩，马小娜，等.刘渡舟教授治疗胃痛十二法[J].吉林中医药，2013，33(6)：559

闫军堂，刘晓倩，马小娜，等.刘渡舟治疗咳嗽十法[J].辽宁中医杂志，2013，40(9)：1772

闫军堂，刘晓倩，王冬，等.刘渡舟教授治疗胸痹心痛十法[J].辽宁中医药大学学报，2013，15(9)：69

闫军堂，孙良明，刘晓倩，等.刘渡舟教授治疗肝炎胁痛十法[J].中华中医药学刊，2013，31(5)：1056

闫军堂，孙良明，刘晓倩，等.刘渡舟治疗黄疸八法[J].辽宁中医杂志，2013，40(1)：28

燕茹，马文辉.试论刘绍武对《伤寒论》厥阴病的辨析[J].山西中医，2013，29(7)：43

杨建猛，林丽珠.朱丹溪与张景岳对噎膈的认识.吉林中医药，2013，33(7)：651

Z

张爱民，沈创鹏，胡正刚，等.岭南伤寒名家陈庆保《伤寒类篇》学术思想概略[J].辽宁中医药大学学报，2013，15(1)：118

张灿玾，张鹤鸣.温病的治疗法则[J].天津中医药大学学报，2013，32(2)：65

张佳丽，刘密，刘金枝，等.《世医得效方》灸法浅议[J].福建中医药，2013，44(3)：48

张健荣，李民，孙学娟.温病热毒血瘀证证型治法探析[J].中医研究，2013，26(11)：8

张昆.《医宗金鉴》灸法特色探析[J].中华中医药杂志，2013，28(1)：49

张仁岗.从《经方实验录》看曹颖甫对仲景学说之发扬[J].中国中医药现代远程教育，2013，11(13)：2

张志强，王燕平，杨利.中医药学“学派意识”钩沉[J].北京中医药大学学报，2013，36(2)：232

郑春素.《温病条辨》苦辛温法应用探释[J].长春中医药大学学报，2013，29(2)：191

郑春素.从病机探讨温疫的治疗方法[J].长春中医药大学学报，2013，29(4)：565

钟远，申春悌.孟河医派主要学术思想探析[J].辽宁中医药大学学报，2013，15(2)：128

朱为坤.洪基与《摄生总要》[J].福建中医药大学学报，2013，23(6)：65

左玉静，朱建贵，王玉玲.《万病回春》头痛病案赏析[J].吉林中医药，2013，33(2)：198

(三)医史文化

【概述】

2013年医学史研究主要涉及疾病史、诊疗史、方药史、医事制度、医学人物、医学文物、医学社会史等方面。

1. 疾病史

张金中等考察了明代以前医家对胁痛的认识和治疗,以宋代为界分为2个阶段:宋以前,胁痛被视为疾病的伴发症状,医家多从寒论治,用药常选肉桂、附子等温热之品,这与重视阳气的传统观念有关;宋以后,尤其是金元时期,胁痛日渐被视为独立病证,其病因病机的认识渐趋丰富,治法从注重散寒转向注重行气,并最终形成了胁痛的辨证治疗思路。反映出宋金元的医学革新精神对具体疾病认识的影响。

单联喆等通过整理研究明清山西史志中与疫病相关的史料记载,认为明清时期山西疫病流行成因有三:一是自然灾害因素,如旱、大寒、大热、蝗、雨、雪、霜、雹等;二是山西的地理气候;三是社会因素,其中饥荒是疫病发生的重要因素,国家的政治经济状况与疫病流行有密切关系。陈旭指出瘟疫对社会的影响,既有它的致病,还有它对社会民众心态的影响。通过史料分析,认为明代瘟疫肆虐之际,社会民众心态有消极心态和积极心态两种。前者如恐惧、无助、消沉、迷信等,后者则有理智、慰藉、感恩、振作等。消极心态的存在,无助于社会对疫情的有效应对,甚至会加重疫情的危害;而积极的心态,则有助于疫情的缓和或控制,也有利于疫后社会生产生活秩序的重建。

2. 诊疗史

周玉祥等认为,去腐法经历代医家的不断发展、充实,成为中医外科的特色治法,但20世纪后,重金属伤害人体事件日益受到重视,故含砷、汞、铅等成分的去腐药物逐渐被禁用,然数千年先贤们的宝贵经验不应由于因噎废食而湮没、消失。樊云等对明清医籍之胸腹按诊手法进行系统总结,认为明清胸腹按诊法不及宋元前昌盛,却仍有大量记载。并指出《厘正按摩要术》中的胸腹按诊法源自日本腹诊术的说法不确切。欧阳珊婷等认为,中医早期的诊脉与经脉病候关系密切,二者与针灸治疗是同步发展的。将"诊脉"理解为诊察多部位动脉与腧穴,手下诊察到的脉象是针灸治疗的最主要的指导因素。并倡用诊察经脉的知识与演进历史来解读《内经》的针灸治疗内容。

梁杏等将中医脉学在西方译介与传播的历程划分为3个阶段:脉学西传初期,即片段译介时期(约1650～1707),具有西医学背景的传教士出于个人兴趣片段译介脉学典籍,通过介绍不同于欧洲医学脉诊的中医脉学,意图取长补短、弥补欧洲医学脉诊技术的不足之处、实现东方诊脉术与欧洲诊脉术的交流融合;完整译介时期(1735～1932),译者们开始以脉学典籍原文为底本翻译,力求保留中医学文化特色,再现脉学典籍原貌并纠正第1时期译文纰漏;创新发展时期(1981～　),脉学译介事业全面繁荣,译介者多为西方中医师,他们借助当代脉学研究成果、结合自身临床经验和研究成果,译介作品从跨文化视角挖掘、继承中医古典脉学理论,探索传统中医脉学的现代科学理解与应用,体现着翻译与研究紧密结合。

谭刚认为,由于自然环境、医疗卫生条件、生活习惯等多方面因素的影响,近代以来内蒙古地区蒙古族居民常罹患疾病,既有鼠疫等烈性传染病,也有梅毒、沙眼等慢性传染病,还有胃病、风湿病等一般慢性疾病。多种疾病的高发,尤其是鼠疫的肆虐和性病的流行,极大地影响了近代以来蒙古族人口的增长速度,也严重阻碍了内蒙古地区社会经济的发展。李董男等认为,晋隋唐时期在疫病病因方面,除继承前代的社会因素、气候失常等观点外,提出了时行之气、疠气(乖戾之气)等重要观点。这一时期,对疫病病机的认识主要有热邪伤阴、热毒动血、毒气传心、发斑(烂胃发斑、温毒发斑、热毒发斑)、动风(热极动风、阴虚生风)等。《诸病源候论》《备急千金要方》《外台秘要》等明确指出疫病中的一部分具有传染性,并对其传染方式、传染强度等进行了初步探究。上述认识奠定了后世疫病病因病机理论的基础,对疫病病因病机理论的发展产生了极为深远的影响。

3. 本草史

王鹏等指出早期的"忍冬"等名称，并非专指忍冬花部，早期本草文献并未提及花部入药，且无"金银花"之名，不能作为现今中药金银花的原始出处，质疑第九版《中药学》教材等著述之相关内容。而首次出现"金银花"药名的文献应为宋《苏沈良方》，首次记载单以忍冬之花入药的文献为宋代《外科精要》。

谢晋等对历代本草著作有关中药掺伪的记载进行了梳理考察，总结了历代药材的掺伪现象、掺伪品种及掺伪手段。指出造成中药掺伪的根本原因，一是医药分家，医不识药，商家职业操守淡漠；二是以药物产地论优劣而不仔细辨别真伪的做法起到一定的消极作用。杨环等发现"十八反"歌诀所涉药物主要来源于南北朝时期陶弘景的《本草经集注》，而歌诀体裁的表述形式则出现在宋金元时期，《儒门事亲》与其他医籍中记载的歌诀并非同源。明代在宋金元时期形成的"十八反"歌诀基础上，又对歌诀所涉药物进行了阐释和补充，相反药物增多，歌诀篇幅加长。《儒门事亲》的"十八反"歌诀在清代之后传播最广，成为迄今最为人熟知的中药禁忌歌诀。

4. 医学人物

宋珍民认为，孙思邈生年"581 年"和"541 年"之旧说，均有明显漏洞，考证发现孙氏当生于公元 560 年；卒年既往有"永淳说"和"永徽说"，考证认为卒年较为合理的表述为："孙思邈约卒于调露二年/永隆元年(680)"，或"孙思邈卒于 680 年±1 年"。袁冰等考证了宋代名医陈言的宗谱及籍贯。陈言的籍贯历来有争议，主要有青田人、栝苍人、莆田人、景宁人等诸说。作者将《陈氏宗谱》中的记载与相关史料参研后发现：依据《陈氏宗谱》中的记载和中国传统习俗，推测陈言的籍贯为浙江省乐清县。陈言在《三因极一病证方论·序》中所署"青田鹤溪陈言无择"的原因，据《陈友芝医案续集》一书中释为青田鹤溪是其出生地。因此，在相关史料缺乏的情况下，应尊重陈言亲署。

孟永亮等在广泛查阅史书的基础上，对北宋校正医书局的重要官员进行了较为系统的研究，本年度共发表学术论文 4 篇，内容包括：① 林亿生平考证。② 掌禹锡生平考证。③ 孙奇、孙兆兄弟生平考证。④ 任"提举校正医书"一职的 3 位官员研究。自校正医书局成立以来，共有 3 位朝廷高官兼任提举校正医书一职，韩琦为首任，范镇、钱象先后接任。并对校正医书局的长官提举一职进行考证，内容包括提举官的来历、校正医书局的隶属关系、首任提举韩琦建言校正医书的背景、提举校正医书局人员的演变等。

5. 医学社会史

潘秋平指出兴盛的巴蜀文化、稳定的政治环境、繁荣的经济、发达的地方医学教育、丰富的药材资源为当地医学的繁荣创造了条件。涂雪峰等指出中国传统医德与中国传统思想文化发展的历史轨迹是同步的，从中吸取传统医德的精华，重新认识传统医德的现代价值，对于完善现代医德规范、协调医患关系、培养新时期优秀医务人员有着重要的启示意义。《寻乐堂日录》为清代中州理学家窦克勤日记，其中有与病痛、治疗相关内容，张博研究发现，窦克勤认为秉持理学观念而形成的精神力量可以战胜病痛，内心的平静及加强道德修养能达到养生的目的，同时排斥佛道等借助外在神秘力量疗病与养生的观念。然而，日常生活中窦克勤的行为并不完全符合他的观念，往往依据实用主义原则对相似的疗病行为采取迥异的态度。此外，他还通过由疗病产生的邀神行为，塑造家族成员的纯孝形象。窦克勤日常生活中的疗病观、生命观等都受到理学观念很大的影响，由此可加深对清代士人群体的认识。黄鑫等选择广升远"定坤丹"、千芝堂"千芝保坤丹"、圣术堂"妇科救苦丹"、瑞生药房"妇女调经白带散"、佛慈制药厂"十灰丸"、凌阁大药房"妇女幸福汤"等几款"御生堂"中医药博物馆藏民国妇科药品包装盒及用药进行了介绍。认为其体现了民国时期妇科商品广告及用药的特点，既想要遵从古方，又想从中体现出西方科学渗透后带有"科学"的印记，同时，形式多样，印刷精美，广告词语文白夹杂，也体现了当时印刷技术的进步。

（王振国　张　蕾　刘　鹏）

【中医药文化的内涵与核心价值研究】

1. 中医药文化的内涵

胡真等对中医药文化的内涵与外延进行了界定，认为中医药文化是中华民族优秀传统文化中体现中医药本质与特色的精神文明和物质文明的总和,它以中国传统哲学、文学、史学为基础;由中医药精神文化、行为文化、物质文化三个方面构成,包含中医药文化理念、文化实践、文化环境三个层面;体现中医药的人文属性;具有塑造中医药文化核心理念和价值观念,形成中医药学思维方式和认知,揭示中医药学规律,影响中医药事业传承与发展和增强中华民族文化认同与自信,扩大中华文化影响力的功能。中医药文化的外延十分广泛,它以中医典籍、中医名家、中医文物、中医史迹为研究对象和载体,以中医药文化哲学基础和文化根源,中医名家名著的文化思想和名家风范,中医道德观念,中医行为规范,中医药文化传承与创新等为研究内容。王旭东认为中医文化的基本范畴是：价值观上强调整体的价值,认知方式上强调事实的认定而不注重本原的识别,思维上采用辩证逻辑为主的直觉式思维——表明中医是用另一双眼睛在看世界,是在以整体的人为起点、以宇宙为终点的大环境中得出的以现象为目标的综合学科体系。

2. 中医药文化的核心价值

陈少宗认为中医学的核心价值体系包括五个方面的内容：天人相应、道法自然的养生保健思想,即尊重规律的养生保健思想;治未病的思想,即预防重于治疗的思想;自然、顺势、调节的思想,即非对抗治疗的思想,这一优势主要体现在疾病初期和恢复期,在疾病暴发期则主要是辅助治疗作用;精神内守,病安从来的思想,即精神、心理状态与健康密切相关的思想;医乃仁术,医心近佛,乃苍生大医的思想,即医生自身的道德要求及对患者人文关怀的思想。申俊龙等认为中医药文化核心价值应该包括四个方面：① 生命价值方面,道法自然的宇宙观和自然观,重视正气、中和平衡的生命观、生活观,燮理阴阳、身心共养、形神兼具、动静相宜、重预防的顺势适时养生观、治未病思想等,这些观念的普及与传播,对现代社会公众健康素养的提升有极大的促进作用。② 思想价值方面,中医药学的价值判断、思维方式、认知方式等,仍是对现代人类思维和实现的重要补充,其蕴含的仁、和等思想,不仅可以促进人的和谐发展,而且促进社会的和谐发展,优化社会发展模式。③ 科学价值方面,中医是多学科知识的整合,体现了生命整体观、有机观、动态观,这是对现代医学的补充和丰实,有利于转化医学和整合医学的发展。④ 伦理价值方面,以人为本、济世活人的价值理念,大医精诚、淡泊名利的精神,是医务工作者永恒的道德追求。

（刘　鹏）

【中医学身体观研究】

刘鹏对中医学身体观的内涵及其主要特点进行了系统阐述,认为中医学身体观是中医学对人体生命的综合认识。身体作为医学立论的基础和最终落脚点,与传统文化中儒家、道家等其他领域的身体观相比较,传统的中医学身体观更加注重对“形神统一生命体”本身的关注,即更加注重对构成生命躯体各基本要素的关注,如脏腑、形体官窍、精、气、血、津液等等。传统文化其他领域的身体观往往把个体生命的身体作为一个既定的、无须详尽阐发的整体,在此基础上重点论述个体生命与自然、社会间的关系,个体生命间的关系,以及处理各种关系的原则和方法,对观念的论述要远远大于对身体本身的讨论。医学则把对身体的讨论作为基础,在讨论的过程中既借鉴和体现了传统文化各领域所共有的一般身体观,又在一定程度上或多或少影响了传统文化一般身体观的内涵与发展。中医学身体观的内容既包括中医学所特有的对身体生命本身的认识,如脏腑学说、精气血津液学说等等,又包括对传统文化一般身体观的理解和融入,如对身体社会属性、自然属性的论述等等。而且,传统中医学对身体的理解与诠释,又影响了整个传统文化对身体的理解,在一定程度上形成了整个传统文化对身体结构及功能理解的基础。中医学身体观具有重时空、重循环、重功能、重联系的特点,可将其主要特点概括为以下四个方面：天人相应,贵在和合——时空的身体;天道周行,如环无端——循环的身体;体用兼备,重在释用——功能的身体;内外相系,各部相连——联系的身体。

（刘　鹏）

【中医教育史研究】

云南医学堂是清代官办的医学堂,系列教材《医学正旨择要》由时任教官的陈子贞等学者编写。李梦华等认为,该学堂重视中医人才唯物自然观的培养,以科学自然观作为指导思想,将抽象、玄奥的中医理论生动融于教材,使习医者乐于接受。教学以《内经》《难经》《伤寒杂病论》等经典构成学术核心,还收罗历代中医理论;二者有机结合,既强调经典医著的传承性,也表明广泛涉猎中医诸家的重要性。教学内容汇集天文、地理、人文等知识，更彰显中医自身多学科融合的特点。

广东中医药专门学校和广东光汉中医专门学校，是广东成立时间最早、持续时间最长、影响最大的两所中医学校。郭强撰文研究民国时期广东中医药学校的三种喉科讲义：古绍尧的《广东中医药学校喉科学讲义》、邬宝杰的《广东光汉中医学校喉科讲义》和钟锦涛的《广东光汉中医学校喉科讲义》。它们在国内同类讲义中编写较早，汇集编写者学术心得与临证经验，系统地将喉科72症的症状、病因病机、治法、方药分条论述，易于学生掌握。三种喉科讲义显现岭南中医喉科的较早教育专业化水平，其编写体例与现今教材非常相似。

（杨奕望）

【卫生用品与医药文化】

张苇航对我国古代传统的常用清洁用品进行了概述，其中包括① 潘沐：即淘米水，又称米泔水，不仅指淘洗稻米的水，也包括淘洗粟、稷、粱等其他粮食的水；不仅可用来洗头，还可用来洗脸、洗身，并有润泽须发的功效，还作为内服药物、溶剂或炮制方法被广泛记载并应用。② 洗石：洗石当是一种具有碱性而细腻的石头，既可以通过搓洗去除死皮，又能溶解污垢。如将“洗”理解为其洗足的本义，那么这种“洗石”主要用来洗脚。③ 澡豆：亦写作藻豆，是中国古代最具代表性的洗浴用品，相当于现代的肥皂。其出现的时间不早于东汉，时至隋唐，澡豆仍是上层社会才能使用的高档物品，并常作为贡品。澡豆的配方作为医方被记录，《千金方》《太平圣惠方》《普济方》等方书均有专篇记载。④ 皂荚：《神农本草经》已载有皂荚一药，但至晋代陶弘景《名医别录》始载其“可为沐药，不入汤”。在魏晋南北朝时期，皂荚是常见的洗涤用品，主要用来洗手和洗衣，亦可用来洗脸。李时珍在《本草纲目》“皂荚”条下另外记载了一种“肥皂荚”，两种植物同目同科，但种属略有差别，以前的文献中对二者不作细分，造成了混乱。

傅维康介绍了古代口香糖的历史。其在中国古已有之，前身是口香剂。宋代《太平御览》中即有汉桓帝以鸡舌香赐与大臣以除口臭的记载。东汉《神农本草经》推许“水苏”的“辟口臭”功效，晋代《肘后卒救方》介绍用豆蔻、细辛研末含口中，能香口辟臭。唐代《千金翼方》记载用香薷煎汁口含，去口中臭气，称赞薄荷“令人口香气洁”。中国古代，用口香剂加工制成口香糖，最迟在唐代就已出现。《备急千金要方》的“七窍病”专卷内，提到对口臭病的治疗，宜“常服含香丸”。例如用芎劳、白芷、橘皮、桂心、枣肉五味药研末，加蜜炼成糖丸，可在“食前食后常含之”。宋代《太平圣惠方》与《圣济总录》收载了相当多的口香剂与口香糖丸。其中有一种“含香圆”，是采用鸡舌香、藿香、零陵香等15味药研为细末，加蜜炼制而成，有生津去腻、香口除臭、消炎固齿等作用。

陈顺杰回顾了我国首种中药针剂“柴胡注射液”的产生及发展轨迹。其始创于抗日战争时期的太行山革命根据地，1941年，由利华药厂研究室主任韩刚提出了用柴胡制作针剂的主张和设计方案，并牵头研制成功了柴胡针剂，名为“发热仃注射液”。1954年武汉制药厂对“柴胡注射液”进行了科研和临床应用，经过病毒、生物组织药理学等科学实验，认为其确有治疗的实际意义。且经临床应用后认为其对普通感冒和流感的退热功效超过了一般对症解热药，对疟疾退热作用明显，应用中未见特殊副作用，并可安全用于儿童和孕妇。“柴胡注射液”的成功研制带动了全国中药注射剂的研制工作。上世纪50年代中期到60年代初期，上海等地研制出“茵栀黄注射液”、“板蓝根注射液”等20余个品种。在70年代“大搞中草药运动”中曾制出上千种中药注射液，进入八九十年代，随着《中药注射剂研究技术指导原则》的出台，中药针剂进入管理规范化、制法高技术化、指标定量化时期，出现了“刺五加注射液”及“双黄连”注射剂。进入21世纪以来，我国中药针剂的发展进入单体化制备阶段。2007年12月，《中药、天然药物注射剂基本技术要求》发布，为中药注射剂再评价提供了重要依据。2010年版《中国药典》对所有中药注射剂品种，增加了重金属和有害元素限度标准，这对于解决中药注射剂的安全性问题起到积极的作用。目前，中药针剂正在逐步走出国门，走向世界。

僧海霞对唐宋时期敦煌地区的药酒基酒进行了考证。唐宋时期的敦煌地区酒类众多，名称各异，选作药酒基酒与直接饮用的酒形成鲜明的对比，有所侧重地反映出各自的特性。它们是不同历史时期或者同一历史时期的不同表述习惯，不同名称之间仍然存在着一定的对应关系。它们同为麦酒，其区别在于酿制工艺的不同。麦是蒸馏酒出现之前敦煌高档酒的主要原料，尤其是药酒的酒基原料。另对唐宋时期敦煌地区的药用醋进行了考证，认为唐宋时期的敦煌地区，麦醋是药用醋的主流。它在古医方中临床应用很普遍，医方中使用的各种称谓，是不同历史时期或者同一历史时期的不同习惯表述，从不同侧面来诠释其品性和文化特征。其中部分名称已游离出南北朝时期醋所界定的概念范围。个别名称被后世误判，缘于它自身的佚失及其在实践中被广泛取代等因素。

高驰等对宋代医学各科应用香药方的现象进行了分析。宋代方剂大量使用香方，涉及领域十分广泛，加之政府参与，也为医药行业制定了一系列配方制剂的原则。至于临证各科，当时医家则根据每一科的不同特点，以及每种香药各自不同的特性，辨证论治，配伍组方，来发挥香药在不同疾病中的优势。由于宋时香药已普及成为日用品，香方制剂具有服用便利的特点，加之宋政府对香方的大力推广，造成香药滥用成风现象非常明显。后世以朱丹溪为代表的医家，对此加以抨击，力陈其弊。此后，无论在政府层面还是医生层面，对香方的使用，重新回归理性与慎重。

(李　从　刘　鹏)

【宋代文化名人与医学研究】

王永恒等认为，宋徽宗有较高的艺术修养，信奉道教，喜欢医学，不仅对中医有较深的造诣，在位期间还采取一系列有利于医药发展的举措。北宋初年，中央医官承袭唐制，设翰林医官院，掌管卫生行政，设立了官药局，是官方经营的药业机构。庆历年间设太医局，专掌医学教育。校订《证类本草》，编纂《太平惠民和剂局方》《圣济总录》，而且宋徽宗还亲自撰写《圣济经》。

孟永亮等考证，林亿为开封人，约出生于北宋真宗咸平、景德年间(998～1007)；景祐元年(1034年)中书判拔萃科，除两使幕职官；嘉祐二年(1057年)七月诏入秘阁；林亿为仁宗朝枢密使高若讷之次婿；他曾有诗作保存于世。嘉祐二年八月成为北宋校正医书局的重要成员，历仁宗、真宗、神宗三朝，十余年间，校勘医籍成就突出，官职屡有升迁。孟氏等还认为，孙奇、孙兆兄弟二人为北宋校正医书局重要成员，但史书中关于其生平事迹的记载较少且零散，目前亦鲜有人研究。通过发掘史料，发现孙氏兄弟为河南卫州人，后客居河阳，二人约生于真宗大中祥符九年(1016年)前后。孙奇于神宗元丰八年(1085年)致仕，卒年不详，累官至朝散大夫，12年间参校医书9部，因校书而名垂史册；孙兆最晚卒于元丰八年(1085年)，累官至将仕郎、殿中丞，16年中参校医书2部，以医术而流芳百世。孙氏兄弟在医籍校正方面，功绩显著，为保存和传承古代医籍做出了重要贡献。

(张志峰)

【近代西医东渐之研究】

于赓哲等撰文提出，在西学东渐和科学主义深入人心背景下，即便古典医学的拥护者也不自觉地受到西方医学的巨大影响，从而形成如此之思维模式：在对西医强大压力进行反弹时，传统医界实际依照西医的样式反复阐明自身的“科学性”，在站到西医对面的同时也成为其映像。对待所谓迷信问题时，除了有简单的回避之外还有从心理学等角度出发所做的“科学解释”，讨论者即便意见完全相左也有一个共同点——他们在以西医为标准衡量古典医学。民众心目中“西医治标，中医治本”的观念，一方面是对西医快速疗效的承认，另一方面是对中医价值的重新阐释。近百余年来，国人对于中国古代手术的重新审视也可以反映此类问题，面对西学的侵迫，中医界不仅有迎合或回避，也有信心的重建，一旦其中有与近代医学理念相契合的个案，往往就成为中国传统医学成就的象征和骄傲。由不相信其真实性到骄傲弘扬，国人近二千年来对待华佗外科手术的态度是一个典型例证。在医学分科、药典问题上也可看到西学影响的痕迹，无论是强调中国分科之古老，还是强调《新修本草》是“世界上第一部药典”，其实都在有意无意以西学为衡量标准，并且“套用”西学的观念。

王银泉等以科学译介为主线，以人物活动为中心，以标志性事件而非朝代更迭为界线，对明末清初入华耶稣会士的科学翻译活动进行全新分期。提出以1687年法国洪若翰、张诚、白晋、李明、刘应这5位“国王的数学家”抵华作为耶稣会士科学译介活动的分水岭，强调法国耶稣会士此后确立的优势地位，并论述他们所取得的突出成就及其对中西文化科技交流的重要影响。

张爽则以近代名医、医学家丁福保为例，展现清末民初西医东渐与中医学的发展。丁福保心怀振兴中国医学之志，置身改进中医；曾赴日考察医学，翻译出版《丁氏医学丛书》，成立“中西医学研究会”，刊发《中西医学报》，致力医疗慈善事业，建立“丁氏医院”、“上海虹桥疗养院”等。丁氏主张取法日本，以西医改良中医，致力中医的科学化转变。

（杨奕望）

【医事制度研究】

冯卓慧等通过研究唐开元年间的《医疾令》，结合唐代律法《唐律疏议》，对唐代医政管理制度、医学教育制度、医生资格考试制度、公费医疗制度、药物管理制度、传染性疫疾的防治制度和违反诸制度及医疗犯罪的惩治法律等方面进行研究并认为：① 医学教育方面。明确规定医科、按摩科、咒禁科、针科的设置，并规定医学学生来源、教师任职资格；教学方法上，在熟读经典后分业学习，规定医科与针科学生的必读教材，学习的侧重点由专业而定；规定医学学生的学制、考试制度、选任制度及学费缴纳制度，以及各州的医学教育和任职制度。② 药物管理方面。《医疾令》规定了药物的采集与收购、京都专设药园、各州对中央药物的输送、药物制作等管理制度。③ 公费医疗制度。唐代实行有限公费医疗制度，规定享受公费医疗待遇的范围，并有明确医师巡诊时的食宿安排。④ 对违反医疗法行为的法律制裁。《唐律疏义》中相关法律 12 条，包括有关医药制造、销售违法犯罪的惩治，以及对违反《医疾令》治疗病患的法律惩治。

夏逸群等认为，明代医药机构设置主要分为中央医药行政管理机关、宫廷及王府医药机构以及民间与地方医药组织三部分，形成了具有明代特色的世医制度和弃儒从医的社会风气，保障了医学人才的数量，提升了医生队伍的整体文化素养。方传明等认为，御医的产生是随着专制政权的产生而产生的。先秦时御医的来源主要是医官；从秦到南北朝时期，御医的来源又多了征辟，征辟的对象就是那些有师承、有名望的民间医生；自隋唐以降，御医的主要来源是官办医学机构的培养和征辟。历代御医地位比较低下，史上医生品阶最高者当推明代太医院院使许绅，其被封为太子太保、吏部尚书，官居一品。御医的工作是为帝后妃嫔诊病、配药，提供保健意见等。所诊患者的生理、病理、疾病谱和包含精神因素的疾病谱与布衣的具有很大差别。诊治经过较难，用药谨慎，讲求圆机活法。

夏媛媛总结了公医制的形成过程：① 公医制的提出。针对于民国时期医疗卫生资源的缺乏，一些有识之士提出了公医制的设想和建议，是我国公医制的雏形。② 公医制的论证。当时学者分别从公医制的实施意义和具体实施方法进行了论证，提出了较为详细的指导意见。论证中很大一部分是有关医学课程设置、医学人才培养模式、医学教育布局的讨论，旨在建立相应的医学教育制度与之配套，保障公医制的顺利实施。③ 公医制的试验。个别医学院校开始了公医制的试验，如 1934 年成立的省立江苏医政学院，针对当时流行的黑热病开办了农村医药初级服务训练班；1937 年夏季镇江针对疟疾的流行开办了防疟训练班，均取得较好效果。④ 公医制的初步成型。民国政府于 1940 年公布了公医制方案《公医学生待遇暂行办法》，此后国民党五届八中全会通过了《实施公医制度以保证全民健康案》，将公医制度确立作为国家卫生行政的目标之一。国民政府卫生署颁布政令，在国内部分地区推行公医制，并将公医制度纳入《中华民国宪法》。限于多种现实因素，公医制度以失败告终，但推动了卫生行政事业与医学教育事业发展。

（张　蕾）

[附] 参考文献

C

陈少宗. 中医科学与中医文化有关问题的思考[J]. 医学与哲学，2013，34(4A)：1

陈顺杰. 中国第一种中药针剂[J]. 武汉文史资料，2013，(8)：39

陈旭. 明代民众面对瘟疫的心态[J]. 中华医史杂志，2013，43(2)：88

F

樊云，齐凤军，刘建民，等. 浅论明清时期中医古籍中胸腹按诊手法的运用[J]. 光明中医，2013，28(4)：768

方传明,李怡. 御医概说[J]. 北京中医药,2013,32(1):38

冯卓慧,王霖冬. 从唐开元《医疾令》看唐代的医疗法[J]. 西安财经学院学报,2013,26(1):102

傅维康. 中国古代的“口香糖”[J]. 中华医史杂志,2013,43(1):8

G

高驰,朱建平. 宋代香方与医学[J]. 中华中医药杂志,2013,28(5):1597

H

黄鑫,黄涛. “御生堂”中医药博物馆藏民国妇科药品包装盒[J]. 中华医史杂志,2013,43(1):54

L

李董男,潘桂娟. 晋隋唐时期疫病病因病机探讨[J]. 中医杂志,2013,54(3):184

李平,张建英,李梦华. 清代云南医学堂中医教学观初探[J]. 光明中医,2013,28(3):617

刘鹏. 中医学身体观的内涵及特点[J]. 南京中医药大学学报(社会科学版),2013,14(4):133

刘鹏. 中医学身体观解读[M]. 南京:东南大学出版社,2013

律正严,裴永兰. 幼而徇齐之我见[J]. 医药前沿,2013,(21):342

M

孟永亮,梁永宣. 北宋校正医书官孙奇、孙兆考述[J]. 辽宁中医药大学学报,2013,15(11):205

孟永亮,梁永宣. 北宋校正医书局林亿生平探析[J]. 北京中医药大学学报,2013,36(6):383

孟永亮,梁永宣. 北宋校正医书局掌禹锡生平考述[J]. 中华医史杂志,2013,43(1):57

孟永亮,梁永宣. 提举校正医书三长官—韩琦、范镇、钱象先考释[J]. 中华医史杂志,2013,43(4):238

O

欧阳珊婷,柳长华. 诊脉与经络病候及针灸治疗的关系[J]. 中华医史杂志,2013,43(3):192

P

潘秋平. 两宋时期巴蜀医学繁盛原因[J]. 安徽中医学院学报,2013,32(3):4

S

单联喆,梁峻. 明清山西疫病流行相关因素[J]. 中华医史杂志,2013,43(1):50

单联喆,梁峻. 清代山西疫病流行时空规律研究[J]. 中国中医基础医学杂志,2013,19(2):124

僧海霞. 唐宋时期敦煌地区美发文化透视[J]. 中医药文化,2013,8(3):36

僧海霞. 唐宋时期敦煌地区药用醋考[J]. 中医杂志,2013,54(14):1248

申俊龙,马洪瑶. 中医药文化核心价值传承与传播的语境及路径分析[J]. 中医杂志,2013,54(24):2076

宋珍民. 孙思邈生年新证[J]. 中华医史杂志,2013,43(1):9

T

谭刚. 近代内蒙古地区疾病流行与蒙古族社会变迁[J]. 中华医史杂志,2013,43(2):95

涂雪峰,傅琛. 中国传统医德的历史嬗变及其现代价值[J]. 中医药管理杂志,2013,21(7):662

W

王鹏,周扬,付先军,等. 金银花的文献出处及相关药用名称药用部位考证[J]. 中华医史杂志,2013,43(3):144

王旭东. 中医文化价值的基本概念及研究目标[J]. 医学与哲学,2013,34(4A):8

王银泉,胡大平. 明清入华耶稣会士科学译介活动新论[J]. 云南大学学报(社会科学版),2013,12(4):89

王永恒,冯伟,周计春. 宋徽宗对中医学的贡献[J]. 中医学报,2013,28(2):303

X

夏逸群,张成博. 明代医药机构设置与世医制度浅析[J]. 山东中医药大学学报,2013,37(2):143

夏媛媛. 民国时期公医制的形成过程及其对医学教育的影响[J]. 南京医科大学学报(社会科学版),2013,54(1):18

谢晋,王德群. 古代中药掺伪考[J]. 中华医史杂志,2013,43(9):262

Y

杨环,范欣生,卞雅莉,等. 中药“十八反”歌诀源流[J]. 中华医史杂志,2013,43(2):76

于赓哲,梁丽. 古典医学的“西学镜像”[J]. 人文杂志,2013,(10):93

袁冰,杨卫华,曹丽娟. 宋代名医陈言宗谱及籍贯考略[J]. 中医文献杂志,2013,31(1):41

Z

张博. 从理学家窦克勤看清代士人的病痛与治疗[J]. 中华医史杂志,2013,43(6):331

张金中，王振瑞．明代以前医家对胁痛的认识和治疗[J]．中华医史杂志，2013，43(2)：71

张爽．丁福保与近代“西医东渐”[J]．江苏教育学院学报(社会科学)，2013，29(4)：89

张苇航．“浴兰汤兮沐芳”——中国传统清洁用品与医药文化溯源[J]．中医药文化，2013，8(2)：27

周玉祥，陆新瑜，于祥林，等．中医外科去腐方法略论[J]．中华医史杂志，2013，43(1)：18

六、民族医药

【概述】

2013年民族医药的研究内容十分丰富，有文献整理、临床应用、医学理论、药物研究等。

1. 医学研究

（1）文献整理　罗彦慧等从回医药历史研究、理论研究、文献和文化研究、方剂和治疗方法等方面总结了回族医药的发展。提出回医药研究新的突破口应以回医药的历史和现状调查研究为主，用文献搜集和田野调查相结合的方式，梳理历史文献中的回医药信息，并挖掘散落民间丰富的回医药资源，吸纳回族伊斯兰文化，从而理清回医药发展史并构建出回医药的理论体系，以解决回医药学的概念问题，为回医药在医学领域的深入研究奠定基础。和虹研究认为纳西族东巴文医书《聚血》隐含了纳西族朴素的血液生成观念与独特的血液聚集呈周期性循环的理论，是第一部纳西族血液流动（空间）与时间关系的文献，开古代纳西族医学理论的先河。王庆林认为《中国药典》（2010年版）中民族习用药材与成方制剂在品种来源、名称、性味归经、功能主治、使用注意等文字术语的描述上存在不足之处，建议修订并规范。郑蓉等认为要重视民族医药文献的抢救性发掘整理出版工作，这是继承发扬民族医药最基础的工作，是促进民族医药学术交流与传播的重要手段。

（2）理论探讨　胡建山等对水族医药治疗骨折的原则进行了整理归纳，已初步建立了水族医药在骨伤治疗的理论体系。雅森·米吉提等报道维吾尔族正常及异常人群血清C肽、癌胚抗原（CEA）、糖化血清蛋白含量存在差异，异常血液质型组血清C肽含量偏高可能是异常血液质型人群对糖尿病的易感性较低的原因所在，异常黑胆质型组血清CEA含量偏高可能是这一类型人群易患恶性肿瘤的分子基础。王毅蓉等从组方药物紧凑、剂型单一、炮制简单、植物药为主、药物别名多、药用部位多、常用鲜品、疗法多样和擅用药膳9个方面分析了哈尼族验方的特点。

（3）临床报道　王艺润等介绍了藏医对糖尿病病因、症状的认识及治疗，并从有效成分、新药开发等不同角度综述了现代藏药（含附方）在糖尿病治疗中的应用。阿扎提古丽·沙塔尔等报道用成熟剂、清除剂、联合用药等维吾尔药物治疗异常黑胆质型良性卵巢上皮性肿瘤30例，结果B超检查囊肿消失或明显缩小。马红梅等用壮药“乳腺消癖汤”（舞草、益母草、糯米条、小木通、丝瓜络、橘核等）治疗乳腺增生46例，治疗3个月经周期，结果总有效率为97.8%（45/46）。李莉等采用壮药班氏抗炎1号（鸡血藤、苏木、三七、马鞭草、忍冬藤、莪术等）保留灌肠治疗湿热瘀结型盆腔炎性后遗症40例，对照组40例采用西药治疗。15 d为1个疗程，治疗3个疗程后，两组有效率分别为92.5%（37/40）、72.5%（29/40），组间比较$P<0.05$。治疗后症状积分、体征积分改善比较，治疗组明显优于对照组（$P<0.01$）。金丽娟等报道蒙西医结合治疗溃疡性结肠炎46例，治疗4周后，总有效率为100%。库力木汗等采用哈医乌特热玛加塔热特勒克疗法治疗盆腔炎150例，经治10～15 d后，总有效率为95.6%（72/75）。索南卓玛等研究认为藏医烟尔灸法治疗“隆偏盛型失眠症”的疗效优于传统方法。

2. 药学研究

（1）品种资源　余华丽等报道畲族药用蕨类植物品种共24科31属37种1变种，初步查清了畲族药用旋类植物资源及分布情况。郑希龙等报道海南万宁市黎族传统药用植物共有202种，分布于80科171属，其中草本植物最多（81种，40.1%），其次为灌木（53种，26.2%）、乔木（36种，17.8%）和藤本（32种，15.8%）。叶或枝叶的使用频次最高（143次，46.3%），其次是根或根茎（73次，23.6%）、全草或全株（56次，18.1%）。万定荣等对有毒民族药的概念与范畴、资源种类、主要科属特点、毒性成分类别及应用进行研究，并就加强有毒民族药的研究与应用提出建议。杜远等报道四川平武白马藏区共有85个科223种中草药和22个偏验方，可用于治疗跌打损伤。

(2) 质量标准　田成旺等采用薄层色谱法对川西獐牙菜药材进行定性鉴别，并用HPTLC测定其主要活性成分獐牙菜苦苷、芒果苷、当药醇苷和齐墩果酸的含量。王晶晶等研究发现，藏药熏倒牛药材显微结构中导管、腺毛及非腺毛较多，可见纤维束散在或成束分布，存在花粉粒，叶表皮细胞中可见气孔等结构，平均含水量为9.80%，木犀草素平均含量为0.745 mg/g。冷英莉等报道维药金锁昆都尔片在定性鉴别中木香烃内酯在0.03～0.07 mg/ml范围内呈良好线性关系(r=0.999 5)，平均回收率为99.31%，RSD为0.62%；去氢木香内酯在0.06～0.14 mg/ml范围内呈良好线性关系(r=1)，平均回收率为99.33%，RSD为0.70%。刘华钢等报道壮药笔管草的薄层色谱，与山柰素对照品在同一位置显相同颜色的荧光斑点；HPTLC定量分析中，山柰素线性范围为0.049～0.539 μg(r=0.999 8)，平均回收率为98.41%，RSD=1.78%。雷沛霖等报道壮药茉莉花的鉴别方法专属性强，槲皮素和山柰素分别进样量在0.400 8～3.206 4 μg和0.040 3～3.225 6 μg范围内，与HPTLC峰面积呈良好线性关系。苏青等报道广西不同产地10批壮药血党均具有相同的性状、显微及TLC色谱特征，浸出物5.1%～10.75%，水分9.201%～12.3%，总灰分5.2%～7.8%，酸不溶性灰分0.1%～0.5%。徐荔等报道傣药黑面神植物来源明确，显微鉴别和薄层色谱鉴别的重现性好、专属性强，水分、总灰分、酸不溶性灰分、浸出物限度设定合理，急性毒性试验结果LD_{50}为123.87 g生药/kg。旦增曲培报道藏药材鸭嘴花与2个代用品(仟毛婆婆纳、赛北紫堇)中的成分在色谱中显有相同颜色的斑点。

(3) 化学成分　孙洁等报道从蒙古黄芪分离得到14个化合物，分别鉴定为红车轴草素、芒柄花素、芒柄花素-7-O-β-D葡萄糖苷、毛蕊异黄酮、毛蕊异黄酮-7-O-β-D葡萄糖苷、(6aR,11aR)-3-羟基-9,10-二甲氧基紫檀烷、(6aR,11aR)9,10-二甲氧基紫檀烷-3-O-β-D-葡萄糖苷、黄芪皂苷Ⅰ、乙酰黄芪皂苷Ⅱ、黄芪皂苷Ⅱ、异黄芪皂苷Ⅱ、腺嘌呤、β-谷甾醇、胡萝卜苷。从蒙古黄芪中主要分离得到是黄酮类和皂苷类化合物。晏永明等报道从彝药日本琵琶甲虫 *Blaps japonensis* 中分离得到9个化合物，分别鉴定为N-乙酰基多巴胺(1)、(-)N-acetylnoradrenaline(2)、1,4-diacetamidobutane(3)、N,N′-pentane-1,5-diyldiacetamide(4)、(1H-indol-3-yl)oxoacetamide(5)、吲哚酸(6)、吲哚醛(7)、deoxyuridine(8)和胸苷(9)。化合物6对HL-60、SMMC-7721、A-549、MCF-7和SW480细胞株有显著抑制作用。许良等报道首次从蒙药森登-4汤中分离得到6个化合物，通过波谱解析鉴定它们的结构为杨梅素、阿魏酸、2α,3β-双氢杨梅树皮素没食子酸酯、2α,3β-双氢杨梅树皮素、槲皮素、苯甲酸。顾青等报道从藏药镰形棘豆 *Oxytropis falcata* 乙醇提取物中分离得到了5个化合物，分别为7-甲氧基二氢黄酮(1)、7羟基二氢黄酮(2)、2′,4′-羟基查耳酮(3)、2′,4′-二羟基-4-甲基查尔酮(4)、N-(2-苯乙基)肉桂酰胺(5)。用四甲基偶氮唑盐比色法表明化合物3具有较好的抗肿瘤活性，对5种肿瘤细胞的增殖具有明显的抑制作用。IC_{50}分别为68.60、169.67、105.88、175.18、172.37 μmol/L。其中化合物5为首次从该种属中分离得到。

(4) 药理作用　王志旺等报道0.150～0.300 g/kg的甘肃产藏药五脉绿绒蒿总黄酮能降低CCl_4、TAA或AP诱发肝损伤小鼠的血清ALT和AST($P<0.01$)，提高CCl_4或TAA诱发肝损伤小鼠肝组织SOD与GSH-Px的活性($P<0.05$,$P<0.01$)，降低CCl_4或AP诱发肝损伤小鼠肝组织MDA的含量($P<0.01$)；同时在0.075～0.300 g/kg甘肃产藏药五脉绿绒蒿总黄酮的肝损伤保护作用显示出一定的量效关系。

(陈仁寿　程　旺)

【藏族医药研究】

1. 理论研究

仁增多杰等探讨了现存最早的藏医药著作《月王药诊》中的尿诊法理论，认为在公元8世纪时藏医尿诊技术基本成熟，建立了独具特色的尿诊技术体系，其理论是以寒热学说和三因学说为理论基础，以五源学说和五行学说为哲学基础。《月王药诊》尿诊法既是一部译作，又是一部整合医学的代表。姚晓武等对藏医文献中有关尿诊所涉及的尿液采集、观察、诊断的方法进行了系统整理，并指出目前尿诊研究存在的问题。端智认为传统藏医文化具有兼容并蓄的学术体系、因地制宜的应用方式以及生死随缘的医疗观念三点特质,并认为对于生态语境的适应性、对于佛教文明的继承性以及对于现代科技的整合性,是藏医学的发展源泉。桑吉才让从藏医的季节与日常起居养生、天人相应与养生、食养及心身养生四个方面探讨了藏医的养生理论。姚晓武从“真布病”临床分型、临床表现、治疗方法及调养护理等方面总结了藏族医家向·初称江楚治疗该病的学术思想和临床经验。邱建智报道,藏医方剂配伍是通过六味、八性、十七效、三化味有机组合进行组分,临床施药绝大部分是由数味药物组成的复方,具有多靶点、多环节、整体性调节机体的特点。

2. 实验研究

熊天琴等研究发现,甲嘎松汤(干姜、豆蔻、肉豆蔻)有一定的保肝作用,与 Nrf_2 激活剂叔丁基对苯二酚有协同效应,能纠正 Nrf_2 持续激活导致的细胞损伤。红梅等研究发现,玛奴西汤颗粒(藏木香、悬钩木、宽筋藤、干姜)能显著延长小鼠的痛阈值($P<0.01$),显著减少小鼠的扭体次数($P<0.05$)、自主活动($P<0.05$)和站立次数($P<0.01$),并且明显缩短戊巴比妥钠阈下睡眠剂量诱导小鼠入睡潜伏期($P<0.01$),增加入睡个数。张燕等研究发现,藏药小檗皮对四氧嘧啶所致糖尿病模型小鼠血糖有明显降糖作用,对正常小鼠血糖无明显作用。薛浩等报道藏药哇夏嘎对治疗组与模型组大鼠脑组织 MMP－9 表达在脑缺血再灌注损伤后均有不同程度升高,并在起病 24～48 h 到达高峰,且治疗组凋亡细胞数目、MMP－9 的表达水平均低于同一时间点的模型组,差异均具有统计学意义($P<0.05$)。

3. 药材资源研究

曹雨虹等认为藏药的炮制因其特定的原料、独特的工艺和神奇的效果显示出浓厚的民族特色和丰富的内涵,越来越为国内外研究者所重视。但由于炮制原料的选取局限且复杂、药材短缺、炮制工艺不完备、对炮制品的文献研究和实验研究不够重视,以及藏药炮制品质量标准的缺失严重影响了藏药炮制的发展。提出应采用现代科学的研究方法,加强藏药炮制的文献研究及实验研究,努力完善藏药炮制品的质量标准,使藏药炮制在保持传统炮制特色的条件下更加具有科学性。端智等提出政府在制定藏药临床实验法规时应考虑到藏药的特殊性、藏药生产企业应理解和积极参与藏药新产品的开发、藏药新药研发与临床试验中应认真处理好藏医药继承与创新之间的辩证关系。卢杰等对拉萨市濒危藏药植物种类、含水率、生物量及资源量进行调查研究,认为濒危藏药植物种类多、分布不均、蕴藏量大、经济价值高,建议更新藏药植物濒危等级、加强科学研究、实现资源的可持续开发利用。

(李永亮)

【蒙族医药研究】

1. 理论研究

其贺力嘎报道蒙医学从基础理论到专论都渗透着数字元素,如蒙医学经典著作《四部医典》就用数字“四”命名,主要医学理论分为四部、八支、十一点、十五会、四要,将人体的主要物质分为三根,将人体整个新陈代谢的过程称为“七精素的转化”、将疾病的外因分为四况、将疾病的入侵途径归类为“六径”等。布仁达来总结建国以来蒙医药古籍文献收集、整理基本情况,并指出蒙医药学发展既要有扎实的古籍文献传统知识,又要注重现代研究方法。王晓华等分析了蒙医学与中医学对病因认识的异同,发现二者病因理论在实践中经过长期发展和演变,逐渐形成了各具特色的理论体系。虽然认识方法和认识特点有诸多相似之处,但差异仍是明显的。特布沁等提出要在新的历史条件下实现蒙医药现代化,除了注重蒙医药学的科学文化属性,还应注重人文文化属性。

包勒朝鲁等介绍了蒙医方剂配伍原则及原理、传统剂型、服药方式等基本理论。恩杰等报道了表面解剖学在蒙医施术要害部位体表定位研究中的应用,并制作出体表标准图谱。包格日勒等从正常尿液、病尿和死症尿的诊察阐述蒙医的尿诊法。布图雅等探讨了内源性气体信号分析与蒙医“赫依”之间的相关性,揭示了“赫依”的部分物质基础。

2. 临床及实验研究

乌日图探讨了蒙医传统银质器具在刮痧疗法中的应用,认为银制器具属冷器具,导热性能好,有较强的杀菌能力,具有活血化瘀、清热止痛、祛黄水、改善和调节气血运行等功能,且疗效确切、价格低廉、操作简便的优点。秀兰等用蒙医理论分析乳腺增生病的病因病机,认为乳腺增生病属于蒙医学"七素布日勒都森病"范畴。苏荣高娃报道蒙药伊赫汤治疗药物过敏，是在蒙医学三根学说理论指导下，以"赫依(气)-希拉(热)-巴达干(寒)"理论对"药物过敏"应用独特"三根调节法"(抑"赫依"、清"希拉"、祛"巴达干")进行有效治疗。特木其乐总结了阿古拉的学术思想与临床经验，并介绍了其自拟方萨乌日勒(以额尔敦乌日勒、嘎日迪-13味为君药)，用于治疗萨病的急性期和恢复期。巴特金等总结了蒙药解酒药物如诃子、干姜、土木香、当归、黑冰片，解酒处方如毛勒日达布斯-4、伊赫哈日-12的解酒功效。韩额尔德木图等研究发现内蒙古自治区呼和浩特市及周边地区慢性心衰以赫依、齐素交搏型居多，其次是巴达干、赫依偏盛型。

米热古丽·卡米力等研究发现，艾菲提蒙汤(菟丝草、卡布尔诃子、西青果、毛诃子、玫瑰花、清泻山扁豆等)在3.3～13.0 g/kg剂量范围内，可明显降低实验性动脉粥样硬化家兔血清中总胆固醇(TC)、甘油三酯(TG)、高密度脂蛋白-胆固醇(HDL-C)、丙二醛(MDA)含量，升高血清中超氧化物歧化酶(SOD)、过氧化氢酶(CAT)、谷胱甘肽过氧化物酶(GSH-Px)、NO水平。李岚等研究发现，古日古木高、中、低剂量组不同程度抑制CCl_4损伤后血浆中谷丙转氨酶(ALT)和谷草转氨酶(AST)的异常增高，提高血清和肝脏中SOD活性，减少MDA形成，降低小鼠肝脏MDA含量，并降低肝组织的NO，升高血浆中总蛋白、白蛋白水平，减轻肝脏疏松化及脂肪变性。表明古日古木对CCl_4所致急性肝损伤有一定的保护作用。纳仁高娃等研究发现，蒙药复方特润舒都乐石油醚提取物能抑制炎症细胞中TNF-α、IL-6以及IL-1β等细胞因子的活化，具有明显的抗炎作用。

3. 药物研究

海潭等通过对比中蒙"草本类"药物以及交叉品种药用部位间的异同点，发现《四部医典》记载中蒙交叉使用的漏芦花、秦艽、茵陈、黄柏等10种药材的药用部位不同。阿里穆斯等报道内蒙古地区分布有50多种蒿属药用植物，中药和蒙药植物资源在种类组成、分类群、药用部位、功能、生活型、生态类型及其地理分区特征等方面均有显著的异同性，同时普遍存在"同物异名"、"异物同名"现象。

何春龙等报道蒙成药德都红花七味丸用薄层色谱法鉴别斑点清晰，分离度良好，且阴性无干扰；含量测定中羟基红花黄色素A峰形好，分离度符合要求，羟基红花黄色素A在0.186 0～32.64 μg/ml范围内具有良好的线性关系(r=0.999 2)，平均加样回收率为102.2%，RSD为0.72%。包勒朝鲁等报道了石花炮制品的药材性状、显微特征以及水分、总灰分和浸出物的含量。

(李永亮)

【蒙药德都红花-7味散治疗肝损伤的实验研究】

娜日苏等将60只大鼠随机均分为正常对照组、模型组、秋水仙碱组、德都红花-7味散(红花、麻黄、天竺黄、木通、蓝盆花、地丁等)高低剂量组，观察德都红花-7味散对实验性肝纤维化大鼠肝功能和纤维化的影响。结果，与模型组比较，德都红花-7味散高、低剂量组均能改善大鼠肝功能、纤维化指标和病理学改变($P<0.05$)，炎症活动度及纤维化程度均降低($P<0.05$)。巴图德力根等研究发现，与空白组比较，德都红花-7味散高低剂量组吞噬率和吞噬指数明显升高($P<0.05$)，脾淋巴细胞培养液吸光度OD值明显升高($P<0.05$)；与模型组比较，德都红花-7味散高低剂量组血清IL-1、IL-6含量均明显降低($P<0.05$)。研究还发现，德都红花-7味散能够明显改善CCL_4所诱导实验性肝纤维化组织病理变化，降低透明质酸、层粘连蛋白、Ⅲ型前胶原、Ⅳ型胶原和IL-1、IL-6、肿瘤坏死因子含量，具有抗肝纤维化作用。韩志强等研究发现，德都红花-7味散能明显改善CCl_4引起慢性大鼠肝损伤组织病理改变，其机理可能与抗脂质过氧化、提高Na^+-K^+-ATP酶活性、改善肝线粒体钠泵功能有关。包玉华等研究表明，德都红花-7味散对D-半乳糖胺所致小鼠急性肝损伤具有保肝降酶作用，并能够明显增加小鼠胆汁分泌量，增强小鼠腹腔巨噬细胞吞噬功能，对ConA诱导的淋巴细胞增值有促进作用。

(李永亮)

【壮族医药研究】

1. 理论研究

覃文波等从壮医"毒"之定义、"毒"致痛的病因病机、"毒"致痛的分类三方面阐述壮医"毒"致痛说，将"毒"致痛分类为痧毒痛、瘴毒痛、蛊毒痛、风毒痛、湿毒痛、中毒痛(根药中毒、根东洋中毒、图腾河中毒、其他毒中毒)6 种,并介绍 6 类痛症的常用内服药物、外治法及其止痛机理。韦金香研究了毒理论、毒与妇科病的关系、毒理论在妇科中的运用三个方面,认为壮医常用清热祛湿解毒药、调气解毒兼顾补虚、擅长调气解毒外治法、综合疗法能提高壮医妇科临床的疗效。王柏灿总结了壮医湿毒理论研究,认为湿毒致病主要与地理气候有关,"湿毒"是风湿痹病的病因之一,黄疸、肝炎、鼻渊、肛门湿疹、腰椎间盘突出症的发病与湿毒有关,湿毒治疗有药线点灸、药物竹罐疗法、熨浴、壮药等方法。宋宁报道壮医"三气同步"的天人自然观,认为是壮医基础理论的核心思想之一,同于中医学"整体观念"。人如做到"三气同步"、平衡、和谐则健康无病,不同步、失衡则变生诸病,临床治疗时要强调三气的"通"、"动"、"衡"。宋氏还报道壮医气血的概念、内涵及其关系,提出平衡气血治则治法,阐述壮医的理法方药体系。洪宗国等论述了壮医伤病的概念与诊断方法,总结了正骨疗法、经筋疗法、药线点灸、鲜药疗法等壮医伤病的特色治疗方法,介绍了各类治疗创伤的方剂与常用药物。还论述了壮医治疗虚病,研究了不同虚病的病因、病理和临床症状、治疗方法及常用补虚药。

2. 临床及实验研究

唐红珍等将 150 例超重、肥胖患者随机均分为两组,分别采用壮医调气畅龙内服方(五指牛奶、土茯苓、土人参、山菠萝、黄花倒水莲、罗汉果等)和西药赛尼可胶囊治疗,30 d 为 1 个疗程。治疗 2 个疗程后,治疗组总有效率为 92.0%(69/75),对照组为 88.0%(66/75),组间比较无显著性差异。两组治疗后肥胖指征、血脂均明显降低,且治疗组更显著($P<0.05$,$P<0.01$)。朱红梅将 200 例甲状腺机能亢进症患者随机均分为两组,分别采用壮医灯心草灸疗法和口服他巴唑治疗,15 次为 1 个疗程。治疗 4 个疗程后,两组总有效率分别为 91.0%(91/100)、79.0%(79/100),组间比较$P<0.05$。侯田培等采用壮医莲花针背廊拔罐法治疗变应性鼻炎患者 30 例,取肺俞、大椎、定喘、项棱穴、壮医加脊穴等,隔天 1 次,15 次为 1 个疗程。叩刺部位包括循路叩刺(依龙路、火路)和循点叩刺(如肺俞、大椎、定喘、至阳等)。对照组 30 例采用辅舒良鼻喷雾剂,1 次/d,治疗 30 d,两组总有效率分别为 86.7%(26/30)、76.7%(23/30),组间比较无显著性差异。治疗后两组生活质量评分分别为(55.73±6.73)、(60.10±8.38),较治疗前明显降低($P<0.05$),且治疗组明显优于对照组($P<0.05$)。

王志萍等研究发现,妇雅净提取物高、中剂量能够较好的抑制二甲苯引起的小鼠耳肿胀($P<0.01$),高剂量抑制冰醋酸致小鼠毛细血管通透性增加($P<0.05$),高、中、低剂量均能抑制小鼠棉球肉芽增生($P<0.01$)。张青青等观察发现,将壮药香花护乳凝胶剂(檀香、野菊花等)涂于白色家兔背部完整及破损去毛皮肤,结果无明显局部刺激性。倪玲等研究发现,广西壮药姜三七能剂量依赖性改善雌、孕激素负荷大鼠子宫色泽、肿胀以及结节,减轻雌、孕激素负荷大鼠子宫重量,减小子宫系数,降低子宫平滑肌层厚度。梁宁等研究表明,依山红对于 CCL_4 所致小鼠急性肝损伤具有一定的保肝降酶作用,且醇提物优于水提物。

3. 药物研究

庞宇舟等收集了壮医治疗气道病方剂 187 首,建立了方剂数据库,并运用关联规则分析壮医气道病方剂用药和配伍规律。结果,在所用的 227 种壮药中,排名前 10 位的高频药物为山芝麻、枇杷叶、石仙桃等,使用总频次为 1 122 次。符合最小支持度和置信度的二联规则集 11 条,三联规则集 7 条,四联规则集 4 条。黄岛平等测定广西 12 个不同产地的土垅大白蚁菌圃多糖的单糖组成,结果发现均含有甘露糖、鼠李糖、半乳糖醛酸、葡萄糖、半乳糖、木糖、阿拉伯糖,10 批样品中半乳糖醛酸相近,说明不同产地来源的土垅大白蚁菌圃多糖含有的单糖组分是基本一致的,且大部分样品的品质较优,对鉴别土垅大白蚁菌圃和评估不同产地土垅大白蚁菌圃药材的质量有重要意义。

(胡　菲)

【回医香药研究】

回医香药疗法是利用回药中芳香性动植物药来防治疾病,增进身心健康的医疗保健方法。近年来临床研究越来越多。

徐静等对目前仅存的一部十分珍贵的回回医药典籍《回回药方》中具有生肌功效方剂的概念、命名、用法及使用特点进行研究,阐明回医方剂与用药特色,多采用回药与华化的海药并用。在 20

首方剂中，所用药物 74 种，其中属于回药有 36 种，使用频率较高的药物有兀沙吉、安咱鲁的、檐木阿黑云、没药、飞古刺、密陀僧、咱刺弯。所用的赋形剂有鸡子清、醋、赛的油、黄蜡、兔儿毛，具有回族特色。李婷婷等对 101 首回药治疗脑卒中方剂进行筛选和整理，发现单味药物胡椒、荜拔、撒法郎、安息香、没药等香药出现的频次较多。并对其中部分药材阿拉伯名与中草药名一一对应，将同一药材的不同阿拉伯名进行统一，同时对香药的使用情况进行考证。

马晓燕介绍了闻香疗法、熏香疗法以及药袋疗法 3 种回医香药疗法。闻香疗法常用的香药有檀香、沉香、艾叶、菖蒲、樟脑、山苍子等，均可配制用于熏、蒸、佩、挂、洒等。熏香疗法主要有醋香法、药熏法和烟熏法。药袋疗法包括香袋疗法、药枕疗法以及肚兜疗法。徐保宁等介绍了回医香药常用的外用剂型，主要有膏剂、糊剂、贴剂、舔剂、露剂、熏洗剂、熏香剂等。

薛新民等介绍了回医香药在复发性口疮、疱疹性口炎、口腔念珠菌病、口腔白斑病等口腔黏膜病中的应用。周波等研究了回回甘松饮（甘松、枸杞、没药、芸香、香芋草、松蕈等）防治湿温病的作用。认为其具有以湿重于热为主、能宣上畅中泄下的治疗特点。并通过实验发现，回回甘松饮能够显著降低湿热证大鼠血清 G－CSF 水平，升高 NO 水平。李娟等研究发现，回医善用香药治疗脑血管疾病，芳香开窍回医回药调控血脑屏障通透性可对脑缺血神经细胞损伤发挥保护作用。

（胡　菲）

【土家族医药研究】

1. 基础研究

洪宗国从土家族来源与演化史、生存环境、经济和科技发展水平等方面探索了土家医药思想源流，认为土家医药根植于土家文化与大中华文化，擅用术数，在一气整体观、阳主阴从阴阳观、三元结构理论方面均较中医有所发挥，形成土家医药哲学内核，应用于生理病理与药理。虽然土家族医药发展水平低于中医药，但在疾病的治疗方法与药材的应用方面富有特色。田华咏等应用文献整理，对不同时代土家族医药的内涵、概念、特点、特色、外延进行总结与提炼，阐明土家族医药发展规律、理论框架及体系。梁正海总结了土家族治病用药的特点，主要有疗病类型和治疗效果与药物生长的空间对应关系、人体组织器官与药物形状在治疗上的对应性、用药时的现采现用以及治疗过程中的药物道具化四个方面。并在此基础上认为应从文化视角认识民间医药知识的科学性，为民间医药知识的传承和发展营造一个良好的环境。

2. 临床研究

奚胜艳等总结象国鼎教授治疗胃脘痛、肝硬化的经验。治疗胃脘痛遵循“同病异治”等中医辨证论治法则，认为消化系统疾患用药切忌偏寒偏热，寒温互用为宜，临证中常以百合与乌药、黄连与吴茱萸、肉桂与黄连等寒温相配药对为主，并随证化裁来治疗胃脘痛，取得明显疗效。认为肝硬化常见病机要素为湿、瘀、气滞等，且肝硬化患者大多存在营养欠佳的情况，因而治疗的全过程注重运用“扶正消癥”之法。对于临床常见的脾肾阳虚、瘀热内结、气虚寒胀等证，处方中多运用黄芪、白术、干姜、甘草等补中健脾扶正之品，使湿去胀除正而不虚，并常配伍枳实、柴胡、青皮、陈皮等理气行气药，使得补而不碍胀消。治疗上还常结合早期 LC 的病机，多采用上下分消湿瘀以除胀满之策，喜用中满分消丸（汤）。杨湘跃介绍了土家族外治法在外科疾病中的应用，包括药物疗法、拔罐疗法、麝针疗法、瓦针疗法、放血疗法、烧灯火、烧灸法、药浴疗法、熏蒸疗法及挑背筋法。

3. 药物资源研究

熊鹏辉报道了石门县境内的土家族珍稀赶火败毒药，有金钱吊葫芦、七叶一枝花、八角莲和九龙胆 4 种药物的形态特征、生长环境、资源分布、性味归经、主治功效以及土家治验方。并在全国第四次中药资源普查中，采用实地调查和走访相结合的方法，对湘西北石门县中药资源进行了调查，发现湘西北土家药材开喉箭的基源植物有 3 种，即紫金牛科朱砂根、百两金和红凉伞。

（田　娟）

【民族医药治疗关节炎的临床及实验研究】

吴刚等应用关联规则研究苗医治疗风湿类疾病用药规律。结果，在治疗风湿类疾病的 348 首验方中共使用 217 种药物 1 901 频次。其中，使用频次在 15 次以上的依次为见血飞、鸡血藤、威灵仙、八角枫、松节等 40 味苗药；关联规则方法分析出以类风湿性关节炎/白三七、风湿性关节炎/松节、风湿腰痛/川续断为典型的症/药关联 15 例;置信度在 15%以上的药对松节/威灵仙、鸡血藤/松节、见血飞/鸡血藤等 105 对。尹智功等采用瑶医药饼(断肠草、大黄、黄柏、两面针、宽筋藤、威灵仙等)外敷联合加味茵陈宣痹汤(防己、苍术、茵陈、黄柏、牛膝、薏苡仁等)治疗 30 例急性痛风性关节炎,并与秋水仙碱组 30 例作对照。治疗 1 周后,治疗组患者的关节疼痛及压痛、关节红肿及关节活动障碍的减轻程度及血尿酸值和血沉值的下降程度均优于对照组($P<0.05$),且不良反应低于对照组($P<0.05$)。叶一萍等予畲药小香勾合刺络拔罐治疗急性痛风性关节炎患者,具有较好的疗效,且无明显胃肠道反应。斯琴高娃等将 70 例膝关节骨性关节炎患者随机均分为两组,予玻璃酸钠关节内注射疗法,治疗组在此基础上行蒙医银针加热疗法。1 次/周,治疗 5 次。结果,与治疗前比较,治疗组 Lysholm 膝关节评分和疼痛 VAS 评分均有明显改善($P<0.05$),且治疗组优于对照组($P<0.05$)。

杨本扎西等根据藏医辨证将 175 例类风湿性关节炎患者分为热、寒性两组,热性又随机分为治疗 1 组(37 例)、2 组(40 例),寒性又随机分为治疗 3 组(49 例)、4 组(49 例)。各组药浴药物配方均用热性水柏枝、小叶杜鹃、刺柏、大籽蒿、麻黄。治疗 1 组:口服药:七味宽筋藤散、十八味党参丸、十五味乳鹏散、风湿止痛散。外治理疗:青鹏涂剂用温开水调匀后涂于肿胀疼痛局部。治疗 2 组:口服药:七味宽筋藤散、十八味党参丸。外治理疗:青鹏涂剂与九味青鹏散用温开水调匀后涂于肿胀疼痛局部。寒性治疗 3 组:口服药:五味润疆汤散、安置精化散、二十五味儿茶丸、二十五味驴血丸。外治理疗:五味甘露加买麸皮、麻渣等炒热敷于肿胀疼痛局部。艾灸:选阿氏穴施灸,特别是趋于变形的关节部位。治疗 4 组:口服药:五味润疆汤散、二十五味儿茶丸。外治理疗与艾灸同治疗 3 组。疗程为(60±5)d。结果,4 组的总有效率分别为 94.6%(35/37)、95.0%(38/40)、95.9%(47/49)、98.0%(48/49),无显著差异($P>0.05$),各组与治疗前比较均有显著差异($P<0.05$)。

邢沙沙等将 60 只大鼠随机均分为正常组、模型组、甲氨蝶呤组、壮药龙钻通痹方(飞龙掌血、大钻、八角枫、两面针、青风藤、九龙藤等)高中低剂量组,结果发现,龙钻通痹方各剂量组均可提高实验性关节炎大鼠模型抗炎因子 IL-4、IL-10 水平,与其他组比较,差异有显著性($P<0.05$)。张青槐等研究发现,龙钻通痹方能显著降低大鼠血清 TNF-α、γ-干扰素水平($P<0.05$ 或 $P<0.01$),其作用优于甲氨喋呤($P<0.05$ 或 $P<0.01$)。姚合梅等研究表明,苗药验方(透骨香、见血飞、黑骨藤、追风伞、大风藤、艾纳香等)皮部熏洗的干预,对骨关节炎模型大鼠的痛行为及膝关节活动有明显的改善作用。可通过上调软骨增值细胞核抗原及转化生长因子 $β_1$ 的表达,促进软骨细胞的增殖,加速软骨的修复,达到防治目的,且熏洗法治疗比单独运用熏法、洗法效果更明显。

(田　娟)

[附]　参 考 文 献

A

阿里穆斯,庄丽,李亚伟,等.内蒙古蒿属药用植物资源调查及其在中药与蒙药中的应用比较[J].辽宁中医杂志,2013,40(4):770

阿扎提古丽·沙塔尔,来提帕·买买提.维医药治疗良性卵巢上皮性肿瘤[J].中国民族医药杂志,2013,19(6):24

B

巴特金,吴超群,朝鲁巴根,等.蒙药解酒作用的研究进展[J].中国民族医药杂志,2013,19(4):57

巴图德力根,韩志强,娜日苏.德都红花-7 味散对 CCl_4 诱导实验性肝纤维化疗效和 IL-1、IL-6、TNF-α 的影响[J].中国免疫学杂志,2012,28(4):316

巴图德力根,徐艳华,韩志强,等.德都红花-7 味散对猪血清诱导慢性肝纤维化大鼠 IL-1、IL-6、TNF-α 及对小鼠脾淋巴细胞、巨噬细胞的影响[J].中药药理与临床,2013,29(1):116

包格日勒,色音宝音.浅谈蒙医对尿液的诊察[J].中国民族民间医药,2013,22(6):13

包勒朝鲁,乌兰图雅,那生桑.蒙药材石化炮制品质量标准研究[J].现代中药研究与实践,2013,26(2):63

包勒朝鲁,乌兰图雅,那生桑.论蒙医方剂学基本理论[J].中华中医药杂志,2013,28(7):1954

包玉华，巴图德力根，乌恩宝音，等. 德都红花-7味散保肝利胆及调节免疫功能的实验研究[J]. 中华中医药学刊，2013，31(7)：1575

布仁达来. 蒙医药古籍文献的整理与研究[J]. 中国民族医药杂志，2013，19(5)：68

布图雅，佟红霞. 内源性气体信号分子与蒙医赫依的相关性探讨[J]. 中国民族医药杂志，2013，19(2)：5

C

曹雨虹，顾健，谭睿，等. 藏药炮制特色及现存问题分析[J]. 中华中医药学刊，2013，31(4)：753

D

旦增曲培. 初探藏药3种“巴夏嘎”的成分[J]. 中国民族医药杂志，2013，19(4)：23

杜远，杨瑶珺，孙志蓉，等. 四川平武白马藏族骨伤科用药的调查整理[J]. 中国民族医药杂志，2013，19(4)：26

端智. 藏医文化的现代解读[J]. 青海师范大学学报(哲学社会科学版)，2013，35(2)：78

端智，孙泰俊，娘毛才. 浅析我国临床研究法规对藏药生产机构的影响——以青海省为例[J]. 中国民族医药杂志，2013，19(5)：39

E

恩杰，斯钦图. 论表面解剖学在蒙医施术要害部位体表定位研究中的应用[J]. 时珍国医国药，2013，24(3)：765

G

顾青，蔡银娜，杨光明，等. 藏药镰形棘豆的化学成分及其抗肿瘤活性研究[J]. 中国实验方剂学杂志，2013，19(11)：72

H

海潭，松林. 蒙药与中药交叉品种的药用部位对比探讨[J]. 中国民族医药杂志，2013，19(6)：41

韩额尔德木图，孟永梅. 慢性心衰的蒙医辨证分析研究[J]. 内蒙古医学杂志，2013，45(5)：544

韩志强，巴图德力根，娜日苏，等. 蒙药德都红花-7味散对慢性肝损伤大鼠肝组织SOD、MDA及肝线粒体钠钾ATP酶活性的影响[J]. 中华中医药学刊，2013，31(5)：1076

何春龙，王焕芸，莎日娜. 蒙成药德都红花七味丸中红花的质量标准研究[J]. 现代中药研究与实践，2013，26(2)：67

和虹. 纳西族东巴文医书《聚血》的发现与浅析[J]. 中国民族民间医药，2013，22(4)：1

红梅，陈秋红，王志瑾，等. 藏药玛奴西汤颗粒镇痛镇静作用的实验研究[J]. 时珍国医国药，2013，24(2)：373

洪宗国. 土家医药思想特色[J]. 中南民族大学学报(自然科学版)，2013，32(3)：30

洪宗国，邓小莲. 壮医伤病论[J]. 中南民族大学学报(自然科学版)，2013，32(1)：36

洪宗国，邓小莲. 壮医虚病论[J]. 中南民族大学学报(自然科学版)，2013，32(2)：55

侯田培，黄贵华，黄谨明，等. 壮医莲花针背廊拔罐法对30例变应性鼻炎患者生活质量的影响[J]. 中国中西医结合杂志，2013，33(5)：705

胡建山，李溥，李文忠，等. 水族医药骨伤临床实践与理论构建的系统研究[J]. 北京中医药，2013，32(5)：358

黄岛平，苏青，黄瑞松，等. 不同产地壮药土垅大白蚁菌圃多糖中单糖组分的测定与品质评价[J]. 时珍国医国药，2013，24(5)：1175

J

金丽娟. 蒙西医结合治疗溃疡性结肠炎46例临床观察[J]. 中国民族医药杂志，2013，19(3)：23

K

库力木汗，加依娜古丽·尔斯别克. 哈医乌特热玛加塔热特勒克疗法治疗盆腔炎150例疗效观察[J]. 中国民族民间医药，2013，22(2)：3

L

雷沛霖，黄瑞松，苏青，等. 壮药茉莉花质量标准研究[J]. 中药材，2013，36(5)：731

冷英莉，孙桂琳，陈菊. 维药金锁昆都尔片的质量标准研究[J]. 现代中药研究与实践，2013，26(2)：59

李娟，刘敬霞，刘洋，等. 回医芳香开窍方药调控血脑屏障的意义和研究进展[J]. 辽宁中医杂志，2013，40(8)：1719

李岚，马丽杰. 古日古木对小鼠CCl_4急性肝损伤模型的影响[J]. 内蒙古中医药，2013，32(11)：46

李莉，杨意兰，余昭胜，等. 壮药班氏抗炎1号保留灌肠治疗湿热瘀结型盆腔炎性疾病后遗症临床观察[J]. 新中医，2013，45(1)：100

李婷婷，董琳，陈国霆，等. 回药治疗脑卒中方剂收集整理[J]. 中国中药杂志，2013，38(14)：2412

梁宁，卢汝梅，李兵，等. 壮药依山红对四氯化碳所致急性肝损小鼠保肝作用研究[J]. 大众科技，2013，15(11)：114

梁正海. 论土家族疗病用药的四大特点[J]. 贵州师范大学学报(社会科学版)，2013，(3)：71

刘华钢，梁美艳，宁带连，等. 壮药笔管草的质量标准研究[J]. 广西中医药，2013，36(2)：57

卢杰，兰小中. 拉萨市珍稀濒危藏药植物资源调查研究[J]. 中国中药杂志，2013，38(1)：127

罗彦慧,方华林.百年回医药研究述评[J].回族研究,2013,(3):111

M

马红梅,马玲,莫智珍.壮药“乳腺消癖汤”治疗乳腺增生46例临床观察[J].江苏中医药,2013,45(7):35

马晓燕.回医香药疗法[J].中国民族民间医药,2013,22(9):1

米热古丽·卡米力,阿布都吉力力·阿不都艾尼,窦勤,等.艾菲提蒙汤对动脉粥样硬化家兔血脂及抗氧化酶的影响[J].中药药理与临床,2013,29(1):124

N

纳仁高娃,王纯洁,黄丽华.蒙药特润舒都乐提取物抗炎作用研究[J].动物医学进展,2013,34(5):67

娜日苏,巴图德力根,韩志强,等.德都红花-7味散对实验性肝纤维化大鼠肝功能和纤维化的影响[J].中医杂志,2012,53(24):2122

倪玲,刘成军,韦世秀,等.广西壮药姜三七对雌/孕激素负荷大鼠子宫肌瘤的影响[J].时珍国医国药,2013,24(1):128

P

庞宇舟,蒋祖玲,宋宁,等.基于关联规则的壮医气道病用药组方规律研究[J].中国中医基础医学杂志,2013,19(10):1190

Q

其贺力嘎.蒙医学的数字文化探讨[J].中国民间疗法,2013,21(8):50

青拉姆.藏药治疗中风后遗症108例临床疗效观察[J].中国民族民间医药,2013,22(4):8

邱建智.藏药学基础理论与方剂配伍规律的探析[J].西部中医药,2013,26(1):64

R

仁增多杰,才让南加.《月王药诊》中尿诊法理论探讨[J].四川中医,2013,31(6):21

S

桑吉才让.藏医养生保健学初探[J].中国民族医药杂志,2013,19(7):66

斯琴高娃,董秋梅,那仁满都拉.蒙医银针加热配合玻璃酸钠注射液治疗膝骨关节炎35例[J].环球中医药,2013,6(4):286

宋宁.壮医“三气同步”自然观的内涵及其应用[J].中医杂志,2013,54(14):1183

宋宁.壮医气血理论的理论基础与临床应用[J].中华中医药杂志,2013,28(1):35

苏青,梁子宁,黄瑞松,等.壮药材血党质量标准研究[J].中国民族医药杂志,2013,19(3):30

苏荣高娃.蒙药伊赫汤治疗药物过敏经验[J].中国民族民间医药,2013,22(8):2

孙洁,张蕾,张晓拢,等.蒙古黄芪的化学成分研究[J].现代药物与临床,2013,28(2):138

索南卓玛,公保吉.藏医烟尔灸法治疗“隆偏盛型失眠症”的临床应用[J].中国民族民间医药,2013,22(4):9

T

覃文波,李凯风,邓汝铭,等.壮医“毒”致痛说浅析[J].中国民族民间医药,2013,22(4):5

唐红珍,宋宁,刘鹏.壮医调气畅龙内服方对超重、肥胖的疗效[J].中国实验方剂学杂志,2013,19(9):291

特布沁,白长喜.蒙医药现代化应注重蒙医药人文文化和科学文化的有机融合[J].内蒙古医科大学学报,2013,35(S1):198

特木其乐.名老蒙医阿古拉学术思想及临床经验整理[J].中国民族医药杂志,2013,19(1):16

田成旺,张铁军,蒋伶活.藏药川西獐牙菜的质量标准研究[J].中国实验方剂学杂志,2013,19(4):75

田华咏,田兰,梅之南.土家族医药文献调研与整理[J].中国民族医药杂志,2013,19(6):48

W

万定荣.中国有毒民族药资源种类概况及其研究应用中有关问题[J].中华中医药杂志,2013,28(2):297

王柏灿.壮医湿毒理论研究概况[J].中国民族医药杂志,2013,19(5):67

王晶晶,景明,李炀,等.藏药熏倒牛质量标准研究[J].中国中医药信息杂志,2013,20(4):48

王庆林.《中国药典》(2010年版)民族习用药材统计与分析[J].中国实验方剂学杂志,2013,19(12):345

王庆林,程友斌.《中国药典》(2010年版)少数民族药成方制剂处方统计与分析[J].中成药,2013,35(3):639

王晓华,宝龙.蒙医学与中医学对病因认识的异同[J].中医药学报,2013,41(5):4

王艺润,赵存花,汪满江措,等.藏医藏药对糖尿病的认识与治疗[J].中国民族医药杂志,2013,19(10):33

王毅蓉,赵永刚.哈尼族验方特点浅析[J].中国民族民间医药,2013,22(6):9

王志萍,夏星,黎芳,等.壮药妇雅净提取物经皮给药抗炎作用的研究[J].时珍国医国药,2013,24(3):612

王志旺,王瑞琼,郭玫,等.甘肃产藏药五脉绿绒蒿总黄酮对小鼠实验性肝损伤的保护作用[J].中国实验方剂学杂志,2013,19(2):206

韦金杏.壮医毒理论在妇科临床中的应用[J].中国民

族民间医药,2013,22(5):5

乌日图.浅谈蒙医传统银制器具对刮痧疗法中的作用机理[J].时珍国医国药,2013,24(2):430

吴刚,田振华,许召林,等.关联规则应用于苗医治疗风湿类疾病用药规律的研究[J].时珍国医国药,2013,24(2):447

X

奚胜艳,王大伟,赵晖,等.土家族名医向国鼎教授辨证论治肝硬化验案探析[J].中华中医药杂志,2013,28(4):979

奚胜艳,赵晖,王大伟,等.土家族名医向国鼎教授寒温药并用为主治疗胃脘痛验案举要[J].中华中医药杂志,2013,28(9):2641

香虹.蒙药治疗布氏杆菌病37例临床观察[J].中国民族民间医药,2013,22(2):9

邢沙沙,庞宇舟,张青槐,等.壮药龙钻通痹方对实验性关节炎大鼠模型抗炎因子IL-4、IL-10的影响[J].中国民族医药杂志,2013,19(12):44

熊鹏辉.石门县土家珍稀赶火败毒药[J].中国民族医药杂志,2013,19(3):29

熊鹏辉.石门县土家珍稀赶火败毒药之二[J].中国民族医药杂志,2013,19(5):35

熊鹏辉,董森珍,沈美英,等.湘西北土家族开喉箭的基源调查[J].中国民族民间医药,2013,22(14):13

熊天琴,李红侠,陈元元,等.甲嘎松汤对肝损伤的保护作用研究[J].中药药理与临床,2013,29(1):132

秀兰,张彬.用蒙医理论分析乳腺增生病的病因病机[J].中国民族民间医药,2013,22(11):1

徐保宁,王文苹,隋宏.回医香药外用剂型简述[J].宁夏医科大学学报,2013,35(11):1193

徐静,杨丽娟,高如宏.《回回药方》中具有生肌功效的方药浅析[J].时珍国医国药,2013,24(3):700

徐荔,彭霞,王娟,等.傣药材黑面神药材质量标准研究[J].中国民族医药杂志,2013,19(1):35

许良,高扬,刘妍,等.蒙药森登-4汤抗炎镇痛有效部位及其化学成分的研究[J].时珍国医国药,2013,24(1):1

薛浩,刘宁,谷有全,等.藏药哇夏嘎对大鼠脑缺血再灌注损伤保护机制的研究[J].四川中医,2013,31(3):54

薛新民,贺晓慧,罗彦慧,等.回医香药在治疗口腔黏膜病方面的应用[J].山西中医学院学报,2010,11(6):69

Y

雅森·米吉提,阿衣古丽·玉努斯,哈木拉提·吾甫尔,等.维吾尔医学不同体液分型人群血清C肽、癌胚抗原、糖化血清蛋白含量比较及其意义[J].中华中医药杂志,2013,28(7):2081

晏永明,董小萍,李艳,等.彝药日本琵琶甲虫的化学成分及其细胞毒活性[J].中草药,2013,44(3):269

杨本扎西,彭毛东主,辛措吉,等.藏医治疗类风湿性关节炎的临床疗效评价研究[J].中国民族医药杂志,2013,19(5):18

杨湘跃.土家医外治法在外科疾病中的应用[J].中国民族医药杂志,2013,19(1):22

姚合梅,王政,崔瑾,等.苗药验方皮部熏洗对骨关节炎大鼠软骨细胞凋亡与增殖的影响[J].浙江中医药大学学报,2013,37(7):893

姚晓武.藏医向·初称江楚治疗“真布病”临床经验的整理研究[J].中国民族民间医药,2013,22(11):2

姚晓武,徐士奎,柏秀英,等.藏医尿诊理论体系研究纵览[J].中国民族民间医药,2013,22(10):1

叶一萍,王法明,李慧珍.畲药小香勾合刺络拔罐治疗急性痛风性关节炎疗效观察[J].浙江中医杂志,2013,48(2):108

尹智功,刘江,肖敬,等.瑶医药饼外敷联合茵陈宣痹汤治疗急性痛风性关节炎临床观察[J].中国中医药现代远程教育,2013,11(4):13

余华丽,李建良,雷后兴.畲族药用蕨类植物资源调查[J].中国民族医药杂志,2013,19(4):36

Z

张青槐,庞宇舟,邢沙沙,等.壮药龙钻通痹方对关节炎大鼠模型致炎因子TNF-α、IFN-γ的影响[J].中国医疗前言,2013,8(21):9

张青青,余胜民,黄琳芸,等.壮药香花护乳凝胶剂皮肤刺激性实验研究[J].时珍国医国药,2013,24(2):300

张燕,孟宪丽,岳丽珺,等.藏药小檗皮对糖尿病模型小鼠血糖水平影响的初步研究[J].现代生物医学进展,2013,13(19):3619

郑蓉,王梅.论民族医药文献发掘性整理出版[J].中国中医基础医学杂志,2013,19(7):750

郑希龙,戴好富,刘寿柏,等.海南黎族药用植物资源调查研究——以万宁市黎族为例[J].中国民族医药杂志,2013,19(4):20

周波,梁爽,徐全壹,等.回医香药回回甘松饮辨治湿温病举要[J].中国民族医药杂志,2013,19(8):28

周波,徐全壹,梁爽,等.回回甘松饮对温病湿热证大鼠G-CSF和NO的影响[J].内蒙古中医药,2013,32(6):123

朱红梅.壮医灯心草灸治疗甲亢疗效机理研究[J].中国民族医药杂志,2013,19(3):7

七、港澳台中医药

【香港中医药】

1. 临床研究

麻子仁丸是历史悠久的治疗热秘的有效方剂，香港浸会大学卞兆祥课题组自 2006 年开始先后获得两项香港食物及卫生局资助课题，并与香港中文大学合作，使用循证医学研究方法进行麻子仁丸治疗慢性功能性便秘的量效关系、临床疗效及安全性研究。研究结果发表于 2011 年 1 月《美国胃肠病杂志》上。为了进一步完善麻子仁丸治疗实热型功能性便秘的循证医学证据，现正在香港浸会大学，与香港中文大学医学院合作进行第三阶段随机双盲双模拟对照研究，将麻子仁丸组与传统治疗便秘的西药及安慰剂做比较，该研究将为麻子仁丸的临床疗效验证提供更充分的证据，目前该研究正在进行中，已发表了研究方案。

临床研究从开始到完成大致可以分为设计、实行、报告和评价 4 个阶段。由世界卫生组织领导建立的全球临床试验注册制度和制订实施的《随机对照试验报告统一规范》(简称 CONSORT)是目前提高临床研究质量强有力的措施，其中规范了临床研究的报告。自 2001 年发表了 CONSORT，陆续有修订版(Schulz KF 等报道)及扩展版(Campbell MK 等报道)。除了规范的临床研究报告外，高质量的临床研究和研究设计是最关键的因素，因为临床研究方案是临床研究设计的基础。Chan AW 等拟定了"规范临床研究方案内容"2013(简称 SPIRIT 2013 声明)，详细说明了临床研究方案报告条目的内容和要求。自 2007 年开始，由 115 位临床研究相关专家组成的 SPIRIT 工作小组通过多次会议和调研，经过反复修改，形成 2013 SPIRIT 条目清单以及声明与详述并发表在《内科学年鉴》。SPIRIT 中文工作组将该声明翻译成英文，经过 6 个步骤，修改共计 5 稿，在 SPIRIT 研究小组授权下发表中文版，旨在推动临床研究方案公开透明，提高临床研究工作者、杂志编辑、研究评审者及公众对临床研究方案的重视，促进中国临床研究质量的进一步提升(Zhong LD 等报道)。

失眠是都市常见病且在香港发病率逐年上升。Yeung WF 等报道，香港大学钟家辉领导的研究团队系统回顾了中药和针灸治疗失眠的现状及症候分布。在 227 个研究中有 17 916 位患者参与研究，共有 87 个中医证型，其中最常见的证型为肝郁脾虚，而中药复方最常用的有归脾汤、安神定志汤和酸枣仁汤。针灸治疗方面，最常用的穴位是神门、印堂、三阴交、百会、安眠及四神聪。

2. 实验研究

(1) 中药化学及中药质量控制研究　Han QB 等建立了两相液态萃取法分离提取乌头中乌头碱类化合物的方法。Liang Z 等采用 laser microdissection 联合 UPLC 的方法，建立了大黄的特征化学识别模式。Tang Y 等采用 UPLC - qTOF - MS 方法，分析了穿龙薯蓣和黄山药的化学成分，建立了鉴别两种植物的特征指纹图谱。Wong KL 等利用 DNA 指纹的方法，分辨出龙胆及其相似品，并建立了标准 DNA 谱图。Fan LL 等利用 HPTLC - DAD - ESI - TOF - MS 技术分辨出大罗伞的两个相似种属 *Fordiae Cauliflorae* Radix 和 *Millettiae Pulchrae* Radix。Li M 利用 LAMP 技术，建立了白花蛇舌草标准图库。Liang Z 等鉴定了半夏、张叶半夏和水半夏的化学成分，为半夏类药材的质量控制提供新方法。Jaiswal Y 等比较了印度和中国的不同炮制方法对乌头类植物化学成分的影响，发现中国传统炮制方法效果最好。Zhan JY 等分析了酒制白芷和酒制川芎的化学成分，利用 PCA 分析方法，发现 ferulic acid、butylphthalide、Z - butylidenephthalide、senkyunolide A 和 Z - ligustilide 的 5 种成分是区分两种药材的主要特征。Kwok KY 等利用 HPTLC 方法对黄连解毒汤的 14 个主要化学成分进行了定量分析，为黄连解毒汤的质量控制提供了新标准。Chen J 等结合化学成分分析和生物活性分析方法，鉴定了不同产地的大枣活性成分，并对不同成熟程度的大枣活性成分也进行了分析。Liu J 等分析了不同产地的紫苏中 rosmarinic acid 的含量，建立了紫苏的质量控制方法。Zhang WL 等利用化学和生物测定的方法，分析了当归补血汤中的主要成分，为当归补血汤的质量控制和生产提供了依据。Yi T 等结合化学成分分析和生物活性分析方法，考察了五指毛桃中活性成分的含量和抗氧化作用，并指出 3′- hydroxyl group of luteolin 是其主要的抗氧化成分。Xie C 等利用药代动力学和基因组学相结合的方法，建立了四物汤的质量控制体系。

（2）肿瘤　Kwan HY 等研究发现 oridonin 具有脂肪酸合成酶抑制作用，对肠癌具有一定治疗作用。Yue GG 等从水朝阳旋覆花 *Inula helianthus-aquatica* 中分离出抗肿瘤化合物 bigelovin，实验证明该化合物能够抑制肿瘤血管新生，并具有免疫调节作用。Zhang JY 等通过比较，发现 quercetin 和 acacetin 在 6 种黄酮类化合物中抗肿瘤作用最强。其中 quercetin 能够诱导鳞状细胞癌细胞线粒体膜电位下降，从而释放细胞色素 C，活化 caspases 通路，引起细胞凋亡。Wang D 等通过活性成分分离的方法，从鸡血藤中分离出抑制 LDHA 的新型抑制剂，发现 epigallocatechin 是鸡血藤抗乳腺癌的活性成分。Wang D 等发现植物提取物中常见的化合物 isoliquiritigenin 是通过调节血管内皮细胞 VEGF 受体活性，从而达到抑制血管新生的作用。Luo KW 等利用小鼠乳腺癌转移模型，发现天然产物 zoledronic acid 可以显著降低肿瘤生长速度，并抑制肿瘤细胞转移到肺和肝。zoledronic acid 的用药剂量非常低，可以作为一种新型的抗癌药在临床上应用。Wang N 等发现 Timosaponin AIII 诱导的细胞凋亡受自噬所调控，而且其诱导的自噬能够引起内源性凋亡抑制剂 XIAP 的降解。Tse AK 等发现活性化合物 cryptotanshinone 能够诱导肿瘤细胞中 TRAIL 受体Ⅱ的表达，而且不受细胞类型的影响，抑制该蛋白的表达能够降低 cryptotanshinone 的作用。

（3）老年性疾病　Xian YF 等发现天然产物生物碱 isorhynchophylline 能够保护神经元细胞 PC12，这种作用于 Akt 通路的激活相关。Maiwulanjiang M 等发现维药 Song bu li decoction 可以减少由于氧化应激引起的神经元细胞凋亡。Ng CF 等发现天麻提取物可抑制神经元细胞氧化应激和凋亡，具有保护神经元细胞的作用。Xu M 等认为黄芩中的黄芩苷能够清除氧自由基，保护神经元细胞免受超氧化物的攻击。Wang Z 等研究发现赤芍药中的主要成分 paeoniflorin 通过作用于多条细胞凋亡相关通路起到保护神经元的作用。Wang Z 等比较了两个同分异构体 paeoniflorin 和 albiflorin，发现两者均有保护神经元细胞的作用，但仅有前者能够降低细胞内钙离子浓度，抑制钙离子通道的活性，提示即使是相似的分子结构化合物也具有不同的作用机理。Xian YF 等比较了黄柏的两个源植物 Cortex Phellodendrichinensis 和 Cortex Phellodendriamurensis，发现两种植物能够抑制神经元细胞凋亡。Xu SL 等研究了黄酮类化合物影响神经元突触蛋白分泌的作用，发现包括 catechin、luteolin 和 isorhamnetin 在内的黄酮类化合物不仅能够促进突触蛋白的分泌，也可以促进神经元细胞的分化，对治疗神经退行性疾病有一定的效果。Chu PH 等的研究表明，枸杞多糖具有保护视神经的作用。

（4）炎症与免疫调节　Yue GG 等应用人血单核细胞作为模型，研究灵芝多糖的免疫调节作用，发现灵芝多糖能够促进单核细胞的免疫功能，加快细胞因子 TNF-α、IL-10 和 TGF-β 的表达，增加 CD_{14}^{+} 细胞群数量。Li LF 等从玉红牛肝菌中发现了两个的化合物 1-ribofuranosyl-s-triazin-2(1H)-one 和 pistillarin。结果这两个化合物均能够抑制免疫细胞分泌促炎性因子，产生免疫抑制的作用。Du CY 等发现玉屏风散具有双向调节作用。在非炎性情况下能够刺激促炎性细胞因子的表达和分泌，而在炎性情况下又能够有效地抑制炎性分子的过度表达。

（5）循环系统和血管生成　在血管生成方面，Yu X 等利用斑马鱼和人 HUVEC 细胞模型，发现淫羊藿具有抑制血管新生的活性，以淫羊藿为主药的二仙汤也具有较强的抑制血管新生的作用，该作用于其抑制细胞内通路 Erk1/2 和 Akt 相关。Liu J 等研究含有黄芪和大黄的自组方的促血管新生的能力，发现该方能够促进 Akt MAPK 等通路的活性和表达，从而促进血管生成。Leung SB 等发现红景天苷能够降低同型半胱氨酸诱导的内皮细胞功能紊乱，这种作用与该化合物降低 ROS 水平，抑制 NOX2 基因表达相关。

(6) 其他　Zhu KY 等研究了中药复方开心散抗抑郁的作用机制,发现开心散能够增强脑星形细胞中神经因子 NGF、BDNF 和 GDNF 的表达,且这种作用并不依赖于蛋白通路或 ER 受体而产生作用。Chan BC 等发现天然的黄酮类化合物地奥司明和香叶木素在抑制耐甲氧西林金黄色葡萄球菌的作用上具有协同效应,推测这种协同效应是因为 ABC 蛋白被抑制所产生。Szeto YT 等研究发现小建中汤能够保护抑制氧化应激造成的 DNA 损伤,这种作用在方剂单味药材中是没有的,说明小建中汤中的各个组分具有协同效应。Xiao HT 等研究了火炭母的止呕作用,发现 ellagic acid 和 corilagin 是其中主要的活性成分。Zhang M 等发现厚朴酚可通过抑制钙离子通道活性发挥抑制小肠肌肉蠕动的作用。Tsang SW 等发现天然产物大黄酸能够抑制慢性胰腺炎中纤维化的发生,这种作用可能与 TGF-β 通路相关。

(王　宁　钟丽丹)

【台湾中医药】

1. 基础研究

苏奕彰以德尔菲法订出六淫证型的诊断基准:风证 20 项(恶风、头痛、身痛等)、寒证 30 项(恶寒、形寒、寒战等)、暑证 19 项(恶热、发热、大汗等)、湿证 37 项(低热、乏力、神昏等)、燥证 16 项(皮肤干燥、身痒、鼻干等),火证 47 项(恶热、发热、胸部灼热等)。谢庆良探讨梗塞型脑中风急性期患者证型与其预后的关系,发现其发病原因以风、痰和气虚为主,气虚型患者的预后较好。张宏州筛选了 92 名脂肪肝患者,辨证分为无明显证型、痰湿内阻型、肝胆湿热型、肝郁气滞型、肝肾阴虚型、脾肾亏虚型和瘀血阻络型。痰湿内阻型、肝胆湿热型较无明显证型患者脂肪肝指数明显升高。肝胆湿热型患者谷丙转氨酶(ALT)异常上升。肝郁气滞型、瘀血阻络型、肝肾阴虚型、脾肾亏虚型患者脂肪肝相关指标无明显特异性。高甘油三酯血症、高密度脂蛋白降低,成为脂肪肝是否需要介入治疗的重要临床鉴别指标。陈方周检测 60 名健康受试者接受热刺激(左手浸到 45℃水中维持 2 min)和冷刺激(左手浸到 7℃的水中维持 2 min)前后左右手前臂的温度、肱动脉血压、心跳、心律变异与桡动脉压力波。发现热刺激降低桡动脉增大系数,表明减少左心室负荷;冷刺激增强桡动脉增大系数,表明增加左心室负荷;桡动脉频谱能量因皮肤温度的刺激而改变,这些变化集中在高频段(10～50 Hz)。戴承杰收集肺癌、大肠直肠癌与乳癌患者在化疗前、化疗第 1、3、6 个月与结束后 1 个月的经络能量、中医体质量表评估、症状、生理检验值与生活品质资料,结果① 整体经络能量与阴虚体质量表呈正相关($r=-0.275, P<0.05$),但个案的经络平均能量与阳虚或痰瘀体质得分均无显著相关($r=-0.267, P=0.053$; $r=-0.192, P=0.168$)。② 患者恶心、呼吸急促、纳差或口干等症状严重度越高,整体经络能量越低($r=-0.333$; $r=-0.338$; $r=-0.317$; $r=-0.276, P<0.05$)。③ 患者心跳越快时,整体经络能量越低($r=-0.298, P<0.05$)。④ 红细胞或红细胞压积值越高,整体经络能量越高($r=0.360, P<0.01$; $r=0.287, P<0.05$);中性粒细胞值越高,整体经络能量越低($r=-0.423, P<0.01$)。⑤ 身体生理功能或活力越好,整体经络能量越高($r=0.335$; $r=0.343$; $P<0.05$)。郭正典等分析对照组及太极拳组各 30 名受测者的脉搏波及心电图,发现太极拳组运动之后与正常对照组右手食指动脉脉搏波谐波在 nPh1、nPh2、nPh7、nPh8 参数上有显著差异,太极拳组运动前后脉搏波频谱变化没有差异。黄升腾比较正常人与系统性红斑狼疮(SLE)患者练习八段锦 1 个月后脉波血液流变学的变化,发现练习八段锦对于正常人心理及生理均有显著改善;对于 SLE 患者虽在心理及生理上的变化未统计意义,但对于身体疼痛及一般感觉则有显著改善。

2. 医史文献研究

刘淑铃等对《神农本草经》的中品药和下品药拉丁名与药效进行了本草考证。统计了孙星衍、孙冯翼所辑中品药收载的 114 种药物,结果① 可供日常食用的药物有:干姜、百合、海藻、龙眼、梅实、粟米、黍米、薤。② 未确定基原者:紫参、肤青。③ 各药物具有相同基原者:干姜—生姜、蠡实—马蔺子、积雪草—雷公根、秦茮—花椒、紫葳—凌霄花、白棘—酸枣、凝水石—寒水石、天鼠屎—夜明砂、乌贼鱼骨—海螵蛸、蜚廉(蠊)—蟑螂、蟅虫—地鳖虫。孙氏所辑下品药收载有 103 种药物,结果① 许多药物皆有毒性,如乌头、半夏、大黄、莨菪子、藜芦、钩吻、恒山、大戟、狼牙、羊踯躅、商陆等,曾被列于《本草纲目》草部毒草类。

② 未确定基原者：藿菌、羊桃、乌韭、药实根。③ 一物数名且具有相同基原者：乌头—附子—天雄、恒山—蜀漆—腐婢—赤小豆。④ 有名无实：粉锡。萧晴颖从医史、本草文献等角度辨析了红参、白参的起源，发现从汉迄宋都是用白参，但有虫蛀的问题。宋代时高丽为了防虫蛀，发明了蒸煮制造红参的方法，之后中国明、清两代亦采用蒸煮加工制作红参，更易储存且方便使用。明代后，临床医家发现红、白参功效不同，拓展了红参温补的疗效。李威寰等借助历代本草、方书典籍等文献材料，并运用历史药物地理学、训诂等方法，对官桂的名实进行考证。结果显示，官桂与菌（箘）桂、筒桂于名实之间相承，异名而同物。“官”为“管”之通假，官桂当是无骨、正圆如竹之筒（管）状而薄卷、筒卷者，由小枝皮的薄卷至重卷的二、三重卷者，甚至大枝皮厚嫩的三重者为良。

3. 临床研究

（1）内科　李建莹等将60例原发性高血脂症患者随机分为治疗组（红曲胶囊、寿美降脂一号加益生菌干酪乳杆菌）30例与对照组（寿美降脂一号加安慰剂）30例。结果① 治疗8周后，两组的低密度脂蛋白和总胆固醇均较第0周降低，但组间比较无统计学意义；治疗组骨钙素与纤维蛋白原的改变较对照组明显，虽未达统计上差异，但有改变的趋势。② 治疗12周后，治疗组平均舒张压降低2.7 mmHg，对照组平均舒张压增加4.4 mmHg，组间比较有统计学意义。③ 加入益生菌干酪乳杆菌反而抵消掉红曲的抗凝血功能。提示寿美降脂一号可有效降低总胆固醇及低密度脂蛋白，但加上益生菌干酪乳杆菌无加乘作用。

（2）妇科　苏珊玉以问卷方式收集产后4～6周妇女的生活饮食、中药服用情况等。结果发现，产后服用1～4帖生化汤及十全大补汤可升高血红蛋白；服用1～3周杜仲可降低子宫大小及子宫腔大小，减少恶露天数；服用中药总天数在15 d以上的产妇，阴道及泌尿道感染率较低。提示产后坐月子期间规范特殊生活行为及特殊饮食，再配合中药对产后身体恢复、生活品质提升有助益。陈燕惠选取产后有腹痛、恶露不净现象的产妇，给予口服生化汤5 d，结果显示生化汤对产后宫缩、腹部疼痛有明显改善。王品涵等将更年期综合症患者分为高剂量组（龟鹿二仙胶200 mg/d）、低剂量组（龟鹿二仙胶100 mg/d）和安慰剂组（每日服用淀粉），连续服用2个月。结果① 高剂量组血中雌激素浓度显著上升（$P<0.05$），促卵泡激素三组间无显著差异。② 高、低剂量组比安慰组在临床症状方面均有改善（$P<0.05$），但低剂量组的治疗效果更好，尤其在改善潮热、盗汗及心悸症状方面。高铭侦等用中药穴位外敷治疗痛经，将香附、延胡索、当归、川芎、蒲黄、五灵脂等药物制成药饼，敷贴于关元穴及神阙穴下方。于每次月经前5 d开始敷贴至经行第3天停止，每晚贴敷8 h，1 d1次。敷贴3个月经周期后，经期腹部疼痛程度减轻，下腹胀、下腹痉挛痛、容易疲倦等生理不适均有一定减轻。

（3）针灸　叶柏岩等评估电针刺足三里、上巨虚穴位组对气血倾移的效应。将46例准备接受泌尿道内视镜手术的受试者随机平分为电针刺组与假针刺组，接受30 min的针刺介入，于针刺前后测量心率、血压与中心体温。结果，电针刺组针刺后体温的上升与假针刺组比较有统计上的意义（$P=0.007$）。认为生命征象参数可作为气血分布倾移状态的初步评估参考，电针刺足三里、上巨虚穴位组对于气血倾移至体腔有一定的效应。刘耕豪等收集了65例接受针灸治疗的脑中风患者，比较其针刺前后神经学损伤的恢复程度及日常生活功能的改善程度，运用子群分析及多项式线性回归寻找最适族群及针刺时机的优势。结果① 针刺治疗对脑中风患者的神经学损伤及日常生活自理能力有改善，尤其是梗塞型患者的日常生活功能以巴氏量表评估可进步7.3分（$P=0.003$）。② 对中等严重度的患者，发病后4周内接受针刺治疗在神经损伤修复方面效果更加显著，其脑中风量表分数可减少4.384分（95%信赖区间：$-8.003\sim-0.765$，$P=0.019$）。

4. 中药研究

（1）中药资源　吴金滨对枇杷细胞悬浮震荡培养过程中养分消耗与二次代谢产物之间的动力学进行研究，并探讨两者之间的交互作用与相互关系。结果① 在28 d的培养中，蔗糖在前2 d快速分解为葡萄糖与果糖，第18 d消耗殆尽；磷酸盐在第10 d消耗殆尽；镁、钙离子在培养前期没有明显变化，18 d后开始快速下降。② 第10 d细胞重量增加开始加快；18 d后细胞重量停止增加，进入细胞生长老化期。③ 当导电度低于4 μm/cm，或碳源消耗殆尽时，细胞开始快速的消耗培养液中的钙离子与镁离子，细胞重量停止增加并迅速的累积二次代谢产物含量。④ 利用生物反应器培养可缩短生长周期、产生更多的细胞与二次代谢产物。

(2) 药材鉴定　李宜融对市售 10 种易混淆及误用的种子类中药(沙苑子、南鹤风、赤豆、车前子、青葙子、菟丝子、蛇床子、地肤子、冬葵子、北五味子)进行基原鉴定，鉴定方法为外观形象、组织镜检的特征鉴别，高效液相色谱分析与薄层色谱分析，DNA 序列分析鉴定等。结果，沙苑子与紫云英、南鹤虱与华南鹤虱、赤豆与赤小豆及木豆、地肤子与藜、冬葵子与苘麻子均有混淆现象。罗竣隆等对台湾市场和原产地收集的 52 个黄芩药材，用 70%甲醇萃取，高效液相层析条件为 C18 管柱(4.6×150 mm，2.7 μm)，移动相为乙腈及 0.25%甲酸混合溶液以流速 0.5 ml/min 梯度冲提。MS/MS 分析以负离子模式进行全质量扫描，各个层析峰的紫外线和质谱数据透过标准品及对照文献后共鉴定出 16 个成分。罗氏等通过鉴别辛夷清肺汤、龙胆泻肝汤、黄连解毒汤中的黄芩，来确定黄芩的基原。罗氏等还以超高效液相层析串联四极杆/飞行式质谱仪(LC-Q-TOF/MS)的方法建立银杏叶萃取物与白果仁的指纹图谱。所有药材与市售制剂检体均以 70%甲醇萃取，再取部分萃取液进行水解。高效液相层析条件为 C18 管柱(3.0×150 mm，2.7 μm)，移动相为水和甲醇均含 0.01%的甲酸水溶液，混合溶液以流速 0.5 ml/min 梯度冲提。质谱条件选择负离子模式，并以标准品及文献的分子量对照确认，分别建立银杏叶萃取物与白果仁水解前后的成分表。结果在白果仁中发现银杏内酯 J 与白果内酯为其它文献未记载。本方法可鉴别银杏叶萃取物与白果仁药材成分 LC-Q-TOF/MS 的差异，并可在未经水解的检体鉴别出市售银杏相关制剂中所含的银杏叶萃取物或白果仁。吕康祖等收集 28 种栀子药材及 22 种栀子制剂检体，进行 DNA 的抽取与纯化，利用 Nested PCR 扩增 ITS 片段，并以自动分析 DNA 序列。所有检体的 DNA 序列，除了位置 153 的盐基外都是一致的。

(3) 中药化学　黄慧琪等从东方肉穗野牡丹(*Sarcopyramis nepalensis*)的酒精萃取物中分离纯化得到 17 个化合物，包括 6 个黄酮类化合物、1 个三萜类化合物、3 个脱镁叶绿酸类化合物、2 个醇类化合物以及 5 个其他化合物。通过细胞杀毒活性测试后显示，化合物 pheophorbide a methyl ester 和 methyl (10S)-hydroxypheophorbide a 对 KB 和 Hela 癌细胞株有杀毒效果，其 ED_{50} 值分别为 3.8～5.2 μg/ml 和 3.4～4.2 μg/ml；化合物 quercetin、quercetin-3-O-α-L-rhamnoside、isorhamnetin-3-O-β-D-glucoside 与 caffeic acid 在清除自由基活性测试中显示具良好的抗氧化活性。疏伟杰等从含羞草根部分离得到 2 个新的二萜化合物，对酵母菌和细菌均具有抗菌活性，对厚皮马拉色菌的抗菌活性最强，其次为白色念珠菌和金黄色葡萄球菌，抑菌圈在 12～16 mm 的范围内。

(4) 中药药剂　江淑端以品质管理指标成分含量及总生菌数为安定性指标，进行六味地黄丸制剂的安定性试验。结果① 采用特殊制程设计可有效得到高含量的六味地黄丸的指标成分丹皮酚(Paeonol)，但若没有配合特殊赋形剂的运用，无法有效控制该成分的挥发，造成制剂的安定性不佳。② 直接采用含 paeonol 药材粉末进行配方制造时，其 paeonol 的安定性显著优于先抽出成分再直接加回制剂的设计。③ 直接采用生药粉末调制制剂时，不易控制制剂的总生菌数。江伯源在固液比(1∶5)、萃取温度(100℃)、萃取时间(1 h)条件下，进行麻黄汤萃取液微胶囊造粒试验。结果显示，麻黄汤微胶囊粒子具有较高膨润力、较低溶解度，在 pH1.5 及 7.5 模式溶离试验中其溶离率比中药及生药粉末低，具有延缓释出的效果。詹道明等以挤压搓圆方法制备六味地黄丸新圆粒剂型，并将其与赋形剂羟丙甲基纤维素压制成锭剂，然后以 23 复因子设计来探讨不同参数的圆粒及锭剂剂型的溶离曲线。结果发现，制备的六味地黄丸圆粒呈现出良好的可压缩性，经由压锭过程形成较坚硬和紧密的结构，药物有较缓慢的初始释出速率，并得到更好的安定性。余哲仁等以微过滤膜(0.45 μm)及 4 种超过滤膜(UK 200，UK 50，UP 20 and UK 10)处理小柴胡汤，评估膜处理对小柴胡汤萃取液澄清度与抗氧化能力的影响。结果显示，因较少的总固形物可通过膜，因此透流液具较高的澄清度，含较多的活性成分如总酚、柴胡总皂甙、甘草甜素与黄芩甙。透流液的抗氧化力包括清除自由基、还原力与总抗氧化力均高于原药，尤其是以 UK 10 膜处理的小柴胡汤。

(5) 中药炮制　张文德利用核磁共振仪测定

各种黄精炮制品的指纹图谱，配合主成分分析统计法（PCA），寻找其关联性与差异性。结果① 蒸制黄精的 PCA 与未炮制生黄精有明显差异，但蒸制 5～9 次的结果是相似的，提示五蒸五晒后的黄精化学成分已趋与一致与稳定。② 多次炮制的黄精样品对体内的树突细胞无明显的免疫活性与毒性。③ 制黄精对正常大鼠的免疫力提升有明显作用；对免疫力低下的大鼠，以生黄精提升 CD_4^+ 的浓度效果较好。王静琼以杜仲中的有效成分松脂醇二葡萄甘和绿原酸为主指标成分，检测炒制前后的成分变化，并用 LC～Mass 观察指纹图谱的变化。结果① 生杜仲内含有松脂醇二葡萄甘和绿原酸的含量比炒制品高。② 温度越高、时间越长则指标成分含量越低，但总多酚含量却增高。③ 炒制过程中加水或加盐水，指标成分含量下降程度较少，但与盐度无成正相关。④ 利用 LPS 刺激人类软骨细胞及兔子膝关节产生发炎现象的试验模式发现：生品润制 4 h，切片后 40℃下烘干，药材与清水为 100 ∶ 35 的湿润 10 min，180℃下滚筒翻炒 1 h 的样品，指标成分下降较少，多酚总含量提高，且抗关节炎作用最强。邓正贤试图建立神曲规格化菌种发酵过程，以蛋白酶、淀粉酶与脂肪酶为活性指标，以黄曲霉素污染为负指标，筛选优良发酵菌组，最后选定大陆的中药饮片有限公司所生产的神曲（代号 SQTCM）为菌种分离与纯化对象，细菌菌株经生理生化分析及 16S rDNA 序列分析，确定为革兰氏阳性杆菌芽孢杆菌科（Bacillaceae）沙芬细菌 Bacillus safensis，丝状真菌为毛霉科（Mucoraceae）伞枝梨头霉真菌 Lictheimia ramose。结果显示，最佳反应温度为 40～50℃，最佳发酵时间为 7～10 d，以脂肪酶活性最好，达 285.5±4.9 mU/g。伞枝梨头霉真菌为神曲药材中首次分离出的优势菌株，且无黄曲毒素污染的疑虑。陈锦树筛选分离出可经诱导分泌高单宁酶活性的 Aspergillus oryzae NCH－42 为试验菌株，分别接种于厚朴、金银花、瓜蒌仁、甘草及丹参的药液中进行固态发酵，探讨较适发酵条件及发酵前后中药机能性的变化。结果① Asp. oryzae NCH－42 均能以各自药液为生长基质，＜30℃、加水量为 1 ∶ 6 进行发酵 5 d，对 7 株受测病原菌可得较广泛的抑菌谱；其中金银花与瓜蒌仁经发酵后可提升其甲醇萃取物抑制革兰氏阴性菌的能力，尤其对大肠杆菌明显增加抑制能力。② 各药液经发酵后的抗氧化能力及总多酚含量均有不同程度的提升，表明经 Asp. oryzae NCH－42 转化后可提高药液中机能性成分的释出。③ 发酵后均可降低药液中的单宁含量。④ 经 HPTLC 分析图谱显示发酵后甘草药液可得较高浓度的杨梅素，金银花药液可得较高浓度的咖啡酸，丹参药液可得较高浓度的芦丁，表明药液发酵后具有提升再利用的效果。

（6）中药药理　季军男探讨鱼腥草抗单纯疱疹病毒（HSV）的作用，结果① 鱼腥草可抑制第一型单纯疱疹病毒（HSV－1）、第二型单纯疱疹病毒（HSV－2）和抗阿昔洛韦的 HSV－1。② 将鱼腥草初萃取物按照分子量分成 1 000 Dalton 以下、1 000～3 000 Dalton 之间、3 000 Dalton 以上 3 个部分，发现皆具有抗病毒的成分，以 1 000 Dalton 以下作用最强。③ 鱼腥草对人类喉癌 HEP－2 细胞株及肺癌细胞 A549 有很低的毒性，可抑制 HSV 在 HEP－2 以及 A549 细胞中的感染。④ 鱼腥草经由直接和病毒颗粒作用从而抑制病毒进入细胞；病毒进入细胞后，鱼腥草经由抑制细胞 NF－KB 活化而减少 NF－KB 结合至 HSV 的 ICP0 基因启动子，从而抑制 HSV 的复制。王苑春研究蚤休抗肠病毒活性及其免疫调节机制，发现蚤休 95%乙醇萃取物：① 对肠病毒 71 型（EV71）及克沙奇 B3 型（CVB3）均显示出良好的对抗活性，其抑制作用包括预防病毒感染、直接杀死病毒（或抑制病毒吸附于宿主细胞）及抑制病毒的复制。② 对感染 EV71 及 CVB3 的宿主细胞，显著增加 IL－6 及降低 IL－8、IL－1β（仅对感染 EV71 的宿主细胞）的含量，对其他细胞激素（IL－2、TNF－α、INF－γ）及一氧化氮等则无影响。③ 对 EV71 或 CVB3 的抑制作用与 IL－6 的增加有高度相关性；IL－1β 及 IL－8 的减少可减缓宿主细胞免疫反应造成的严重致病性。表明蚤休 95%乙醇萃取物兼具致死病毒及减缓宿主免疫致病性的双重功效。

温晓薇评估盐酸小檗碱奈米微脂体对人类肝癌的抑制能力。细胞实验表明：① 在浓度为 5 μg/ml 下，对正常肝细胞 Clone 9 无显著伤害，但可使肝肿瘤 HepG2 细胞存活率下降至 50%。② 加入 HepG2 细胞中会造成线粒体膜电位下降、半胱氨酸蛋白酶 3 活性表现增加，细胞出现 Sub－G1 期。显示盐酸小檗碱奈米微脂体是以半胱氨酸蛋白酶线粒体依赖途径促使 HepG2 细胞进入细胞凋亡。动物实验表明：其可抑制肝肿瘤生长，对生物体无明显副作用，且经包合后可增加在体内的循环时间。李珮端在体外试验发现甘草酸、甘草次酸、甘草水煎剂及芍药甘草汤皆显著减少P-糖蛋白(P-gp)在细胞中的蓄积，显示其为P-gp的诱导剂；甘草酸、甘草次酸及高浓度的芍药甘草汤皆显著增加多药耐药相关蛋白2(MRP2)在细胞中的蓄积，显示其为MRP2的抑制剂。这些现象与体内动力学交互作用的结果相符。汪贵珍以系统生物学研究平台探讨中草药防治败血症的病理生理与治疗机理，发现血管内皮细胞受到细菌内毒素刺激后，直接或间接改变核转录因子(NF-κB)上游Pias1基因及SPA6蛋白质的活性，及其下游基因(IL-1RN、IL-1β及CD_4^+)及蛋白质(IL-6及MCP-1)的表现；并引起抗发炎、抗细胞程式性死亡及抗氧化基因及蛋白质的表现。针对特定标的基因与蛋白质研究，发现灵芝、肝炎草、厚叶铁线莲、金丝草等中草药成分具有保护作用。其中，灵芝的部分纯化物具有双向的免疫调节作用，肝炎草与金丝草的抗发炎活性成分为新化合物，厚叶铁线莲成分具选择性抗炎作用。吴永昌以细胞存活率测试与克隆形成测定测试中草药复方及单味药萃取物对人类肝癌细胞株HepG2的毒杀与生长抑制作用，结果① 大建中汤与小建中汤具有抗肝癌细胞增生的作用。② 箭叶凤尾草水萃物与其活性成分Kaempferol 3-O-α-L-rhamnoside-7-O-β-D-glucopyranoside具有抗肝癌活性，其水萃物可造成HepG2细胞周期停滞于G2/M期，并引发caspase相关的细胞凋亡。项千芸利用功能性基因体学平台研究中药免疫调控机制，结果① 在NF-κB基因转殖鼠中，淋巴组织的位置与NF-κB冷光讯号的位置呈现高度相关性，提示冷光讯号的强度可以反应活体内NF-κB的活性。② 脂多糖可诱导小鼠体内NF-κB的活性，山栀子、黄连、黄柏可降低LPS所诱导的NF-κB活性，山栀子的主成份栀子素可藉由降低IL-1β及肿瘤TNF-α的产生、影响干扰素介导蛋白及趋化因子配体相关基因的表现，从而抑制LPS所诱导的发炎反应。徐松锟以人肺癌细胞株A549及H1299筛选抗癌中药，结果① 桑叶、白花蛇舌草、桃仁对癌细胞生长无显著影响，半枝莲、丹皮、泽兰在中、高浓度时可抑制癌细胞生长，连翘、薄荷、金银花在高浓度时有效。② 薄荷、白花蛇舌草、泽兰可抑制表皮生长因子受体(EGFR)的表现与磷酸化，薄荷、白花蛇舌草可抑制A549细胞中蛋白激酶B(AKT)的磷酸化。陈荣秀研究具有护肤作用的中药，结果① 牛蒡子、容水沉香、荷叶、紫苏叶、金银花、山楂、牡丹皮、覆盆子、榄仁叶具有较佳的清除DPPH自由基效果，以榄仁叶效果最优。② 荷叶、紫苏叶、金银花、牡丹皮、榄仁叶、菟丝子具有较强的紫外线吸收效果。③ 菟丝子、容水沉香、柿叶、覆盆子、榄仁叶具DNA保护效果。④ 血竭、柿叶及牡丹皮的保水能力较佳。⑤ 牡丹皮的萃取物对于金黄色葡萄球菌具中度活性的抑菌作用。⑥ 决明子、莲子心、樟芝、覆盆子、木香较具有细胞毒性及刺激性。温国庆对台湾产葡萄科植物抑制基质金属蛋白酶及弹力蛋白酶进行了研究，结果① 广东山葡萄茎、细本山葡萄茎、崖爬藤叶与茎、金香葡萄茎及蜜红葡萄茎有很好的DPPH抗氧化活性。② 广东山葡萄茎、白蔹根、崖爬藤叶与茎、细本山葡萄茎、金香葡萄茎及蜜红葡萄茎的50%乙醇萃取物均具AAPH抗氧化活性且与剂量及时间呈正相关，尤以广东山葡萄茎及白蔹根比维生素C佳。③ 白蔹根对MMP-1,9具抑制活性，崖爬藤茎及叶对MMP-1,3,9具抑制活性，蜜红葡萄茎对MMP-1,3具抑制活性、且对Ⅰ型前胶原具促进活性，金香葡萄茎对MMP-9具抑制活性，台湾乌敛莓茎可抑制MMP-9活性，台湾乌敛莓叶可抑制MMP-1,3,9活性。郑静枝探讨内皮细胞受损时蜂胶成分(CAPE)的抗炎功效，结果① CAPE对内皮细胞的毒性极低，若事先以CAPE处理，可明显抑制由γ-干扰素所诱导的信号转导与转录激活因子1(STAT1)的Tyr701及Ser727磷酸化现象，且呈剂量相关性，但对于JAK1及JAK2的磷酸化则无明显抑制作用。② CAPE进一步抑制具有STAT偶合体连接的趋化因子IP-10的启动子活化，IP-10基因表现及蛋白质的分泌也受到明显抑制。③ T细胞沾粘到内皮细胞的多寡会经由干扰素的诱导而增加，此反应也被CAPE预处理而压制。李连滋等探讨山竹萃取物主要活性成份α-山竹素在老鼠肝星状细胞(HSC-T6)的作用，进而评估其在四氯化碳诱发老鼠肝纤维化的作用。结果① α-山竹素可降低所有纤维化刺激因子(血小板原性生长因子、肿瘤坏死因子-α、转变增长因子-β1和脂多糖)在HSC-T6细胞刺激所导致的α-SMA的生成，尤其是LPS。② 在四氯化碳诱发老鼠肝纤维化试验中，经口先期投与100 mg/kg山竹提取物可明显抑制血清ALT、AST的增加并显著降低纤维化的程度。表明α-山竹素可降低发炎引起的肝纤维化，机制是抑制纤维生成、抗发炎和抑制HSC-T6细胞系功能的综合结果。游进益等探讨虎杖根部乙醇萃取物(PcE)抑制EB病毒潜伏期膜蛋白质1(LMP1)的功能。结果① EB病毒阳性，B95-8细胞经由PcE处理会因为剂量增加及作用时间延长而导致细胞存活率下降。② PcE能够藉由抑制Rta的表现，进而有效抑制LMP1基因，BNLF1的转录及蛋白质的表现。③ 流式细胞仪分析结果发现B95-8细胞经由PcE处理，会增加停滞在sub-G1期的细胞数，同时细胞呈现细胞凋亡的特征。

(7) 方剂研究　苏珊玉的研究发现沙参麦冬汤(SMD-2)可降低接受放射线及化学治疗的头颈部癌病人血液中的Cu/Zn及Cu/Se的比值，明显改善生活品质如身体功能、角色功能、情绪功能、社会功能以及疲劳、疼痛、恶心呕吐、食欲不振、便秘、呼吸困难、食欲不振等症状。李珍珍探讨市售小柴胡汤与防风通圣散对于间质性肺炎的作用及机制，结果① 给予台湾顺天堂与仙丰公司生产的小柴胡汤及防风通圣散24 h后，会抑制人类肺部纤维细胞增生、人胶原蛋白Ⅰ型)mRNA及MMP-9的表现，增加转化生长因子-β(TGF-β)诱发肺部纤维细胞增生、human collagen type Ⅰ mRNA的表现，增加MMP-9的表现，抑制金属蛋白酶组织抑制剂1的表现。但香港香兰公司生产的小柴胡汤及防风通圣散并不增加TGF-β诱发的肺部纤维细胞增生。② 成熟小鼠每日喂食建议剂量1倍与2倍的小柴胡汤及防风通圣散28 d后，不会引发间质性肺炎。③ 间质性肺炎小鼠喂食建议剂量1倍与2倍的小柴胡汤及防风通圣散21 d后，无明显增加肺部发炎及纤维化的情形。杨贤鸿进行疏经活血汤与抗凝血药的中西医交互作用研究，结果单服疏经活血汤不影响纽西兰白兔的凝血作用，与华法林同时喂服时凝血作用的相关因子活化部分凝血活酶时间及凝血酶原时间明显延长，此现象在疏经活血汤停服3 d后回复到正常值。表明疏经活血汤并用华法林会增强华法林的抑制凝血作用。魏正宗评估龟鹿二仙胶改善骨关节炎的有效性与安全性，发现骨关节炎患者服用12周后无明显副作用，也无显著疗效，但对于体质阴虚的骨关节炎患者有改善的趋势。

(黄　颖)

[附] 参考文献

C

Campbell MK, Elbourne DR, Altman DG, et al. CONSORT statement: extension to cluster randomised trials[J]. British Medical Journal, 2004, 328(7441): 702

Chan AW, Tetzlaff JM, Altman DG, et al. SPIRIT 2013 statement: defining standard protocol items for clinical trials[J]. Annals of Internal Medicine, 2013, 158(3): 200

Chan BC, Ip M, Gong H, et al. Synergistic effects of diosmetin with erythromycin against ABC transporter over-expressed methicillin-resistant Staphylococcus aureus (MRSA) RN4220/pUL5054 and inhibition of MRSA pyruvate kinase[J]. Phytomedicine, 2013, 20(7): 611

Chen J, Li Z, Maiwulanjiang M, et al. Chemical and biological assessment of Ziziphus jujuba fruits from China: different geographical sources and developmental stages[J]. Journal of Agricultural and Food Chemistry, 2013, 61(30): 7315

Chu PH, Li HY, Chin MP, et al. Effect of lycium barbarum (wolfberry) polysaccharides on preserving retinal function after partial optic nerve transection[J]. PLoS One, 2013, 8(12): e81339

陈方周. 中医诊断方法标准化之研究(2-1)子计划二：寒热脉象诊断标准化研究：冷加压与热应力试验对桡动脉脉波之影响[J]. 中医药年报，2012，1(1)：56

陈锦树. 台湾常见中药及其废弃物经Aspergillus oryzae NCH-42固态发酵处理对其机能性成分之研究[J]. 中医药年报，2012，1(10)：427

陈荣秀. 中草药在皮肤保养品之应用开发[J]. 中医药年报，2012，1(10)：518

陈燕惠. 妇女在更年期或产后服用中药制剂对体内总代谢体之影响(2～2)[J]. 中医药年报，2012，1(3)：405

D

Du CY, Choi RC, Zheng KY, et al. Yu Ping Feng San, an ancient Chinese herbal decoction containing

Astragali Radix, Atractylodis Macrocephalae Rhizoma and Saposhnikoviae Radix, regulates the release of cytokines in murine macrophages[J]. PLoS One, 2013, 8(11): e78622

戴承杰. 接受化学治疗癌症病患之中医诊断：以经络能量诊察为基础(2~1)[J]. 中医药年报,2012,1(1): 146

邓正贤. 建立安全有效神曲发酵制程最佳化的研究[J]. 中医药年报,2012,1(10): 200

F

Fan LL, Yi T, Xu F, et al. Characterization of flavonoids in the ethomedicine Fordiae Cauliflorae Radix and its adulterant Millettiae Pulchrae Radix by HPTLC-DAD-ESI-IT-TOF-MSn[J]. Molecules, 2013, 18(12): 15134

G

高铭侦,钟莹慧,杨淑龄. 中药药物穴位外敷治疗痛经之疗效初探[J]. 中医药杂志,2013,24(1): 85

郭正典,吕万安. 太极拳对中老年人脉波频谱之效应[J]. 中医药年报,2012,1(1): 310

H

Han QB, Tang WL, Dong CX, et al. An interesting two-phase solvent system and its use in preparative isolation of aconitines from aconite roots by counter-current chromatography[J]. Journal of Separation Science, 2013, 36(7): 1304

黄慧琪,黄士元,梁羽涵,等. 台湾产东方肉穗野牡丹之化学成分研究[J]. 中医药杂志,2013,24(1): 1

黄升腾. 八段锦对于正常人及红斑狼疮患者在脉波血液流变学上的表现[J]. 中医药年报,2012,1(1): 325

J

Jaiswal Y, Liang Z, Yong P, et al. A comparative study on the traditional Indian Shodhana and Chinese processing methods for aconite roots by characterization and determination of the major components[J]. Chemistry Central Journal, 2013, 7(1): 169

季军男. 鱼腥草抗单纯疱疹病毒作用机制之研究[J]. 中医药年报,2012,1(3): 158

江伯源. 中草药微胶囊造粒技术及品质改善之评估[J]. 中医药年报,2012,1(10): 478

江淑端. 中药(查验登记)药品安定性试验基准之探讨与改善方法研究计划[J]. 中医药年报,2012,1(5): 311

K

Kwan HY, Yang Z, Fong WF, et al. The anticancer effect of oridonin is mediated by fatty acid synthase suppression in human colorectal cancer cells[J]. Journal of Gastroenterology, 2013, 48(2): 182

Kwok KY, Xu J, Ho HM, et al. Quality evaluation of commercial Huang-Lian-Jie-Du-Tang based on simultaneous determination of fourteen major chemical constituents using high performance liquid chromatography[J]. Journal of Pharmaceutical and Biomedical Analysis, 2013, 85: 239

L

Leung SB, Zhang H, Lau CW, et al. Salidroside improves homocysteine-induced endothelial dysfunction by reducing oxidative stress[J]. Evidence-Based Complementary and Alternative Medicine, 2013, 2013: 679635

Li LF, Chan BC, Yue GG, et al. Two immunosuppressive compounds from the mushroom Rubinoboletus ballouii using human peripheral blood mononuclear cells by bioactivity-guided fractionation[J]. Phytomedicine, 2013, 20(13): 1196

Li M, Wong YL, Jiang LL, et al. Application of novel loop-mediated isothermal amplification (LAMP) for rapid authentication of the herbal tea ingredient Hedyotis diffusa Willd[J]. Food Chemistry, 2013, 141(3): 2522

Liang Z, Sham T, Yang G, et al. Profiling of secondary metabolites in tissues from Rheum palmatum L. using laser microdissection and liquid chromatography mass spectrometry[J]. Analytical and Bioanalytical Chemistry, 2013, 405(12): 4199

Liang Z, Zhang J, Wong L, et al. Characterization of secondary metabolites from the raphides of calcium oxalate contained in three araceae family plants using laser microdissection and ultra-high performance liquid chromatography-quadrupole/time of flight-mass spectrometry[J]. European Journal of Mass Spectrometry, 2013, 19(3): 195

Liu J, Wan Y, Zhao Z, et al. Determination of the content of rosmarinic acid by HPTLC and analytical comparison of volatile constituents by GC-MS in different parts of *Perilla frutescens* (L.) Britt[J]. Chemistry Central Journal, 2013, 7(1): 61

Luo KW, Ko CH, Yue GG, et al. Anti-tumor and anti-osteolysis effects of the metronomic use of zoledronic acid in primary and metastatic breast cancer mouse models[J]. Cancer Letter, 2013, 339(1): 42

李建莹,魏正宗. 红曲加上益生菌对降血脂作用之评估[J]. 中医药年报,2012,1(3): 109

李连滋，刘思秀，林孟男，等. 山竹素对老鼠星状细胞生成α-SMA之抑制及其对老鼠肝纤维化之预防作用[J]. 中医药杂志，2013，24(2)：211

李珮端. 中西药交互作用体内—体外试验模型之建立及相关性探讨(2～2)[J]. 中医药年报，2012，1(3)：372

李威寰，李世沧. 官桂名实考证[J]. 中医药杂志，2013，特刊(1)：55

李宜融. 10种市售易混淆及误用药材种子类之基原鉴定[J]. 中医药年报，2012，1(5)：90

李珍珍. 市售小柴胡汤与防风通圣散对于间质性肺炎之作用及机制之探讨[J]. 中医药年报，2012，1(3)：332

刘耕豪，黄悦翔，李宗海，等. 针灸辅助治疗对亚急性期脑中风患者之疗效评估：回溯性研究[J]. 中医药杂志，2013，24(2)：251

刘淑铃，郭昭麟，柯裕仁，等.《神农本草经》下品药拉丁名与药效之本草考证[J]. 中医药杂志，2013，24(1)：65

刘淑铃，郭昭麟，柯裕仁，等.《神农本草经》中品药拉丁名与药效之本草考证[J]. 中医药杂志，2012，23(2)：199

罗竣隆，卢芬铃，刘宜祝，等. 运用LC-Q-TOF/MS建立银杏叶萃取物与白果仁之指纹图谱及其在制剂上的应用[J]. 药物食品分析，2013，21(1)：27

罗竣隆，卢芬铃，刘宜祝，等. 运用液相层析串联质谱方法建立黄芩之指纹图谱及其在中药制剂上的应用[J]. 药物食品分析，2012，20(4)：887

吕康祖，谢咏筌，李蕙君，等. 应用巢式PCR-DNA定序方法鉴别中药制剂中的栀子药材[J]. 药物食品分析，2012，20(4)：974

M

Maiwulanjiang M, Zhu KY, Chen J, et al. Song bu li decoction, a traditional uyghur medicine, protects cell death by regulation of oxidative stress and differentiation in cultured PC12 cells[J]. Evidence-Based Complementary and Alternative Medicine, 2013, 2013：687958

Moher D, Schulz KF, Altman D, et al. The CONSORT statement: revised recommendations for improving the quality of reports of parallel-group randomized trials[J]. Journal of the American Medical Association, 2001, 285(15)：1987

N

Ng CF, Ko CH, Koon CM, et al. The Aqueous Extract of Rhizome of Gastrodia elata Protected Drosophila and PC12 Cells against Beta-Amyloid-Induced Neurotoxicity[J]. Evidence-Based Complementary and Alternative Medicine, 2013, 2013：516741

S

Schulz KF, Altman DG, Moher D, et al. CONSORT 2010 statement: updated guidelines for reporting parallel group randomized trials[J]. Annals of Internal Medicine, 2010, 152(11)：726

Szeto YT, Cheng NF, Pak SC, et al. Genoprotective effect of the Chinese herbal decoction xiao jian zhong tang [J]. Natural Product Communications, 2013, 8(3)：389

疏伟杰，何姣青. 由含羞草根部得到两个新的二萜类抗菌成分[J]. 中医药杂志，2013，24(2)：223

苏珊玉. SMD-2合并手术后放射线及化学治疗头颈部癌病患对血中微量元素Cu/Zn及Cu/Se之比值与生活品质与中医体质之随机取样二期临床试验评估以及SMD-2对舌癌、口腔癌之细胞株及小鼠免疫之机转探讨[J]. 中医药年报，2012，1(3)：284

苏珊玉. 产妇坐月子的生活饮食型态与产后短期生活品质、身体恢复及身心状况之间相关研究(2～1)[J]. 中医药年报，2012，1(1)：385

苏珊玉. 产妇坐月子的生活饮食型态与产后短期生活品质、身体恢复及身心状况之间相关研究(2～2)[J]. 中医药年报，2012，1(1)：456

苏奕彰. 以德菲法探讨中医临床证型诊断基准——六淫证型(2～2)[J]. 中医药年报，2012，1(1)：1

苏奕彰. 以德菲法探讨中医临床证型诊断基准——六淫证型[J]. 中医药年报，2011，1(1)：353

T

Tang Y, Yi T, Chen H, et al. Quantitative comparison of multiple components in Dioscorea nipponica and D. panthaica by ultra-high performance liquid chromatography coupled with quadrupole time-of-flight mass spectrometry[J]. Phytochemical Analysis, 2013, 24(4)：413

Tsang SW, Zhang H, Lin C, et al. Rhein, a natural anthraquinone derivative, attenuates the activation of pancreatic stellate cells and ameliorates pancreatic fibrosis in mice with experimental chronic pancreatitis[J]. PLoS One, 2013, 8(12)：e82201

Tse AK, Chow KY, Cao HH, et al. The herbal compound cryptotanshinone restores sensitivity in cancer cells that are resistant to the tumor necrosis factor-related apoptosis-inducing ligand[J]. The Journal of Biological Chemistry, 2013, 288(41)：29923

W

Wang D, Tan QR, Zhang ZJ. Neuroprotective effects of paeoniflorin, but not the isomer albiflorin, are associated with the suppression of intracellular calcium and calcium/calmodulin protein kinase II in PC12 cells[J]. Journal of Molecular Neuroscience, 2013, 51(2)：581

Wang D, Wong HK, Feng YB, et al. Paeoniflorin, a natural neuroprotective agent, modulates multiple anti-apoptotic and pro-apoptotic pathways in differentiated PC12 cells[J]. Cellular and Molecular Neurobiology, 2013, 33(4): 521

Wang N, Feng Y, Zhu M, et al. A novel mechanism of XIAP degradation induced by timosaponin AIII in hepatocellular carcinoma[J]. Biochimica et Biophysica Acta, 2013, 1833(12): 2890

Wang Z, Wang N, Han S, et al. Dietary compound isoliquiritigenin inhibits breast cancer neoangiogenesis via VEGF/VEGFR-2 signaling pathway[J]. PLoS One, 2013, 8(7): e68566

Wong KL, But PP, Shaw PC. Evaluation of seven DNA barcodes for differentiating closely related medicinal Gentiana species and their adulterants[J]. Chinese Medicine, 2013, 8(1): 16

汪贵珍. 以系统生物学研究平台探讨中草药防治败血症之病理生理与治疗机转——以灵芝为例,结合基因体学、蛋白质体学与生物资讯学之研究(3～3)[J]. 中医药年报,2012,1(4): 1

王静琮. 杜仲炮制研究及工厂规范制订[J]. 中医药年报,2012,1(9): 289

王品涵,李怡秋,吴奕慧,等. 龟鹿二仙胶治疗更年期综合症之临床评估[J]. 中医药杂志,2012,23(2): 165

王苑春. 蚕休抗肠病毒活性及其免疫调节机制之研究[J]. 中医药年报,2012,1(3): 188

魏正宗. 红曲加上益生菌对降血脂作用之评估(2～2)[J]. 中医药年报,2012,1(3): 130

魏正宗. 教学医院成立中药临床试验中心[J]. 中医药年报,2012,1(11): 1

温国庆. 台湾产葡萄科植物应用于抗光老化化妆品之开发——抑制基质金属蛋白酶及弹力蛋白酶之探讨[J]. 中医药年报,2012,1(10): 580

温晓薇. 黄连及盐酸小檗碱奈米微脂体的抗人类肝癌细胞作用之分析与细胞凋亡机制之探讨[J]. 中医药年报,2012,1(3): 222

吴金滨. 中草药资源永续使用之探讨研究——建立枇杷细胞悬浮培养之研究[J]. 中医药年报,2012,1(10): 1

吴永昌. 人类癌症基因体以验证探讨抗癌中草药子计划一、中草药调节生长因子及其接受器基因对抗肝癌机制的探讨(2～1)[J]. 中医药年报,2012,1(4): 50

吴永昌. 人类癌症基因体以验证探讨抗癌中草药子计划二、中草药调节生长因子及其接受器基因对抗肝癌机制的探讨(2～2)[J]. 中医药年报,2012,1(4): 69

X

Xian YF, Lin ZX, Ip SP, et al. Comparison the neuropreotective effect of Cortex Phellodendri chinensis and Cortex Phellodendri amurensis against beta-amyloid-induced neurotoxicity in PC12 cells[J]. Phytomedicine, 2013, 20(2): 187

Xian YF, Lin ZX, Mao QQ, et al. Isorhynchophylline protects PC12 cells against beta-amyloid-induced apoptosis via PI3K/Akt signaling pathway[J]. Evidence-Based Complementary and Alternative Medicine, 2013, 2013: 163057

Xiao HT, Tsang SW, Qin HY, et al. A bioactivity-guided study on the anti-diarrheal activity of Polygonum chinense Linn[J]. Journal of Ethnopharmacology, 2013, 149(2): 499

Xie C, Wang Z, Wang C, et al. Utilization of gene expression signature for quality control of traditional Chinese medicine formula Si-Wu-Tang[J]. AAPS Journal, 2013, 15(3): 884

Xu M, Chen X, Gu Y, et al. Baicalin can scavenge peroxynitrite and ameliorate endogenous peroxynitrite-mediated neurotoxicity in cerebral ischemia-reperfusion injury[J]. Journal of Ethnopharmacology, 2013, 150(1): 116

Xu SL, Zhu KY, Bi CW, et al. Flavonoids induce the expression of synaptic proteins, synaptotagmin, and postsynaptic density protein-95 in cultured rat cortical neuron[J]. Planta Medica, 2013, 79(18): 1710

Xu SL, Zhu KY, Bi CW, et al. Flavonoids, derived from traditional chinese medicines, show roles in the differentiation of neurons: possible targets in developing health food products[J]. Birth Defects Research Part C, Embryo today, 2013, 99(4): 292

项千芸. 利用功能性基因体学平台为基础进行中药免疫调控之研究(3～1)[J]. 中医药年报,2012,1(4): 173

萧晴颖,蔡贵花,张贤哲. 红参白参起源辨析[J]. 中医药杂志,2013,24(2): 231

谢庆良. 中医诊断方法标准化之研究(2-1)子计划一: 梗塞型脑中风急性期患者中医证型与其预后关系之探讨[J]. 中医药年报,2012,1(1): 56

徐松锟. 建立抗癌中药筛选平台: 以肺腺癌为例[J]. 中医药年报,2012,1(8): 782

Y

Yeung WF, Chung KF, Poon MM, et al. Prescription of chinese herbal medicine and selection of acupoints in pattern-based traditional chinese medicine treatment for insomnia: a systematic review[J]. Evidence-Based Complementary and Alternative Medicine, 2012, 2012: 902578

Yi T, Chen Q, He X, et al. Chemical quantification and antioxidant assay of four active components in Ficus hirta root using UPLC - PAD - MS fingerprinting combined with cluster analysis[J]. Chemistry Central Journal, 2013, 7(1): 115

Yu X, Tong Y, Han XQ, et al. Anti-angiogenic activity of Herba Epimedii on zebrafish embryos in vivo and HUVECs in vitro[J]. Phytotherapy Research, 2013, 27(9): 1368

Yu X, Tong Y, Huang W, et al. Erxian Decoction, a traditional chinese herbal formula, inhibits angiogenesis in human umbilical vein endothelial cells[J]. Biological & Pharmaceutical Bulletin, 2013, 36(5): 754

Yue GG, Chan BC, Han XQ, et al. Immunomodulatory activities of Ganoderma sinense polysaccharides in human immune cells [J]. Nutrition and Cancer, 2013, 65(5): 765

Yue GG, Chan BC, Kwok HF, et al. Anti-angiogenesis and immunomodulatory activities of an anti-tumor sesquiterpene bigelovin isolated from Inula helianthus-aquatica[J]. European Journal of Medicinal Chemistry, 2013, 59: 243

杨贤鸿. 中药疏经活血汤与西药抗凝血药之中西医交互作用研究[J]. 中医药年报,2012,1(5): 1

叶柏岩,刘耕豪,许逸群,等. 电针刺足三里上巨虚穴位组对气血倾移的效应[J]. 中医药杂志, 2012, 23(2): 235

游进益,陈师莹,陈怡频,等. 虎杖根部乙醇萃取物抑制 EB 病毒潜伏期膜蛋白质 1 的功能[J]. 药物食品分析, 2013,21(1): 20

余哲仁,林美素,翁义铭,等. 膜处理改变小柴胡汤水萃物的物化性、澄清度与抗氧化活性[J]. 药物食品分析, 2013,21(1): 13

Z

Zhan JY, Zhang WL, Zheng KY, et al. Chemical changes of Angelicae Sinensis Radix and Chuanxiong Rhizoma by wine treatment: chemical profiling and marker selection by gas chromatography coupled with triple quadrupole mass spectrometry [J]. Chinese Medicine, 2013, 8(1): 12

Zhang JY, Yi T, Liu J, et al. Quercetin induces apoptosis via the mitochondrial pathway in KB and KBv200 cells [J]. Journal of Agricultural and Food Chemistry, 2013, 61(9): 2188

Zhang M, Zang KH, Luo JL, et al. Magnolol inhibits colonic motility through down-regulation of voltage-sensitive L - type Ca2 + channels of colonic smooth muscle cells in rats[J]. Phytomedicine, 2013, 20(14): 1272

Zhang WL, Zheng KY, Zhu KY, et al. Chemical and biological assessment of angelica roots from different cultivated regions in a chinese herbal decoction danggui buxue tang [J]. Evidence-Based Complementary and Alternative Medicine, 2013, 2013: 483286

Zhong LD, Cheng CW, Chan Y, et al. Chinese herbal medicine (Ma Zi Ren Wan) for functional constipation: study protocol for a prospective, double-blinded, double-dummy, randomized controlled trial[J]. Trials, 2013, 14(1): 366

Zhong LD, Cheng CW, Wu TX, et al. Increasing Protocol Design is the Cornerstone for Overall Improvement of Clinical Trials[J]. Chinese Journal of Evidence-Based Medicine, 2013, 13(12): 1500

Zhu KY, Xu SL, Choi RC, et al. Kai-xin-san, a chinese herbal decoction containing ginseng radix et rhizoma, polygalae radix, acori tatarinowii rhizoma, and poria, stimulates the expression and secretion of neurotrophic factors in cultured astrocytes[J]. Evidence-Based Complementary and Alternative Medicine, 2013, 2013: 731385

詹道明,吴姿慧,蔡东荣,等. 以挤压搓圆法制备传统中药(六味地黄丸)圆粒新剂型之统计适宜化[J]. 药物食品分析,2012,20(4): 908

张宏州. 脂肪肝临床表现与中医证型关系研究[J]. 中医药年报,2012,1(1): 169

张文德. 利用代谢体学建构中药炮制技术科学化规范——黄精药材炮制技术的比较[J]. 中医药年报,2012, 1(9): 243

郑静枝. 蜂胶成分 Caffeic Acid Phenethyl Ester 抑制干扰素于内皮细胞中所诱导的 STAT1 活化及其下游基因表现[J]. 中医药杂志,2012,23(2): 103

八、国外中医药

【国外针灸治疗乳腺癌伴随症状的研究】

Smith C 等[澳大利亚]观察针刺对乳腺癌患者疲乏和康健状态改善的疗效。将至少在一个月前已停止化疗的患者随机分为治疗组 9 例，假针刺组 10 例，等候针刺组 10 例，治疗组选用太溪、俞府、足三里、三阴交、关元、气海穴，留针20 min，1 次/周，治疗 6 次。结果与假针刺组及等候针刺组比较，治疗组在针刺治疗 2 周后疲乏症状明显减少，平均差异为 5.3，95%置信区间为 4.5～6.2，$P=0.05$；而健康状态在针刺治疗 6 周后明显改善，平均差异为 2.7，95%置信区间为 2.1～3.2，$P<0.01$；这些患者在睡眠、情绪与放松等方面也有明显好转。Jeong Y J 等[韩国]研究针刺治疗正接受抗雌激素疗法(服用他莫昔芬或阿那曲唑)的乳腺癌患者的面部潮热症状。患者均处于绝经期前后，潮热症状每周平均出现 3 次或更多次数，伴有轻度至严重程度血管舒缩现象，而且至少在治疗前 4 周已经停止使用激素替代疗法或其它针对潮热的治疗。治疗组 10 例患者共接受 12 次针刺治疗，选用百会、印堂、少府、阴谷、行间穴，每次留针 20±5 min，3 次/周、连续 4 周。结果显示，与治疗前比较，所有患者面部潮热症状的严重程度均有 70%～95%改善，潮热的视觉模拟评分显著改善，同时潮热的严重度也有显著改善(均$P<0.01$)，针刺治疗结束 4 周后这些患者的潮热症状未有加剧。Bokmand S 等[丹麦]研究针刺缓解乳腺癌患者更年期样不适症状(面部潮热与夜眠不安)的疗效。将 94 例患者随机分为针刺组 31 例，假针刺组 29 例，未进行治疗者 34 例。针刺组选用阴郄、太溪、三阴交、太冲等穴，每次留针 15～20 min，1 次/周，疗程为 5 周。结果针刺组有 16 例(52%)潮热症状明显改善，假针刺组有 7 例(24%)潮热症状明显改善($P<0.05$)。与假针刺组比较，治疗组平均潮热视觉模拟评分下降；治疗组在第 5 次治疗后 12 人仍睡眠不安，治疗结束 12 周后 13 例患者诉说睡眠不安(均 $P<0.05$)。Cassileth BR 等[美国]研究针刺治疗乳腺癌患者手术后上肢淋巴水肿的疗效。选取乳腺癌手术和(或)放疗后患侧与健侧臂围长度差异≥2 厘米，且病史 6 个月～5 年的患者 33 例，2 次/周、连续 4 周的针刺，选用肩髎、肩髃、尺泽、中脘、中极、合谷、足三里与三阴交穴，每次留针30 min。结果 11 例(33%)患者的淋巴水肿减低程度≥30%，18 例患者的淋巴水肿降低程度≥20%。患者平均臂周长度差异由治疗前的 4.6±2.2 厘米降为治疗后的 3.7±2.3 厘米。随访发现 4 位患者疗效保持至治疗结束后 4 个月。

（陈业孟）

【国外对气功的研究】

Yeung A 等[美国]收录 14 名华裔美国人重度抑郁症患者，接受为期 12 周的气功干预。习练前、6 周及 12 周测量患者的 17 项汉密尔顿抑郁评定量表(HAM－D17)、临床总体印象的严重程度(CGI)和改进(CGI－I)、生活的享受和质量满意度调查问卷、短表(Q－LES－Q－SF)和多维领悟社会支持量表(MSPSS，含家庭 MSPSS－FA、朋友 MSPSS－FR 和其他满意度 MSPSS－SO)。结果 71%的受试者完成整个试验，气功有效率为 60%，缓解率为 40%，HAM－D17、CGI－S、CGI－I、Q－LES－Q－SF 和 MSPSS 量表治疗前后比较，差异均有统计学意义。提示气功干预在卫生保健与初级护理重度抑郁症患者是可行的。Sawynok J 等[加拿大]在前期的有关 1 级超意返还功对纤维肌痛的对照临床疗效观察试验成果基础上，继续扩展开展 2 级超意返还功对 20 例纤维肌痛的开放性临床疗效观察试验。受试者前 8 周每天练习 2 级超意返还功 60 min 之后，每天持续其他常规锻炼直至 6 个月。练习前、8 周、4 个月及 6 个月，定量测量患者的疼痛(NRS－PI 量表)、影响(纤维肌痛影响量表)、睡眠(PSQI 量表)、生理心理状态(SF－36 量表)和锻炼时间；定性记录患者的满意度、全身性改善情况评价等。结果除 7 名受试者未完成试验外，13 名完成本试验的受试者(65%)在第 8 周且持续到 6 个月疼痛、影响、睡眠及生理状态均有显著改善；其中 7 名练习积极性较高的受试者症状改善疗效最佳。

并且定性检测试验数据提示患者在其他领域的健康状况也有所改善。该扩展临床试验提示纤维肌痛患者认真练习 2 级超意返还功能获显著健康改善。Oh B 等[美国]从 Pubmed、Medline、ProQuest、Science Direct、EMBASE 和 PsycIno 等 6 大数据库检索了至 2011 年末所有关于气功对抑郁症治疗作用的临床随机对照实验，共 10 篇符合要求的文章入选。其中，4 个报道认为气功对治疗抑郁是有效的；2 篇报道认为气功与体育锻炼对治疗抑郁的效果相当；1 个报道认为气功的疗效可与综合性康复治疗相当；其余 3 篇报道认为气功对抑郁无效。相关的文献分析显示气功对治疗抑郁有潜在作用，但并非决定性因素，需要严密设计的实验研究来进一步证明这个观点。Lauche R 等[德国]针对气功对纤维肌痛的疗效作了系统回顾和 Meta 分析。查询 PubMed/MEDLINE、Cochrane 图书馆、EMBASE、PsycINFO 和 CAMBASE 数据库截止至 2012 年 12 月的数据，筛选出气功和其他干预措施相比较的随机对照试验，主要检测指标为疼痛、生活质量，次要指标为睡眠质量、疲劳、抑郁和安全性。试验中共纳入 395 名纤维肌痛患者。分析显示，短期疼痛、生活质量及睡眠质量的改善有低质量证据。与常规护理相比，很低质量证据证明气功能改善纤维肌痛患者的疲劳症状。与其他积极治疗相比，没有证据证明气功疗效有优势。无严重不良事件的报告。该系统评价显示气功可能是纤维肌痛患者的一种有效疗法，但根据证据的质量只能微弱地证明这一点，需要进一步的高质量的随机对照试验证明其长期疗效。

（尚妍妍）

[附] 参考文献

B

Bokmand S & Flyger H. Acupuncture relieved menopausal discomfort in breast cancer patients: A prospective, double blinded, randomized study[J]. The Breast, 2013, 22: 320

C

Cassileth BR, Zee KJ Van, Yeung KS, et al. Acupuncture in the Treatment of Upper-Limb Lymphedema[J]. Cancer, 2013, 119(13): 2455

J

Jeong Y J, Park YS, Kwon HJ, et al. Acupuncture for the Treatment of Hot Flashes in Patients with Breast Cancer Receiving Antiestrogen Therapy: A pilot Study in Korean Women[J]. The Journal of Alternative and Complementary Medicine, 2013, 19(8): 690

L

Lauche R, Cramer H, Hauser W, et al. A systematic review and meta-analysis of qigong for the fibromyalgia syndrome[J]. Evidence-Based Complementary and Alternative Medicine, 2013, 2013: 635182

O

Oh B, Choi SM, Inamori A, et al. Effects of qigong on depression: a systemic review[J]. Evidence-Based Complementary and Alternative Medicine, 2013, 2013: 134737

S

Sawynok J, Lynch M, Marcon D. Extension trial of qigong for fibromyalgia: a quantitative and qualitative study[J]. Evidence-Based Complementary and Alternative Medicine, 2013, 2013: 726062

Smith C, Carmady B, Thornton C, et al. The effect of acupuncture on post-cancer fatigue and well-being for women recovering from breast cancer: a pilot randomized controlled trial[J]. Acupuncture Medicine, 2013, 31(1): 9

Y

Yeung A, Slipp LE, Jacquart J, etc. The treatment of depressed chinese americans using qigong in a health care setting: a pilot study[J]. Evidence-Based Complementary and Alternative Medicine, 2013, 2013: 168784

九、教学与科技研究

(一) 教学研究

【中医经典课程教学方法研究】

对中医经典课程教学方法的研究近来得到广泛重视，其研究主要集中在《黄帝内经》、仲景学说以及温病学说的教学方面，包括对教学理念、课程建设、教学方法以及考核方式的探讨。

关于《内经》教学研究，王小平提出《内经》教学目的应当从单纯的知识灌输转向中医学方法和文化素养的培训。具体内容包括：教学中注重文化背景，分析理论形成的认识方法，厘清核心概念的源流演变，阐明其表述方式的认知背景等，并由此充分发挥中医经典教学所承载的导航作用。朱鹏举等指出在《内经》教学中教师应把握其理论精髓，避免盲从古圣原典与盲从教材两种错误倾向。陈士玉从深化理解旧知识、关联知识比较分析、鉴别各家观点、展示逻辑分析过程与敢于提出问题几方面探讨了如何在《内经》授课过程中培养学生发现问题、探索问题、解决问题的能力。在课程建设方面，高程熙等强调《内经》精品课程建设的重要意义，指出建设过程中多媒体的素材收集和选择是一大难点，应重视现代技术和网络技术在中医经典理论教学中的应用。在具体教学实践上，李迎霞等指出在《内经》授课时宜将原先的单个知识点串联成线，使学生从整体上把握中医的理论知识。陈士玉等认为在《内经》教学中应贯彻诵、解、别、明、彰五个步骤，引导学生由浅入深、夯实基础、逐步提升学习能力，从而领略经典的理论精髓。钱会南对《内经》藏象理论体系的教学方法进行了探讨，认为应该从各篇章论述切入的不同角度展开讲解，重视对藏象内容的梳理比较，并关注对后世医家的影响和中医理论形成的意义，以及藏象理论的临床指导，结合实践运用进行讲解。周杰等指出《内经》的教学当引入实践教学的理念，从参观实践、走出课堂，改变主体、自主讲授，名家传授、提升高度，参与科研、拓展思路，见习临床、学以致用5个方面进行教学方法改革，使实践教学成为课堂教学的有益补充，两者相辅相成，相互为用。董晓英等从案例式教学在《内经》课程中的应用入手，提出古今医案的合理布局可以增强案例式教学效果，强调《内经》案例教学对教师在教学案例的选择、课堂教学设计、临床经验的丰富等方面提出更高要求。在教学效果的评价方面，赵剑波等从影响《内经》课程教学的相关因素、考核方式及效果、课后收获等方面对山西中医学院的学生进行调查，认为应继续强化教与学的有效互动、通过原文培养中医思维、鼓励学生自行积极解决问题以及强化考核方式、增强学习信心。

关于《伤寒论》教学研究，绝大多数研究者皆从理论联系实践角度出发，强调通过教学培养学生的辨证思维和临床能力。孔祥亮等将“一体两翼”的办学理念融入《伤寒论》教学，形成《伤寒论》三段递进式教学模式，用科研成果来充实教学内容，用PBL教学等手段来调动学生主动学习的积极性，同时结合现代医学知识来讲解《伤寒论》病证本质与方药功效，结合人文社会学知识来诠释《伤寒论》文化内涵，强化学生的中医临证辨治思维和实践能力，提高其综合素质。周刚从常变辨证思维、整体辨证思维、动态辨证思维、顺势辨证思维等4个方面举例阐释了《伤寒论》临床辨证思维方法，强调在基于条文学习的前提下，应注重培养学生的辨证思维方法，使《伤寒论》六经辨证体系灵活地应用于临床。在具体教学实践方面，《伤寒论》案例式教学已得到广泛运用。如李赛美等基于案例版《伤寒论》，对广州中医药大学2008级经典方向班进行《经典名医医案》课程自主学习尝试，并对课堂教学方法改革及自主学习需求与条件、收获与设想提出见解。同时又以伤寒论病区真实案例诊治全程为依据，报道该班级开展PBL

教学实践的过程与效果，对案例基本情况、教学设计、教学评价等进行了较全面的介绍，对中医经典课程开展 PBL 教学提出了独到见解。鲁美君等通过教学实践中以案例式教学法贯穿课堂始终、多种教学方法配合应用、改革考核方式等 3 个方面探讨了对《伤寒论》教学临床思维的培养。在具体教学措施和方法上，何丽清等通过山西中医学院的教学实践，从修订完善教学目标、编写系列教材、改革教学方法、规范教学组织管理、加强师资队伍建设以及建立合理可行的教学质量评估体系等方面对构建有特色的《伤寒论》教学模式进行了研究。曲夷从教学内容、教学设计、成绩考核 3 个环节入手，介绍了在《伤寒论》教学中加强学生心力培养的体会。李孝波等分析了形象化教学法的意义及在《伤寒论》教学中的必要性和可行性，并例举教学视频与声音图像的采集、动画制作、模拟演练、还原场景等形式说明其具体应用。

关于《金匮要略》教学方面，研究者主要对案例式教学、讨论式教学等开放式教学方法进行了实践和探讨，认为此类教学方法相比较传统方法而言，更能够调动学生学习的积极性，培养学生独立思考和创新思维，提高学生的临床思路和诊治能力。如李云海等通过《金匮要略》课程教学中传统教学方法和递进式案例教学法的比较研究，分析了“案例式—启发式—互动式”多维教学法的优势。张茂云等在《金匮要略》教学过程中运用“病案模拟—学生诊查—导入原文”三步式教学模式，认为该模式在一定程度上能弥补当前中医经典课程教学与临床脱节的问题，适合在中医经典课教学中推广应用。又基于《金匮要略》中体现的“仲景杂病诊疗体系”(包括病、证、理、法、方药)，探讨了临证思维的建构方法。柴可夫等探讨了在硕士研究生《金匮要略》课程教学中采用 PBL 教学方法的适应性，论述了《金匮要略》PBL 教学法教案的准备与实施方法。刘晓玲等在传统病案教学法的基础上，整合教学及临床各种资源，初步建立了体现中医经典临床思维的《金匮要略》教学案例影像库。

关于《温病学》的教学方面，作为中医经典理论的重要组成部分，其教学亦得到关注与研究。如苏丽清等指出在《温病学》教学过程中，要从课程内容、教学模式、教学方法、临床实践等方面进行适当改革，加强对学生中医临床思维能力的培养，以适应现代中医药高水平临床型人才培养的需要。魏凯峰探讨了《温病学》研究性教学课程体系建设的方法及内容，初步分析了课程建设的要素，包括教材建设、师资建设、教学方法建立、网络教学平台建设、考核方法建设、课程教学评价方法建设等等，为进一步建立中医学研究性教学课程体系进行了有益的探索。赵岩松等在认知理论指导下，进行了构建温病学教学平台的设想和实践，通过专题讲座、影像教学、临床观摩、课堂讨论等多种教学手段结合，加强知觉学习、激发学习动机，从而提高学生的学习能动性。在具体教学方法和教学模式的采用上，展照双等认为可对温病发展史、温病类型、温病与相关概念、温病三焦辨证以及温病治法等内容采用比较归纳法，使其知识条理化、简单化、系统化，便于理解和记忆。郑旭锐等分析了集多种教学方法手段为一体、充分利用多媒体和网络技术、以基础知识讲解与临床技能培训、学习策略结合的创新教学模式在《温病学》教学中的应用，指出该模式对稳固基础知识、增强文化氛围、引导自主学习、加强实践教学等方面均有重要作用。岳冬辉等探讨了易位式教学模式在温病学教学中的应用与实施效果，认为易位式教学理念在温病学课程中的实践能激发学生学习兴趣，使学习从被动接受变为主动探求，充分调动学生学习的自主性与积极性，提高教学内容的实践性和针对性，从而实现以教师为中心向学生为中心的新型教学理念的转变。周丽雅等在教学实践中进行了温病学多元化教学改革与实践，从运用典型病例、联系专题病案讨论、采取对比鉴别法、利用多媒体和实施 PBL 教学法等 5 个方面进行了教学探索。郑春素对《温病学》课程的形成性评价体系构建进行了研究与实践，具体通过教学过程中的观察、座谈、访谈、活动记录、问卷调查、记读书笔记、学生自评、互评等形式对学生的学习行为、学习能力、学习态度和合作精神等进行持续性评价。

另外，在中医临床经典的综合性教学方面，谢忠礼聚焦师资培养问题，分析了中医临床经典课程的理论教学和实践现状，提出要解决中医经典教学中青年教师存在的临床教学能力相对不足的问题，应建设集医疗、教学和科学研究为一体的中医经典医教团队以及相应的实践基地建设。屠燕捷等对新开设的《中医临床经典导读》课程教学进行了探索，认为在教学中可采用案例引导的探究式教学与理论讲授相结合的教学方法，同时注意掌握以学生为中心的提问技巧与课堂上的有效沟通技巧，从而引导学生逐步形成运用中医经典辨证思维分析临床病证的习惯，为后续经典课程和临床各科的系统学习打好基础。

（张苇航）

【临床教学方法研究】

黄敏等在中医院校普外科实习中运用TBL(以团队为基础的教学法)与SP(模拟病人)相结合的教学法。选择普外科常见病种，按照“提纲—分组—讨论—小结”流程开展教学实践。具体为：教师结合学生知识结构，按照教学大纲要求，围绕带教内容，提出若干问题，作为讨论提纲。学生3～4人为1组，由教师提供1名模拟病人。小组成员分工收集患者相关临床资料，专科体检由模拟病人口述。教师给予学生一定时间自学讨论，围绕问题加以思考，教师提供部分参考资料。以问题为基础进行组间讨论，各组学生发言，阐述对提纲中问题及所选病例的看法。学生讨论完毕，由教师提炼总结，以小结形式给出病例诊治方案。马睿杰等介绍了临床路径教学法及其优势，强调了在中医临床教学中引入该教学法的必要性，认为该方法有助于临床医学生接受全新的单病种质量控制观念，锻炼标准化、规范化、科学化的临床思维方式，初步掌握循证医学方法，对获取系统的现代医学知识有着重要作用。李青等在临床护理教学中引入临床路径教学法，将进入中医伤科实习的护生随机分为两组，对照组为传统跟班带教，试验组按照临床路径教学法规范教学。实习结束后对所有护生进行考核。结果表明，试验组在护理基本理论、基本技能、文件书写能力、沟通能力、病人满意度等方面均明显优于对照组。王佳雯等研究了多媒体结合PBL教学模式在中医外科临床见习中的应用效果。将80名参加中医外科临床见习的本科生随机分为两组，进行不同模式的见习带教，并对两组教学质量进行评估。试验组采用多媒体结合PBL教学模式，对照组采用传统教学模式。两组均采用闭卷考核及学习效果问卷调查方式进行评价。结果，试验组闭卷考核成绩优于对照组($P<0.05$)，试验组学习效果问卷调查满意度高于对照组($P<0.05$)。曾平等分析了传统中医骨伤科临床技能教学中存在的问题，指出模拟教学是解决理论与实践相脱节的有效方法。采取现代高端模拟人等临床模拟设备，通过营造骨折、脱位、创伤、休克等临床场景，构建理论授课、操作示范、学生练习、临床考核为一体的临床技能培训模式。吴发胜等认为在中医内科临床教学中应借鉴循证医学模式和观念。指出教师应创新教学观，以循证医学作为终身学习的重要途径，把解决临床实际问题作为实践教学的中心。在教学过程中，注重培养学生自我学习与自我更新知识、发现问题与解决问题的能力。教师可运用EBM模式针对某一临床问题或某一疾病提出问题，建立假设，由学生查阅文献，寻找证据。通过小组讨论加以论证，得出结论。以问题为基础的循证医学教学模式符合医学发展趋势，有助于培养学生临床思维能力，值得在临床教学中推广使用。朱莹等改革传统中医内科见习模式，根据门诊和病房特点，采取不同见习方式。门诊以见习中医内容为主，兼顾西医知识，采用“分阶段实例教学法”。第一阶段，识症辨方。使学生熟悉常见症状的辨识，认识方剂的重要性。第二阶段，识病辨证。着重培养学生运用所学知识辨病辨证的能力。第三阶段，临证试诊。着重培养学生独立处理内科常见病、多发病的能力。病房临床带教强调“以学生为主体，以患者为中心”，针对不同专题建立学习模块，开展PBL教学模式。罗仁等在中医实习医师培养中创用“2244”模式，以实习医师为中心，通过1次查房、1个病例、2个学生(分别扮演上下级医师角色)、4种方法进行查房训练。在查房过程中，由实习医师汇报病历摘要，另一实习医师扮演上级医师补充收集病史，按照临床特点、诊断分析、辨证分析、治疗方案4个步骤进行查房分析。总结病情特点，明确诊断和鉴别诊断，分析中医病因病机，确定证型，制定系统治疗方案。其他实习医师对上述2位医师进行评价，带教教师现场综合点评，全体实习医师完成一份查房分析报告。认为“2244”模式以学生为主体，有利于学生综合分析、判断力、思维方法的训练，加强了临床技能训练，培养了解决临床问题的能力。

（陈慧娟）

【中医药人才培养模式研究】

1. 继承型人才培养

郑玉玲、呼海涛等报道，为了探索师承教育与院校教育的有机结合，河南中医学院开设了仲景学术继承班。该班以培养人文素养高、中医理论功底扎实、中医思维和实践动手能力强的优秀人才为目标，优化课程设置。重视传统文化教育，强化经典学习，增设中医传统技能课程，削减公共课及西医课程比例。积极改革教育教学方法，将启发式、案例式等先进教学理念引入教学中。通过导师制拓展第二课堂，使学生早临床、多临床，实施经典诵读、名家讲座、读书成才等辅助培养措施。鼓励学生开展学术创新、科学研究活动。建立模拟实习医院，增加临床见习、实习，培养学生中医思维和临床能力。组建教学研究机构，为中医传承教育提供学术支撑。制定教学各环节质量标准，建立形成性评价和终结性评价考核体系。黄必胜等报道，湖北中医药大学建立了“中医继承型人才培养模式实验区”，通过开办中医教改实验班，探索院校教育与师承教育结合的模式。将中国传统文化课程纳入中医人才培养必修课体系，重视中医经典教学，构建“双维临床实践教学体系”。实现院校教育与师承教育、班级制与导师制的有效互补。课程设置上，采取先中后西顺序，第一阶段安排中医课程，结合跟师临床；第二阶段学习西医课程，继续强化中医临床实践。以突出中医教学，帮助学生建立中医思维。

2. 国际型人才培养

谢春娥等报道，为了探索国际型中医药人才培养模式，北京中医药大学和新加坡南洋理工大学联合培养“生物—中医”双学士，在教育教学理念、考核体系等方面做了一系列尝试。教育理念方面，注重“以文化解读中医”，增设古代汉语、古典哲学等课程。教学理念崇尚“厚基础，早临床，多临床”。采取本科生导师制，强化导师临床经验传授。在临床实践中学习临床课，实行“观诊、助诊、试诊”三段式临床带教法。考核体系采用“中医临床三段十站考核方案”，即第一阶段为中医基础理论笔试；第二阶段为临床各科专业技能考核，设立内、外、妇、儿、针灸等诊疗站；第三阶段为临床综合能力考核，包括病史采集、体格检查、病历书写、临床思维等。高静等报道，成都中医药大学探索中西医结合中外合作护理人才培养，初步建构了国际化人才培养模式。学制上采取 3＋2 双校园培养(前 3 年在成都中医药大学，后 2 年在维多利亚大学)，要求培养出的学生具有良好的外语应用能力，熟悉中西方文化，兼具中西方护理知识和技能。以此为目标，优化课程体系，增加人文课程及交叉学科课程，强化中医特色护理课程，完善实践教学体系，加大英语教学力度，突出国际护理特色。

3. 创新型人才培养

徐大量等报道，广州中医药大学以培养创新人才为目标，倡导多元化人才培养模式，创立了“中医传统医学人才”、“中医临床实用型人才”、“复合型中药学应用人才”等不同形式的人才培养模式创新实验区。通过组建中医学实验班探索“精英式”人才培养模式；通过产学研合作，探索“订单式”人才培养模式；通过开放实验室、本科创新实验项目，探索科研型人才培养模式。围绕创新人才培养目标，优化课程体系。加强通识教育，注重人文科技教育与专业教育的融通。突破专业壁垒，精心设计基础教育课程。构建专业选修课程体系，科学分化专业方向。

4. 应用型人才培养

朱乔青等探讨了中西医结合临床人才培养新思路——中医见习医生制。该模式在课程体系改革、实践改革基础上，利用“名院、名科、名医”，贯穿“读经典，跟名师，重实践”主线，采取“见习医生制”的临床教学方式。具体方法为：将中医临床基础课分为原文选读、临床应用两部分，原文选读分伤寒、金匮、内经、温病学选读，临床应用整合为中医经典临床应用一门课。中西医临床课程，除开设中医临床导论及讲授部分西医临床课程总论外，其余临床课程均并入中医见习临床课程中，由临床医生床边授课。该模式使临床教学从学校走入医院，从教室走入病房，从大班分为小组，学生角色转变为实习医生，有助于学生融会贯通地学习中西医临床课程。同时，学生有机会师承各科名医，最大限度发挥了“名院、名科、名医”的作用。

(陈慧娟)

[附] 参考文献

C

柴可夫,沈祥峰.在硕士研究生《金匮要略》课程中开展PBL教学法的探讨[J].中医药管理杂志,2013,21(9):935

陈士玉,谷峰,朱鹏举.浅谈“诵、解、别、明、彰”在《内经》教学中的实施[J].国际中医中药杂志,2013,35(2):173

陈士玉.《内经》教学中提高学生独立学习能力的几点思考[J].中国民族民间医药,2013,22(12):49

D

董晓英,周杰.古今医案合理布局在《内经选读》教学中的应用[J].中医药导报,2013,19(11):144

G

高程熙,赵博,郭宪立,等.《内经选读》精品课程建设的意义及体会[J].贵阳中医学院学报,2013,35(4):332

高静,杨翔宇,吴晨曦,等.中西医结合护理中外合作人才培养模式的建构[J].中华护理教育,2013,10(1):19

H

何丽清,窦志芳,张瑞卿,等.加强教学改革,提高《伤寒论》教学效果[J].中医药管理杂志,2013,21(2):149

何丽清.构建我院《伤寒论》教学模式,注重中医经典的传承[J].贵阳中医学院学报,2013,35(2):14

呼海涛,詹向红,王振亮,等.院校教育与师承教育相结合培养中医人才模式的探索与实践[J].中医药管理杂志,2013,21(3):256

黄必胜,舒劲松,黄琼霞.建立实验区,构建适应中医药学术继承和发展的人才培养模式[J].湖北中医药大学学报,2013,15(5):77

黄敏,金维捷,杨晓冬,等.TBL结合SP教学法应用于中医院校普通外科临床教学初探[J].中国中医药现代远程教育,2013,11(4):88

K

孔祥亮,吴中平,何新慧.“一体两翼”讲《伤寒》[J].河南中医,2013,33(1):1

L

李青,李朝霞.临床路径教学法在中医筋伤科护理教学中的应用[J].护理研究,2013,27(7):2025

李赛美.基于案例版《伤寒论》的自主学习方法尝试与思考[J].中国中医药现代远程教育,2013,11(13):102

李赛美,罗方波,彭万年.《伤寒论》PBL教学尝试与评价[J].中国中医药现代远程教育,2013,11(14):52

李孝波,邓晓鹏,窦志芳,等.形象教学法在伤寒论教学中的应用[J].中医教育,2013,32(2):75

李云海,林连美.《金匮要略》课程“案例式—启发式—互动式”多维教学方法体系研究[J].中国医药导报,2013,10(27):134

刘晓玲,李季,雷旭杰.《金匮要略》教学案例影像库的建立探讨[J].世界中医药,2013,8(3):345

鲁美君,张友堂,孙敏.对《伤寒论》教学临床思维培养的探讨[J].国际中医中药杂志,2013,35(12):1090

罗仁,王天,聂晓莉.基于“2244”教学法的临床教学查房模式[J].南方医学教育,2013,(3):39

M

马睿杰,林咸明,陈晓军.中医临床教学的改革与探索[J].光明中医,2013,28(5):1062

Q

钱会南.《内经》藏象教学探讨[J].中国中医药现代远程教育,2013,11(11):4

曲夷.伤寒论教学中的心力培养[J].中医教育,2013,32(4):45

S

苏丽清,赵国荣,李鑫辉,等.《温病学》教学应注重培养学生的中医临床思维能力[J].中国中医药现代远程教育,2013,11(24):88

T

屠燕捷,郭永洁,杨爱东.《中医临床经典导读》之教学探索[J].上海中医药大学学报,2013,27(2):8

W

王佳雯,潘一滨,陈红风.多媒体结合PBL教学模式在中医外科临床见习中的应用初探[J].世界中医药,2013,8(9):1115

王小平.论内经教学目的及实现对策[J].中医教育,2013,30(1):76

魏凯峰.中医《温病学》研究性教学课程体系构建探讨[J].辽宁中医药大学学报,2013,15(1):90

吴发胜,岳桂华,张爱珍,等.循证医学在中医内科临床教学应用中的展望[J].中国医药指南,2013,11(20):74

X

谢春娥,赵翠芳,张小会,等.从“生物—中医”双学位

模式谈国际型中医临床人才的培养[J]. 中医药管理杂志，2013,21(7)：701

谢忠礼. 中医经典教学中青年教师临床实践若干问题探讨[J]. 中医药管理杂志，2013,21(10)：1073

徐大量. 自主创新视域下的高等中医药教育人才培养模式研究[J]. 西北医学教育，2013,21(3)：435

Y

岳冬辉，周丽雅，陈凤芝，等. 易位式教学模式在温病学教学中的探索与实践[J]. 中医教育，2013,32(3)：27

Z

曾平，秦刚，廖小波，等. 模拟教学在中医骨伤科专业临床技能训练中应用的探讨[J]. 大学教育，2013,(4)：60

展照双，张思超. 比较归纳法在《温病学》教学中的应用[J]. 湖南中医杂志，2013,29(8)：92

张茂云，牟宗毅. 关于构建《金匮要略》"病案模拟—学生诊查—导入原文"三步式教学模式的实践与思考[J]. 辽宁中医药大学学报，2013,15(6)：102

张茂云，牟宗毅. 基于"张仲景杂病诊疗体系"的中医本科生临证思维建构[J]. 中医学报，2013,28(10)：1485

赵剑波，穆俊霞，晋钰丽，等.《内经选读》教学调查及分析[J]. 国际中医中药杂志，2013,35(5)：471

赵岩松，刘果，于河，等. 温病学临床教学平台构建的设想[J]. 中医教育，2013,32(5)：30

郑春素. 温病学形成性评价体系的构建与实践[J]. 光明中医，2013,28(6)：1284

郑旭锐，董正华，惠毅. 创新模式在中医创新实验班《温病学》教学应用探析[J]. 河北中医，2013,35(9)：1439

郑玉玲，詹向红，呼海涛，等. 中医传承教育人才培养模式的思考与探索[J]. 中医教育，2013,30(1)：8

周刚. 浅谈《伤寒论》课程教学中常用的辨治思维方法[J]. 山西中医，2013,29(9)：53

周杰，赵文景. 中医经典课程《内经选读》实践教学方法探析[J]. 中医药导报，2013,19(11)：136

周丽雅，岳冬辉，陈凤芝. 温病学多元化教学方法改革与实践[J]. 辽宁中医药大学学报，2013,15(7)：23

朱鹏举，陈士玉，谷峰.《内经》教学应做到两个不盲从[J]. 中国民族民间医药，2013,22(5)：121

朱乔青，应航，姚定国. 新时期中西医结合医学人才培养模式探讨——中医见习医生制临床教学实践[J]. 浙江中医药大学学报，2013,37(2)：199

朱莹，邹君君. 中医大学内科学临床见习教改方法初探[J]. 湖南中医杂志，2013,29(5)：103

(二)科技研究

【中西医结合研究的理论与方法学思考】

弓箭等论述了中西医结合研究中存在的一些问题。首先，由于对中西医学的本质差异认识不清，不论是当年的中西医汇通，还是半个多世纪的中西医结合，在中西医的关系上，既没有在理论上认识清楚，更没有在实践上产生根本性的成果。重要原因之一是对中西医学术内涵的差异均缺少准确深刻的认识。长期以来，大多数的研究均限于中西医概念原理的机械比附，最终的结论都似是而非，经不起时间的考验。现代中西医结合的研究，除了指标高级复杂之外，其思想方法还是在重复汇通派的局限，并没有实质的进步，对实现中西医结合的目标而言没有多大意义。中西医学的概念、原理、诊治原则等，其学术内涵是不等值的，中医学的范畴没有西医范畴那样的实证内涵，所以用西医(甚至包括任何科学技术)任何水平的指标都不能说明中医理论概念的学术实质。中西医学的差异不仅是医学理论和技术的差异，其背后还有更为深刻的思想文化差异。其次，对中西医结合必然性的理论研究薄弱。原因在于对中西医结合是否存在客观必然性缺少充分的研究。中西医结合是一项伟大的科学文化事业，涉及的问题既深刻又复杂，必须对中西医结合的合理性与必然性展开深入广泛的理论研究，从而使中西医结合得到正确理论的指导。第三，对中西医结合的内涵却没有获得一致的认识，尤其是没有将中西医结合的目标和具体中西医两法治病两者相区别。中西医结合的目标是明确的，就是两种医学体系合二为一，形成统一的医学体系。为了实现这一目标，就要从各方面展开中西医结合的研究活动。而与这一目标无关的活动，尽管也用了两法治病，但是却不应属于中西医结合研究范畴。弓氏针对目前中西医结合研究的思路与方法进行了分析，认为在科研命题选择及设计方面均有待改进。如果以严格的科学态度总结分析中西医结合工作，一方面应该承认做了大量的探索，得出了众多研究结果；另一方面也应该承认，至今还没有取得突破性的中西医结合研究成果，在任何领域都没有实现中西医结合的预期目标。表现为，未得出可以通贯中西医的理论结论、未出现可以推广和疗效统一的临床诊治规范、未产生中西医共用而无差别的技术成果。肖锋刚等指出中西医两法并用是中西医结合临床研究的最普遍的形式，但是中西医两法并用的结果在学术上存在太多的未知，在实践上也存在潜在的风险。同时，如果不对这两法并用结果进行深入的学术研究，其对汇通融合中西医学体系而言则缺少意义和价值。

戴恩来从中西医结合模式的探索与形成、病证结合的内涵、优势互补原则 3 个方面对构建中西医结合的临床基本模式进行探讨。关于中西医结合模式的探索与形成，认为构建起“病证结合，优势互补”的中西医结合临床模式，是对中西医结合历史的总结与传承，具有一定的临床实践意义。病证结合的优点就在于点面结合，总体把握，兼顾个体。从而能在整体而系统的层面认识疾病，这是单纯的西医、中医均无法做到的。要深入全面地把握疾病的普遍性与特殊性的关系，就必须做到宏观与微观、整体与局部、病原的致病性与机体反应性的三结合。优势互补是病证结合法则在治疗方法上的体现或者延续。熊航等指出中西医结合从中西医汇通派出现开始，无论在学术理论还是实践技能上都还没有真正的结合在一起，更没有产生新的理论体系，只能算是用中医、西医两种方法治病。认为中西医理论是两种不同的理论，二者的世界观和方法论存在着巨大差异，至今还没有找到能够消灭这种差异的公理性依据。所以，目前中西医在理论上始终无法真正结合。而“病证结合”模式本身只是一个方法学课题，是中西医诊治方法、手段的联合，是两种思维模式的整合，并非结合。熊氏提出应注意防止以下两种不良倾向：一是用时髦的名词术语代替和解释传统中医理论，出现问题的虚假解决；二是把西医作为评价知识或方法价值的唯一标准，以分析方法代替综合方法，以还原方法代替系统方法，以白箱方法代替黑箱方法，中医只是西医研究的一种材料，而不是一个不同范式的知识体系，从而降解和忽略了中医可能具有的价值。认为应该提倡在传统中变革，在继承中创新，同时要注重在观念更新与务实研究并进，理论研究与实验研究相结合，基础研究与应用研究相转化，只有这样来发展中医才是比较稳妥的。

邸宏杰等从科学人文主义的角度，论证中西医结合的必要性和正确性，认为中西医结合是中医现代化的必经之路，同时指出任何一门学科都可以追溯到其哲学时期，不同的只是其理论体系成为科学之后从哲学母体脱离的时间差异。从医学发展史来看，中医脱离哲学成为科学的脚步比西方医学等科学要慢，但是可以据其特征，预计其科学化的可能性。邸氏认为，中医学存在跨学科成分。中医并不像西方医学那样讨论分子之间的相互作用，而是将人看做阴阳并存的整体，并且用调节阴阳的方式整体医治。科学化走在前面的心理学，用元素和构造的特征来剖析人类的意识和行为，那么中医西学也可以让中医药的成分明晰，用现代科技精确治疗疾病。从某种程度上来说，要想中医现代化，中西医结合是必要的，也是客观条件下的唯一出路。但是，需要关注科学化所带来的弊端。首先，中西医结合是使中医国际化的必经之路，但并不是说就要摒弃中医理论中优秀的理论成果。其次，就像科学主义心理学的弊端一样，中医与西医不能单纯地关注人的“物性”，更不能对疾病采取单纯的“物性”治疗。西医在诊疗过程中，缺乏人文关怀，而中医在这方面可给予更多关注。西医是主体—客体的诊疗过程，而中医是主体—主体的诊疗过程，这一过程能给予患者更多的慰藉，即中医关注“人性”的一面。在中西医结合过程中，不能抛弃人文关怀，而要发扬这种传统，使医患保持和谐关系。总之，中西医结合的过程，是一个取长补短的过程，尽管中间充斥着两种文化的矛盾与冲突，但人文与科学走向科学人文主义是必然的过程。

（邸若虹）

【中医临床研究方法探讨】

刘保延提出真实世界的中医临床科研范式，即以人为中心，以数据为导向，以问题为驱动，医疗实践与科学计算交替，从临床中来到临床中去的临床科研一体化的科研范式。该范式继承了中医研究的基本模式，融合现代临床流行病学、循证医学、统计学和信息科学等概念、理论和技术，经过多年研究，成功开发出“中医临床科研信息共享系统”，解决了中医临床经验数字化、数据化以及管理、利用临床复杂数据的方法和关键技术，同时也较好地解决了“共享系统”在推广应用中的工程实施问题。“中医临床科研信息共享系统”建立了标准的中医术语系统，在此基础上通过结构化电子病历系统采集临床数据，通过中央随机数据管理系统采集理想世界临床数据，通过中医科学数据平台提供古文献和现代中医科学数据，通过患者报告结局量表产生疗效评价数据，最后通过数据预处理、分析挖掘系统获取、产生中医辨证论治个体化诊疗规律。共享系统包括中医药科学数据平台、“患者报告结局（PRO）”测量量表体系、数字化中医临床术语系统、高度结构化的中医电子病历系统、中医临床研究中央随机系统、数据管理系统、中医大数据的管理与利用系统。以上系统大多已先后在150多家医院的相关科室应用，积累40多名老中医临证经验医案，中医、中西医结合治疗冠心病、糖尿病、中风、肿瘤病历数据10余万份，开展相关临床研究近200多项。目前该系统已经成为16家国家中医临床研究基地的关键技术平台之一。谢雁鸣等将实效研究与中医临床研究相结合，认为中医学的基本特点与实效研究的特点有相似之处。中医临床实效研究应关注实际效果的设计与评价，效力评价是实现效果评价的基础。“十一五”国家科技支撑计划中医药领域项目涵盖重大疾病中医综合治疗方案的示范研究、疑难病中医干预及疗效评价研究、中医治疗常见病研究，部分实施方案发挥中医综合调节和辨证论治的优势，运用中药、针灸、推拿、手法等不同的干预措施，形成综合治疗方案或疾病预防方案，纳入、排除标准更为宽泛，试验设计和评价更贴近于“真实世界”。试验设计方面，实用性随机对照试验、队列研究、注册登记研究、上市后再评价研究、远期随访研究均属于实效研究的范畴；疗效评价方面，应尽量选择病死率、病残率、生存质量等重要结局，进行多元结局指标的测量。

朱向东等指出中医临床疗效评价模式的问题是中医药发展的瓶颈。中医思维应该是中医临床疗效评价的基石。认为判定中医药的疗效，应该运用中医思维对病象、证象、正邪斗争的态势，人体正气抗病出现的反应进行全面分析，特别是经过合理的辨证治疗后病人出现的各种抗邪反应，更应该运用中医思维进行科学的分析和辨识，去伪存真，进行实事求是的判定，才能真正捕捉到“趋佳”和“向愈”的实质，而不致被假象所迷惑。强调思维方式的转变是中医临床疗效判定的关键，指出“正向思维”是西医、中医判定临床疗效的主要依据，“反向思维”是中医判断临床疗效的重要方面。朱氏还从取象思维角度探讨了中医临床疗效判定的3个方面：医患共同体察病人的7种能力，医患共同勘对5种生命条件，医患共同检验精、气、神三宝。赵琼等对古代文献和现代期刊文献中关于中医疗效评价的内容进行梳理并对两者的异同点进行了归纳。相同点：①两者都体现了中医学整体观和辨证论治两个基本特点。②现代中医关于疗效评价的方法依然贯穿有传统中医临床疗效评价的方法与指标。③两者都重视根据治疗前后证候对比评价疗效。④都包含了生存质量的内容。不同点：①古代中医疗效评价运用阴阳五行、运气学说判断疗效，这些内容在现代疗效评价体系中已经很少见到。②现代中医疗效评价时会经常利用西医指标与方法评价中医临床疗效。③虽然古代中医疗效评价体系中包含了生存质量的内容，但与现代中医所提及的生存质量测评方法还是有着本质的差别，现代中医所用的生存质量测评方法大都是简单引用西医学生存质量量表去测评。④现代中医疗效评价体系中会借鉴循证医学的内容去对中医药疗效进行评价。张帆等认为系统论指导下的综合评价是中医疗效评价的最适方法一。即运用多个指标对多个标的进行评价，明确每个评价标的的最适宜指标群及其评价效力，对其进行指标权重的排序。评价过程不是逐个指标顺次完成的，而是通过一些特殊方法将多个指标的评价同时完成。在综合评价过程中，根据指标的重要性进行加权处理，评价结果不再是具有具体含义的统计指标，而是以指数或分值表示标的“综合状况”的排序。以此可构建起既体现中医自身治疗特色与优势，又与现代诊疗模式相适应的，涵盖患者报告结局指标、终点结局指标、中医证侯指标、生存质量指标、安全性指标和卫生经济学指标等多维的中西医结合临床疗效评价指标体系。谢晴宇等提出将中医临床路径的流程设计与决策知识相结合，把开放的建模理念引入到中医临床路径系统研发中，构建了中医临床路径工作流系统模式图。认为该模式区别于传统的临床路径医嘱单，强调运用动态、时序化的流程来集成诊疗数据，链接决策知识，构成复杂的认知网络，为后续的方法学评价提供临床素材。认为中医临床路径实践在思维层面需要的是源头活水，是充满人文气息的理性思考；在组织管理层面，需要的是严谨的方法学设计和流程质量控制；在政策法规方面，有赖于行业规范的调整，让医院有动力去降低医疗成本，推动优势疗法的涌现。

（李永健）

【交叉学科知识在中医药研究中的应用】

田甜等提出了本体的概念及其在中医药领域应用的现状，指出中医药领域本体建立的意义在于推动中医知识的数字化和规范化进程，而难点在于中医药学科本身的复杂性及中医药学概念的不规范和多重性。本体技术作为一种新的知识组织工具，可以多维度、可视化、动态地表示和组织中医知识和相关的信息资源。构建中医药学本体，应该符合中医学的思维方式。田氏尝试用人工智能技术，通过构建语义网络来将各个概念的定义、关联准确、完整、忠实地表现出来，以解决本体构建过程中的问题。认为中医本体作为中医信息处理的重要基础，在科研、教学、辅助诊断、电子病例、新药开发等多个方面均有良好的应用前景。屈华等以《伤寒论》中医经典传承为目的，针对《伤寒论》存在大量非结构化知识、概念和概念间关系的高度复杂性的问题，在形式概念分析和概念格的基础上发展出属性偏序结构图的生成方法，并建立了《伤寒论》方剂、中药量效和方证的属性偏序结构图。通过对这类结构图的分析，显示了很好的频次、聚类和关联特征，并能够层次化、结构化和可视化地进行知识表达和知识发现。基于严密的形式概念分析数学理论和属性偏序结构图原理的多层次复杂概念网络生成方法，初步建立了中医经典传承知识发现的理论基础，可有效并合理地描述多层次中医复杂概念和概念层次，为下一步开展基于方证对应的中医经典辨治疑难病专家系统的研究工作奠定基础。张博等指出，理解中药方剂与病证的生物学基础是中医药现代研究的一个重点，随着系统生物学等交叉学科的兴起，以生物分子网络为切入点的网络药理学和网络医学有望系统地刻画中医药的整体性特征，从一个新的视角阐释中医证候的生物学基础和中药方剂的药效物质基础。网络药理学用于中医药转化医学研究是一个既传统又年轻的领域，不仅要求该领域的研究思路符合中医理论与实践，而且在应用过程中还面临诸多挑战。基于生物分子网络的系统分析方法与中医学的思维与实践存在交汇之处，有效弥补了中医基础研究与临床转化的沟壑。

张萍等通过将中医与以物理学为代表的自然科学进行对比可发现,中医与其他自然科学类似,同样选择了自然界存在的客观事物进行研究。中医选择了人体的生命现象为研究对象,生命现象的客观存在性和临床疗效是中医科学性的坚实基础。中医学的研究方法特征与现代物理有相通之处。中医学的某些观点已经被现代实验所证实,但还有不少部分尚无法被证实或证伪。中医试图从宏观、整体、系统的角度思考自然世界,并以此为基础,建立了大量依托于各个单元协作组合而产生的参量概念,如经络、穴位等。在大量实践活动的基础上,中医学构建了从整体和系统角度出发的独特的理论体系。现代物理尤其是量子力学的最新进展揭示了中医学的理论并非不科学,甚至说是其部分与现代科学最前沿的看法有相同之处。刘颖等基于代谢组学的概念和常用分析技术,总结了代谢组学与中医阴阳五行、藏象、经络学说、病因病机及防治原则的关系,论述了代谢组学在中医药中的应用并提出几点思考。认为整体性思路的代谢组学技术与中医基础理论研究相结合会使传统医学的研究更加标准化、规范化和透明化,并希望在中医循证医学方面探索出新的思路与方法。黄欣荣指出中医通过其整体思维而实现了整体性、关联性这两个复杂系统的重要特征,继而形成了经络相连、阴阳平衡、整体调理这些复杂性科学的先进理念和手段。通过辨证论治而实现了复杂系统的自主性、多样性和涌现性等特征。在整体观的视野下,通过辨证论治来达到辨识病因,并通过方剂、针灸诸多疗法来实现患者的康复。认为中医药理论是具备了复杂性理论的几乎所有特征,因此是一种在复杂性科学理论正式提出之前的朴素复杂性理论形态。中医注重临床实践,从实践到理论,从下(实践)到上(理论)的研究范式,可以称之为"实境范式",为当今的复杂性科学研究提供了一种具有悠长历史的真实研究案例。认为中医不属于简单性科学范式,因此难于融入西方近现代科学体系之中,难于与西医相融合成一个学科体系。从复杂性科学的视野看,中医不但不是伪科学,反而是未来科学发展的新方向和新典范。复杂性科学的思维与方法对中医药融入世界科学洪流中具有巨大的意义,而中医药理论和实践对复杂性科学也具有重要的理论和实践意义。

(邸若虹)

[附] 参考文献

D

戴恩来.病证结合,优势互补——构建中西医结合的临床基本模式[J].甘肃中医学院学报,2013,30(3):91

邸宏杰,徐家华.科学人文主义与中西医结合[J].卫生职业教育,2013,31(11):7

G

弓箭,肖锋刚,常存库.中西医结合研究存在的主要问题[J].医学与哲学,2013,34(4A):17

H

黄欣荣.复杂性科学与中医[J].中医杂志,2013,54(19):1621

L

刘保延.真实世界的中医临床科研范式[J].中医杂志,2013,54(6):451

刘颖,周红光,吴勉华.代谢组学应用于中医基础理论现代化研究的思考[J].山东中医药大学学报,2013,37(2):96

Q

屈华,李赛美,洪文学,等.基于多层次复杂概念网络表示原理的《伤寒论》群结构知识发现方法研究[J].中华中医药杂志,2013,28(5):1241

T

田甜,高思华.本体在中医药学领域的应用现状及展望[J].中华中医药杂志,2013,28(6):1832

X

肖锋刚,弓箭,常存库.中西医结合两法并用的状态及意义[J].中医药信息,2013,30(2):126

谢晴宇,孟庆刚,王永炎.中医临床路径实践模式的思考[J].北京中医药大学学报,2013,36(1):5

谢雁鸣,魏戌,王永炎.实效研究与中医临床研究[J].中国中医基础医学杂志,2013,19(2):139

熊航,王玉来,郭蓉娟,等.关于中西医结合的思考[J].云南中医学院学报,2013,36(6):87

Z

张博,李慧颖,李梢.网络药理学:中医药与转化医学研究新途径[J].转化医学研究(电子版),2013,3(3):1

张帆,刘光辉,张哲,等.有关中医临床疗效评价指标的思考[J].中华中医药学刊,2013,31(6):1285

张萍,竺炯.从西方物理学与中医的对比看中医的科学性[J].时珍国医国药,2013,24(8):1968

赵琼,闫卫红.关于古今中医疗效评价的理论探讨[J].中医杂志,2013,54(11):983

朱向东,梁永林,王燕.从中医思维角度探讨中医临床疗效评价问题[J].中华中医药杂志,2013,28(1):152

记　　事

一、学 术 会 议

▲ 全国中医妇科流派学术研讨会在广州举行 2月22～23日，由广东省中医药学会和广州中医药大学第一附属医院主办，广药集团白云山中一药业协办。首批全国中医妇科流派传承人—岭南罗氏妇科传承工作室同时启动。

▲ 骨伤流派传承工作研讨会在北京举行 3月23日，辽宁华山正骨、上海石氏伤科、平乐郭氏正骨、襄阳何氏正骨、宁夏张氏回医正骨、北京清宫正骨等15个骨伤流派传承工作室的专家代表进行学术交流。

▲ 第十一次全国老年医学学术会议在武汉召开 4月19～21日，由中华医学会老年医学分会(下称老年医学分会)主办。来自全国各地的老年医学及相关专业的学者专家参与了会议，对老年医学学科建设、中国健康老年人标准等老年医学学科建设问题进行了探讨，并就学科热点问题作了学术报告。会议对此次学术报告中获奖的青年医师进行了颁奖表彰。

▲ 中国男科医学大会在北京召开 4月20～21日，由中国中西医结合学会男科专业委员会、美国加州生殖医学协会、中国性学会性医学专业委员会共同发起举办，来自全国23个省市和美国、英国等地的三百余位医师出席了会议。大会收到来自中国、美国、英国等地的男科学术论文90余篇，涵盖前列腺疾病、整形、性功能障碍、男性更年期疾病、不育症等诸多方面内容。

▲ 2013年卷《中国中医药年鉴(学术卷)》编委会暨审稿会议在上海召开 4月22～24日，国家中医药管理局办公室副主任徐皖生，上海市卫生局中医发展办主任郑锦，中国出版协会年鉴工作委员会副会长、上海市年鉴学会会长朱敏彦，以及《中国中医药年鉴(学术卷)》编委、特邀编委和学科编辑约60人出席。《年鉴》编委会办公室主任王兴伊主持会议，常务副主编刘平致开幕词，常务副主编张如青汇报2013卷《中国中医药年鉴(学术卷)》编纂工作以及编委换届、新任编委情况，并表达了对资深编委的感谢，常务副主编余岚介绍了上海辞书出版社对《中国中医药年鉴(学术卷)》出版工作情况。会议期间编委们审阅了各栏目稿件，就《中国中医药年鉴(学术卷)》的文献来源、编纂形式、学术精神及发行量等进行了研讨，并建议国家中医药管理局增加对《年鉴》扶持力度，在部分高校及科研院(所)将《年鉴》发稿纳入考核范围，建立《年鉴》网站，网页包含《年鉴》内容检索引擎、《年鉴》相关新闻动态、《年鉴》投稿系统等，以期提高《年鉴》影响力及发行量。

▲ 关幼波诞辰100周年纪念大会暨中医肝病学术研讨会在北京召开 5月18～19日，由首都医科大学附属北京中医医院主办。国家中医药管理局副局长于文明出席，关幼波提出的肝病立法方药，如"治肝十法"、"退黄三要则"等，至今仍在有效指导临床应用。

▲ 海峡两岸中医药研讨会在厦门召开 6月16～17日，由国家中医药管理局和厦门市人民政府共同主办。海峡两岸中医药界知名专家、学者及企业界450余名代表参会，国家卫生和计划生育委员会副主任、国家中医药管理局局长王国强出席开幕式。

▲ 中医男科新进展暨陈文伯学术研讨班在北京举行 6月22日，由北京鼓楼中医医院"陈文伯名医传承工作室"主办。北京中医药大学附属东直门医院、中国中医科学院广安门医院、中日友好医院等单位的8名男科专家分别介绍其经验及研究成果。

▲ 第八次全国中西医结合男科学术会议在开封举行 8月23～25日，由中国中西医结合学会男科专业委员会主办，河南省中医院和河南省中西医结合男科专业委员会共同承办。大会收到专题报告课件30个，论文391篇，其中男性不育120篇，前列腺疾病87篇，性功能障碍90篇，男性杂病77篇，不孕不育77篇。

▲ 第九次中医急诊学术研讨会暨急诊分会换届改选会议在连云港举行 8月24日，由中华中医药学会主办、中华中医药学会急诊分会承办。参会代表近200人，就中西医结合诊治耐药菌感染和慢阻肺急性发作、如何提高中医急诊疗效、中

医参与突发公共卫生事件、中医应急体系建设等进行交流及研讨。会议选出新一届委员会，王融冰任主任委员，孙塑伦、杜怀堂、钱英、符为民、李乾构等任顾问委员，王永炎、晁恩祥为名誉主委。

▲ 世界中医药学会联合会神志病专委会成立暨第一届学术年会在哈尔滨举行 8月29日，学术年会围绕中医神志病学的创新与发展为主题，就中医神志病临床诊疗标准化与客观化研究、神志病预防、诊疗及症候演变规律，神志病中西医结合治疗方法等进行了交流与探讨。黑龙江神志医院院长赵永厚当选为专委会会长，浙江省立同德医院院长冯斌任秘书长，国家自然科学基金委员会生命科学部中医学与中药学学科专家王昌恩，北京安定医院专家王彦恒被聘请为顾问。

▲ 第十七次全国儿科中西医结合学术会议在杭州萧山举行 9月4～6日，由中国中西医结合学会儿科专业委员会主办，萧山中医院、杭州市中医药协会和萧山中医药学会联合承办。来自全国16个省、自治区、直辖市的100余位中西医结合儿科学界的专家、学者参会并进行了学术交流及研讨。与会专家认为，某些感染、呼吸系统疾病如哮喘、免疫系统疾病如过敏性紫癜、内分泌系统疾病如甲状腺功能低下和性早熟等以单纯西医治疗并不十分理想的疾病，采用中西医结合的方法综合治疗，能取得单纯中医或单纯西医治疗所不可比拟的效果。

▲ 中国骨科医学大会暨国际骨科专家高峰论坛在北京召开 8月9～11日，由美国加州医学会、中国中西医结合学会骨伤科分会、中华医学发展研究会共同举办。全国23个省市以及美国、英国等地的300余位医师出席了大会，收到骨科医学论文90余篇。

▲ 第十二届国际针灸学术研讨会在天津召开 9月14日，由天津中医药大学第一附属医院与天津市针灸学会共同主办。中国工程院院士石学敏、中国科学院院士韩济生、中国针灸学会副会长朱兵等专家及来自美国、德国、澳大利亚等30多个国家和地区的400名代表参加了会议。

▲ 首届回医药学术交流会在北京召开 9月27日，由北京市民族事务委员会、北京市中医管理局、宁夏中医药(回医药)管理局主办。国家中医药管理局副局长马建中，以及来自国内回医药研发与回族文化传播等相关领域的180余位专家、学者参加了会议，大会收到学术论文52篇。

▲ 2013中华中医药学会编辑出版年会暨慢病防控优秀论文交流会在张家港举行 9月28～29日，国家中医药管理局副局长吴刚，江苏省卫生厅副厅长兼中医药管理局局长陈亦江，中华中医药学会副会长兼编辑出版分会主委李俊德，以及全国各期刊、出版社的负责人、专家约150人出席。全国100多家杂志参与了中医药期刊交流展示。100余篇论文分别参加了编辑年会、慢病防控会议的交流。

▲ 2013全国中西医创面修复高层论坛在天津举办 10月11日，由中华中医药学会外科分会主办，天津中医药大学第一附属医院承办。国内多位研究创面修复的中医与西医界专家、学者出席会议并表示，中医与西医创面修复相互参与、相互融合，将汇聚一支理论水平高、实践能力强的创面修复专家队伍，共同推动中国创面修复研究的发展。同时，成立"中华中医药学会外科分会创面修复临床评价专业学组"，"中华医学会外科创面修复专科联盟成员"在天津中医药大学第一附属医院外科挂牌。

▲ 首届全国骨科微创外固定关键技术推广应用学习研讨会在北京举行 10月12日，由中国中医科学院望京医院主办。来自全国骨伤界的150余位专家、学者出席会议并作了"继往开来、创立中国特色的骨科微创治疗体系"、"下肢畸形与残缺外科治疗新技术"、"新型肱骨外科颈夹板的研发与临床验证"等21场专题演讲。

▲ 国际气功科学研讨会在上海举行 10月18～19日，由上海中医药大学、上海市中医药研究院主办。来自中国、法国、加拿大等国及港台地区的气功养生专家、传统功法流派传人、医疗气功专业人士、气功爱好者与受益者150余人参加了会议。会议分"大会论文交流"与"气功功法交流"两部分，收到论文47篇，其中43篇收入论文集。

▲ 第五届心身医学国际论坛在北京广安门医院召开 10月18～20日，由北京中医药学会、中国中医科学院广安门医院等主办。日本九州大学心身医学科须藤信行、广安门医院赵志付、北京大学人民医院刘梅颜、海军总医院李秀玉、北京中医医院张捷等介绍以刚柔辨证治疗胆囊炎、心脏神经官能证等常见心身疾病的经验，以及就心血管科的精神心理关注、肝郁与抑郁、中医整体观与心身医学等主题最新进展分别进行了交流。

▲首届世界脊诊整脊医学联盟大会暨全国脊诊整脊技术学术委员会换届大会在天津召开 10月19～20日,来自全国各地及美国、新加坡、马来西亚、韩国、日本的专家、代表共500余人参加了会议。会议选举天津北辰北门医院院长王遵来任联盟主席兼执行主席,并就整脊手法治疗脊柱病的最新进展、微创技术在脊柱疾病中的应用、民营医院管理与发展进行了探讨。

▲高健生和庄曾渊从医五十年研讨会在北京中国中医科学院眼科医院举办 10月25日,来自全国各地的几十名中医眼科专家就眼科最新学术成果进行交流研讨。

▲第30次全国中医儿科学术大会在济南举行 10月26日,由中华中医药学会主办,中华中医药学会儿科分会、山东中医药大学附属医院承办。全国29个省、市、自治区的500余名儿科专家参加会议并就儿科临床热点问题,以及中医新思维、方法、技术的最新研究进行了交流。

▲第十七届全国药史本草学术研讨会在蕲春召开 10月31日,中国中医科学学院副院长黄璐琦、香港浸会大学赵中振、广州中医药大学附属中山医院梅全喜、中国中医科学院医史文献研究所肖永芝等应邀作学术报告。

▲王焘学术思想研讨会在陕西眉县召开 10月31日,由中国民族医药学会和陕西省中医药科技开发研究会主办。

▲国际健康论坛暨《中华医学百科全书》2013主编年会在北京召开 11月8～9日,第67届联合国大会主席武克·耶雷米奇、国际健康与环境组织主席王彦峰等,以及来自世界各地的学者、专家、企业家700余人出席了会议。

▲世界中医药学会联合会中药专业委员会换届会议暨保健食品国际学术会议在北京召开 11月3日,世界中医药学会联合会主席佘靖及来自海内外11个国家和地区的90余名代表参会。龙致贤当选为第三届中药专委员会理事会会长,曹俊岭任秘书长。会议邀请美国国立卫生研究院(NIH)基金资深评审专家钱肃凡就如何撰写NIH基金标书进行了培训指导。

▲世界中医药学会联合会护理专业委员会成立大会暨首届中医护理学术国际研讨会在南京召开 11月9日,世界中医药学会联合会主席佘靖,江苏省卫生厅副厅长、省中医药局局长陈亦江及来自美国、加拿大、葡萄牙等19个国家与地区的中医护理界专家进行了学术研讨。南京中医药大学护理学院院长徐桂华当选为首届护理专委会会长。

▲泰山学术论坛在济南山东中医药大学举行 11月16～17日,由山东省教育厅主办、山东中医药大学承办。论坛以"中医学术流变与跨文化传播"为主题,中国科学院院士陈凯先作"当代中医药学的作用和地位"学术报告,黑龙江中医药大学副校长程伟、中国中医科学院孟庆云、黄龙祥等专家就中医学术流变与跨文化传播作专题学术报告。

▲国医大师陆广莘学术思想研讨会在北京举行 11月29日,陆广莘作了"以人为本创生性实践的生生之学"主题发言,国家中医药管理局原副局长诸国本、中国中医科学院中医基础理论研究所原所长孟庆云等发表专题演讲。

▲全国第十六次中医药文化学术研讨会与中华中医药学会中医药文化分会换届在北京召开 12月5～6日,由中华中医药学会主办,中医药文化分会承办,中国中医药出版社协办。中国中医药出版社社长王国辰当选为主任委员,北京中医药大学张其成为名誉主任委员,北京中医药大学教授钱超尘等9人为学术顾问。141位专家学者对中医药文化传承、传播、发展及其相关问题深入研讨。

二、中 外 交 流

▲ ISO秘书长考察中医药标准化工作 2月22日，国际标准化组织（ISO）中央秘书处秘书长罗博·斯蒂尔先生考察了中医药国际标准化工作。罗博·斯蒂尔先生对受邀来访表示感谢，肯定了ISO/TC249秘书处为中医药国际标准工作所做出的努力并希望取得更大成就。

▲ 韩国正统针灸学会学员到甘肃学习针灸 3月11日，韩国正统针灸学会10名学员赴甘肃省中医院开始了为期3周的中医针灸学习，旨在拓展中韩双方在传统医疗技术和学术交流领域的合作。

▲ 李大宁率团访问美国、巴哈马 3月3日，国家中医药管理局副局长李大宁率团访问美国、巴哈马。访美期间，代表团与希伯来健康养老中心就美国持续照料退休社区（美国养老社区，CCRC）发展状况及与中国合作等相关事宜进行会谈，并初步达成了合作意向。

▲ 2013国际中医药学术交流大会在旧金山市举办 3月18日，由北京市华夏中医药发展基金会协办，与“第84届美国国医节”大型庆典活动同时举行。来自中医药学术界、针灸界、中医院校、医疗器械及关心支持中医药的各国人士与会汇聚。

▲ 第16届日中友好针灸研修之旅研讨会在京举办 3月28日，日本东方出版社社长野濑真主持了会议，中医药专家马继兴、李经纬、余瀛鳌、钱超尘等100余人出席。

▲ 中法中医药合作委员会第五次会议在法国巴黎召开 4月22～23日，委员会中方主席王国强率中方代表团出席会议，并代表国家中医药管理局与法国巴黎公立医院集团签署《在中医药领域合作的框架协议》。外交部（驻法国使馆）、国家食品药品监督管理总局、国家中医药管理局等中方委员会成员单位代表及中国科学院院士陈凯先等中方委员会成员20多人参团与会。法国社会事务与卫生部部长马丽索·杜兰，法国科学院终生秘书长卡特琳娜·布雷西尼亚克，委员会法方主席、法国工程院名誉主席弗朗索瓦·基诺等出席会议。

▲ 中新签署中医药合作计划书 5月15日，新加坡卫生部代表团访问国家中医药管理局，在中新中医药合作委员会会议上，国家卫生和计划生育委员会副主任、国家中医药管理局局长王国强与新加坡卫生部及人力部政务部长许连碹，签署中新中医药合作计划书，双方将在中医药科研、教育、管理等领域加强交流合作。

▲ 甘肃与乌克兰基辅州合作培养中医药人才 6月19日，应乌克兰基辅州政府邀请，甘肃省中医药及卫生合作项目考察团一行赴乌克兰在基辅与州政府代表会谈并达成多项共识。甘肃省卫生厅厅长刘维忠和基辅州卫生厅副厅长亚历山大代表双方正式签署合作框架协议，建立定期交流互访机制。乌克兰国立医科大学和甘肃中医学院初步达成在互换学生、中医药科研及联合在乌建立岐伯中医学院等方面开展合作的意向。

▲ 北京中医药大学与慕尼黑工大续签合作协议 6月24日，北京中医药大学与德国慕尼黑工业大学合作协议续签仪式在慕尼黑举行。双方还就深化中医科研和临床领域合作等议题进行了座谈。

▲ 王国强会见吉尔吉斯斯坦代表团 6月26日，国家卫生和计划生育委员会副主任、国家中医药管理局局长王国强会见了来华访问的吉尔吉斯斯坦卫生部国务秘书苏优姆巴耶娃、吉外交服务局局长伊尔萨利耶夫、吉政府建设和区域发展署副署长玛姆别托夫一行。国家中医药管理局副局长于文明陪同出席并主持工作会谈。中吉双方达成共识：同意由中国国家中医药管理局与吉尔吉斯斯坦卫生部签署政府部门间的中医药合作谅解备忘录，共同成立中医药合作工作组，两国对应机构执行某一方面的具体合作。

▲ 富布赖特项目访问团到陕西中医学院附属医院参观交流 7月5日，为加强国际间的医学交流与合作，由宾夕法尼亚州立大学、圣爱德华大学、哥伦比亚特区大学等美国各大院校代表组成的富布赖特项目访问团一行18人，到陕西中医

学院附属医院进行参观与交流。

▲ 上合组织官员赴陕西中医学院附属医院访问交流　7月10日，来自俄罗斯、吉尔吉斯斯坦、乌兹别克斯坦、塔吉克斯坦、哈萨克斯坦5个上海合作组织成员国从事医药行政管理、医疗、教学、科研等工作的19名官员到陕西中医学院附属医院进行访问与交流。

▲ 中澳合建国际中医药研究中心　7月24日，"中澳国际中医药研究中心"澳方揭牌仪式在澳大利亚皇家墨尔本理工大学举行。该中心为国家中医药管理局批准，依托广东省中医院、广东省中医药科学院与澳洲皇家墨尔本理工大学建立的首个国际中医药研究中心，旨在"进行高影响力的传统与补充医学研究，服务民众的循证卫生保健"。

▲ 中瑞签署中医药合作计划书　7月29日，国家中医药管理局副局长于文明，以及国家中医药管理局国际合作司、传统医药国际交流中心有关负责人与来访的瑞士联邦 Mediqi AG 集团(聚英欧洲中医诊疗中心集团)杜力·巴多拉董事长和克劳迪欧·麦茨董事长一行会谈并签署新一轮中医药合作计划书。于文明肯定了中瑞合作以来所取得的成绩，希望双方能继续加强交流合作，国家中医药管理局会密切关注中瑞双边合作进展及合作成果。

▲ 第十三次中韩传统医学协调委员会会议在北京召开　7月31日，国家卫生和计划生育委员会副主任、国家中医药管理局局长王国强与韩国保健福祉部次官李永灿就两国进一步扩大推动传统医药产业领域合作，继续促进民间传统医学学术与人员交流，加强在国际平台的合作等签署备忘录。

▲ 中美开展JCI中医院质量标准研究　8月5日，广东省中医院陈达灿与美国贸易发展署东亚区主任 Geoffrey Jackson 先生作为双方代表在北京签订协议，双方约定共同开展中医院临床质量监控研究项目，美国贸易发展署将提供资金用于该项研究。主要以广东省中医院为工作参照点，IBM-JCI 团队共同收集信息，评估医院责任人对质量的理解和对上述3块功能区域流程标准化的接受程度，藉此评估医院技术能力。根据 JCI 和试点中医院报告的方案形成研究市场开发前的评估报告，作为建立中医院质量管理架构和相关标准重要的参考依据。国家中医药管理局国际合作司司长王笑频和美国驻华使馆商务处参赞 Val Huston 分别作为中美双方见证人在该协议上签字。

▲ 王国强会见世卫组织总干事陈冯富珍　8月21日，国家卫生和计划生育委员会副主任、国家中医药管理局局长王国强在北京会见了世界卫生组织总干事陈冯富珍一行。王国强表示，愿继续加强双方合作，促进中西医结合及中医药在海外发展，共同帮助非洲国家开展疾病防治和卫生体系建设，实现联合国千年发展目标做出更大贡献。

▲ 中医系列讲座走进墨西哥　8月31日，墨西哥中国文化中心与重庆市文广局省部合作项目——重庆中医大师、国家级非遗传承人刘光瑞系列讲座，在墨西哥国立自治大学外国语言中心开讲。此次讲座是10场系列讲座的第一讲，由墨西哥中国文化中心与墨西哥国立自治大学孔子学院合作举办。

▲ 第四期亚洲区域中医药教育高级师资研修班在天津中医药大学开班　9月9日，来自印尼、马来西亚、新加坡、泰国、越南、蒙古等7国的13名传统医药领域的专家学者，在该校进行为期两周的学习和交流。

▲ 中吉两国签署中医药领域合作谅解备忘录　9月11日，国家卫生和计划生育委员会副主任、国家中医药管理局局长王国强与吉尔吉斯斯坦卫生部长迪娜拉·萨基姆巴耶娃，在吉尔吉斯斯坦首都比什凯克签署了《中华人民共和国国家中医药管理局与吉尔吉斯共和国卫生部关于中医药领域合作谅解备忘录》，并就落实备忘录细则以及双边合作共同在吉建立中医医疗机构举行正式会谈。

▲ 王国强率中医药代表团访问俄罗斯　9月12～16日，应俄罗斯莫斯科州政府邀请，国家卫生和计划生育委员会副主任、国家中医药管理局局长王国强率团访问俄罗斯。其间与莫斯科州州长沃罗比约夫举行会谈并签署会谈纪要，双方商定将开展中医药各领域的交流与合作，共同推荐相关机构在莫斯科州开展中医医疗合作。代表团还应俄国防部邀请，与俄国防部第一副部长查理科夫会谈，对方表达了与中方开展中医药医疗领域合作的强烈愿望，使俄方军人能享受中医药特色和优势。王国强表示将支持推动在俄建立中医药中心一事。

▲ 第十届世界中医药大会暨世界中医药学会联合会成立十周年庆典在旧金山举行 9月21～22日，由世界中医药学会联合会主办。世界中医药学会联合会主席佘靖，中国驻旧金山总领事馆总领事袁南生，以及来自世界各地的中医药专家学者及企事业机构的1 000余名代表参会。世界中联第三届第五次理事会与第四次监事会会议同期召开。

▲ 马建中会见波兰代表团 10月16日，国家中医药管理局副局长马建中在北京会见来访的波兰药品、医疗器械和生物制品注册总局副局长马钦·克拉克斯基一行。波方表示愿意为中药产品在波兰注册提供尽可能的支持，并安排波兰专家学者访华，学习中医药知识。国家中医药管理局科技司、国际合作司相关同志参加会见。代表团还参观访问了北京中医药大学东方医院等中医药机构。

▲ 以岭医药研究院与英国卡迪夫大学联姻 10月20日，英国卡迪夫大学——以岭医药研究院医药研究中心在北京成立。国家中医药管理局副局长于文明，英国卡迪夫大学校长、主席Professor Colin Riordan，中国工程院院士吴以岭、程书钧等出席揭牌仪式。中心将进一步开展养正消积胶囊抗肿瘤的靶点研究、联合开发新的抗肿瘤药物。同时教学、研究人员定期交换、交流，联合举办国内外学术会议推广新成果、新技术。

▲ 王国强会见马其顿卫生部代表团 10月21日，国家卫生和计划生育委员会副主任、国家中医药管理局局长王国强在北京会见了来访的马其顿卫生部部长尼科拉·托多罗夫一行。双方达成共识，将在马其顿高校设立中医课程，加快中马双方在中医药教育和中药产品方面的合作进程。双方将通过派出中方教师赴马教学和接受马方师资队伍来华进修两个途径，尽快在马其顿相关大学开展中医药，尤其是针灸教学，推荐成都中医药大学与马其顿相关大学建立合作关系。

▲ 马其顿总统伊万诺夫到成都中医药大学附属医院参观访问 10月23日，马其顿总统伊万诺夫一行在外交部欧洲司参赞亓玫，四川省外事办、四川省中医药管理局、成都中医药大学等领导陪同下，参观访问了成都中医药大学附属医院。伊万诺夫邀请成都中医药大学附属医院代表及中医药专家到马其顿卫生部及相关大学访问，希望双方能就中医药知识和技能开展进一步学术交流。

▲ 岐黄中医学院在乌克兰医科大学挂牌 10月30日，甘肃中医学院与乌克兰国立医科大学在乌克兰首府基辅市签署合作框架协议，设立“岐黄中医学院”并挂牌。根据双方签署的协议，甘肃中医学院与乌克兰国立医科大学今后将借助岐黄中医学院这一平台，共享教育及科研资料，共同合作出版科研成果，联合创办科学期刊。

▲ 马建中率团访问澳大利亚和斐济 10月31日～11月7日，应澳大利亚中医针灸协会和斐济卫生部邀请，国家中医药管理局副局长马建中率中医药代表团于对两国进行工作访问。访澳期间，代表团出席了世界针灸学会联合会第八届会员大会和学术大会。访斐期间，马建中与斐济卫生部部长尼尔·夏尔马相互交流了本国传统医学发展情况，表达了在该领域开展合作的共同愿望。

▲ 世界针联第八届针灸学术大会在悉尼会展中心开幕 11月2日，由世界针灸学会联合会和中国中医科学院共同主办，澳大利亚针灸中医协会承办。国家中医药管理局副局长马建中，世界针联高级顾问、中国中药协会会长房书亭，以及来自世界各地近40个国家和地区约100个世界针联团体会员组织的代表和观察员共822名出席。世界针灸学会联合会第八届会员大会同期召开，33个国家和地区的76名代表被选举成为第八届世界针灸学会联合会执行委员会委员。会上通过了将每年11月16～22日定为“世界针灸周”的提案。

▲ 中国中医科学院望京医院与墨西哥东南针灸医学协会签署合作协议 11月9日，墨西哥东南针灸医学协会暨拉丁美洲耳针协会与望京医院就教学合作达成协议，并正式签署合作协议书。同时，望京医院与墨西哥东南针灸医学协会和东方脉搏(北京)信息技术有限责任公司共同签署了有关网络培训、专题理论讲座、临床见习为主要内容的教学合作协议书。

▲ 2013新加坡国际中医药高层论坛在新加坡大巴窑中医学院举行 11月16～17日，来自中国、德国、新加坡等国的100余位专家学者参加论坛。论坛围绕“中医药临床新进展”的主题展开研讨，中国中医科学院首席研究员、973首席科学家仝小林作了“经方在糖尿病及并发症中的应用”

的专题演讲。

▲ **黑龙江中医药大学与俄医学院签署合作协议** 12月6日，黑龙江中医药大学与俄罗斯阿穆尔国立医学院在哈尔滨举行教育交流合作协议签约仪式。根据协议，双方于2014年7月互派5至10名学生到对方学校进行为期3周的临床实习。

▲ **中国中医科学院与俄罗斯莫斯科州政府开展中医医疗合作** 12月30日，双方成立中俄合作中医诊疗中心并在莫斯科州和中国中医科学院西苑医院同时挂牌。西苑医院将定期选派中医专家赴俄开展中医诊疗服务，俄方所需中医药品、保健品由西苑医院供应。

三、动 态 消 息

▲《东医宝鉴》英译本正式发行 1月4日，国家社科基金重大项目《中医典籍研究与英译工程》最新成果、中国社会科学院重大出版项目《东医宝鉴》(英译本)由社会科学文献出版社出版，并于1月上旬正式发行。

▲ 夏桂成荣获“白求恩奖章” 1月7日，在全国卫生工作会议上，卫生部、人力资源社会保障部和国家中医药管理局领导向中医系统唯一的白求恩奖章获得者江苏省中医院主任中医师夏桂成颁发了奖章和证书，同时对上海中医药大学附属曙光医院、山西中医学院附属医院等32家中医(民族医)系统单位以及中国中医科学院广安门医院路志正、北京中医药大学东直门医院王耀献等获全国卫生系统先进集体、先进工作者进行了表彰。

▲ 2013年全国中医药工作会议在北京召开 1月10日，由国家中医药管理局组织。卫生部党组书记张茅，国家中医药管理局吴刚、于文明，李大宁、马建中、王志勇及各司办和局直单位领导，解放军总后勤部卫生部医疗管理局、各省(区、市)主管中医药工作的卫生厅(局)长等参加会议。会议总结2012年中医药工作，分析面临的形势，部署2013年主要任务，解放思想、改革创新，凝聚共识、振奋精神，改进作风、真抓实干，全力推进中医药事业科学发展。卫生部副部长、国家中医药管理局局长王国强在会上提出，中医药作为独特的卫生资源，重要的经济、科技、文化和生态资源，应该也能够为全面建成小康社会作出贡献，要将中医药融入经济建设大局。会上对第四批全国老中医药专家学术经验继承工作项目、第二批全国优秀中医临床人才研修项目先进单位和个人及全国基础中医药工作先进单位进行了表彰。

▲ 首届中国中医药非遗保护发展论坛在太原举办 1月13日，由文化部非遗司、中国中医科学院、中医药文化研究中心、中国医史文献研究所、山西省文化厅、山西省中医药管理局主办。300余位学者、专家就探究我国中医药行业健康发展方向、实现非物质文化遗产医药项目的保护与发展等进行了研讨。

▲ 第七届全国名中医临床经验传承论坛暨中国民间中医医药研究开发协会名中医学术研究专业委员会换届大会在北京举行 1月12～13日，国家中医药管理局医政司司长许志仁当选新一届主任委员，国医大师陆广莘任名誉主任委员。

▲ 果德安荣获美国植物药委员会最高荣誉奖 2月1日，美国植物药委员会在美国加州隆重举行庆典活动及颁奖仪式，表彰果德安在中草药化学和分析研究领域所做出的具有重要意义的研究工作及发表的大量论文。果德安是唯一获得该奖的亚洲华人学者。

▲ 2012年中医药十大新闻揭晓 2月1日，由国家中医药管理局新闻办公室和中国中医药报社共同主办，康美药业股份有限公司协办。中医药十大新闻分别是：

1. 中医药事业发展“十二五”规划颁布实施，重大项目扎实推进。

2. 中医药积极参与医改，国家实施基层中医药服务能力提升工程。

3. 中医药服务贸易纳入国家贸易发展战略。

4.《藏医药大典》《中国军事本草》出版发行。

5.《中医药标准化中长期发展规划纲要》颁布实施。

6. 首批64家学术流派传承工作室确定。

7. 中药首次以药品进入欧洲市场。

8. “养熊取胆”、“打通任督二脉”2个中医药话题引发社会关注。

9. 首批15种中医药文化科普图书向公众推荐。

10. 中医药应急救治体系初步形成，应对突发公共事件能力提升。

▲ 82家医院被命名为“全国综合医院中医药工作示范单位” 2月1日，由卫生部、国家中医药管理局和总后勤部卫生部联合开展的全国综合医院中医药工作示范单位创建活动，经过自评、评估推荐、专家审核、社会公示等程序，最终决定命名首都医科大学宣武医院等82家单位为“全国

综合医院中医药工作示范单位”。示范单位称号即日生效，有效期5年。北京市，首都医科大学宣武医院；河北省，涉县医院、香河县人民医院；内蒙古自治区，内蒙古医学院附属医院、内蒙古包钢医院、内蒙古科技大学包头医学院第一附属医院、内蒙古科技大学包头医学院第二附属医院；辽宁省，中国医科大学附属第一医院、辽宁医学院附属第一医院；吉林省，榆树市医院、桦甸市人民医院；黑龙江省，黑龙江省农垦总局总医院；上海市，上海市同济医院、上海市第五人民医院、浦东新区公利医院、普陀区利群医院；江苏省，南通市第一人民医院、苏北人民医院、射阳县人民医院；浙江省，台州市第一人民医院、富阳市人民医院、绍兴县中心医院、义乌市中心医院、嘉兴市第一医院；安徽省，界首市人民医院、合肥市第一人民医院、铜陵市人民医院；福建省，仙游县医院、厦门大学附属中山医院、南平市第一医院；山东省，济南市第五人民医院、淄博市第一医院、济宁市第一人民医院、中国石化集团胜利石油管理局胜利医院；湖北省，十堰市红十字医院、荆门市东宝区人民医院、湖北省肿瘤医院、武汉市中心医院、武汉市第五医院；湖南省，湖南省马王堆医院、南华大学附属第一医院、长沙市第四医院、澧县人民医院；广东省，中山大学孙逸仙纪念医院、广州医学院附属第三医院、广东医学院附属医院、广州市红十字会医院、深圳市罗湖区人民医院、东莞市塘厦医院；广西壮族自治区，南宁市第二人民医院、柳州市工人医院、河池市第三人民医院、浦北县人民医院、武鸣县人民医院；重庆市，重庆市第三人民医院、重庆市第九人民医院、南川区人民医院；四川省，内江市第二人民医院、自贡市第一人民医院、安县人民医院；贵州省，贵州省人民医院、思南县人民医院；云南省，大理市第一人民医院；陕西省，西安市儿童医院、西安市第八医院、咸阳市中心医院、神木县医院、府谷县人民医院；甘肃省，酒钢医院、酒泉市第二人民医院、通渭县人民医院、康乐县人民医院；宁夏回族自治区，银川市第二人民医院、中卫市沙坡头区人民医院、石嘴山市第一人民医院；新疆维吾尔自治区，阿克苏地区第一人民医院；军队系统，沈阳军区第208医院、北京军区北戴河疗养院、兰州军区兰州总医院、济南军区青岛第二疗养院、南京军区第454医院、空军载人离心机医学训练基地。

▲ 全国标准化工作会议在北京召开 2月21日，国家质量监督检验检疫总局、国家标准化管理委员会对2013年“中国标准创新贡献奖”获奖单位(组织)和个人进行了表彰。全国政协副主席、科技部部长万钢，国家质量监督检验检疫总局局长支树平等出席颁奖仪式。

▲ 国家食品药品监管局药品审评中心发布《2012年度中国药品审评报告》 2月28日，截至2012年底，新批中药37个，包括中药新药21个、改剂型14个、仿制药2个，其中，九味熄风颗粒为首个用于治疗小儿抽动症的中药复方药物；批准中药药物临床研究39个，包括临床试验37个，生物等效性试验2个；受理新注册申请6 919个(以受理号计)，其中，受理中药新申请共519个。

▲ 王李名珍王定一中西医药研讨会在香港举行 3月6～8日，国家中医药管理局国际合作司、香港食物与卫生局、香港卫生署以及香港东华三院王李名珍王定一中医药研究与发展基金创办人王定一夫妇、历届东华三院主席、顾问，来自两岸四地的中医药医疗、教学和产业界近200人参会。

▲ 国家卫生和计划生育委员会正式组建 3月16日，根据国务院总理李克强提名，经过十二届全国人大一次会议第六次全体会议投票表决，决定李斌为国家卫生和计划生育委员会主任。

▲ 广东率先成立中医药标准化专委会 3月20日，广东在全国率先成立地方中医药和中西医结合的标准化专业委员会。2013年度国家中医药标准研究推广基地培训项目“广东省中医药标准化培训班”同期举行。

▲ 安徽中医学院更名为安徽中医药大学 3月21日，国家教育部复函安徽省政府，同意安徽中医学院更名为安徽中医药大学。

▲ 国家食品药品监督管理总局正式挂牌 3月22日，新组建的国家食品药品监督管理总局由张勇任局长、党组书记。

▲ 北京中医药大学校友会上海分会成立 3月22日，北京中医药大学校长徐安龙、副校长靳琦以及来自上海的近50名校友参会。上海中医药大学副校长刘平到会祝贺，上海中医药大学袁秀荣教授当选上海分会会长。

▲ 针灸名家胡荫培百年纪念会在北京举行 3月24日，国家中医药管理局、北京中医管理局、中国针灸学会、北京针灸学会、北京市东城金针研究学会及胡荫培先生亲属等200余人出席了纪念会，国医大师贺普仁发来贺词。

▲“三棱针”技术规范获中国标准创新贡献奖 3月28日,由天津中医药大学针灸学院完成的“国家标准·针灸技术操作规范 第4部分 三棱针”获得中国标准创新贡献奖二等奖。三棱针技术操作规范,对确保针灸操作安全、提高针灸疗效、临床推广应用以及促进国际间推广交流具有重要意义。

▲2013中国—东盟传统医药高峰论坛和第五届中国(玉林)中医药博览会在玉林市国际会展中心开幕 4月12日,来自中国和东盟国家政府部门官员,以及传统医药学术团体、院校、企业代表260余人参加了论坛和药博会。1 300余家企业及5 000余客商参会参展。

▲国家明确中药二氧化硫残留标准 4月27日,国家药典委员会完成对国家药品标准的修订,其中,明确中药材及饮片二氧化硫残留标准。中药材及饮片(矿物来源的中药材除外,下同)中亚硫酸盐残留量(以二氧化硫计)不得过150 mg/kg,山药、牛膝、粉葛、天冬、天麻、天花粉、白及、白芍、白术、党参等10种中药材及其饮片中亚硫酸盐残留量(以二氧化硫计)不得过400 mg/kg。

▲王国强等被任命为国家卫生和计生委副主任 4月27日,国务院任命王国强、马晓伟、陈啸宏、王培安、刘谦、尹力、崔丽(女)、徐科(女)为国家卫生和计划生育委员会副主任。

▲第二届中药质量鉴定技术研修班在澳门举办 5月13日,由中国科学技术交流中心和澳门特区政府科学技术发展基金共同主办、澳门大学和澳门科技大学承办。

▲针灸国际标准新闻发布会在北京召开 5月14日,《针灸针》《耳穴名称与定位》《艾灸操作规范》和《头针操作规范》4项针灸国际标准发布。世界针灸学会联合会主席邓良月、副主席刘保延等出席发布会。

▲北京中医药大学举行中医内科学临床学系成立大会 5月17日,国家中医药管理局人事教育司巡视员、副司长洪净,北京中医药大学校长徐安龙,副校长王庆国,以及各教学医院、职能部门负责人,中医内科教研室与临床科室主任及教师、相关学科的教研室主任约80余人参加了会议。

▲首家肿瘤专家远程会诊中心在北京安定门中医医院成立 5月20日,由中国民间中医医药研究开发协会名中医学术研究专业委员会、北京中西医结合学会肿瘤专业委员会、中北卫科癌症医学研究院等机构联合主办。国家中医药管理局副局长吴刚出席启动仪式。

▲新疆维吾尔药材及特有植物数据库建成 据《中国中医药报》5月23日报道,中科院新疆理化技术研究所建成维吾尔医常用药材及新疆特有植物化合物样品数据库。该数据库分为药材、方剂、疾病等7个子数据库。用户可以输入植物名称、编号、结构式、分子式等进行查询。

▲首届国际中西医结合慢病管理论坛在香港召开 5月31日,由广东省中医药学会、广东省中医院、广东省中医药科学院、香港中西医结合医学会等单位承办。来自国内外慢病管理相关领域约200位专家、学者们就如何通过有效的慢病管理,让慢性非传染性疾病患者康复回归社会等问题,进行交流和讨论,并从不同的角度深入探讨了未来中西医结合慢病管理的工作方向。

▲世界中医药网络联盟成立大会在北京召开 6月2日,由世界中医药学会联合会主办,世界中医药网、世界中联网络技术(北京)有限公司承办。国家中医药管理局副局长李大宁,世界中医药学会联合会主席佘靖、副主席李振吉,中国互联网协会副理事长黄澄清,中国科学院院士陈可冀,中国中药协会会长房书亭等出席大会。联盟是自愿结成的国际网站组织,旨在通过各国(地区)中医药网站互联互动,实现全球中医药信息资源共享。

▲第三届973中医理论专题专家组在北京成立 6月14日,专题专家组专家及部分首席科学家和在京中医药行业相关代表共50余人参加。国家卫生和计划生育委员会副主任、国家中医药管理局局长王国强,科技部副部长陈小娅出席会议并为专家组成员颁发聘书。专家组由15位科学家组成,中国中医药国际合作中心李振吉任组长,上海中医药大学校长陈凯先院士和中国中医科学院常务副院长刘保延研究员任副组长。

▲第五届中医药国际贡献奖在北京揭晓 6月29日,何鲁丽、王国强、佘靖、于文明、王志勇等出席颁奖典礼,国务院副秘书长丁向阳、澳大利亚西悉尼大学阿伦·本树森荣获个人奖,中国国家标准化管理委员会国际合作部荣获团体奖。

▲第一期中医医院职业化管理高级研修班在北京开班 7月6日,由国家中医药管理局主办,中国中医科学院承办。国家卫生和计划生育

委员会副主任、国家中医药管理局局长王国强，国家中医药管理局副局长马建中，中国中医科学院党组书记王志勇，中国中医科学院院长张伯礼参加开班仪式，78名三甲中医医院院长接受职业培训。

▲ 中美中医药合作战略座谈会在北京召开 7月19日，国家中医药管理局副局长于文明出席会议，提出要以产学研结合为抓手促进中美中医药合作发展。与会专家及相关机构和企业代表，就目前已有的中美合作经验进行交流总结。

▲ 中国药品监督管理研究会在北京成立 7月19日，中国药品监督管理研究会成立并举办第一届全国会员代表大会，全国政协委员、原国家食品药品监督管理局局长邵明立当选会长。

▲ 中医学术流派传承工作室启动建设项目会在广州召开 7月29～30日，国家中医药管理局副局长李大宁出席会议。会上部署了中医学术流派传承工作室建设工作，成立了国家中医药管理局中医学术流派传承推广基地及理事会，并组织与会代表就如何完成中医学术流派传承工作室建设任务进行讨论。

▲ 第五次中医膏方大会在上海举行 8月10日，由中华中医药学会主办，中华中医药学会膏方分会筹委会、上海中医药大学附属龙华医院、山东东阿阿胶股份有限公司承办。来自全国350余名中医师进行了膏方处方开具、制备工艺规范的培训和交流。

▲ 中医药文化与产业博览会及“第二届中国道地药材论坛”在北京展览馆举办 8月10～12日，30多家中药饮片企业参展。金世元、王孝涛、张世臣、杨明会等中医药名家出席开幕式，来自中国中医科学院、首都医科大学以及中药企业的专家代表就中药资源普查及动态监测、道地药材与无硫加工、道地药材GAP基地建设和现代化中药房建设等问题进行了交流研讨。

▲ 香港食物及卫生局局长访问国家中医药管理局 8月12日，国家卫生和计划生育委员会副主任、国家中医药管理局局长王国强在北京与率团来访的香港食物及卫生局局长高永文一行会面。双方就共同推动中医药标准化建设、科学研究、人才培养等领域合作交换了意见与看法。国家中医药管理局副局长于文明，国家中医药管理局国际合作司、人事教育司等部门负责人陪同会见。

▲ 全国卫生援外工作暨援外医疗队派遣50周年会议在北京召开 8月15日，会议表彰了30个全国援外医疗工作先进集体、59个先进个人，长春中医药大学附属医院获全国援外医疗工作先进集体，上海中医药大学附属岳阳中西医结合医院主治医师李昌植、浙江中医药大学主任中医师褚海林、福建中医药大学附属人民医院院长刘建忠、江西省中医学院附属医院主任医师许金水、湖北省丹江口市第一人民医院主任中医师王大军获全国援外医疗工作先进个人。

▲ 第十二届国际现代化中医药及健康产品展览会在香港举行 8月16日，由香港贸易发展局和现代化中医药国际协会主办，国家中医药管理局副局长李大宁出席。139多家参展商，分6个展馆。同时举办了“中医药防治肿瘤研究最新进展研讨会”、“香港第九届国际研究生中医药研讨会”及“香港贸发局美食博览”、“香港贸发局香港国际茶展”等活动。

▲ 中国卫生信息学会中医药信息化专业委员会成立大会暨中医药信息化工作座谈会在石家庄召开 8月23日，国家中医药管理局副局长吴刚出席。国家中医药管理局规划财务司副司长武东当选为主任委员，局办公室副巡视员陈伟当选为秘书长。北京、河北、福建、深圳等地专家委员进行了经验交流。

▲ 海峡两岸医卫媒体交流座谈会在北京举行 8月29日，两岸医药卫生媒体代表就如何有效传播科学健康知识以及未来两岸媒体合作设想等进行了交流，并对海峡两岸在中医药领域的进一步沟通、交流表示了期待。

▲ 全国中医药养生产业发展论坛在北京举办 9月6～8日，由中华中医药学会主办、藏象集团股份有限公司承办。国内知名养生企业就养生规范政策标准制定、落实，行业趋势以及未来发展的创新模式等进行了探讨。

▲ 教育部高等学校中医学类专业教学指导委员会工作会议在兰州举办 9月21日，由教育部高等学校中医学类专业教学指导委员会主办、甘肃中医学院承办。来自教育部、国家中医药管理局、教指委等相关单位的领导、专家及全国36所高等院校的教育工作者，就共同推进中医高等教育改革，提高中医药人才培养质量等进行了

探讨。

▲**“弘扬大医精神 抵制不正之风”高峰论坛在北京举行** 9月23日,国家卫生和计划生育委员会副主任崔丽、中国医师协会会长张雁灵等出席会议,全国人大常委会副委员长陈竺给论坛发表视频讲话。会上,60位医生被评为大医精神代表,3位中医人入选。

▲**2013年山清世界传统医药博览会暨山清世界药膳烹饪大赛在韩国山清郡东医宝鉴村举行** 9月6日,中国药膳研究会会长沙凤桐率中国代表团参赛。中国代表团的8支参赛队在比赛中,荣获7个奖项,其中南京同仁堂健康酒店代表队获大赛大奖。

▲**全国回医药学术论坛暨中国民族医药学会回医药分会筹备成立大会在吴忠举行** 9月11～13日,国家中医药管理局副局长、中国民族医药学会会长马建中出席。会上选举田丰年为中国民族医药学会回医药分会理事会会长。

▲**第四届中医药现代化科技大会在成都召开** 9月26～27日,由科技部、国家卫生和计划生育委员会等13个国家部委与四川省政府共同主办,全国政协副主席、科技部部长万钢担任大会主席,四川省省长魏宏担任组委会主任。期间举办“中医药国际协作与发展政府论坛”等8个主题分会、4场专题交流以及“现代中药与生物医药成果转化项目对接洽谈会”等活动。

▲**北京中医药大学校友会内蒙古分会在包头成立** 9月28日,北京中医药大学副校长靳琦等出席,内蒙古自治区卫生厅中蒙医管理局局长于连云、包头市卫生局副局长彭晓东到会祝贺,来自内蒙古的近30名校友参会。包头市120指挥中心总指挥靳虹当选为会长、包钢医院马亚琴当选为秘书长。

▲**中国针刀医学技术创新联盟在北京成立** 10月12日,由北京中医药大学、北京世华针刀中医医院等40余家单位共同发起。其目的是以针刀医学发展需求为基础,以提升针刀医学技术创新为目标,大力推进针刀医学技术产业化。

▲**2013年中医急诊高峰论坛在北京开幕** 10月12日,由北京中西医结合学会、北京市中医急危重症质量控制中心、北京中医药大学东直门医院、首都医科大学附属北京中医医院主办。与会专家一致认为,中医急诊在公共卫生服务中的作用至关重要。

▲**国家中医药管理局确定全国名老中医药专家传承工作室建设项目专家名单** 10月14日,2013年全国名老中医药专家传承工作室建设项目专家共144人。其中北京市7人(鼓楼中医医院张士杰、曹洪欣,朝阳区中医医院金伯华,首都医科大学附属北京中医医院柯薇君、周乃玉、宋祚民、孙伯扬);天津市4人(天津中医药大学第一附属医院曹克光,天津中医药大学第二附属医院李今垣、李永成,南开医院崔乃强);河北省3人(石家庄市中医院郭纪生、王淑玲,邯郸市中医院高社光);山西省4人(山西中医学院附属医院贾六金,太原市中医医院王有奎,山西省中医院王晞星、冯五金);内蒙古自治区3人(内蒙古国际蒙医医院包景荣、乌苏日乐特,内蒙古中医医院张铎);辽宁省5人(中国医科大学附属盛京医院关娴清,大连医科大学附属第一医院齐清会,辽宁中医药大学附属医院谭毅,辽宁中医药大学附属第二医院王春林、李中宇);吉林省4人(长春中医药大学附属医院于凯成、赵振昌,吉林省中医药科学院李莹,吉林中西医结合医院李吉平);黑龙江省4人(黑龙江省中医药科学院张佩青、滕义和,黑龙江中医药大学附属二院张金良,黑龙江中医药大学附属一院刘建秋);上海市10人(上海中医药大学附属龙华医院林水森、王庆其、吴银根、邱佳信,上海中医药大学附属曙光医院王灵台、丁学屏,上海中医药大学附属岳阳中西医结合医院东贵荣,上海市中西医结合医院奚九一,上海市中医医院虞坚尔,复旦大学附属肿瘤医院于尔辛);江苏省6人(江苏省中医院汪受传,江苏省中西医结合医院徐荷芬,无锡市中医医院赵景芳,徐州市中医院孙凤霞,苏州市中医医院何焕荣,海安县中医院夏治平);浙江省5人(富阳市中医骨伤医院张玉柱,浙江省中医院徐锡山,浙江省立同德医院魏克民,浙江中医药大学附属第三医院方剑乔,绍兴市中医院常青);安徽省4人(安徽中医药大学第一附属医院胡国俊、鲍远程,马鞍山市中医院范绍荣,亳州市华佗中医院杨从鑫);福建省3人(福建中医药大学附属人民医院陈长华,福建中医药大学附属第二人民医院肖定远,福州市中医院谢宝慈);江西省4人(江西中医药大学附属医院刁军成,江西中西医结合医院熊墨年,景德镇市中医院黄夏雨,万安县中医院彭学礼);山东省6人(山东中医药大学中鲁医院张志远,烟台毓璜顶医院田文,潍

坊市中医院张奇文，山东省中医药研究院附属医院金伟，山东中医药大学第二附属医院董建文，山东中医药大学附属医院宋爱莉）；河南省 6 人（洛阳市第二中医院乔保钧，河南中医学院第三附属医院唐宋，河南中医学院第一附属医院张东岳，郑州东方肿瘤医院邵梦扬，河南护理职业学院附属医院关思友，郑州市大肠肛门病医院宋光瑞）；湖北省 4 人（湖北省中医院张晓星、李同生，武汉市中西医结合医院杜健民，荆州市中医医院黄祥武）；湖南省 6 人（湖南中医药大学第一附属医院李传课、程丑夫，湖南省中医药研究院附属医院刘炳凡、蔡光先、蒋士生，湖南中医药大学第二附属医院刘贵云）；广东省 8 人（广东省中医院刘茂才、罗笑容，广州中医药大学第一附属医院欧阳惠卿、陈基长，广东省第二中医院吕雄，深圳市中医院李顺民，广东省中西医结合医院老昌辉，珠海市第二人民医院刘敏如）；广西壮族自治区 2 人（广西中医药大学第一附属医院陈慧依、朱少廷）；海南省 1 人（海口市中医医院傅汝梅）；重庆市 3 人（重庆市中医院王仁强、曾定伦，江北区中医院欧阳作理）；四川省 5 人（内江市中医医院胡国栋，洪雅县中医医院祝之友，眉山市中医医院周建国，安岳县中医医院廖洪韬，阿坝州藏医院夺机卓玛）；贵州省 3 人（贵阳中医学院第一附属医院董湘玉、戴永生、吴文尧）；云南省 4 人（云南省中医医院陈乔林、苏藩、赵淳，迪庆州藏医院柏玛丹增）；西藏自治区 3 人（西藏自治区藏医院索朗欧珠，那曲索县藏医院旦松扎巴，那曲地区藏医院阿加）；陕西省 3 人（陕西省中医医院曹利平，陕西中医学院附属医院李彦民，西安市中医医院张素清）；甘肃省 3 人（甘肃中医学院附属医院许自诚，兰州中医骨伤科医院郭宪章，甘南州藏医院杨宏权）；青海省 2 人（青海省中医院巴卓玛，青海省藏医院南拉卡）；宁夏回族自治区 2 人（宁夏回族自治区中医医院张凤武，银川市中医医院焦天才）；新疆维吾尔自治区 2 人（和田地区维吾尔医医院沙依甫汗·吐尔迪艾合买提，昌吉州中医医院何复东）；中国中医科学院 10 人（西苑医院麻柔、聂莉芳、王书臣、周文泉，广安门医院姚乃礼、庄国康、许铣，中国中医科学院眼科医院高健生、庄曾渊，中国中医科学院针灸研究所吴中朝）；北京中医药大学 5 人（北京中医药大学东直门医院臧福科、孟宪坤，北京中医药大学尉中民、鲁兆麟、刘景源）。

▲ 2013 年中药上市后再评价国际大会在北京召开 10 月 17 日，国家中医药管理局副局长王志勇，中国科学院院士陈可冀，中国工程院院士李连达等，以及来自美国、英国，中国香港、澳门等国家和地区的专家、学者共 400 余人出席。大会成立世界中医药学会联合会中药上市后再评价专业委员会。

▲ 首届中医佛典高级研修班在北京开班 10 月 20 日，由北京中医药大学和嵩山少林寺联合主办，全国 16 个省市 40 多位学员入学。研修班采取学院教育与师徒传授相结合的形式，凡按规定修完全部学分，符合学位授予标准者，将授予北京中医药大学硕士学位。

▲ 王琦获 2013 年何梁何利奖 10 月 30 日，何梁何利奖基金 2013 年度颁奖大会在北京举行，46 位国内科技界的杰出人才获奖，北京中医药大学终身教授、博士生导师王琦获科学与技术进步奖。

▲ 世界中医药学会联合会成立 10 周年座谈会在北京召开 10 月 30 日，由世界中医药网承办，美国美孕医疗集团协办。全国人大常委会前副委员长何鲁丽、国家中医药管理局副局长吴刚等领导及学者共 150 人出席。

▲ 全国“中医药科技查新”暨“方剂数据汇交”培训会议在长沙召开 11 月 4 日，由中国中医科学院中医药信息研究所主办，湖南省中医药研究院文献信息研究所承办。会议邀请福建中医药大学研究生部林丹红、湖南省中医药研究院文献信息研究所陆惠民等多位专家，就大数据时代的中医药信息学发展趋势、中医药查新工作的起源、历史、现状及规范化、拓展与延伸等进行专题讲座。

▲ 第四届藏医药研修班在北京藏医院结业 11 月 11 日，来自全国四大藏区以及北京、山西五台山等地的 76 名藏医，经过 11 天的学习，获得第四届全国藏医药高级研修班结业证书和国家一类继续教育学分。本次培训邀请西藏藏医学院副教授嘎务，以《晶镜本草》为教材，讲授了 1 350 种藏药材的药味、药效、鉴定等知识。

▲ 北京中医药大学校友会宁夏分会在银川成立 11 月 16 日，北京中医药大学副校长靳琦等出席，宁夏近 80 名校友参会。宁夏回族自治区卫生厅中医药管理局原局长王忠和当选为宁夏分会会长，宁夏医科大学中医学院副院长刘敬霞、药

学院系主任隋宏当选为秘书长。

▲ 首届"世界针灸周" 在北京举行 11月16～22日,由世界中医药学会联合会、中国中医科学院针灸研究所、中国针灸学会、北京中医药大学主办,中国中医科学院针灸医院、北京广安中医门诊部承办。16日在中国中医科学院和北京中医药大学同时举行展览;18日在中国中医科学院举行庆祝世界针灸周确立暨纪念"中医针灸"申遗成功3周年专家座谈会。

▲ 中澳中医药国际联合研究中心获国家级认定 11月29日,科技部颁发了《2013年度国家级国际联合研究中心认定的通知》,经各级组织部门推荐及科技部专家评审,中国中医科学院西苑医院"中澳中医药国际联合研究中心"获此认定。

▲ 第六届南方医药论坛在广州举行 12月4日,由中国医药物资协会南方医药合作组织、中华大唐医药协会等单位主办。来自全国医药工业、商业、连锁药店等界别的企业家、行业专家共600人参会。以"新政策、新趋势、新模式"为论坛主题,与会代表们进行了深入的探讨和交流。

▲ 北京中医药大学校友会福建分会在厦门成立 12月7日,北京中医药大学党委书记吴建伟、副校长靳琦及来自福建的80余名校友参会。厦门市中医院脑病科主任林安基当选为会长,福建中医药大学药学院院长褚克丹等4人当选为副会长,徐丽林当选为秘书长。

▲ 于文明会见香港慈善机构联合代表团 12月10日,国家中医药管理局副局长在北京会见了来访的香港慈善机构联合代表团一行。代表团由香港博爱医院、仁爱堂、仁济医院、青松观和圆玄学院五大慈善机构组成。国家中医药管理局相关司室人员陪同会见。

▲《中华大典·医药卫生典·药学分典》出版 12月13日,《中华大典·医药卫生典·药学分典》出版发行。《药学分典》主编为中国中医科学院中国医史文献研究所研究员、中国本草研究领域学科带头人郑金生,成书15册2 170万字,药图21 059幅,收药4 302种。《中华大典》1992年启动编纂,全书分为24典110多个分典,收录两万多种古籍。

▲ 于文明会见香港大学中医药学院院长劳力行 12月27日,国家中医药管理局副局长于文明在北京会见了来访的香港大学中医药学院院长劳力行一行。双方围绕中医学生培养模式、香港大学中医专业学生临床实习基地建设和加强两地中医药科研合作等问题交换了意见。劳力行希望内地对港大中医药学院发展给予更多支持。

索　　引

主题词索引

A 艾敖

艾菲提蒙汤/治疗应用 401a
艾滋病/中西医结合疗法 56a /预防和控制 56a
敖朗黑布/化学 238b

B B八巴白败班斑版半包保北本鼻萆扁便冰丙补不

Bell's 面瘫/针灸疗法 188b
八段锦 208b
巴布剂/投药和剂量 309b
巴豆/生产和制备 329a
巴戟天/生产和制备 329a
白蒺藜皂苷/药理学 164b
白芍总苷胶囊/治疗应用 172b
败丹黄灌洗液/治疗应用 171b
班秀文 48a
斑蝥/生产和制备 327a
版本研究 377a
半夏白术天麻汤/治疗应用 355a
半夏泄心头/治疗应用 355a
包合物/生产和制备 310b
保真汤/治疗应用 60b
北柴胡/生产和制备 329a
本草考证 391a
鼻窦炎，慢性/中西医结合疗法 171b
鼻康片/药理学 171a
鼻敏片/药理学 170b
鼻炎，变应性/中西医结合疗法 170a /预防和控制 170a
鼻炎片/治疗应用 170a
鼻渊舒/治疗应用 171b
鼻渊通窍颗粒/治疗应用 171a
萆薢渗湿汤/治疗应用 106a
扁桃体炎，化脓性，急性/中西医结合疗法 166a
便秘，功能性，小儿/中药疗法 122b /中医外治疗法 122b/按摩疗法 204a
冰香散/药理学 54b
丙肝冲剂/治疗应用 60a
补肝益肾活血汤/治疗应用 169a
补骨脂/生产和制备 327a
补肾安胎冲剂/治疗应用 109a
补肾化痰调经汤/治疗应用 105b
补肾健脾方/治疗应用 58a
补肾清解汤/治疗应用 107b
补肾清透方/治疗应用 58a
补肾柔肝方/治疗应用 111a
补肾益气健脾方/治疗应用 169a
补肾育宫汤/治疗应用 105b
补肾育胎汤/治疗应用 109a
补益营卫方/治疗应用 374a
补中益气丸/治疗应用 61a
不育症，男性/中药疗法 144a

C 苍藏草茶柴肠超陈澄痴虫川刺催痤

苍耳散/治疗应用 171b
苍耳子/生产和制备 327b
苍耳子滴鼻剂，复方/药理学 171a
藏医烟尔灸法 398b
草乌/生产和制备 327b
茶黄素衍生物/药理学 55a
柴桂温胆汤/治疗应用 95b
柴胡/生产和制备 329b
柴胡桂枝干姜汤/治疗应用 355a
柴胡疏肝汤/药理学 355b

柴苓汤/治疗应用　168b
肠易激综合征/针灸疗法　185b
超临界 CO_2 流体萃取/方法　306b
超声提取/方法　306b
陈皮利咽合剂/药理学　166a
澄江学派/历史　194a
痴呆,血管性/中药疗法　96b
虫草抗痨胶囊/治疗应用　61a
川椒方/药理学　165a
刺法研究　177b　180b
刺五加注射液/药理学　165b
催乳汤/治疗应用　109a
痤疮/中药疗法　136a

D　大带丹胆当德滴抵癫电东多

大黄乌梅汤灌肠/治疗应用　57a
大孔吸附树脂/生产和制备　308b
大麻药/生产和制备　329b
带脉/利用　105a
带状疱疹/针灸疗法　192a　/中药疗法　131b
丹参滴丸,复方/治疗应用　168b
丹参三七混合液/药理学　167a
丹参注射液/治疗应用　60b
丹红化瘀口服液/治疗应用　168b
胆蒲通脉胶囊/治疗应用　95b
当归拈痛汤/治疗应用　141a
当归四逆汤/治疗应用　92b
德都红花-7味散/治疗应用　401b
滴丸/生产和制备　310a
抵当汤/药理学　168a
癫痫,小儿/中药疗法　123a　/中西医结合疗法　123a
电子鼻技术/利用　234b
《东坡养生集》　373a
多囊调经汤,复方/治疗应用　110a
多指标评价,中药炮制工艺/利用　326a

E　恶耳二

恶性肿瘤并发抑郁/中药疗法　69a　/情志疗法　69a　/音乐疗法　69a
耳聋,感音神经性/中药疗法　165b
耳聋,突发性/中西医结合疗法　169b
耳聋2号煎剂/治疗应用　170a
二补助育汤/治疗应用　113b
二仙丸,加味/治疗应用　78a

F　防仿肥肺分妇附复腹

防治糖尿病中药/药理学　337b
仿生提取/方法　307a
肥胖/针灸疗法　186b
肺癌/中西医结合疗法　65a
肺疾病,阻塞性,慢性/中西医结合疗法　78b
肺结核/中西医结合疗法　60b
肺炎,小儿/中药疗法　119b　/中医外治疗法　119b　/中西医结合疗法　119b
肺炎,支原体,小儿/中药疗法　120b　/中西医结合疗法　120b
肺与大肠相表里　27a
分子生物学技术/利用　216a
妇春Ⅰ号/治疗应用　108a
附子/生产和制备　327b
附子楮实汤/治疗应用　86b
复聪汤Ⅰ号口服液/药理学　165b
复元汤/治疗应用　168b
腹水,肝硬化/中西医结合疗法　86b

G　改干肝葛狗枸骨固龟鬼桂

改善神经细胞凋亡/药物作用　339b　340a
改善缺血性脑损伤/药物疗法　362b

改善胰岛素抵抗/药物疗法 364a
干眼症/中西医结合疗法 169a
肝癌/中西医结合疗法 67b /中药疗法 67b
肝炎,丙型,慢性/中西医结合疗法 59b /中医病机 59b /诊断 60a
肝炎,乙型,慢性/中西医结合疗法 54a,57b /中医病机 57b /诊断 58b /预防和控制 54a
肝炎,重症/保留灌肠疗法 57a /中西医结合疗法 57a
肝硬化,肝炎,乙型,慢性/中西医结合疗法 54b
葛根/生产和制备 329b
狗脊/生产和制备 328a
枸杞提取物/药理学 168b
骨骼系统/药物作用 337a
骨性关节炎/中医外治疗法 157b /中药疗法 157b
骨折,股骨粗隆间/中医外治疗法 153a /中药疗法 153a
骨折,桡骨远端/中医外治疗法 152a
骨折,胸腰椎/中医外治疗法 154a /中西医结合疗法 154a
骨折/护理 213a
骨质疏松/中药疗法 156b /中西医结合疗法 156b
固体分散体/投药和剂量 310b
龟鹿调经汤/治疗应用 111b
龟息功法 208a
鬼针草叶/治疗应用 169a /药理学 169a
桂枝挥发油/药理学 55a

H 何红厚呼虎化还黄回混藿

何首乌/生产和制备 330a
红藤汤/治疗应用 108a
厚朴/化学 238a
呼吸系统/药物作用 335a
虎杖/生产和制备 328a
化湿行瘀清热方/治疗应用 172a
还脑益聪颗粒剂/治疗应用 374b
黄斑变性,年龄相关性/中药疗法 168a /中西医结合疗法 168a
黄斑祛湿方/治疗应用 168a
《黄帝内经》 378b
黄褐斑/中药疗法 134a
黄精/生产和制备 328a
黄连/生产和制备 330a
黄连解毒汤/药理学 355b
黄芪桂枝口服液/治疗应用 165a
黄酮类/分析 238a
《回回药方》 402b
混合痔/中药疗法 139a
藿朴夏苓汤/治疗应用 90a

J 脊济加甲肩煎简健姜浆胶焦角结睫解金经荆颈九灸聚卷

脊柱炎,强直性/中西医结合疗法 96a
《济阳纲目》 327b
加压减压提取/方法 307b
甲嘎松汤/治疗应用 400a
甲瘤方/治疗应用 355b
肩关节周围炎/中医外治疗法 155a /中药疗法 155a /按摩疗法 204a
肩手综合征/针灸疗法 187b
煎煮提取/方法 306b
简单比较,中药炮制工艺/利用 323a
健黄饮/治疗应用 112b
健脾抑瘤汤/治疗应用 67b
"姜醋"/治疗应用 109b
浆细胞性乳腺炎/中药疗法 137a
胶囊剂/投药和剂量 309a
焦虑症/中西医结合疗法 97b
角膜炎,单纯疱疹病毒性,复发性/中西医结合疗法 165a
结肠炎,溃疡性,口服,灌肠/中药疗法 83b
结膜炎,过敏性/中药疗法 165a
睫状体平坦部滤过术/利用 164b
解毒化瘀颗粒/治疗应用 57b
金匮肾气汤/治疗应用 358a /药理学 358a

金匮肾气丸/治疗应用 170a
金莲花/化学 238b
金纳多注射液/治疗应用 169b
金银花/化学 238a
经络研究 177a
荆芥挥发油/分析 55a
颈椎病/中医外治疗法 158a /中药疗法 158a
九味镇心颗粒/治疗应用 97b
灸法文献 193b
灸法研究 177b
《聚血》 398a
卷柏/生产和制备 328a

K 开抗颗咳克口苦坤

开喉剑喷剂/治疗应用 61b,166b
抗病原微生物中药/药理学 338b
抗流感/药物疗法 363b
抗衰益智胶囊/治疗应用 374b
抗血管性痴呆中药/药理学 339a
抗炎中药/药理学 337b,340a
抗氧化/药物作用 339a
抗肿瘤中药/药理学 338a
颗粒剂/生产和制备 309a
咳嗽,小儿,慢性/中药疗法 119a
克比奇羚羊角胶囊/治疗应用 166b
口腔扁平苔藓/中西医结合疗法 172a /诊断 172a
口腔溃疡,复发性/中药疗法 166b
口疡清方/药理学 166b
苦参素胶囊/治疗应用 59b
苦碟子注射液/治疗应用 167a
坤泰胶囊/治疗应用 105b

L 蓝狼类李痢莲凉林临灵苓流龙罗

蓝芩口服液/治疗应用 172a
狼毒/生产和制备 328b
类风湿关节炎/针灸疗法 191b
李玉奇 46a
痢疾/预防和控制 55a
莲/化学 238b
凉血解毒方/治疗应用 57a
林亿 394a
临床教学方法 424a
灵芝/化学 238a
苓桂术甘汤,加味/治疗应用 85a
流感,甲型 H1N1/中药疗法 54b /中西医结合疗法 54b /预防和控制 54b
龙胆泻肝汤/治疗应用 171b
龙血竭片/治疗应用 167a
罗仙子/生产和制备 330a

M 麻玛迈脉慢蒙孟泌密免明膜

麻黄细辛附子汤/药理学 55a
麻疹/诊断 55b
玛奴西汤颗粒/治疗应用 400a
迈之灵片/治疗应用 167a
脉络膜新生血管,实验性/中药疗法 164a
慢性盆腔疼痛综合征/按摩疗法 201b
慢性疲劳综合征/针灸疗法 187a
慢性阻塞性肺疾病/针灸疗法 182a
蒙药伊赫汤/治疗应用 401a
孟河医派/历史 386b
泌尿生殖系统/药物作用 336b
密蒙花方/治疗应用 168b
密蒙花提取物/药理学 169b
密蒙花总黄酮/药理学 169b
免疫系统/药物作用 337b
明睛颗粒/投药和剂量 164a
膜过滤/方法 308a

N　内纳脑宁凝牛女

内质网应激/药物作用　342a
纳米粒/利用　312b
脑梗死,急性/中西医结合疗法　95a
脑炎,乙型,流行性/中西医结合疗法　55b
宁神益智方/治疗应用　371b
凝胶膏剂/投药和剂量　309a
牛蒡子苷/药理学　168a
女性压力性尿失禁/针灸疗法　191a

P　P盘喷盆皮枇脾片贫葡

PI3K/Akt 通路/药物作用　344a
盘龙七片/治疗应用　96a
喷雾干燥/方法　306a
喷雾剂/投药和剂量　309b
盆炎丸/治疗应用　355a
皮肤溃疡,慢性/中药疗法　130b
枇杷叶/生产和制备　330b
脾胃病/中医药疗法　387b
片剂/投药和剂量　346b
贫血,癌性/中药疗法　68b
贫血,再生障碍性,慢性/中西医结合疗法　88b
葡萄膜炎/中西医结合疗法　164b

Q　启杞气潜芩秦禽青清

启明丸/治疗应用　168a
杞藿饮/治疗应用　374a
杞菊润目贴/药物作用　169b
气功,国外　420b
潜阳封髓丹/治疗应用　171b
芩蒿滴鼻剂/药理学　170b
秦艽/生产和制备　225a
秦皮滴眼液/治疗应用　169a
禽流感/预防和控制　55a
青光眼/中药疗法　164b
青藤碱/药理学　170b
清肝通窍汤/投药和剂量　170a
清火消斑汤/治疗应用　90a
清热散瘟口服液/治疗应用　61b

R　热人乳润弱

热毒宁注射液/治疗应用　61b
人才培养　424b
乳腺癌伴随症状/针灸疗法　420a
乳腺增生病/中药疗法　138a
润目灵颗粒/治疗应用　169a
弱视,斜视性/中药疗法　165a

S　三沙山伤烧摄参深肾生圣失湿石视手疏腧双水四宋素速孙

三七/生产和制备　328b
三仁汤/治疗应用　90a
沙参麦冬汤/药理学　355b
《伤寒杂病论》　383a
伤寒、副伤寒/预防和控制　55b
烧伤/中药疗法　142a
摄涕止衄汤/药理学　171a
参苓白术散/治疗应用　60b
参麦合剂/药理学　60b
深静脉血栓/中药疗法　140a　/中西医结合疗法　140a
肾脏病,慢性/中西医结合疗法　87a
生血丸/治疗应用　68b
圣愈五子汤/治疗应用　111a
失眠/按摩疗法　/针灸疗法　189b,201b
湿疹/中药疗法　132b
石斛/生产和制备　328b
石辛含片/治疗应用　172b

视明宝颗粒/药物作用　165a
视神经萎缩/中药疗法　168b
视网膜病变,糖尿病性/中药疗法　168b　/中西医结合疗法　168b
视网膜静脉阻塞/中药疗法　166b　/中西医结合疗法　166b
视网膜脱离,术后视网膜下积液/中西医结合疗法　164a
手足口病/中药疗法　61b　/保留灌肠疗法　61b　/中西医结合疗法　61b
手法机制　201a,202b
疏风凉血补肾方/治疗应用　89a
疏风宣肺抗流感方/药理学　55a
疏肝清热通络方/治疗应用　93a
疏络散结汤/治疗应用　69a
腧穴研究　177a
双百口服液/治疗应用　61a
双花清胃汤/治疗应用　166b
水蛭/生产和制备　328b
四君子汤/药理学　359b
四物汤/治疗应用　169a
宋徽宗　394a
《素问病机气宜保命集》　211a
速效耳净灵/治疗应用　165b
孙奇　394a
孙思邈　390a
孙兆　394a

T　调胎台太糖桃藤体萜通推

调节神经递质中药/药理学　339b
调节受体功能中药/药理学　339b
胎宝汤/治疗应用　108b
台湾中医药　410a
太极拳/方法　209a
糖尿病,2 型/中西医结合疗法　90a
糖尿病/针灸疗法　183b
糖尿病并发症/针灸疗法　183b
糖尿病周围神经病变/中西医结合疗法　92b
糖尿病足/中药疗法　141a　/中西医结合疗法　141a
糖网明/药物作用　168a
桃花四物汤/治疗应用　355a　/药理学　355a
藤黄/生产和制备　330b
体质学说　211a
萜类/分析　238a
通脉化瘀汤/治疗应用　167a
通窍活血汤/治疗应用　170a
通乳汤/治疗应用　109b
推拿手法/利用　202b

W　万微维卫胃温五

万应胶囊/治疗应用　166a
微波提取/方法　306b
微粉粉碎/方法　306a
微囊/投药和剂量　311b
微球/投药和剂量　311b
微乳/投药和剂量　312a
微丸/投药和剂量　311a
维康颗粒/治疗应用　371b
卫生用品/历史　393a
胃癌前病变/中药疗法　82b
胃病/针灸疗法　184b
胃炎,慢性,小儿/中药疗法　122b
胃炎,萎缩性,慢性,口服,静脉滴注/中药疗法　82a
温病/中医药疗法　383b
温肺止流丹/药理学　171a
温阳解毒化瘀颗粒/投药和剂量　57b
五龙颗粒/治疗应用　166a

X　西犀香消小效心辛新猩醒盱絮玄血薰寻荨训

西洋参/化学　238a
西医东渐　395b

犀角地黄汤/药理学 355b
香港中医药 408a
香菊胶囊/治疗应用 171a
消化系统中药/药理学 336a
消化性溃疡/护理 213b
小柴胡汤/治疗应用 54b,59b /药理学 356a
小胶质细胞/药物作用 343b
效应面法,中药炮制工艺/利用 323b
心肌炎,病毒性,小儿/中药疗法 121b /中西医结合疗法 121b
心血管系统/药物作用 335a
心脏病,肺源性/中西医结合疗法 79b
辛芷鼻敏胶囊/药理学 170b
新安医学/历史 385a
新剂型/投药和剂量 309a
猩红热/预防和控制 55b
醒鼻凝胶剂/投药和剂量 170b
盱江医学/历史 384a
絮凝澄清/方法 308a
玄驹胶囊,复方/治疗应用 113a
血管生长因子/药物作用 341a
血管生成抑制因子/药物作用 341b
血塞通注射液/治疗应用 167a
血小板减少性紫癜,特发性,小儿/中药疗法 123a
血小板减少症,免疫性/中西医结合疗法 89a
薰鲁香/化学 238b
《寻乐堂日录》 390b
荨麻疹/中药疗法 133a /中西医结合疗法 133a
训诂学 377b

Y 牙亚咽颜厌养腰医胰抑益阴茵银玉育愈原月运

牙周炎,慢性/中西医结合疗法 166b
亚健康状态 373a
咽炎,慢性/中药疗法 171b /中西医结合疗法 171b /中医病机 171b
咽炎方/治疗应用 171b
颜德馨 50a
厌食,小儿/按摩疗法 205a
养阴润肺益气健脾汤/治疗应用 61a
养正消积胶囊/治疗应用 66a
腰肌劳损/中医外治疗法 155a /中药疗法 155a
腰椎间盘突出症/中医外治疗法 159a /中药疗法 159a
医事制度 395a
胰腺炎,重症/中药疗法 143a /中西医结合疗法 143a
抑郁,脑卒中后/中西医结合疗法 95b /中医疗法 95b
抑制血管生成/药物作用 341a
益气温阳方/治疗应用 166a
益肾固本方/治疗应用 57b
益肾化湿颗粒/治疗应用 87b
益肾毓麟汤/治疗应用 108b
阴阳五行学说 25b
茵陈蒿汤/治疗应用 357a /药理学 357a
银屑病/中药疗法 135a /中西医结合疗法 135a
银杏叶提取物/治疗应用 169b
玉屏风散/药物作用 165a
育泡饮/治疗应用 112b
愈障生血汤/治疗应用 88b
原花青素/药物作用 164a
《月王药诊》 399b
运气学说 26b

Z 皂针正证支脂指质中朱竹注驻壮滋紫自

皂苷类/分析 238a
针刺麻醉 179a
针刺镇痛 179a
针灸,国外 420a
针灸机理 178b
针灸流派研究 179b
正交试验,中药炮制工艺/利用 323a
证候动物模型 31b
支气管哮喘/针灸疗法 181a
脂肪肝,非酒精性/中药疗法 84b

脂质体/投药和剂量　316a
指纹图谱,中药炮制品/利用　325b
质量标准,中药炮制品/利用　325b,326b
质谱联用/利用　324a
中耳炎/中药疗法　165b
中风/护理　212b
中风后遗症/针灸疗法　187b
《中国药典》 398a
中枢神经系统中药/药理学　337a
中药/毒性　38b,339a
中药安全性评价　232b
中药材的宏观认识　216a
中药材/解剖学和组织学　223a
中药采收期　221a
中药道地性　220a
中药分离纯化/方法　308a
中药分离和提纯/方法　238b
中药分子鉴定技术/利用　217b,233b
中药归经研究　38a
中药化学成分/解剖学和组织学　239b
中药挥发油成分/解剖学和组织学　283a
中药硫黄熏蒸/投药和剂量　222a
中药酶提取/方法　313b
中药内在属性的关联研究　42a
中药炮制理论　40a,325b
中药炮制品/毒性　324b　/化学　326b　/药理学　324b
中药配伍禁忌　39b,40b
中药气味研究　38a
中药闪式提取/方法　313a
中药升降浮沉研究　38b
中药特征指纹图谱技术/利用　233a
中药效用理论　39a,40a
中药药代动力学　339a
中药药性理论研究　38a
中药遗传多样性　218b
中药制药技术/利用　306a
中药质量评价　231a
中药资源调查　218b
中药资源生理生态学　217b
中药资源再生技术　218a
中医翻译　390a
中医教育学/历史　392b
中医经典课程教学方法　422a
中医临床路径　430a
中医临床研究方法　429a
中医外科学/历史　390a
中医文献研究方法　379b
中医学身体观　392b
中医药文化　390b
朱丹溪　387b
竹叶兰/化学　238b
注射剂/投药和剂量　310a
注意缺陷多动障碍,小儿/中药疗法　123b　/中西医结合疗法　123b
驻景方/药理学　164a
壮药龙钻通痹方/治疗应用　404b
壮医“毒”致痛说　401b
壮医莲花针背廊拔罐法　402a
滋水平肝宁心汤/治疗应用　112a
滋阴利肺汤/治疗应用　61a
滋阴清热育卵方/治疗应用　111b
紫癜,过敏性/中西医结合疗法　89b
自微乳/投药和剂量　312a

2014卷《中国中医药年鉴》(学术卷)特邀编委名单

一、特邀副主任编委:

1. 乾坤集团董事局　刘鸿业主席
2. 大连华立金港药业有限公司　谢恬总经理

二、特邀常务编委:

1. 辽宁中医药大学　杨关林校长
2. 贵州师范大学　乙引副校长

三、特邀编委(排名不分先后):

1. 长春中医药大学　校长宋柏林
2. 天津中医药大学　高秀梅常务副校长
3. 陕西中医学院　周永学院长
4. 江西中医药大学　吴晓明校办主任
5. 遵义医学院　石京山校长
6. 南方医科大学中医药学院　吕志平院长
7. 湖南中医药高等专科学校　郭争鸣校长
8. 安徽中医药高等专科学校　赵国胜校长
9. 四川中医药高等专科学校　金虹副校长
10. 重庆三峡医药高等专科学校　谭工副校长
11. 成都中医药大学附属医院　钟森院长
12. 贵阳中医学院第一附属医院　孙波院长
13. 广西中医药大学附属瑞康医院　梁健院长
14. 湖南中医药大学第二附属医院　熊辉院长
15. 江苏省中医药研究院　王佩娟副院长
16. 广州中医药大学附属骨伤科医院　谢华民院长
17. 徐州市中医院　王培安院长
18. 辽宁省血栓病中西医结合医疗中心(沈阳市第二中医医院)　赵凯院长
19. 萍乡市中医院　林家坤院长
20. 天水市中西医结合医院　杨国栋副院长
21. 武汉市黄陂区中医医院　彭建明院长
22. 深圳市龙岗区中医院　胡世平院长
23. 兖矿集团有限公司总医院　殷晓轩副院长
24. 重庆市北碚区中医院　尹平院长
25. 安徽中医药大学中西医结合医院　何光远院长

26. 平阳县中医院　张美稀院长
27. 苏州市中西医结合医院　陆治平院长
28. 南通良春中医医院　朱婉华院长
29. 新疆石河子市中医医院　刘珀董事长
30. 无锡市龙砂医学流派研究所　顾植山所长
31. 天士力控股集团有限公司董事局　闫希军主席
32. 上海和黄药业有限公司　周俊杰总经理
33. 上海市诗丹德生物技术有限公司　谢天培董事长

江西中醫藥大學

江西中医药大学创建于 1959 年。50 多年来，特别是改革开放 30 多年来，学校始终坚持“为中医药事业发展服务，为地方经济发展和社会全面进步服务，为国家需要服务”的办学宗旨，弘扬“惟学、惟人、求强、求精”的校训，以“培养适应社会进步和中医药事业发展需要，具有市场竞争力的实践型、创新型、创业型人才”为目标，努力办好人民满意的大学，先后多次获得全国和全省党的建设和思想政治工作先进高校、全国大学生暑期社会实践活动先进单位，是全国绿化模范单位、江西省文明单位。

江西中医药大学是一所江西省人民政府直辖的普通高校。从诞生起，学校先后历经了江西中医进修学校、江西中医专科学校、江西中医学院、江西中医药大学，以及由原江西医学院、江西中医学院合并组建的江西医科大学等几个历史发展时期。

江西中医药大学是中央统战部、国家民委、教育部指派的对口支援西部的高校，是全国医药院校中唯一的“少数民族高层次骨干人才医学类硕士研究生（预科）基础培训基地”。

学校是教育部批准的首批有资格接受外国留学生的高等院校之一。通过广泛开展国际学术交流与合作，与 20 多个国家和地区的科研、医疗、教育机构建立了长期的合作关系。近年来学校实现了跨越式发展，各项事业均达到了前所未有的高度。学校的综合办学实力和竞争力明显增强，办学质量和为国家、区域服务的能力显著提高，国际影响力大幅度提升。

学校校园（湾里校区）占地面积 1644.79 亩，是目前国内校园面积最大的中医药高等院校。现有 2 所直属附属医院，8 所非直属附属医院。学校拥有各类学生 2 万余人，其中，全日制本科生 10620 人，研究生 1005 人，留学生 393 人。学校拥有在职教职工 1064 人（不含附属医院）。学校教师队伍中，专任教师 789 人，其中教授 144 人，有全国优秀教师 7 人、全国卫生系统先进个人 1 人、全国中医药专家学术经验继承工作指导老师 38 人、第十届国家药典委员会委员 5 人、江西省首届高等学校“井冈学者”特聘教授 2 人、江西省主要学科学术带头人培养对象 1 人、入选江西省“赣鄱英才 555 工程”13 人、享受国务院特殊津贴专家和省政府特殊津贴专家共 66 人、江西省省级优秀教师 20 人、江西省名中医 28 人、江西省新世纪“百千万人才工程”人选 24 人、博士生导师 24 人。本科生和研究生层次教育涉及医学、理学、工学、管理学科、社会学科、人文学科等 6 大学科门类，拥有博士学位授权一级学科点 2 个，拥有硕士学位授权一级学科点 4 个、硕士学位授权二级学科点 34 个，省级示范性硕士点 2 个，博士后科研流动站 1 个，本科专业 21 个。学校现有省部级重点实验室 10 个、国家级工程研究中心 2 个，是全国中医药院校中唯一拥有 2 个国家级工程研究中心的学校。近 5 年，共承担国家重点基础研究发展计划（“973”计划）、国家高技术研究发展计划（“863”计划）、国家自然科学基金、国家“十一五”科技支撑计划等国家级项目 137 项，省部级项目 326 项，年均科研经费 6004.92 万元。近 5 年，共获得国家发明专利授权 56 项、新药证书 9 项、计算机软件著作权 3 项，有 28 项成果获省部级以上奖励，其中国家科技进步二等奖 2 项，省级科技进步一等奖 4 项。

学校倡导并践行“赢在终点”为核心的教育理念，引领人才培养模式改革与创新，先后开展了科研实践班、双惟实践班等一系列教育教学改革实践。拥有国家级人才培养模式创新实验区 1 个，国家级高等学校实验教学示范中心 1 个，国家级大学生校外实践教育基地 1 个，国家级本科专业综合改革试点 1 个，教育部高等学校特色专业建设点 3 个，国家级精品课程 2 门，国家双语示范课程 1 门，国家教学团队 1 个，国家中医药管理局重点学科 18 个、江西省一级学科高水平学科与“十二五”重点学科 5 个。两项教学改革研究项目分别于 2001 年、2009 年获得教育部国家教学成果二等奖。

学校始终坚持以推动中医药事业进步为使命，在中药药剂、针灸推拿等学科领域形成了突出优势。研发的中药制药系列关键技术和设备被 100 多家企业采用，产生了良好的经济社会效益。原始创新成果——“热敏灸”理论和技术，揭示了针刺穴位和灸疗穴位的差异，开创了内源性热敏调控治疗疾病的新途径，显著提高了艾灸的临床疗效，有力缓解了老百姓看病难、看病贵的难题，成为国家行业建设标准并在上海世博会上向全球推广，开创了“北看天津针、南看江西灸”的格局。

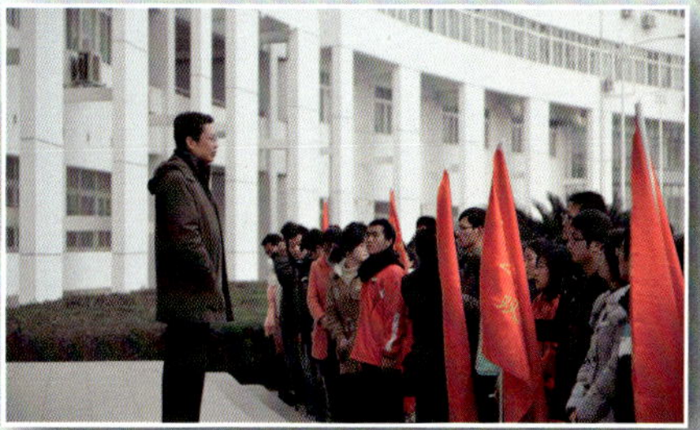

▲ 中国教育电视台深度报道：“老刘”和“双惟班”的故事

【学生培养】2013 年学校获批国家级中药学实验示范中心、药学专业综合改革实验区、国家级大学生校外实践教育基地各 1 项。获得江西省教改课题 26 项，编著 5 部教材获省级优秀教材奖。成功举办第四届教学标兵比赛，8 名教师喜获“教学标兵”。组织教师参加江西省和全国首届高校微课教学比赛，获全国首届微课比赛优胜奖 1 项、江西省首届微课比赛一等奖、二等奖各 1 项。组织 3 名教师参加全国高等中医药院校青年教师教学基本功竞赛，1 人获二等奖，2 人获优秀奖。以市场和学科发展为导向，开展了新一轮本科专业培养方案修订工作。成功承办教育部高等学校中药学类专业人才培养模式改革现场经验交流会及研讨会。

2013 年学校共招收本专科新生 3020 人，生源质量得到显著提高，江西本省本科二批第一志愿率为 100%，外省第一志愿率为 96.2%，创历史新高。成功获批江西中医药大学大学生创新创业园项目，获资助经费 20 万元；获批大学生创新创业训练计划 45 项，其中国家级项目 20 项，省级项目 25 项，资助经费 45 万元。落实就业工作“一把手工程”，开展了演讲比赛、简历大赛、模拟招聘会、毕业生经验交流会、考研交流会等一系列就业指导活动。经江西省教育厅组织的第三方调查认证，学校 2013 届本科生就业率为 90.31%，考研升学率 19.82%，均位居江西省本科院校最前列。

2013 年学校招收统招硕士生 348 人，其中专业学位型硕士生 152 人、学术型硕士生 196 人，招收少数民族高层次骨干人才强化班学员 147 人。研究生就业率达 93.3%，获第十届“华为杯”全国研究生数学建模竞赛二等奖。

2013 年成人教育共录取新生 4409 人，同比增长 58%；共有 1316 名成人学生毕业，180 名学生被授予成人学士学位。2013 年共举办“走进西部”县级医院骨干医师培训班、全省县级中医临床技术骨干培训等各类培训 6 期，培训学员 675 名，获培训经费 125.23 万元，学员满意度达 95% 以上。开展“县级中医院西医人员西学中培训”，培训学员 327 名。2013 年培训保健按摩师、公共营养师等技能人才 1245 人，同比增长 25%，95% 以上的学员通过鉴定获得国家职业资格证书。

学校独立学院顺利通过江西省教育厅规范验收工作组预验收，得到充分肯定和高度评价。2013 年招收学生 1590 人，报到率达 95.2%，名列江西省独立院校第三名；毕业 1381 人，学生就业率、考研录取率分别达 85.66% 和 13.76%，均位居江西省独立院校第一名，荣获“全省就业工作优秀单位”。

【科学研究】学校牵头组建的“江西民族传统药现代科技与产业发展”协同创新中心获批建设，由此学校拥有了 2 个省级协同创新中心；获批建设“江西省传统中药炮制重点实验室”。2013 年共获得各级各类项目 130 项，资助经费共计 6601 万元。其中国家级项目 29 项，经费 3867 万元。2013 年获批人文社科类项目 25 项，其中教育部人文社科基金项目 4 项，并实现音乐学、心理学高水平研究项目零的突破。学校获江西省自然科学二等奖和江西省科技进步三等奖各 1 项，获江西省高等学校科技成果奖 7 项，其中一等奖 2 项，二等奖 5 项。2013 年承担企事业单位委托项目 12 项，合同经费 341.7 万元。

【学科建设】扎实推进省级重点学科建设，顺利完成中医学、中药学 2 个江西省高水平学科以及药学、中西医结合、公共管理 3 个江西省“十二五”重点学科的中期检查。积极开展校级重点学科中期检查工作，通过学科自查、专家检查和意见反馈，不断加强校级重点学科建设。出台《江西中医药大学关于重点学科经费支持出国（境）学习实施办法（试行）》等制度，编印《江西中医学院重点学科建设管理文件汇编》，加强规范管理。启动 2013 年重点学科青年教师培养计划资助项目，投入经费 80 万元，立项资助 63 个项目。承办多个高水平学术会议，扎实推进中医脉诊学术研究交流。召开盱江医学研究会成立大会暨第一次学术研讨会，学校盱江医学研究进入新的历史阶段。

【人才队伍建设】受聘“井冈学者”特聘教授 2 人；刚性引进博士研究生 14 人，柔性引进高层次领军人才 2 人、续聘 2 人；被列为 2013 年度（第十七批）江西省主要学科学术和技术带头人培养对象 1 人；被确定为 2013 年度（第七批）江西省青年科学家培养对象 1 人；申报入选“赣鄱英才 555 工程”人选 4 人、战略创新团队 1 个；获批领军人才培养计划人员 2 人，青年拔尖培养计划人选 1 人；组织开展各类人员培训 10 余次，派出 680 人次参加国（境）内外访学、研修培训；66 名教师申请在职攻读博士学位。

【对外交流】成功举办第四届全国青年发展论坛暨首届“江中·远志杯”全国高等中医药院校大学生课外学术科技作品竞赛，全国 23 所中医药院校的领导、专家学者、青年领袖近 200 人参加，反响良好。签订协议与英国安格利亚鲁斯金大学在生物工程、心理治疗等专业方向进行合作；与芬兰东芬兰大学、瑞典针灸学院、智利圣地亚哥大学、新西兰中医学院等院校签署合作框架协议；与台湾大仁科技大学、香港浸会大学等院校就学术交流、学生互派等合作达成了意愿；获批全省唯一具有对港免试招生资格的院校。

【基本建设与服务支撑】按照“高效率用完、高质量用好、高要求用廉”的工作原则，学校扎实推进化债资金项目。截至 2013 年底，化债资金项目实施工作领导小组会议通过项目审批的采购金额达 4.574 亿元，其中完成招标 3.8869 亿元，完成比例达 86.88%；已签订合同金额达 3.608 亿元，占预算总额的 80.65%；已支付款项为 1.1876 亿元，占预算总额的 26.55%。通过化债资金项目实施，重点打造了一批行业领先、国内一流、国际接轨的高层次科研平台、高标准教学平台和高起点公共平台，为建设高水平、有特色的中医药大学进一步奠定了坚实基础。

学校后勤管理部门创新管理方式，提高师生满意度。推行“后勤啄木鸟行动实施方案”，发放调查问卷 1800 份，对后勤服务态度、服务质量、满意度进行测评；向学生发放《后勤温馨服务提示卡》15000 份，向老师发放《后勤服务手册》1300 份。地毯式排查近 2000 间宿舍，完成相应维修项目。进一步改善校园环境，修建了两条行政楼景观道，改造兴湾大道护坡色带 800 米，硬化了食堂周边地面，方便师生停车。

【年度工作亮点】2013 年 4 月 18 日，教育部致函江西省政府，同意学校更名为“江西中医药大学”；6 月 15 日，江西省政府正式批复学校更名。9 月 26 日，学校隆重举行更名揭牌仪式，江西省副省长朱虹为“江西中医药大学”揭牌。

2013 年 7 月 19 日，国务院学位委员会下发《关于下达 2008-2015 年立项建设博士、硕士学位授予单位及其授权学科名单的通知》；8 月 6 日，江西省人民政府学位委员会下发《关于下达我省新增博士、硕士学位授予单位及其授权学科名单的通知》，经国务院学位委员会第三十次会议审议批准，学校被确定为博士学位授予单位，中医学、中药学两个学科为博士学位授权一级学科，覆盖了这 2 个主干学科的全部二级学科。

学校正式成立了岐黄国医书院。学校投入 4400 万元建设资金，在完成机构设置、项目选址、建设规划、师资选聘、培养方案、设备采购等一系列工作基础上，首届 21 名学生于 9 月 5 日入学。

学校陈日新教授的论文《灸之要，气至而有效》获得“2012 年中国百篇最具影响国内学术论文”殊荣，该项评选的范围为 2008-2012 年 5 年间的全国中文论文，分布在 81 个机构中，江西省仅此 1 篇论文入选，极具分量。

学校贯彻落实中央、江西省委的统一部署，在江西省委第十六督导组的悉心指导下，学校牢牢把握“为民务实清廉”主题，紧紧围绕“照镜子、正衣冠、洗洗澡、治治病”总要求，精心组织，周密安排，认真扎实地组织开展了为期半年的党的群众路线教育实践活动，全校 25 个基层单位党委（党总支、直属党支部）、148 个基层党支部、3100 多名党员全程参加了活动，取得了良好成效。学校的学习风气明显好转，党员干部思想认识进一步提高；群众观念明显强化，党员干部工作作风进一步转变；宗旨意识明显增强，党群干群关系进一步密切；育人氛围明显增浓，学校教风学风进一步优化；中心工作明显推进，学校内涵建设进一步提升；制度建设明显加强，反对“四风”机制进一步完善。江西省委“活动办”《简报》，人民网、江西日报、中国中医药报、江西卫视、江西人民广播电台、中国江西网、江西教育电视台等新闻媒体多次对学校教育实践活动进行了宣传报道。

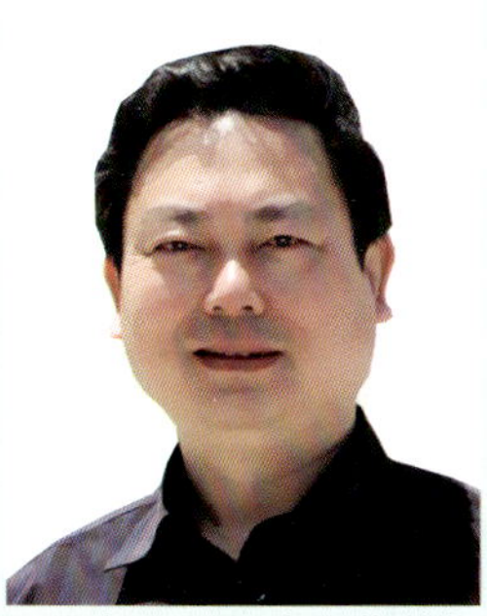

▲吴晓明 江西中医药大学

吴晓明 男，1959 年 12 月出生，中共党员，江西中医药大学党办、校办主任，教授。

吴晓明教授于南昌大学马克思主义基础理论专业毕业，浙江大学研究生院思想政治教育专业结业，长期从事高校管理工作、宣传思想工作、高等教育研究及中医药文化研究，主管学校年鉴编纂工作及各方面年鉴报送材料的撰稿、审稿工作，发表相关论文数十篇，主持过若干省级科研课题，参加过一系列中医药管理、发展、学术研讨、文化研讨会议，熟悉高校工作及本校各方面情况，参与《中国中医药年鉴》（学术卷）特邀编委的工作。

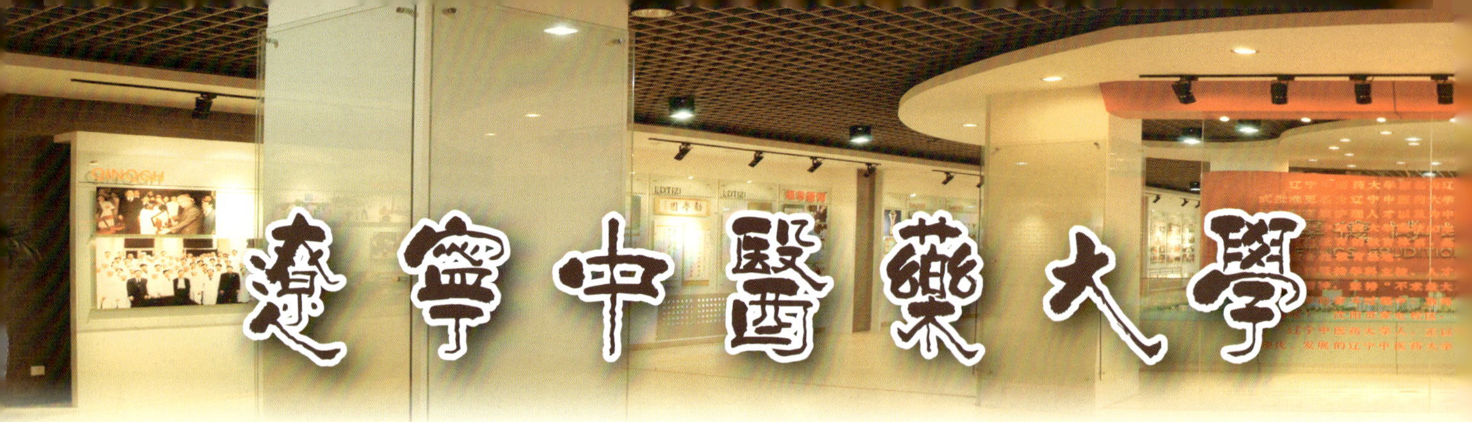

遼寧中醫藥大學

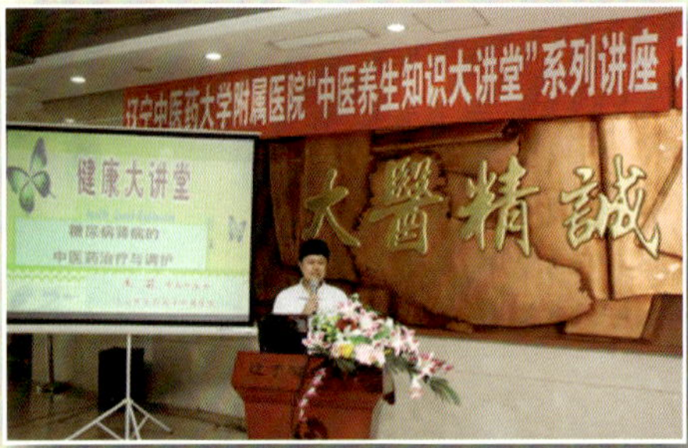

▲ 中医讲堂

学校成立于1958年，主校区位于省会城市沈阳，分校区位于大连和本溪，初步形成“南药北医中产业”的发展格局，是辽宁省唯一一所培养中医、中药、针灸推拿、中西医临床医学、高级护理和医学相关类人才的高等院校，2013 年组建成立辽宁省中医药科学院。学校先后获得全国教育纪检监察先进集体、全国创先争优先进基层党组织、辽宁省先进基层党组织、辽宁“五一”奖状等多项荣誉称号。

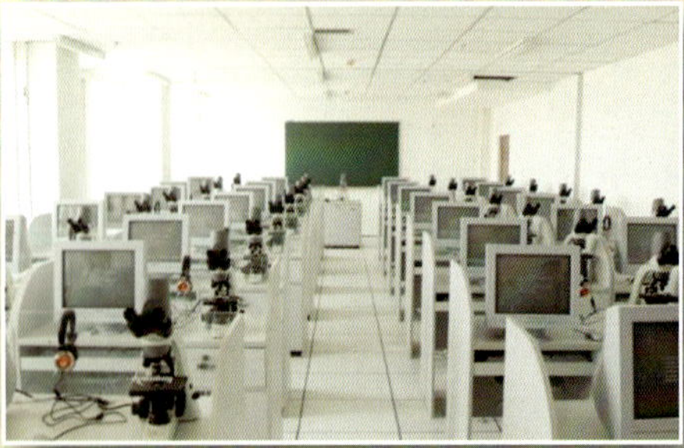
▲ 实验室

学校设置医、理、工、管、文5个学科门类，19 个本科专业，现有在校生万余人，下设 17 个学院、4 所直属附属医院、2 个教学部、2 个教学实验中心、3 个研究院、6 个研究所、2 所图书馆。有 1 个国家重点学科、26 个国家中医药管理局中医药重点学科、3 个省一流学科，7 个省高等学校重点学科、5 个省“提升高等学校核心竞争力特色学科建设工程”立项学科、21 个省中医药重点学科；3 个博士后科研流动站、3 个一级学科博士学位授权学科、3 个一级学科硕士学位授权学科。现有 1 名“973 计划”首席科学家，1 名国家名师、1 名国医大师、26 名国家级名中医、18 名全国老中医药专家学术经验继承指导教师，1 人入选“辽宁省院士后备人选培养工程”，8 名省级教学名师、5 名省级专业带头人；“新世纪百千万人才工程”国家级人选 3 人，享受国务院政府特殊津贴专家 42 人，卫生部有突出贡献中青年专家 3 人。有 1 个国家中医临床研究基地、2 个国家临床药理基地、3 个国家中医药管理局重点研究室、11 个国家中医药管理局科研三级实验室、22 个省重点实验室及工程中心，承担和完成国家重大科研项目数十项。2014 年，学校中医脏象理论及应用省部共建教育部重点实验室顺利通过验收，实验室总面积达到 7420 平方米，规划建设了 3890 平方米 SPF 级实验动物中心。目前实验室具有 4 个稳定的研究方向，6 个实验平台及 25 个功能单元，实验仪器设备总值达 7000 余万元，承担完成“973”计划、国家自然科学基金、国家科技支撑计划、国家重大新药创制专项等课题 60 余项；发表科研论文 500 余篇；出版学术专著、教材 50 余部；获得省、市级科技奖励近 80 项。4 所直属附属医院，共有 11 个国家卫生部临床重点专科，20 个国家中医药管理局重点专科，31 个省重点专科；分别增具辽宁省中医院、辽宁省中医药研究院、辽宁省肛肠医院、辽宁省中西医结合医院名称，附属医院康复中心暨辽宁省中医院慢病医院，积极发挥康复、养生、保健、疗养等服务功能。在文化传承创新方面，学校打造一批具有中医药特色的科普教育基地，“一堂四馆”，即中医文化大讲堂、医史馆、人体生命科学馆、校史馆、中药标本馆，面向社会广泛传播中医文化知识。

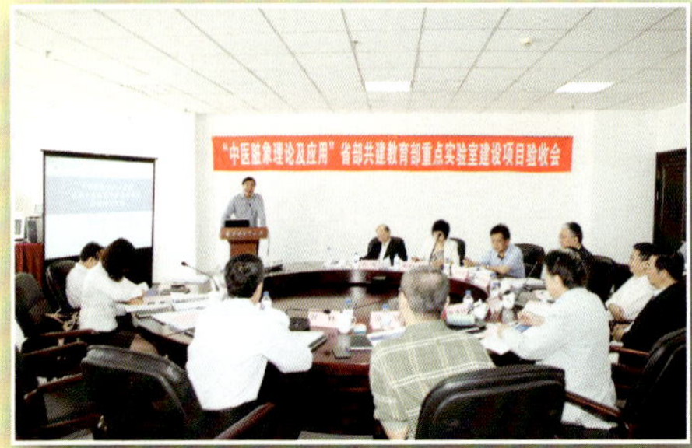
▲ 省部共建教育部重点实验室建设项目验收会

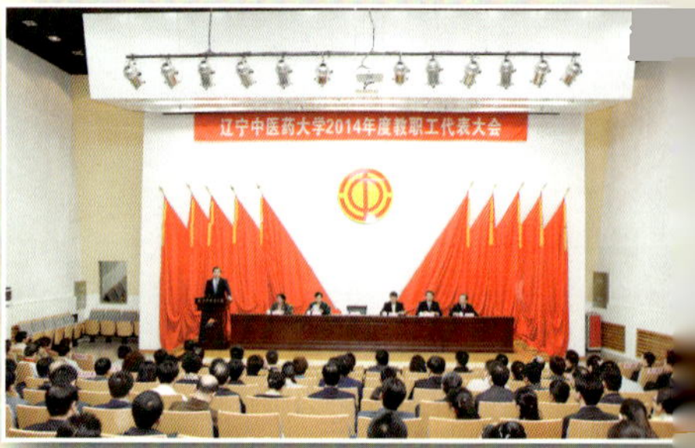

▲ 2014教职工代表大会

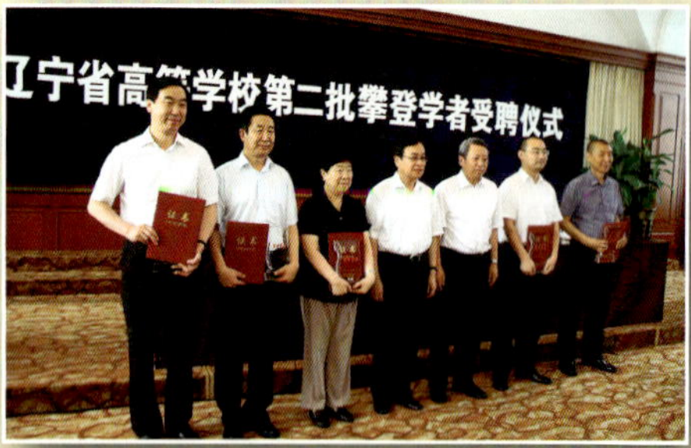
▲ 攀登学者

辽宁中医药大学本着“不求最大，但求最强”的办学理念，实施“学科立校、人才强校、科技兴校”战略，全面加强内涵建设，在振兴辽宁老工业基地方面发挥了应有的作用，为祖国中医药事业的传承和发扬做出了重要的贡献，正向着高水平教学研究型中医药大学的建设目标而努力奋斗！

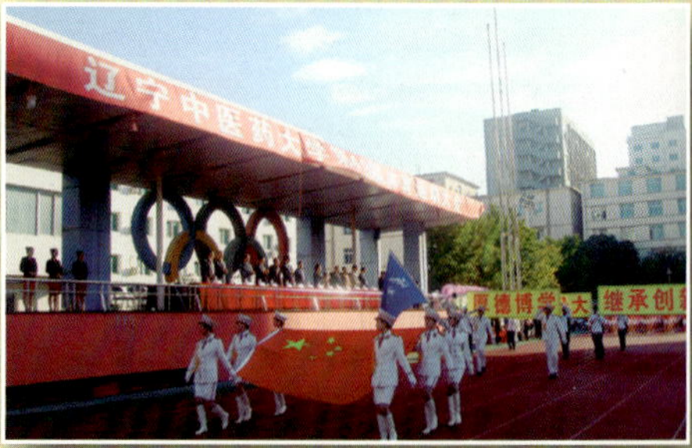
▲ 运动会

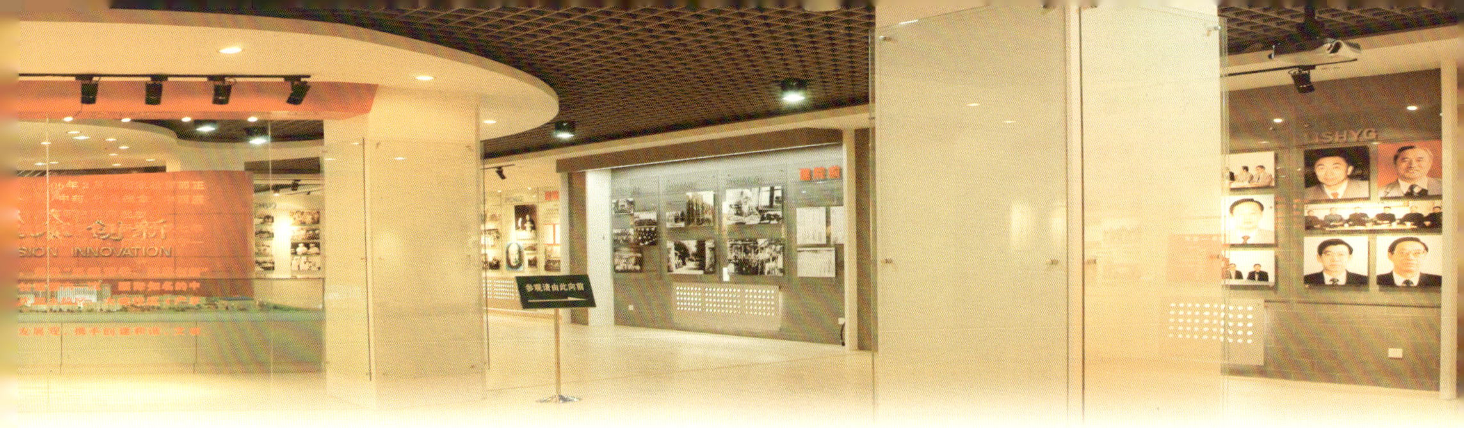

杨关林 男，锡伯族，1962年10月生，黑龙江省肇东人，农工党党员，教授，主任医师，博士研究生导师，辽宁中医药大学校长。农工党中央教育工作委员会主任，农工党辽宁省委副主委，辽宁省人大常委。本科就读于北京医学院（现北京大学医学部），1988年研究生毕业于辽宁中医学院（现辽宁中医药大学）。历任心血管科医师，心电监护科主任，干诊科主任，医务科科长，辽宁中医药大学附属医院副院长、院长，辽宁中医药大学副校长。

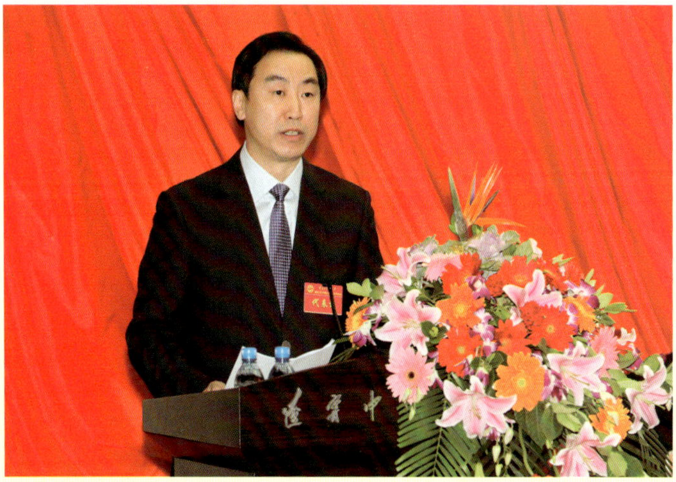

▲ 杨关林 在学校教代会上讲话

杨关林教授为国家“973计划”首席科学家，国家中医药管理局重点专科（心血管）学术带头人，省重点学科（中西医结合临床）学科带头人，中西医结合临床专业博士点学术带头人，享受国务院政府特殊津贴，辽宁省名中医，辽宁省高等学校攀登学者，辽宁省院士后备人选，辽宁省第二批领军人才；兼任中华中医药学会常务理事、老年病分会会长，世界眼针医学研究中心学术委员会主任委员，国家中医药管理局血脉病重点研究室主任，中国中西医结合学会理事，世界中医药学会联合会教育指导委员会副会长，全国高等中医药教材评审委员会中西医临床医学专业教材评审委员会副主任委员，辽宁省中西医结合学会会长，辽宁省医师协会副会长，辽宁省中医药学会副会长，辽宁省康复医学会副会长等。先后获得全国优秀科技工作者、卫生部有突出贡献中青年专家、中国医师奖、辽宁省百千万人才工程“百人层次”等荣誉称号。

杨关林从事医疗、教学、科研、管理工作近30载，始终艰苦奋斗，高瞻远瞩，不仅学术造诣深厚，临床经验丰富，科研能力卓越，而且工作作风严谨，管理能力突出，在学科建设和人才培养上硕果累累。擅长中西医结合防治心脑血管疾病、老年病，中医药临床药效评价关键技术研究等，尤其擅长冠心病、心衰、高血压病、心律失常等疾病的治疗。始终视保护病人生命为第一要任，潜心研究，创新性地提出“从痰瘀论治动脉粥样硬化”的学术观点，丰富了“痰瘀论治”理论，并以此展开了动脉粥样硬化中医病机探悉和防治策略的研究，研发防治动脉粥样硬化的新制剂化瘀祛痰颗粒剂，获得国家发明专利。2013年，杨关林担任首席科学家的国家“973”项目“脾主运化、统血”等脾脏象理论研究项目，实施期为5年，研究经费2300万元，这是辽宁省首家以省属高校作为第一承担单位组织实施的国家“973”项目，该项目实施2年来，揭示基于“脾主运化、统血”等脾脏象理论对健康和疾病的作用规律及调控机制，以及“从脾论治”相关疾病（冠心病心绞痛、功能性胃肠病、血小板减小性紫癜）的临床疗效机制和规律，为提高相关疾病的辨证论治水平提供科学支撑等方面取得了阶段性成果。此外，他在国内率先提出“血脉病”概念，创新发展了中医基础理论；主编学术专著9部，发表学术论文77篇；主持科技部重大新药创制项目1项、“十一五”支撑计划1项、科技部行业公益项目1项。获得辽宁省科技进步一等奖1项、二等奖3项、三等奖3项；辽宁省教学成果一等奖1项、二等奖1项；中华中医药学会科学技术奖3项、学术著作奖1项、科普著作奖1项。自担任研究生导师以来，已培养博士后7人，博士生17人，硕士生115人。他所带团队被授予“辽宁省高校创新团队”及“辽宁省高校本科优秀教学团队”称号。

▼ 杨关林校长担任加中传统医药国际论坛主席主持大会

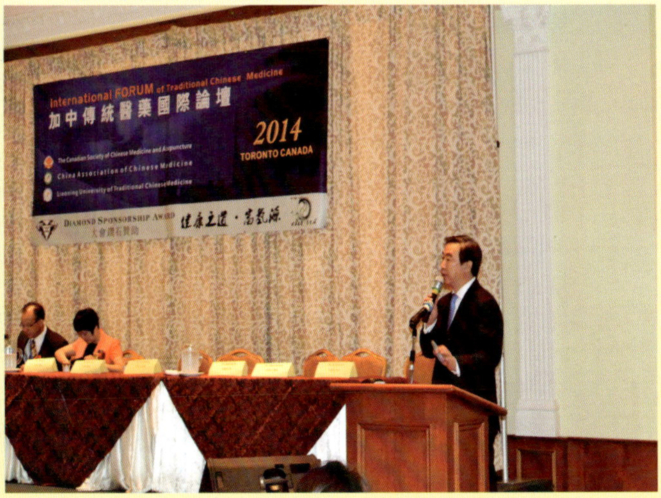

在杨关林率领下，学校获批组建辽宁省中医药科学院，这是学校发展史上具有里程碑意义的重大事件，通过整合全省中医药科技资源与力量，构建中医药自主创新平台，加快中医药科技创新人才的培养，促进中医药创新成果转化和产业化。杨关林同时担任中医脏象理论及应用省部共建教育部实验室主任，经过两年的建设周期，实验室在原有面积基础上扩建3000余平方米，实验室总面积达到7420平方米，规划建设了3890平方米SPF级实验动物中心。目前实验室具有4个稳定的研究方向，6个实验平台及25个功能单元，实验仪器设备总值达7000余万元。承担完成“973”计划、国家自然科学基金、国家科技支撑计划、国家重大新药创制专项等课题60余项；获得省、市级科技奖励近80项，该实验室现已通过教育部重点实验室验收。2014年，杨关林组织召开了加中传统医药国际论坛，并作为大会主席进行主题报告。

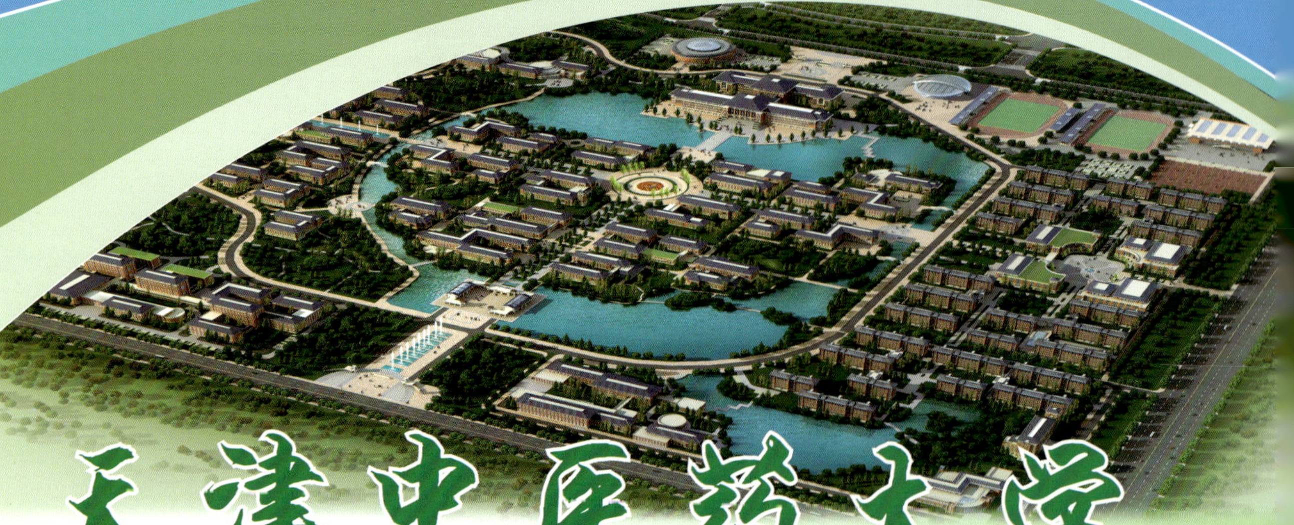

天津中医药大学

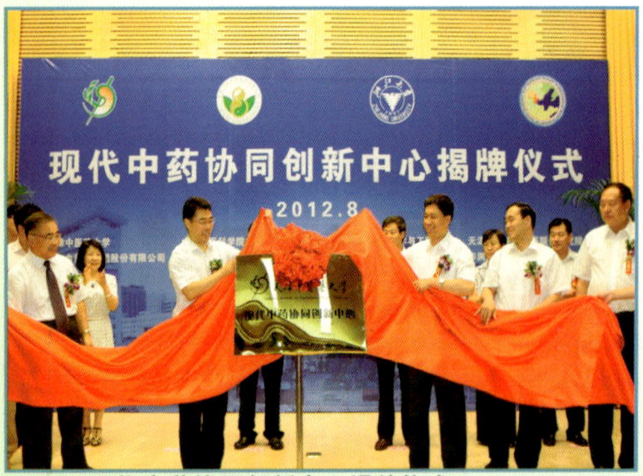

▲ 现代中药协同创新中心揭牌仪式

天津中医药大学始建于 1958 年，2006 年正式更名为天津中医药大学。1992 年经国家教委批准，加挂中国传统医药国际学院校牌，是教育部高等学校中医学、医学人文素质教学指导委员会主任委员单位和世中联教育指导委员会主任委员单位。正在建设中的新校区座落于天津市静海县团泊湖畔，占地 2600 余亩，建筑面积 60 余万平方米，将建设成为全国最大的中医药博物馆、中药植物园，全国最先进的中医药科技园及中医药国际教育中心。

学校有教职工约 4000 人，具有高级专业技术职称教师 1000 人。本科在校生 7800 余人，硕博研究生 3100 余人，留学生及港澳台侨生 2000 余人。学校拥有针灸推拿学和中医内科学国家级重点学科 2 个、国家中医药管理局重点学科 23 个、天津市"十二五"重点学科 5 个。建有天津市现代中药实验室——省部共建国家重点实验室、国家科技部中药现代化科技产业基地（天津）——现代中药研究中心、国家级国际联合中心——中意中医药联合实验室、教育部方剂学重点实验室、现代中药发现与制剂技术教育部工程研究中心、天津市组分中药技术工程中心、天津市重点实验室 3 个、国家中医药管理局三级科研实验室 14 个、国家中医药管理局重点研究室 2 个、市卫生局重点研究室 8 个。学校有中医学、中药学、中西医结合 3 个博士后科研流动站，3 个一级博士点，25 个二级博士点和 46 个二级硕士点；拥有附属医院 6 家，临床教学基地 43 家。

▼ 现代中药制药质量控制技术高级研修班

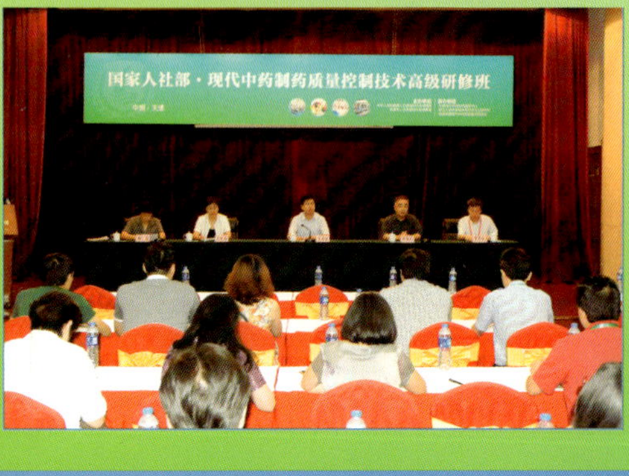

学校有中国工程院院士 3 名，国医大师 2 名，还有教育部长江学者奖励计划特聘教授、国家杰出青年科学基金获得者、万人计划、新世纪"百千万人才工程"、教育部新世纪优秀人才、卫生部有突出贡献中青年专家、人事部有突出贡献中青年专家等一批高层次人才。

为贯彻落实教育部"高等学校创新能力提升计划"（简称"2011"计划）的重大举措，率先建成现代中药协同创新中心，由天津中医药大学牵头，联合中国中医科学院中药研究所、浙江大学药学院中药科学与工程学系、天津国际生物医药联合研究院等科研院所，天士力制药集团股份有限公司、山东步长制药股份有限公司、石家庄以岭药业股份有限公司、华润三九医药股份有限公司等大型中药制药企业，于 2012 年 3 月共同组建。

"优势互补，协同攻关，重点突破，整体提升"是协同创新中心的宗旨，采取了"1+3+X"的创新合作模式，围绕中药产业结构调整与转型发展的重大需求，针对影响制约中药产业发展的共性问题，开展科学研究与成果转化。形成了以组分中药新药研发、中药资源高质量开发利用、中药制药工艺优化、中药安全性基础研究、中药大品种二次开发和国际化为重点方向，整合优势力量、协同攻关。目前，协同创新中心已经汇聚专业研发人员 600 余名，其中院士 4 人，国家杰出青年、国家千人计划、长江学者等顶级优秀人才 50 余人，形成人才聚集高地。拥有国家重点学科 2 个，获批国家科技部创新人才培养示范基地、教育部创新团队等 11 支高层次专业研究团队，大型仪器 1000 余台，可供中药研发实验室面积 6 万余平米，牵头单位天津中医药大学新校区产学研联合基地新增建设面积将达到 5 万平米，可进一步满足中心进行协同创新、集群研发的软硬件需要。

协同创新中心成立以来承担国家科技支撑计划、973 计划等国家级课题 300 余项，纵横向经费达 10 亿元。年均发表学术论文 2500 余篇，其中 SCI 收录 400 余篇，年均申请专利 150 余项，其中发明 80 余项，PCT 进入美国、欧盟、日本等国家和地区。中心作为中药行业产业的核心和纽带，发挥人才、学科、科研"三位一体"创新能力，进一步加强专业技术的交叉融合，知识和成果的集成转化，对区域经济发展和行业科技进步发挥着重要的辐射和带动作用。

近些年来，学校科技成果数量和水平均有大幅度提升。荣获国家科学技术进步奖 8 项，其中一等奖 2 项，二等奖 6 项；省部级科技奖励 40 余项；荣获国家级教学成果奖 5 项。2014 年，学校作为第一完成单位，历经 8 年联合攻关，完成了"中成药二次开发核心技术体系创研及其产业化"项目得国家科技进步一等奖。该项目围绕做大做强药品种的重大需求，分析制约中成药品种做大的因素，张伯礼院士带领课题组率先提出了中二次开发研究策略，经历理论创新、技术突破广应用，构建了中成药临床准确定位、药效物体系统辨析、网络药理学、工艺品质调优和数全程质控等五大核心技术体系。该项目从解决药品种个性化难题起步，聚焦于突破中成药二发共性关键核心技术，开辟了中药制药技术升径，研究成果无缝转化，对中药产业提质增效了引领支撑作用。本项目具有原创性，拥有自识产权，获 19 项发明专利及 7 项软件著作权，论文 150 篇，SCI 收录 91 篇。本项目完成的 3中成药品种二次开发，销售额过亿元品种由 3 加到 12 个，2013 年销售额达 50 亿元，累计销

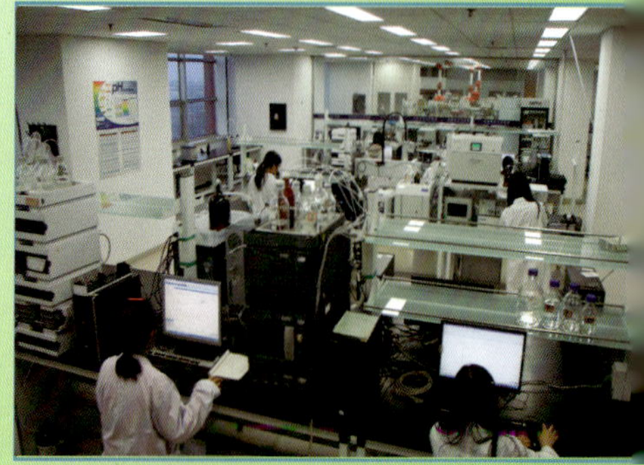

▲ 实验室平台

超过 200 亿元。项目技术已在全国 19 个省市推应用于近百家中药企业。通过推广实施中药二次发战略，培育了中药大品种群，提高了中药行业中度，过亿元中药品种增长了 3 倍，年累计销售达 1200 亿元。中药二次开发引领了中药产业创发展方向，推动了中药产业技术升级换代，促进药产业向科技型、高效型和节约型转变。

实践证明中成药二次开发是一条投入少、见快、创新驱动中药产业跨越发展的有效途径，不能推动调整产业结构、转变经济发展方式，同时务医改、惠及民生，可为重大疾病防治提供安全效、质优价廉的药物，对保障我国医改成功，促进物医药产业发展，将起到重大推动作用，产生了大经济效益和社会效益。

学校以"进德修业，继承创新"为校训，以点学科建设和中医药对外教育为特色，以科学研协同转化为优势，以中医药学为主，医、理、文、工、教育等多学科协调发展。坚持"传承与创新同，科研与服务并举，以质量求内涵，全面协调展"方针，建设高水平、外向型、国内一流、国际名的教学研究型中医药大学。

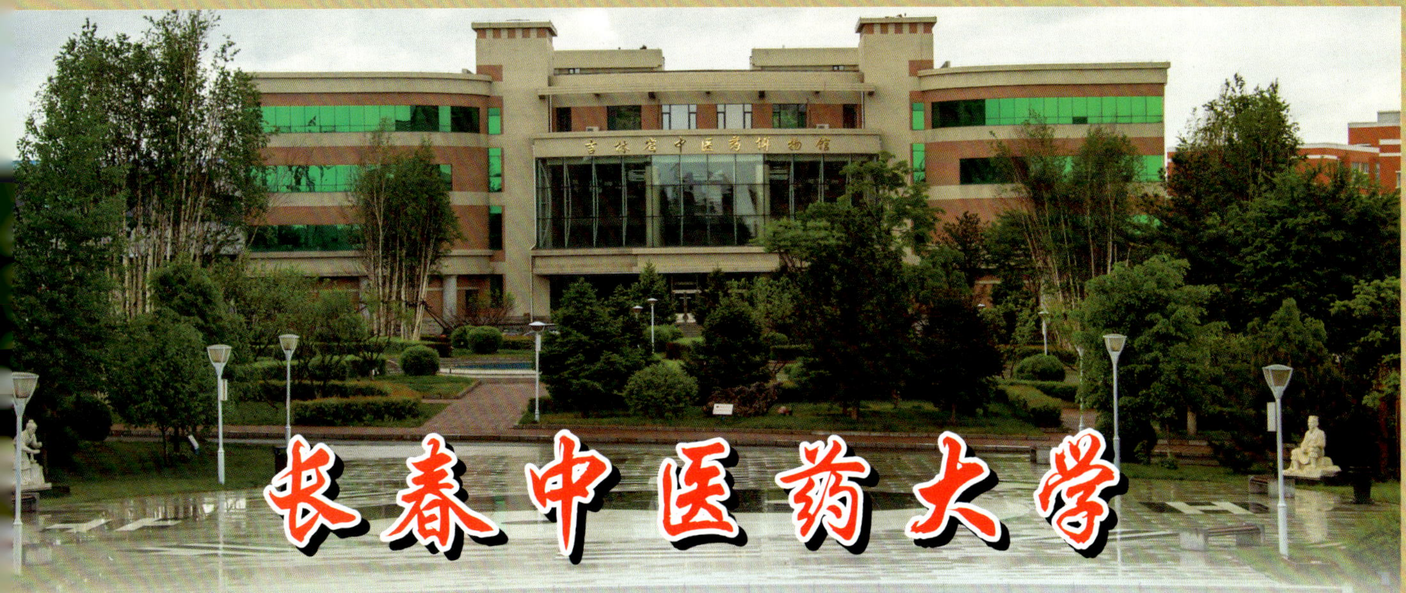

长春中医药大学

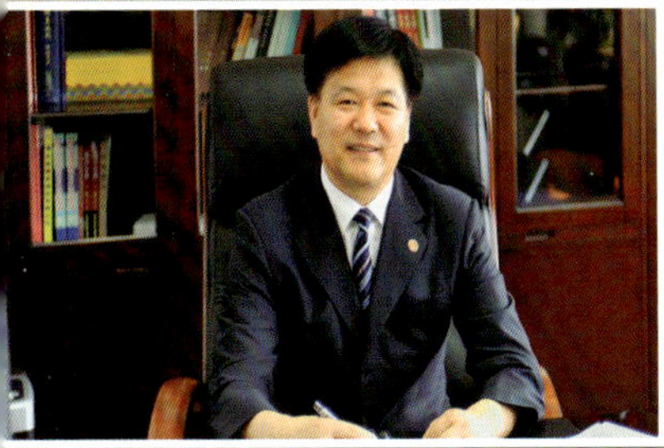

▲ 宋柏林 长春中医药大学校长

宋柏林 男，1962年2月出生，中共党员，教授，医学博士，博士研究生导师。现任长春中医药大学校长；兼教育部高等学校公共卫生与全科医学教学指导委员，中华中医药学会医院管理分会副会长、推拿专业委员会副主任委员，中国针灸学会针灸推拿结合专业委员会副主任委员，全国高等中医院校骨伤教育研究会及中国人才研究会骨伤人才分会副会长，世界中医药联合会伦理审查委员会理事会副会长，吉林省中西医结合学会会长，吉林省中医药学会推拿专业委员会主任委员、中医院管理专业委员会副主任委员，吉林省卫生政务信息与新闻宣传工作理事会副理事长，《中国医院管理》杂志常务理事，《中国现代医生杂志》编委，科技部奖励评审专家，国家自然科学基金委员会评议专家，卫生部"健康中国2020战略规划研究专家"，中华中医药学会科技评审专家，李时珍医药创新奖评审专家，吉林省科技厅奖励评审专家，吉林省政府第三届决策咨询委员，长春市第十三届人大代表。

长春中医药大学前身为1958年创办的长春中医学院，2006年更名长春中医药大学。历经50余年的辛勤耕耘、孜孜以求和创新发展，学校形成了"启古纳今，厚德精术"的校训；形成了"坚持以中医药学科为主体，走学研产结合之路，主动服务地方经济建设和社会发展"的办学特色；形成了博士、硕士、学士授权的办学层次；形成了本科教育、研究生教育、高职教育、继续教育、留学生教育等培养高等中医药人才的教育体系，已经成为吉林省唯一一所以中医药学科为主，医、理、工、管、文等多学科协调发展、具有鲜明办学特色和广泛社会声誉的省属重点大学。50多年来，学校为国家培养输送了4万余名毕业生，校友遍及海内外，为国家和吉林省的经济社会发展提供了坚实的人力和智力支撑。

▼ 学校承办世界中医药联合会理事会

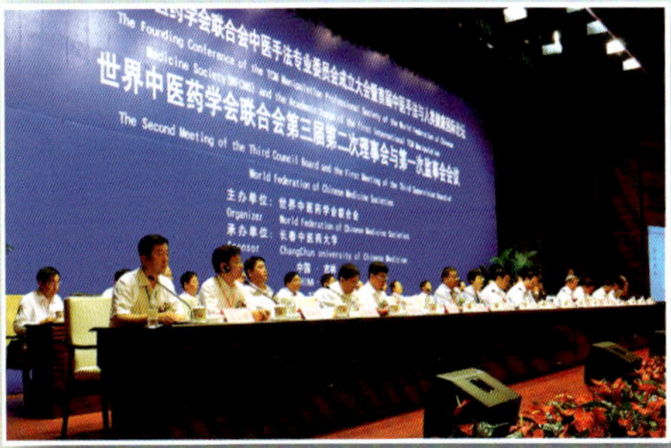

进入新世纪以来，学校紧紧抓住难得的发展机遇，创造性地开展工作。在充分发挥自身的品牌、学科和人才优势的基础上，励精图治、科学发展，实现了内涵建设与外延建设的齐头并进，取得了多项具有标志性意义的成就：净月新校区建成并投入使用；成为博士学位授权单位；中医学、中药学两个一级学科在全国具有博士学位授权一级学科整体水平评估中位居第7名、第9名；成为省属重点高校；更名为长春中医药大学；建立了中医学、中药学博士后流动站；教育部本科教学工作水平评估获得优秀；与省政府共建吉林省人参科学研究院；成为国家中医临床研究基地；中医学成为一级学科博士学位授权单位；任继学教授荣获"白求恩奖章""国医大师""吉林骄傲"称号；学校获得了国家中西部高校基础能力建设工程项目，跻身于国家中西部高校百强行列；学校被评为全国毕业生就业典型经验高校。

学校占地面积54.7万平方米，建筑面积41.2万平方米。主校区坐落在净月经济开发区，毗邻净月潭国家森林公园。学校现有本科专业18个，硕士学位授权点30个，一级学科博士学位授权点2个，博士后流动站2个，博士后创新工作站1个。全日制在校生10864人。校本部现有教职工990人，具有高级专业技术职务人员365人，其中正高级专业技术职务人员124人、副高级专业技术职务人员241人。享誉全国的终身教授6人；博士生导师51人，硕士生导师248人；国家"白求恩奖章"获得者1人，"国医大师"获得者2人，国家"973"首席科学家1人，长白山学者3人，长白山技能名师1人，国家级优秀教师4人，享受国务院特殊津贴者29人，国

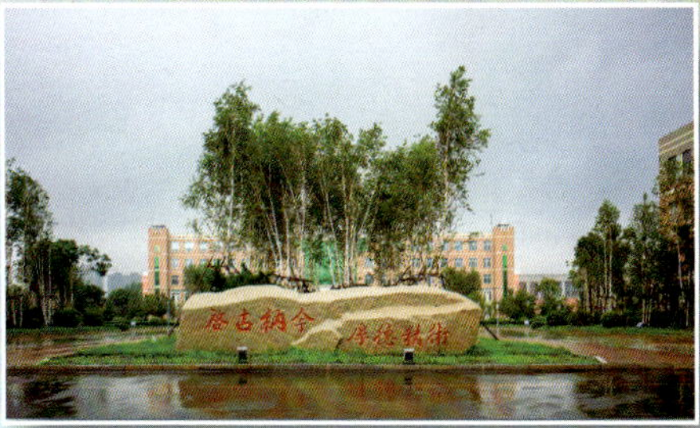

▲ 校训石

家及省级有突出贡献的中青年专家16人。入选教育部新世纪优秀人才计划2人；吉林省资深高级专家1人、吉林省高级专家5人，优秀专业技术人才1人，教学名师奖获得者6人；被批准为省教育厅新世纪优秀人才计划4人，新世纪首席教授1人，吉林省名中医29人，吉林省第三届创业先锋1人，吉林省特等劳动模范2人。

学校现有"十一五"国家级特色专业建设点4个、省级品牌专业建设点3个，"十二五"省级特色专业8个；国家级精品课程3门，省级精品课程23门，省级优秀课程41门，省级优秀教学团队12个；主编国家"十一五"规划教材13部、主编教育部"十二五"规划教材4部、主编国家"十二五"行业规划教材25部；国家级人才培养模式创新实验区1个，国家级大学生文化素质教育基地1个，省级实验教学示范中心5个；有省部级重点学科22个；有省部级以上科研平台23

▼ 时任省长巴音朝鲁莅临学校指导

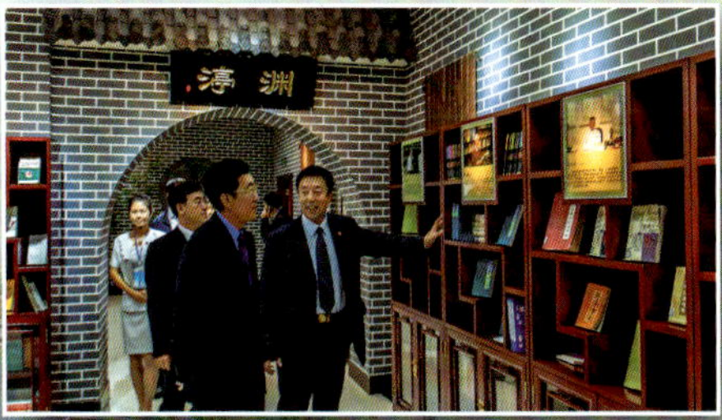

个，其中国家级中医临床研究基地1个，国家科技部国际科技合作基地1个，国家地方联合工程研究中心1个，国家生物产业基地医药中试平台1个，教育部省部共建重点实验室1个；省校共建吉林省人参科学研究院1个。学校教学科研仪器设备总值20581万元。馆藏图书103万册，有一批学术价值很高的珍、善本典籍。出版发行《长春中医药大学学报》《吉林中医药》等学术期刊。学校是教育部首批批准招收国外留学生的中医药院校，留学生培养涵盖本科生、研究生教育两个层次。学校广泛开展国际学术交流与合作，多次主办中医药国际学术会议，与多个国家和地区的高校与研究单位保持着长期的友好往来。

站在新的历史起点上，长春中医药大学正在继往开来，科学发展，追求卓越，续写华章，不断将学校事业做精做特做强，为把学校早日建成在国际上有广泛影响、在省属高校中优势突出、具有鲜明办学特色的国内一流教学研究型中医药大学而共同努力。

安徽中医药大学

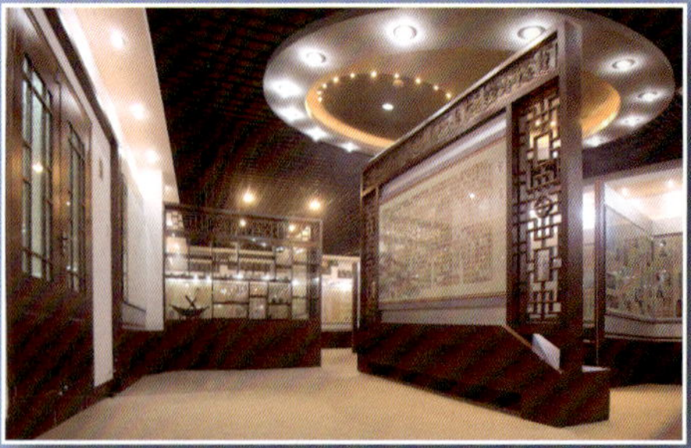

▲ 新安医学文化馆

安徽中医药大学是一所以中医药学科为主，相关学科协调发展，办学层次齐全，优势特色鲜明的中医药高等学府，是国家中医临床研究基地、国家中药现代化科技产业（安徽）基地、国家中医药国际合作基地、国家药品临床研究基地、硕士研究生推荐免试单位。

学校以人才培养为第一要务，坚持“弘扬新安医学，培育中医人才”的办学特色，人才培养质量不断提高。现有 2 个国家级教学团队、3 个省级教学团队，1 门国家级精品课程、16 门省级精品课程。学校注重办学特色的彰显，深入推进教学改革，举办新安医学教改实验班，在临床专业建立客观化结构考试中心。2010 年开始与长春、福建 2 所中医药大学开展相互交流培养学生；设立大学生课外科技创新与创业基金；开展“百人获奖、千人参与、万人受益”的大学生知识技能竞赛和“挑战杯”等各级各类竞赛活动。近 5 年来，学校共有学生 200 余人次在学术科技与创新创业领域获省部级以上表彰和奖励 70 余项（其中获全国大学生管理决策模拟大赛特等奖 1 次、全国“挑战杯”大学生创业计划竞赛三等奖 1 次、全国“挑战杯”大学生课外学术科技作品竞赛三等奖 2 次）。近 5 年来，先后获国家级、省级质量工程项目 100 余项，国家级教学成果奖 1 项，省级教学成果特等奖 1 项、一等奖 4 项。

学校大力推进科技强校战略，积极促进教学水平与人才培养质量的提高。近 5 年来，学校共承担各级各类项目 1400 余项，其中承担国家“973”计划、“863”计划、科技支撑计划、自然科学基金等国家级项目 90 项，科研经费 2 亿余元；取得研究成果 300 余项，获得省部级以上科技奖励 27 项（其中国家科技进步奖 2 项）。现有 4 个省级科技创新团队，24 个省级以上重点实验室及工程（技术）研究中心。建立了安徽省中药材科技产业战略联盟。成功举办中医药科技创新与新安医学研究国际论坛、针灸经络 50 年回顾与展望国际学术研讨会等有较大影响的国际学术会议。学校被国家科学技术部授予“全国科技特派员工作先进集体”称号，被国家中医药管理局授予“中医药科技管理工作先进集体”称号。

▼ 新安医学文化馆

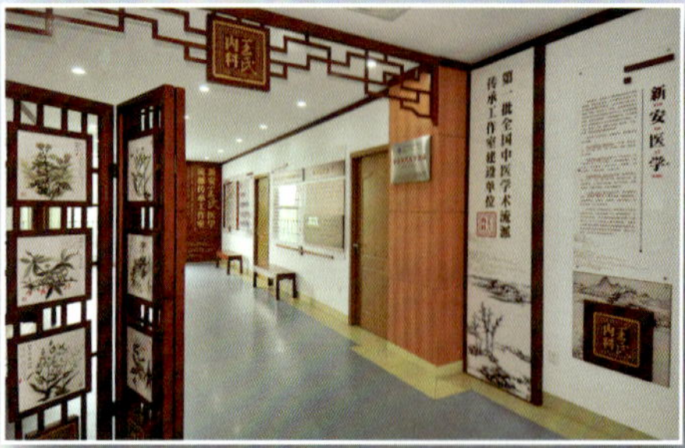

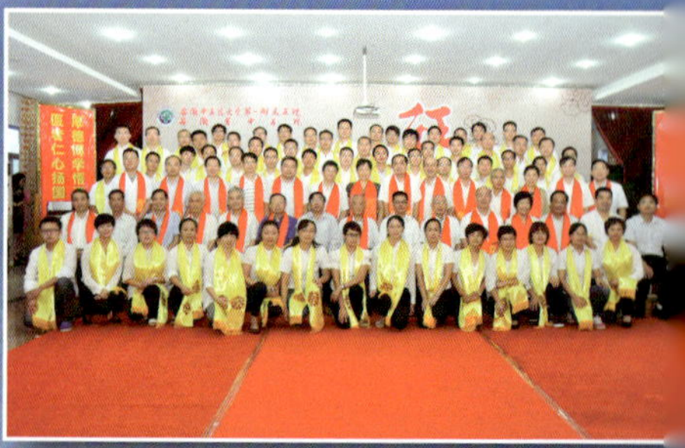

▲ 拜师仪式

学校不断加强产学研用合作，服务地方经济社会建设能力不断增强。学校与黄山、亳州、绩溪、舒城等市县人民政府签订全面合作协议，与河南宛西、江苏康缘、深圳三九等国内知名中医药企业签订战略合作协议，建有亳州济人药业等 22 个产学研合作基地，开展 50 多项技术服务，服务地方经济社会发展的能力不断提升。积极为政府在出台有关中医药发展规划和相关政策方面提供决策咨询，学校在国家中药现代化科技产业（安徽）基地建设中作出了积极贡献。第一附属医院作为全省最大的三级甲等综合性中医医院，多次派出医疗队奔赴四川灾区开展卫生援建工作；第二附属医院作为全国首家三级甲等针灸专科医院，积极支援基层中医院建设；中西医结合医院是国家第三批重点建设的中西医结合医院，神经病学研究所附属医院是一所国内外有影响的以“肝豆状核变性诊治”为优势的专科医院，国医堂是一所以纯中医方式为主要医疗手段的医疗单位，成为开展社会服务的重要力量。

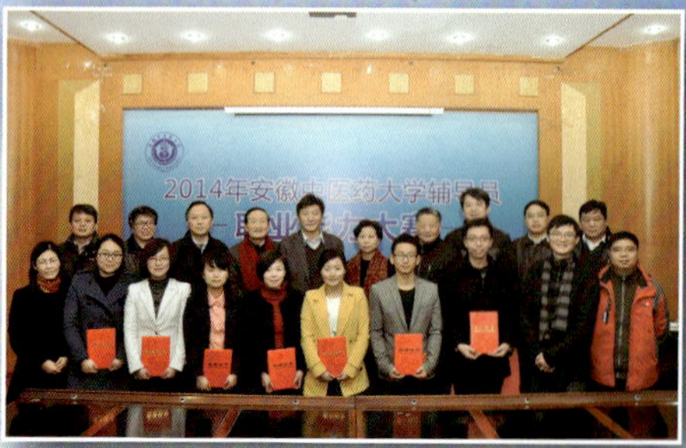

▲ 辅导员职业能力比赛

“十二五”期间，学校以邓小平理论、“三个代表”重要思想和科学发展观为指导，坚定中医信念，弘扬中医精神，秉承“至精至诚、惟是惟新”的理念，实施“质量立校、人才兴校、科技强校、特色弘校、文化塑校、和谐融校”的办学方略，围绕特色，强化优势，提升质量，着力培育“精诚是新”中医药人才，构筑安徽中医药协同创新高地，弘扬“北华佗南新安”中医药文化，引领安徽中医药事业产业发展，建成富有特色、卓有贡献、高水平有影响的中医药大学，为建设美好安徽、服务人民大众健康做出更大贡献。

▼ 王键校长门诊

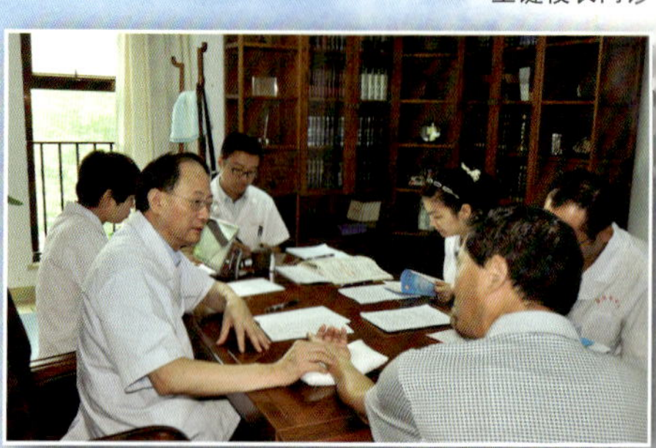

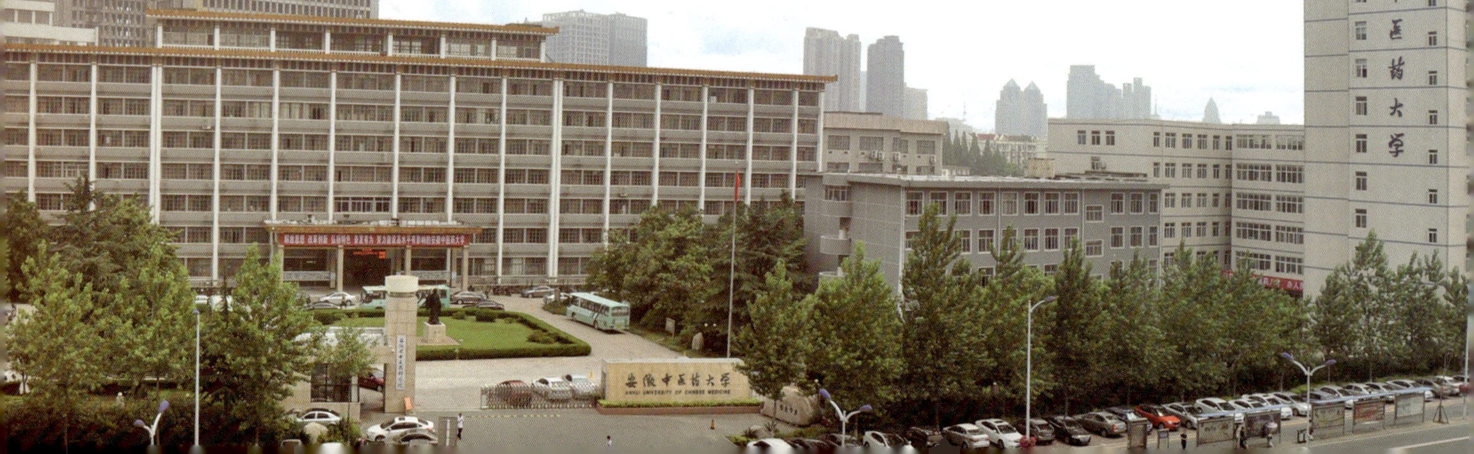

南京中医药大学中药炮制平台

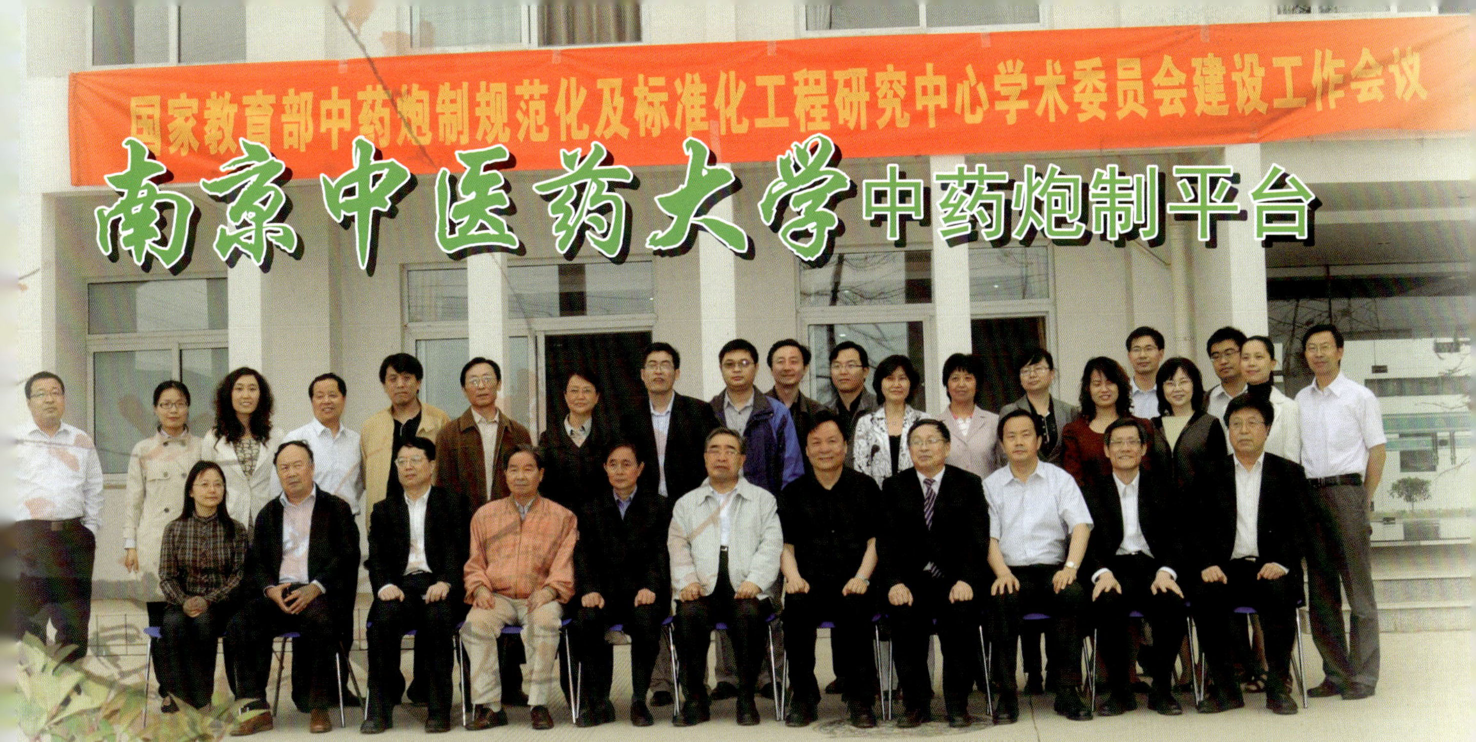

南京中医药大学中药炮制平台依托于国家中医药管理局中药炮制学重点学科，现有教授 5 名，副教授 6 名，博导 4 名，硕导 9 名，享受国家政府津贴专家、国家级有突出贡献的中青年专家、全国百千万人才工程第一、二层次 1 人；江苏省有突出贡献的中青年专家 2 名；江苏省优秀科技工作者 1 名，江苏省“333”人才工程第二、三层次 3 人，江苏省高校跨世纪学术带头人 1 名；江苏省高校“青蓝工程”中青年学术带头人 1 名，优秀青年骨干教师 1 名；ISO/TC249 国际标准化组织／中医药标准技术委员会国际注册专家 1 名。中药炮制学是学校国家级重点学科中药学中最具优势的二级学科，自 1985 年起连续 3 次承担全国中药炮制师资培训班，并于 1986 年、1994 年分别开始招收中药炮制专业硕士、博士研究生，是全国最早设立中药炮制专业硕士、博士学位授予点的学科。1996 年中药炮制学获江苏省高校二类优秀课程，2004 年获江苏省高校一类优秀课程，2009 年被评为国家教育部精品课程，2013 年被入选国家教育部精品资源共享课程。平台目前拥有国家教育部“中药炮制规范化及标准化工程研究中心”，科技部“中药饮片质量标准技术平台”，国家中医药管理局“中药炮制标准重点研究室”，江苏省“中药炮制重点实验室”“产学研基地——南京海昌中药集团”等优质资源。近年来共承担各级各类课题 56 项，其中国家自然科学基金课题 14 项，国家级课题 9 项，省部级课题 20 项，研究经费达 2405 万元；获得省部级奖 2 项；申请专利 26 项，授权 20 项；发表论文 337 篇，其中 SCI 57 篇，主编出版专著及教材 7 部。获得省部级科技进步奖 3 项。培养硕士研究生 200 余名，博士研究生 30 余名。

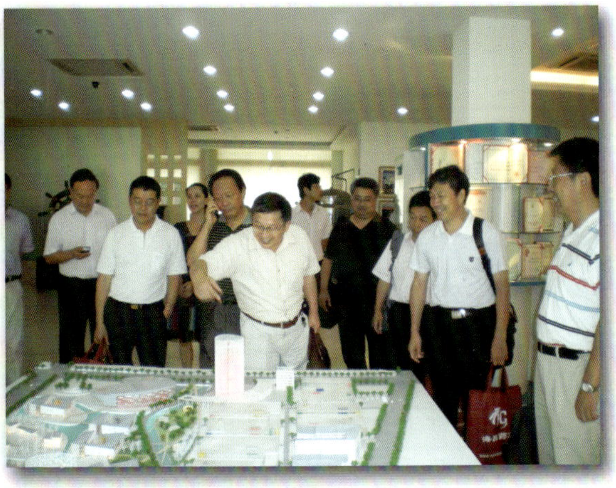

▲ 蔡宝昌教授介绍产学研基地

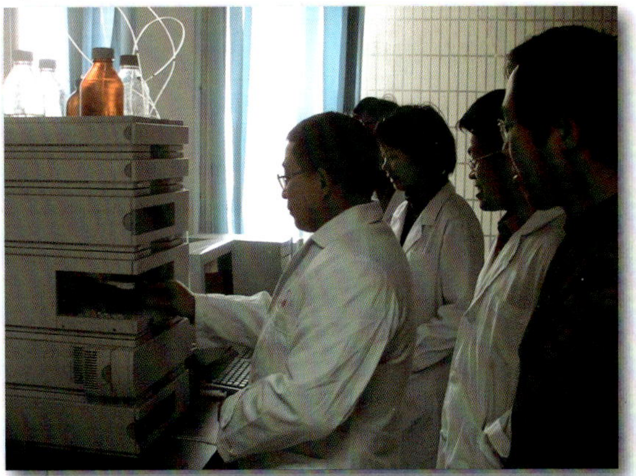

▲ 蔡宝昌教授在工作中

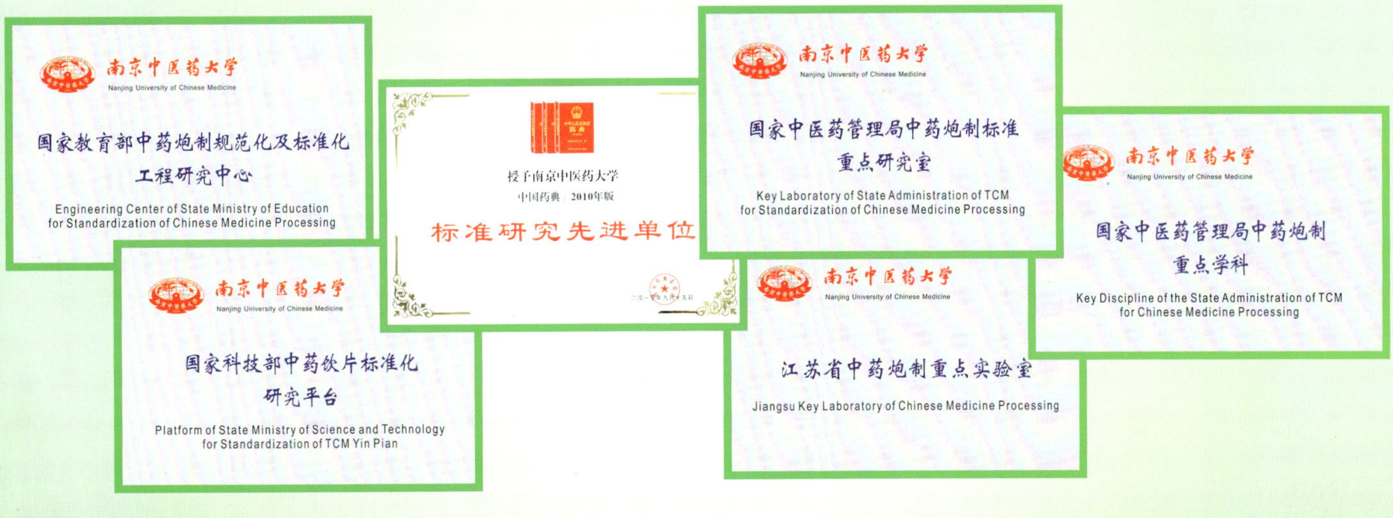

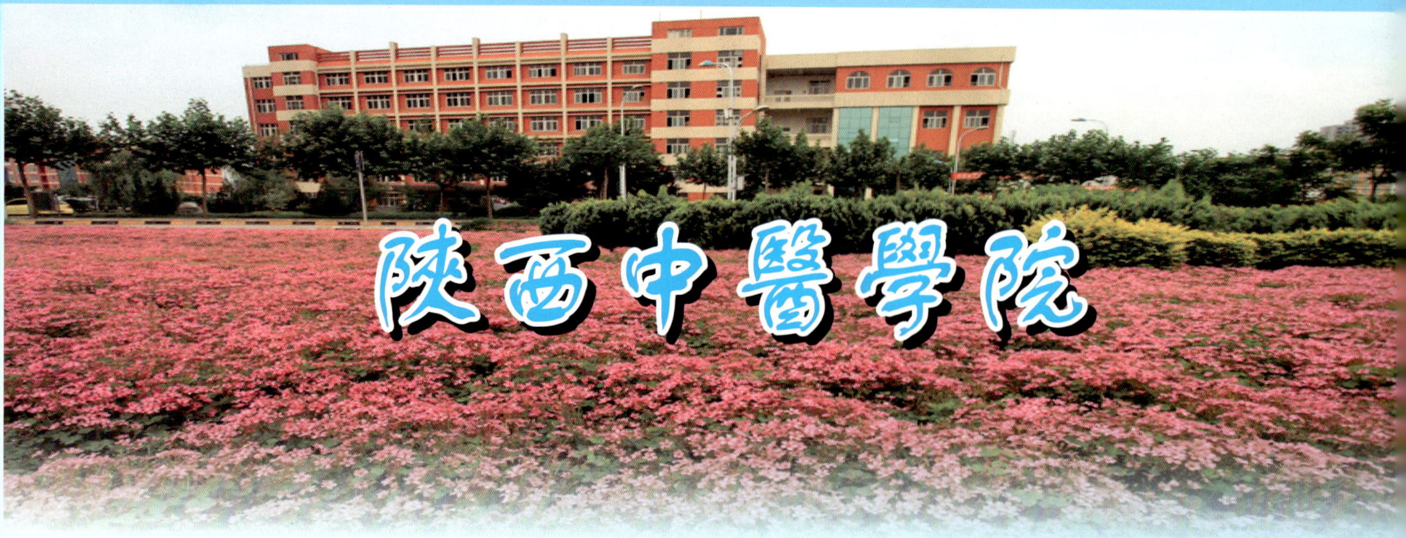

陕西中醫學院

陕西中医学院前身是 1952 年创建于西安的西北中医进修学校，1959 年升格为陕西中医学院，1961 年迁至咸阳，是陕西省唯一一所培养高级中医药人才的普通高等院校，是 1978 年中共中央 56 号文件确定的全国 8 所重点建设中医院校之一，是国务院学位委员会批准的首批硕士学位授权单位。学校占地面积 1300 亩，分南（新校区）、北两个校区。南校区位于陕西省西咸新区沣西新城世纪大道中段。学校现有基础医学院、第一临床医学院（下设中医系、中西医临床医学系）、第二临床医学院（下设临床医学系）、药学院、继续教育学院等 5 个二级学院，有针灸推拿系、护理系、医学技术系、公共卫生系、人文科学系、英语系、体育部、社会科学部等 8 个教学系部，有 2 所直属附属医院、15 所非直属附属医院、1 家制药厂、1 个陕西医史博物馆。学校开设中医学等 21 个本科专业及 1 个高职专业。现有 5 个硕士学位授权一级学科，招收 28 个二级学科领域及方向招收研究生。具有临床医学（中医药类）、中药学硕士专业学位授权点，以及同等学力申请硕士学位授予权。学校成立 60 年来，涌现了西北唯一的“国医大师”张学文教授、世界非物质文化遗产中国针灸传承人郭诚杰教授、全国著名伤寒与肾病专家杜雨茂教授为代表的一批在全国有重要影响的名医名师名家，为国家培养了 5 万余名高级中医药人才。

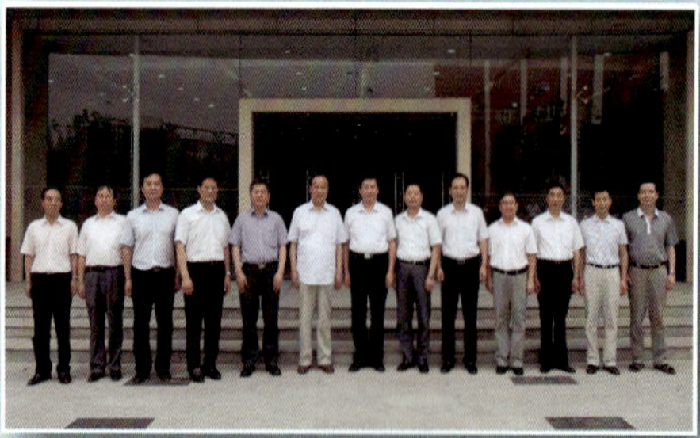

▲ 庄长兴副省长一行来我校调研

【大事记】

副省长庄长兴一行莅临学校调研工作。学校牵头建设的“陕西中药资源产业化协同创新中心”入选“陕西省 2011 协同创新中心”。附属医院获批设立陕西省博士后创新基地。

【教育教学】

药学等 4 个本科专业成功获批。中医学专业成为首批国家级专业综合改革试点项目，针灸推拿学和医学检验技术 2 个专业成为第二批省级专业综合改革点。“针灸推拿学教学团队”被评为 2013 年省级教学团队；“制药工程实验教学示范中心”被评为 2013 年省级实验教学示范中心；“针灸推拿人才培养模式创新实验区”被评为 2013 年省级人才培养模式创新实验区；中药化学等 6 门课程被评为 2013 年度省级精品资源共享课程。陕西中医学院附属医院成功申报并获批陕西省高等学校首批博士后创新基地。学校申报的“陕西中医学院 —— 陕西海天制药有限公司药学实践教育基地”。学校获批省级“中医药科普教育基地”。

【师资队伍建设】

2013 年新增享受国务院政府津贴专家 1 人、三级教授 3 人、16 位专家获批为“第二届陕西省名中医”。国家第一批中医药传承博士后合作导师 2 人，推荐优秀科技工作者 7 人，青年科技奖 3 人。2013 年引进 95 名优秀硕博士（含两所附属医院），进一步改善了学校的人才队伍结构。完成第二期“百名人才工程”人才的遴选工作，遴选 17 名特聘教授、16 名学术带头人和 50 名骨干教师，遴选了学校十大名师 5 人、十大名医 11 人。学校支持 12 名教师在国内大学提高学历（其中博士 4 名，硕士 8 名），5 名青年教师到国内外大学访问学习，组织第二届“国医大师”申报工作。

【学科建设】

学校成立了陕西中医学院学科建设办公室，健全一系列制度，出台相关配套措施，进一步加强学科建设。方剂学、中医肺病、中医脾胃病三个学科已获批准为省中医管理局重点学科，获得财政建设资金 150 万元。中医文化学重点学科通过家中医药管理局“十二五”中医药重点学科建设规划答辩会并通过教育厅验收。

【科研及科技产业工作】

“陕西中药资源产业化协同创新中心”被认定为首批省级“2011 计划”协同创新中心；聘请中国中医科学院针灸研究所所长朱兵教授为学校特聘教授，成立了“针药结合创新研究中心”。学校组建医学科研实验中心。“中医药文化传承与发展研究基地”2013 年顺利通过省教育厅组织的立项验收。2013 年全校共申报各级各类项目 34 次，获批立项各级各类项目 123 项，纵向项目到账科研经费达 1501 万元。全校共承担横向课题 12 项，合同经费达到 2518 万元。国家自然科学基金年中标项目数量首次突破两位数。2013 年全校共申报国家自然科学基金项目 74 项，其中青年基金 28 项，面上项目 45 项，国际交流项目 1 项，中标 11 项，总经费 453 万元，创历史新高。全校完成国科金结题 5 项，进展报告 15 项。“陕西中医学院科技产业基地项目”稳步实施，征地测绘工作基本完成。制药厂完成新版 GMP 认证工作和新厂征地任务，启动了企业股份制改制工作，改制方案获上级批准。制药厂全年实现销售回款 4982 万元，较 2012 年增长 575 万元，增长率为 13%。

【医疗工作】

2013 年附属医院李彦民教授被授予国家级名老中医称号，获得建设经费 50 万元。肿瘤科申报国家临床重点专科，获得建设经费 300 万元。名医馆、科教大楼、肝病大楼已经落成并投入使用。全年医院业务收入达 4.3 亿元，增长率达 19.7 %。门诊接诊 28 万余人次，出院人数 2.9 万人，病床使用率 106.9%，手术 8206 人。第二附属医院继续发挥品牌科室效应，突出专科特色，中医脾胃病学和肿瘤科分别荣获陕西省中医药重点学科建设项目和重点专科建设项目，共获得建设资金 80 万元。全年实现业务总收入 3.01 亿元，门诊诊疗人数 304185 人次，出院 30760 人次，患者平均住院日 8.9 天，中西医结合治疗率门诊 66.99%、住院 58.5%，药品占业务收入的 26.79%。

【党的建设】

学校成功召开了学校第五次党代表大会，大会选举产生了新一届学校领导班子，并对学校未来 5 年发展建设作出科学规划。学校党委按照中央、省委和高教工委的统一部署，开展了以为民务实清廉为主要内容的党的群众路线教育实践活动。选配处科级干部 38 人，选派 6 名干部参加省上举行的处级干部培训班，并对全校处级干部进行了集中培训。2013 年学校共发展预备党员 384 人。积极配合陕西省委第三巡视组对学校开展巡视工作。

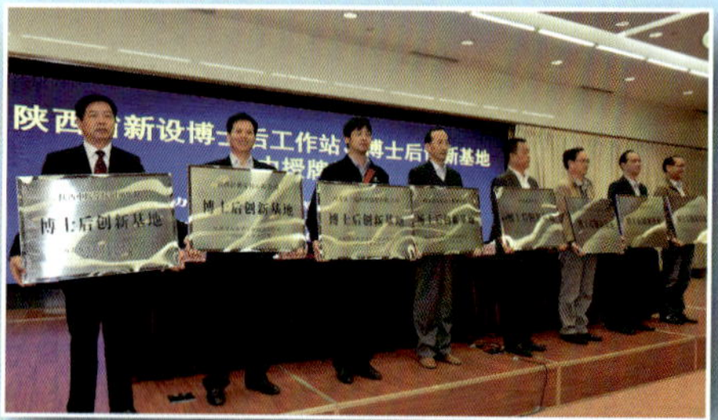

▲ 附属医院获批博士后创新人才基地

【学生工作】

学校办理各类国家及社会奖助学金、生源地贷款等资助项目共计 3000 万元，比 2012 年增加 100 万元。组织开展毕业生就业专场小型招聘会 63 场，成功举办了陕西省医药类毕业生就业洽谈会，总体就业率较往年稳中有升。2013 年我校毕业生总人数共计 2193 人，本科就业率 92.2%，专科就业率 78.92%，硕士研究生就业率 87.4%。

【合作交流】

2013 年学校与商洛市人民政府签订战略合作协议，完成了中医药服务贸易重点项目的申报工作，接待国（境）外代表团来访团组 10 多批约 60 多人，10 名同学代表学校参加了省优秀大学生赴韩国交流团，茹意等 6 名同学获得“新加坡政府护理专科奖学金”。

▼ 2012.10.29.学校护理系五名应届新生首次获得新加坡护理奖学金

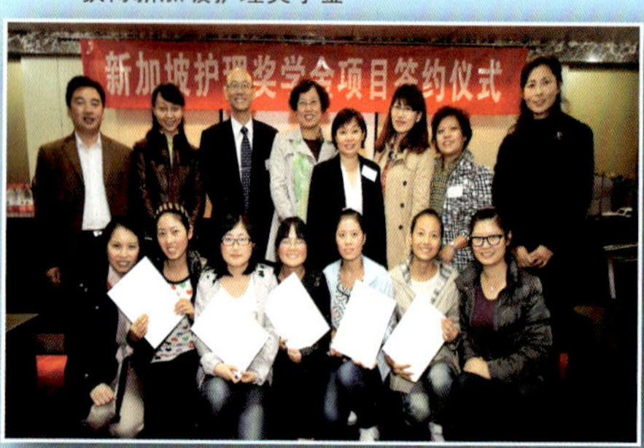

【重要荣誉】

2013 年，学校荣获省社会管理综合治理委员会办公室、中共陕西省委高等教育工作委员会、陕西省教育厅、陕西省公安厅授予的陕西省“平安校园”称号。学校被国家中医药管理局评为“第四批全国老中医药专家学术经验继承工作先进管理单位”。附属医院脑病科被国家中医药管理局评为“全国中医医院优质护理服务先进病房”，护理部主任荣获“全国中医医院优质护理服务先进个人”称号。

遵义医学院

基础药理省部共建教育部重点实验室

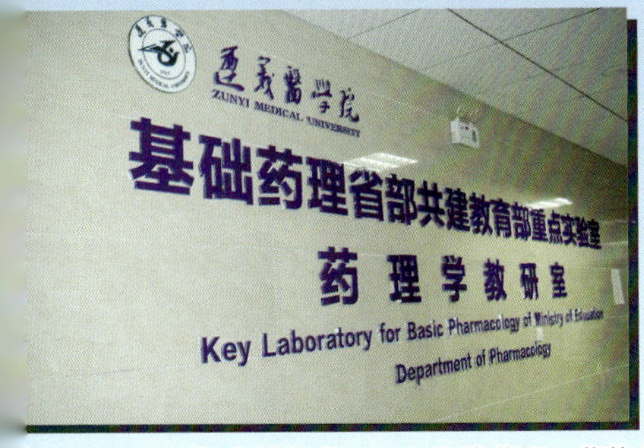

基础药理省部共建教育部重点实验室位于遵义医学院新蒲校区综合实验楼内，占地面积达4000平方米，建有500平方米的SPF动物实验室，配置药理学相关研究大型设备总价值约2000万元，拥有神经药理、心血管药理、药物代谢与药物毒理学等多个研究技术平台，教学科研条件良好。该实验室依托于遵义医学院药理学学科，是该学科的科研教学基地。

遵义医学院药理学学科诞生于1949年，由我国著名药理学家、一级教授张毅创建。在六十余年的发展历程中，秉承团结进取的优良传统，弘扬严谨治学的学风，经过刘国雄、黄燮南、石京山等几代人的继承和发扬，该学科在人才培养和科学研究等方面取得长足发展。该学科是1955年首批面向全国招收硕士研究生的学科之一，1978年恢复研究生教育制度后，为首批面向全国招收硕士生的学科，1981年获得首批硕士学位授权点。1992年被评为首批贵州省重点学科，2001年开始与其他高校联合培养博士研究生，2003年复评时被评为贵州省优秀重点学科。2003年药理学课程被评为首批“贵州省精品课程”，2009年被复评为“贵州省优秀精品课程”，同年与贵州百灵企业集团制药股份有限公司合作，建立“贵州省新药药理与毒理研究生教育创新基地”。2010年被评为“贵州省医学创新基地”子基地，2011年被评为首批“贵州省特色重点学科”，2012年获批“国家重点(培育)学科”。目前开设“药理学”“临床药理学”“药理学进展”等课程。自1978年以来，共招收培养硕士100余人、博士6人。

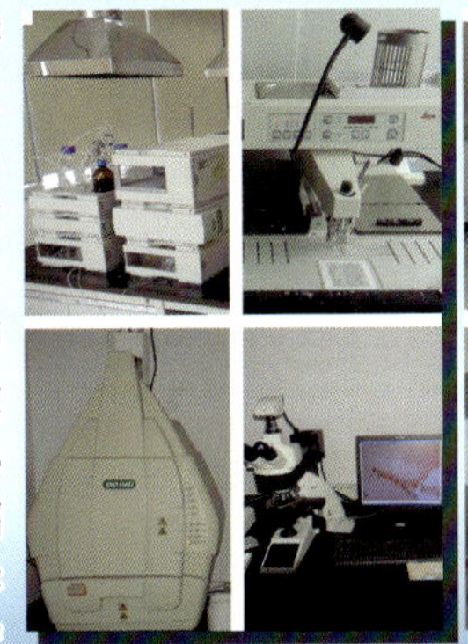
▲ 实验仪器

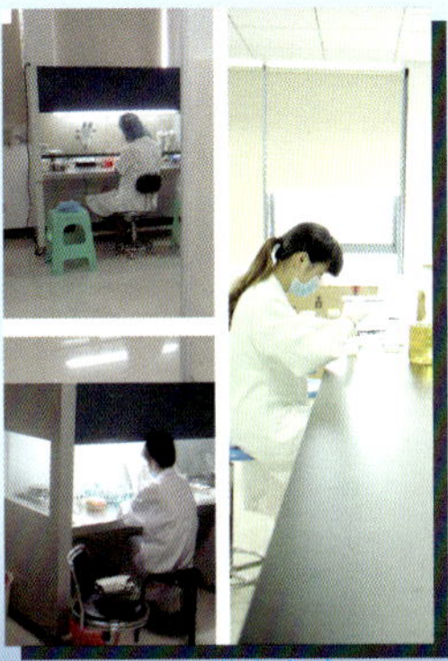
▲ 学生实验

实验室有一支年龄结构、职称结构、学缘结构合理的团队，是一个充满朝气、认真负责、富有创新精神的团队。其中教授9名、副教授6名(包括高级实验师1名)、讲师14名、助教3名。拥有教育部“长江学者和创新团队发展计划”创新团队1个(“老年痴呆的发病机制及防治研究”团队)、贵州省科技创新团队1个、贵州省教学团队1个、贵州省核心专家1名、省管专家2名、教育部新世纪优秀人才支持计划入选者2名、国务院特贴专家2名。2008年该学科团队被评为首批“贵州省科技创新团队”，2009年被评为“贵州省高等学校省级教学团队”。

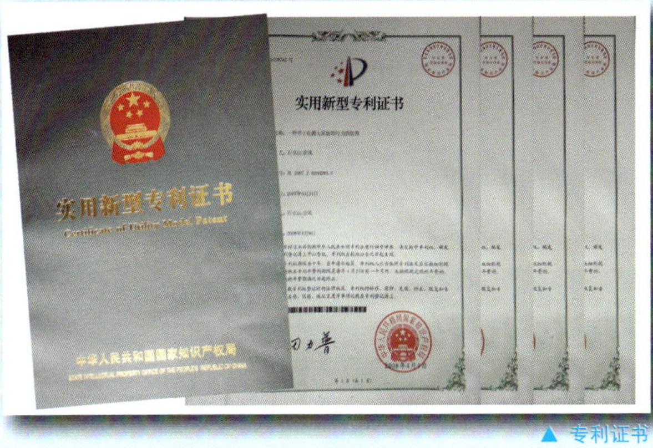

▲ 专利证书

通过多年积累和技术的不断完善，该学科充分利用全省中草药资源丰富这一优势，形成了主要以民族药为研究对象且具有明显学科交叉融合为特征的三个长期稳定的研究方向，即：神经药理学、心血管药理学、药物代谢与药物毒理学，并逐渐形成了“重应用、重交叉”的学科特色。尤其在民族药的药理研究方面取得了显著成效。先后对全省主要民族药钩藤、淫羊藿、石斛、天麻、吴茱萸、毛蒟等主要活性部位及成分用于防治中枢神经系统疾病、心血管系统疾病研究及部分活性成分的药物代谢动力学研究，对含有砷、汞重金属的安宫牛黄丸、万胜华风丹等进行了增效减毒研究。

2007年以来，该实验室承担“973”前期项目1项、国家自然科学基金8项、教育部项目2项、省重大专项1项、其他各级纵向项目60余项，总经费1600余万元。获授权国内发明专利4项、实用新型专利1项。发表学术论文200余篇，其中SCI收录70余篇。获贵州省科技进步一等奖1项、二等奖1项、三等奖3项，其他各级奖励23项。

实验室的目标是立足贵州、面向全国，建设成为具有国内先进水平的中药现代化产业的重要研发基地，高素质实用型人才的重要培养基地，和国内外学术交流基地，从而更好地为全省和周边地区的高水平、深层次药理学研究服务，为贵州省制药企业的药物研发服务，为地方经济发展服务。

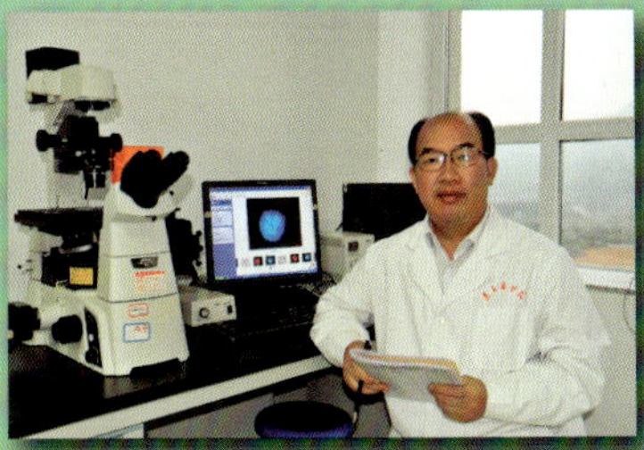
▲ 石京山 遵义医学院院长兼党委副书记

石京山 男，1959年生，中共党员，二级教授，贵州省核心专家、兼职博士生导师，国务院特殊津贴获得者。1982年、1989年分别获得遵义医学院学士学位和硕士学位，1996年毕业于复旦大学医学院(原上海医科大学)，获博士学位。1999年2月—2000年3月作为访问学者前往瑞典哥德堡大学研究神经生物与神经药理学，2001年3月至7月进修于清华大学。现任遵义医学院院长兼党委副书记，基础药理省部共建教育部重点实验室主任；兼中国药理学会神经精神药理专业委员会常委、中华医学会贵州省分会及贵州省药学会副会长、贵州省科学技术协会常委、贵州省中药现代化专家组专家、首批贵州省科技创新人才团队领衔人，国家自然科学基金、国家“863”项目和国家科技进步奖评审专家。先后被评为“贵州省优秀科技工作者”“科技部中药现代化科技产业基地建设十周年先进个人”以及“全国优秀科技工作者”。

主要从事神经药理学研究，先后将贵州省道地中药材淫羊藿、金钗石斛等的有效成分用于中枢神经系统退行性变疾病，特别是阿尔茨海默病、帕金森病防治的研究已取得阶段性成果。获“贵州省科技进步成果奖”一等奖1项、二等奖2项、三等奖3项，“遵义市科技进步奖”一等奖1项，获批国家发明专利4项、实用新型专利1项，申请国家发明专利2项(实审中)。先后主持“国家自然科学基金”4项，“973”前期专项课题1项，以及中央财政部“中央－地方共建基础药理实验室项目”等省部级以上课题20余项。近5年来发表SCI收录论文10余篇，核心期刊收录30余篇。作为主编、编委或参编的教材共计10余部。目前为*Aging Cell*, *Journal of Alzheimer's disease*, *Amino Acids*, *Acta Pharmacol Sin*等10余家杂志的审稿人，国内《中华预防医学杂志》《中国新药与临床杂志》等编委。

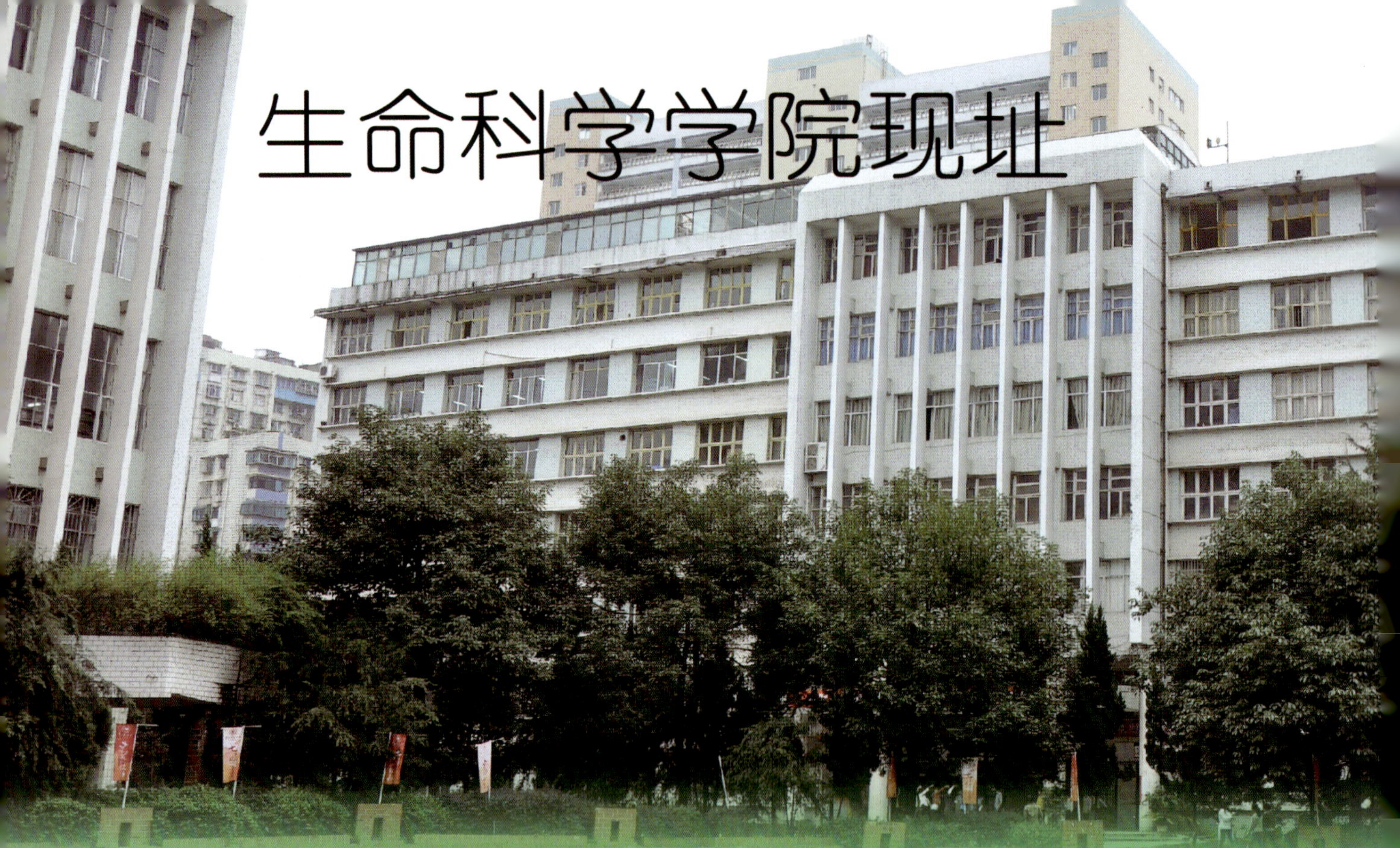

贵州師範大學生命科學學院

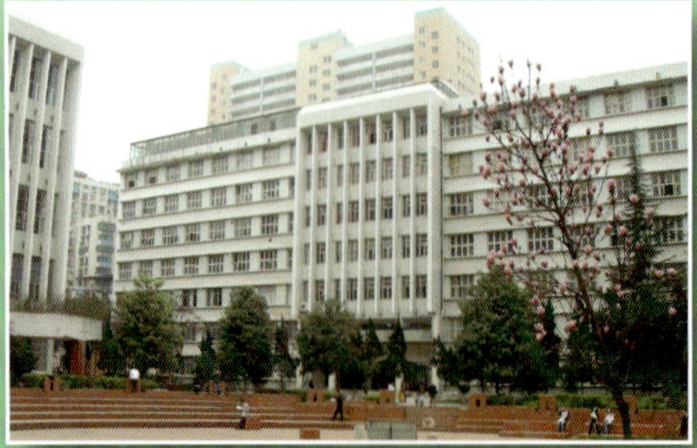

▲ 生命科学学院大楼

贵州师范大学生命科学学院成立于2008年9月，是由具有50多年办学历史的传统生物科学专业及现代生命科学前沿专业生物技术和生物工程专业构成的新兴学院，专门从事基础生命科学及现代生物技术和生物工程的教学、研究和产业开发。现任院长乙引，书记王亚筑。学院现有在册教职工75人，专任教师57人，其中教授17人，副教授（及相当）36人，讲师4人；博士28人，在读博士10人，讲师5人；2012年引进博士2人，在职教师考取博士5人。在职称结构上，教授占任课教师总数的29.8%、副教授占63.2%、讲师占7%；在学历层次上，博士、硕士比例分别达到49.1%和42.1%；在学缘结构上，非本校毕业比例

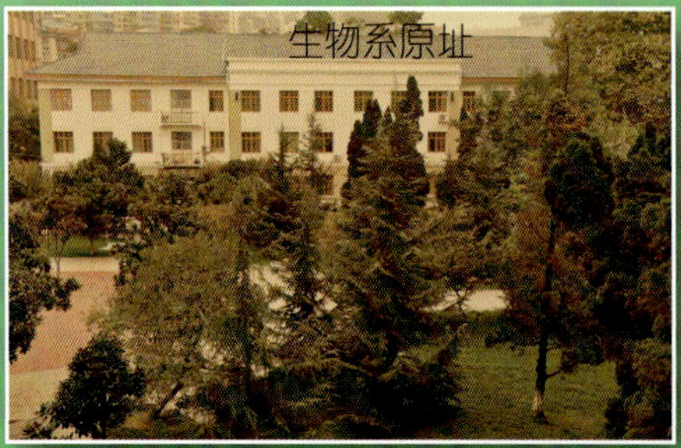

▲ 生物系原址

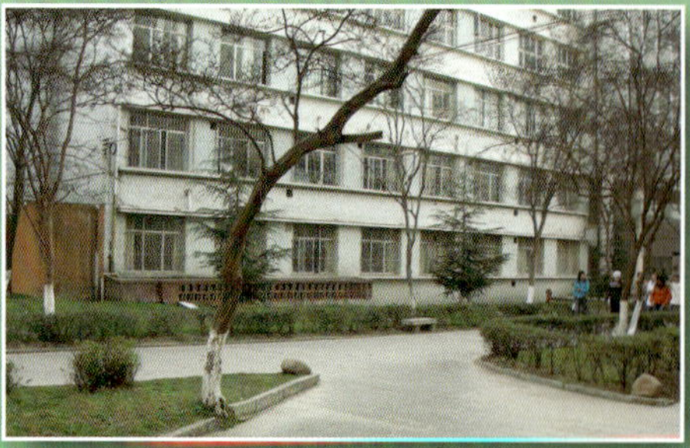

▲ 学院一角

达到89.5%。由于良好的师资队伍，2012年生命科学学院获得了教育部科技创新人才团队，实现了学校在国家级创新团队方面零的突破。此外，学院还拥有教育部高等学校生物科学与工程教学指导委员会委员1人，多人先后获得"全国师德先进个人"、国务院政府特殊津贴、省管专家、省级教学名师、"省五四青年奖章"、"省青年科技奖"、"省优秀青年科技工作者"、"省优秀教师"和"省优秀党务工作者"等荣誉和称号，生物技术核心课程教学团队获校级优秀教学团队。

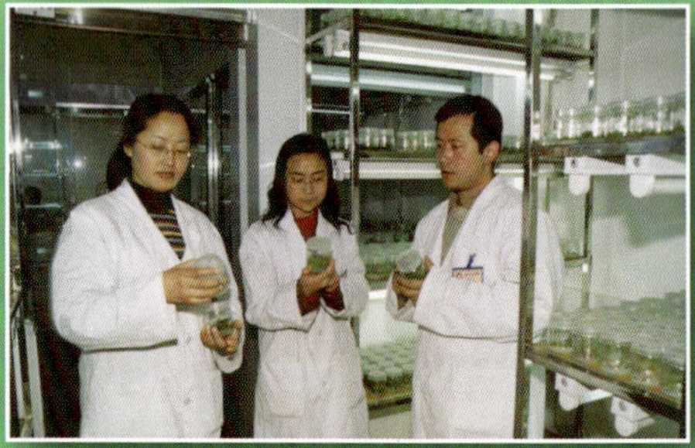

▲ 乙引教授工作中

学院设有1个省级重点学科（植物学），1个国家级本科示范专业（生物科学），1个省级本科示范性专业（生物

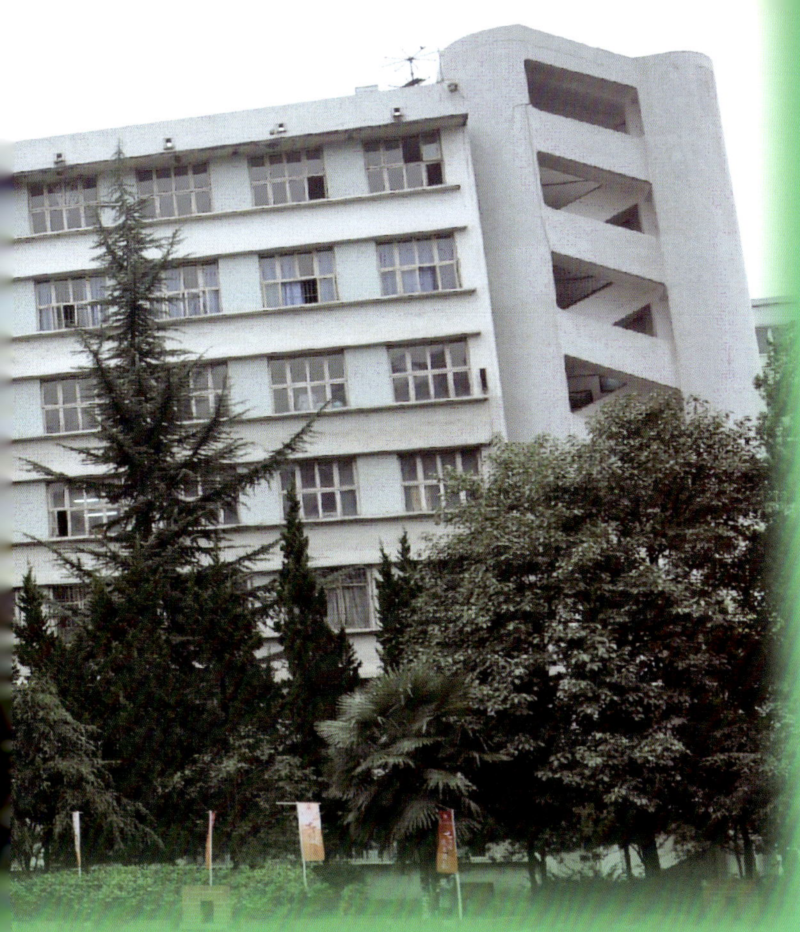

技术）。6 个专业可招收培养硕士生，1 个专业可招收培养教育硕士；4 个专业可招收本科生，1 个专业可招生自考学生，3 个专业可招生函授、业余学生。在校本科生992人，硕士研究生152人。

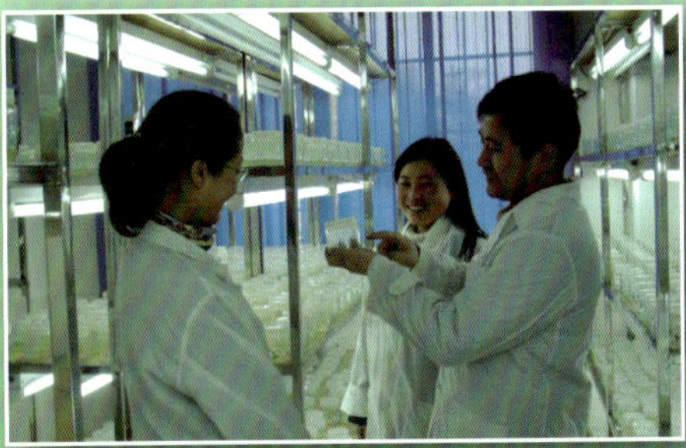

▲ 乙引教授介绍石斛快速繁殖情况

学院现有 8000 多平方米的教学科研用房和 1500 多万元的现代生物学实验仪器设备，学院资产近 2000 万元。拥有 3 个省级评估合格实验室（生物科学基础实验室、生物技术基础实验室和生物工程专业实验室），2 个校级重点实验室（分子生物学和植物遗传育种实验室）。近 5 年来，先后主持国家自然科学基金、教育部新世纪人才计划等国家、省部级科研项目 60 余项，发表 SCI、核心期刊论文 100 余篇，获省部级奖 10 项，年均科研经费 200 余万元。学院的出路在市场、生命在特色、活力在机制、建设在人才、发展在拼搏。瞄准学术前沿，倡导学术优先，打造一流学科，强调合作精神，努力培养基础扎实、综合素质高、实践能力强、具有创新精神的生命科学研究领域高级专门人才，实现学院跨越式发展。

▼ 乙引教授在考察石斛种植情况

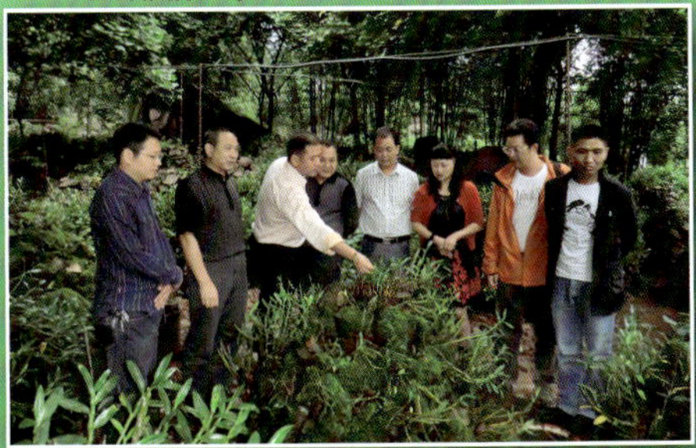

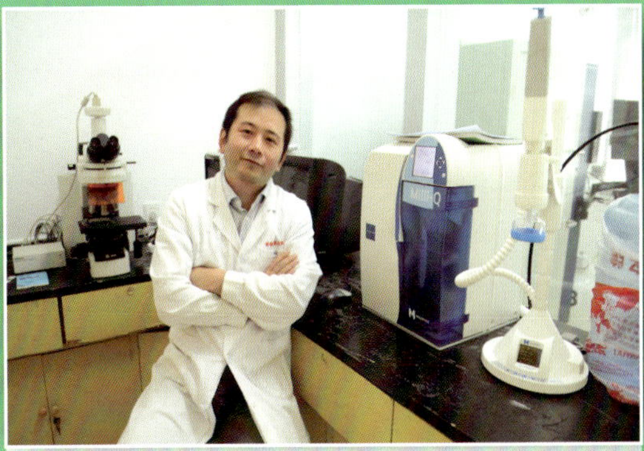

▲ 乙引 贵州师范大学副校长

乙引 男，1967 年生。南京大学植物学学士、生态学博士，中国科学院上海植物生理研究所博士，贵州师范大学教授，贵州省省管专家，教育部高等学校教学指导委员会委员，中国植物生理学会理事，贵州省植物学副理事长，贵州省植物生理与发育调控重点实验室主任。2012 年领衔喀斯特山地生物多样性保护与可持续利用创新团队入选教育部“创新团队发展计划”。

近年来，重点开展贵州道地中药材种植和喀斯特植物嗜钙机制研究。先后主持喀斯特森林喜钙植物嗜钙机理及其环境适宜性、中医药疗效及安全性基本问题研究、黔药用石斛 ISSR 指纹图谱比较研究、金钗石斛等 7 种药材规范化种植和野生保护抚育关键技术研究及应用示范等国家自然科学基金、国家科技支撑计划项目、教育部骨干教师人才专项基金等国家和省部级项目 30 余项。在植物对喀斯特环境适应性研究方面，创造性地提出高钙累积是喀斯特喜钙植物对环境干旱和营养亏缺适应的重要途径；在兰科植物石斛研究方面，完成了贵州所有石斛物种的组织培养再生植株研究和大规模悬浮培养研究，包括金钗石斛（Dendrobium.nobile）、铁皮石斛（D.candidum）、环草石斛（D. loddigesii）、马鞭石斛（D. fimbriatum）和束花石斛（D.chrysanthum）等 5 种药用石斛。同时，分离得到了对石斛生长具有促进作用的内生真菌，该项研究为省内领先。

获得了金钗石斛的 DNA 指纹图谱和 HPLC 指纹图谱。发表学术论文 150 余篇，出版专著 2 部。先后获贵州省高等教育教学成果一、二等奖各 1 项，获第八届贵州省青年科技奖，获“全国师德先进个人”称号。

乾坤集团
QIAN KUN GROUP

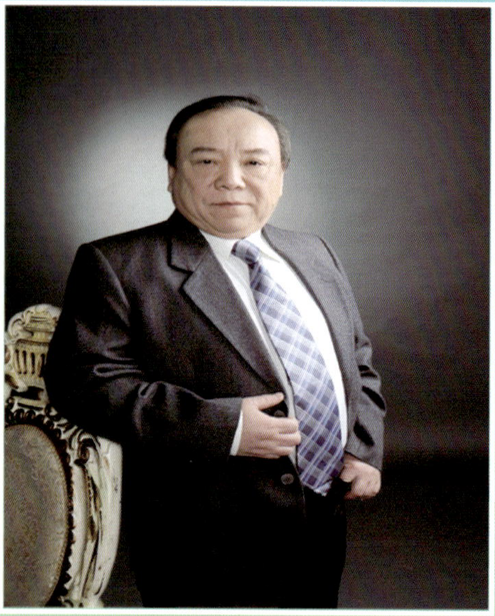

乾坤集团董事会主席刘鸿业

刘鸿业 中西医结合主任医师，《中国中医药年鉴（学术卷）》邀副主任编委、中国抗癌协会委员、青岛市市北区人大代表、青岛市善总会监事。40多年来潜心研究中西医结合治疗方法，与中国医学科院、中国中医研究院、中国心电学会等机构的全国著名专家学者反复讨，共同研制抗癌系列中医药辨证施治方案，30余年共治疗36800多次，取得了较大成效；并创造了血液稀释平衡辅以中医传统的中西结合独特疗法，对脑血栓、偏瘫、高脂血症、老年脑萎缩、冠心病、肌梗死、风湿性心脏病等病症有独特疗效。

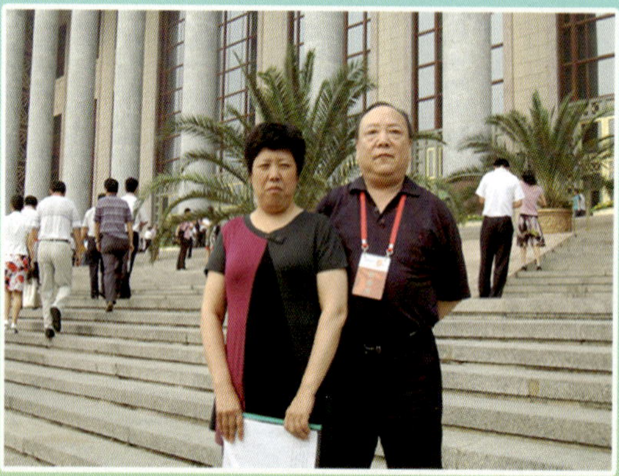

2009年7月刘鸿业先生在北京人民大会堂参加中华慈善总会颁奖大会。荣获“中华慈善突出贡献人物奖”

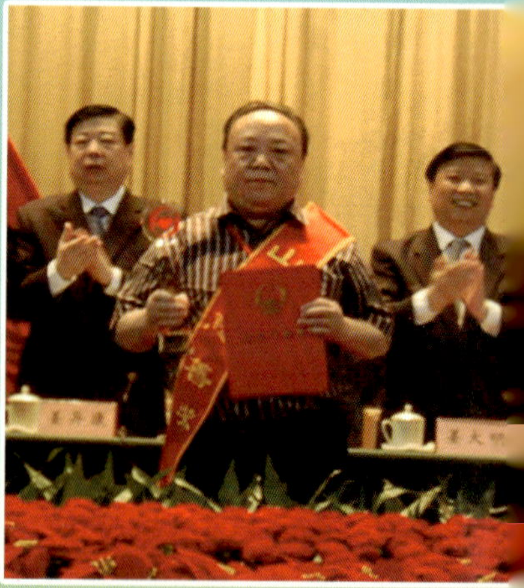

山东省委书记姜异康、省长姜大明为荣获“最具爱心捐赠个人”刘鸿业先生

刘鸿业还是一位慈善家，自1991年开始创办医院以来，在为众多患者解除痛苦的同时，更为一些困难的退休老工人、低保户、残疾人等困难群众减免一部分医疗费用，2002年来他率先向青岛市慈善总会提出开设慈善门诊，给困难患者以医疗慈善援助，且10余年来从未间断。2008年3月24日首次与青岛市慈善总会签订了3000万元“慈善冠名基金”协议，将基金5%年增值部分的150万元用于医疗慈善援助，并连续签了4年协议，2012年6月签订了5000万元的冠名基金，2014年分别与市北区慈善总会、李沧区慈善总会签订了各1000万元的“慈善冠名基金”协议，至2014年“慈善冠名基金”已达到2.7亿元，且并以每年1亿元的速度增长。10余年来其创建的乾坤集团已为困难群众进行医疗慈善援助了4280多万元。充分体现了其高度的社会责任感，为构建和谐社会作出了贡献。

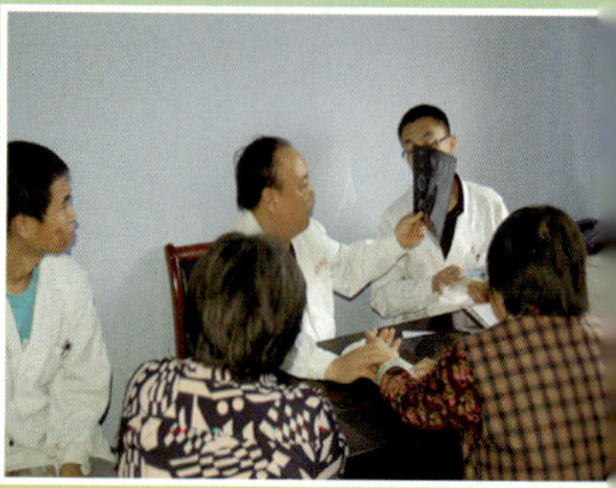

刘鸿业先生认真分析患者的病症

2006年乾坤集团荣获青岛市慈善奖，2009年5月刘鸿业被山东省慈善总会评为“最具爱心捐赠个人”，2009年7月荣获“中华慈善突出贡献个人奖”，2009年8月被青岛市民网络投票评选为“十大青岛好人”，2011年6月乾坤集团被评为青岛市“十大民营慈善企业之星”，2014年评为“中华慈善突出贡献个人奖”。

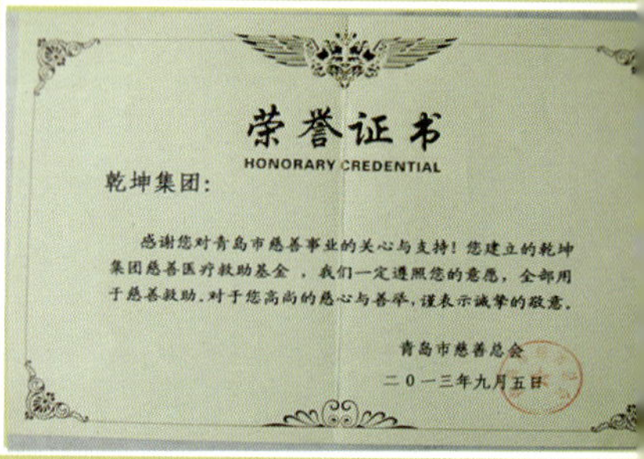

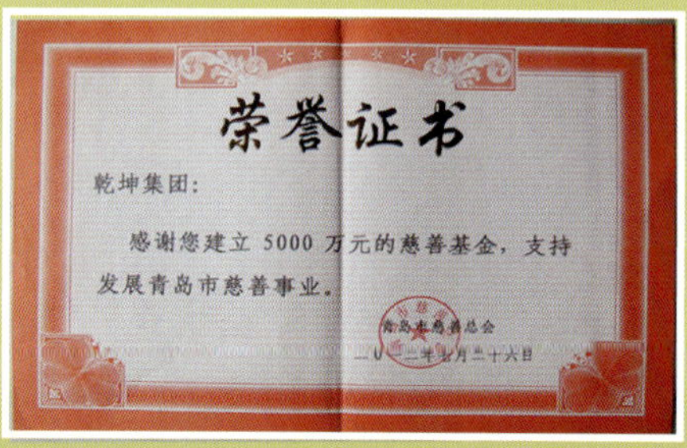

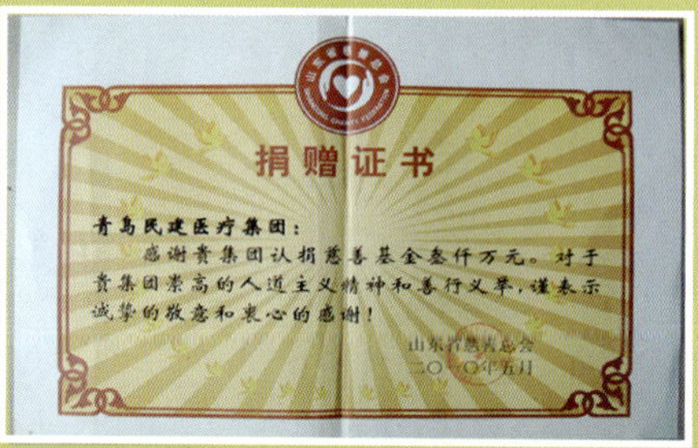

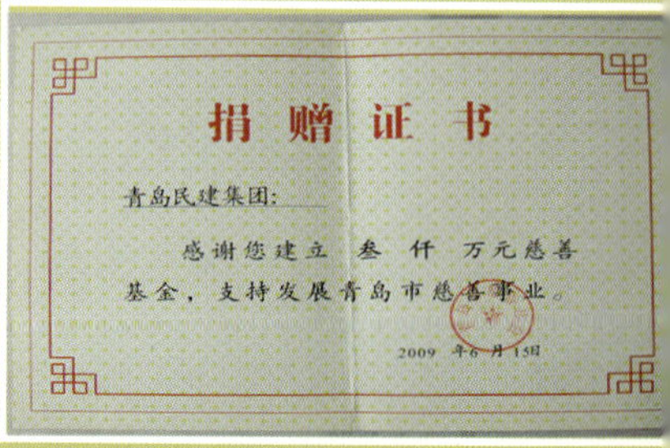

大连华立金港药业有限公司

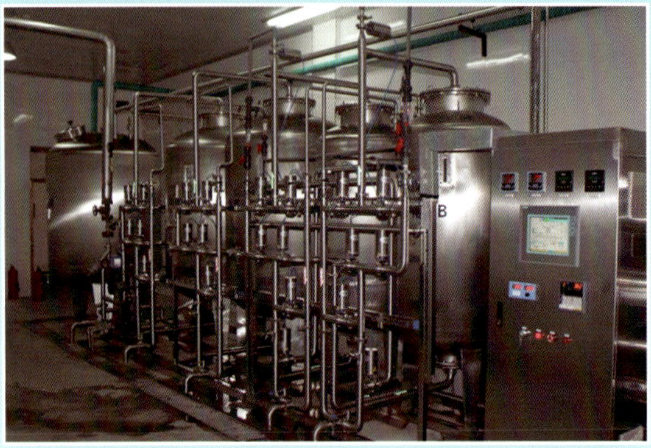

▲ 全世界第一条脂质体靶向抗癌药物产业化生产线（金港榄香烯）

大连华立金港药业公司位于北方明珠大连市金州新区。拥有通过新版 GMP 认证的大容量注射液车间、小容量注射剂车间、口服液车间及原料药车间。现有产品包括三大类：1. 抗肿瘤植物药：具有自主知识产权的**金港榄香烯脂质体系列靶向抗癌药**，包括榄香烯原料药、榄香烯注射液（脂质体）、榄香烯口服乳（脂质体）等；2. 治疗原发性和继发性血小板减少症植物药：**金港血康口服液**；3. 治疗儿童智力结构陷缺症及老年性痴呆良药：**金港精苓口服液**等。还有多个在研的具有自主知识产权的国家一类和二类新药。金港药业建成了全世界第一条脂质体靶向抗癌药物产业化生产线，是我国脂质体靶向制剂、载药乳剂和抗癌植物药的产业化摇篮及龙头企业。

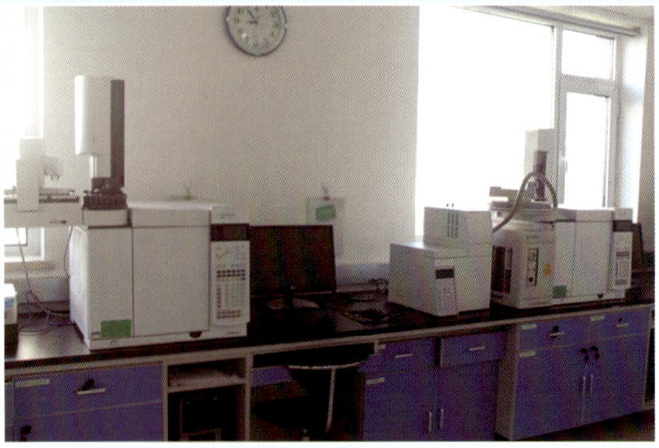

▲ 金港榄香烯脂质体质量控制先进仪器

金港药业坚持走拥有自主知识产权、填补国内空白的技术创新之路。公司现有注册品种 60 余种，拥有国内外发明专利 20 多项。金港榄香烯注射液（脂质体）、金港榄香烯口服乳（脂质体）是金港药业独家生产的原研专利抗癌新药，是国家发改委抗肿瘤药物高技术产业化示范工程项目，国家“十五”“十一五”“十二五”攻关项目。金港榄香烯（注射液、口服乳）2009 年列入《国家医保药品目录》，2004 年进入《国家基本药物目录》。经循征医学系统评价证实：金港榄香烯注射液和榄香烯口服乳对肺癌、肝癌、脑瘤（包括脑转移癌）、食管癌、胃癌、肠癌、鼻咽癌、骨转移癌、胰腺癌、白血病、膀胱癌、妇科肿瘤及癌性胸腹水等恶性肿瘤安全有效，尤其在延长生存期、提高生存质量、抗转移复发等方面与化疗药比较有明显优势，与放疗化疗联用有增效减毒作用，近期还发现金港榄香烯有逆转化疗药和分子靶向药耐药的作用。金港榄香烯脂质体系列靶向抗癌药物基础研究 2008 年获教育部科技进步一等奖，金港榄香烯脂质体系列靶向抗癌药物临床研究 2009 年获中国中西医结合学会科学技术奖一等奖，金港榄香烯脂质体系列靶向抗癌天然药物产业化技术及其临床应用 2012 年荣获国家科技进步二等奖，2013 年金港榄香烯又被科技部、商务部、环保部等部委列入“国家重点新产品”。

▼ 金港榄香烯脂质体质量控制先进仪器

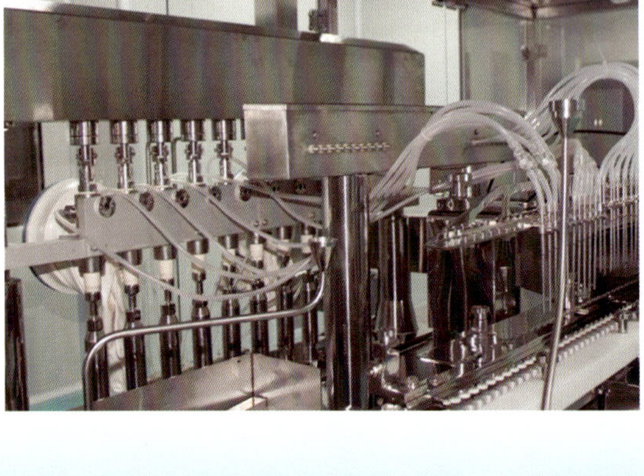

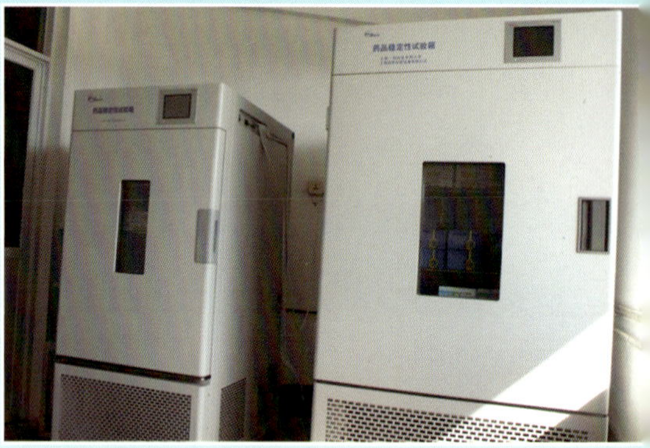

▲ 金港榄香烯脂质体质量控制先进仪器

金港药业建立了富有特色的专业化、学术化营销服务体系。秉承学术营销、科研营销、服务营销的理念，围绕肿瘤患者遇到的问题，推出脂质体系列靶向抗癌药：除榄香烯注射液（脂质体）之外，还推出了安全、有效、使用更方便的金港榄香烯口服乳（脂质体），让病人出院后继续方便地进行抗癌康复治疗，抗复发转移；为解决放化疗中出现的血小板减少症，推出升血小板特效植物药金港血康口服液；为指导癌症患者的饮食和心理问题，建立癌症防治与康复教育交流平台，为患者提供更好的治疗与康复服务。金港药业成立多项爱心慈善基金，已资助全国贫困研究生 200 多位，全程资助大连市贫困中小学生 30 多位；帮助山区 1000 多户农民种植提取抗癌药榄香烯的中药材，使每个农户年均增加收入 2 万多元，使金港药业成为一个有社会责任感的企业，得到了社会各界的高度赞誉。

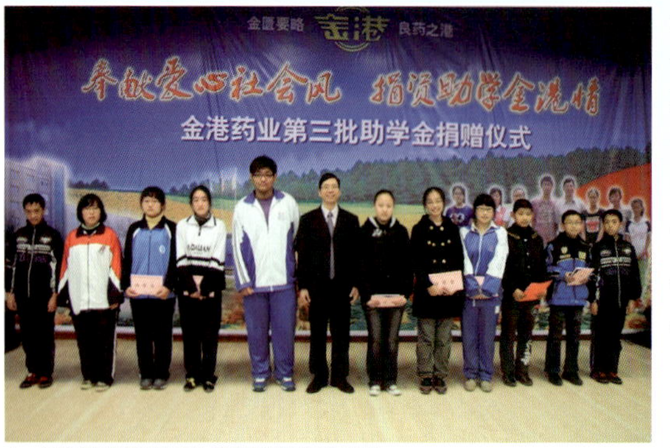
金匮要略
金港
良药之港
奉献爱心社会风 捐资助学金港情
金港药业第三批助学金捐赠仪式

▲ 金港榄香烯脂质体质量控制先进仪器

金港人正以实际行动实践着自己的使命——**为医生提供良药、为病人解除疾苦、为社会创造价值、为健康做出贡献！**

（更多信息请浏览网站：http://www.holleykingkong.com）

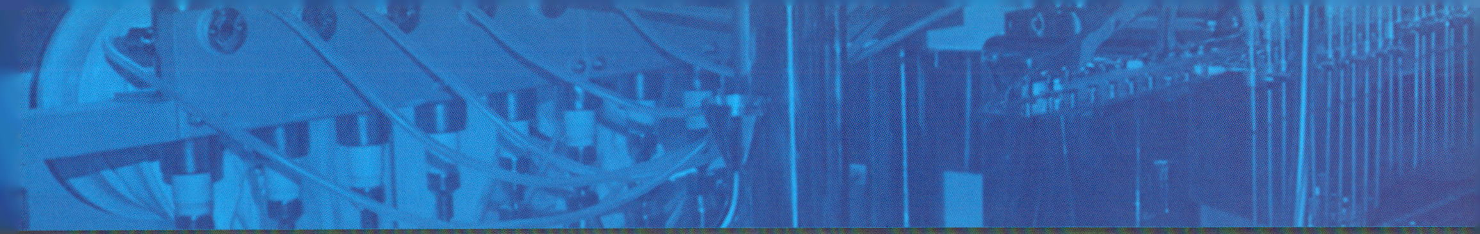

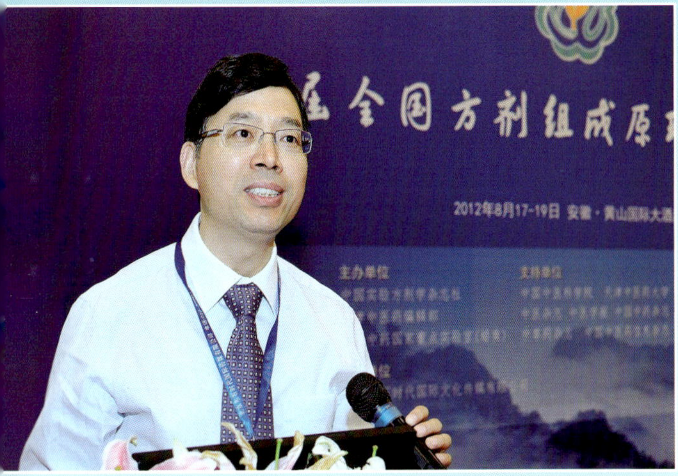

▲ 谢恬教授做学术报告

谢恬 男，1961年12月生，1992年加入农工民主党，990年获医学博士学位，教授、研究员、教授级高工，享受国务院特殊津贴专家，浙江省突出贡献中青年专家，浙江省“151”人才导师，杭州师范大学生物医药研究所所长，南京中医药大学、成都中医药大学、上海中医药大学、北京大学肿瘤医院、广东药学院客座教授、博士生导师。

▼ 谢恬教授在实验室指导研究生

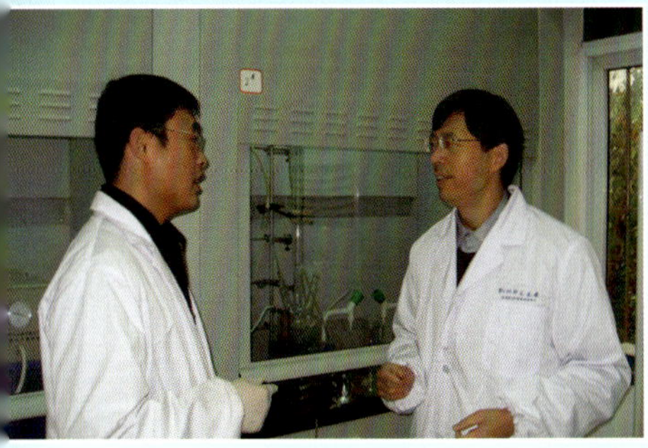

从事中西医结合转化医学、中药学、脂质体靶向抗癌药物、绿色化学、制药工程等领域研究、教学和产业化30余年，注重产学研结合，重视中西医结合、医学与药学结合、实验与临床结合、研究与产业化结合。获美国、欧盟及中国发明专利30余项，创新提出“分子配伍”理论研发新药（现代中药），研发成功新药十多个。主持完成的“榄香烯脂质体系列靶向抗癌天然药物产业化技术及其应用”荣获国家科技进步二等奖，其他成果获教育部一等奖、中国中西医结合学会一等奖、杭州市人民政府二等奖、浙江省人民政府三等奖。

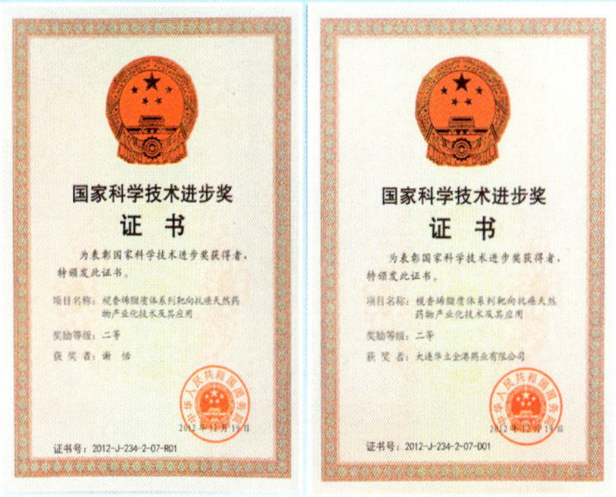
国家科学技术进步奖
证　书
为表彰国家科学技术进步奖获得者，特颁发此证书。
项目名称：榄香烯脂质体系列靶向抗癌天然药物产业化技术及其应用
奖励等级：二等
获 奖 者：谢　恬
2012年12月19日
证书号：2012-J-234-2-07-R01

国家科学技术进步奖
证　书
为表彰国家科学技术进步奖获得者，特颁发此证书。
项目名称：榄香烯脂质体系列靶向抗癌天然药物产业化技术及其应用
奖励等级：二等
获 奖 者：大连华立金港药业有限公司
2012年12月19日
证书号：2012-J-234-2-07-D01

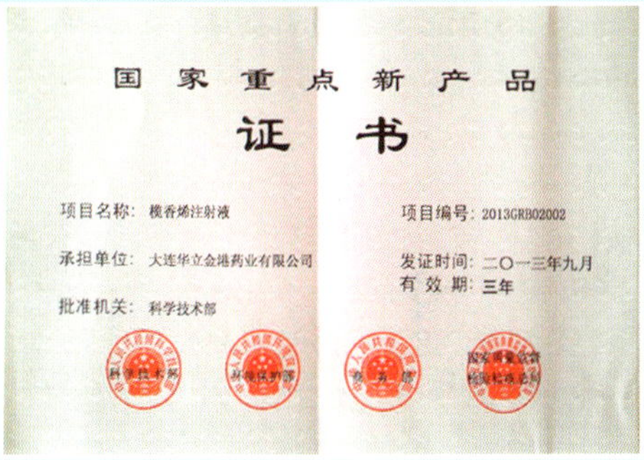
国 家 重 点 新 产 品
证　书
项目名称：榄香烯注射液
项目编号：2013GRB02002
承担单位：大连华立金港药业有限公司
发证时间：二〇一三年九月
有 效 期：三年
批准机关：科学技术部

兼任国家科学技术奖评审专家，教育部科学技术奖评审专家，中华中医药学会科技奖评审专家，中国中西医结合学会科技奖评审专家、中药学专业委员会副主任，中国抗癌协会常务理事，中华中医药学会肿瘤分会副主任、中成药分会副主任，中国医师协会中西医结合肿瘤专家委员会副主任；《中国中医药年鉴（学术卷）》特邀副主任编委，《中国实验方剂学杂志》《世界中西医结合杂志》《肝癌》等杂志副主编，《中国中西医结合杂志》《中国肿瘤临床》《中国中药杂志》等杂志编委。

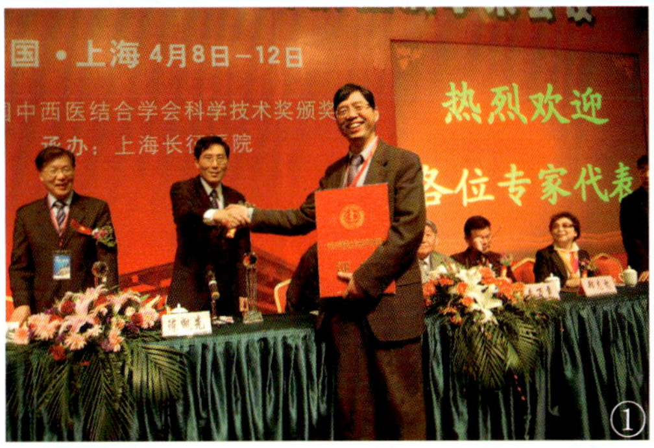

①

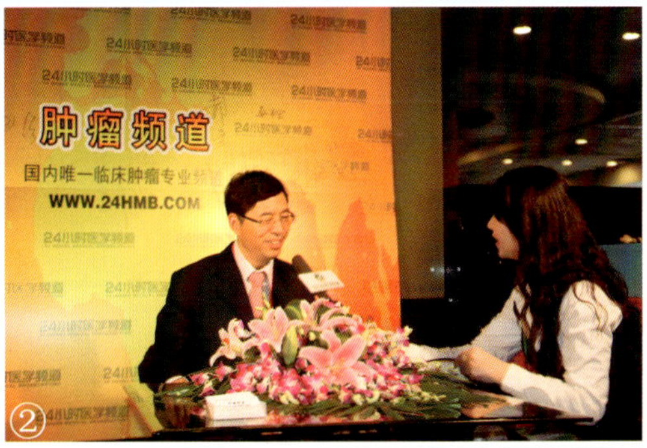

②

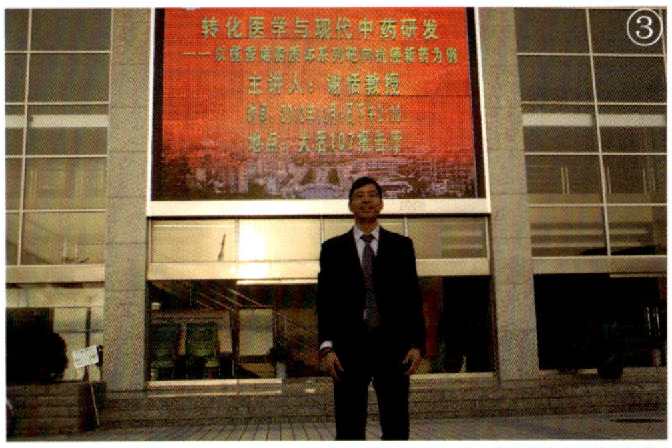

③

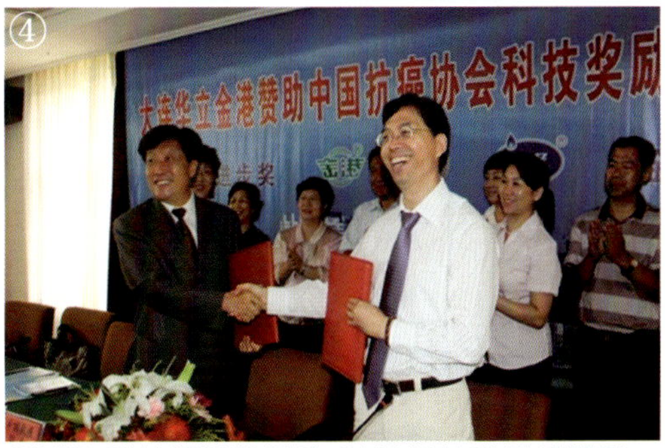
④

①谢恬教授荣获中国中西医结合学会科技奖一等奖-陈凯先院士颁奖　②接受肿瘤频道记者采访　③谢恬教授回母校南京中医药大学作学术报告　④金港药业资助中国抗癌协会科技进步奖

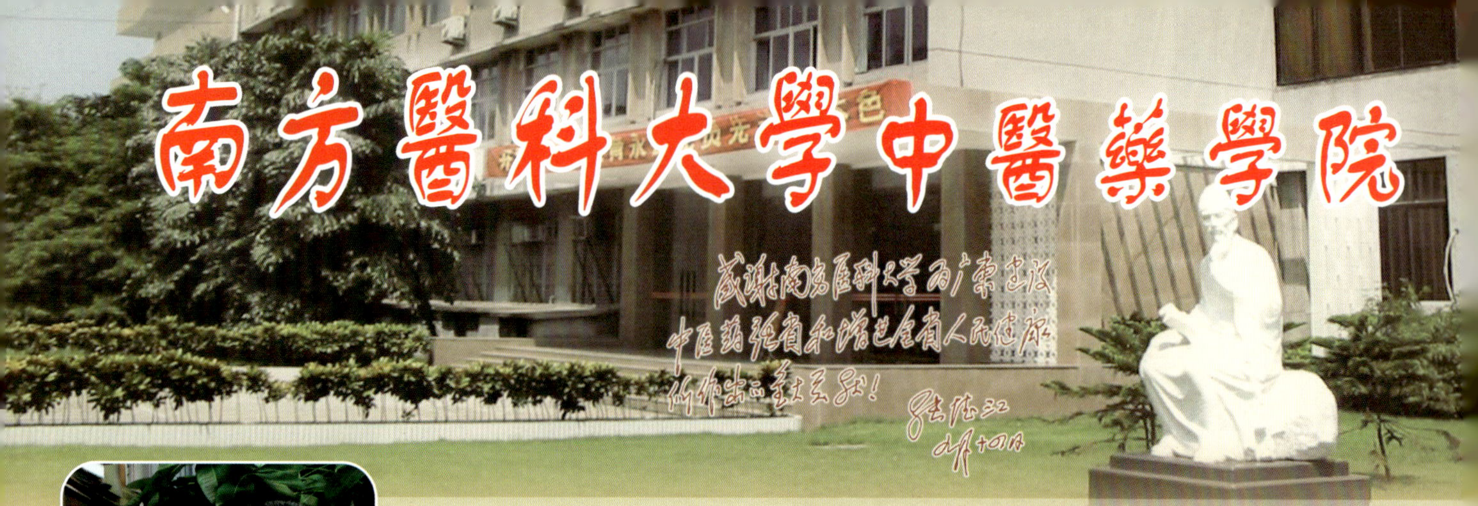

南方醫科大學中醫藥學院

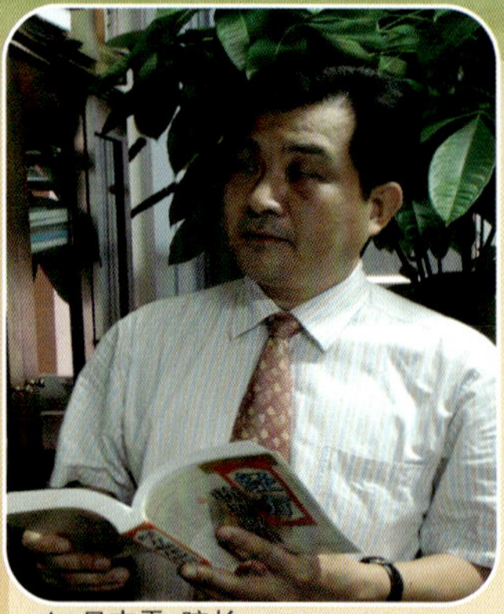

▲ 吕志平 院长

吕志平 教授、主任医师、博士生导师，现任南方医科大学中医药学院院长、南方医科大学中西医结合研究所所长、南方医科大学中西医结合博士授权点和中西医结合博士后流动站负责人、广东省重点专科肝胆专科带头人，是南方医科大学附属中西医结合医院、附属南方医院中西医结合肝病学科学术带头人，全国优秀教育工作者，国家名老中医师承制导师，广东省名中医，教育部国家重点学科、特色学科中西医结合临床学科带头人，广东省重点学科中西医结合学科带头人，国家中医药管理局三级实验室分子生物学实验室负责人，教育部中西医结合内科学教学团队带头人。

兼任国家教育部中医教育指导委员会委员，中华中医药学会常务理事，中国中西医结合学会常务理事、中医基础理论专业委员会副主委，中国医师协会中西医结合医师分会常务理事，中国中西医结合教育工作委员会副主委，中国中西医结合科研院所工作委员会副主委，广东省中医药学会副会长、中医络病专业委员会主任委员、中医肝病专业委员会副主委，广东省中西医结合学会副会长，广东省高等教育学科学位评议组成员。

先后主持国家自然科学基金重点项目、国家科技重大专项、国家支撑项目、军队重大科研项目等 20 余项，获中国中西医结合学会科技成果一等奖 1 项，中国中西医结合学会中西医结合贡献奖，中国中西医结合学会、军队及省部级科技二等奖 5 项、主编全国高等医学院校教材《中西医结合导论》等 3 部，发表中文期刊论文 170 多篇，SCI 文章 7 篇，其中 *Caveolin-1 is essential for protecting against binge drinking-induced liver damage through inhibiting reactive nitrogen species* 在世界肝脏病学顶级杂志美国 *Hepatology* 上发表（IF 12.003）。获国家发明专利 2 项。主编出版专著 22 部（册）。

南方医科大学中医药学院座落在风景秀丽的广州市白云山东麓，其前身为中国人民解放军第一军医大学中医系，始建于 1975 年 7 月。1986 年成立全军中西医结合研究所，1997 年 3 月更名为中医药研究所，1998 年批准建立中医医院，是系、所、院合一的编制体制，也是全军唯一的集教、研、医为一体的培养全军中医、中药、中西医结合高级人才基地。2005 年 6 月学校转制后成立中医药学院。2006 年，广东省委省政府关于建设中医药强省决定中明确提出“支持南方医科大学发挥中西医结合学科群优势，建设一所投资多元、医教研一体，国内一流水平的南方中西医结合医院”。学院、医院实行“院院合一”模式。中西医结合医院已通过三级甲等中医医院的评审。

一、学科门类齐全

学科布局上涵盖中医学、中药学和中西医结合三个一级学科，19 个二级学科。拥有博士后流动站 1 个（中西医结合），一级学科博士学位授权学科 2 个（中西医结合和中药学），硕士学位授权点 5 个。有国家重点学科 1 个、国家中医药管理局重点学科 6 个，国家中药临床药理基地 1 个，国家中医药管理局科研三级实验室 3 个，广东省攀峰重点一级学科 1 个，广东省重点实验室 1 个，广州市中药品种开发中心 1 个。在教育部网站上公布的 2007 年中国大学研究院各二级学科 A++ 级学校排行榜中，学校中西医结合临床医学排名第二（共 67 个）；在《中国大学评价》课题组公布的 07 中国大学研究生院医学各一级学科 A++ 级学校排名中，学校中西医结合医学学科排名第四（共 71 个）。同时中西医结合被确定为学校四大重点建设的技术平台和四大特色学科群之一。2008 年由该学科牵头组织的“疑难病证中西医结合诊疗方案优化及新制剂研发”项目，成功进入广东省省“211 工程”三期重点建设项目。

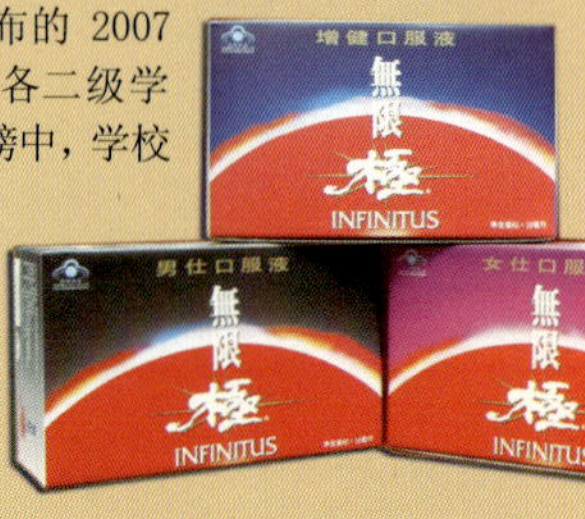

二、师资力量雄厚

现有专任教师 130 人，其中教授 28 人、副教授 29 人，副教授以上占 47%；博士学位 49 人，硕士学位 61 人，硕士学位以上占 79%。其中有全国老中医药专家学术经验继承工作指导老师 4 人；博士生导师 26 名、硕士导师 43 名；拥有一支由国家有突出贡献中青年专家、全国优秀教师、全国优秀教育工作者、广东省教学名师等优秀人才组成的骨干队伍。担任省部级以上学术任职 96 人次，国家级学会主委 2 人、副主委 28 人，省级学会主委 4 人、副主委 45 人。

三、教学优势明显

中医药学院现承担中医学、中药学、中西医结合医学三个一级学科的博士后、博士、硕士、本科、专科多层次教学及培训任务。学院有国家特色专业 1 个，国家级教学团队 1 个，国家精品课程 1 门，广东省名牌专业 2 个，广东省高校实验教学示范中心 2 个，广东省精品课程 2 门，广东省精品视频公开课 1 门，广东省级精品资源共享课 1 门。学院已形成了以本科生和研究生培养为主体、留学生培养为特色，以中西医结合为教学模式、学历教育和继续教育相结合的人才培养体系。先后为军队和地方培养中医药人才 2500 余人，其中包括 25 个国家和地区的留学生 300 余人，目前在校生近 2000 人。

四、科研成果

2004 年，转制以来，和参学院主持与各类科研课题 350 余项，获科研经费 7000 多万元。其中“863”课题 1 项、“973”课题 1 项、国家科技重大专项（重大新药创制）2 项、国家“十一五”科技支撑计划课题 2 项、国家自然科学基金 80 项、教育部博士点基金 5 项。省级以上课题 80 余项，市厅级以上课题 150 余项。发表统计源期刊以上科研论文 2000 余篇，其中 SCI 收录论文 150 余篇。取得国家发明专利 70 余项。开发中药新药 2 个，并已成功转化。获得各类科研成果 18 项，其中省部级科技奖励一等奖 2 项，二等奖 4 项。

五、新药研发强劲

学院在中药新制剂、新剂型，中医急症新药研方面处于国内先进水平。在国际上第一个研制成中粉针剂双黄连，并成功用于工业化生产，获国家发专利；首创抗轮状病毒感染疾病新药葛根芩连微丸国内首创中药袋泡剂剂型。研制的三九胃泰、正天丸金关片、壮骨关节丸原是南方制药厂（三九集团）主打产品，由康臣药厂生产的尿毒清产值超过十几元，研制的无限极保健系列口服液现在还是李锦保健食品有限公司的主要上市产品，补脾益肠丸是李济药厂的重要产品，益元口服液、无限极系列口服液等保健品年销售额逾 2 亿元，创造了巨大的经济效益和社会效益。

新药研究储备品种较多，适用范围广。连番止泻胶囊、都梁软胶囊、五虎口服液已获得国家新药证书。在研的有保肝宁颗粒、肝泰粉针剂、顺天胶囊、妇宁软胶囊、急泻康胶囊等 30 余个品种，部分品种已完成临床前研究。

六、医疗特色鲜明

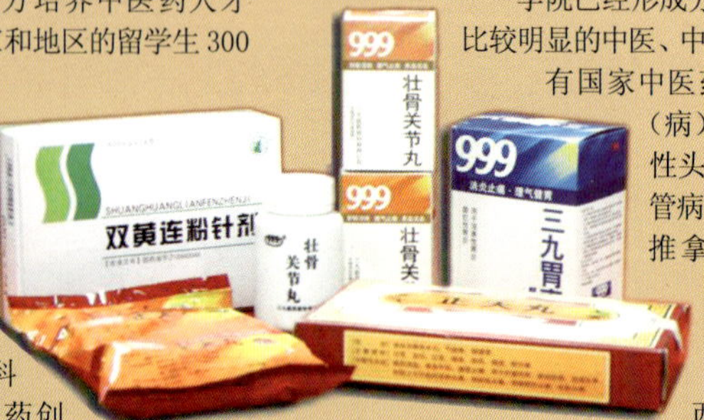

学院已经形成分科比较齐全、特色比较明显的中医、中西医结合诊疗体系。有国家中医药管理局重点专科（病）4 个（中西医结合慢性头痛、中西医结合心血管病、中医风湿病、针灸推拿）；国家中医药管理局治未病中心 1 个；广东省中医药局重点专科 2 个（中西医结合脾胃病、中西医结合肝病）。在中医药防治肾病、脑病、风湿病、脾胃病、肝胆病、老年心血管病、慢性软组织损伤、退行性骨关节病和中西医结合治疗肿瘤等疑难杂症方面在省内外享有较高声誉。目前，中西医结合医院通过三级甲等中医医院的评审，已展现良好的发展前景。

湖南中醫藥高等專科學校

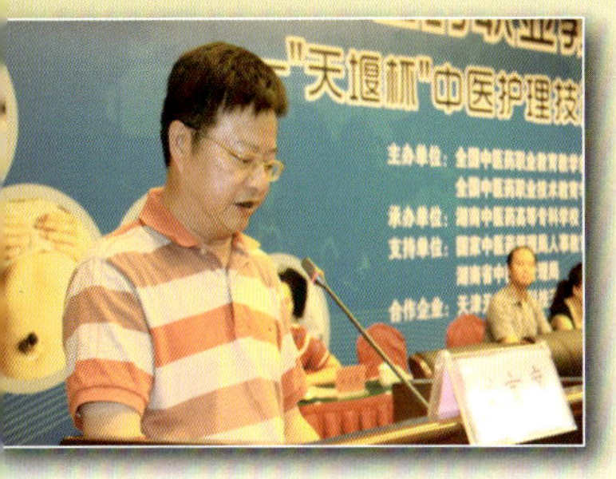

▲ 郭争鸣 湖南中医药高等专科学校 校长

郭争鸣 男，汉族，中共党员，湖南医学院临床医疗系毕业，医学学士，湖南中医学院中西结合研究生课程班结业，生理心理学教授。1983年担任株洲卫校生理学和心理学教师，1985年任教研组长，1987年任湖南省中医药学校教务副科长，同年晋升为讲师；1993年任教务科长并晋升高级讲师；1997年任后勤副校长；2000年任学校党委书记、副校长；2004年任湖南中医药高等专科学校党委副书记、教学副校长，同年平转副教授，2006年晋升为教授；2009年12月任校长。

坚持深入教学、科研一线，每年担任教学任务均在200学时左右，主持厅级以上的科研课题6项。先后主编、参编教材教参15部。在各级各类刊物上发表科研、教学和管理论文35篇。负责主讲的"医护心理学"课程2006年被评为省级精品课程。牵头负责的"基础医学教学团队"获2010年省级优秀教学团队。在生理学和心理学领域中有一定的学术地位，为中国中医心理学会理事，湖南省生理科学会常务理事，湖南省心理卫生协会常务理事，湖南省中西医结合学会常务理事。先后获得省市和学校各种表彰奖励30多项；先后两次评为株洲市双文明建设先进个人，4次荣立卫生厅二等功。

校址：湖南省株洲市芦淞区芦淞路136号
电话：0731-28519008 28519148
28519048
传真：0731-28519168
邮编：412012
电子邮箱：hnzyygzb@163.com
网址：www.hntcmc.net

学校于2004年经教育部批准成立，是由湖南省卫生厅、湖南省教育厅管理的公立全日制普通高等专科学校，地处全国两型社会综合配套改革试验区、中南地区最大的交通枢纽——株洲市，是湖南省中医药实用型技能性人才的主要培养基地。学校实行党委领导下的校长负责制，实行校系二级管理；现有直属附属医院1家，松散型附属医院3家。

1.招生就业 双获先进

2013年大专新生报到2170人，到校率达89.63%，远远高于全省高职高专平均水平；新增五年制大专新生414人；全年共招收大中专新生 2902人，办学层次进一步优化，被教育厅授予招生工作先进单位。2013年学校有1845名大专生毕业，年终就业率达91.60%，实现毕业生就业人数持续增加。麦可思数据公司调研结果显示：学校2012届毕业一年后的就业率为96.4%，比全国高职院校毕业半年后（90.4%）高6.0个百分点。被省教育厅授予毕业生就业工作"一把手工程"优秀单位。

2.科学研究 增量提质

2013年学校各级各类课题立项64项，比去年增长49%，全国教育科学"十二五"规划课题1项，省教育科学规划课题7项，省卫生厅课题2项，省中医药管理局课题8项（其中2项重点），其他省市校级课题46项。科研经费投入169万元，比去年增长31%。发表论文147篇，其中核心期刊刊发20篇，比去年增长33%；结题28项，获中华中医药学会科技成果三等奖1项，市社会科学成果三等奖 1项，湖南省教学成果二等奖 1项。

3.师资队伍 优化合理

坚持人才强校战略，围绕学校重点专业、特色专业和新建专业，引进高职称、高学历、高技能的专门人才充实师资队伍。2013年度正式录用19人，其中副高职称2人；顺利晋升正高6人，副高14人。选拔2013学年度访问学者共4名；申报青年骨干教师共7名；在职读博4人，读硕5人。王德瑜教授被评为湖南省卫生系统"225工程"领军人才。

4.专业学科 打造精品

按照"突出特色，打造品牌，注重培育，整体发展"的专业建设总体思路，确定各专业的主体功能。中药类做大，中医类做强，护理类做细，相关医学类做实，形成鲜明的专业特色群。增设公共卫生管理和食品药品管理两个专业。血液净化、重症监护、中医护理、涉外护理等专业方向正在积极探索之中，学校专业建设逐步形成新格局。推拿学科作为国家中医药管理局重点建设学科通过了规划认定，正在抓紧建设之中。

5.教学资源 共建共享

充分发挥数字资源库作用，大力推进无纸化机考，制定了无纸化考试题库申报书和验收标准，共建56个题库，5门课成功进行了机考和智能组卷。2013年学校获湖南省信息化试点学校。根据精品资源共享课程建设要求，国家、省、校级精品课程建设同步推进，共立项48门课程为校级精品资源共享课程；"医护心理学"等4门省级精品课程通过评审复查；王德瑜教授的国家级网络精品课程"推拿手法技术"成功升级为国家级精品资源共享课程。2013年有16位主编，35位副主编和参编参与国家卫计委和人民卫生出版社中医药高职高专第三轮规划教材建设项目。

▼ 学校承办全国中医护理技能大赛

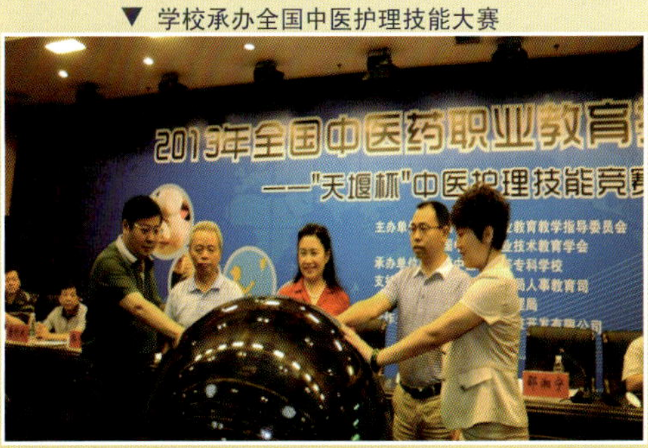

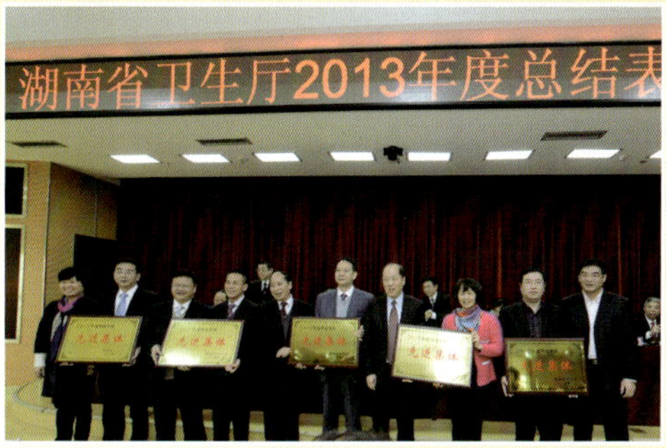

▲ 2013年学校获得湖南省卫生厅年度考核先进集体

6.校外基地 互利双赢

完善校企合作人才培养模式，促进校内学习与实际工作的"无缝"对接，实现"五融合"人才培养模式。2013年先后有张家界、岳阳、长沙、衡阳等地市中医院相继新增为学校临床教学基地；天士力湖南民生、中和制药有限公司为药学实习基地；与台湾罗丽芬集团、岳阳秀媛堂生物有限公司、千金湘江制药厂和老百姓大药房继续签订"订单班"。千金药业与学校合作的人才培养示范基地获教育厅立项，康保系大学生创新平台获教育厅立项。

7. 人才培养 质量提升

学校积极探索专科医学人才培养模式，与多家企业、医院签定了合作办学协议，开办了订单式培养班；与附属医院联合实施"1+2"人才培养模式，株洲伤科医院和千金药业2013年均被评为湖南省校企合作人才培养示范基地。2013年全国中医护理大赛在学校举行，学校大专选手包揽前四名，双双获得高职、中职组团体一等奖。学校代表湖南省在全国中药传统技能大赛再次夺魁。冠军王义崇免试进入湖南中医药大学"专升本"深造。2013年荣获"解剖学"全省统考第1名，学校还获得2013年基层卫生人才培训先进单位。全国护士执业资格考试通过率达99.7%，遥遥领先于全国56.7%的通过率。

8.党的建设 引领全局

2013年，学校深入开展了"为民务实清廉"为主题的党的群众路线教育实践活动，取得了阶段性的成果。2013年9月，省委高校巡视组进驻学校，扎实进行了为期1个月工作，有效地促进了学校的建设和管理。党委召开全校"七一"党员大会，表彰先进，发展了一批新党员。同时启动了创建省直文明单位活动和节能示范单位。2013年学校再次获得湖南省卫生厅年度绩效考核先进集体。

9.校园文化 唱响主题

邀请杰出校友回学校与在校师生一起畅谈"中国梦 我的梦"。邀请最美护士何遥慧回母校做"立足岗位 学习雷锋"主题演讲报告会，给予大学生学习生活正能量。中医药文化艺术节组织开展了辨药大赛、中草药标本制作大赛等10余个富有中医药特色的活动项目。一年一度的体育艺术节，凝聚了集体主义协作精神，丰富了师生业余生活。"5·12"国际护士节文艺晚会，弘扬南丁格尔精神，展现文明护生风采。学校在《健康报》《中国职业技术教育》《人民网》和《新华网》等国家级媒体发表新闻报道4篇，湖南教育电视台、《湖南日报》等省市主流媒体发表正面报道73篇。

安徽中醫藥高等專科學校

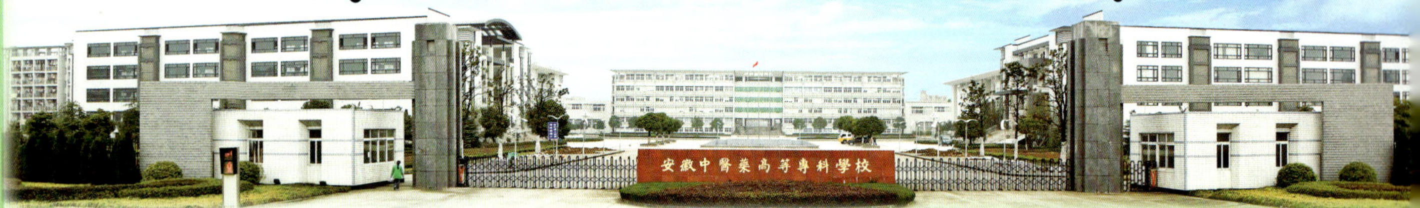

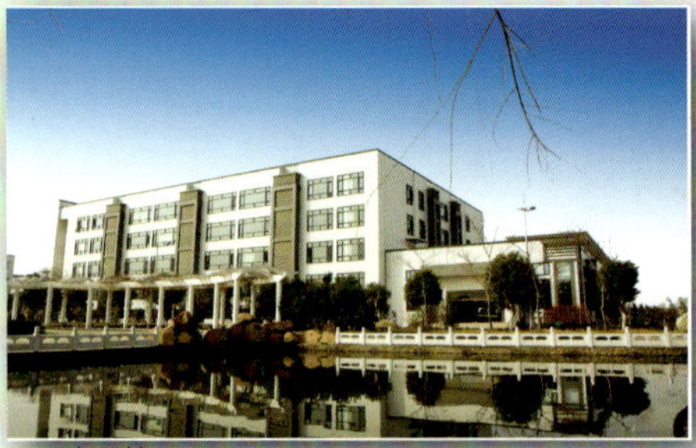
▲ 办公楼

安徽中医药高等专科学校的前身是始建于1960年的芜湖市中医学校；2001年，学校升格并于次年经教育部批准，在全国同类院校率先更名为高等专科学校。为整合卫生教育资源，壮大学校实力，2006年，市政府将芜湖市中医医院成建制划归学校作为其直属附属医院。经过50多年的建设与发展，学校已经成为具有鲜明中医药特色的地方性高等院校。2010年，学校在高职高专院校人才培养工作评估中获得“优秀”等次，成功创建了“安徽省示范性高等职业院校”。

▼ 第二教学楼

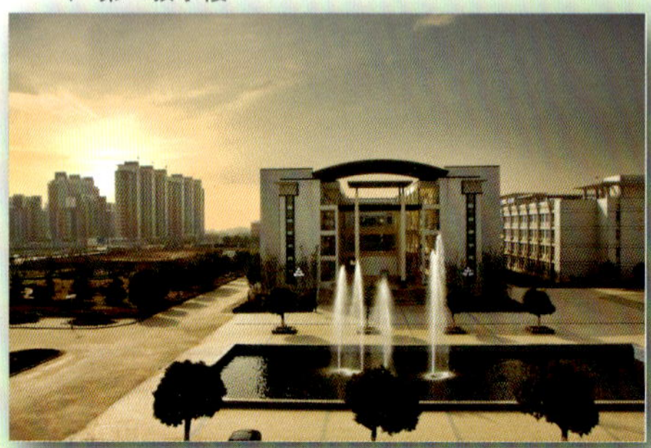

学校现为教育部中医药职业教育教学指导委员会副主任委员单位、全国中医药职业技术教育学会常务副理事长单位、全国中医药高职高专教育教材建设指导委员会主任委员单位、安徽省中医药学会中医养生保健专业委员会理事长单位、安徽省药学会中药材种植（养殖）专业委员会理事长单位。

学校占地面积826亩，总建筑面积29.96万平方米，设有医疗系、药学系、康复保健系、护理系、口腔医学系、基础教学部和思想政治理论课教学研究部等7个教学系部，开设中医学、中医骨伤、针灸推拿、中药、中药制药技术、药学、药品质量检测技术、护理、医疗美容技术等26个专业，面向全国27个省、市、自治区招生，全日制专科在校生9000余人。

学校现有教职医护员工1169人，专任教师528人，其中，副高以上专业技术人员173人，硕士研究生以上学历学位人员175人，全国名老中医4人，全国优秀教师1人。学校还聘任国医大师李济仁、长江学者叶文才等 15 名专家教授为特聘教授、客座教授。

学校下辖4所直属附属医院、1所附属药厂、1个安徽中药资源研究所、1个中药材种植基地、1个天然药用植物园和9所非直属附属医院、25所教学医院以及113家校外实习基地。学校附属中医医院（芜湖市中医医院）创立于1958年，在中医界素有“江南中医一枝花”的美誉，为“全国首批示范中医院”“国家三级甲等综合性中医医院”，医院拥有4个国家级重点中医专科专病、6个省级重点中医专科专病、5个市级重点中医专科。

学校现有中央财政支持实训基地1个，中央财政支持提升专业服务产业发展能力项目2个；省级教学团队4个，省级教改示范专业1个，省级特色专业6个，省级精品课程8门，省级卓越型人才技能计划1项，省级人才培养模式创新实验区1个，省级高职高专专业综合改革试点项目1个，省级示范实验实训中心3个，省级示范实习实训中心1个，省级校企合作实践教育基地1个，省级教学名师3人、教坛新秀5人。“十一五”以来，学校牵头组织了“全国中医药高职高专卫生部规划教材”编写工作，主编卫生部规划教材11部，其中7部教材入选国家级规划教材，2部教材入选教育部普通高等教育精品教材。2013年，学校在第三轮国家卫计委高职高专医药卫生规划教材修订工作中，共有15名主编、35名副主编、50名编者参与教材编写。近年来，学校共承担了各类科学研究项目214项，获得科研成果及奖励48项，其中，省市级以上科研成果奖8项；公开发表学术论文538篇，其中中文核心期刊类论文71篇，5篇被SCI期刊收录；出版专著、教材261部；承担各类教学研究项目57项，其中省级19项、省级重点5项，获得教学成果奖41项，其中省级教学成果奖13项。学校主办的《现代中药研究与实践》为中国科技核心期刊，影响因子0.639，是国内研究中药材生产和质量管理领域最有影响的学术期刊之一。

学校的办学成绩获得上级党委、政府充分肯定和社会各界广泛赞誉。2006年，安徽省委组织部、宣传部和省委教育工委授予学校“先进基层党组织”光荣称号；2008—2010年，安徽省高等学校毕业生就业工作委员会连续三年授予学校“安徽省高校毕业生就业先进集体”称号；2009年，安徽省就业工作领导小组授予学校“全省就业工作先进单位”称号；2010年，安徽省教育厅、财政厅确定学校为“省级示范性高职院校”建设单位；2011年，安徽省教育厅授予学校“安徽省创新创业教育示范校”称号，安徽省人力资源和社会保障厅授予学校大学生创业孵化基地“首届安徽省AA级创业孵化基地”称号；在连续三年荣获“安徽省高校毕业生就业工作先进集体”的基础上，2011和2012连续两年被安徽省高等学校毕业生就业工作委员会授予“安徽省高校毕业生就业工作标兵单位”称号。

50年多来，学校秉承“厚德、博学、济世、日新”的校训，坚持“以人为本，尚德重技，创新服务，特色发展”的办学理念，在中医药专业建设、应用型人才培养、中医药对外交流、中医药产业研发以及服务地方经济和社会发展等方面，形成了独特的优势，为国家培养了3万余名中医药应用型人才。当前，学校正进一步解放思想，同心同德，抢抓机遇，科学发展，努力提高人才培养质量和提升办学层次。

▼ 第一教学楼

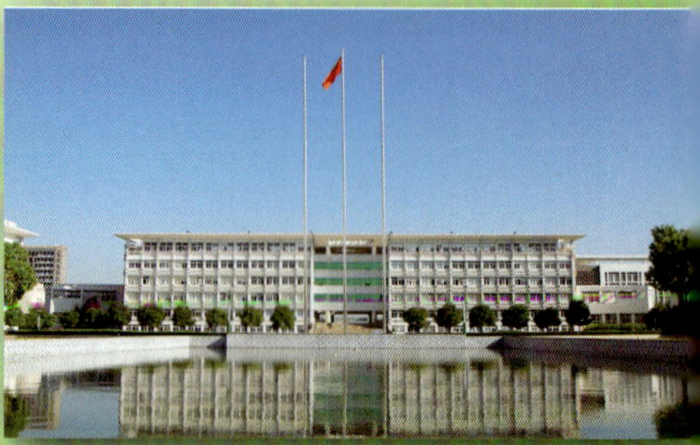

▼ 赵国胜校长

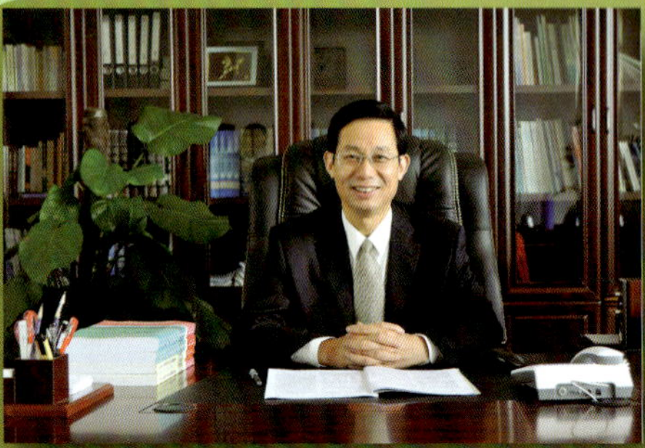

赵国胜，男，1957 年 8 月出生，中共党员，教授。1983 年毕业留校，1988 年起历任皖南医学院基础医学部副主任、学院党委组织部副部长、人事处副处长、基础部党总支书记、教务处处长等职；2005 年 7 月调任安徽中医药高等专科学校校长、党委副书记。

社会兼职：全国中医药职业教育教学指导委员会副主任委员、全国中医药职业技术教育学会常务副理事长、全国中医药高职高专教育教材建设指导委员会主任委员、中国职教学会院校科研教研工作研究会副主任委员、全国医学高职高专教育临床医学分会副主任委员、中国病理生理学会大中专教育工作委员会副主任委员、安徽省病理生理学会副理事长、安徽省中医药学会副理事长等。

▼ 中医美容实践教学

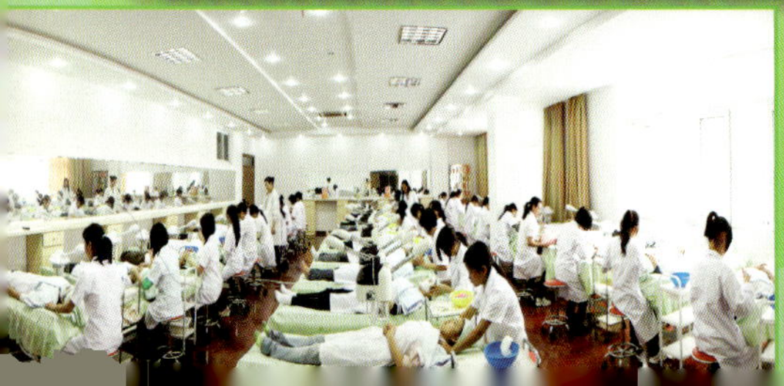

▼ 推拿实践教学

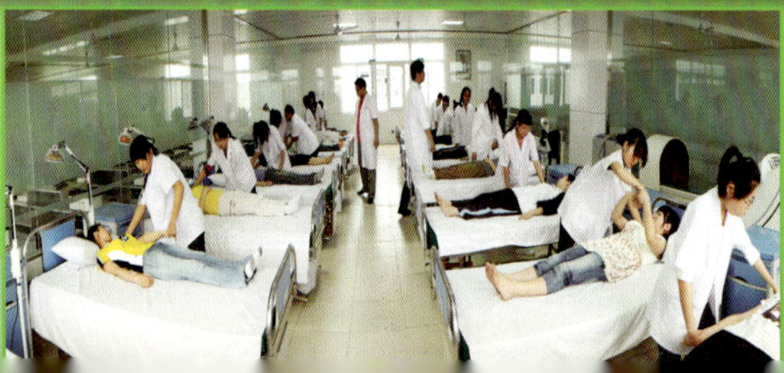

▼ 太极拳

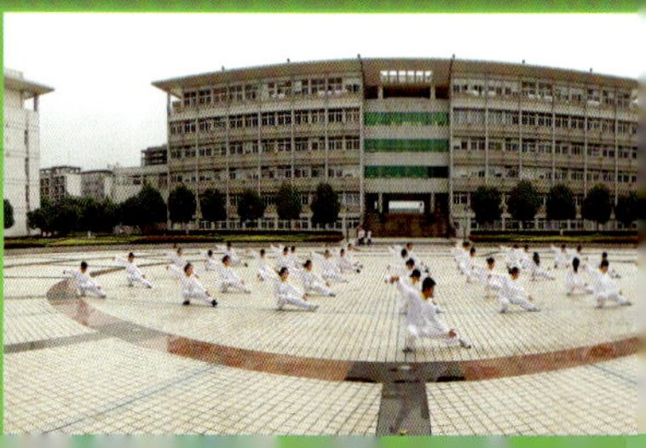

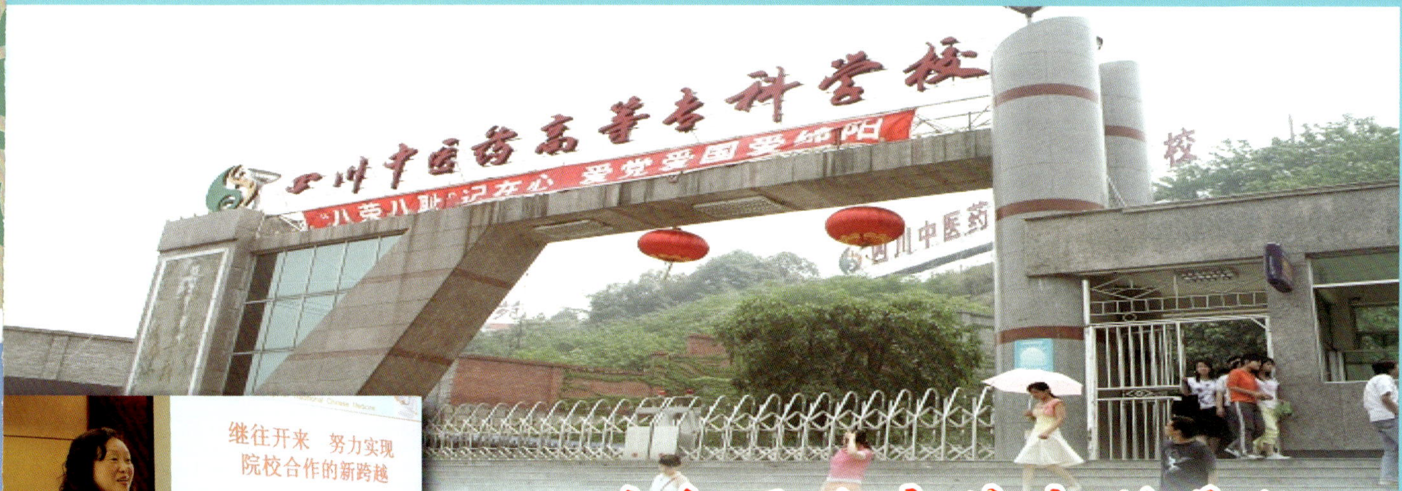

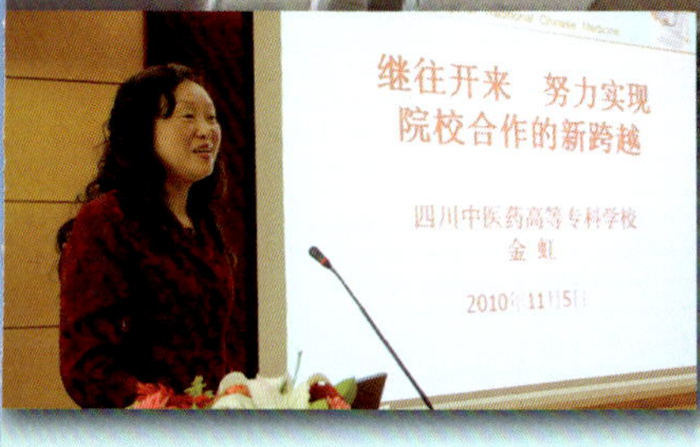

▲ 金虹　四川中医药高等专科学校副校长

金虹 1963年生，重庆人，教授。中国药学会高级会员，国家执业药师，绵阳市药学会副会长，绵阳职业教育研究中心学术委员会副主任委员，绵阳市中医药学会副秘书长，《中草药》杂志编委及特约审稿专家。1985年毕业于成都中医学院，先后在绵阳市中医药研究所、绵阳市药检所任副主任药师；2002年引进西南科技大学生命科学与工程学院任副教授，从事研究生和本科教学与科研工作，任食品与制药工程系主任；2009年6月任四川中医药高等专科学校副校长，中药学专业带头人，学校“现代中药技术课程组”教学团队负责人、第二届“教学名师”，绵阳市2012年度优秀教师。

主讲“药用植物学与生药学”“药物分析”“中药制剂分析”等课程，多次获校级“优秀教学质量奖”。主要研究方向为中药活性成分及其开发应用，主持主研国家自然科学基金、省教育厅、省中医药管理局和市科技局等教学及科研课题20多项，其中获市级以上科技成果奖6项，市级社会科学成果及校级教学成果奖各1项，发表学术论文30余篇，其中在《中国中药杂志》《中草药》等核心期刊发表16篇，《酶解法制备银杏叶提取物及其抗辐射损伤试验》《石菖蒲体外抑酶活性的研究》等多篇论文分别在第三届中医药现代化国际科技大会、中国药学会学术年会等国际及全国学术会议交流。目前正主研科技部创新基金项目“平武天麻总苷、多糖活性组分的提取及高值化利用”的研究，主持绵阳市科技项目“川麦冬资源的开发与利用研究”和四川省教育厅自然学科重点项目“基于酶抑制作用的石菖蒲活性成分的研究”。

四川中医药高等专科学校

四川中医药高等专科学校是2006年经教育部批准成立的一所全日制公办普通医学高等专科学校，实行省市共建，以绵阳市管理为主的管理体制。学校位于绵阳市中国科技城，占地755亩，在编教职工447人，其中具有高级专业技术职务126人；具有硕、博士学位73人，有绵阳市名中医2人。另聘请行业企业一线优秀专业技术人员790人为学校兼职教师，现有在校学生8200余人。

学校从2006年升专时设置的临床医学类、护理类、药学类3个专业类别、6个专业，发展成覆盖临床医学类、护理类、药学类、医学技术类、卫生管理

▼ 实验课

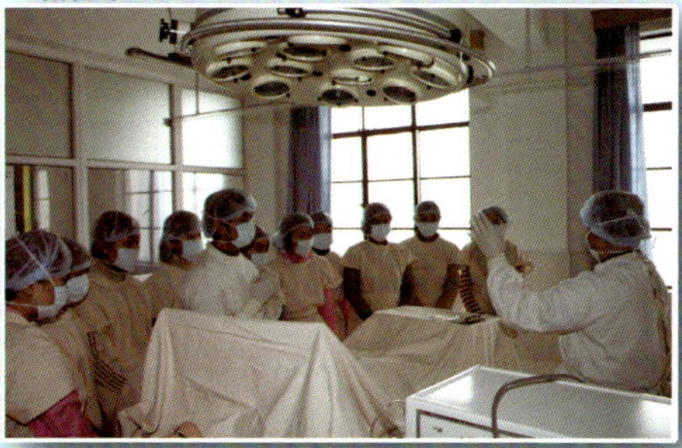

类、制药技术类、农业技术类、市场营销类8个专业类别，包含中医、中医骨伤、中药制药技术、医疗美容技术、康复治疗技术、针灸推拿、医学检验技术、中药、公共卫生管理、口腔医学技术、临床医学、助产、护理、中草药栽培技术、医药营销共计15个专业，面向全国14个省（直辖市、自治区）招生。

学校将科学研究和科技服务作为提高教师素质的关键环节之一，升专以来逐步完善科研管理制度，加大科研经费的投入，设立校级科研基金并积极参与各级各类科研项目的申报。近年来，有70余项科研项目获得立项。其中“院校和校企合作构建针推专业开放式实践课程教学体系研究”“中医药职业院校教学方法与教学手段改革的研究——基于实训的高职高专基础护理学教学模式改革研究”获得国家中医药管理局　“十二五”中医药教育教学改革研究课题立项资助；“绵阳市中医医疗状况调查”“《医录便览》详注”“蒲辅周学术思想及临床经验研究”获得四川省中医药管理局专项资助；“基于酶抑制作用的石菖蒲活性成分的研究”“三氧化二砷抗胰腺癌的分子机制及复方研究”“利用氢核磁共振法研究不同等级麦冬差异”及“李杜诗作中的医药文化研究”获得四川省教育厅立项。此外，学校还与相关企业积极开展横向合作。与绵阳市一康制药有限公司合作研究“平武天麻总苷、多糖活性组分的提取及高值化利用”增强一康制药有限公司研发实力并使该企业获得国家科技型

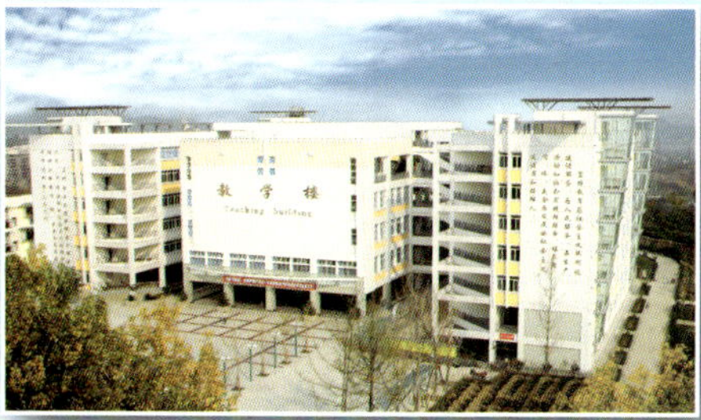

▲ 教学楼

中小企业技术创新基金资助。学校附属二院提供技术为绵阳百信医院配制“合欢神调合剂”等7种中药新制剂，获批为医疗机构制剂。学校针推保健系协助四川常乐足道服务有限公司解决其技术操作缺乏规范和完整技术程序的问题，帮助其制定了企业“踩背保健”“足浴保健”“按摩保健”等技术操作规范。升专以来，学校教师出版教材和专著共34部；发表论文600余篇，部分论文在核心期刊发表，或收录于SCI，EI；获得省级科技进步奖3项、市级科技进步奖8项。

学校义不容辞地承担了弘扬中医药文化，普及中医药知识，宣扬传统文化，促进中医药教育事业发展的重要责任，多次组织教师开展常见病防治义

▼ 实验楼

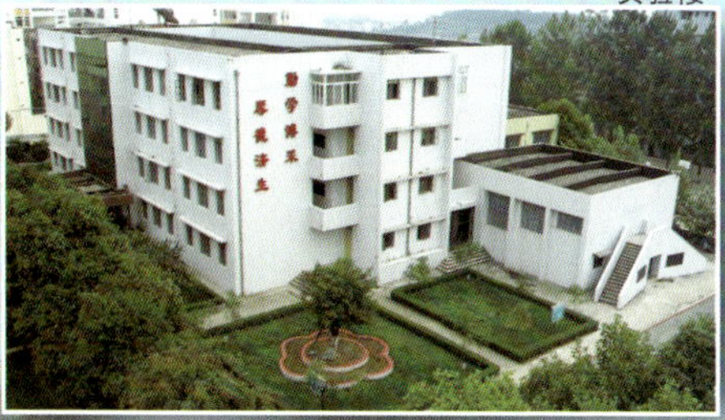

务咨询活动、中医药中国行义诊、咨询、中医推广等活动。自2010年起举办中医药文化节，以“认识中医中药、发掘伟大宝库”为主题，开展中医药论坛、“爱我中华、扬我中医”演讲比赛、中医药文化体验、社区义诊、中药标本鉴定大赛、中药标本盆栽展、大学生征文及学术研讨会、推拿手法技能大赛等一系列活动。

学校秉承“德馨、技精、博学、笃行”的校训，扎实开展医药卫生人才的培养工作，先后毕业学生近5万名，为国家特别是四川培养了大批医疗、预防、康复保健服务和卫生管理人才，如今，他们大多数已成为四川特别是川西北地区各级各类医疗、康复、卫生管理机构中的骨干力量，为区域经济社会和医药卫生事业发展做出了突出贡献。

广州中医药大学附属骨伤科医院

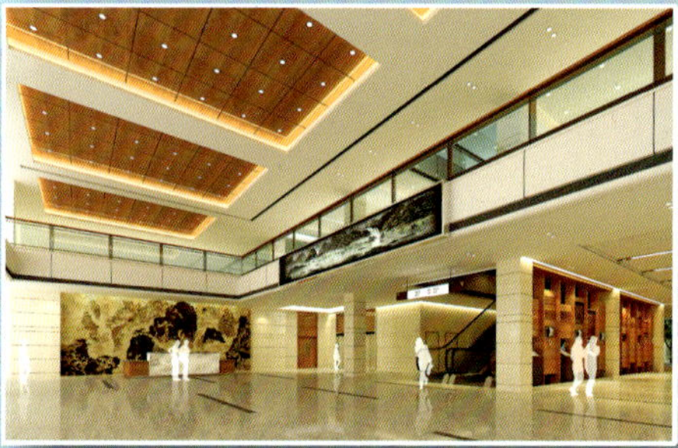

▲ 大堂效果

广州中医药大学附属骨伤科医院是华南地区唯一一所集医教研为一体、以中医骨伤科诊疗特色的医科大学附属骨伤科专科医院。医院坚持科学发展观，牢牢把握正确的办院方向，统一全院干部职工的思想，确定医院建设目标。院领导始终把新院的发展作为第一要务，经充分论证，制定完善《广州中医药大学第三附属医院（广东省中西医结合骨伤科医院）建设方案》，新院按三级甲等医院的标准，建设成为以中西医结合骨伤科为主体、相关专科配套、具有明显特色的现代化中西医结合医院，总设置床位1200张。以新院为载体使医疗、教学、科研各项工作全面发展，成为全省乃至全国高水平的中西医结合骨伤科医疗中心。医院从建院以来，将艰苦创业、自强不息的文化精神贯穿在医院整体建设中，将医院文化及中医药文化建设相结合，发扬“医者仁心 大医精诚”精神，精中强西，构建和谐医院。

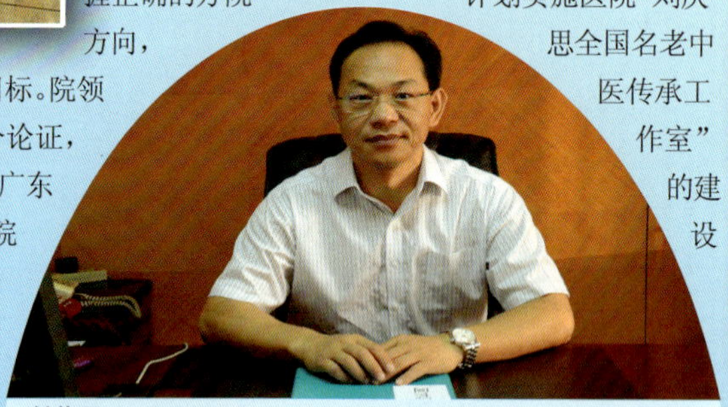

谢华民 从事中医药教育、党务和思想政治工作以及医院管理25年多，爱祖国和人民，拥护中国共产党的领导，热爱中医药事业，爱岗敬业，遵纪守法，有高度的事业心和责任感，对中医药工作充满热忱。能认真贯彻省委、省政府关于建设中医药强省的决定，积极实施“三名两进”工程，竭力推动中医药文化的继承传播，工作业绩显著。现任广州中医药大学附属骨伤科医院（第三附属医院、第三临床医学院）院长，广州中医药大学社会医学与公共事业管理硕士研究生导师。

历任全国高等中医药教育学会中医护理教育分会副理事长、全国中医药职业教育学会理事、广东省中等中医药职业技术教育学会副主任委员、广东省中医药学会理事、广东省中医医院医学伦理委员会副主任委员等。主持及主要参与国家级、省级和厅局级等科研课题8项，发表学术论文10余篇。

多次荣获广州中医药大学“优秀党员”“优秀党务工作者”以及各种先进工作者称号，并被评为2009-2010年广州市社会治安综合治理先进工作者。主编的新世纪全国高等中医药院校创新教材《中医临床护理学》于2009年8月被全国高等中医药教材建设研究会评为“新世纪全国高等中医药优秀教材”。

历任广州市海珠区第十四届、第十五届人大代表。

医疗

根据医院创“三甲”之要求，拟定了医院综合目标管理考核计划，制定了《医院综合目标管理制度》，作为年度的重点工作。在综合目标管理检查的同时，联合药学部，重点监控临床用药及治疗情况，拟定合理检查、合理用药、合理治疗的管理制度。每月对全院医生“合理检查、合理用药、合理治疗”执行情况以及病历完成情况进行检查，及时杜绝安全隐患。2013年3月，为满足患者的就医需求，医院开设了骨科夜诊服务。

科研

医院骨质疏松医疗中心荣获中国老年学学会骨质疏松委员会“先进集体奖”、刘庆思教授荣获中国老年学学会骨质疏松委员会“终身成就奖”、黄宏兴教授荣获中国老年学学会骨质疏松委员会“突出贡献奖”。认真按计划实施医院“刘庆思全国名老中医传承工作室”的建设工作，已出版专著1部，举办广东省中医药局继续教育项目1项。由医院负责的骨质疏松方面的研究是广州中医药大学“211工程”重点学科中医骨伤科学的重要组成部分，医院按照重点学科建设的要求，整合相关的资源，凝练学科研究方向，积极配合重点学科的建设。医院关节病科、创伤科、脊柱病科、康复科、血液病科、脑病科、妇科共7个专科成为广东省“十二五”中医重点（特色）专科建设项目。

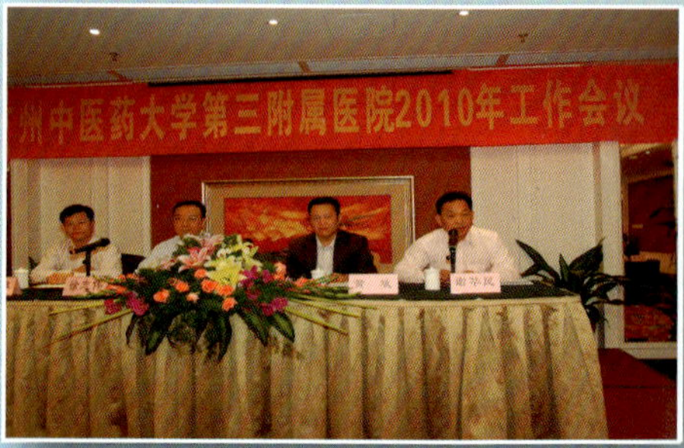

▲ 谢华民院长发言

教育

医院所属的第三临床医学院全年共承担理论大课14门课程891学时。在读研究生70人，新招收研究生28人（包括港澳台生1人）。新招收硕士研究生24人，博士研究生4人。在教学管理上进一步加强临床实践教学管理工作，推进临床实践教学水平；重视对教师的道德修养、学术素养及创新精神的培养，全面提升教师队伍素质；积极开展各项教学活动，全方位提升学生知识素养；利用学科特色和优势，加强研究生教育；教学管理工作进一步规范化、科学化、常规化。

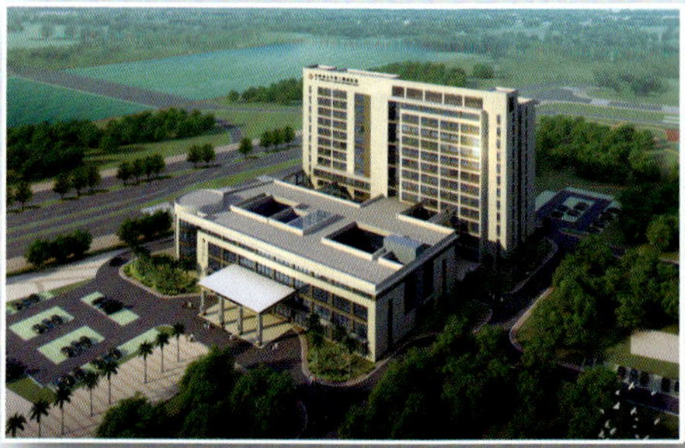

▲ 外观鸟瞰效果图

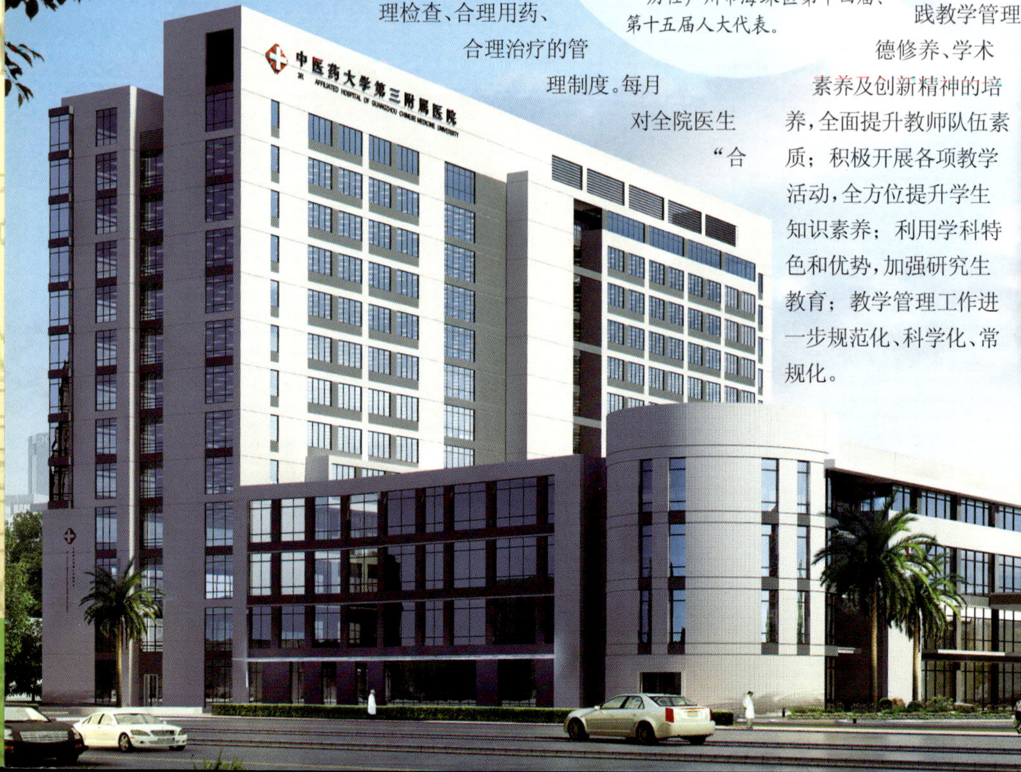

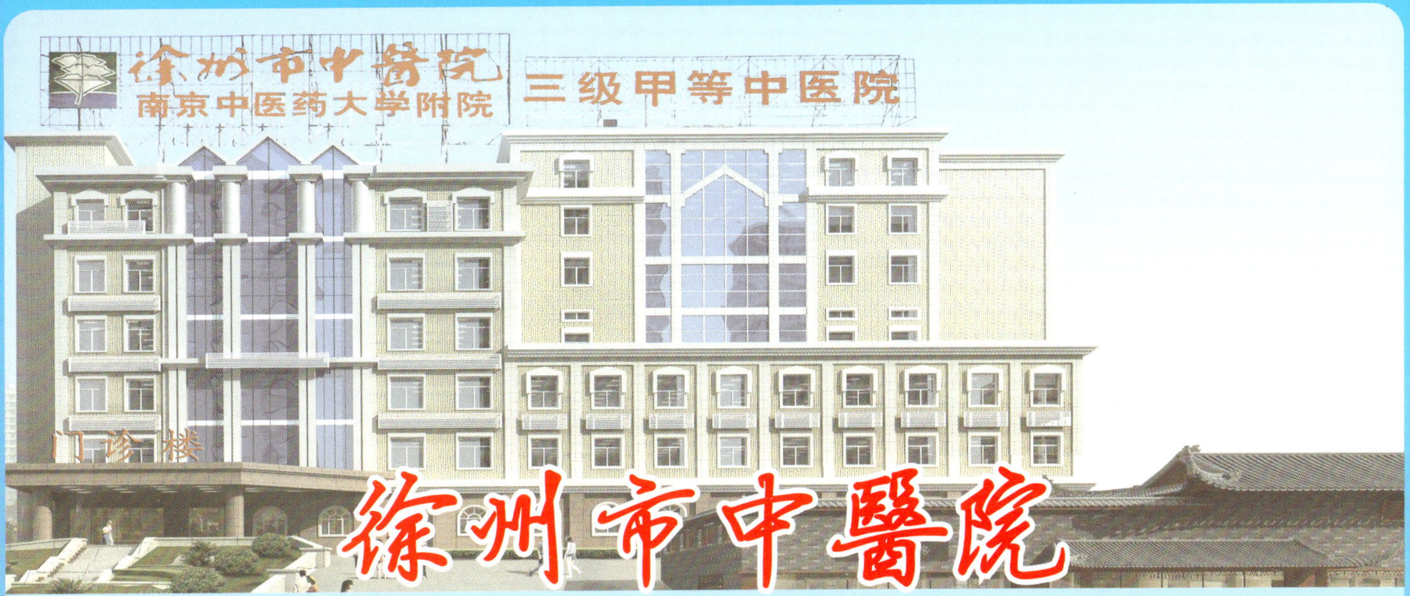

徐州市中醫院

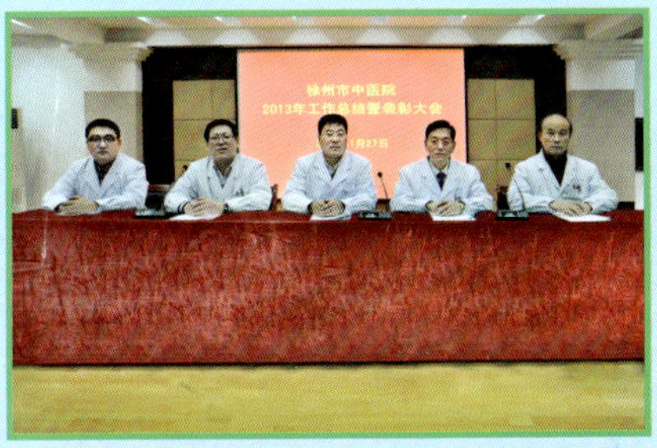
▲ 团结奋进的院领导班子

徐州市中医院始建于1956年，是一所集医疗、保健、康复、教学、科研、社区卫生服务于一体的国家三级甲等中医院，南京中医药大学附属医院，江苏省首批基本现代化中医院；连续两年进入全国地市级城市医院竞争力百强。

医院占地面积2.4万平方米，建筑面积4.6万平方米，门诊设26个临床科室、15个医技科室、80个专科专病门诊，住院部设22个病区，实开1200张病床，年出院病人逾2.5万人次，年门诊量逾155万人次。院外开设了养生堂、普济药店、中医特色社区卫生服务中心和一个年产值3000万元的中药制剂中心。

医院人才济济，现有职工1128人，卫技人员953名，中高级职称人员369名，省、市名中医13名，硕士研究生导师6名，博士研究生10名、硕士研究生87名，全国名老中医工作室指导老师2人，国家优秀中医临床人才1人，省级优秀临床人才2人，省“333工程”重点人才2人，省中医领军人才及拔尖人才2人等。

医院制定了“技术专科化、专业化，服务精品化、人性化，标准数字化、国际化，经营品牌化、高效化，管理系统化、科学化，发展社会化、集约化”的发展战略。始终坚持突出中医特色，走专科发展之路，实现了重点专科率先发展，群体发展。目前，医院26个临床科室，有国家、省、市级重点专科32项（次）。心血管科为国家中医药管理局中医临床重点专科；皮肤科为卫生部财政部国家临床重点专科（中医专业）建设专科和国家中医重点建设单位；针灸科为国家中医药管理局重点专科建设单位；护理学为国家中医重点专科培育单位；中医药预防保健与康复临床能力为国家中医药管理局重点专科建设项目；心血管科和肛肠科为江苏省中医临床重点示范专科；心血管科、针灸科、肛肠科和皮肤科为江苏省中医重点专科；中医皮肤病学为江苏省中医重点学科建设单位；中医肛肠病学为江苏省中医重点学科培育单位；中医外科、风湿科为江苏省重点专科建设单位；肛肠科为徐州市优势学科和诊治中心，肛肠科和针灸科为徐州市医学重点学科；心血管科、针灸科、肛肠科、皮肤科、肾病科、脾胃病科、呼吸科、肾内科为徐州市中医临床重点专科；妇科、骨伤科和肿瘤内科为徐州市中医临床重点建设专科。此外，还拥有眼科、耳鼻喉科、口腔科、儿科、推拿科、男性病科、不孕不育科、生殖助孕科、康复医学科、重症医学科、急救中心、老年病科、介入科、普外科、脑外科、肿瘤外科、泌尿外科、胸心外科等一批中医特色突出，中西医结合显著的特色诊疗科室。医院获批21项省级二类医疗技术准入资质，列全市第三位，全省中医系统第二位。医院参加国家中医药管理局22个重点专科优势病种攻关协作组。

医院拥有日立核磁共振、飞利浦128层螺旋CT，DSA、岛津数字减影X线机、全套消化内镜、腹腔镜、经皮肾镜、输尿管镜、德国拜耳全自动生化分析仪等大型设备100件（套）。

医院坚持科教兴院，参与了国家“973”计划项目、国家科技支撑计划、全国中医药行业科研专项项目、江苏省科技厅课题，多次获得省市中医药科技进步奖，医院网站创办的网络医院被评为江苏省2011年“中医药十大新闻”。

医院先后荣获全国卫生系统先进集体、全国中医药文化建设试点单位、全国服务质量满意文明单位、全国最佳百姓放心示范医院、江苏省基本现代化中医院、江苏省文明单位、江苏省卫生系统先进集体、江苏省用户满意服务明星单位、江苏省中医药文化建设示范单位、徐州市人民满意医院、徐州市文明单位、徐州市卫生系统先进集体等荣誉。

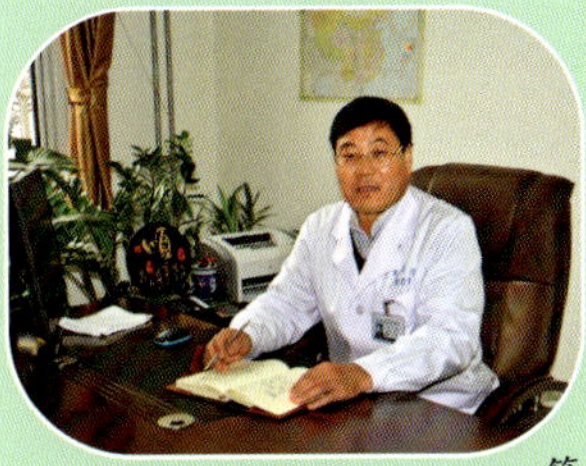
▲ 王培安院长

王培安 男、汉族、出生于1965年、中共党员，研究员，毕业于澳大利亚弗林德斯大学医院管理专业，研究生学历，现任徐州市中医院院长、党委副书记。

王培安同志长期从事医院管理和卫生行政管理工作，在创新医院发展战略，拓展学科建设思路，强化科学管理理念等方面成就显著。其先后担任徐州市卫生局基层卫生与妇幼保健处处长、医政处（保健处）处长，徐州市中心医院副院长，徐州市妇幼保健院院长、党委副书记；江苏省医院协会第二、三届妇幼保健院分会委员会副主任委员；徐州市医院协会第五、六届副会长、秘书长，徐州市中医学会副会长（常务）。曾多次被评为市卫生系统先进工作者、优秀党员、优秀领导干部。

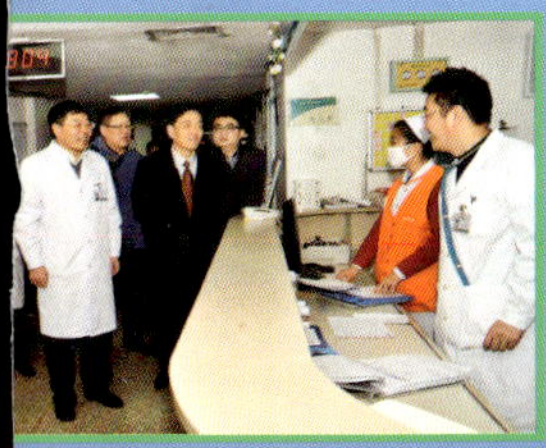
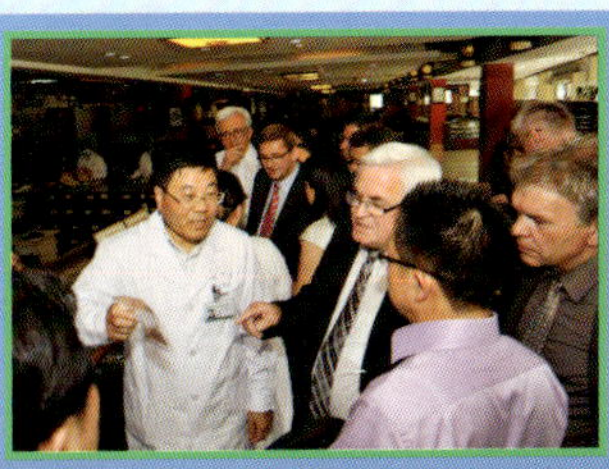
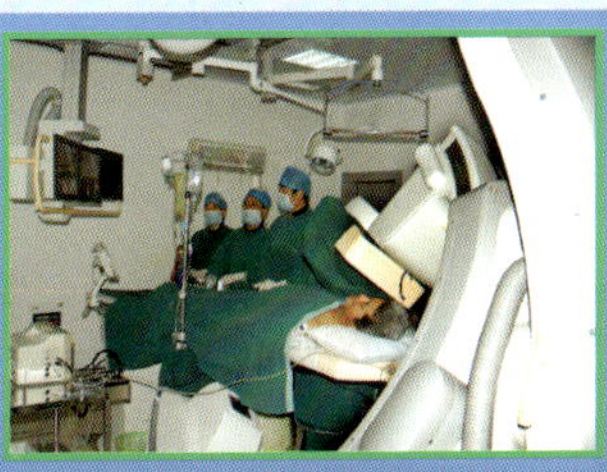
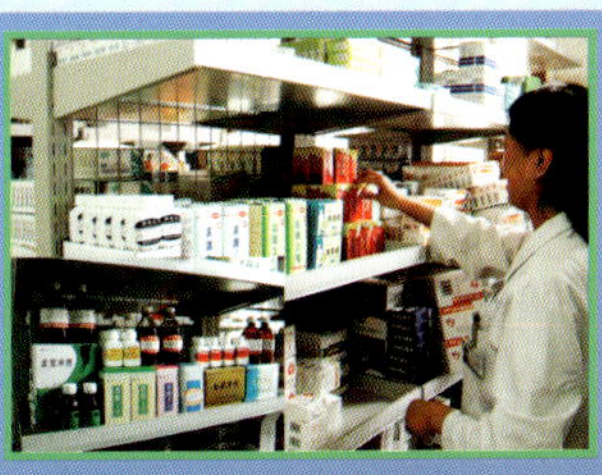
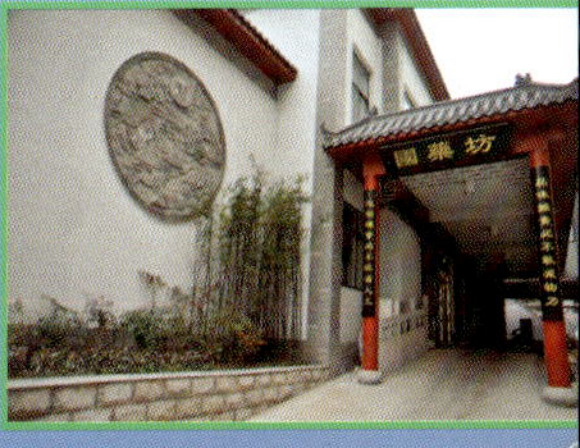

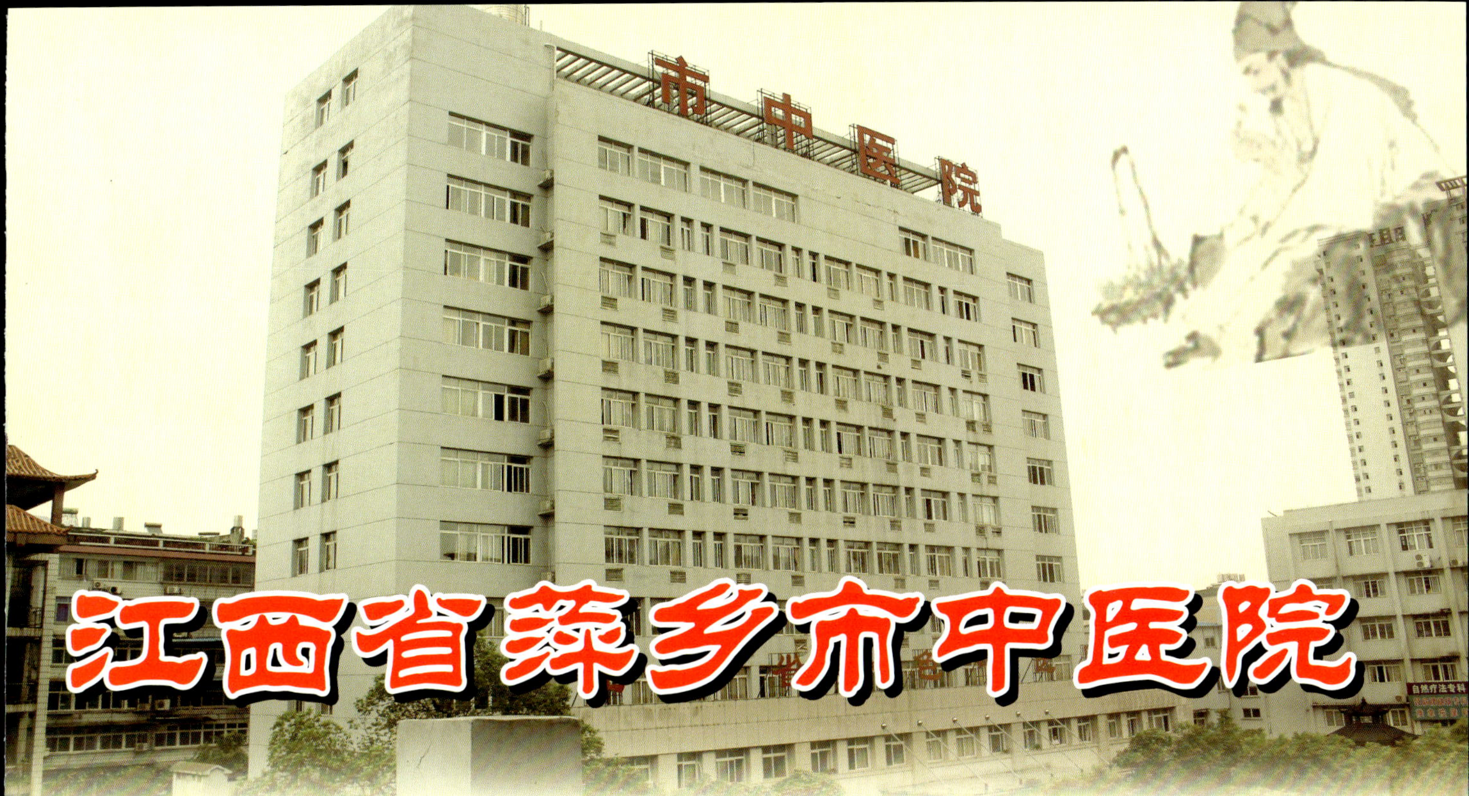

江西省萍乡市中医院

萍乡市中医院创建于1956年，“文革”期间被撤并，1979年复建，经过几代人的努力，发展成为一所中医药特色突出的现代化中医医院。1996年被评为三级乙等中医医院、国家级示范中医院，2004年获得江西省“群众满意医院”称号，2009年江西省卫生厅评定为江西省三级甲等中医医院，2011年获得江西省“特色中医医院”称号。2012年获国家中医药管理局三级甲等中医医院，是江西中医药大学临床教学基地。

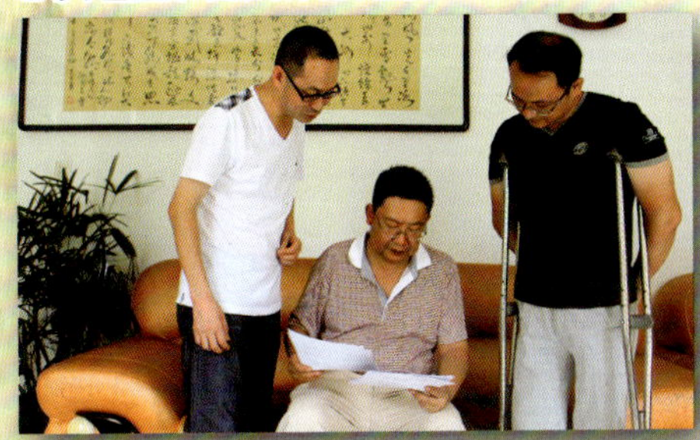

▲ 林家坤教授指导博士生、硕士生

医院现有在职职工529人，其中卫生技术人员441人，占医院职工总数的71%；注册执业医师190人，其中中医类108人，占62%；有主任中医师13人，主任医师1人，主任中药师1人，副主任中药师1人，副主任中医师19人，副主任医师7人，副主任护师3人，副主任技师1人。医院占地面积32亩，编制床位400张、实际开放床位430张。

开设一级临床科室29个：脑病科（中风病科）、肿瘤科、糖尿病科、心血管病科、脾胃病科、老年病科、肾病科、肝胆病科、神志病科、骨伤科、椎间盘病专科、外科、肛肠科、泌尿外科、重症医学科、妇产科、急诊科、针灸科、康复科、推拿科、口腔科、眼科、耳鼻喉科、皮肤科、儿科、麻醉科、感染性疾病科、预防保健科。设有药械科（下设药学部、医学装备管理部）、医学检验科、输血科、病理科、放射科、磁共振室、CT室、功能科、手术室、营养科等医技科室。拥有磁共振、双排CT，64排CT，DR2台、四维彩超、大C臂机、全自动生化分析仪、大型微波治疗仪、康复系统成套设备、中医四诊（体质）仪等大型诊疗设备。肿瘤科开展“海扶刀”技术、“热灌注技术”、“粒子射频消融技术”、肿瘤介入治疗。心内科已经开展了心脏支架植入技术。

萍乡人文底蕴丰厚，中医名家辈出。医院历年来重视中医药学术传承，现有国务院特殊津贴获得者1人，省政府特殊津贴获得者1人，全国优秀临床研修人才1人，全国名老中医药专家学术经验继承第一、二、三、四、五批指导老师7人、学术继承人12人。2013年经国家中医药管理局批准成立了王德祖名中医工作室。

医院中医药学术氛围浓厚，读经典、做临床，积极参与临床科研和学术总结，近年来先后出版了《伤寒方证研究》《张仲景方剂研究》《坤园笔谈》《中医临床手册》《坤园杂谈》《坤园论谈》《睡眠知要—失眠的整体疗法》《中医诊疗规范》《王德祖医学三书》等多部学术专著。学科建设长抓不懈，糖尿病专科被确定为国家中医药管理局重点专科，神志病专科被列为国家中医药管理局“十二五”重点专病培育项目，拥有全国名老中医药专家传承工作室1个，江西省中医药重点专科7个，是国家中医药管理局制剂能力建设单位，国家中医药管理局中医药治疗艾滋病定点单位，江西省糖尿病临床基地，江西省特色中医医院。

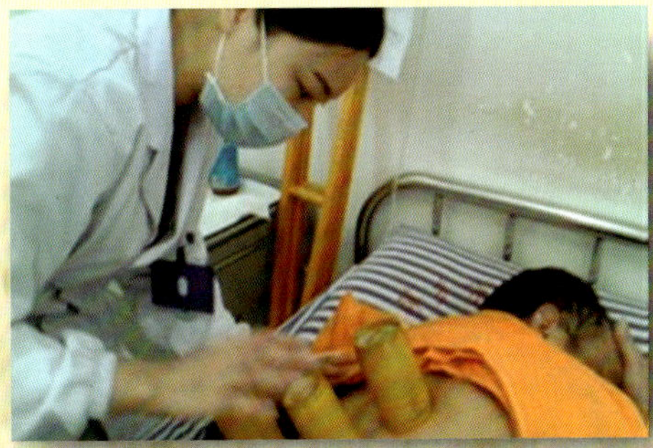

▲ 中医护理操作

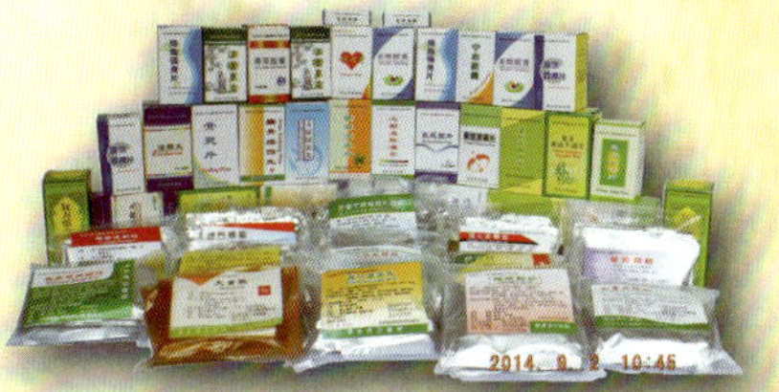

▲ 医院中药制剂产品

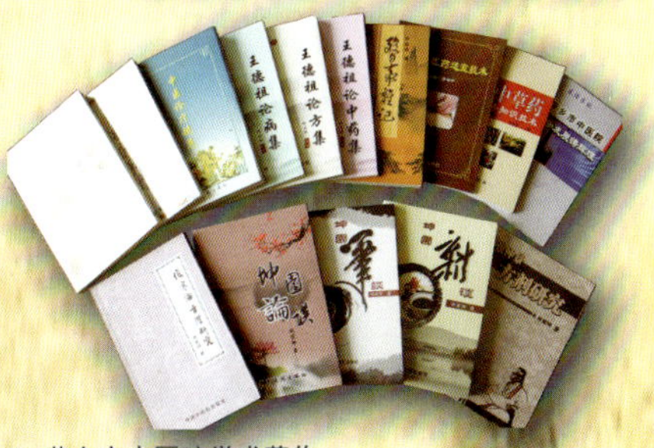

▲ 萍乡市中医院学术著作

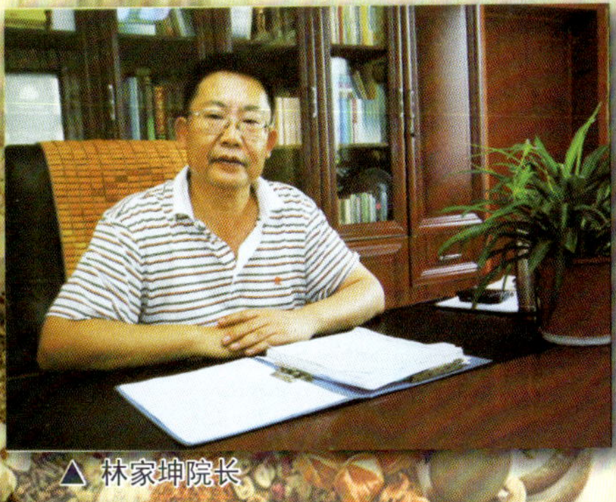

▲ 林家坤院长

林家坤 男，1962年出生，毕业于江西中医学院，获学士学位。萍乡市中医院院长，主任中医师，江西中医药大学教授，硕士研究生导师，南京中医药大学博士研究生导师，省政府特殊津贴获得者，国家中医药文化建设先进个人，江西省中医药学会理事，江西省医院管理学会中医医院管理专业委员会常务委员，江西省萍乡市中医药学会副会长，江西省名中医，第五批全国中医药专家学术经验传承指导老师。

大学毕业后一直从事中医临床工作，主攻肾病、肝病的中医药治疗，近年来致力于糖尿病、高脂血症等代谢性疾病临床诊疗、科研工作和中医养生法的研究。

国学功底深厚，学以致用，出版国学著作《读国学谈管理》。

从事中医临床工作30年，国家中医药第四批名老中医药专家学术继承人，师从全国名中医王德祖。潜心研究《伤寒论》20多年，主持或参与主持省市级科研课题多项，在中外学术期刊发表学术论文百余篇，先后出版医学专著13部，其中包括《伤寒论方证研究》《张仲景方剂研究》《坤园笔谈》《坤园杂谈》《坤园论谈》《中医临床手册》《中医诊疗规范》；收集全国名中医王德祖经验，主编《王德祖医学三书》。现担任国家中医药管理局“十一五”重点建设专科——糖尿病专科的学术带头人，研究采用中医养生、药膳、情志疗法综合防治糖尿病，临床实践倡导糖尿病肾病从“风”入手，临床运用虫类药搜风、贝类药平风、草类药熄风，研制出糖肾1号、2号、3号等投入临床使用。提出采用中医养生、药膳、情志疗法结合综合开展2型糖尿病中医药社区防治。主持研制的“贺普丁增效剂”“心脑血脉通”等制剂用于临床，临床疗效满意。

甘肃省天水市中西医结合医院（天水市第二人民医院）始建于1939年11月，经过70余年的发展，现已成为一所集医疗急救、公共卫生、科研教学、康复理疗、健康检查、职业病防治为一体的国家重点中西医结合医院、地市级中西医结合三级甲等综合医院和甘肃中医学院附属天水中西医结合医院。年门诊诊疗30余万人次、出院病人23000余人次、开展手术4600多台次。医院核定病床1030张，现有在职职工1200余人，其中正高职称26人，副高职称87人，中级职称207人，享受国务院特殊津贴专家1人，“甘肃省‘555’创新人才工程人才”1人，甘肃省中青年学术技术带头人2人，甘肃省优秀专家1人，甘肃省名中医4人，天水市领军人才2人，“天水市‘222’创新人才工程市级学术技术带头人”10人，天水市名中医3人。全院58个科室，其中临床科室32个，职能科室17个，医技科室9个。现有国家中医药重点专科1个、重点建设专科1个，省级中医药重点专科4个，市级医疗卫生重点学科12个。是甘肃省普外专业委员会腹腔镜外科学组天水培训基地，甘肃省天水腔镜诊疗培训中心，甘肃省肝胆胰外科研究所天水分所，兰州大学临床医学院肿瘤防治中心天水分中心，中国—巴基斯坦友好医院（甘肃省首家中外友好医院）。

医院先后荣获“全国卫生先进集体”“全国计划生育先进集体”“全国百姓放心医院”“全国百姓放心示范医院”“全国文化科技卫生‘三下乡’先进集体”，甘肃省卫生系统“医德医风先进集体”“省级价格计量信得过单位”“省级文明单位”“全省卫生系统精神文明建设先进单位”“甘肃省万名医师支援农村卫生工程先进支援单位”等10余项省级以上殊荣。

医院拥有国内先进的德国西门子256层双源炫速CT、德国西门子全数字化通用型平板血管造影系统（大C）、直线加速器、磁共振成像系统、西门子双板DR、直接数字化X线成像系统（DR）等大型医疗设备300余台件。医院先后有“中国围产儿出生缺陷监测及高发出生缺陷病因学探讨”等90余项科研成果获得部、省、市科技成果进步奖，“祛风湿药褥”等3项发明获国家专利，在省级以上刊物发表学术论文1000余篇。

近年来，原卫生部部长高强，副部长王陇德、曹荣桂、殷大奎、陈啸宏、王国强、尹力及副省长罗笑虎、冯健身、咸辉等领导先后赴院视察指导工作，对医院各项工作给予了充分的肯定。

展望未来，该院正以三级甲等中西医结合医院为新的起点，讲团结协作，重学术氛围，求服务质量，创医院特色，使医院真正成为一所专科优势明显、临床疗效显著、管理科学规范、示范带动作用突出的全国重点中西医结合医院和全国百姓放心示范医院，为百姓健康贡献力量。

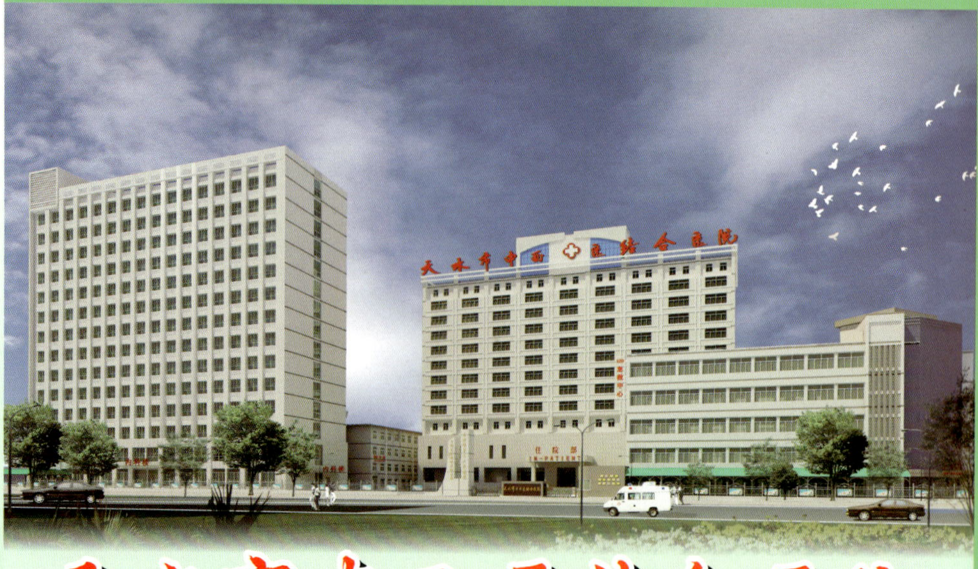

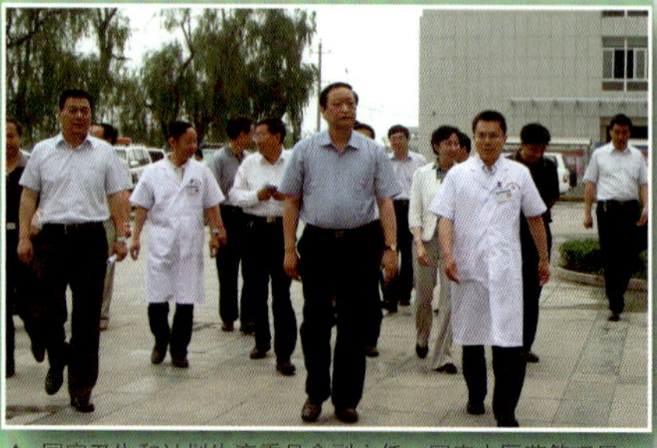

▲ 国家卫生和计划生育委员会副主任、国家中医药管理局局长王国强赴院调研

天水市中西医结合医院

杨国栋 男，1959年10月出生，中共党员，研究生学历，天水市中西医结合医院副院长、党委委员，中西医结合内科副主任医师，是甘肃省名中医和市级名中医，甘肃省中医药学会优秀工作者，甘肃省卫生行业精神文明建设先进个人，天水市市领军人才，天水市“222创新人才工程”学术技术带头人，天水市精神文明先进工作者，天水市首届扶残助残志愿者，兼任《中华实用中西医结合》杂志特邀编辑、《中华综合医学》特邀编委、《中华中西医结合杂志》专家编委、《天水中医》编委、中华中医药学会会员、中国中西医结合学会会员、中国文化研究会传统医学专业委员会专委、甘肃省中医药学会理事、甘肃省中西医结合学会常务理事、甘肃省医疗教育集团第一届理事会常务理事、甘肃省络病专业委员会副主任委员、甘肃省心脑血管病专业委员会委员、甘肃省虚证与老年病专业委员会副主委、甘肃省中西医结合急救专业委员会副主委、甘肃省康复医疗学会理事、天水市“治未病”研究会副会长、天水市伏羲中医药文化研究会副会长兼秘书长、天水市科技顾问团医疗卫生专业组顾问、甘肃省市级中医药师承教育工作指导老师、政协天水市麦积区第六届委员会委员。

他酷爱中医，精研细读《黄帝内经》《伤寒论》《金匮要略》《温病条辨》等经典著作，他学习记取了省名中医刘东汉、裴正学、刘国安、余元泰等教授的经验与特色，铭记裴正学教授“西医诊断、中医辨证、中药为主、西药为辅”的十六字方针、刘东汉教授“凭脉辨证，凭证用药，以西医诊断为依据，以中医辨证论治为准绳，师古而不泥古，参西而不背中”的诊治方略，践行“不读伤寒论，终是门外人”的信条，尊崇“熟读王叔和，不如临证多”的训诫，在临床上坚持“中西医并重”的思想方针，充分发挥中医药“简、便、廉、验”特色优势，在应用现代影像及临床检验等高精医疗设备检查分析的基础上，对临床疑难病症诊治能够灵活应用中西医结合方法治疗、突出中医特色、临床辨治讲究理、法、方、药进行施治，疗效满意，颇获好评。

他重视疾病的诊治与追访，积累了大量的科研资料及临床经验。总结撰写了《中医药对免疫学的认识及临床意义》《张仲景“伤寒论”方证学术思想研究》《中西医结合临床思路与方法总结研究》《裴正学教授中西医结合学术思想初探》《中西医结合治疗脑卒中临床观察研究》《中西医结合治疗急性病毒心肌炎临床疗效观察》《刘东汉教授中医药临床与学术思想研究》《益肺宁心汤治疗肺心病疗效观察》等文章40余篇。先后主持完成

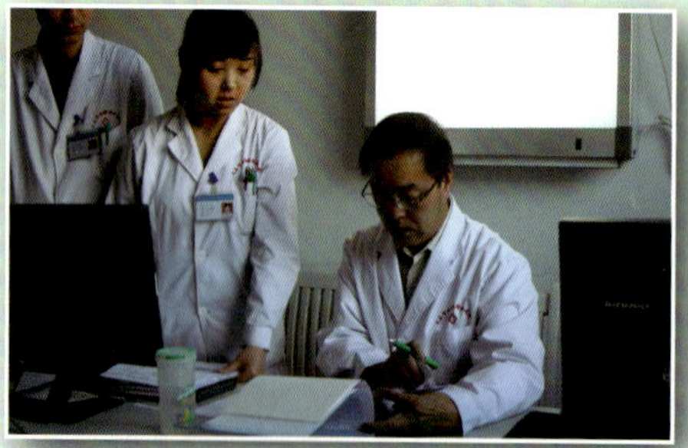

▲ 杨国栋副院长工作中

“心衰宁颗粒临床研究”“养精还神降粘颗粒治疗中老年病症及改善血液流变学临床研究”“祛风湿止痛药褥临床研究”等10余项临床科研项目，分别获得甘肃省皇甫谧科技进步二等奖2项、三等奖1项，甘肃省级科技进步三等奖1项，天水市级科技进步一等奖2项、二等奖3项、三等奖1项；撰写专著2部，主办省级以上继教项目10余项。

他坚持行政管理与临床业务齐抓并举，坚持两手抓、两手硬，改革讲效率、医疗讲疗效是硬道理。先后组织实施了医院人事分配制度改革行政后勤竞岗试点工作，带头创建“省级文明单位”“省级物价计量信得过单位”“全国百姓放心医院”“全国百姓放心示范医院”“三级乙等医院晋等达标”“天水市中西医结合医院申报、评估、验收”“省级重点专科的创建”“市级安全先进单位”和“全国第二批10所重点中西医结合医院建设”项目计划的拟定申报与创建组织实施，能够敏锐捕捉发展机遇，组织管理思路清晰，制定方案措施切合实际，能吃苦耐劳，顾全大局，谦虚谨慎，刻苦勤奋，时时刻刻讲党性、讲政治、讲正气，严于律己，清廉勤政，不计较个人得失，上下内外协调联系，坚持原则，作风纯朴，顽强拼搏，踏实认真，团结群众，构建和谐，以人为本，德行仁善，富于进取，求实创新，深受广大职工及社会的好评。

30多年来，无论是门诊还是病房，他热情待患，审慎求因，仔细诊查、中西兼顾、标本兼治、证病结合、药症相符，疗效验应，每年诊治数百病人，无医疗纠纷和事故发生。他博极医源，精勤不倦，继承创新，师古不泥，牢记为人民服务、救死扶伤的宗旨，为人民群众的医疗保健及中西医结合事业的发展倾尽所能。

▼ 血液净化中心

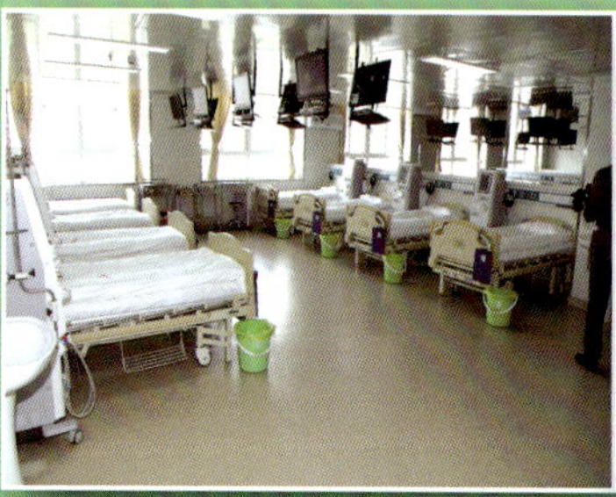

▼ 重症医学科

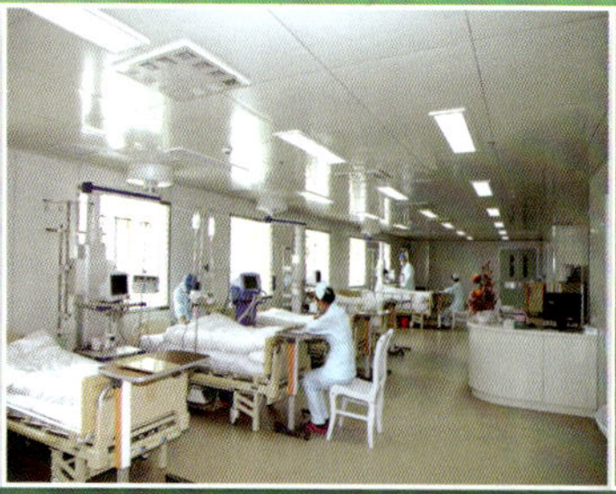

▼ 新生儿重症监护室

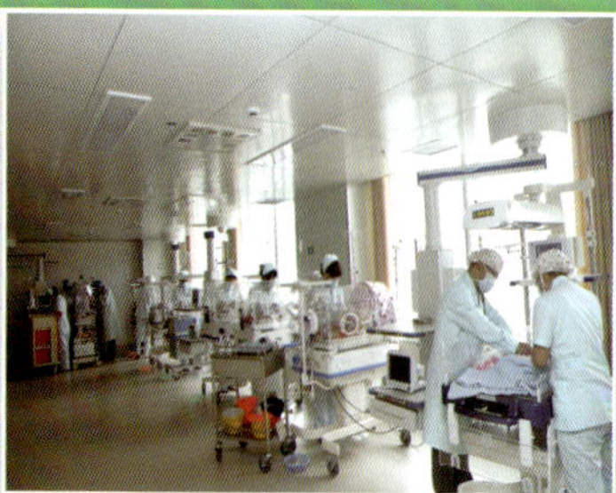

▼ 美国医学专家团来院学习交流

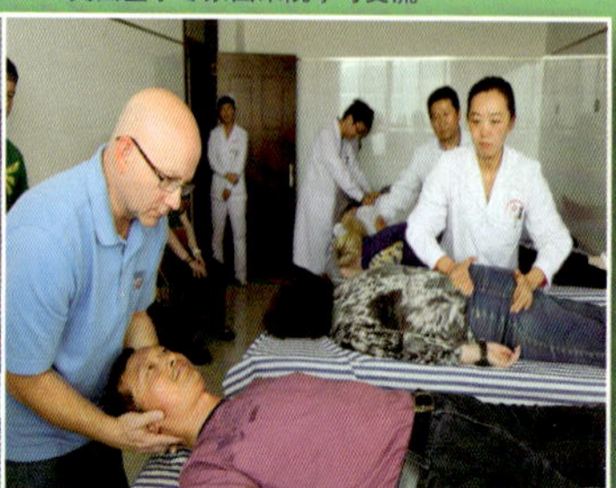

市黄陂区中医院整体规划鸟瞰图

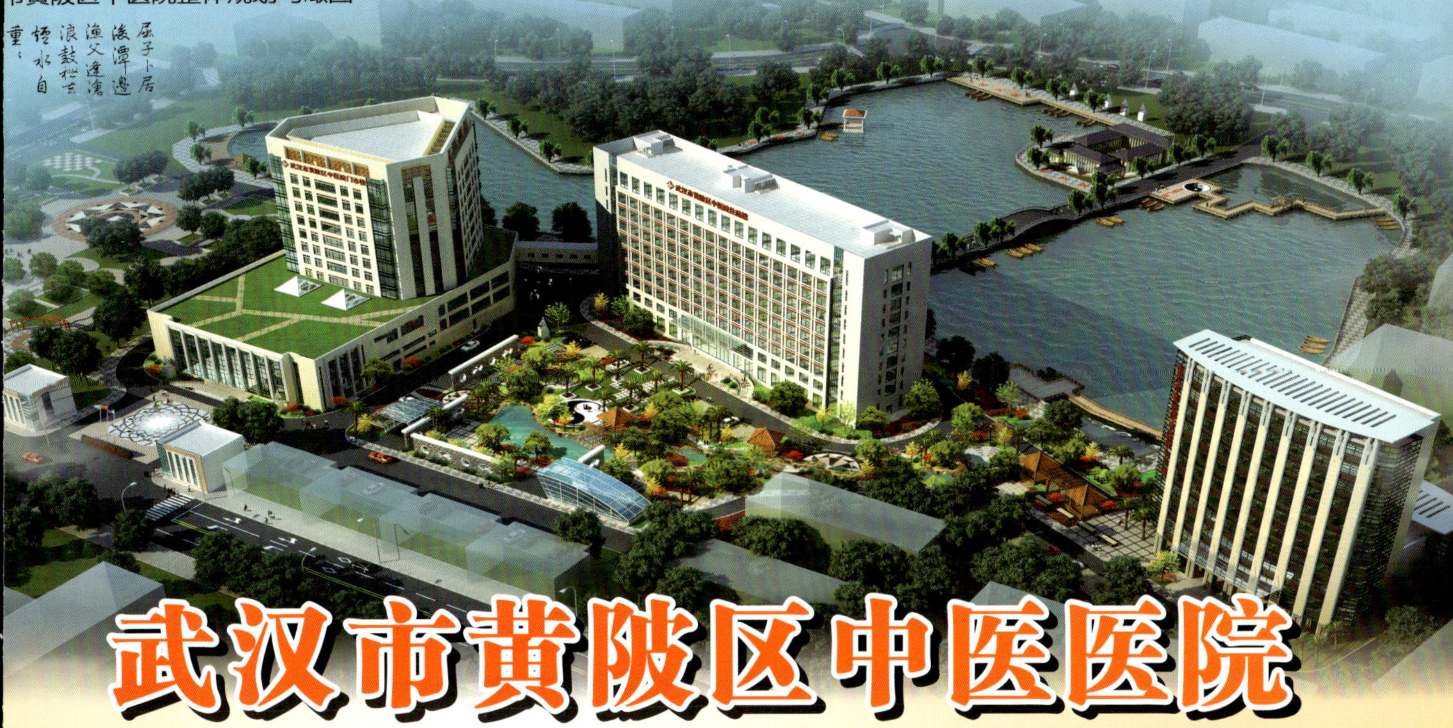

武汉市黄陂区中医医院

黄陂区中医医院坐落于“陂邑十景”之一的铁锁龙潭旁，四季风景怡人。是武汉地区唯一一所拥有“全国县级示范中医医院”称号和黄陂首家三级甲等医院殊荣的大型医院。

医院编制床位800张。设有心血管病科、脑病科、肺病科、肿瘤科、脾胃科、肾病科、外一科、外二科、妇产科、骨伤一科、骨伤二科、儿科、针灸科、肛肠科、康复理疗区等30个一级科室，其中脑病科、心血管病科、骨伤科、针灸科为“十二五”省级重点专科；妇科、肛肠科为“十二五”市级重点专科；2014年老年病科被授予“武汉市工人先锋号”称号。

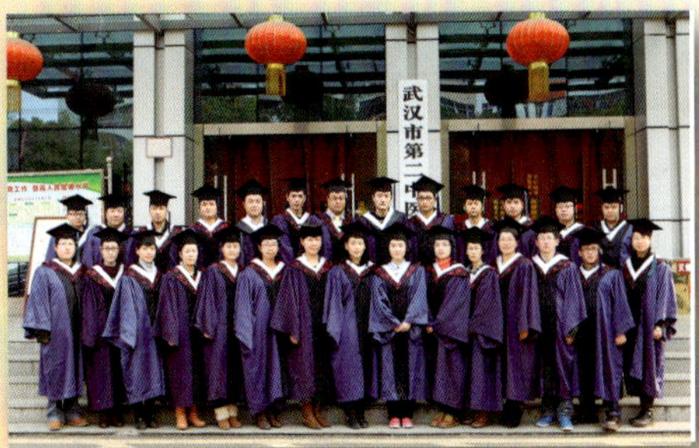

▲ 黄陂区中医院研究生团队

医院为湖北中医药大学教学医院，北京中医药大学东直门医院协作单位，湖北中医药大学硕士研究生培养基地。

医院现有人员612人，其中专业技术人员510人，高级职称94人，中级职称149人；研究生学历35人，本科学历219人，副院长王友明入选第三批全国优秀中医临床人才研修项目培养对象，外科彭建明，心血管病科陈朝金、王友明，脑病科高正主等正高级专家为湖北中医药大学硕士研究生导师。医院不仅有湖北省知名中医段世彪、武汉市知名中医杜献琛坐诊，还常年聘请全国知名中医涂晋文教授、张介眉教授带徒坐诊。

医院就医环境温馨舒适、设备先进，有全省一流的住院大楼以及设备一流的层流手术室。医院拥有核磁共振成像系统、双排CT，CR，DR数字成像系统、500毫安X线机、透析机、全自动生化分析仪、电视腹腔镜、电子胃镜、电子结肠镜等一批高精尖设备，50余台（套）中医诊疗设备，以及煎药收膏系统、床头呼叫系统、中心供氧系统、弱电智能化中央空调新风系统等。

医院秉承“仁和、精术、继承、创新”的院训，坚持“秉承中医传统、弘扬奉献精神、铸造卓越品牌”的发展战略和“严谨术精、态度至诚、德业同行、阳光温馨”的管理理念，以“生命至上、构建和谐、优质高效、追求卓越”的宗旨，全力打造百姓信赖医院。

2013年，医院被省卫生计生委批准加挂武汉市第二中医医院；经专家评审被国家中医药管理局批复为黄陂区首家“三级甲等中医医院”，被湖北省卫生计生委评为湖北省中医药文化建设示范单位。黄陂区中医药事业发展又登上了一个新的台阶。

同年，医院联合六指卫生院、长岭卫生院、木兰卫生院、姚集卫生院、蔡店卫生院、蔡榨卫生院、王河卫生院和环城社区卫生服务中心共9家医院组成医疗联合体。

2014年，结合医疗卫生体制改革重点，转型为健康管理联合体，与基层医疗卫生机构签定双向转诊协议，乡镇卫生院将其接诊病情较重或因设备技术原因不能确诊或疗效不佳的病人转至中医院治疗；中医院收治对口乡镇卫生院的病人，需要后期康复的，则将其转至相应卫生院继续治疗，形成优势互补，缓解群众看病难、看病贵问题。

同时黄陂区中医医院为8家卫生院提供业务指导和技术支持，组织专家团队下乡坐诊、查房，提升基层医疗机构的服务水平。医院不断改革创新，利用健联体的辐射力，为基层医疗机构送去贴敷膏药，让更多百姓在家门口就能享受到“冬病夏治”活动；并下乡开展义诊和咨询活动，为各类人群制定不同的健康计划，制定系列健教处方，广泛宣传健康生活方式的重要意义和中医“治未病”理念，以“健联体”方式切实为老百姓的健康服务。

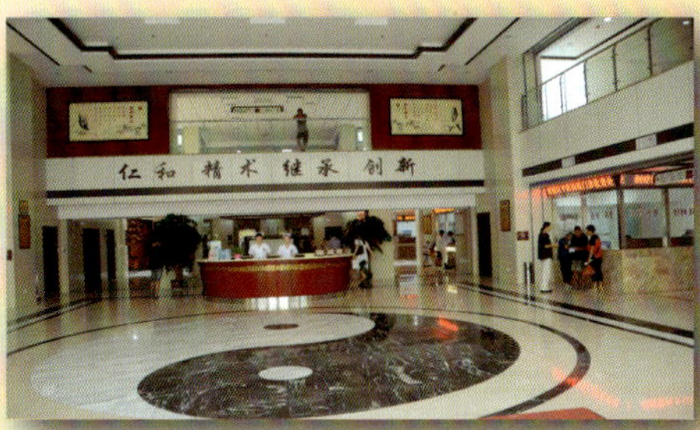

▲ 门诊大厅

医院成立了健康管理中心，设置中医养生保健门诊和心脑血管专科门诊，将社会“医、养结合”模式逐步推广到养老服务的体系中，与“老来乐”老年公寓联合打造“湖北省健康管理试点医养结合示范单位”，创新开展“医、养结合”健康管理模式。

医院新内科大楼正式投入使用，开放床位由原来的450张扩大到800张，缓解了黄陂区目前患者住院难的状况。同时医院正式挂牌成为湖北中医药大学教学医院和硕士研究生培养基地，加入了北京中医药大学东直门医院中医战略联盟，挂牌为北京中医药大学东直门医院协作单位。

▼ 硕士研究生导师

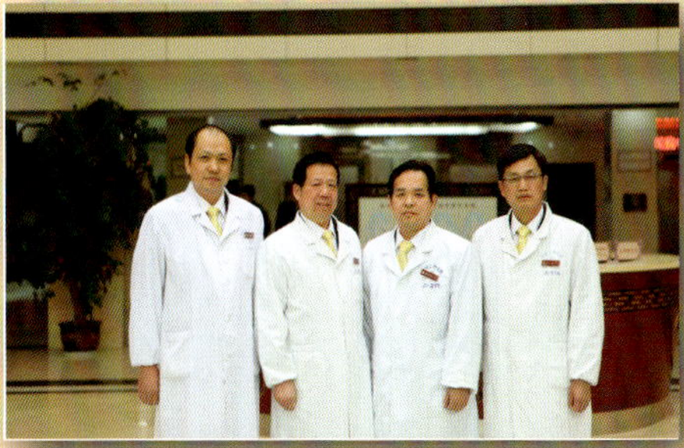

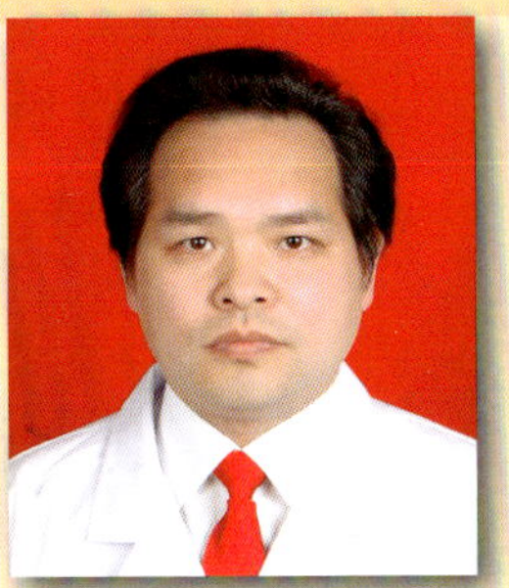

▲ 彭建明 黄陂区中医医院院长

彭建明 男，1963年6月出生，主任医师、教授，毕业于湖北医科大学、大学本科学历，现任黄陂区中医医院院长，湖北中医药大学硕士研究生导师。是黄陂区外科学术带头人，曾在北京协和医院、解放军总医院、上海瑞金医院等国家著名院校进修学习，清华大学医院管理高级研修班毕业。目前有1项省级科研已立项正在进行中，1项市级科研已验收、1项市级科研正在进行中，有7篇论文在国家核心杂志发表。是中国中西结合外科学会委员（全省区县级唯一一人）、湖北省外科学会委员（全市远城区唯一一人）、武汉外科学会常委、武汉中西结合腔镜学会副主任委员、武汉腹腔镜学会委员、湖北中医药大学外科教授、《中国实用医学杂志》编委、《中国医学研究杂志》编委；2007年黄陂区首届科技优秀人才，2007年黄陂区首届优秀拔尖人才，2009年获武汉市政府专项津贴，2011年获湖北省卫生先进个人荣誉，曾连续7年被评为优秀共产党员、黄陂区党代表，2012年被评为全市新城区科技界唯一三级正高职称；2012年4月当选为黄陂区青春励志人物。

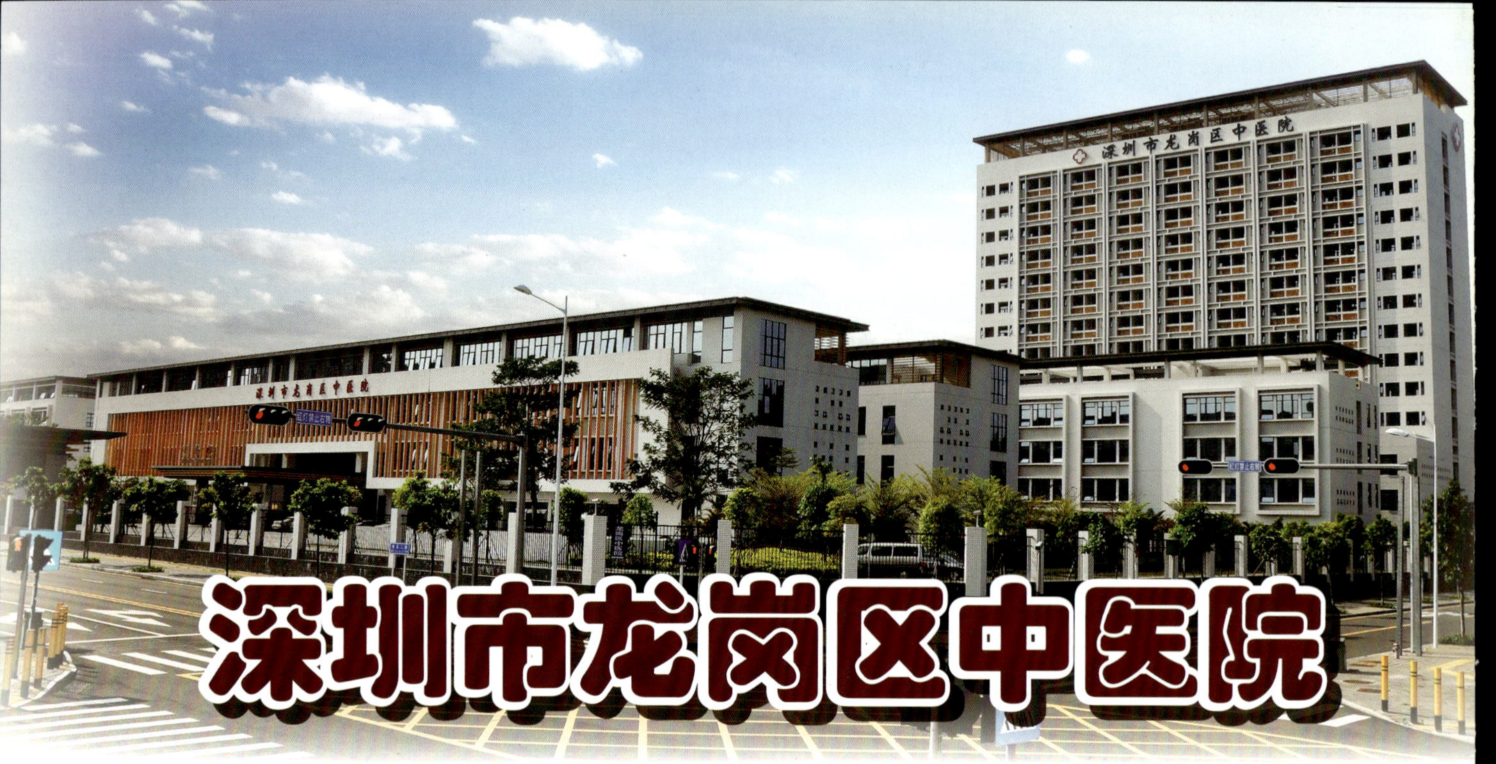

深圳市龙岗区中医院

龙岗区中医院于2012年12月28日正式开业，是深圳市龙岗区唯一一家公立中医院。是北京中医药大学东直门医院的战略联盟医院，广州中医药大学的教学实习医院，广东省中医院的协作医院，深圳市中医适宜技术培训基地，深圳市中医药学会中医传染病（肝病）专业委员会、中医优生优育委员会、中医科普专业委员会主委挂靠单位。

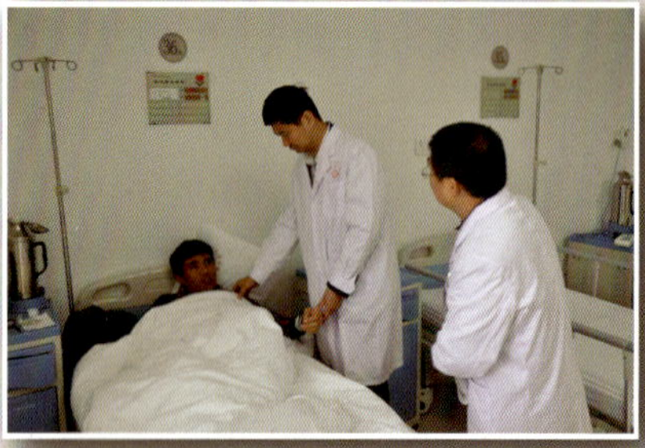

▲ 胡世平院长带队行政查房

医院占地面积6万平方米，总建筑面积8万平方米，设置床位数为500张，储备用地近8000平方米。该院广纳贤德才俊，依靠人才强院。目前有广东省名中医2名，深圳市名中医2名；高级职称医务人员51人；博士13人，博士后1人，博士生导师1人。现有设备总值近五千万元，包括飞利浦DR，64排螺旋CT、数字胃肠机、高档彩超，全自动生化分析仪等。

目前医院开放临床医技科室37个，其中市级特色专科5个。龙岗区中医院中医治疗率达到80%以上，是深圳市中医特色最浓厚的公立中医院。医院有肝病科、针灸推拿科、治未病中心、中医儿科、疼痛科、中医妇科、中医骨伤科等一大批专科特色浓郁的重点科室和颇具特色的专科疗法。

科研教学方面，医院在开业一年半时间内获得广东省中医药局科研资助课题立项3项，深圳市科创委科研资助课题立项1项，深圳市卫生局科研非资助课题立项2项，龙岗区科技局科研课题立项7项。2014年成功申报省市级中医继续教育项目共18项，是深圳市5家公立中医院项目最多的单位。

医院业务突飞猛进，开业一年半来，每季度业务量均按两位数递增，实现开业初期跨越式发展。医院以提高医疗质量和服务水平为目标，着力突出中医药特色优势，同步提高综合医疗服务能力，积极推进内涵建设，夯实医院基础，全院广大医务员工牢记使命，勤奋工作，社会影响力不断扩大。

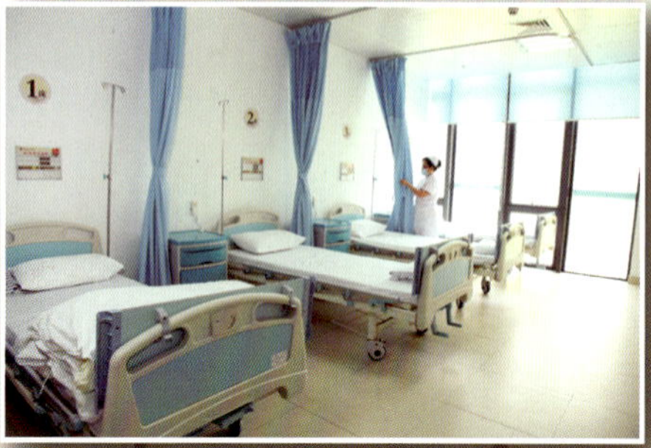

▲ 病房

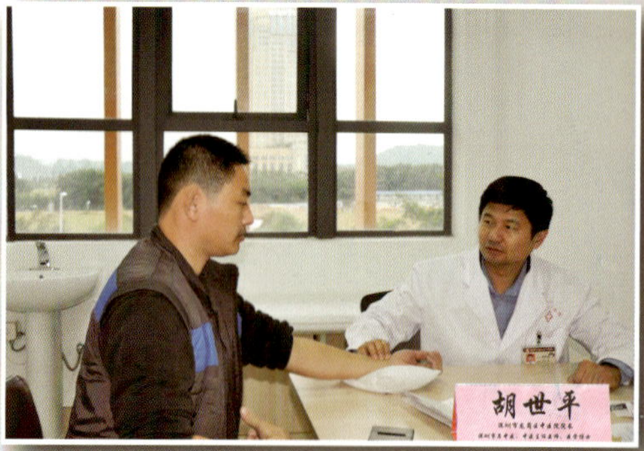

▲ 胡世平院长坐诊

胡世平，主任医师，院长，广州中医药大学教授、硕士生导师，首批深圳市名中医、医学博士，毕业于广州中医药大学。深圳市中医药学会副会长、传染病（肝病）专业委员会主任委员，深圳市中西医结合学会常务理事。

擅长运用中医药治疗慢性乙型肝炎、脑动脉硬化症和其他内科常见病、多发病和疑难杂症，如肝硬化、胃肠疾病、男性功能障碍、女子不孕症，及脉管炎、静脉炎、动脉硬化闭塞症等周围血管疾病，并在多年的潜心研究与临床实践中形成了独特的学术思想体系，包括“慢性乙肝从正虚邪恋立论，突出中医辨证治疗”“正虚血瘀是脑动脉硬化的基本病机”等。创立了“肝敷康”穴位敷贴的内病外治法，对慢性乙肝有显著疗效；开发研制了治疗乙肝的国家级新药（国药准字B20020282号）及治疗呼吸系统疾病的新药（豫卫药健字Z35号），研制了“柴芪益肝颗粒”“通脉灵”“溶栓通络丸”等协定方，并取得了良好的疗效。

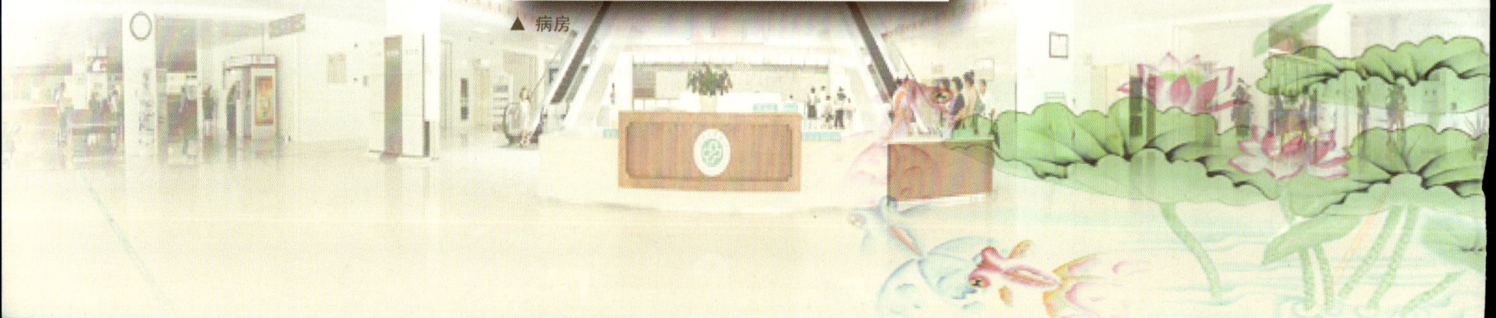

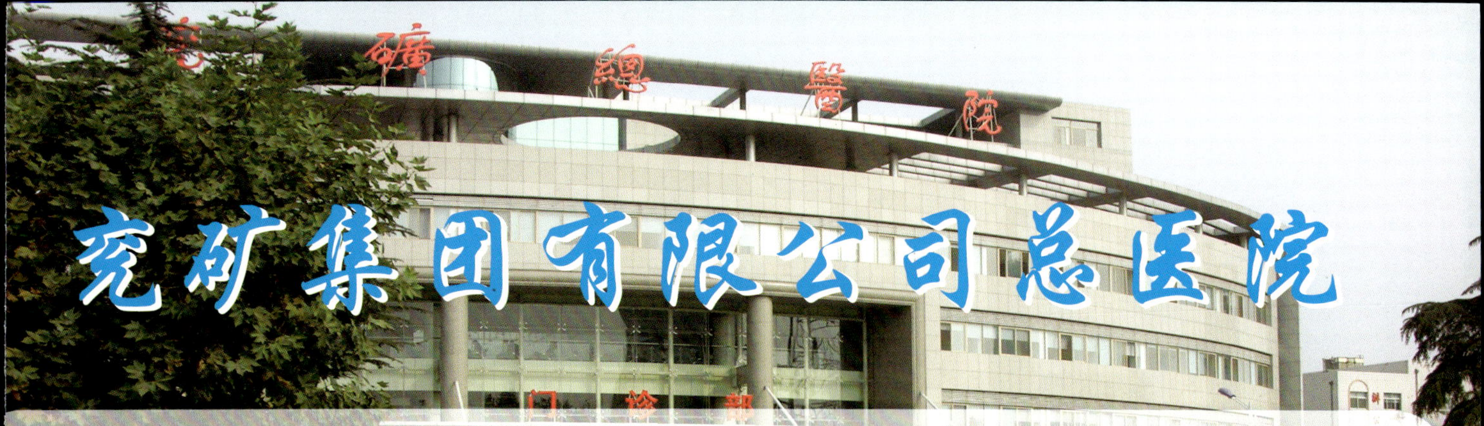

兖矿集团有限公司总医院

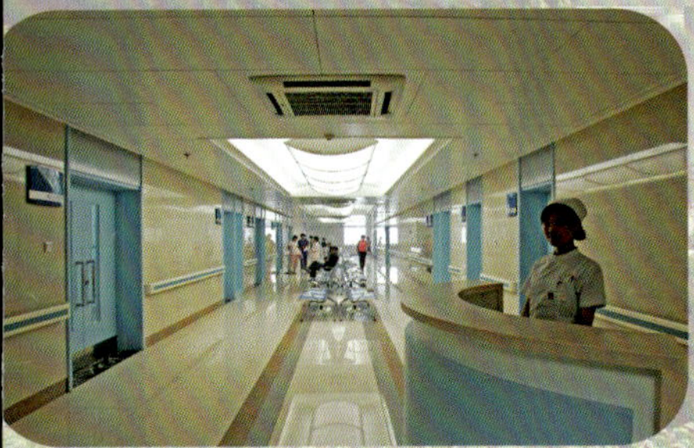
▲ 医院内部

兖矿集团总医院隶属于兖矿集团，创建于1972年9月，是当地唯一一家具有综合医疗服务功能的国家三级甲等医疗服务机构。开放床位1100张，职工1658人。其中，卫生医技人员占全院总人数的79.56%。医院所在社区人口120多万，服务半径约100公里，医院占地200余亩，建筑面积9.3万平方米，总资产5.7亿元。医院有3.0 T核磁共振、电子直线加速器、多座位高压氧舱、螺旋CT、多排CT，ECT、全自动生化分析仪、DR、高档彩超、大型X线机、DSA西门子智能机器人等万元以上的医疗设备1535台（件）。设有56个诊疗科室，其中，中医科为山东省中医药大学硕士研究生培养基地；山东省综合医院中医药工作示范单位；普外科、骨科、放化疗科、心内科、消化内科、神经内科、检验科、中医科、急诊科、感染疾病科、烧伤整形科是济宁市重点专科（专业）。下设3个分院和13家社区卫生服务站，并特设劳动卫生职业病、结核病和妇幼保健3个防治所。医院现有高级专业技术人员225人、中级专业技术人员645人，具有硕士博士学位71人。年门诊量73万人次以上，年出院病人3.5万余人次。经过40年的建设与发展，医院已成为一所集医疗、急救、教学、科研、预防、职业病防治为一体，专科特色突出的现代化国家三级甲等综合医院。是国家宫颈癌防治定点医院，济宁医学院、华北煤炭医学院等十几所医学院校的教学医院；济宁市新农合、城镇职工、居民、工伤保险定点医院。医院与北京中医药大学东直门医院、解放军总医院、卫生部中日友好医院、首都医科大学地坛医院、山东省立医院、齐鲁医院等建立了友好协作关系，这些医院定期派专家来院技术指导。

建院40年来，全院干部职工牢记为矿区及周边企业安全生产服务、为人民群众身体健康服务的宗旨，坚持以病人为中心、以质量为核心，走科技兴院、质量强院、文化建院、诚信立院之路，服务无止境、热情到永远。树立建设现代化一流大医院的远大目标，争创人才一流、技术一流、设施一流、服务一流的综合性医院。

医院始终坚持以病人为中心、以质量为核心、服务大众、奉献社会，通过实施“四零工程”（医患零距离、服务零投诉、诊疗零差错、科室零纠纷），开展“三好一满意”、先看病后付费、优质护理服务、“星级服务窗口”竞赛、温馨医院创建、“安康杯”劳动竞赛、青春笑脸等活动，各项工作有了长足的发展，整体面貌日新月异，在业界树立了良好品牌形象。先后被评为全国煤炭工业先进集体、全国百家“三好一满意”示范医院、全国医疗保健服务质量优秀示范医院、全国诚信示范医院、全国医疗质量信得过优秀医院 、全国综合医院中医药工作示范单位、山东省综合医院中医药工作示范单位、山东省中医药养生治未病中心、2010年度山东省百姓口碑最佳荣誉单位、山东省优质医疗服务示范单位、山东经济文化强省建设先锋集体 、山东省健康体检工作先进集体、山东省和谐发展示范医院、2012年度济宁市医疗管理工作先进单位、济宁团市委优秀青年志愿者先进集体；连续六年获得集团公司先进基层党委、“四好”领导班子和优秀单位称号。

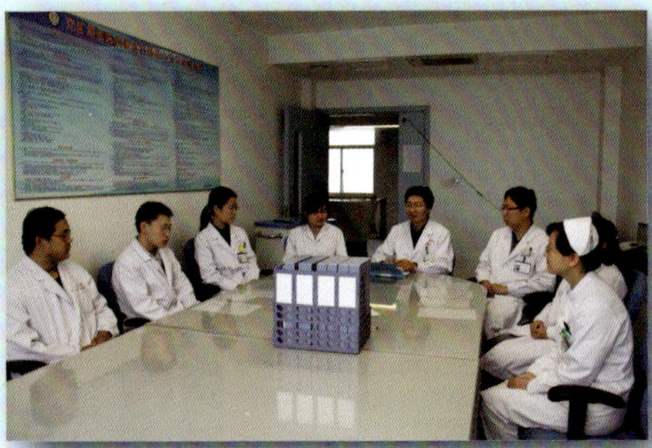
▲ 召开科室会议

殷晓轩 兖矿集团有限公司总医院副院长，山东中医药大学硕士研究生导师、济宁医学院中医学兼职教授，全国中医专家委员会常务委员、济宁市中医药学会理事、中华医学会继续教育学会青年委员、中国医师协会肿瘤专业委员会委员、山东中医药学会肝病专业委员会委员、山东中西医结合学会肝病专业委员会委员、山东中西医结合学会康复专业委员会委员、山东中西医结合学会心理学专业委员会委员、济宁市中医药学会肝病专业委员会主任委员、济宁市中医药学会脉学专业委员会副主任委员，《中华临床医学杂志》常务编委。

分管医院教学科研、东院区和20个社区的医疗安全、主持中医科、康复科的科室建设工作，全面完成科室医疗任务，门诊量、出院病人和经济收入较往年有了大幅度提高。在集团公司领导和医院领导的支持鼓励下，经过科室成员共同努力，中医科已逐渐成为集中医治疗、康复治疗、针推理疗、治未病与养生指导和中药配送为一体的综合性科室。现在科室已成为具有崭新健康理念的、现代化的、又不失传统中医学精髓的集医疗、养生、

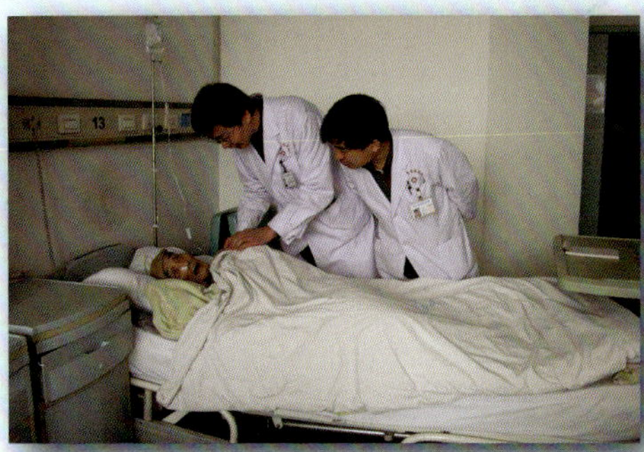
▲ 查房

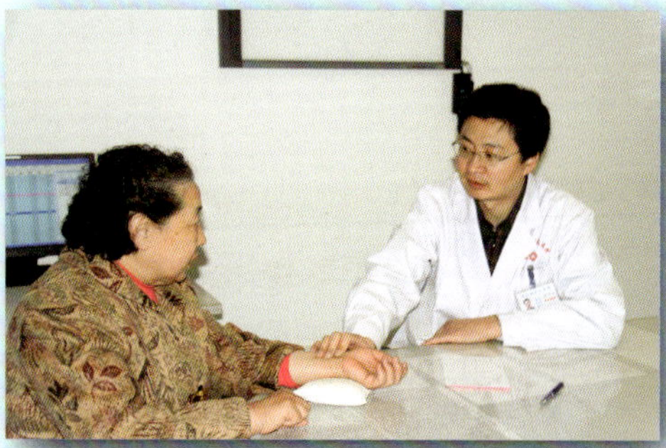
▲ 殷晓轩副院长坐诊

科研和教学为一体的中医药服务单位。

多年来，对中医内科学消化系统疾病作了深入的专题研究，能在临床中灵活运用中医辨证方法，仔细遣方用药。在肝病的中医药治疗上，强调随症加减，坚持环节用药，注重阶段用药，将宏观辨治与局部微观用药相结合，总结出“治肝九法”等一系列行之有效的治疗方法和规律，取得良好的临床疗效。

积极参与科研攻关，撰写学术论文10余篇，获国家医学技术专利3项、参与撰写专著书籍2部；以主要研究者身份参与完成了省级“十一五”公关课题，获山东省科技进步三等奖；参与完成了兖矿集团立项科研课题，获兖矿科技进步三等奖；参与国家“十一五”科技重大专项研究，山东省中医局课题，济宁市“十二五”重大专项课题等。先后获兖矿第二、三、四、五届优秀学科带头人、兖矿优秀医务工作者、兖矿首届道德模范提名、兖矿第二届廉洁奉献道德模范、济宁市中医工作先进个人、济宁市名中医药专家、济宁市优秀名中医以及医院级别的诸多荣誉。

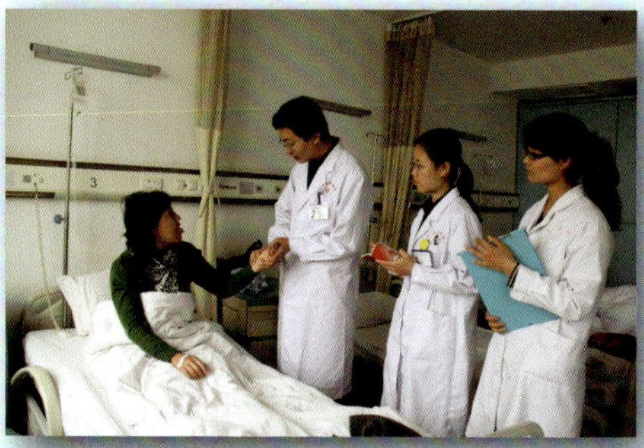
▲ 殷晓轩副院长临床带教

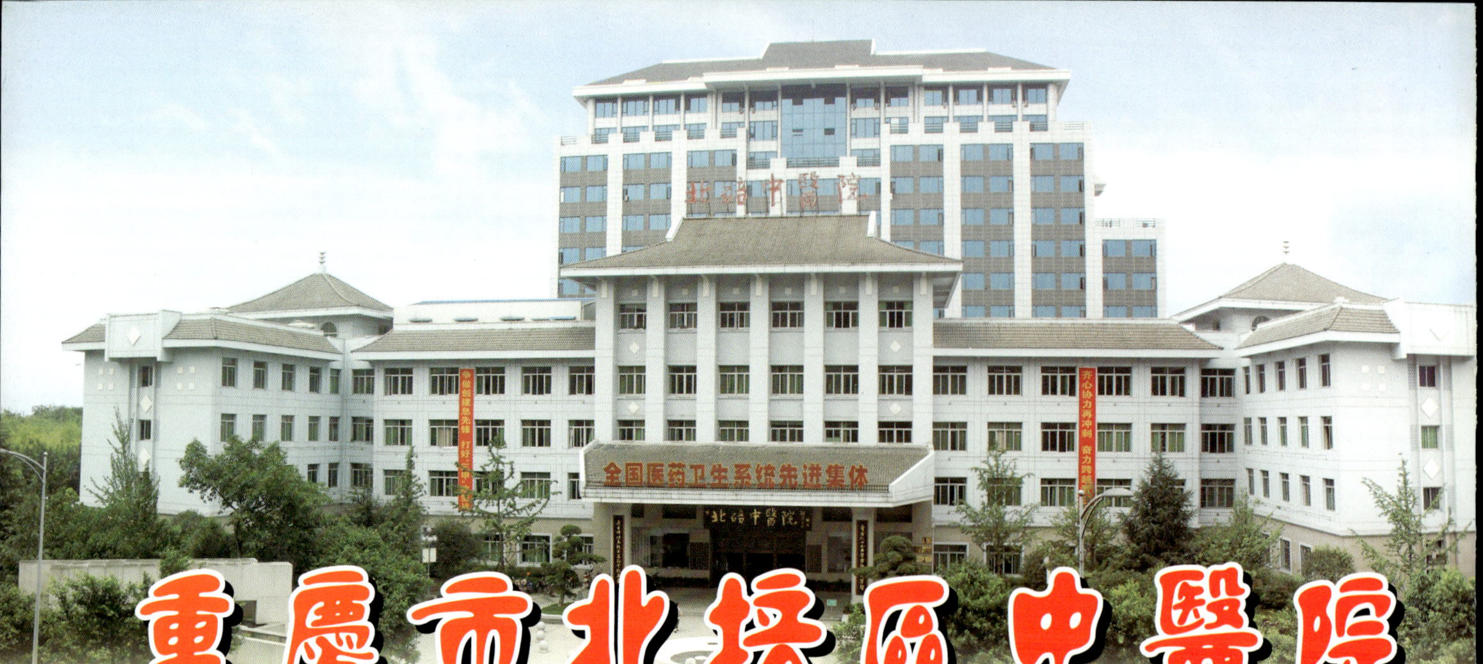

重慶市北碚區中醫院

北碚区中医院始建于1953年，座落于素有“都市花园、人文福地、宜居之城、两江新秀”美誉的重庆市北碚城区内，是一所学科设置齐全、技术力量雄厚、中医特色突出、设备配套先进，集中医医疗、教学、科研、预防保健和康复于一体的三级甲等中医医院；是广州中医药大学附属医院，成都中医药大学、重庆医科大学、西南大学药学院等多家高校的教学医院，广东省中医院协作医院；是全国中医药继续教育基地、教育部“本科教学工程”国家级大学生校外实践教育基地和重庆市中医住院医师规范化培训基地。先后荣获全国医药卫生系统先进集体、全国中医药文化建设先进单位、重庆市十佳医院、重庆市文明单位等多项殊荣。

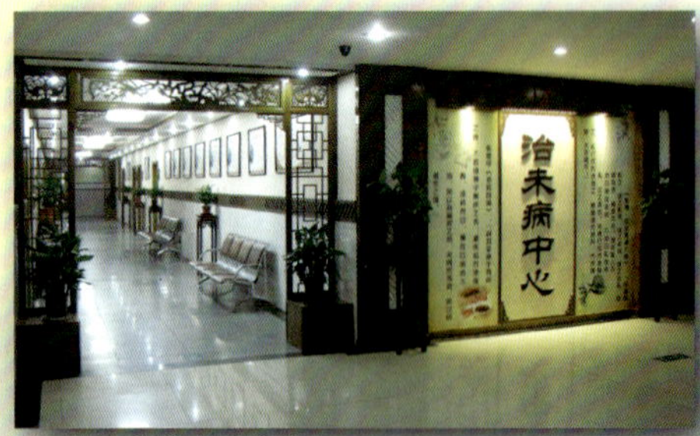

▲ 全国第四批“治未病”预防保健服务试点单位

医院占地60亩，业务用房面积4.8万平方米，固定资产总值2.88亿元，编制床位470张，开放床位710张。开设内科、外科、妇（产）科、儿科、针灸科、推拿科、治未病科等临床科室29个和医技科室10个。年门诊35万人次，出院2.2万人次。

医院技术力量雄厚。在全院在岗职工869人中，本科及以上学历348人，其中博士5名，硕士44名；专业技术人员697人，其中高级专业技术人员67人，中级专业技术人员139人；有全国师带徒导师2名、学术继承人8名，市级师带徒导师2名、学术继承人4名，区级师带徒导师21人、学术继承人34人，广州中医药大学硕士生导师6名，全国优秀基层中医1名，西部之光访问学者1名，跨世纪学科带头人1名，重庆市高级中医药人才2名，重庆市高级中医药人才培养对象4名，重庆市名老中医1名，重庆市优秀青年中医1名，北碚区名中医15名。

医院专科特色突出。拥有国家临床重点专科建设项目2个（脑病科、耳鼻喉科）、国家中医药管理局“十二五”重点专科建设项目1个（耳鼻喉科）、国家中医药管理局“十一五”重点专病1个（中风病）、国家级中医药特色专科4个（耳鼻喉科、骨伤科、针灸科、肺病科）；重庆市中医重点专科6个（脑病科、耳鼻喉科、骨伤科、心血管科、肿瘤科、肾病科）；市级中医药特色专科1个（针灸科）；区级重点专科1个（脾胃病科）；治未病中心是全国第四批“治未病”预防保健服务建设试点单位，并承担中医预防保健于康复能力建设项目。中药制剂室是重庆市中医药科研二级实验室，拥有制剂批文品种60个、自主知识产权品种19个。

医院科研成效显著。作为国家“十一五”科技支撑计划重大项目课题分中心，建有国家中医药管理局中医药科研二级实验室1个，近3年立项科研课题21项、结题13项，获科研成果9项、国家专利3项，研制的“冰莲清咽喷雾剂”获批为三类新药，发表论文134篇，主编专著1部，参编专著2部。

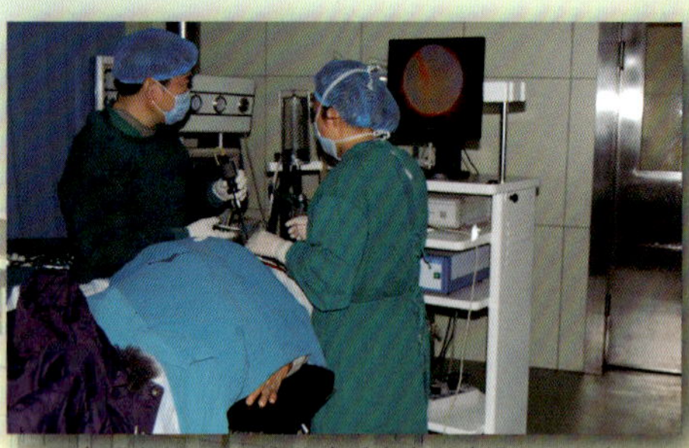
▲ 耳鼻咽喉科——国家临床重点专科建设项目科室

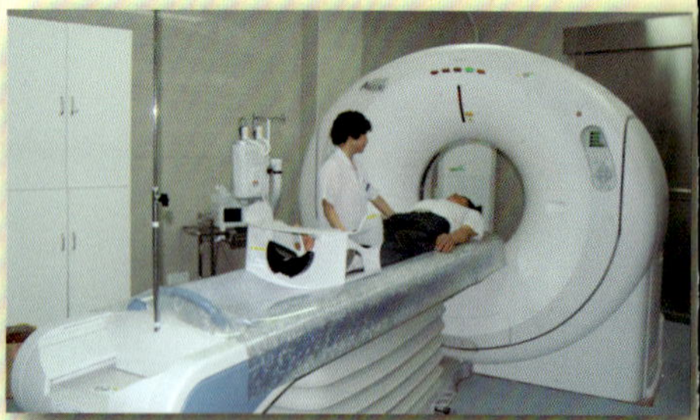
▲ 日本东芝64排128层螺旋CT

医院中医药文化氛围浓厚。作为全国中医药文化建设先进单位，全院职工牢固树立大医精诚的核心价值观，《员工手册》人手一册，悬挂院徽统一形象，高唱院歌凝聚精神，奉行院训规范行为，印制读本传播文化，被誉为“重庆中医的一张名片”。国家卫计委副主任、国家中医药管理局局长王国强视察医院时给予了“印象深刻、不虚此行，认真总结、值得推广”的高度评价。

医院医疗设备先进。拥有美国通用GE Signa HDe 1.5 T超导磁共振（MRI）、日本东芝64排128层螺旋CT、日本日立彩超、美国GE彩超、日本奥林巴斯电子胃肠镜系统、日本潘太克斯胃肠镜系统、美国贝克曼全自动生化分析仪、体外冲击波碎石机、美国史赛克腹腔镜系统、500 ma X线机和中医经络检测仪、美国/IL全自动血凝分析仪等一大批先进诊疗设备。

面对未来，医院将始终坚持“文化铸魂、品牌立院、发挥特色、群众满意”的办院宗旨，继续秉承“病人至上、优质服务”的办院理念和“弘扬国粹、自强不息”的医院精神，不断推进继承创新，充分发挥特色优势，努力打造“管理规范化、人才精英化、科室特色化、设备现代化、服务人性化、环境园林化”的现代化综合性“三甲”中医医院，为人民的健康事业，播撒杏林春晖！

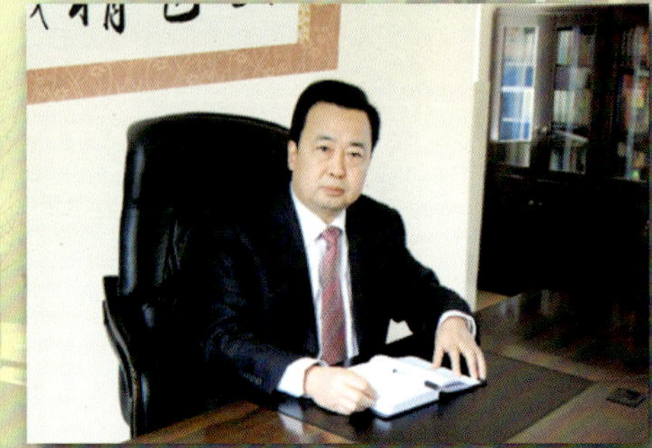
▲ 尹平　北碚区中医院 院长

尹平 男，汉族，重庆北碚人，中共党员，西南大学经济与现代管理研究生。现任北碚区中医院院长；兼中华中医药学会医院管理分会常委，重庆市中医药行业学会副会长，为广州中医药大学硕士研究生导师，北碚区第八届、第九届、第十届、第十一届党代会代表。

自2007年担任医院院长以来，团结带领全院干部职工，以持续改进医疗服务质量为重心，全面加强医院内涵建设为重心，不断提高人民群众健康水平为核心，举全院之力修建住院大楼，聚全院之智创建“三甲”医院，在医院改革、规范管理、人才培养建设、学科建设、科技创新、医疗质量、行风建设、医院文化等方面取得了长足的进步和发展。2012年，有着60年历史的北碚区中医院成功晋级“三甲”医院，因其管理有方，成绩卓著，先后荣获了“全国中医药系统创先争优先进个人”“全国中医药急诊急救能力先进个人”“重庆市卫生系统抗震救灾先进个人”“重庆市西部大开发工作先进个人”“重庆市优秀共产党员”等称号。

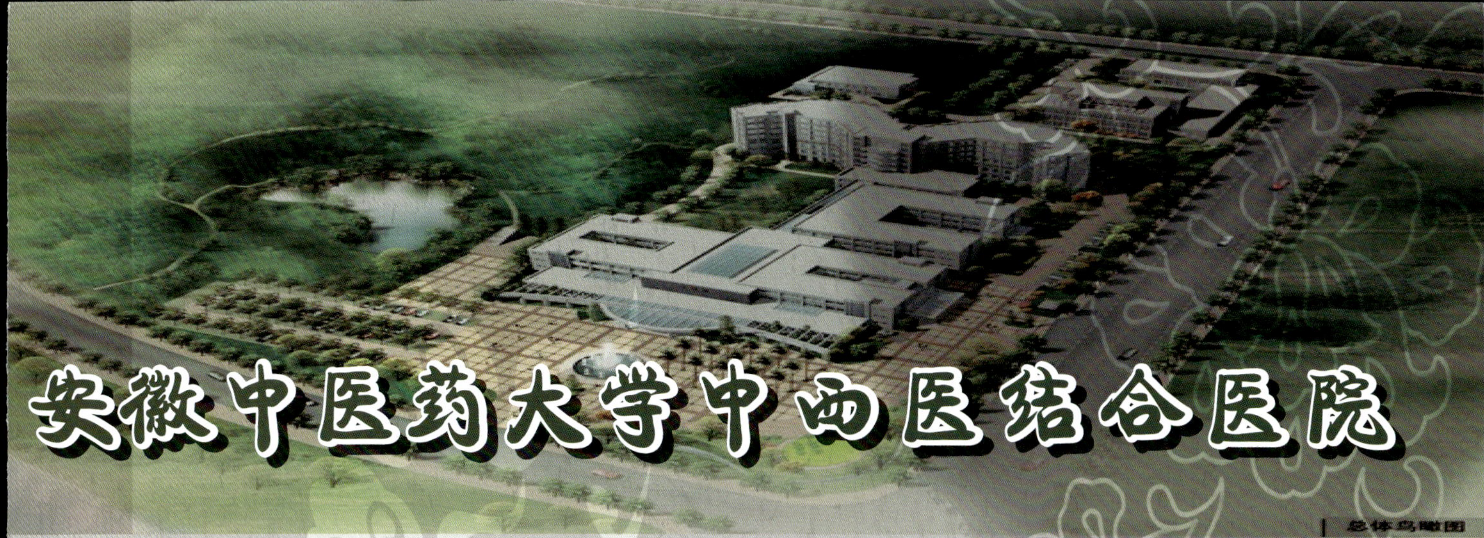

安徽中医药大学中西医结合医院

总体鸟瞰图

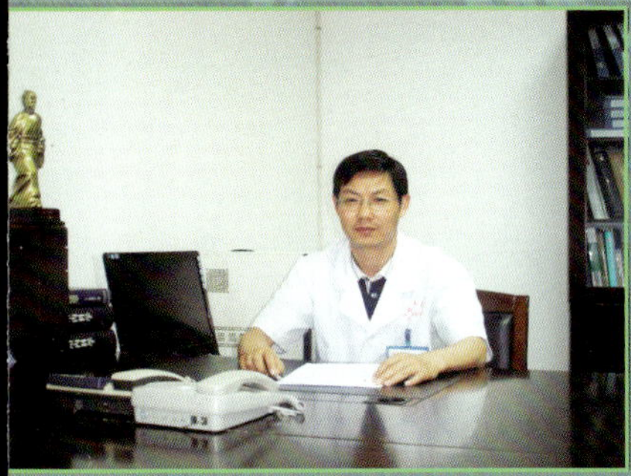

何光远院长

何光远 院长，主任医师，硕士研究生导师。现为国家中医药管理局"十二五"推拿重点专科学术带头人，安徽省中医药管理局针灸推拿重点专科学术带头人、国家名老中医李业甫教授推拿名医工作室学术继承人。

兼任民进安徽中医药大学支部主委、民进安徽省委科技与医卫工作专门委员会副主任、中华中医药学会推拿专业委员会副主任委员、安徽省中医药学会推拿专业委员会主任委员、安徽省中医药学会常务理事、安徽省灸法研究会副会长、安徽省老年学研究会副会长、中国中西医结合学会养生学与康复医学专业委员会常务委员、安徽省针灸学会理事、中华医学会安徽分会物理医学与康复学第七届委员会常务委员、中国老年学学会第五届理事会理事、中华中医药学会医院管理分会常委。担任《安徽中医药大学学报》第四届编委会委员，《中华中西医临床杂志》《医学综述》第三届编委会委员，《中国中医药年鉴(学术卷)》特邀编委。

近年来，主持并参加国家自然科学基金、国家中医药管理局、省卫生厅、省教育厅、省科技厅等10余项科研课题研究，获省科技成果奖 1 项。发表医学论文 10 余篇，主持编写《推拿学》、《运动系统常见疾病临床检查图解》、《中国疾病相关基因与基因诊断》、《中医康复学》(普通高等教育"十一五"国家级规划教材暨新世纪全国高等中医药院校康复医学专业创新教材)、《实用小儿推拿》、《实用美容推拿》6 部医学专著及教材，参编《推拿学》、《推拿手法学》(普通高等教育"十二五"国家级规划教材新世纪全国高等中医药院校规划教材) 2部国家级规划教材。

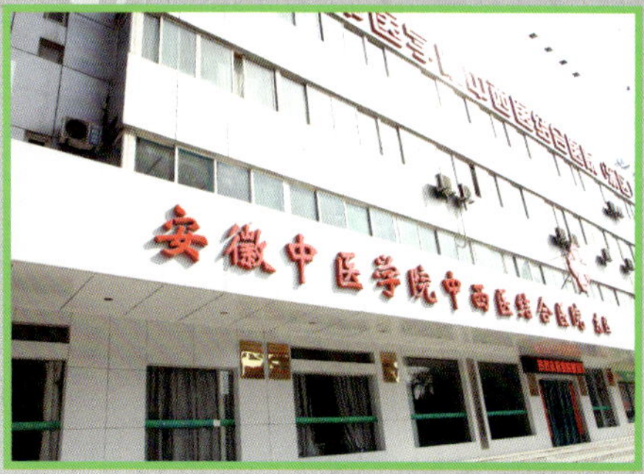

东院

医院成立于2003 年，隶属于安徽中医药大学，目前分东西两个院区。医院是省、市城镇职工医保定点医院，合肥市居民医保定点单位，合肥市工伤医保定点医院，安徽省新型农村合作医疗定点医院，全国推拿专业委员会副主任委员单位，安徽省推拿专业委员会主任委员单位，安徽省灸法研究会副会长单位。2012 年医院被确立为全国第三批重点中西医结合医院建设单位，目前医院正在筹建三级甲等规模的安徽省中西医结合医院暨安徽中医药大学第三附属医院，医院新址位于合肥市史河路 45 号（原安徽中医药大学西区），占地 97 亩。安徽省人民政府已批复同意在医院基础上组建成立安徽省中西医结合医院，面向社会开展中西医结合医疗、预防、保健、救护和康复工作。

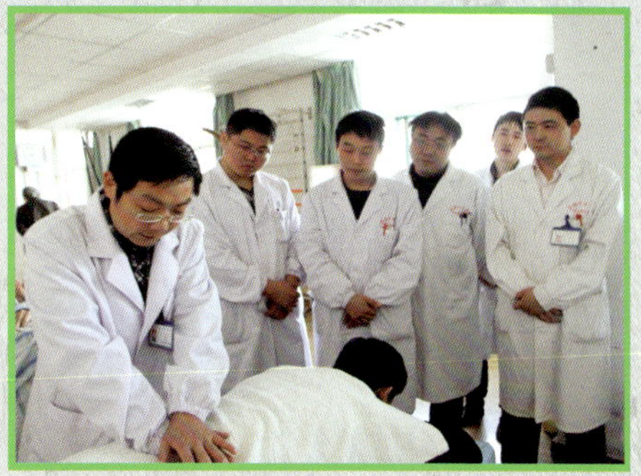

何光远院长临床带教

医院拥有一批省内外著名专家、教授及名老中医，其中国家级名老中医 1 人，安徽省名老中医工作室指导老师 2 人，硕士研究生导师 10 余人，博士、硕士研究生 30 余人。设有内科、外科、针灸科、推拿科、骨伤科、康复科等多个临床科室，其中李业甫推拿名医工作室为全国名老中医传承工作室建设单位，推拿科是国家中医药管理局"十二五"重点专科建设科室，针灸推拿科是安徽省"十二五"中医重点专科，针灸科为合肥市卫生局第三周期特色专科建设单位。

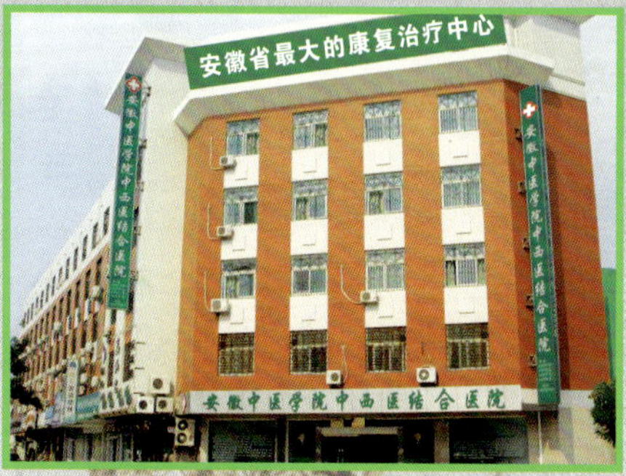

西院

医院拥有先进的意大利 esaote 全身多普勒彩超、德国 STORZ 腹腔镜、膝关节镜、胃镜、肠镜、全自动生化分析仪、高压氧舱、体外碎石机、脑彩超、C 臂机及中医诊疗设备等中西医诊疗设备。

医院始终秉承"精诚精术 为仁为和"的院训，坚持"省内一流、国内显著影响、特色鲜明的现代化中西医结合医院"的发展目标，坚持"传承岐黄之道 发展中西医结合事业"的宗旨，坚持"文化塑院、仁德扬院、特色弘院、科技强院"的发展战略，立足中西医结合事业，不断提升医院社会参与度、贡献力和影响力，更好地服务安徽省公共医疗事业。

医院地址：新址：安徽省合肥市史河路45号
东区：安徽省合肥市敬亭山路1号（胜利广场东侧200米） 西区：安徽省合肥市青阳南路1号（青阳路与贵池路交叉口
24小时健康热线：0551-65169198 62839969 医院网址：http://www.ahzxy.com

平阳县中医院

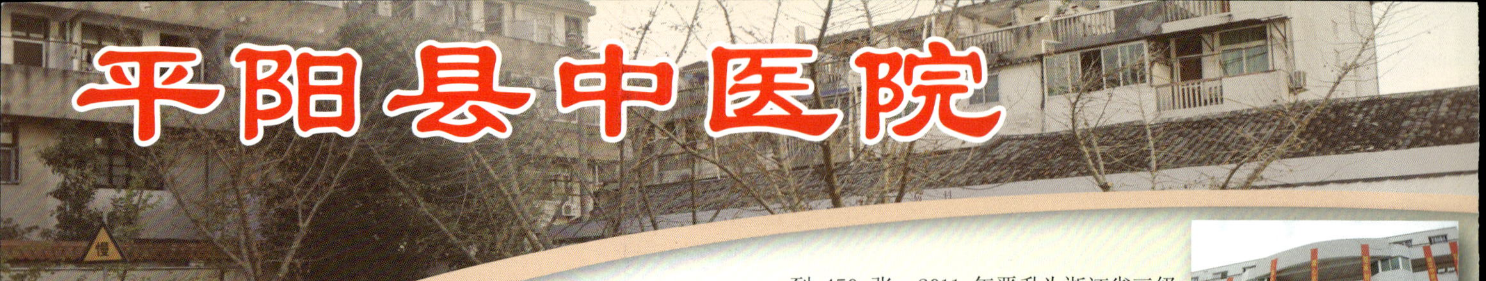

▼ 平阳中医院外景

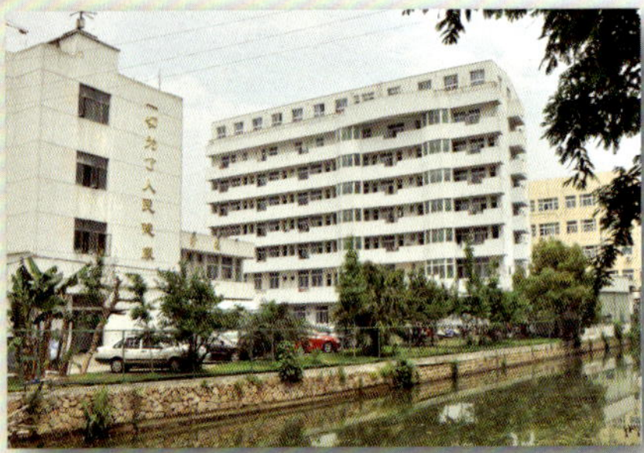

平阳县中医院坐落在美丽的鳌江镇七星桥畔，是一所集医疗、康复、教学、科研为一体的国家三级乙等中医医院，江西中医药大学教学医院，浙江省首批中医“名院”建设单位。

医院于1991年3月17日正式开诊。1992年通过省标一级乙等医院的评审，并经浙江省卫生厅（浙卫〔1992〕263号）批准，核定床位增加到100张；1995年行政楼建成投入使用；1997年被授予“县级文明单位”；2001年新病房大楼建成投入使用并通过“放心药房”的达标验收；2002年在全市医疗机构中率先通过ISO 9001：2000国际质量管理体系认证，同年档案工作通过省级达标；2003年开卫生医疗机构改革的先河，兼并平阳县第三人民医院，使有效的卫生资源得到很好的组合，并顺利通过从合并磨合期到融合期的过程；2004年被授予“市级文明单位”，核定床位增加到250张；2005年以高分通过二级甲等中医医院的评审；2006年成为江西中医学院教学医院，标志着平阳县中医院真正成为集医疗、康复、教学、科研为一体的二级甲等中医医院；2007年被确定为浙江省首批中医“名院”建设单位；2010年，经省卫生厅批准，核定床位增加到450张；2011年晋升为浙江省三级乙等中医医院；2012年晋升为国家三级乙等中医医院。

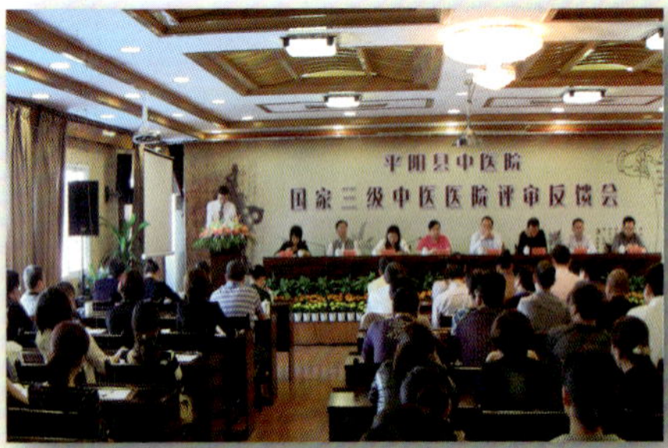

▲ 创建国家三级乙等中医医院反馈会现场

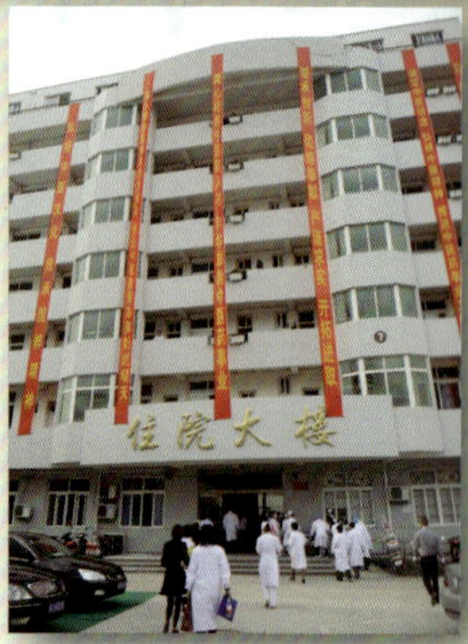

▲ 住院部大楼

医院目前占地面积9112平方米，建筑面积16404平方米。核定床位450张，截至目前实际开放床位489张，2013年年门诊量66万余人次，年出院病人12540人次，年业务收入2.065亿元。现有职工603人，其中高级职称52名，中级职称149名；配有16排CT，CR，C臂、彩超、电子内窥镜、全自动生化分析仪、免疫发光机、血透仪、钼钯X射片机、进口胃肠机等先进医疗仪器。设有急诊科、ICU、内科、外科、儿科、妇产科、骨伤科、肿瘤科、针灸科、推拿科、皮肤科、眼科、耳鼻喉科、口腔科、肛肠科、康复科、神志病科、麻醉科、感染科、治未病科等一级临床科室20个、12个病区及12个医技科室，2个国家级农村医疗机构特色专科、1个省级专科。

医院全体员工时刻牢记办院宗旨，“取中西医之精华，为人民健康服务”，努力使医院在技术水平、中医特色、服务水平等方面再上一个新台阶。

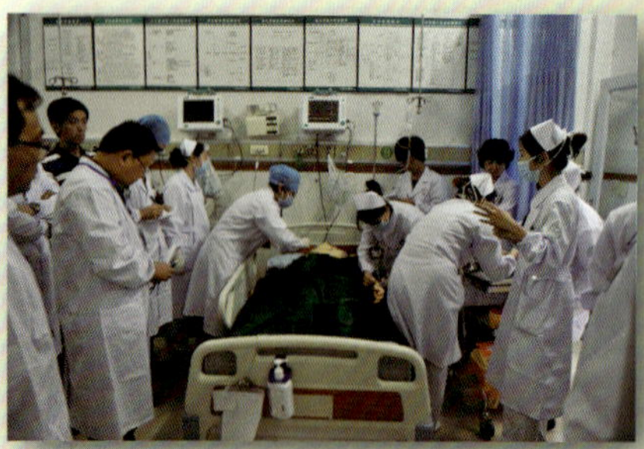

▲ 抢救培训现场

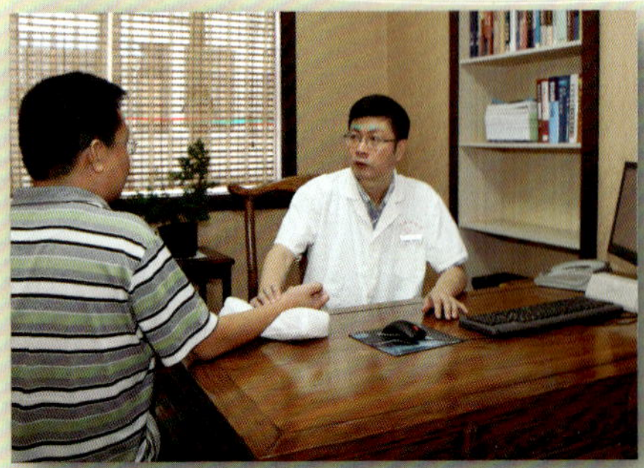

▲ 张美稀 院长

张美稀 男，医学硕士，主任中医师，江西中医药大学兼职教授。平阳县首届十大名医，温州市名中医。1990年7月毕业于浙江中医学院中医系。

1998年被省中医管理局确定为浙江省中青年中医临床学科带头人培养对象，1999年5月至2000年4月在上海中医药大学附属曙光医院急诊科和肝病研究所进修。2002年5月通过省卫生厅组织的考核，被授予浙江省中医临床技术骨干称号；2007年12月被温州市卫生局评为优秀中青年中医；2008年5月和2011年9月分别被评为平阳县第六、第七轮专业技术拔尖人才。2003年被中共温州市组织部与人事局确定为温州市“新世纪551人才工程”第二梯队培养对象，2005年12月通过考核被评为优秀人才。2006年6月获温州医学院医学硕士学位。主持县、市、厅级课题共3项，获县科技进步一等奖2项，在省级以上专业杂志发表论文18篇（一级文章5篇），其中一篇被国际权威文献检索机构美国*CHEMICAL ABSTRACTS*收录。温州市第十二届、十三届自然科学优秀论文共2项。由其带头的脾胃病专科2007年7月分别被国家中医药管理局、浙江省中医药管理局评为重点建设专科。县政协第十一届、第十二届委员。县第十五届人民代表大会代表。现担任的学术职务有：浙江省中医药学会肝病分会、脾胃病分会委员，温州市中医药学会理事、肝胆脾胃专业委员会副主任委员，温州市中西医结合学会理事，平阳县中医药学会会长，学术上主攻病毒性肝炎、脂肪肝、萎缩性胃炎的中西医结合诊治。

蘇州市 中西醫結合 木瀆人民 醫院

苏州市中西医结合医院（苏州市木渎人民医院）始建于1958年，是一所公立医院，集医疗、教育、科研、预防保健、社区卫生服务为一体的三级中西医结合医院创建单位，江苏省卫生厅认定的住院医师规范化培训基地，南京中医药大学教学医院，同时也是苏州卫生职业技术学院、无锡卫生职业技术学院、盐城卫生职业技术学院、安徽卫生职业技术学院等院校的教学实习基地。同时也是江苏省价格诚信单位、江苏省群众满意的医疗卫生机构、苏州市卫生系统文明单位、四星级健康医院。

医院占地面积55.1亩，业务用房总建筑面积45000平方米，另有建筑面积 19600 平方米的外科住院楼在建。现有正式职工792名，卫技人员720名，其中高级职称83名，研究生以上学历42名。设临床、医技科室36个，配备护理单元的病区15个，目前开放床位516张，服务苏州市西南片约60万人口。

▼ 中医特色门诊

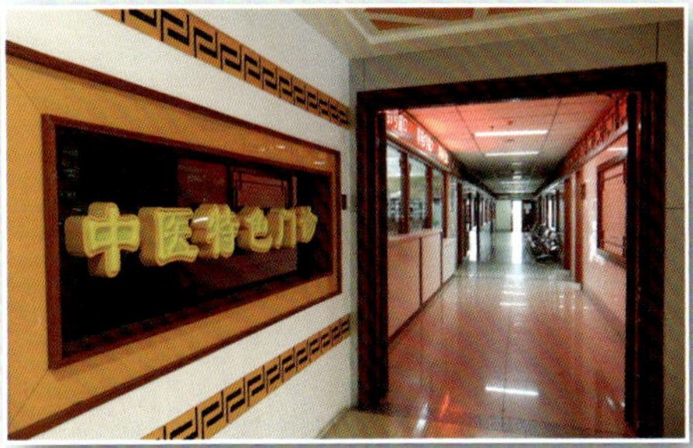

医院有市、区级临床重点专科8个，市级重点专病1个。其中，骨科是苏州市临床重点专科，心内科、呼吸内科、重症医学科、肾病科、肝病科、肿瘤科、神经外科等七个科室为吴中区临床重点专科，蛇咬伤专病是苏州市中医临床重点专病，感染性疾病科是吴中区定点单位。

医院拥有1.5 T核磁共振、64排螺旋CT、彩色多普勒超声诊断系统、高压氧舱、800 ma C臂机等大型医疗设备，并拥有DR，500 ma多功能数字胃肠机、血液透析机、电子胃肠镜、呼吸机、腹腔镜、关节镜、前列腺汽化电切镜、震波碎石机、全自动生化分析仪等一系列先进医疗设备。

医院除传统的中西医结合治疗蛇咬伤、尿毒症患者的血液透析治疗、有机磷农药中毒的抢救、心内科和肿瘤科的介入治疗、儿童哮喘的规范化治疗等优势项目外，近年来，积极探索和引进新的医疗技术，如开展腹腔镜下直肠癌根治术、腹腔镜胆道镜双镜联合下胆总管切开取石术、关节镜下半月板部分切除术、人工LARS韧带重建术、微创式人工髋关节置换术、脑动脉瘤夹闭术等高难度手术。2013年医院与同济大学附属杨浦医院

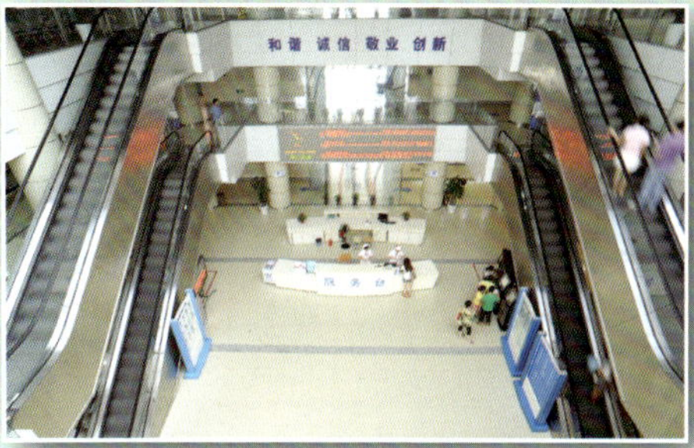

▲ 宽敞明亮的门诊大厅

合作成立苏州妇科微创合作中心，在子宫肌瘤和妇科盆底疾病的微创治疗方面具有显著技术优势。

医院开设了中医内科、中医妇科、针灸理疗科、骨伤科、肛肠科等门诊科室，建有肾病科、肝病科、肿瘤科、老年康复科等病区。开展针灸、拔罐、理疗、推拿、牵引、穴位贴敷、穴位注射、中药灌肠、中药熏洗、骨折手法整复、中药外敷等多项中医治疗技术。医院拥有全国优秀中医临床人才1名，江苏省农村优秀中医临床人才1名，苏州市十大健康养身专家1名；另有近10名专家任省、市级中医学会、中西医结合学会理事及专业委员会委员；15名中医药专家受聘南京中医药大学兼职教授、副教授。

医院积极开展新技术、新项目。近3年来，获苏州市医学新技术奖1项，吴中区科技进步三等奖5项，获区卫生局医学新技术二等奖4项、三等奖7项，多项新技术、新项目填补了吴中区技术空白。全院发表论文170篇，其中在核心期刊上发表21篇，SCI 2篇，获奖论文有36篇，开展市级以上课题4项。

▼ 中医诊室

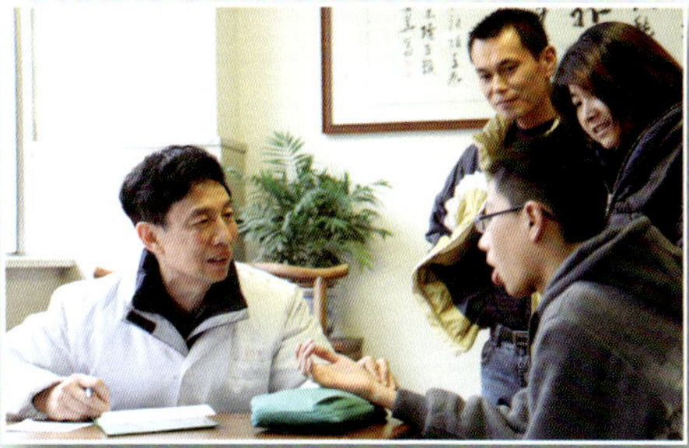

医院本着"和谐 诚信 敬业 创新"的院训精神，以崇德、敬业之心关爱患者，提供人文医疗；以求精、创业之力追求技术，缓解患者痛苦；创造和谐、诚信的医疗环境。努力将医院建设为技术先进、服务卓越、管理一流的，具有示范水平的现代化三级中西医结合医院。

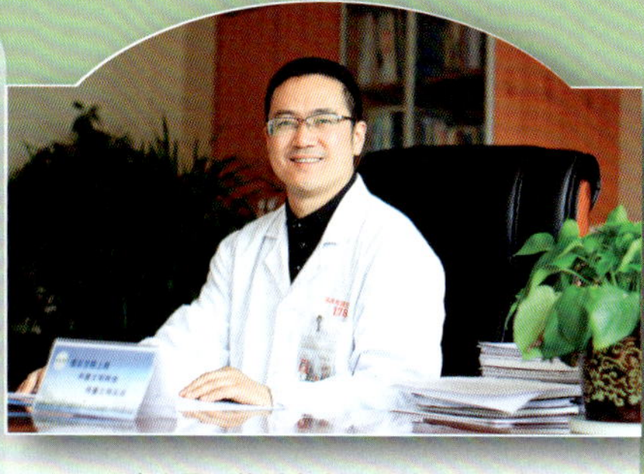

▲ 陆治平　苏州市中西医结合医院院长

陆治平　男，1971年7月出生，苏州人，中共党员，1990年8月参加工作，临床医学、法律本科及医院管理硕士学历。现任苏州市中西医结合医院（苏州市木渎人民医院）院长、党委书记，骨科副主任医师；兼江苏省中西医结合学会疼痛专业委员会委员，苏州市中西医结合学会痛症专业委员会主任委员，苏州市医学会骨质疏松与骨矿盐疾病专业委员会常务委员。

在新医改的大潮中，陆治平院长带领全院职工努力探索公立医院改革举措，积极制定医院中长期发展战略规划，以加强人才队伍和重点学科建设、提高医疗质量和医疗服务水平、推行医院全成本核算、实施综合目标管理和绩效考核等举措为切入点，大胆尝试医院内部运行机制的改革，在提高医院运行效率和社会效益等方面都起到了较大作用。审时夺度，勇于抓住机遇，于2013年将医院发展方向由综合性医院调整为中西医结合方向，并成为三级中西医结合医院创建单位，实现了医院历史上成功的转型升级。

在从事医院管理的同时，没有放弃临床工作，2005年其与同事共同立项开展的课题"旋入式自锁髓内钉在四肢长骨骨折中的应用"获得了吴中区科技进步二等奖。近年来在省级以上期刊上发表专业论文3篇。

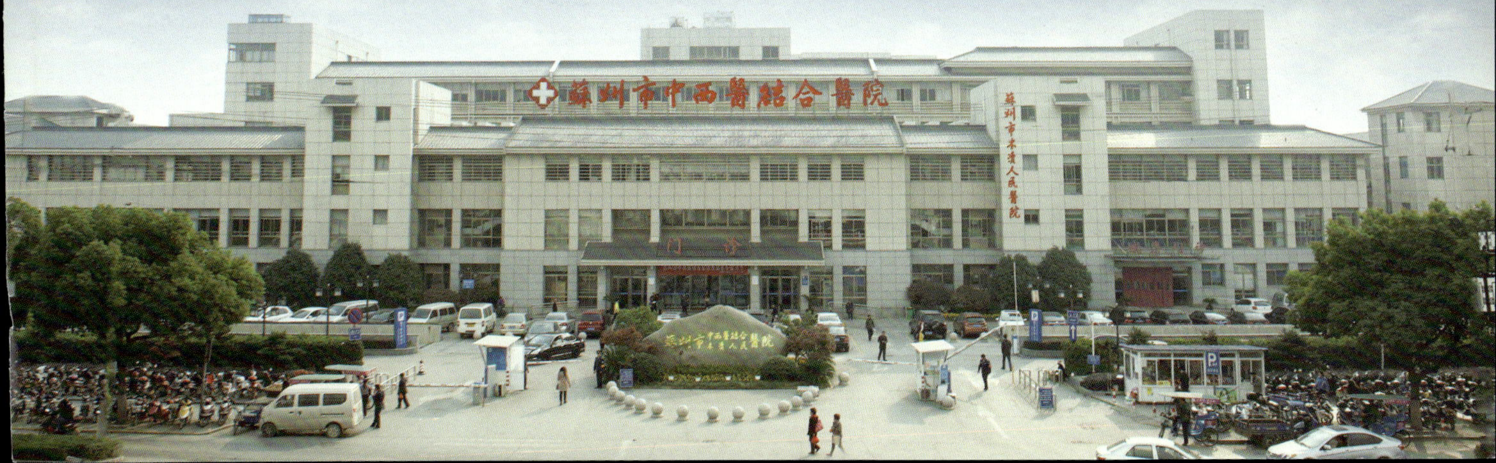

武汉市新洲区骨伤专科医院

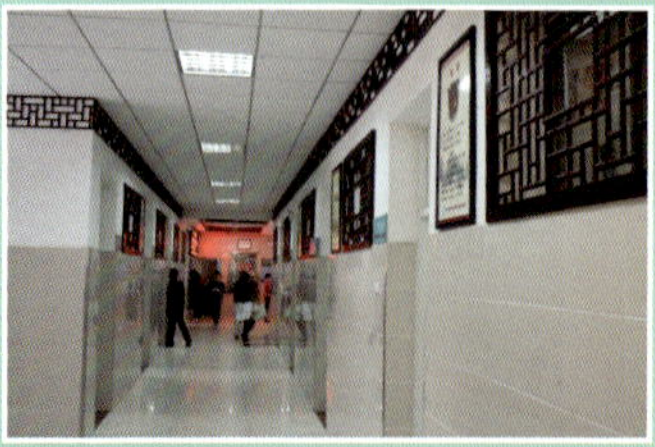

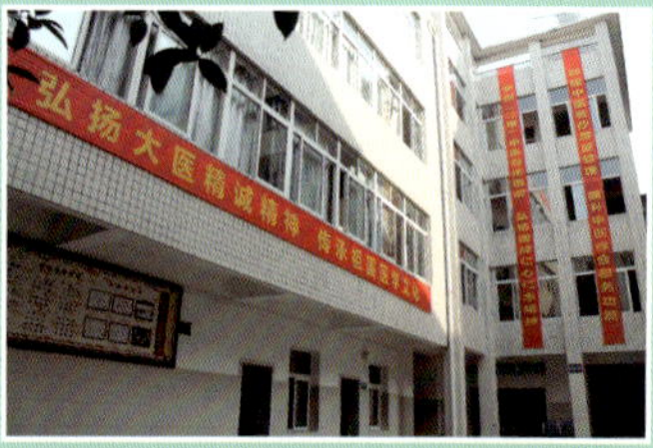

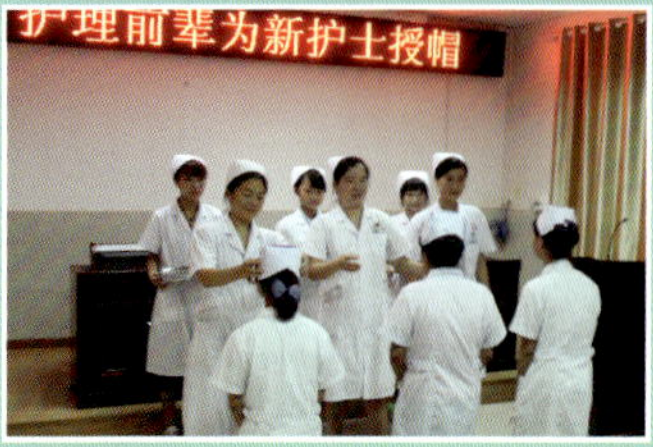

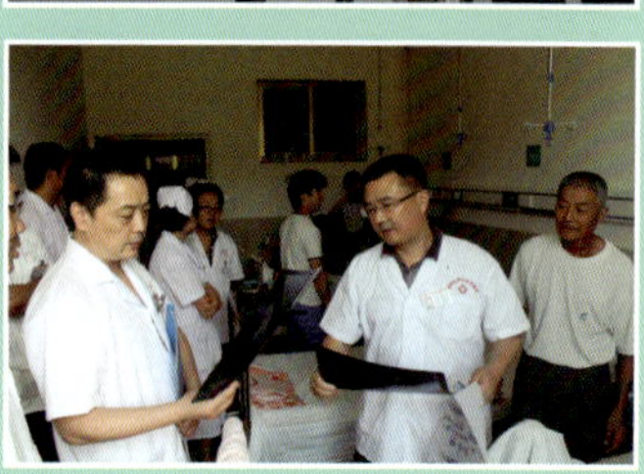

武汉市新洲区骨伤专科医院是一所中医特色浓厚的专科医院，始建于1987年，历经20余年的创业和发展，现已成为湖北省中医骨伤重点专科。2014年6月11日湖北省卫计委审核批准为“二级甲等”中医骨伤医院。医院致力于科研、业务建设，拥有一支合理的人才梯队，有各类专业技术人员95人，其中省、市级中医名医各1名，高级卫技人员6人，中级卫技人员26人，专科技术跨入省、市先进行列，2013年医疗业务收入2572万元，比去年同期增长29%；共完成门诊量40516人次；收治住院病人数4025人次，其中75%的四肢骨折病人是采用中医传统手法复位、杉树皮固定，治愈率高。是城镇职工医保定点医疗机构和新洲、红安、团风、麻城等区县市新型农村合作医疗定点医院。

医院秉承湖北名医刘楚樵的精湛医术、崇高医德。坚持“以人为本，特色兴院”的宗旨，在治疗四肢骨折、脱位、扭伤、挫伤、软组织损伤、骨质增生、老年性腰、腿、关节疼痛等病，突出中医辨证论治，中药内服外敷，运用传统中医手法复位、杉树皮夹板固定，充分发挥中医中药优势，取得了满意疗效。四肢骨折病人75%是采用中医传统手法治疗，其治疗费用仅是西医外科手术治疗费用的1/10，彰显了中医“简、便、验、廉”的特点，深受广大患者青睐，医疗业务以每年20%递增。

医院不断传承创新传统中医药学，研发了一系列疗效确切，效尤价廉的院内制剂，目前生产的“桃红接骨合剂”、“舒松液”、“风湿Ⅰ号”等5个中药制剂应用临床，临床疗效显著，享誉周边团风、大悟，红安、麻城等县市。

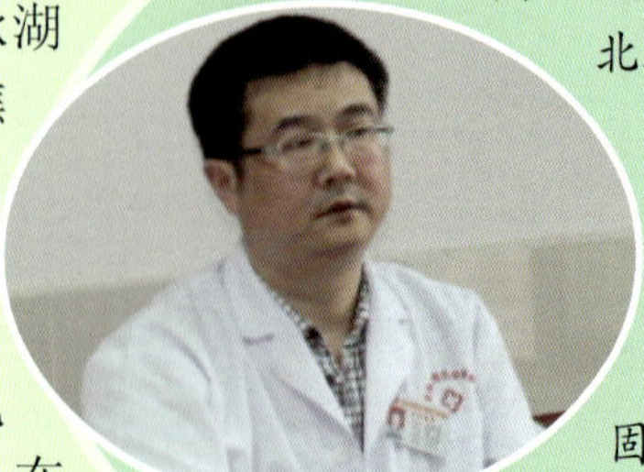

许建国

男，46岁，本科学历，中共党员，中医副主任医师，现任湖北省武汉市新洲区骨伤专科医院院长，湖北省中医药学会骨伤科专业委员会委员、骨质疏松专业委员会常委。长期从事骨伤科的临床和科研工作，有扎实的中医理论基础和现代医学知识，具有丰富的临床经验，擅长解决本学科较复杂、较疑难病证的诊治，特别是运用传统中医手法复位、杉树皮夹板固定，治疗四肢骨折，疗效显著，深受广大患者欢迎。在中西医结合治疗骨病（骨质疏松）等方面有较深入的研究。主持参与市，区级科研课题多项，在国内各级学术期刊上发表医学论文30多篇。

医院始终坚持科技兴院、人才强院的办院宗旨，提倡科技创新，以科技进步促专科发展。近5年来，医院狠抓医疗质量、专科建设，努力培养科技型人才；全面实施电子病历，切实提升医疗质量，促进医院精细化、规范化、信息化建设再上新台阶；积极推行专科优势病种临床路径和治疗方案，治疗率达到95%以上；在诊疗同时，积极总结临床经验，已在专业核心期刊上发表论文60余篇，不断提升学科建设水平和专科影响力。

医院通过改扩建，核定编制床位120张，实际开放床位100张，设有10个临床科室（包括一间百级层流手术室），4个医技科室。技术力量雄厚，医疗设备先进，拥有磁共振，DR放射机、C臂机、床边X光机、骨折治疗仪、多功能牵引床，激光治疗仪等设备，为骨伤疾患精确诊治打下良好基础。医院环境优美，管理规范，是伤筋折骨患者康复治疗的理想场所。

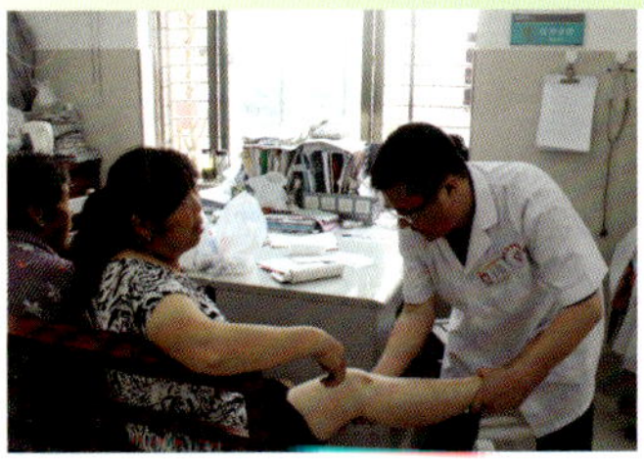

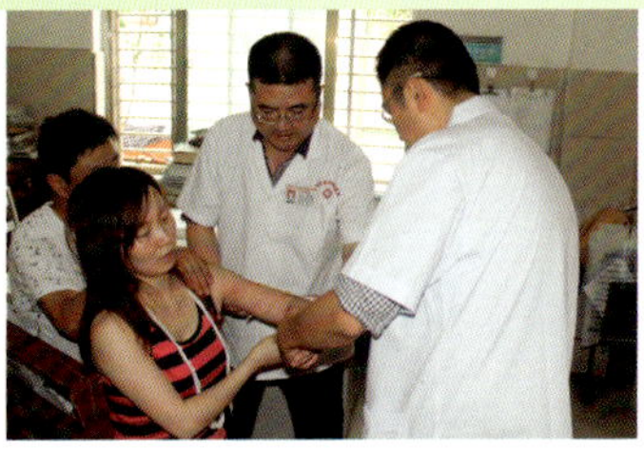

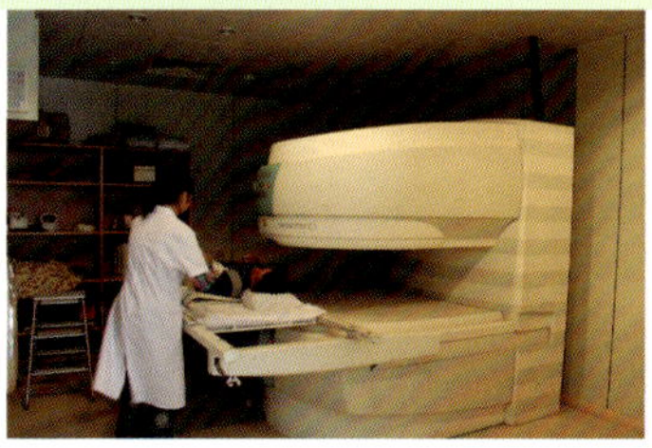

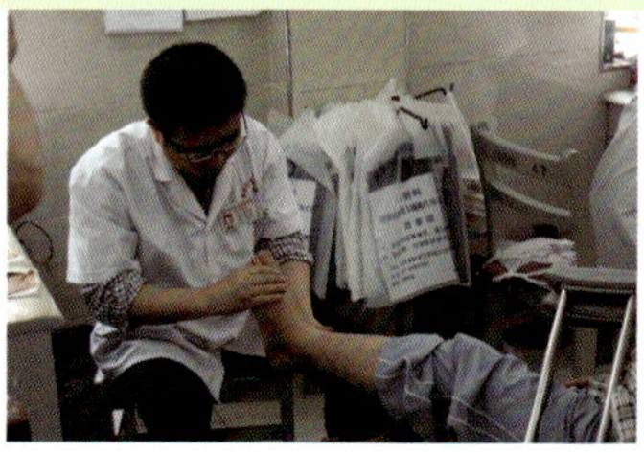

南通良春中医医院

南通良春中医医院成立于 2006 年 9 月 21 日，由首届国医大师朱良春教授和他的学术继承人朱婉华教授领衔创办，为南通市医保定点单位，于 2012 年 1 月被南通市卫生局正式批准为二级中医医院。

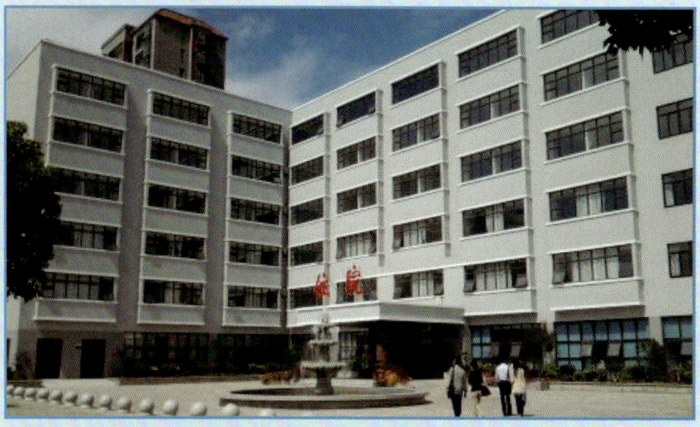

▲ 医院正门

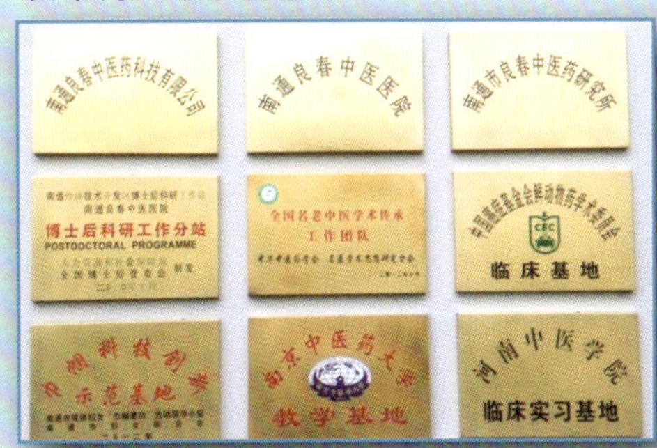

▲ 医院名称

良春中医医院一直秉承着董事长朱良春“经验不保守、知识不带走”的传承理念，积极努力与各大院校、学术团体等开展交流与合作，现已成为中国中医科学院中医临床基础医学研究所博士后流动工作室（站），南京中医药大学、河南中医学院临床实习基地和中国癌症基金会鲜药学术委员会临床基地。2014 年 3 月 18 日，又与国家中医药管理局中国中医药科技开发交流中心签署合作意向书，并启动了“全国名老中医经验、名方、特色诊疗技术传承促进工程”。

良春中医医院设有门诊部、住院部、中医保健与康复中心、良春中医药研究所和虫类药博物馆，风湿病科、肿瘤科、中医保健与康复科是医院的特色科室。

风湿病科为国家中医重点专科，全国痛风协作组组长单位。以辨证与辨病相结合、标本兼治、善用虫药为治疗法则，对类风湿关节炎，强直性脊柱炎，痛风，颈、胸、腰椎退变，椎间盘突出，椎管狭窄，骨关节炎，红斑狼疮，干燥综合征，皮肌炎，硬皮病，白塞病，间质性肺炎，肺纤维化等风湿病有确切的疗效。所研制的益肾蠲痹丸经检验证明，是众多治疗类风湿关节炎中成药中唯一对骨质破坏有修复作用的中成药；所创立的“益肾蠲痹法治疗风湿病”技术，2005 年被国家中医药管理局定为全国科技成果推广项目，2010 年 8 月被列入南通市非物质文化遗产保护名录。

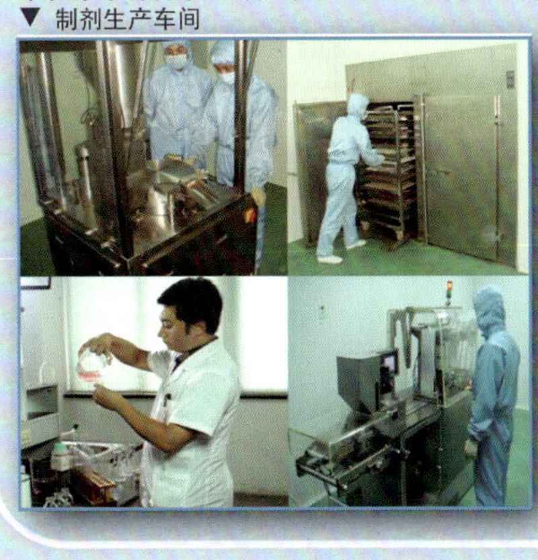

▼ 制剂生产车间

肿瘤科为江苏省肿瘤重点专科“十二五”建设单位。良春中医医院的学术团队采用扶正消癥法，选用鲜动物药内服、外用相结合的中医药综合治疗方法，临床证明有缓解症状、稳定病情、增强体质、提高生活质量、延长生存期的作用。

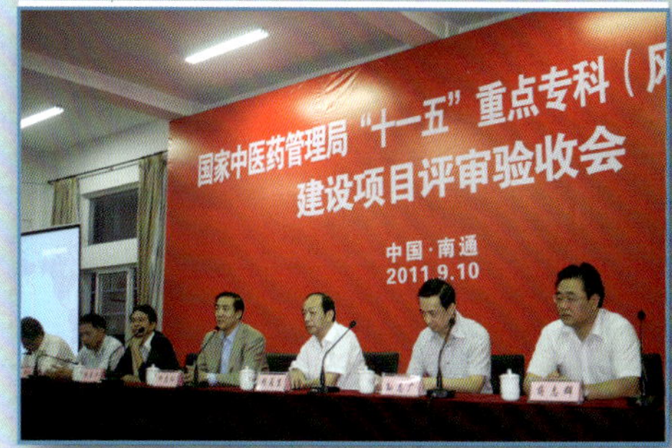

▲ 2011年9月21日通过国家中医药管理局“十一五”风湿病重点专科验收

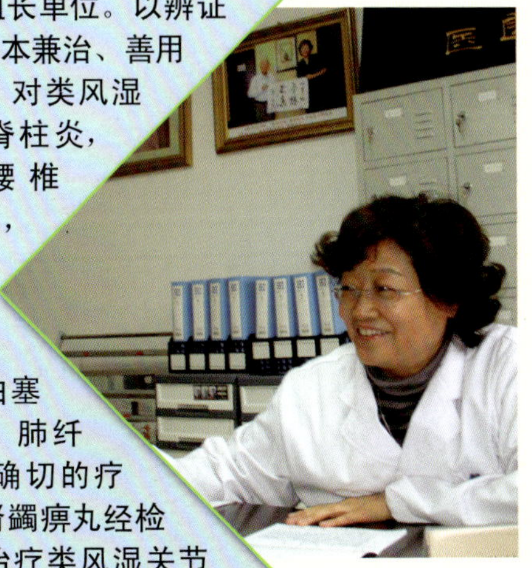

朱婉华

1949年出生，我国首批国医大师朱良春教授的学术继承人。毕业于南京中医学院，硕士，主任中医师。南通良春中医医院院长，南通市良春中医药研究所所长；南京中医药大学中医内科学硕士研究生指导教师，安徽中医药大学兼职教授、河南中医学院兼职教授。兼中华中医药学会风湿病分会副主任委员、名医学术思想研究会副主任委员，中国癌症基金会北京鲜药研制中心副主任委员，中国中西医结合防治风湿病联盟副主席，中国中医药研究促进会肿瘤专业委员会副主任委员，世界中医药学会联合会风湿病专业委员会常务理事，澳门中国中医药文化研究促进会资深专家委员会副主任委员，海峡两岸医药卫生交流协会风湿免疫病学专家委员会常务委员、中西医结合专业委员会常务委员。

朱婉华教授从医40年，善于继承和创新，在整理国医大师朱良春教授经验的基础上，在中医药治疗风湿病、肿瘤领域已形成自己独特的临床治疗体系。在风湿病领域已有7个项目获得部、省、市级科技成果进步奖，并研发国家级新药益肾蠲痹丸；参加过14部著作和5部大型工具书的编写。在各级各类杂志发表学术论文50余篇，其中20余篇获国际、国内优秀论文奖。主持和参与完成科技部“十五”重点攻关项目2项、“十一五”科技支撑计划课题2项，江苏省科技支撑计划1项，为国家中医药管理局全国痛风协作组组长。

良春中医医院还建有 2800 平方米达到 GGP 标准要求的制剂用房，生产浓缩益肾蠲痹丸，扶正蠲痹Ⅰ、Ⅱ等 21 种有自主知识产权的医院制剂。在生产环境和生产质量上，严格按照制剂标准执行。

创办迄今，良春中医医院一直秉承着“自强不息、止于至善”的敬业精神，坚持中医特色，发扬专病专科优势，中药使用率达 90%以上，病员遍及全国各地包括港、澳、台地区及英国、美国、法国、德国、澳大利亚、新加坡、马来西亚、新西兰、日本、韩国、泰国、越南等国，受到海内外患者的赞誉。路漫漫其修远兮，良春中医医院将一如既往，以“仁心仁术”为办院宗旨，将祖国传统医学发扬光大！

地址：南通经济技术开发区上海东路68号
邮编：226009
电话：0513-85966258 18962991880(办公室)
传真：0513-85966269
E-mail：ntlczyyy@163.com
网　址：www.jszlc.com

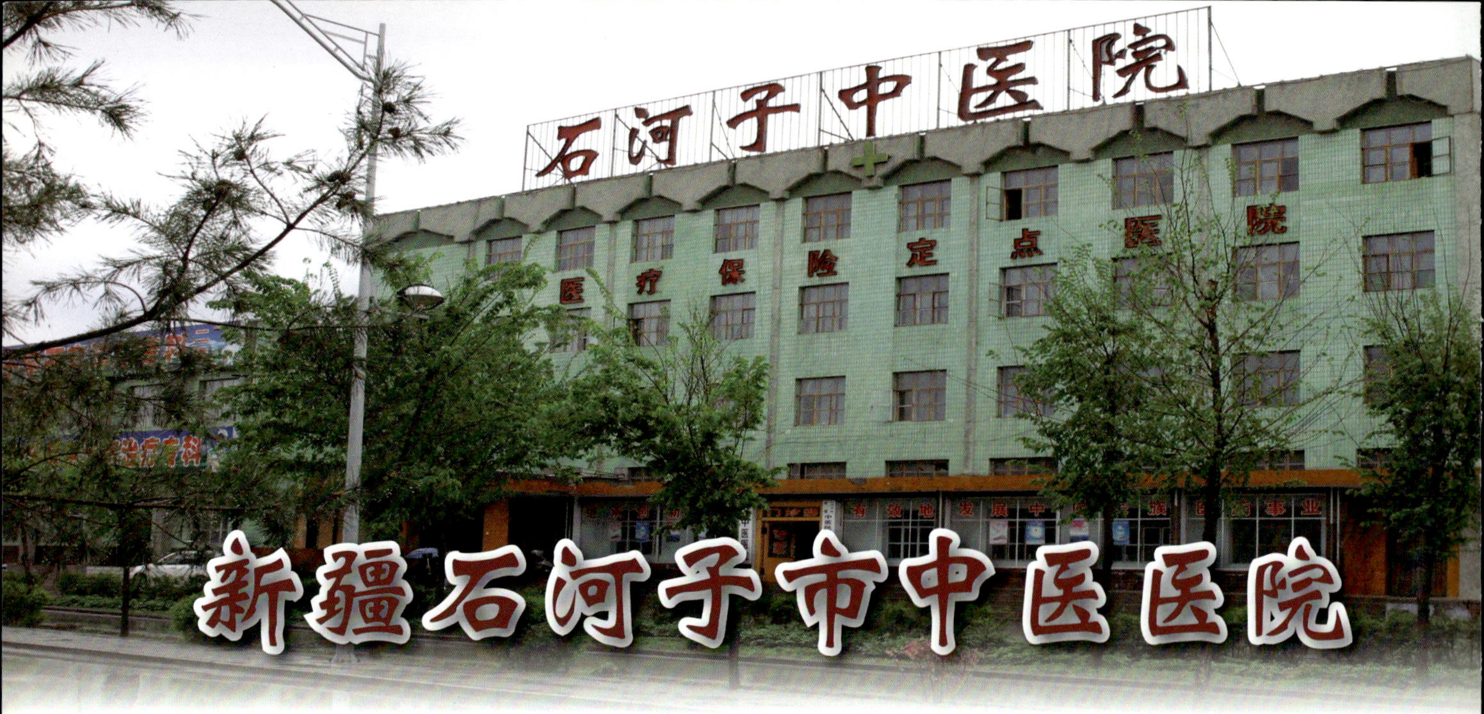

新疆石河子市中医医院

新疆石河子市中医医院始建于 1986 年 12 月，2000 年 10 月经政府批准改制为民办非企业单位；是由自治区卫生厅批准、民政厅注册登记的“ 二级综合性中医院 ”、兵团首批医疗保险定点医院，也是集中医医疗、预防、教学、科研、康复为一体的综合医疗单位。先后被被自治区民政厅授予“ 自治区民办非企业先进单位 ”“ 创先争优先进单位 ”“ 规范化建设自治区级 4A 单位 ”；被国家民政部先后授予“ 全国民办非企业先进单位 ”“ 全国先进社会组织 ”；经国家中医药管理局批准为“ 全国优秀民营中医院 ”；多年被师市及街道办事处授予“ 诚信单位 ”及“ 先进基层党组织 ”等荣誉称号。

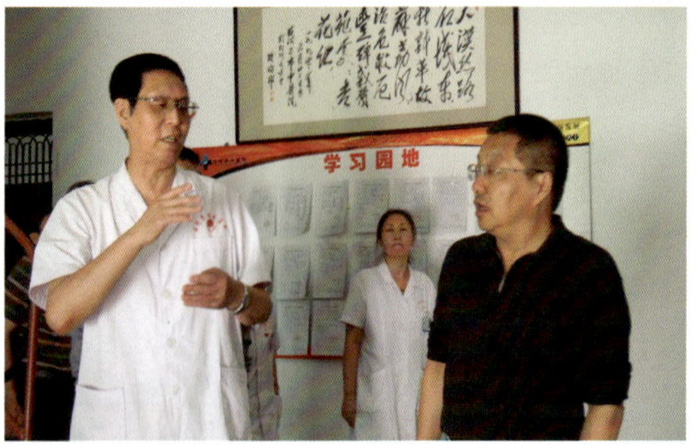
▲ 刘珀董事长工作中

医院现有职工 160 余人，其中卫技人员占 90% 以上，副高以上职称 12 人，中级职称 20 余人，建立了以中医老专家为核心，由自治区、垦区知名专家和来自北京、江西、陕西、青海、长春、成都等地的八大院校中医本科毕业生组成的医生队伍，在医务人员结构上形成了老、中、青三结合的完善体系。新疆名老中医石河子市中医医院名誉院长刘纪元副主任医师的继承人，其子刘珀主任医师继承发展了祖传秘方，研制的“ 肾泰脾康 ”浸膏片，具有补肾健脾、颐养阴精、抗疲劳、增强免疫力等特殊功效，该药获国家专利，被列为国家级开发项目，作为院内制剂受到了广大患者的好评。

医院现拥有门诊部和住院部两座大楼，医技楼和老年康复中心大楼经有关部门批准正在动工修建并对原门诊楼进行全面整修，门诊部科室设置齐全，除开设了具有传统中医特色的中医内科、针灸推拿科、肛肠科、风湿科、泌尿科、软伤疼痛科、妇科、老年心血管病科、咳喘病科等多个专科外，还配备了现代化 B 超仪、计算机 X 线摄影系统（CR）、大生化分析仪、心电监护仪、24 小时动态心电图等 30 多种仪器。

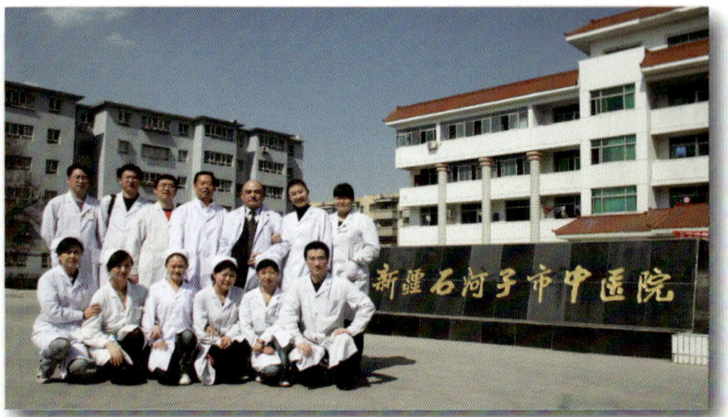

▲ 医护团队

住院部为患者提供全方位、多层次的优质服务，是集治疗、保健与修养为一体的最佳场所。设有内一科、内二科、内三科、针灸病房、骨伤科和肛肠科，共有病床编制 150 张，配备现代化医疗服务设施，住院病人的所有医疗、配药、收费等项目均实行了计算机电子化统一管理，安装了快捷、安全的呼叫应答装置，保证了医疗的及时到位。医院提供的标准病房，均有电视、电淋浴器、卫生间等现代化的生活保障设施，一流的房间设施可与本地任何一家医院相媲美，还专为患者设置了医疗专用电梯，极大地支持和方便了医疗及患者。医院餐饮部为配合治疗，特开设餐饮服务，妥善解决了患者的营养膳食，为患者的康复提供了有力的保证。

医院坚持突出中医特色，党团组织和领导班子健全。从建院开始就把疗效作为医院生存的关键，把医疗质量作为取得疗效的关键，把医德医风作为保证医疗质量的关键，把科学管理作为良好医德医风的关键，把以人为本作为科学管理的关键。医院坚持在“ 振兴中医，发展事业，防病治病，患者至上，科学兴院，走向世界 ”的宗旨指导下，抓好五个关键，以病人为中心，一切为了病人。自 2013 年以来每日住院病人已在平均 300 人以上，石河子垦区人民已经信任这家百姓医院。社会以多种方式关心、支持、完善这座正在发展中的戈壁明珠上的中医院。

刘 珀主任医师，现任新疆石河子市中医医院董事长，新疆保元堂中医民族医药研究院院长。刘珀主任医师自幼随其父新疆名老中医刘纪元副主任医师学习中医药。从事中医药工作 40 余年来努力挖掘祖国医学宝库，大胆实践，撰写学术论文 60 余篇，参与了 8 部中医著作的编写。1995 年他被中国文化研究会传统医学专业委员会聘任为全国副主席、新疆区域执行主席，担任《世界传统医学大系》副总编辑。曾于 1994 年至 2014 年间 15 次赴美国参加世界传统医学大会。《轩镇食疗》《肾泰脾康的研究》《净府汤治积癖》《追风散治头痛》和《肾泰脾康健脑长寿》等学术论文获得国际金杯一等奖 2 次、二等奖 3 次、三等奖 2 次。1997 年在法国“ 世界中医学会年会 ”上获国际二等奖，2001 年在香港举办的“ 世界大城市卫生首脑暨医学论坛 ”会议上“ 肾泰脾康增强免疫力抗疲劳的研究 ”获“ 卓越医家 ”学术奖。其论文除在《新疆中医药杂志》《四川中医》《中医杂志》上登载外，也曾在中国香港和美国的医学杂志上刊登。

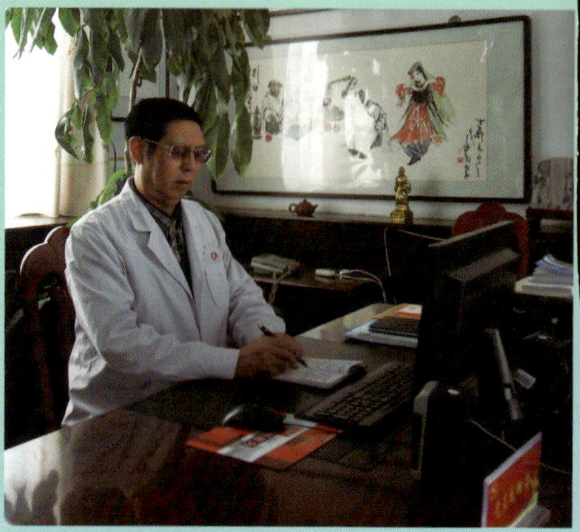
▲ 刘珀　新疆石河子市中医医院董事长

他积极从事中医药科研工作，获得国家知识产权局授予发明专利 2 项。“ 肾泰脾康片 ”曾在新疆等地的 14 家医院临床应用，并曾在美国、法国、日本、韩国、泰国及中国台湾、香港地区进行过交流和推广。2007 年新疆生产建设兵团正式将“ 肾泰脾康药技 ”确定为兵团级（省级）非物质文化遗产保护项目。

2001 年被国际名人研究中心评估授予“ 世界杰出人士 ”称号，2005 年被国家邮政部批准载入中国邮政发行“ 世界杰出人士 ”肖像邮票。2004—2006 年连续被评为优秀人大代表。其以满腔的热忱，精神饱满地参与各种社会活动，实现自己的崇高理想，发挥自己的才能，努力服务于社会，为祖国中医药事业奉献一生。

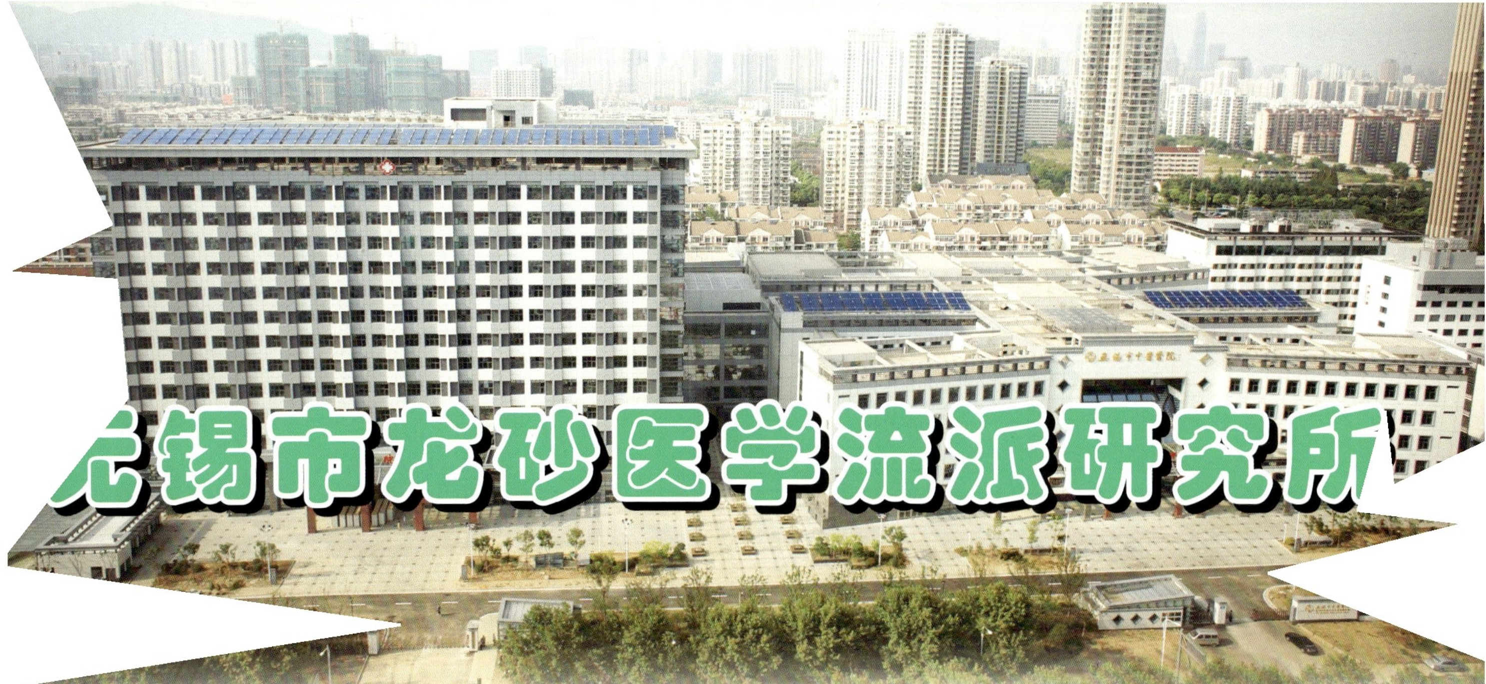

无锡市龙砂医学流派研究所

无锡市龙砂医学流派研究所设置在无锡市中医医院，是2013年3月由无锡市编委批准设立的中医学派研究机构，与无锡市中医医院、无锡市中医骨伤中心、无锡市中医药研究所实施“一套班子，四块牌子”的管理模式。医院聘请江阴柳宝诒四传弟子、国家中医药管理局“龙砂医学流派传承工作室”代表性传承人兼项目负责人、中华中医药学会五运六气研究专家协作组组长顾植山教授为所长，南京中医药大学基础医学院名誉院长、博士生导师、经方家、国家中医药管理局“龙砂医学流派

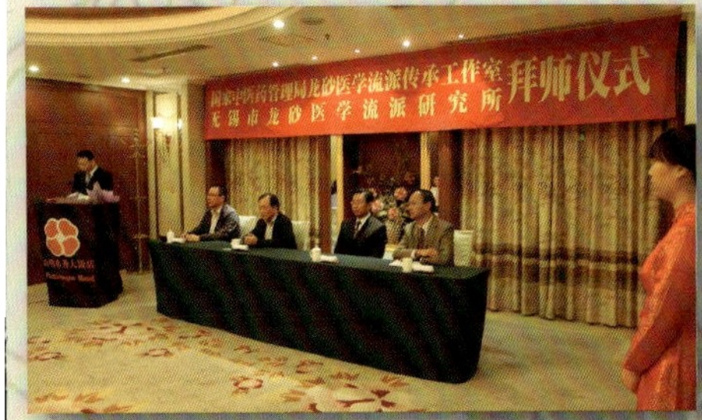

▲ 拜师仪式

传承工作室”代表性传承人黄煌教授为首席专家，中华中医药学会心病分会副主任委员、无锡市“名医”、市中医内科首席医师、无锡市中医院党委副书记兼副院长、博士生导师陆曙为常务副所长；并特聘朱良春、颜德馨两位国医大师为终身名誉所长。

无锡市龙砂医学流派研究所下设办公室，有工作人员5名；设有五运六气、经方、医史文献、“中医疫病预测预警的理论方法和应用研究”等学术科研研究小组，14名中医骨干为专（兼）职研究成员；设有“龙砂医学特需诊疗区”“名医堂”等诊疗场所，建有“龙砂医学流派展示馆”等文化传播场所。

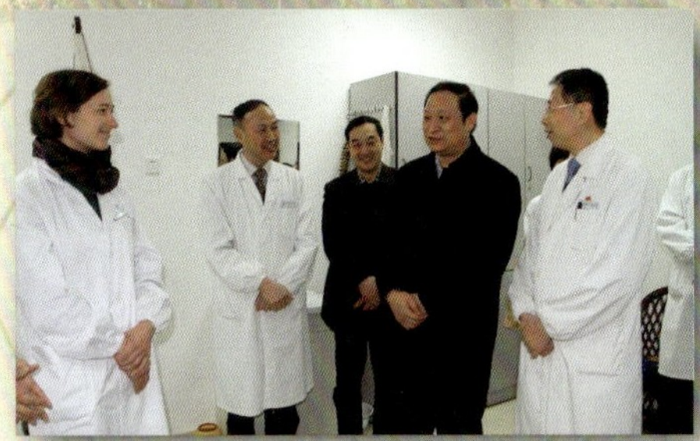
▲ 国家卫生和计划生育委员会副主任、国家中医药管理局王国强局长检查指导工作

无锡市龙砂医学流派研究所以弘扬中医药传统文化，整理发掘无锡历代中医药名家的经典文献和学术思想，优化无锡地区中医药学术资源，探索中医药科研合作模式为目标，以研究、整理、发掘历代中医药名家的史料、医案、文献，促进无锡中医药学术传承，提升无锡市中医药学术水平和科研水平，提高临床疗效为主要任务。通过建立“五运六气”专家活动基地、开展中医药学术理论研讨活动等方式，拓展无锡中医在全省乃至全国的影响力，推动中医药事业又好又快发展。2013年，无锡市中医医院13名骨干分别与顾植山、黄煌

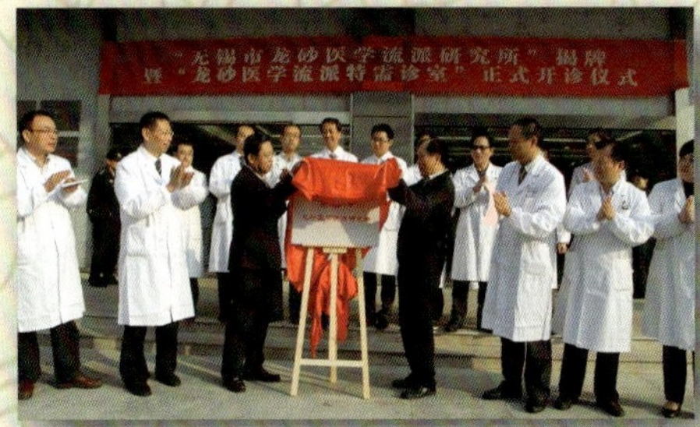

▲ 无锡市龙砂医学流派研究所揭牌仪式

两位导师结成师承关系，成为龙砂医学流派新一代传承人。

无锡市中医医院始建于1954年10月，是一家集医疗、教学、科研、预防、保健、康复为一体的三级甲等综合性中医院，南京中医药大学附属医院。建有国家博士后科研工作站、院士工作站、国家中医药科研二级实验室（心血管病）等平台；医院具备国家药物临床试验机构资质，6个专业获得GCP资格认定。医院是全国数字化医院试点示范单位和全国中医医院信息化示范单位。建有国家临床重点

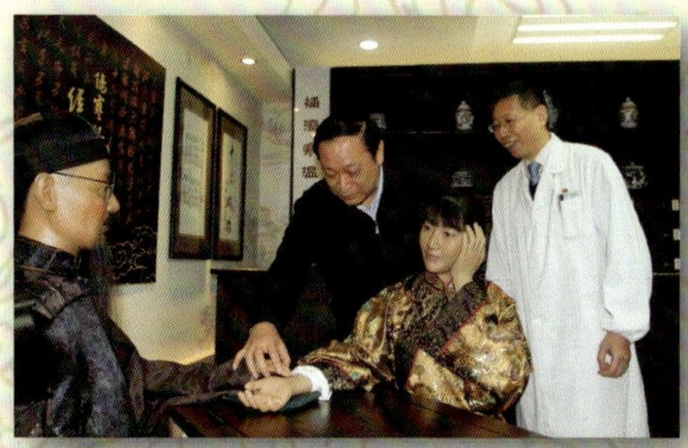
▲ 国家卫生和计划生育委员会副主任、国家中医药管理局王国强局长检查指导工作

专科建设单位1个，国家中医药重点专科2个、重点专科建设单位3个。建有国家中医药管理局“黄氏喉科疗法流派传承工作室”及吴新欲、赵景芳、朱世楷等3个“全国名老中医传承工作室”。黄氏喉科、刘氏骨伤疗法、丁氏痔科疗法、杜氏金针手法、龙砂医学诊疗技术先后入列市级非物质文化遗产项目名录。医院2013年9月迁至中南西路8号新址。新址地处锡城西南部，湖滨路与中南西路交界处，毗邻滨湖新城。医院总投资近11亿元，占地108亩，总建筑面积16多万平方米。2014年上半年门急诊量60万人次，出院病人1.22万人次。

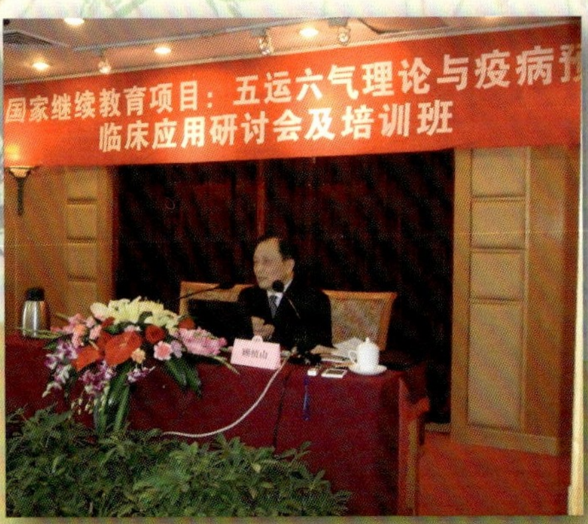

▲ 顾植山教授

顾植山 安徽中医药大学教授。江阴柳宝诒四传弟子。1979年被安徽省政府作为“特别优秀”的中医药人材选调到安徽中医学院任教，1986年中国中医研究院文献研究班毕业。历任国家中医药管理局《中华本草》学术编委、新世纪全国高等中医药院校规划教材《中医文献学》主编、教育部“十一五”规划教材《中医文献学》主审、国家中医药管理局特别专项课题“运用五运六气理论预测疫病流行的研究”课题组组长、国家“十一五”科技重大专项“中医疫病预测预警方法研究”负责人等。

现任国家“十二五”科技重大专项“中医疫病预测预警的理论方法和应用研究”课题组组长、国家中医药管理局中医学术流派传承推广基地理事会理事、国家中医药管理局龙砂医学流派传承工作室代表性传承人兼项目负责人、中华中医药学会五运六气研究专家协作组组长、无锡市龙砂医学流派研究所所长、江阴市致和堂中医药研究所所长等。

顾植山教授全面继承了龙砂医学善用五运六气理论、重视伤寒六经经方、擅长膏方调体养生的流派特色，特别在五运六气的研究方面，为全国这一领域的学术带头人，享誉国内外。

临床方面在中医内科、妇科杂病、老年病及诸多疑难杂病的治疗等方面均有较高造诣。

出版独著和主编著作7部，发表学术论文80余篇。

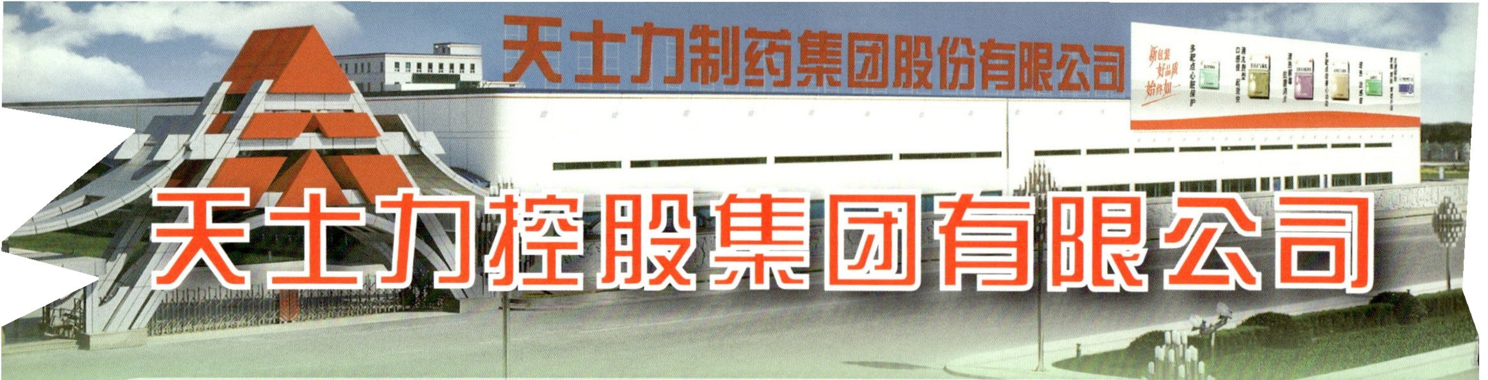

天士力控股集团有限公司

天士力控股集团有限公司创建于1994年，是以大健康产业为主线，以生物医药产业为核心，以健康产业和医疗康复、健康养生、健康管理为两翼的高科技国际化企业集团。

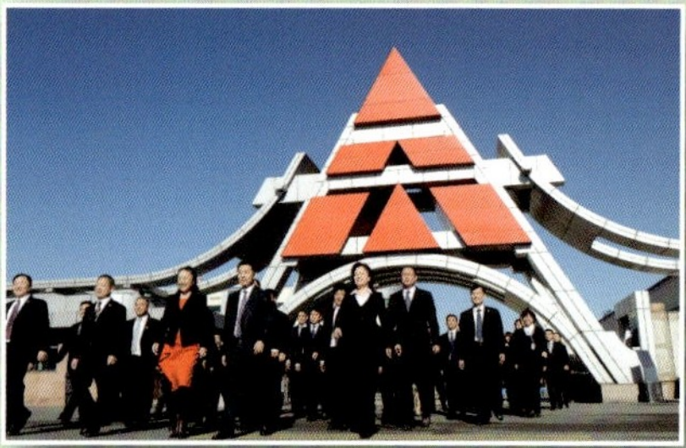

▲ 天士力正门

集团成立以来，始终秉承"追求天人合一，提高生命质量"的企业理念和"创造健康，人人共享"的企业愿景，坚持打造中药现代化、国际化第一品牌，打造大健康产业领先品牌，不断推进大健康产业持续快速发展。2013资产总额262亿元，销售额240亿元，实现利税36亿元。

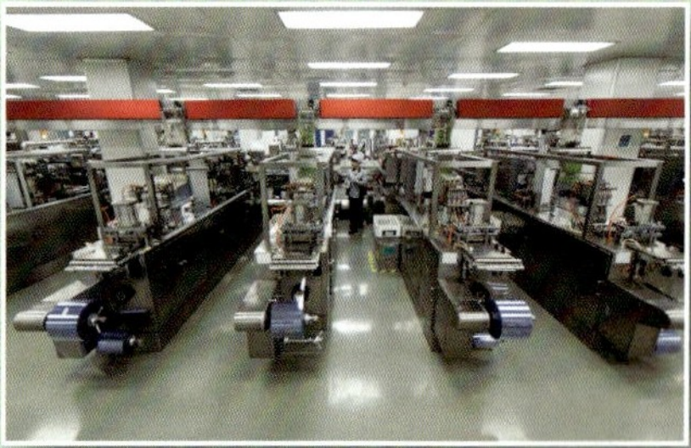

▲ 复方丹参滴丸外包装生产线

天士力集团积极倡导、推动和实践大健康五大体系的建设，即：树立大健康理念体系、普及大健康教育体系、创新大健康技术体系、发展大健康产业体系、完善大健康服务体系，围绕让人们"生得优、活得长、病得晚、走得安"的人生期望目标，全力打造"五个一"工程，即：做好一盒药、一瓶水、一杯茶、一樽酒、规划设计一套健康管理方案，努力成为大健康产品的创造者、大健康管理方案的设计者、大健康文化的践行者。

▼ 复方丹参滴丸内包装生产线

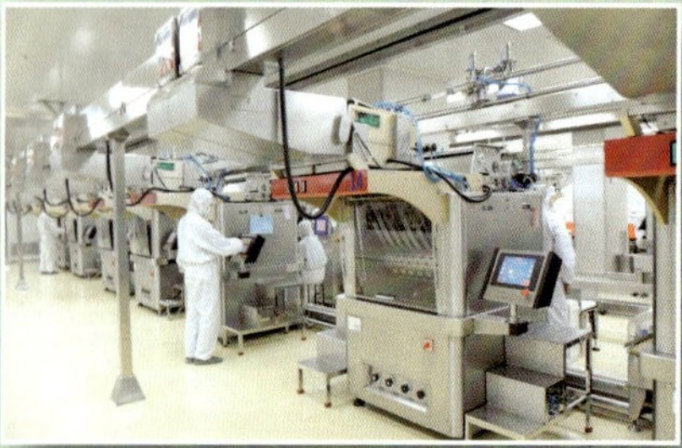

天士力生物医药产业立足科技创新、管理创新，形成了医药产业产品研发体系、技术研发体系、先进制造体系、营销服务体系，开发培育了复方丹参滴丸、养血清脑颗粒、芪参益气滴丸、益气复脉等系列现代中药，替莫唑胺、右佐匹克隆片等特色化学药，注射用生物一类新药普佑克等医药产品集群。其中最具代表性的现代中药复方丹参滴丸于2010年顺利完成了美国FDA（食品和药品管理局）Ⅱ期临床试验，目前正在全球开展Ⅲ期临床试验。

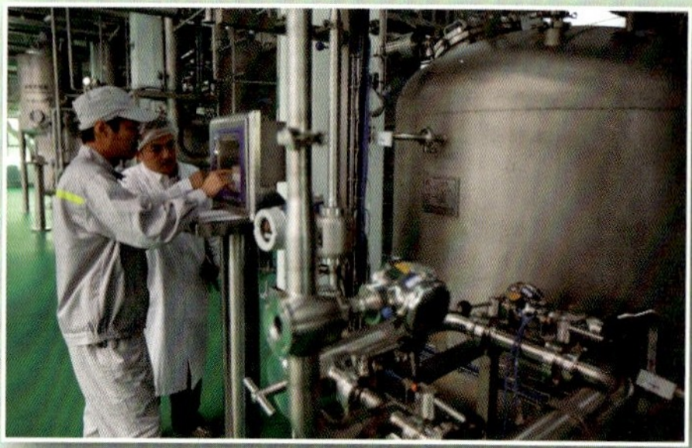

▲ 天士力现代中药数字化提取中心

借助于生物医药领域的技术优势，紧紧抓住关系到健康生活的核心要素，天士力以科技创新为先导，以优势资源开发为基础，逐渐向健康产业扩展，为大健康行业发展注入了新的活力。目前已形成以"国台"为品牌的现代白酒产供销体系，并积极探索健康葡萄酒产业发展；形成以"帝泊洱"为品牌的生物普洱茶、健康饮用水产品系列；保健品、功能食品的产业群也不断完善；稳步发展以湖南湘雅博爱康复医院为启航的医疗康复、健康养生与健康管理。

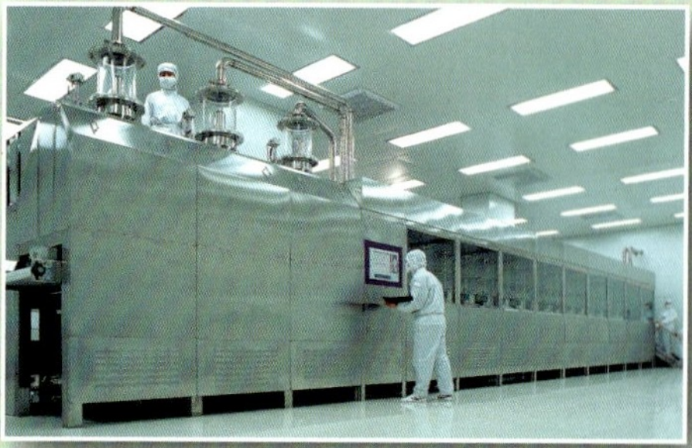

▲ 天士力拥有自主知识产权的大型数字化滴丸生产线

企业先后承担国家"863"计划、"973"计划、"十一五""十二五"重大新药创制专项等重大科研课题近百项。连续三届获得"全国精神文明建设先进单位"，先后获得"高新技术企业""创新型企业""全国劳动关系和谐企业""全国创建学习型组织先进单位""全国民主管理厂务公开先进单位"等荣誉称号。

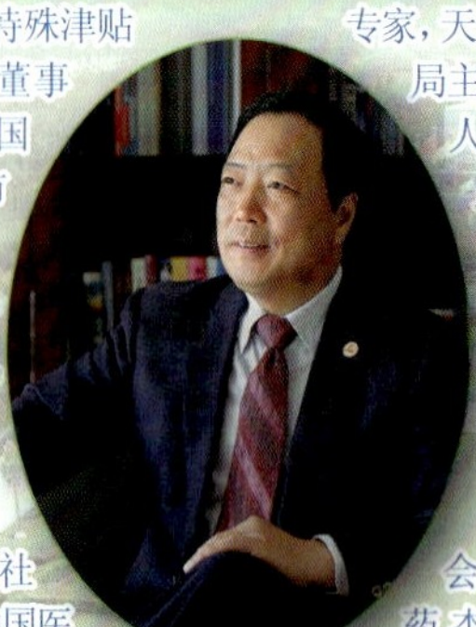

闫希军 博士，主任药师，国务院特殊津贴专家，天士力创始人。现任天士力控股集团党委书记、董事局主席，天士力研究院院长。第十一届、第十二届全国人大代表，第十四届、第十五届、第十六届天津市人大代表；兼任全国工商联第十一届执委会常委、中国光彩事业促进会副会长、中国药学会科普工作委员会副主任委员、中医药标准化专家技术委员会委员、天津市上市公司协会会长、天津市药学会副会长、中医药世界联盟董事局主席等职务。

获得全国劳动模范、优秀中国特色社会主义事业建设者、全国中药系统劳动模范、中国医药杰出企业家、中国优秀民营科技企业家、天津市特等劳动模范、天津市"十一五"期间最有影响力劳动模范、天津市劳动模范、天津市技术创新带头人等多项荣誉。

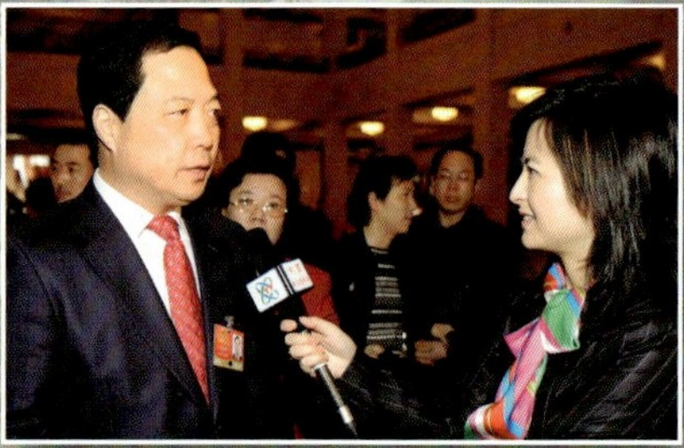

▲ 闫希军参加2009全国两会接受采访

曾获国家科技进步三等奖，军队科技进步二等奖，天津市科技进步一等奖、二等奖以及国家级企业管理创新成果一等奖等奖项。荣获军队二等功1次，三等功4次。

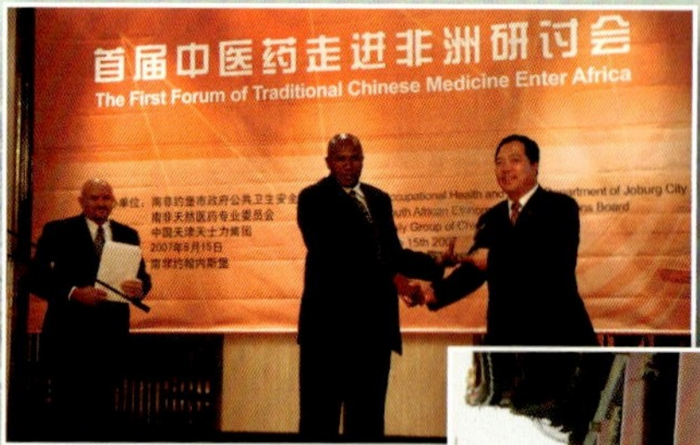

▲ 南非天然医药专业委员会主席Dr. IssacKekana授予天士力集团董事长闫希军"传统医药杰出贡献奖"

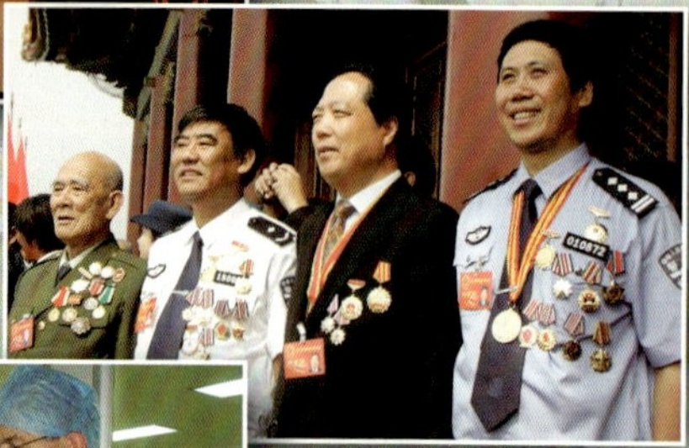

▲ 2007年8月闫希军参加全军英模大会在天安门上合影

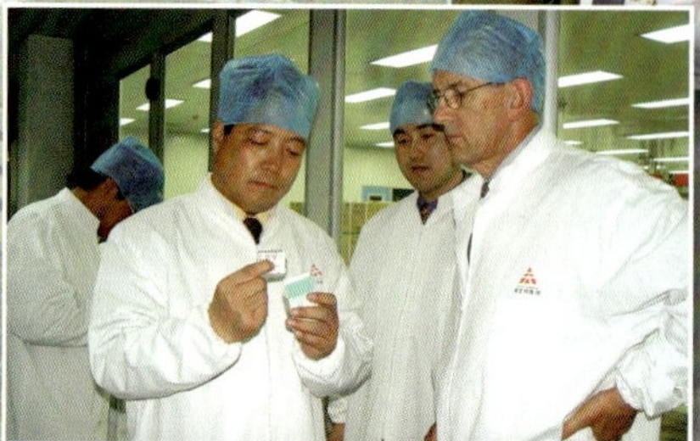

◀ 天士力集团董事长闫希军陪同美国药审专家考察天士力现代中药城

Shanghai Hutchison Pharmaceuticals
上海和黄药业

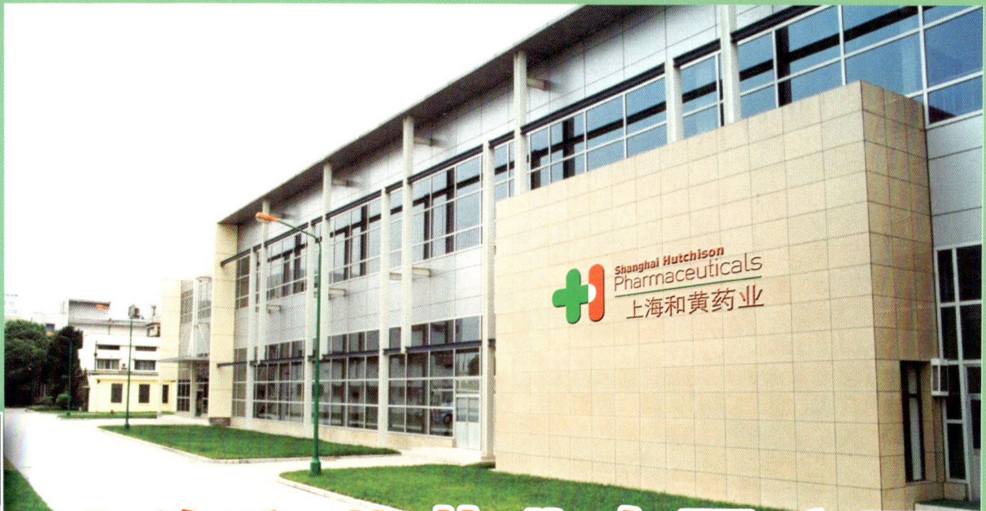

上海和黄药业有限公司

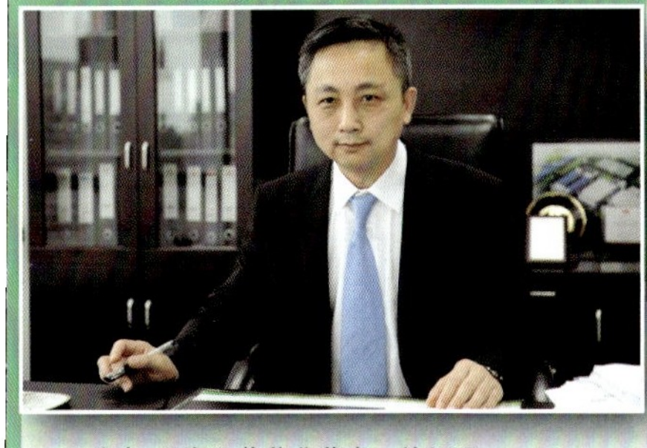

▲ 周俊杰 上海和黄药业董事、总经理

周俊杰 上海和黄药业董事、总经理，长三角医药企业社会责任优秀企业家，上海市领军人才，中国中药协会副会长，中国非处方药物协会副会长，中国医师协会医师道德建设委员会委员，上海医药行业协会副会长，上海中药行业协会副会长，普陀区第十四届、第十五届人大代表。

周俊杰具有多年跨国医药企业工作经验，在企业管理、产品研发及市场营销等方面积累了丰富经验。上海和黄药业是香港李嘉诚先生和上海药材有限公司共同投资组建的上海首家中药制药合资企业。周俊杰自加入上海和黄药业以来，坚持“基础研究与临床应用研究”及“科技创新与学术推广”的有效结合，不断应用先进的科学技术和方法，坚持产品二次开发，提升产品科技内涵和产品品质。特别是对国家中药保密品种麝香保心丸的现代科学研究取得了显著成绩，分别进行了麝香保心丸化学物质组学、系统生物学、促进治疗性血管新生、网络药理学、循证医学、临床注册登记等现代创新研究，并于2012年荣获“上海市科技进步一等奖”。麝香保心丸销售额从合资前的约6千万元人民币增长到2013年的近10亿元人民币，更成为了“药效物质基础清楚、作用机理明确、临床安全有效、质量稳定可控”的现代中药，为推动中药国际化迈出了重要一步。

强强联手的中药制药企业

上海和黄药业有限公司成立于2001年8月，是由李嘉诚先生旗下和记黄埔（中国）有限公司与上海医药集团股份有限公司，在原上海中药制药一厂的基础上，共同投资组建的上海首家中药合资企业。和黄药业首创产品32个，拥有丸剂、片剂、注射剂等各种剂型和“上药”牌注册商标及麝香保心丸、胆宁片、生脉注射液等70个知名中成药产品。公司秉承“创新传统中药，服务和谐社会”的宗旨，在传承经典中药产品的基础上，投入大量资金，不断应用国际最先进的科学技术和方法，对传统中药产品进行二次开发，不断推进中药现代化。

▼ 上海和黄药业与中国医师协会长期合作，关注医疗公益事业

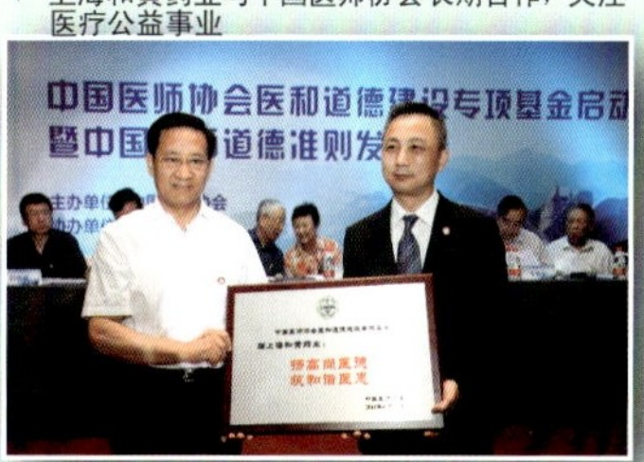

创新传统中药

上海和黄药业不断致力于传统中药的创新研究与开发，其中，核心产品麝香保心丸的相关研究得到上海市中药现代化项目、国家“十一五”科技支撑项目、国家重大新药创制项目及国家自然科学基金等专项支持，发表相关学术论文800余篇，其中SCI论文20多篇，影响因子达9.283，申请专利12项，入选国家中药保密品种，荣获上海市科技进步一等奖。

麝香保心丸源于宋代名方苏合香丸，是第一个被证明具有促进缺血心肌血管新生的中成药；物质基础研究从麝香保心丸中分离得到95个化合物及30个入血成分，明确了其物质组分构成及分子结构；系统生物学通过基因组学、代谢组学从分子水平阐述了麝香保心丸治疗冠心病、抑制心肌梗死的作用机制；网络生物学采用分子网络来研究麝香保心丸多成分多靶点防治冠心病的作用机理；2010年，由复旦大学附属中山医院、华山医院牵头启动了麝香保心丸随机、双盲、安慰剂对照的多中心大规模循证医学研究。

▼ 麝香保心丸是中成药创新的典范，荣获2012年度“上海市科技进步奖”一等奖

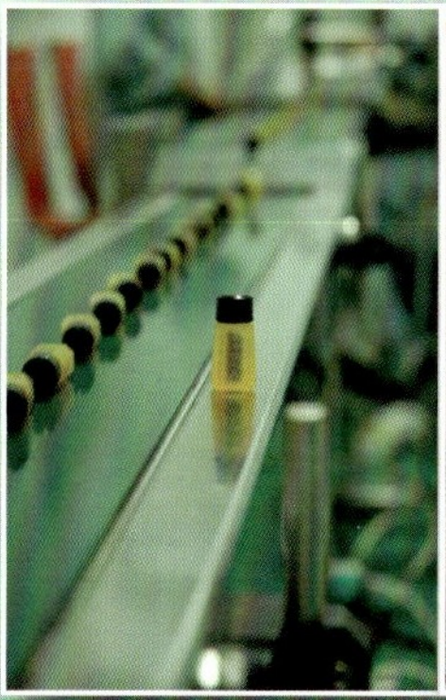

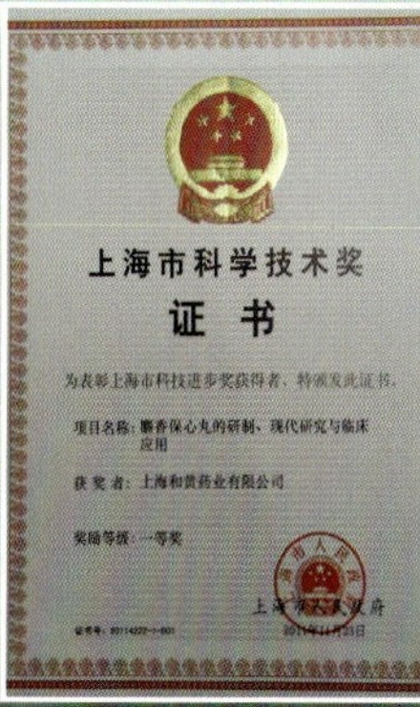
上海市科学技术奖
证书
为表彰上海市科技进步奖获得者，特颁发此证书。
项目名称：麝香保心丸的研制、现代研究与临床应用
获奖者：上海和黄药业有限公司
奖励等级：一等奖
上海市人民政府

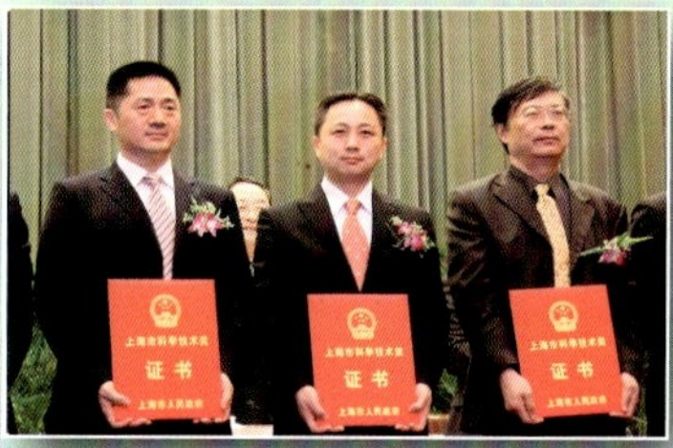

▲ 周俊杰总经理（中）代表公司上台领奖

通过对传统中药产品进行二次开发，运用现代科学技术方法、手段，阐明复方中药的药效物质基础和作用机理，使其成为药效物质清楚、作用机理明确、临床安全有效、质量稳定可控、具有自主知识产权的现代中药。目前，麝香保心丸已经成为全国知名的中药大品种，全国销量最大的中药微粒丸制剂，成为治疗冠心病、心绞痛最常用的经典中成药。

▼ 上海和黄药业“人参规范化种植基地”挂牌

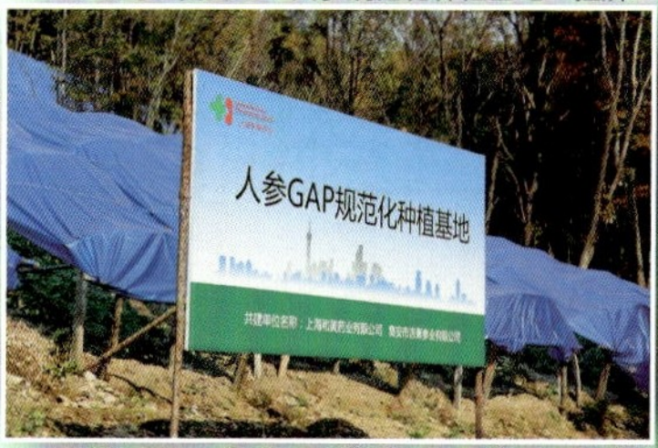

服务和谐社会

作为一家从事健康产业的公司，上海和黄药业勇于承担企业社会责任，热心社会公益事业。2006年起与中国医师协会携手开展“新世纪的医师执业精神——医师宣言”“心希望工程——医患携手社区健康干预”等社会公益项目，2013年，与中国医师协会共同设立“医和”道德建设专项基金。同时，和黄药业还持续开展对智障儿童及孤寡老人的定期关爱活动、援建上海和黄药业希望小学、向贫困地区捐助“和黄书屋”等一系列社会公益活动。

▼ 和黄希望小学捐助仪式

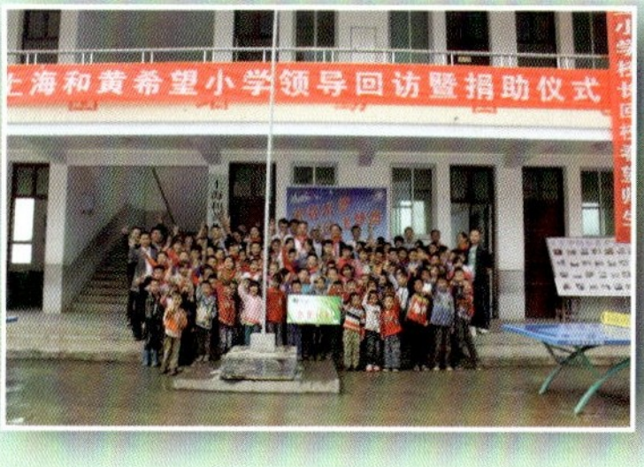